ADVANCED PRACTICE
PALLIATIVE NURSING

ADVANCED PRACTICE PALLIATIVE NURSING

SECOND EDITION

EDITED BY

Constance Dahlin

Patrick J. Coyne

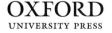

OXFORD
UNIVERSITY PRESS

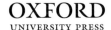

Oxford University Press is a department of the University of Oxford. It furthers
the University's objective of excellence in research, scholarship, and education
by publishing worldwide. Oxford is a registered trade mark of Oxford University
Press in the UK and certain other countries.

Published in the United States of America by Oxford University Press
198 Madison Avenue, New York, NY 10016, United States of America.

© Oxford University Press 2023

Library of Congress Cataloging-in-Publication Data
Names: Dahlin, Constance, editor. | Coyne, Patrick J., 1957– editor.
Title: Advanced practice palliative nursing / [edited by] Constance Dahlin and Patrick J. Coyne.
Other titles: Advanced practice palliative nursing (2016)
Description: Second edition. | New York, NY : Oxford University Press, [2023] |
Includes bibliographical references and index.
Identifiers: LCCN 2021034903 (print) | LCCN 2021034904 (ebook) |
ISBN 9780197559321 (hardback) | ISBN 9780197559345 (epub) |
ISBN 9780197559352 (online)
Subjects: MESH: Hospice and Palliative Care Nursing—methods |
Advanced Practice Nursing—methods
Classification: LCC R726.8 (print) | LCC R726.8 (ebook) |
NLM WY 152.3 | DDC 616.02/9—dc23
LC record available at https://lccn.loc.gov/2021034903
LC ebook record available at https://lccn.loc.gov/2021034904

DOI: 10.1093/med/9780197559321.001.0001

Printed by Sheridan Books, Inc., United States of America

We dedicate this second edition to all palliative APRNs who step in every day to promote access to quality care for individuals with serious illnesses and support family caregivers. You provide excellence in palliative care and promote palliative care equity and inclusion to diverse populations with unique needs. As palliative© APRNs, you create new programs and initiatives across clinical, educational, research, policy, and payment settings, forge new roles, develop new programs, conduct palliative research and quality improvement initiatives, create new technologies, and steer social justice within palliative care. We know it takes courage, knowledge, skills, strength, energy, and support to do this work.

CONTENTS

PREFACE

A palliative care textbook is always a labor of love. It symbolizes one's passion and commitment to the specialty. The ability to accomplish such a textbook is only through collaboration, patience, a sense of humor, and a north star of excellence and quality. The first edition of *Advanced Practice Palliative Nursing* was born out of the fact that there was no specific textbook for palliative APRNs. Prior to its publication, many seasoned APRNs learned content along the way and applied it to the APRN role. The goal of the first edition was to capture the uniqueness of the role, as well as validate and codify practice and ground the role the evidence, practice, and research. Each chapter was led by a practicing APRN to assure authenticity. Since that time, we have been thrilled from the outpouring of support for *Advanced Practice Palliative Nursing* as many APRNs said it met their need and their practice.

We recognize that we need to assure education and resources to the cadre of APRNs who will need to practice both primary and specialty palliative nursing. APRNs will need to develop new roles, lead new programs, and care for many populations across all health settings. The world and practice environment has changed considerably since the first edition. The APRN role continues to be the fastest growing segment of healthcare, and there will be a burgeoning of care for older adults. The current social construct puts more emphasis on the role of palliative care in crises including infectious disease such as the COVID-19 pandemic, humanitarian crises from conflicts, and natural disasters such as fires, floods, earthquakes, hurricanes, and the like. And the emphasis on health equity is urgent in palliative care, an issue brought to the forefront by the disparities illuminated by COVID-19 and structural racism.

Our plan had been to initiate the next edition in late 2022, as we were in the middle of other projects. However, the pandemic changed everyone's plans and it changed ours. We immediately thought to revise this edition, knowing that palliative APRNs were answering the call of the pandemic in many ways. They were particularly on the frontlines since palliative care expertise was needed to support patients in the crisis. We put out a call to authors and were pleasantly surprised when many said this would be a great diversion and provide some normalcy in a chaotic world. We were even more thrilled that 32 new chapter authors stepped in. To assure authenticity to each chapter, it was a requirement that the lead author of each chapter was an APRN currently in practice. Many of the authors APRNs are certified in advanced hospice and palliative nursing (ACHPN). It was a joy to coach and mentor them to succeed in the production of their chapters. We are grateful for all authors' contributions and appreciate the sharing of their expertise.

As a result, this textbook provides the essential knowledge and attitudes to improve skills and practice in palliative nursing to assure quality care. We hope it serves as a foundation for advanced practice palliative nursing practice. It is intended for the graduate nursing student as well as the novice, advanced beginner, and competent palliative APRN to support their specialty palliative care practice. It is also intended to support all APRNs in their provision of primary palliative care. We also hope it promotes role delineation and development within the spectrum of APRN practice. Finally, it is directed to nurse educators to help support their learners in primary and specialty palliative nursing and offer a curricular resource in preparing the next generation of palliative APRNs. We hope the reader will find the knowledge helpful to their practice and appreciate that it reflects current practice and research.

Constance Dahlin and Patrick J. Coyne

ACKNOWLEDGMENTS

We are grateful for the support and understanding of our families as we follow our passion to further the field. We thank Dr. Betty Ferrell for her previous editorship.

DISCLAIMER

To avoid repetitive information in the references, please note that all online material was accessed and is current as of October 1, 2021.

CONTRIBUTORS

Katharine Adelstein, PhD, ANP-BC, PMHNP-BC
Assistant Professor of Nursing
School of Nursing
University of Louisville
Louisville, KY, USA

Elizabeth Archer-Nanda, DNP, APRN, PMHCNS-BC
Manager
Behavioral Oncology Program
Norton Healthcare
Louisville, KY, USA

Alice Bass, MSN, APRN, CPNP-PC
Pediatric Nurse Practitioner
Nationwide Children's Hospital
Columbus, OH, USA

Vanessa Battista, DNP, MBA, MS, CPNP-PC, CHPPN, FPCN
Senior Nursing Director of Palliative Care
Dana Farber Cancer Institute
Boston, MA, USA

Kelly Baxter, DNP, FNP-BC, ACHPN
Founder & CEO
Baxter Palliative Consulting, LLC
Wakefield, RI, USA;
Adjunct Faculty
Salve Regina University
Newport, RI, USA

Sarah Bender, MPH, MS, AGPCNP-BC, ACHPN
Nurse Practitioner
Brookdale Department of Geriatric and Palliative Medicine
Mount Sinai
New York, NY, USA

Barton T. Bobb, MSN, FNP-BC, ACHPN
Palliative Nurse Practitioner
Virginia Commonwealth University Health System
Richmond, VA, USA

Brittany Bradford, MSN, ACNP-BC
Nurse Practitioner
Department of Women's Health—Breast Cancer Survivorship
City of Hope National Medical Center
Duarte, CA, USA

Jeannine M. Brant, PhD, APRN, AOCN, FAAN
Executive Director of Nursing Science & Innovation
City of Hope Medical Center
Duarte, CA, USA

Abraham A. Brody, PhD, GNP-BC, ACHPN, FAAN, FPCN
Associate Director
Hartford Institute for Geriatric Nursing
Associate Professor
New York University Rory Meyers College of Nursing
New York, NY, USA

Kathleen Broglio, DNP, ANP-BC, ACHPN, CPE, FPCN, FAANP
Nurse Practitioner, Section of Palliative Medicine
Associate Professor, Geisel School of Medicine at Dartmouth
Dartmouth-Hitchcock Medical Center
Lebanon, NH, USA

Marcia J. Buckley, MSN, ANP-BC, OCNS, ACHPN
Senior Nurse Practitioner
Palliative Care Consultation Service
University of Rochester Medical Center—Strong Memorial Hospital
Associate Professor of Clinical Nursing
University of Rochester School of Nursing
Adjunct Faculty
St. John Fisher College
Rochester, NY, USA

Penelope R. Buschman, MS, PMHCNS-BC, FAAN
Assistant Professor of Clinical Nursing
School of Nursing
Columbia University
New York, NY, USA

Beth Carlson, MS, PA-C
Ventricular Assist Device Coordinator
Facilitator for Advanced Communications
University of Rochester Medical Center—Strong Memorial Hospital
Rochester, NY, USA

Joan G. Carpenter, PhD, NP-C, GNP-BC, CRNP, ACHPN, FPCN
Assistant Professor
University of Maryland School of Nursing
Baltimore, MD, USA;
Palliative Nurse Practitioner
Coastal Hospice and Palliative Care
Salisbury, MD, USA;
Health Scientist
Corporal Michael J. Crescenz VAMC
Philadelphia, PA, USA

John Chovan, PhD, DNP, CNP, PMHNP-BC, ACHPN
Associate Professor of Nursing
Chair, Department of Nursing
Chief Nurse Administrator
Otterbein University
Westerville, OH, USA

Kimberly Chow, DNP, MBA, ANP-BC, ACHPN
Director of Advanced Practice Providers
Lightyear Health
Walnut Creek, CA, USA

Joan "Jody" Chrastek, DNP, RN, FPCN, CHPN
Coordinator
Pediatric Advanced Complex Care
Fairview Home Care and Hospice
Minneapolis, MN, USA

David Collett, MSN, AGACNP-BC, ACHPN
Nurse Practitioner
Brookdale Department of Geriatrics and Palliative
Medicine Mount Sinai
New York, NY, USA

Carrie L. Cormack, DNP, APRN, CPNP, CHPPN
Assistant Professor
Lead Palliative Care Faculty
College of Nursing
Medical University of South Carolina
Charleston, SC, USA

Nessa Coyle, PhD, APRN, FAAN
Palliative Care and Ethics Consultant
New York, NY, USA

Patrick J. Coyne, MSN, ACNS-BC, ACHPN, FCPN, FAAN
Program Director, Palliative Care
Medical University of South Carolina
Charleston, SC, USA

Natasha Curry, MS, ANP-C, ACHPN
Nurse Practitioner
Palliative Care Services
UCSF at San Francisco General Hospital and
Trauma Center
San Francisco, CA, USA

Constance Dahlin, MSN, ANP-BC, ACHPN, FPCN, FAAN
Palliative Nurse Practitioner
Mass General Brigham—Salem Hospital
Salem, MA, USA;
Co-Director
Palliative Care APP Externship
Charleston, SC, USA

Jamil Davis, DNP, MSN-Ed, FNP-C, PMHNP-BC, MAC
Program Coordinator of PMHNP Program
PhD Candidate
Valdosta State University College of Nursing and Health Sciences
Valdosta, GA, USA

Susan M. Delisle, DNP, ANP-BC, PMHNP-BC, ACHPN
Nurse Practitioner
Columbia University Medical Center/Harkness Pavilion
New York, NY, USA

Katherine E. DeMarco, DNP, MSHS, APN, FNP-BC, ACHPN
Palliative Care Consultant
Mountain Lakes, NJ, USA

Nicole DePace, MS, GNP-BC, APRN, ACHPN
Director Palliative Care Services
NVNA and Hospice
Norwell, MA, USA

Alma Y. Dixon, EdD, MSN, MPH, RN
President
Volusia Flagler Putnam Chapter, Inc.
National Black Nurses Association
Silver Spring, MD, USA

Erin Donaho, MS, ANP-C, CHFN, CHPN
National Cardiac Care Specialist
Seasons Hospice & Palliative Care
Houston, TX, USA

Jennifer Donoghue, MS, ARNP, AGNP-BC, ACHPN
Nurse Practitioner
Palliative Care
Advocate Illinois Masonic Medical Center
Chicago, IL, USA

Denice Economou, PhD, CNS, CHPN
Associate Adjunct Professor
School of Nursing
UCLA
Los Angeles, CA, USA

Tonya Edwards, MS, MSN, FNP-C
Nurse Practitioner
Palliative Care & Rehabilitation Medicine
UT MD Anderson Cancer Center
Houston, TX, USA

Bonnie D. Evans, MS, GNP-BC, ACHPN
End of Life Doula, LLC
Bristol, RI, USA;
Adjunct Faculty
Rhode Island College School of Nursing
Providence, RI, USA

Beth Fahlberg, PhD, MN, RN
Founder and Creative Director
Palliative Nursing Network
Monona, WI, USA

Hannah N. Farfour, DNP, APRN, AGNP-C, ACHPN
Palliative Nurse Practitioner
Mayo Clinic School of Medicine
Rochester, MN, USA

Betty Ferrell, PhD, MA, RN, FAAN, FPCN, CHPN
Director and Professor
Division of Nursing Research & Education
City of Hope Comprehensive Cancer Center and Beckman
Research Institute
Duarte, CA, USA

Patricia Maani Fogelman, DNP, MSN, FNP-C, ACHPN
System Medical Director
Palliative Medicine
Guthrie Clinic
Sayre, PA, USA

Helen Foley, MSN, AOCNS, ACHPN
Senior Clinical Nurse Specialist
Seidman Cancer Center
University Hospitals Cleveland Medical Center
Cleveland, OH, USA

Mallory Fossa, MSN, CPNP-PC, CCRN, CHPPN
Nurse Practitioner
Connecticut Children's
Division of Pain and Palliative Medicine
Hartford, CT, USA

Alice C. Foy, MSN, GNP-C
Nurse Practitioner
Palliative Care and Hospice Service, Geriatrics and Extended
Care Service
VA Puget Sound Health Care System
Seattle, WA, USA

Jennifer Gentry, DNP, ANP-BC, ACHPN, FPCN
Nurse Practitioner
Palliative Care Consult Service
Duke University Hospital
Clinical Associate Professor
Duke School of Nursing
Durham, NC, USA

Janine A. Gerringer, MSN, CRNP, FNP-C
Nurse Practitioner
Geisinger Health
Danville, PA, USA

Rosemary Gorman, MS, AGPCNP-BC, ACHPN
Advanced Practice Nurse
Monmouth Medical Center
Long Branch, NJ, USA

Marian Grant, DNP, APRN, ACNP-BC, ACHPN, FPCN
Senior Regulatory Advisor
The Coalition to Transform Advanced Care
Washington, DC, USA

Joanne M. Greene, MSN, MA, APRN, CPNP-BC, ACHPN
Pediatric Nurse Practitioner
Pediatric Palliative Care
The University of Texas MD Anderson Cancer Center
Houston, TX, USA

Amy Corey Haskamp, MSN, PCNS-BC, CPON, CHPPN, APRN
Pediatric Palliative Care
Riley Hospital for Children at Indiana University
Health
Indianapolis, IN, USA

Jaime Hensel, MSN, APRN, FNP-BC, ACHPN
Nurse Practitioner
Department of Pain Medicine, Palliative Care &
Integrative Medicine
Children's Hospitals and Clinics of Minnesota
Minneapolis, MN, USA

Erica J. Hickey, MSN, FNP-C, ACHPN
Clinical Instructor
School of Medicine
University of Colorado
Denver, CO, USA

Rikki N. Hooper, MBA, MSN, FNP-BC, ACHPN
Chief Clinical Officer
Four Seasons Palliative Care
Flat Rock, NC, USA

Mimi Jenko, DNP, APRN, PMHCNS-BC, CHPN
Faculty
School of Nursing
Greenville Technical College
Greenville, SC, USA

Faith Kinnear, MSN, APRN, CPNP-AC
Nurse Practitioner
Palliative Care Team and Critical Care Medicine
Baylor College of Medicine/Texas Children's Hospital
Houston, TX, USA

Timothy W. Kirk, PhD
Professor of Philosophy
City University of New York, York College
New York, NY, USA;
Ethics Consultant
MJHS Hospice and Palliative Care
New York, NY, USA

Lauren Koranteng, PharmD, BCPS
Clinical Pharmacy Specialist
Memorial Sloan Kettering Cancer Center
New York, NY, USA

Katherine Kyle, DNP, AGNP-C, CHPN
Nurse Practitioner
Palliative Care/General Internal Medicine
Medical University of South Carolina
Charleston, SC, USA

Kerstin Lea Lappen, MS, ACNS-BC, ACHPN, FPCN
Clinical Nurse Specialist
Palliative Care
Livio Helath Group
Minneapolis, MN, USA

Ann Laramee, MS, ANP-BC, ACNS, CHFN, ACHPN, FHFSA
Nurse Practitioner
Departments of Palliative Medicine and Cardiology
University of Vermont Medical Center
Burlington, VT, USA

Kathleen O. Lindell, PhD, RN, ATSF, FAAN
Associate Professor
Mary Swain Endowed Chair in Palliative Care
College of Nursing
Medical University of South Carolina
Charleston, SC, USA

Janice Linton, DNP, APRN, ANP-BC, CCRN, ACHPN
Assistant Professor
Palliative Nurse Practitioner
Ron and Kathy Assaf College of Nursing Nova Southeastern University
West Palm Beach, FL, USA

Sarah Loschiavo, MSN, APRN, FNP-C, ACHPN
Program Director
Oncology Supportive Care
Carole and Ray Neag Comprehensive Cancer Center
UConn Health
Farmington, CT, USA

Polly Mazanec, PhD, ACNP-BC, AOCN, ACHPN, FPCN, FAAN
Visiting Associate Professor
Francis Payne Bolton School of Nursing
Case Western Reserve University
Cleveland, OH, USA

Julia McBee, MSN, CPNP-PC
Nurse Practitioner
Hassenfeld Children's Hospital at NYU Langone
Pediatric Advance Care Team
New York City, NY, USA

Donna E. McCabe, DNP, GNP-BC, PMHNP-BC
Hartford Institute for Geriatric Nursing
New York University Rory Meyers College of Nursing
New York, NY, USA

Melissa McClean, MSN, ANP-BC, ACHPN
Medical Director
Community-Based Palliative Care
Capital Caring Health
Falls Church, VA, USA

Kerrith McDowell, MSN, AGPCNP-BC
Nurse Practitioner
Palliative Care
Duke University Health System
Durham, NC, USA

Matthew McGraw, DNP, ANP-BC, CNP, ACHPN
Nurse Practitioner
Community Palliative Care
Allina Health
Minneapolis, MN, USA

Marlene E. McHugh, DNP, FNP-BC, AGACNP-BC, ACHPN, DCC, FPCN
Associate Professor
School of Nursing
Columbia University
Nurse Practitioner
Montefiore Medical Center
New York, NY, USA

Paula McKinzie, MSN, ANP-BC
Associate Clinical Director
Duke Regional Palliative Care
Nurse Practitioner
Duke Regional Hospital
Durham, NC, USA

Joseph Albert Melocoton, MSN, NP-C, AOCNS
Nurse Practitioner
Division of Palliative Medicine
VA Greater Los Angeles Healthcare System
Los Angeles, CA, USA

Kate Meyer, MSN, AGNP-BC, CNP
Nurse Practitioner
Allina Health
St. Paul, MN, USA

Ember S. Moore, MSN, AG-ACNP-BC, ACHPN
Nurse Practitioner
Section of Palliative Medicine
Dartmouth Hitchcock Medical Center
Lebanon, NH, USA

Cecilia R. Motschenbacher, DNP, APRN, FNP-C, ACHPN
Nurse Practitioner
Hematology Oncology
Kaiser Permanente
Olympia, WA, USA

Karen Mulvihill, DNP, APRN, FNP-BC, ACHPN
Network Director
Palliative Care Services
Nuvance Health System
Danbury, CT, USA

Ryan Murphy, MSN, AGNP-C, ACHPN
Palliative Nurse Practitioner
St. Joseph's Health
Paterson, NJ, USA

Victoria Nalls, PhD, GNP-BC, ACHPN, CWS
Director of Education
Capital Caring Health
Falls Church, VA, USA

Jessica Nymeyer, MBA, MSN, AGACNP-BC, ACHPN, CCRN
Palliative Nurse Practitioner
Calvary Hospital
Bronx, NY, USA

James C. Pace, PhD, MDiv, APRN, FAANP, FAAN
Dean and Professor
Valdosta State University College of Nursing and
Health Sciences
Valdosta, GA, USA

Judith A. Paice, PhD, ACHPN, FAAN
Director, Cancer Pain Program
Division of Hematology-Oncology
Northwestern University, Feinberg School of Medicine
Chicago, IL, USA

Shila Pandey, MSN, AGPCNP-BC, ACHPN
Nurse Practitioner
Supportive Care Service
Memorial Sloan Kettering Cancer Center
New York, NY, USA

Kristyn Pellecchia, MSN, PMHNP-BC
Clinical Director
Advanced Practice Nursing
Psychiatric Nurse Practitioner
Senior Medical Associates
San Diego, CA, USA

Kathy Plakovic, MSN, ARNP, FNP-BC, ACHPN, AOCNP
Palliative Nurse Practitioner
Seattle Cancer Care Alliance
Teaching Associate
Department of Medicine, Division on Oncology
University of Washington
Seattle, WA, USA

Chari Price, MSN, AGNP-BC, ACHPN
Director of Community Palliative Care
Four Seasons Hospice
Flat Rock, NC, USA

Robert David Rice, PhD, MSN, RN, NEA-BC
Chief Nurse—Research, Innovation, and
Development
Designated Learning Officer—Workforce
Development
VA Greater Los Angeles Healthcare System
Los Angeles, CA, USA

Maggie C. Root, MSN, CPNP-AC, RN, CHPPN
PhD Student
School of Nursing/Graduate School
Vanderbilt University
Nashville, TN, USA

Jamie Lee Rouse, DNP, AGNP-BC
Nurse Practitioner
Four Seasons
Flat Rock, NC, USA

Adrienne Rudden, DNP, ACACNP-BC
Palliative Nurse Practitioner
Brookdale Department of Geriatrics and Palliative Medicine
Mount Sinai
New York, NY, USA

Rachel Rusch, MSW, MA, LCSW
Clinical Social Worker
Division of Comfort and Palliative Care
Children's Hospital Los Angeles
Los Angeles, CA, USA

Gina Santucci, MSN, APRN, FNP-BC
Nurse Practitioner
Palliative Care Team
Texas Children's Hospital
Houston, TX, USA

Nicole Sartor, MSN, APRN, CPNP-PC, CHPPN
Children's Supportive Care Team Coordinator
Department of Palliative Care
University of North Carolina Children's Hospital
Chapel Hill, NC, USA

Renata Shabin, MSN, APRN, AGPCNP-BC, ACHPN
Nurse Practitioner
Palliative Care Team
NYU Langone Medical Center
New York, NY, USA

Traci Sickich, MSN, APRN, FNP-BC, ACHPN
Palliative Care Practitioner
Providence Medical Center
Anchorage, AK, USA

Robert Smeltz, MA, NP, ACHPN, FPCN
Assistant Director and Nurse Practitioner
Palliative Care Program
Bellevue Hospital
New York, NY, USA

Brooke Smith, MSN, APRN, FNP-BC, ACHPN
Nurse Practitioner
Department of Palliative Care
Medical University of South Carolina
Charleston, SC, USA

Kira Stalhandske, DNP, FNP-C, ACHPN
Adult Palliative Nurse Practitioner
Michigan Medicine
University of Michigan School of Nursing
Ann Arbor, MI, USA

Angela Starkweather, PhD, ACNP-BC, CNRN, FAAN, FAANP
Professor & Associate Dean for Academic Affairs
School of Nursing
University of Connecticut
Storrs, CT, USA

Lisa A. Stephens, MSN, APRN, ANP-BC, ACHPN, FPCN
Lead Nurse Practitioner
Associate Program Director, Interprofessional
Fellowship
Section of Palliative Medicine
Dartmouth-Hitchcock Medical Center
Lebanon, NH, USA

Ann Quinn Syrett, MSN, FNP-C, ACHPN
Lead Nurse Practitioner
Adult Palliative Care Consultation Service
University of Rochester Medical Center—Strong
Memorial Hospital
Associate Professor of Clinical Nursing
University of Rochester School of Nursing
Rochester, NY, USA

Cheryl Ann Thaxton, DNP, APRN, CPNP-BC, FNP-BC, CHPPN, ACHPN, FPCN
Associate Clinical Professor
DNP Program Director—College of Nursing
Texas Woman's University
Denton, TX, USA

Charles Tilley, MS, ANP-BC, ACHPN, CWOCN
Hospice and Palliative Nurse Practitioner
Calvary Hospital and Hospice
New York, NY, USA;
Assistant Director of Simulation
NYU Rory Meyers College of Nursing
New York, NY, USA

Lorie Resendes Trainor, MSN, ANP-BC, CNP, ACHPN
Clinical Manager/Nurse Practitioner
Commonwealth Care Alliance
Boston, MA, USA

Carolyn White, MSN, NP-C, FNP-BC, GNP-BC, ACHPN
Lead Nurse Practitioner
Palliative Medicine
Centra Health Palliative Care
Lynchburg, VA, USA

Phyllis B. Whitehead, PhD, MSN, CNS, ACHPN, PMGT-BC, FNAP, FAAN
Clinical Nurse Specialist
Clinical Ethicist
Carilion Health System
Associate Professor
Carilon School of Medicine
Virginia Tech
Roanoke, VA, USA

Dorothy Wholihan, DNP, AGPCNP-BC, ACHPN, FPCN, FAAN
Clinical Professor and Director
Palliative Care Specialty Program
Meyers College of Nursing
New York University
New York, NY, USA

Clareen Wiencek, PhD, ACNP-BC, ACHPN, FAAN
Professor and Director of Advanced Practice for MSN
Program
School of Nursing
University of Virginia
Charlottesville, VA, USA

Brenna Winn, MSN, APRN, FNP, NP-C
Nurse Practitioner
GraceMed Health Clinic
McPherson, KS, USA

Devon S. Wojcikewych, MD
Associate Professor
Department of Internal Medicine
Virginia Commonwealth University Health System
Richmond, VA, USA

SECTION I

THE PALLIATIVE APRN

1.

PALLIATIVE APRN PRACTICE AND LEADERSHIP

PAST, PRESENT, AND FUTURE

Constance Dahlin and Patrick J. Coyne

> ### KEY POINTS
>
> - The foundational principles of nursing and palliative care are synergistic. Modern nursing has always focused on alleviating suffering for individuals in health and illness. Palliative care focuses on quality of life.
>
> - All advanced practice registered nurses (APRNs) practice primary palliative care within their practice. Specialty palliative APRNs focus on more complex care for individuals with serious illness.
>
> - Palliative APRNs promote access to palliative care, facilitate evidence-based palliative practices, and deliver safe, quality palliative care across settings and populations.
>
> - Palliative APRN leaders are essential to the evolution of palliative care.

HISTORY OF NURSING AND PALLIATIVE APRNs

As the largest segment of healthcare providers, nurses have a prominent role in the front line of care. Nurses spend the most time with patients and families. This proximity allows for comprehensive assessment of the person and family to facilitate personalized care, implementation and evaluation of the treatment plan, and care coordination. Nurses are uniquely positioned in healthcare to observe family interactions, support a patient's coping, and listen to a patient's inner most thoughts and concerns across many situations. Advanced practice registered nurses (APRNs) are one of the fastest growing segments of nursing and healthcare and will continue to have a growing influence on the accessibility and quality of healthcare.[1,2]

Both nursing and palliative care have evolved to focus on health, wellness, and caring across a continuum.[3] Nurses protect, promote, and optimize human function; prevent illness and injury; and alleviate suffering through their compassionate presence, including individuals coping with actual or potential serious illness.[4] Florence Nightingale and Mary Seacole established nursing practice while caring for soldiers in the Crimean War, many of whom were critically wounded.[5] Thus, the essence of nursing was grounded in caring for gravely ill individuals. When nursing moved to the United States,

Clara Barton of the American Red Cross advanced nursing through the Civil War. Again, nursing practice was based in the care of soldiers wounded in battle.[6]

Nursing has developed in its breadth and scope of practice to include registered nurses (RNs) and graduate-level (master's or doctoral)–prepared specialty nurses. In the mid-twentieth century, four advanced practice nursing roles developed: certified nurse midwife, nurse practitioner (NP), clinical nurse specialist (CNS), and certified nurse anesthetist. These roles play a significant part in hospice and palliative care in the United States today. This textbook highlights how APRNs are leaders in the assurance of high-quality palliative care for all, the delivery of palliative care, the development and administration of palliative programs, advocacy in policy related to palliative care, access to palliative care education, and the development and participation in necessary palliative care research, with an emphasis on nursing.

HISTORY OF HOSPICE AND PALLIATIVE CARE

The modern hospice movement was established in the 1960s in England by Dame Cicely Saunders, a physician who was first a nurse, then a social worker. At St. Joseph's Hospice, Dr. Saunders followed her calling to promote compassionate care to the dying, calling on her background in nursing and social work. She then founded St. Christopher's Hospice to further develop hospice care.[6] These concepts traveled to the United States through the work of Dr. Florence Wald, then dean of the Yale School of Nursing. Dr. Wald developed an expansive nursing curriculum that emphasized the nursing skills necessary for caring for dying patients, specifically pain and symptom management and communication.[7] Dr. Wald stated, "Hospice care is the epitome of good nursing care." She asserted, "It enables the patient to get through the end-of-life on their own terms. It is a holistic approach, looking at the patient as an individual, a human being. The spiritual role nurses play in the end-of-life process is essential to both patients and families."[7] Dr. Wald then founded the Connecticut Hospice, the first hospice in the United States.

In 1982, the Medicare Hospice Benefit was enacted, offering benefits to patients with a terminal illness. Specific *Medicare Hospice Conditions of Participation* (CoPs) directed hospices to offer a certain set of services to patients and families.[8] Within the benefit, nursing has a prominent role as a core service. In programs across the United States, the majority of hospice care is provided by nurses visiting patients' homes. However, in its infancy, the Medicare Hospice Benefit recognized only RN practice. It was not until recently that the Medicare Hospice Benefit even acknowledged that APRNs lead hospice teams and oversee the care of hospice patients. The most recent version of the CoPs (2011) clarifies the role of the APRN.[9]

In addition, when the Medicare Hospice Benefit was started, care of dying patients was marked by a lack of consistency in care provision and little consensus on the defining characteristics of palliative care or quality indicators for adults and children. Even less was known about patients with serious illness. Research from the 1990s confirmed the worst fears about healthcare. *The Study to Understand Prognoses and Preferences for Outcomes and Risks of Treatment* (SUPPORT) demonstrated a failure to honor patients' preferences even when patients were clear about their wishes and preferences.[10] The study found a continued lack of communication between patients and their healthcare providers about end-of-life care. Furthermore, patients who were seriously ill and dying reported high levels of pain and other symptoms, extensive financial stress, and, most importantly, a lack of concordance between care provided and their care preferences. Despite patient preferences to focus on quality of life, aggressive care was often continued despite reduced quality of life.[10] In the intervention arm of the study, nurse-conducted patient interviews did not improve outcomes in aligning care with patient goals. However, there was variation in the SUPPORT study: both APRNs and RNs were used in the intervention which meant variability in communication skills and scope of practice. This may have caused an inconsistency in the interventions for patients and, ultimately, the affected consistency of outcomes.

As the findings from SUPPORT were being disseminated in the mid-1990s, hospice concepts moved into the academic hospital setting in the form of palliative care.[11] This care applied hospice concepts of symptom management, family support, goal-centered care, and quality of life earlier in the care of hospitalized patients. Care first focused on adults with serious and life-threatening illnesses whose care was complicated, as well as on terminally ill patients who were not ready for hospice.[11] Specialty pediatric palliative care then developed as well.

INCEPTION OF PALLIATIVE CARE AND PALLIATIVE NURSING

Pioneer palliative care programs were developed across the country. Many of these palliative care services had a large presence of APRNs.[11] With their enhanced graduate education and scope of practice, APRNs offered a wide range of clinical services to patients and families, such as taking histories, performing physical examinations, developing diagnoses, creating care plans, prescribing medications, and offering treatment options.[11,12] Moreover, many APRNs had been selected as faculty scholars of the Open Society *Project on Death in America* to improve care at the end of life.[13] APRNs

also had prominent roles in program development, research, and education of patients, families, professional colleagues, and health systems. The challenge was ensuring appropriate education and training so that APRNs could move into these roles. The development of the specialty of palliative APRN practice was just beginning. See Box 1.1 for a review of the specialty.

In the early years, most APRNs who moved into palliative care roles had to design their own education and support for clinical decision-making since there were no organized educational plans. Frequently, APRNs learned aspects of a palliative approach through clinical care over months to years. It was often the case of on-the-job skill building while developing individual models of care. Often education, practice expertise, and skills emanated from either oncology nursing or AIDS/HIV nursing, which involved a range of skills associated with symptom control, care at end of life, coping, and bereavement. Other nurses moved from hospice care into palliative care because of shared experience in pain and symptom management, counseling about life-limiting illness, and working with an interprofessional team.

ESSENTIAL REPORTS

The release of essential reports about dying in America influenced palliative advanced practice nursing. The 1997 Institute of Medicine (IOM) report *Approaching Death* described the state of end-of-life care in America.[16] This report recommended the subspecialty of palliative care, reviewed the use of medications for pain and symptom management, supported financial investment in palliative care, and appealed for professional education that included palliative care content in various curricula, textbooks, and training programs.[14]

EVOLUTION OF PALLIATIVE CARE

The Precepts of Palliative Care were released by Last Acts (formerly a Robert Wood Johnson Foundation-funded organization, which was enveloped within the National Hospice and Palliative Care Organization).[15] These precepts reaffirmed the comprehensive approach of palliative care as a specialized area of expertise. *The Precepts of Palliative Care* also stated that care should respect patient choices, affirmed that care utilizes the strengths of the interdisciplinary team, and encouraged the building of palliative care support through financing, outcomes, and research.[15]

In 2002, Last Acts published a seminal document, a state-by-state report card of end-of-life care in America, which captured a fairly bleak picture of palliative care in the United States.[16] It promoted much discussion about a unified response from the palliative care community. This state reporting was subsequently monitored by the Center to Advance Palliative Care. Other significant reports included two IOM reports, *When Children Die* and *Crossing the Quality Chasm*, and a monograph by the National Hospice Work Group and the Hastings Center in association with the National Hospice and Palliative Care Organization (NHPCO) entitled *Access to Hospice Care: Expanding Boundaries, Overcoming Barriers*.[17–19]

1982	Enactment of the Medicare Hospice Benefit
1986	Establishment of the Hospice Nurses Association
1991	Release of American Nurses Association *Position Statement: Nursing and the Patient Self-Determination Act: Supporting Autonomy*
1993	Establishment of National Board for Certification of Hospice Nurses
1994	Establishment of the Open Society-Project on Death in America-to support the leadership development of interdisciplinary faculty, including APRNs, to address barriers to end-of-life care.
	Administration of first examination for hospice nursing offered by National Board for Certification of Hospice Nurses
1995	Release of the *Study to Understand Prognoses and Preferences for Outcomes and Risks of Treatments* (SUPPORT)
1997	Publication of Institute of Medicine Committee on Care at the End of Life *Approaching Death: Improving Care at the End of Life*
	Centers for Medicare and Medicaid Services first recognizes and allows the billable services of a nurse practitioner
	Development of first palliative nursing master's programs for NPs and CNSs
1998	Publication of American Association of Colleges of Nursing *Peaceful Death: Recommended Competencies and Curricular Guidelines for End-of-Life Nursing Care*
	Transition of the Hospice Nurses Association to the Hospice and Palliative Nurses Association (HPNA)
	Transition of National Board for Certification of Hospice Nurses to the National Board for Certification of Hospice and Palliative Nurses (NBCHPN)
1999	Publication of Last Acts *The Precepts of Palliative Care*
	Establishment of the Nursing Leadership Academy for End-of-Life Care to design an agenda for end-of-life care for the nursing profession
2000	Publication of the Institute of Medicine Committee on Palliative and End of Life Care *When Children Die: Improving Palliative and End-of-Life Care for Children and Their Families* and *Crossing the Quality Chasm: A New Health System for the 21st Century*
	City of Hope National Medical Center and American Academy of Colleges of Nursing collaborate to create the End-of-Life Nursing Education Consortium (ELNEC), which develops a nursing curriculum for care at end of life and partners.
	Publication of *HPNA Statement on the Scope and Standards of Hospice and Palliative Nursing Practice* (2nd ed.)
2001	Publication of *Advanced Practice Nurses Role in Palliative Care: A Position Statement from American Nursing Leaders*, supported by Promoting Excellence in End-of-Life Care
	Creation of *HPNA Professional Competencies for the Generalist Hospice and Palliative Nurse*
	Publication of *Oxford Textbook of Palliative Nursing* (1st ed.)
2002	Publication of HPNA and ANA *Scope and Standards of Hospice and Palliative Nursing Practice* (3rd ed.)
	Creation of *HPNA Competencies for the Advanced Practice Hospice and Palliative Care Nurse*
2003	Administration of first palliative and hospice examination for APRNs administered within a partnership of NBCHPN and American Nurses Credentialing Center
2004	Publication of National Consensus Project for Quality Palliative Care *Clinical Practice Guidelines* (1st ed.)
2005	Publication of *Oxford Textbook of Palliative Nursing* (2nd ed.)
2006	Recognition of NBCHPN by the Centers for Medicare and Medicaid Services as a national certifying body for APRNs allowing for practice solely as a palliative APRN, which allows palliative NPs to bill
	Release of *HPNA Position Statement: Value of the Advanced Practice Nurse in Palliative Care* (revised 2010, with name changed to *Value of the Advanced Practice Registered Nurse in Palliative Care*)
2007	Publication of HPNA and ANA *Hospice and Palliative Nursing: Scope and Standards of Practice* (4th ed.)

(continued)

Box 1.1 Continued

2008	Enactment of National Council of State Boards of Nursing Licensure, Accreditation, Certification and Education (LACE) to standardize advance practice nursing across states, defining palliative nursing as an advanced practice nursing specialty, to be added to population-based licensure
2009	Publication of National Consensus Project for Quality Palliative Care *Clinical Practice Guidelines* (2nd ed.)
	Publication of *Core Curriculum for the Advanced Hospice and Palliative Registered Nurse* (1st ed.)
2010	Publication of *Oxford Textbook of Palliative Nursing* (3rd ed.)
2011	Publication of *HPNA Position Statement: The Nurse's Role in Advance Care Planning*
2013	Institute of Medicine forms the Transforming Care at the End-of-Life Committee to review and expand palliative care across healthcare settings.
	Publication of National Consensus Project for Quality Palliative Care *Clinical Practice Guidelines* (3rd ed.)
	Transition of National Board for Certification of Hospice and Palliative Nurses (NBCHPN) to the Hospice and Palliative Credentialing Center
	Publication of HPNA *Core Curriculum for the Advanced Practice Hospice and Palliative Registered Nurse* (2nd ed.)
2014	Publication of the Institute of Medicine *of Dying in America—Improving Quality and Honoring Individual Preferences Near End of Life*
	Inauguration of Cambia Healthcare Foundation Sojourns Leadership Scholars Program funding leadership development for nurses and physicians
	Development of ELNEC for APRNs, which focuses on both clinical care and program development
	Publication of HPNA and ANA *Palliative Nursing: Scope and Standards—An Essential Resource for Nurses* (5th ed.)
	Publication of HPNA *Competencies for the Hospice and Palliative Advanced Practice Nurse*
2015	Release of ANA *Position Statement: Roles and Responsibilities in Providing Care and Support at the End of Life*
	Publication of HPNA *Standards for Clinical Education* to identify essential type of clinical experiences
	Publication of *Oxford Textbook of Palliative Nursing* (4th ed.)
2017	Release of ANA and HPNA *Call for Action: Nurses Lead and Transform Palliative Care*
2018	Publication of National Consensus Project for Quality Palliative Care *Clinical Practice Guidelines* (4th ed.)
	Centers for Medicare and Medicaid Services allows NPs and CNSs to certify home health care
2019	Publication of AACN primary palliative nursing competencies for graduate-prepared nurses, *Graduate Competencies and Recommendations for Educating Nursing Students (G-CARES).*
	Publication of *Oxford Textbook of Palliative Nursing* (5th ed.)
2020	Release of ANA *Position Statement: Nursing Care and Do-Not-Resuscitate (DNR) Decisions*
	Publication of HPNA *Core Curriculum for the Advanced Practice Hospice and Palliative Registered Nurse* (3rd ed.)
2021	Publication of HPNA *Palliative Nursing: Scope and Standards of Practice* (6th ed.)
	Publication of HPNA *Competencies for the Palliative and Hospice Palliative APRN* (3rd ed.)
	Publication of AACN *The Essentials: Core Competencies for Professional Nursing Education*, which requires primary supportive/palliative/hospice nursing education

Adapted from American Nurses Association, Hospice and Palliative Nurses Association. *Palliative Nursing: Scope and Standards of Practice: An Essential Resource for Hospice and Palliative Nurses.* 5th ed.[20]; Dahlin C, ed. *Palliative Nursing Scope and Standards of Practice.* 6th ed.[21]

These reports argued for significant changes in access to palliative care that would promote access for all ages, ensure care in all health settings, and provide services for all progressive chronic, serious, or life-threatening illness and injuries.[17–19]

A significant development in the field was the 2004 release of the National Consensus Project for Quality Palliative Care's (NCP) *Clinical Practice Guidelines*, created by the five major professional organizations dedicated to promoting hospice, palliative, and end-of-life care: the American Academy of Hospice and Palliative Medicine (AAHPM), the Center to Advance Palliative Care (CAPC), the Hospice and Palliative Nurses Association (HPNA),

Last Acts, and the National Hospice and Palliative Care Organization (NHPCO). These guidelines established principles to improve and ensure the quality of palliative care in the United States.[22] They offer a framework for the future of palliative care and continue to serve as a blueprint to create new programs, guide developing programs, and set high expectations for excellence in existing programs. The guidelines set ideal practices and goals that palliative care services should strive to attain rather than setting minimally acceptable practices. The guidelines have three specific aims: (1) to promote quality and reduce variation in new and existing programs, (2) to develop and encourage continuity of care across settings, and (3) to facilitate collaborative partnerships among palliative care programs, community hospices, and a wide range of other healthcare delivery settings.[22–24] Now in its fourth edition, the *NCP Clinical Practice Guidelines* are a collaboration of a wider group of professional organizations dedicated to care of individuals (both children and adults) with serious illness. Moreover, the guidelines stress specialty education, training, and certification; specific to APRNs is the promotion of obtaining advanced certification within hospice and palliative nursing.[24,25]

Later in 2004, the first national meeting on palliative care research was convened in Bethesda, Maryland. The National Institutes of Health (NIH) held the first State of the Science Conference on Improving End-of-Life Care, which put forth statements to formulate future palliative research.[26] The co-chairs who convened the meeting concluded that (1) the definition of end-of-life care was vague and poorly understood and was experienced differently across subgroups of culture, healthcare settings, and disease populations; (2) the vague definition led to poor-quality, fragmented care, and lack of continuity; and (3) research measures and interventions in use were inconsistent and lacked validation.[26] In 2011, the National Institute for Nursing Research (NINR) convened a follow-up meeting that provided a summary of research initiatives and offered innovative methods to develop palliative metrics and measure quality.[27] It also emphasized the need for interdisciplinary research and training.[27] Palliative-focused research continues through the National Center for Palliative Care Research and the Palliative Care Research Cooperative Group.

In 2014, the IOM released its report *Dying in America: Improving Quality and Honoring Individual Preferences Near End of Life*.[28] The report focuses on five areas for quality palliative care: (1) delivery of person-centered and family-focused palliative care, (2) clinician–patient communication and advance care planning, (3) professional education in palliative care, (4) policies and payment for palliative care, and (5) public education and engagement in palliative care.[28] These areas would provide a focus for healthcare improvement and would move care upstream to patients with serious illness rather than focusing just on the end of life. In addition, the report calls for more coordinated and collaborative care that is based in the community. APRNs would have a major role in the implementation of these areas and, more broadly, in moving palliative care into the community.

In 2018, the Commonwealth Fund released the report *Health Care in America: The Experience of People with Serious Illness*. It outlines several important findings: (1) the distress of people with serious illness caused by physical and psychological symptoms and distress; (2) the challenges of care related to insurance coverage, procedures, and conflicting information; and (3) the financial devastation of serious illness. It offers three strategies: (1) assessment of social determinants of health and management of these needs, (2) coordination of care across teams, and (3) affordable care. These have become major themes as palliative care evolves into the future. The APRN has a role in addressing each of these strategies to improve the care of people with serious illness.[29]

QUALITY

There have been several significant events related to the quality of palliative care. APRNs are obligated to ensure the quality of palliative nursing practice, which requires an awareness of these developments and standards and an appreciation of how they affect care delivery, the measurement of quality practice, and education. The National Quality Forum (NQF) is a nonprofit public–private partnership focused on quality care through the adoption of voluntary standards. Its goal is to develop meaningful information about care delivery, including timeliness, efficiency, safety, equality, and patient-centeredness.[30] In 2006, it published *A National Framework and Preferred Practices for Palliative and Hospice Care Quality: A Consensus Report*,[31] which built on the NCP's eight domains of care and put forth 38 preferred practices for hospice and palliative care.

Related to the NQF was the formation of the National Priorities Partnership (NPP). In 2008, the NPP released the report *National Priorities & Goals: Aligning Our Efforts to Transform America's Healthcare*. It identified palliative and end-of-life care as one of the six National Priorities that, if addressed, would significantly improve the quality of care delivered to Americans.[32] In 2010, the NPP convened a palliative and end-of-life care meeting. It developed several areas on which to focus strategies to promote palliative care, including quality improvement stakeholders, insurers, consumer groups, certification groups, professional groups, and educational institutions.[33] In 2012, the NQF developed 14 measures on palliative and end-of-life care.[34]

Within the federal structures of healthcare reporting, work has been done as well. The Measure Applications Partnership (MAP) is a public–private partnership convened by the NQF. MAP was created to provide input to the Department of Health and Human Services on the selection of performance measures for public reporting and performance-based payment programs. Each year the MAP clinician workgroup reviews measures for the government to use in its reporting programs. It continues the work on the measures put forth by the NPP and the previous measures endorsed in 2012.

EVOLUTION OF PALLIATIVE NURSING EDUCATION

Other initiatives are exclusive to nursing. The multifaceted project *Strengthening Nursing Education to Improve End-of-Life Care* was funded by the Robert Wood Johnson Foundation and focused on improving nursing knowledge about end-of-life care.[35] The first component of the project reviewed nursing textbooks for end-of-life content, which was liberally defined as pain and symptom management, care of the dying patient, or spiritual care. This was completed in 1999, and it demonstrated that written content in end-of-life nursing care was nearly nonexistent.[35] One result was *The Oxford Textbook of Palliative Nursing*, originally co-edited by Betty Ferrell and Nessa Coyle. Now in its fifth edition, with Drs. Betty Ferrell and Judith Paice as editors, this nursing text serves as a reference for both the RN and APRN.

The second component of the project examined end-of-life care content in nursing licensing examinations. This resulted in the creation of baccalaureate education competencies in end-of-life care that were disseminated within the American Association of Colleges of Nursing (AACN) document, *Peaceful Death: Recommended Competencies and Curricular Guidelines for End-of-Life Nursing Care*.[36] Previous research had clearly demonstrated that both RNs and APRNs felt they had inadequate preparation in end-of-life care.[37,38] These competencies have served as the basis for nursing education at both the graduate and undergraduate levels. Palliative and end-of-life content questions now appear on the National Council Licensure Examination (NCLEX) and on some national advanced practice certification examinations.

The third component was to support key organizations to improve end-of-life education for nursing. The result was the *Nursing Leadership Consortium on End-of-Life Care*, funded by the Project on Death in America. The goal was to design an agenda for the nursing profession in end-of-life care.[39] The agenda emphasized (1) educating nurse leaders in strategies of planning and managing change and advocacy related to palliative care and end-of-life care; (2) creating a system of support, networking, and mentorship for nurses engaged in leadership and advocacy in palliative and end-of-life care; and (3) developing and implementing innovative strategies to advance the priorities of the Nursing Leadership Consortium on End-of-Life Care.[39]

An important collaboration between AACN and the City of Hope established the End-of-Life Nursing Education Consortium (ELNEC), which created a model of education for nurses.[40] The ELNEC curriculum, which initially focused the 1997 AACN's *Peaceful Death Competencies*, was created to educate nurses at all levels of practice and across all specialties. With a goal of developing a core of expert educators and teaching resources to enhance end-of-life care competency, many versions have been developed over the past 20 years, including core, graduate, oncology, critical care, geriatrics, pediatrics, and veterans.[40] More than 1 million nurses and health professionals have been trained. In 2013, the ELNEC Advanced Practice Registered Nurse Curriculum was developed, with the authors of this chapter serving as consultants for its development. The goal is to offer education to new APRNs entering palliative care. There is a graduate version online as well as a curriculum for Doctor of Nursing Practice (DNP) faculty to teach them how to integrate palliative care into a DNP oncology curriculum. Recently, a curriculum specific to oncology APRNs has been created to help integrate primary palliative nursing skills into advanced oncology nursing practice. Current ELNEC versions include core, critical care, pediatric, geriatric, APRN, DNP palliative oncology, and oncology APRN.[40]

In 2001, an important summit was held of national nursing leaders who represented clinical practice, academia, and research. The goal was to discuss advanced practice nursing in palliative care. The result was the document, *Advanced Practice Nurses Role in Palliative Care: A Position Statement from American Nursing Leaders*, which outlined the unique role of advanced practice nurses (APNs) in palliative care, and a companion monograph of pioneer APNs in the field.[12,41] The position statement acknowledged the APN role in palliative care as a "valuable resource in national efforts to improve care and quality of life for Americans and their families living with advanced, life-limiting illness."[41] These concepts were later woven into HPNA position statements.

Two graduate programs with a focus on specialist palliative nursing emerged early in palliative nursing development.[6] In 1998, Ursuline College in Ohio offered preparation for the palliative CNS and New York University offered a program for the palliative NP. Both of the novel programs promoted specialist practice. The programs were successful for several years. However, in 2008, the National Council of State Boards of Nursing released the Licensure, Accreditation, Certification, and Education (LACE) model to increase the clarity and uniformity of APRN education and practice.[42] The LACE model stated that APRNs must be educated in one of six population foci: (1) family/individual across the lifespan, (2) adult-gerontology, (3) pediatrics, (4) neonatal, (5) women's health/gender-related, or (6) psychiatric/mental health.[42] Thus, APRN education was focused on population-based and primary practice rather than disease-focused specialties. The result was that palliative care was no longer recognized as a primary practice, but as a specialty practice. Thus, both programs needed to revise their curricula, moving away from a primary palliative care focus to meet the population/primary care focus of the LACE model. The LACE model remains controversial because palliative care cuts across all the foci and requires knowledge across the life trajectory of wellness and illness.

PALLIATIVE NURSING AS A SPECIALTY

In 1998, the Hospice Nurses Association embraced palliative care and changed its name to the Hospice and Palliative Nurses Association. In 2002, the *Scope and Standards of Hospice and Palliative Nursing Practice* was published in collaboration with the American Nurses Association.[43] These delineated the actions of RNs, APNs, and APRNs. Each subsequent standard represents the broader scope of palliative nursing for individuals with serious illness, beginning at diagnosis, through treatment and, if preferred by the patient and family, continuing to hospice care, which focuses on the last 6 months of care. Moreover, they reflect the current social, cultural, and political milieu.[20,21] Primary palliative nursing and specialty palliative nursing are described, and the different levels of advanced practice nursing within palliative care are delineated. One is a clinical role, where the APRN practices in the role of CNS, NP, certified nurse midwife, or certified nurse anesthetist. In a nonclinical role, the researcher, administrator, case manager, and educator are delineated as APNs.

To emphasize the practice of APRNs, *Competencies for the Advanced Practice Hospice and Palliative Care Nurse* were first developed in 2002 by the HPNA.[44] They are in their third edition and speak to care across the life continuum from perinatal to geriatric care. They focus on the fact that the principles of advanced practice and nursing process are consistent for all practice, although specific care delivery differs by age group.[45]

In 2006, HPNA developed the *Standards for Clinical Practicum in Palliative Nursing for Practicing Professional Nurses*, which were updated in 2015.[46,47] The goal of the standards is to ensure quality and consistency within palliative nursing education. Specific to advanced practice nursing is that a palliative program must have an Advanced Certified Hospice and Palliative Nurse (ACHPN) who leads the nursing education for graduate practicums and provides mentoring in the role development of an APRN. In addition, it sets the standard that palliative programs offering advanced nursing preceptorships or practicums must have been established for at least 2 years. It emphasizes the importance of using the NCP's *Clinical Practice Guidelines* as a framework for education. Finally, it requires palliative care programs offering APRN practicums or preceptorships to use the *Palliative Nursing: Scope and Standards of Practice* and the *Competencies for the Palliative and Hospice APRN*.

PALLIATIVE NURSING CERTIFICATION

Certification is a measure of specialty practice and serves as public recognition of an APRN's expertise. Within palliative care, nursing was first to develop a specialty hospice nursing certification in 1994, which in 2001 was expanded to include palliative nursing.[6,21] (See Chapter 3, "Credentialing, Certification and Scope of Practice Issues for the Palliative APRN.") This was based on being recognized by ANA as a nursing specialty in 1987. Medicine offered certification in hospice and palliative medicine in 1996, and social work in 2000, followed later by chaplaincy organizations. In 2003, specialty certification at the APRN level was first offered.[48] As a note, palliative care was not recognized as a medical specialty by the American Board of Medical Specialties until 2007. As a collaborative effort between the American Nurses Credentialing Center and the National Board for the Certification of Hospice and Palliative Nursing, the examination necessitated evaluation of the CNS role and the NP role. The role delineation study found that the work in each role was almost identical and therefore only one examination was necessary; this study has been repeated several times with

similar results continuing with one examination. Starting in the early 2000s, many nurses used the ACHPN credential to establish palliative care as their primary practice.

An important milestone was achieved when the Center for Medicare and Medicaid Services recognized the National Board of Certification of Hospice and Palliative Nurses as one of seven recognized national certifications for reimbursement eligibility.[49,50] However, this was short-lived, because implementation of the LACE model no longer allowed palliative care as a primary area of practice.[42] Nevertheless, the role delineation study to determine the difference between CNS and NP practice was recently repeated, and the results again found that the activities were similar, necessitating one examination. To date, more than 2,200 APRNs have obtained the ACHPN credential.[51]

THE PALLIATIVE APRN TODAY

The palliative APRN role has evolved over the past 20 years, more rapidly in adult care than in pediatric care. APRNs are practicing primary palliative care and specialty palliative care across the lifespan, diseases, settings, and roles. Of note, pediatric APRN roles are still evolving because of how pediatric palliative care is billed and the prevalent consultant model of care. In addition, there is a difference in how pediatric care is delivered in designated children's hospitals that may have the luxury of more resources versus community or safety net hospitals that care for children.

There are two roles of advanced practice nursing in palliative care, set forth by the American Nurses Association and described in *Palliative Nursing: Scope and Standards of Practice*. One role is the graduate-level prepared specialty nurse who is educated at the master's or doctoral level but does not practice in the clinical arena.[21, p. 23] The second role is the clinical role, or APRN, educated at a master's degree or higher, working across settings.[21, p. 23] The phrase "advanced practice nurse" is an umbrella term which includes both types of graduate-prepared nurse. Therefore, all APRNs are APNs, but not all APNs are APRNs. Table 1.1 explains the two roles, and Table 1.2 gives information about the settings where APNs practice.

The current state of graduate palliative nursing education is inconsistent. Work has been done to create content guidelines for graduate programs for APRNs wanting to focus on palliative care as a minor or subspecialty. Table 1.3 and Table 1.4 offer resources and guidelines for palliative APRN practice. Several national organizations, such as ELNEC, CAPC, and HPNA, have recognized this gap in education and skill-building. HPNA offers palliative-focused continuing education for all levels of nursing practice. Since 2000, ELNEC has offered 2-day education programs focusing on eight modules. Recognizing the lack of APRN-specific education, in 2013, ELNEC launched a 2-day classroom APRN course focusing on six clinical modules (overview of palliative nursing, pain management, symptom management, communication, loss and grief, the final hours) and four program development models (finances, quality, education, and

Table 1.1 ADVANCED PRACTICE NURSING DESIGNATION, EDUCATION, AND ROLES

APN TYPE	EDUCATIONAL PREPARATION	ROLES
Graduate-level–prepared APN[4,20]	Master's or doctoral degree	Administrator Researcher Case manager Academic educator Policy advocate Ethicist
Clinically educated APRN	Master's, post-master's, doctoral degree	Clinical nurse specialist (CNS) Nurse practitioner (NP) Certified nurse midwife (CNM) Certified registered nurse anesthetist (CRNA)

Table 1.2 ROLES AND SETTINGS FOR PALLIATIVE APRNS

Clinical nurse specialist or nurse practitioner	Hospice, home health agency, clinic, residential facility, skilled care facility, long-term care facility, hospital
Case manager	Insurance company, hospital (acute and rehabilitation), skilled care facility, hospice, home health agency, private practice
Educator	Academic setting, such as school of nursing and/or medicine, hospital, professional organization
Researcher	National research entity, such as National Institutes of Health or National Institute of Nursing Research, academic setting, such as school of nursing and/or medicine, academic medical setting, professional organization
Administrator	Hospice, home health agency, palliative care service
Policymaker	Professional organization, public organization, federal or state legislative body
Ethicist	Healthcare organizations, schools of nursing, professional organizations
Social justice advocate	Professional organizations, public organizations, federal or state legislative bodies, clinical settings (hospice, home health agency, clinics, residential facility, skilled care facility, long-term care facility, hospital, schools, prisons, group homes, rural clinics, etc.), payor settings (insurers and reimbursement entities), academic education settings, professional organization, public organization, federal or state legislative body
Technologist	Telehealth development within organizations, health apps, smart device integration, electronic information storage, health equipment

Table 1.3 PROFESSIONAL ORGANIZATIONAL RESOURCES FOR APRNS

American Nurses Association	*Nursing: Scope and Standards of Practice*, 4th ed. (2021)[4] *Position Statement: Nurses' Roles and Responsibilities in Providing Care and Support at the End of Life* (2016)[52] *Position Statement: The Nurse's Role in Ethics and Human Rights: Protecting and Promoting Individual Worth, Dignity, and Human Rights in Practice Settings* (2016)[53] *Position Statement: Nursing Care and Do Not Resuscitate* (DNR) (2020)[54]
Hospice and Palliative Nurses Association	*Palliative Nursing: Scope and Standards of Practice*, 6th ed. (2021)[21] *Competencies for the Palliative and Hospice APRN*, 3rd ed. (2021)[45] *Position Statement: The Nurse's Role in Advance Care Planning* (2017)[55] *The Hospice and Palliative APRN Professional Practice Guide* (2017)[56]
National Council of State Boards of Nursing	*Consensus Model for APRN Regulations: Licensure, Accreditation, Certification & Education*[42] (LACE) (2008)

Table 1.4 REFERENCES FOR THE PALLIATIVE APRN

National Consensus Project for Quality Palliative Care	*Clinical Practice Guidelines for Quality Palliative Care,* 4th ed. (2018)
National Comprehensive Cancer Network	*NCCN Clinical Practice Guidelines in Oncology (NCCN Guidelines) Palliative Care* (2022)
National Institute of Nursing Research	*The Science of Compassion: Future Directions in End-of-Life & Palliative Care* (2011)
National Quality Forum	*Measure Applications Partnership: Performance Measurement Coordination Strategies for Hospice and Palliative Care Final Report* (2012) *Annual Reports of the Measure Applications Partnership: Various Workgroups: Clinician, Medicaid, Hospital, Post-Acute Care/Long-Term Care, Rural Health*
National Academy of Medicine (Formerly Institute of Medicine)	*The Future of Nursing: Charting a Path to Health Equity* (2021) *The Future of Nursing: Leading Change, Advancing Health* (2011) *Delivering High-Quality Cancer Care: Charting a New Course for a System in Crisis* (2013) *Dying in America: Improving Quality and Honoring Individual Preferences Near the End of Life* (2014)
Oxford University Press	*Oxford Textbook of Palliative Nursing,* 5th ed. (2019) *Communication in Palliative Nursing* (2012) *Textbook of Interdisciplinary Communication* (2014)

leadership), anticipating that APRNs would be leading more palliative care programs.

Outside of fellowships and observerships, there are few clinical experiences for APRNs. Of the few that exist, there are limitations in patient care exposure due to licensure, time, expense, and support for both CNSs and NPs.[57] There are few graduate programs that offer focused palliative care education, subspecialty, or certificate programs at either the master's or doctoral level.[58] Moreover, there are only a handful of APRN fellowships.[59] For pediatric care, there is only one graduate program devoted to pediatric palliative care and one fellowship focusing on developing pediatric expertise. Except for one community-based program, fellowships are offered at academic medical centers, with the majority targeted toward NPs.

The result is that the majority of fellowships are using this training to increase their workforce and retain APRNs rather than promote APRNs as leaders in the field.[57] Nonetheless, it is important to promote consistency in palliative APRN fellowships to assure that, even with the goal of interprofessional work, specific APRN role development and competencies are integrated into curricula. Graduate nursing program faculty with palliative care subspecialties developed consensus-based elements for palliative APRN education at the graduate level. This includes essential content, pedagogy, and competencies for the specialty palliative APRN to enter into practice content after graduation from these programs.[58] In addition, competencies and content have been built for postgraduate palliative APRN fellowships.[59]

Graduate-level–prepared specialty nurses work in indirect roles, such as research, case management, administration, and education. Their settings of practice include academic research or education settings, schools of nursing, professional organizations, specialty clinics, and community settings. APRNs in these roles promote all aspects of palliative care and palliative nursing by developing diverse programs for the public, insurers, and international communities; creating palliative care and nursing educational programs; and performing palliative care and palliative nursing research. Many documents frame such work, including the NQF's *A National Framework and Preferred Practices for Palliative and Hospice Care Quality: A Consensus Report,* the NPP's *Palliative and End-of-Life Convening Meeting Synthesis Report* strategies, and the NCP's *Clinical Practice Guidelines.*[25,31,33] Although specialty palliative certification in these indirect roles does not exist, it is available in related areas, such as RN, administrator, pediatric nurse, or perinatal loss expert.

APRNs making a midcareer change into palliative care may find it a difficult transition. Educational opportunities are limited due to financial constraints, lack of education time, and shrinking education funds. There are also limits imposed by the variations of APRN practice—specifically, licensure variability from state to state makes it difficult for APRNs to cross into other states to obtain direct clinical experience. However, there are immersion programs that offer cost-effective exposure to APRN leaders in quality palliative care programs.[60] One such program, created by APRNs specifically for APRNs, is the Palliative APRN Externship. This is a 1-week program of both didactic and clinical exposure for a small cohort at three sites across the country; it has shown impressive outcomes.[60,61]

APRN ROLES

Social Justice and Health Equity Advocate

The role of APRN as social justice and health equity advocate arises out of the new definition of nursing, one that places advocacy at the forefront for all patients and care. In the past few years, the role of the APRN as social justice and health equity advocate has become increasingly important through the exposure of systemic racial injustice in healthcare. APRNs use their education in community assessment to examine who is being cared for in the community and who is not, and they collaborate with communities to help grow palliative care in underrepresented, underserved, and marginalized communities. APRNs can also foster the next generation of nurses by examining the palliative care workforce in their area and working to promote diversity. Finally, APRNs can work together in other roles to ensure equity and diversity in education, both in content and faculty, research in terms of populations, clinical practice in terms of assuring access for all, and policy to assure access for all.

Research

The role of research allows the APRN full participation to initiate, create, participate in, or lead research projects. This can include quantitative or qualitative research. There are the formal research roles of identifying clinical problems, developing and conducting research studies, and overseeing recruitment and data collection. Other important projects include quality improvement, translating research into practice, using research to create policies and procedures, educating others about the research process, and the use of evidence-based practice. In either type of role, the APRN draws on clinical experience from a patient or clinical perspective, enabling solutions to common palliative care concerns.

Education

The role of educator has both a formal and an informal dimension. Formal academic roles at schools of nursing include tenured faculty positions, such as adjunct professor, assistant professor, associate professor, and professor. Nontenured positions include instructors, lecturers, and adjunct clinical positions. Educator roles may also include educational positions within professional organizations, such as director or coordinator of education for a professional nursing organization or another discipline. Other education roles are present in palliative care and palliative care–related corporations, as with continuing education providers, pharmaceutical companies, or technical assistance companies, such as those providing learning management systems. Finally, there are educational initiatives that offer regional, national, and international opportunities in palliative care and palliative nursing education using the ELNEC curricula. APRN educators must ensure there is understanding of the various aspects of advanced nursing practice. Other aspects of education include palliative care development, APRN roles (role development and scope of practice), palliative care delivery (content, medications, communication, etc.), social context (ethical issues within palliative care), policy, reimbursement, technology, and health equity, to name a few.

Care Manager, Care Coordinator

The role of APRN care manager is found within healthcare organizations, insurers, and private companies. Care managers within hospitals are charged with increasingly difficult post-hospital care planning, with the emphasis on moving patients out of the hospital. In the community, there are more APRN care managers who have the skills to create plans to keep complex patients in the community setting. These may include geriatric specialists, hospice specialists, or case managers within home health, hospice, or specialty programs, such as cardiac disease or pulmonary disease. With an increasingly complex health system and a growing geriatric population, care managers and care coordinators will be needed now more than ever before.

Administrator

The role of the APRN administrator is long established because many APRNs have started and led palliative care programs and palliative care initiatives. APRN administrators are charged with using their leadership skills inherent within the role and integrating skills from their graduate education. In addition, they may manage and coordinate programs depending on the progressiveness of the system in which they work. Similar to the collaborative work of interprofessional clinical care, the APRN administrator must collaborate with colleagues from business, finance, and informational technology to be effective in a leadership or managerial role. As palliative care develops, there are more aspects than just clinical care in which to lead.

Policy Expert

The APRN in policy and advocacy can be found in legislative entities or policy departments of professional organizations, associations, and insurers. Issues to work on include recognition of practice, ability to undertake full scope of practice, autonomy to support the Medicare Hospice Benefit, reimbursement, and prescriptive authority to name a few. Working in policy and advocacy, the APRN collaborates with others to determine strategic processes while also working to develop consistent messaging. The APRN grounds their work from their nursing practice and the public trust in nursing.

Clinical Practice

Within the clinical roles of CNS, NP, certified nurse midwife, and certified nurse anesthetist, many APRNs work in myriad health settings, including telehealth, home, hospice, ambulatory and outpatient clinics, long-term care, skilled nursing facilities, community and rural hospitals, and academic medical centers (see Table 1.2). They have met or been "grandmothered" into the requirements set by the National Council of State Boards of Nursing, or they may have completed a curriculum that combines population-specific issues with pain, palliative, or hospice concepts.

The APRN has two functions: a consultant or a primary care provider. In the consultant role, the APRN offers expertise in the care and management of patients with chronic progressive, serious advanced, or life-limiting illness. In this role, the APRN offers advice but does not write orders, request diagnostic tests, or write prescriptions. Part of the consulting process involves educating colleagues about the appropriateness of moving palliative care upstream to diagnosis. The other part of consulting is performing expert care and offering expert opinion in the physical, psychological, spiritual, and emotional aspects of care. As a consultant, the APRN has limited control over the patient's care; rather, it is hoped that through the collaborative process, recommendations, suggestions, and advice will be followed. In a primary care role, the APRN takes on responsibility for the patient. In this role, he or she is responsible for all aspects of care, from diagnostics to prescriptions, from admission to discharge, and everything in between. As a primary provider, the APRN has more control but a larger burden of care. Patients may require more time and focus.

In addition, the APRN is part of an interdisciplinary team, as required by the definition of specialty palliative care stated in the NCP guidelines. The interdisciplinary team may include physicians, chaplains, nurses, nursing assistants, social workers, physical therapists, occupational therapists, speech and language pathologists, dieticians, pharmacists, volunteers, and bereavement specialists. The team must work collaboratively and capitalize on each member's strengths and expertise. Effective team communication is essential, because this is a clear indicator of quality care and patient and family satisfaction.

THE FUTURE OF PALLIATIVE APRNS INFLUENCING CARE DELIVERY

In the changing healthcare landscape, nurses, particularly APRNs, have been identified as an essential element to improving care and access, particularly as healthcare reform continues.[1,41,57,62,63] The *Promoting Excellence: Advanced Practice Nurse Position Statement* acknowledged early on that APRNs offered promise for managing the changing needs of the aging population. Specifically, APRNs have the skills in clinical practice, education, and advocacy to develop palliative care in novel ways. The 2011 IOM report *The Future of Nursing: Leading Change, Advancing Health* acknowledged the essential contributions of nursing at the bedside and in healthcare redesign with four messages, on which work continues in the *Future of Nursing 2030*[63,64]:

Nurses should practice to the full extent of their education and training.

Nurses should achieve higher levels of education and training through an improved education system that promotes seamless academic progression.

Nurses should be full partners with physicians and other healthcare professionals in redesigning healthcare in the United States.

Effective workforce planning and policymaking require better data collection and information restructure.

Each of these messages has important implications for hospice and palliative advanced practice nursing. APRNs should be practicing to the full extent of their education and training, but also to their scope of practice.

There is much work to be done to promote the APRN role within all types of programs. A more diverse population of nurses should be encouraged to pursue graduate education and training to promote palliative care within primary care practices, specialty clinics, and specialty programs. This promotes health equity, quality care, and access to care. Of note, to ensure quality delivery, there must be more emphasis placed on promoting well-being and resiliency at the individual, team, and organizational levels.[21,65,66,67,68] APRNs offer creative solutions in redesigning healthcare with population-focused initiatives and need to be involved in the development of technology for palliative care of the future. This allows them to create innovative models of care, develop software applications, and assess technological efficacy of care. APRNs may have a major role in workforce redesign and in restructuring care away from the hospital and back into the community where patients and family prefer care. Moreover, this promotes health equity because the *Future of Nursing 2030* promotes care that is patient-, family-, and community-centered. Positions are being created in the community that allow APRNs to use their full range of skills, outside the hierarchy inherent in hospital settings.

The National Academy of Medicine's *Future of Nursing for 2030: Charting a Path to Health Equity* recognizes the constant presence of nursing. The message is that nursing can create a culture of health, reduce health disparities, and improve the health and well-being of both the nurse and the US population in the twenty-first century.[21,64,69] Palliative APRNs are part of the future, working to facilitate changes in clinical care, nurse education, nursing leadership, and nursing–community partnerships.[64]

By the nature of their care, APRNs provide person-centered, family-focused care and engage in expert nurse–patient communication and advance care planning. APRNs are teaching and mentoring the next generation of clinicians, as well as their colleagues and the public, about palliative care. As a reimbursable provider and leaders of palliative care programs, APRNs have an integral role in payment and policies related to palliative care and need an understanding of reimbursement.[70] With the goal of palliative care being to keep patients at home and out of the hospital, APRNs are uniquely qualified and positioned to provide services, particularly in rural and community settings. They practice throughout the country in urban, suburban, community, and rural areas, with a focus on promoting wellness and alleviating suffering for patients and families living with illness. Within their scope of nursing practice, APRNs may diagnose, treat, prescribe for, and manage various health problems.

Within cancer care, there is a mandate for quality palliative care, and APRNs will be necessary to meet the growing demands of care. In 2012, the American Society of Clinical Oncology stated that palliative care should be offered to patients with advanced stages of lung cancer as well as for metastatic disease.[69] In the same year, the American College of Surgeons, in collaboration with the Commission on Cancer, issued a statement that palliative services should be offered to all cancer patients across the cancer trajectory.[69,71] Finally, the 2013 IOM report *Delivering High-Quality Cancer Care: Charting a Course for a System in Crisis* suggests that scope of practice and reimbursement structures be created to promote comprehensive care.[72] With the shortage of oncology physicians, the interdisciplinary team will need to be maximally utilized based on their skills. APRNs will be needed to provide palliative care within oncology care.

In cardiovascular care, there is a new emphasis on palliative care. In 2014, the American Heart Association and the American Stroke Association issued joint guidelines for palliative care in caring for patients with heart disease and stroke.[73] The organizations recognized that palliative care should begin at the onset of such an event. In particular, this includes advance care planning, goal-setting, and family support, in particular for surrogate decision-makers. Given the call for palliative care for all stroke patients, APRNs will have a large role in promoting the use of palliative care and providing it across settings. This will have an impact on the large numbers of nurses in cardiovascular nursing. However, other chronic conditions, such as renal disease, neurodegenerative disease, and dementia have been integrating palliative care into their standards of treatment.

Despite this goal, clinical education and organized training in palliative care are seriously lacking. The NCP's *Clinical Practice Guidelines* offers a structure for future nursing education and research developed and initiated within the realm of advanced practice nursing in all aspects of palliative nursing. The provision of expert advanced palliative nursing requires clinical education and experience. The challenge for palliative APRNs will be developing the skills and knowledge necessary for their roles. For nurses entering a graduate program, there may be palliative care courses in pain and symptom management, advanced illness, and psychological coping. If an APRN is making a midcareer change into palliative care, there is a structure to allow development and mentorship within the palliative APRN role. While interprofessional education is appropriate for content and principles of palliative care, APRNs must receive coaching, mentoring, and education in specific palliative nursing principles and role-specific issues.

Furthermore, it is hoped that more innovative programs will be developed for midcareer transitions into palliative care. There are several examples of APRN-led palliative care programs: a NP–led primary care palliative care clinic,[74] a NP–led palliative care clinic imbedded in a health system,[75] and a CNS–led initiative in an oncology clinic.[76] There is the potential for more community-based models to emerge in which palliative APRNs initiate or play a leading role in development and service delivery.

LEADERSHIP

As the numbers of APRNs grow, leadership will be essential. Leadership is necessary to improve the care of individuals with serious illness. Leadership gives APRNs the influence to guide social, practice, and environmental change. While there are many definitions of leadership, two are germane to palliative care. Kruse states that leadership is "a process of social influence that maximizes the efforts of others toward achieving a goal."[77,78] This definition speaks to the aspects of leaders within a palliative care team focusing on quality care and access. Sullivan and Decker state that "Leadership involves influencing the attitudes, beliefs, behaviors and feelings of others."[10] Leadership in palliative care is about influencing many constituencies. Patients, families, healthcare colleagues, healthcare systems, insurers, legislators, and communities need education on quality palliative care as part of quality healthcare (Box 1.2).

APRNs are increasingly being asked to lead initiatives such as palliative care programs, palliative care teams, policy initiatives, quality outcomes, and organizations.[57,79] Leadership can occur within the areas of clinical practice, management and administration, research, education, policy, quality, health equity, well-being, and technology. Leadership encapsulates various characteristics and skills, including building connections, developing trust, engaging in critical thinking and critical listening, taking accountability and responsibility, communicating effectively, assessing oneself, giving constructive feedback, and negotiating conflict. The challenge is that there are limited leadership resources for APRNs, and most of these focus on management or administration and are expensive. Therefore, leadership is grounded within the NCP *Clinical Practice Guidelines*. APRN leadership includes expertise or continual growth in both evidence-based palliative care and advanced practice palliative nursing and understanding of palliative care models, healthcare principles, and Medicare guidelines. There are many good choices for obtaining leadership development through the programs and resources listed in Box 1.3.

Box 1.2 **APRN LEADERSHIP EXAMPLES**

Designing new strategies to achieve health equity within palliative care by focusing on workforce diversity, culturally sensitive palliative care content, and initiatives to assure palliative care to unserved and underserved populations

Developing, leading, managing, and administrating hospice and palliative care teams across acute care, long-term care, ambulatory, residential, hospice, and home settings for populations across the life trajectory

Role-modeling expert clinical care in acute care, long-term care, ambulatory, residential, hospice, and home settings

Educating colleagues in palliative care principles (what it is; assessment of the physical, psychological, emotional, spiritual, and social domains; program development; quality; communication; and grief and loss) across acute care, long-term care, ambulatory, residential, hospice, and home settings

Participating in and developing research of all aspects of palliative care and nursing and translating evidence into practice

Consulting in patient care issues, program development, and quality issues

Advocating for patients, caregivers, and healthcare professionals in terms of regulations, statutes, laws related to scope of practice, regulatory issues related to hospice and palliative care, advance care planning, pain management, access to care, and reimbursement

Box 1.3 NURSING LEADERSHIP PROGRAMS AND RESOURCES

Programs

American Association of Colleges of Nursing
Leadership Development
https://www.aacnnursing.org/Resources-for-Deans/Leadership-Development

Diversity Leadership Institute
https://www.aacnnursing.org/Diversity-Inclusion/Diversity-Leadership-Institute

Educating Leaders in Academic Nursing
https://www.aacnnursing.org/Academic-Nursing/Professional-Development/Leadership-Development/ELAN

AACN -Wharton Executive Leadership Program
https://www.aacnnursing.org/Faculty/Professional-Development/Wharton-Executive-Program

American Association of Nurse Practitioners
Executive Leadership Program
https://www.aanp.org/practice/professional-development/leadership-program

Cambia Health Foundation
Sojourns Scholar Leadership Program
https://www.cambiahealthfoundation.org/funding-areas/sojourns-scholars-leadership-program.html

Duke and Johnson and Johnson Nurse Leadership Program
https://fmch.duke.edu/community-health/educational-programs/duke-johnson-johnson-nurse-leadership-program

Johns Hopkins Nursing Leadership Academy
https://www.hopkinsmedicine.org/institute_nursing/leadership/

Nursing Leadership Network
NLN Leadership Institute—LEAD and SIMULATION
http://www.nln.org/professional-development-programs/leadership-programs

Robert Wood Johnson Foundation Clinical Scholars Program
https://clinicalscholarsnli.org/

Sigma Theta Tau
Nurse Leadership Academy for Practice
https://www.sigmanursing.org/learn-grow/sigma-academies/nurse-leadership-academy-for-practice

New Academic Leadership Academy
https://www.sigmanursing.org/learn-grow/sigma-academies/new-academic-leadership-academy

Experienced Academic Leadership Academy
https://www.sigmanursing.org/learn-grow/sigma-academies/experienced-academic-leadership-academy

University of Pennsylvania Wharton Nursing Leaders Program
https://executiveeducation.wharton.upenn.edu/for-individuals/all-programs/wharton-nursing-leaders-program/

University of South Carolina Center for Nursing Leadership
https://executiveeducation.wharton.upenn.edu/for-individuals/all-programs/wharton-nursing-leaders-program/

Resources

American Organization of Nurse Leaders Nurse Executive Competencies
https://www.aonl.org/resources/nurse-leader-competencies

American Nurses Association Leadership Institute Competency Model
https://www.nursingworld.org/~4a0a2e/globalassets/docs/ce/177626-ana-leadership-booklet-new-final.pdf

Campaign for Action
Wisconsin Center for Nursing. Leadership Toolkit
https://campaignforaction.org/wp-content/uploads/2015/08/Leadership-Toolkit-WI.pdf

Future of Nursing Campaign for Action (AARP Foundation and Robert Wood Johnson Foundation)
https://campaignforaction.org/about/

Hospice and Palliative Nursing Leadership Resources
https://advancingexpertcare.org/

MENTORING

To ensure the maturity of the field, mentoring is essential. Mentoring is a professional relationship between an individual who is entering a profession, role, specialty, or organization and an individual with more experience who provides support, guidance, assistance, and education. APRNs, as experts and leaders, serve as important mentors to mentees (a novice or protégé) to help them invest in the specialty of palliative nursing, the nursing profession, the field of palliative care, or an organization. Palliative APRNs may be mentors in clinical settings, healthcare settings, professional organizations, healthcare systems, and policy organizations.

Mentoring can be formal, using an application process with established goals, objectives, and a contract, or it can be informal, building mutual respect in a more unstructured process. For the palliative APRN, the mentoring roles include structural, organizational, and career development domains. The domains are educational in terms of the role of the APRN, supportive in terms of a system or organization, or administrative in terms of a leadership role.[57] Again, there is a lack of formal mentoring programs. However, more APRNs are turning to mentor others in an informal structure.

SUMMARY

With their foundational nursing practice and primary palliative care skills, APRNs have more opportunities in emerging models of healthcare. Being the fastest growing sector of healthcare providers and with an emphasis on advocacy, well-being, and health equity, APRNs will be part of the solution to workforce shortages and an aging population. They will be situated in myriad settings in the community, and they must ensure quality access to all populations to reduce health disparities in marginalized or underserved populations, with a focus on patient-, family-, and community-centered care.[64] To promote better care for individuals with serious illness, the APRN's clinical settings include primary care clinics, in-home care for frail elders, and rural practices, as well as accountable care organizations and medical homes and hospitals.

Across these settings, APRNs will prevent unnecessary admissions and promote appropriate, safe, and timely discharges. In determining their roles and responsibilities, key areas for the APRN to survey will include knowledge, role clarification, palliative nursing competence, and a culture that embraces both advanced practice nursing and palliative nursing. Some of the issues APRNs will need to grapple with are (1) the clinical and didactic palliative care education required for clinical roles; (2) licensing, credentialing, and certification for both clinical and nonclinical roles; (3) qualifications to do either primary or specialty advanced palliative nursing; (4) the creation of supportive work environments; and (5) obtaining and ensuring appropriate financial support for their services.

Undoubtedly, the field of palliative care will continue to mature to meet the needs of individuals with serious illness and an aging and sicker population. Specialty palliative APRNs will promote further maturity of the role and create new models of palliative care by building on their knowledge and expertise. Their future is bright as they shape care delivery under health reform.

REFERENCES

1. Auerbach DI, Buerhaus PI, Staiger DO. Implications of the rapid growth of the nurse practitioner workforce in the US. *Health Aff.* 2020;29(2):273–279. doi:10.1377/hlthaff.2019.00686

2. US Department of Health and Human Services, Health Resources and Services Administration, National Center for Health Workforce Analysis. *Projecting the Supply and Demand for Primary Care Practitioners Through 2020.* Rockville, MD: US Department of Health and Human Services. https://bhw.hrsa.gov/data-research/projecting-health-workforce-supply-demand/primary-care-practitioners

3. Lynch M, Dahlin C, Hultman T, Coakley E. Palliative care nursing: Defining the discipline? *J Hosp Palliat Nurs.* 2011;13(2):106–111. doi:10.1097/NJH.0b013e3182075b6e

4. American Nurses Association. *Nursing: Scope and Standards of Practice.* 4th ed. Silver Spring, MD: American Nurses Association; 2021.

5. Dahlin C. *Evolution of Palliative Nursing: Art, Science and Collaboration.* In Levison, J, Fine B. Eds. The Pursuit of Life - The Promise and Challenge of Palliative Care. State College, PA: Pennsylvania State University Press; 2022.

6. Dahlin C, Lynch M. Evolution of the advanced practice nurse in palliative care. In: C Dahlin, M Lynch, eds. *Core Curriculum for the Advanced Practice Hospice and Palliative Registered Nurse.* 2nd ed. Pittsburgh, PA: Hospice and Palliative Nurses Association; 2013: 3–12.

7. Yale Bulletin and Calendar. American academy honors three from YSN. New Haven, CT. 2001. http://archives.news.yale.edu/v30.n11/story9.html

8. Centers for Medicare and Medicaid Services. Medicare Benefit Policy Manual. Chapter 9: Coverage of hospice services under hospital insurance. CMS Publication 100-02, Chp 9, 10, 20.1, 40.1.3. Washington, DC. 2012. http://www.cms.gov/Regulations-and-Guidance/Guidance/Manuals/Downloads/bp102c09.pdf

9. Department of Health and Human Services, Services Centers for Medicare and Medicaid Services. *Transmittal 141: New Hospice Certification Requirements and Revised Conditions of Participation (CoPs).* Washington, DC: CMS Manual System; 2011. https://www.cms.gov/Regulations-and-Guidance/Guidance/Transmittals/2011-Transmittals-Items/CMS1244970

10. SUPPORT Principal Investigators. A controlled trial to improve care for the seriously ill hospitalized patients: The study to understand prognoses and preferences for outcomes and risks of treatment (SUPPORT). *JAMA.* 1995;274(20):1591–1598. doi:10.1001/jama.1995.03530200027032

11. The Robert Wood Johnson Foundation, Milbank Memorial Fund. *Pioneer Programs in Palliative Care: Nine Case Studies.* New York: Milbank Memorial Fund; 2000.

12. Promoting Excellence in End of Life Care. Advanced Practice Nursing: Pioneering Practices in Palliative Care. 2002. https://www.yumpu.com/en/document/view/37527925/advanced-practice-nursing-pioneering-practices-in-dying-well

13. Aulino F, Foley K. The Project on Death in America. *J R Soc Med.* 2001;94(9):492–495. doi:10.1177/014107680109400923

14. Institute of Medicine. *Approaching Death: Improving Care at the End of Life* Washington, DC: National Academies Press; 1997. doi:10.17226/5801

15. Last Acts. *Precepts of Palliative Care.* Washington, DC: Last Acts; 1997.

16. Last Acts. *Means to a Better End: A Report on Dying in America Today.* Washington, DC: Last Acts; 2002.

17. Institute of Medicine. *When Children Die: Improving Palliative and End-of-Life Care for Children and Their Families.* Washington, DC: National Academies Press; 2002. doi:10.17226/10390

18. Institute of Medicine. *Crossing the Quality Chasm: A New Health System for the 21st Century.* Washington, DC: National Academies Press; 2001. doi:10.17226/10027

19. Jennings B, Ryndes T, D'Onofrio C, Baily MA. Access to Hospice Care: Expanding Boundaries, Overcoming Barriers. *Hastings Center Report.* 2003(March-April);Supplement 33(2):S3–S7, S9–S13, S15–S21 passim. PMID: 12762184.

20. American Nurses Association, Hospice and Palliative Nurses Association. *Palliative Nursing: Scope and Standards of Practice—An Essential Resource for Hospice and Palliative Nurses.* 5th ed. Silver Spring, MD: American Nurses Association and Hospice and Palliative Nurses Association; 2014.

21. Dahlin C, ed. *Palliative Nursing Scope and Standards of Practice.* 6th ed. Pittsburgh, PA: Hospice and Palliative Nurses Association; 2021.

22. National Consensus Project for Quality Palliative Care. *Clinical Practice Guidelines for Quality Palliative Care.* Pittsburgh, PA: National Consensus Project for Quality Palliative Care; 2004.

23. National Consensus Project for Quality Palliative Care. *Clinical Practice Guidelines for Quality Palliative Care.* 2nd ed. Pittsburgh, PA: National Consensus Project; 2009.

24. National Consensus Project for Quality Palliative Care. *Clinical Practice Guidelines for Quality Palliative Care.* 3rd ed. Pittsburgh, PA: National Consensus Project for Quality Palliative Care; 2013.

25. National Consensus Project for Quality Palliative Care. *Clinical Practice Guidelines for Quality Palliative Care.* 4th ed. Richmond, VA: National Hospice and Palliative Care Coalition; 2018. https://www.nationalcoalitionhpc.org/ncp/

26. National Institutes of Health. NIH state-of-the-science conference statement on improving end-of-life care. *NIH Consens State Sci Statements.* 2004;21(3):1–26.

27. The National Institute for Nursing Research (NINR). *Executive Summary: The Science of Compassion Future Directions in End-of-Life and Palliative Care Summit.* 2011; Bethesda, MD. https://www.ninr.nih.gov/sites/files/docs/science-of-compassion-executive-summary.pdf

28. Institute of Medicine. *Dying in America: Improving Quality and Honoring Individual Preferences Near End of Life.* Washington, DC: National Academies Press; 2014. doi:10.17226/18748

29. Schneider E, Abrams M, Shah A, Lewis C, Shah T. *Health Care in America: The Experience of People with Serious Illness.* New York: Commonwealth Fund; October 2018. https://www.commonwealthfund.org/sites/default/files/2018-10/Schneider_HealthCareinAmerica.pdf

30. National Quality Forum. Mission and Vision. 2021. https://www.qualityforum.org/about_nqf/mission_and_vision/

31. National Quality Forum. *A National Framework and Preferred Practices for Palliative and Hospice Care Quality: A Consensus Report.* Washington, DC: NQF; 2006.

32. National Priorities Partnership. National Priorities & Goals: Aligning Our Efforts to Transform America's Healthcare. Washington, DC, 2008. http://psnet.ahrq.gov/resource.aspx?resourceID=8745

33. National Priorities Partnership. *Palliative Care and End-of-Life Convening Meeting Synthesis Report.* Paper presented at Palliative Care and End-of-Life Convening Meeting. Washington, DC; 2010.

34. National Quality Forum. *Endorsement Summary: Palliative Care and End-of-Life Care Measures.* Washington, DC: National Quality Forum; 2012.

35. Ferrell BR, Grant M, Virani R. Strengthening nursing education to improve end-of-life care. *Nurs Outlook.* 1999;47(6):252–256. doi:10.1089/jpm.1999.2.161

36. American Association of Colleges of Nursing. Peaceful death: Recommended competencies and curricular guidelines for end-of-life nursing care. Washington, DC.1997; https://eric.ed.gov/?id=ED453706

37. White K, Coyne P, Lee J. Nurses' perceptions of educational gaps in delivering end-of-life care. *Oncol Nurs Forum.* 2011;38(6):711–717. doi:10.1188/11.ONF.711-717

38. White K, Coyne P, White S. Are hospice and palliative care nurses adequately prepared for end of life care? *J Hosp Palliat Nurs.* 2012;14(2):133–140. doi:10.1097/NJH.0b013e318239b943

39. Rushton CH, Sabatier KH. The nursing leadership consortium on end-of-life care: The response of the nursing profession to the need for improvement in palliative care. *Nurs Outlook.* 2001;49(1):58–60. doi:10.1016/s0029-6554(01)70061-9

40. American Association of Colleges of Nursing, City of Hope. ELNEC Fact Sheet. April 2021. http://www.aacnnursing.org/Portals/42/ELNEC/PDF/FactSheet.pdf

41. Promoting Excellence in End of Life. Advanced practice role nursing role in palliative care: A position statement from American nursing leaders. Missoula, MT. 2002. http://www.mywhatever.com/cifwriter/content/41/pe3673.html

42. National Council of State Boards of Nursing, APRN Advisory Committee. APRN regulation: Licensure, accreditation, certification, and education. Chicago, IL. 2008. https://www.ncsbn.org/Consensus_Model_for_APRN_Regulation_July_2008.pdf

43. Hospice and Palliative Nurses Association, American Nurses Association. *Hospice and Palliative Nursing: Scope and Standards of Practice.* Silver Spring, MD: American Nurses Publishing; 2002.

44. Hospice and Palliative Nurses Association. *Competencies for Advanced Practice Hospice and Palliative Care Nurses.* Pittsburgh, PA: Hospice and Palliative Nurses Association; 2002.

45. Dahlin C. *Competencies for the Palliative and Hospice APRN.* 3rd ed. Pittsburgh, PA: Hospice and Palliative Nurses Association; 2021.

46. Hospice and Palliative Nurses Association. Standards for clinical practicum in palliative nursing for practicing professional nurses. 2006.

47. Hospice and Palliative Nurses Association. *HPNA Standards for Clinical Education of Hospice and Palliative Nurses.* 2nd ed. Pittsburgh, PA: HPNA; 2015. https://advancingexpertcare.org/HPNA/HPNAweb/Education/Standards_for_Clinical_Education.aspx

48. Dahlin C. Palliative care program development. *J Palliat Care Med.* 2015;S5(1):1000S1005–1000S1008. doi:10.4172/2165-7386.1000S5008

49. Centers for Medicare and Medicaid Services, Department of Health and Human Services. *Transmittal 75: Nurse Practitioner (NP) Services and Clinical Nurse Specialist (CNS) Services.* Washington, DC: CMS Manual System; 2007. https://www.cms.gov/Regulations-and-Guidance/Guidance/Transmittals/downloads/r75bp.pdf

50. Centers for Medicare and Medicaid Services, Department of Health and Human Services. *Transmittal 219: Nurse Practitioner (NP) Services and Clinical Nurse Specialist (CNS) Services.* Washington, DC: CMS Manual System; 2007. https://www.cms.gov/Regulations-and-Guidance/Guidance/Transmittals/2016-Transmittals-Items/R219BP

51. Hospice and Palliative Credentialing Center. Advanced certified hospice and palliative nurses (ACHPN). 2021. https://advancingexpertcare.org/HPNA/HPCC/CertificationWeb/Certification_Verification.aspx

52. American Nurses Association. Position statement: Nurses' roles and responsibilities in providing care and support at the end of life. Silver Spring, MD. 2016. https://www.nursingworld.org/~4af078/globalassets/docs/ana/ethics/endoflife-positionstatement.pdf

53. American Nurses Association. Position statement: The nurse's role in ethics and human rights: Protecting and promoting individual worth, dignity, and human rights in practice settings. Silver Spring, MD.2016. https://www.nursingworld.org/practice-policy/nursing-excellence/official-position-statements/id/the-nurses-role-in-ethics-and-human-rights/

54. American Nurses Association. Position statement: Nursing care and do not resuscitate (DNR) decisions. Silver Spring, MD. 2020. https://www.nursingworld.org/~494a87/globalassets/practiceandpolicy/nursing-excellence/ana-position-statements/

social-causes-and-health-care/nursing-care-and-do-not-resuscitate-dnr-decisions-final-nursingworld.pdf

55. Hospice and Palliative Nurses Association. Position statement: Advance care planning. Pittsburgh, PA. 2017. https://advancingexpertcare.org/position-statements/

56. Dahlin C. *The Hospice and Palliative APRN Professional Practice Guide* Pittsburgh, PA: Hospice and Palliative Nurses Association; 2017.

57. Dahlin C, Coyne P. The palliative APRN leader. *Ann Palliat Med.* 2018;8(Suppl 1):S30–S38. doi:10.21037/apm.2018.06.03

58. Dahlin C, Ersek M, Wholihan D, Wiencek C. Specialty palliative APRN practice through state-of-the-art graduate education: Report of the HPNA Graduate Faculty Council (SA509). *J Pain Symptom Manage* 2019;57(2):445. doi:https://doi.org/10.1016/j.jpainsymman.2018.12.189

59. Dahlin C, Wholihan D, Johnstone-Petty M. Palliative APRN fellowship guidelines: A strategy for quality specialty practice: Report of the HPNA APRN Fellowship Council (TH300). Abstract for the Annual Assembly. *J Pain Symptom Manage.* 2019;57(2):383. doi:https://doi.org/10.1016/j.jpainsymman.2018.12.029

60. Dahlin C, Coyne P, Cassel J. The advanced practice registered nurses palliative care externship: A model for primary palliative care education. *J Palliat Med.* 2016;19(7):753–759. doi:10.1089/jpm.2015.0491

61. Gentry JH, Dahlin C. The evaluation of a palliative care advanced practice nursing externship. *J Hosp Palliat Nurs* 2020;22(3):172–179. doi:10.1097/NJH.0000000000000637

62. Auerbach D, Staiger D, Muench U, Buerhaus P. The nursing workforce in an era of health care reform. *New Engl J Med.* 2013;203:1470–1472. doi:10.1056/NEJMp1301694

63. Institute of Medicine. *The Future of Nursing: Leading Change, Advancing Health* (vol. 2019). Washington, DC: The National Academies Press; 2011. http://www.nationalacademies.org/hmd/Reports/2010/The-Future-of-Nursing-Leading-Change-Advancing-Health.aspx

64. National Academy of Medicine. *The Future of Nursing 2020–2030. Charting a Path to Achieve Health Equity.* Washington, DC: National Academies Press; 2021. https://nam.edu/publications/the-future-of-nursing-2020-2030/

65. Altillio T, Dahlin C, Remke SS, Tucker R, Weissman D. *Strategies for Maximizing the Health/Function of Palliative Care Teams: A Resource Monograph from the Center to Advance Palliative Care (CAPC).* New York: Center to Advance Palliative Care; 2014. https://media.capc.org/bootcamp-2019/26-capc-monograph-strategies-for-maximizing-the-health-function-of-palliative-care-teams.pdf

66. Perlo J, Balik B, Swensen S, Kabcenell A, Landsman J, Feeley D. IHI White Paper: IHI Framework for Improving Joy in Work. 2017. http://www.ihi.org/resources/Pages/IHIWhitePapers/Framework-Improving-Joy-in-Work.aspx

67. National Academies of Sciences, Engineering, and Medicine. *Taking Action Against Clinician Burnout: A Systems Approach to Professional Well-Being.* Washington, DC: National Academies Press; 2019. https://www.nap.edu/catalog/25521/taking-action-against-clinician-burnout-a-systems-approach-to-professional

68. American Nurses Foundation. Well-being initiative for nurses. 2020. https://www.nursingworld.org/news/news-releases/2020/american-nurses-foundation-launches-national-well-being-initiative-for-nurses/

69. Smith TJ, Temin S, Alesi ER, et al. ASCO American Society of Clinical Oncology Provisional Clinical Opinion: The integration of palliative care into standard oncology care. *J Clin Oncol.* 2012;30(8):880–887. doi:10.1200/JCO.2011.38.5161

70. Mayer AM, Dahlin C, Seidenschmidt L, Dillon H, Brown A, Crawford T, Coyne P. Palliative Care: A Survey of Program Benchmarking for Productivity and Compensation. *American Journal of Hospice and Palliative Medicine*®. February 2022. doi:10.1177/10499091221077878

71. American College of Surgeons, Commission on Cancer. *Cancer Programs Standards 2012: Ensuring Patient-Centered Care* (vol. V1.2.1). Chicago, IL: American College of Surgeons; 2012.

72. Institute of Medicine. *Delivering High-Quality Cancer Care: Charting a New Course for a System in Crisis.* Washington, DC: National Academies Press; 2013. https://www.nap.edu/catalog/18359/delivering-high-quality-cancer-care-charting-a-new-course-for

73. Holloway RG, Arnold RM, Creutzfeldt CJ, et al. Palliative and end-of-life care in stroke: A statement for healthcare professionals from the American Heart Association/American Stroke Association. *Stroke.* 2014;45(6):1887–1916. doi:10.1161/STR.0000000000000015

74. Owens D, Eby K, Burson S, Green M, McGoodwin W, Isaac M. Primary palliative care clinic pilot project demonstrates benefits of a nurse practitioner-directed clinic providing primary and palliative care. *J Am Acad Nurs Practit.* 2012;24(1):52–58. doi:10.1111/j.1745-7599.2011.00664.x

75. Deitrick LM, Rockwell EH, Gratz N, et al. Delivering specialized palliative care in the community: A new role for nurse practitioners. *Adv Nurs Sci.* 2011;34(4):E23–E36. doi:10.1097/ANS.1090b1013e318235834f.

76. Prince-Paul M, Burant CJ, Saltzman JN, Teston LJ, Matthews CR. The effects of integrating an advanced practice palliative care nurse in a community oncology center: A pilot study. *J Support Oncol.* 2010;8(1):21–27. PMID: 20235420.

76. Kruse K. *What Is Leadership?* Jersey City, NJ: Forbes Media; 2013.

78. Sullivan EJ, Decker PJ. *Effective Leadership and Management in Nursing.* 7th ed. London: Prentice Hall; 2009.

79. Dahlin C, Coyne P, Goldberg J, Vaughn L. Palliative care leadership. *J Palliat Care.* 2018;34(1):21–28. doi:10.1177/0825859718791427

FUNDAMENTAL SKILLS AND EDUCATION FOR THE GENERALIST AND SPECIALIST PALLIATIVE APRN

Dorothy Wholihan, Charles Tilley, and Adrienne Rudden

KEY POINTS

- Advanced practice registered nurses (APRNs) provide primary palliative care through integration of basic palliative care interventions with their population-focused practice and through expert board-certified specialty palliative care.

- The Licensing, Accreditation, Certification, and Education (LACE) model of regulatory standards developed by the National Council of State Boards of Nursing defines specialist-level palliative care as an APRN specialty practice, which is defined by professional board certification.

- Current palliative care education for APRNs includes a variety of programs, including master's, post-master's, doctoral, and continuing professional education programs.

CASE STUDY: APRN EDUCATION

Carlos DeLeon has been an acute care registered nurse (RN) working in the medical intensive care unit of a hospital for 4 years. After a surge of COVID cases, he saw too many people die with uncontrolled symptoms and without any support for themselves or their families. He realized he needed a change in his practice and wanted to help people to stay out of the ICU at the end of their lives. During the pandemic, he was exposed to how the palliative care team worked closely with patients and families to manage symptoms and articulate their goals to attain the best outcomes possible. He attended a virtual End-of-Life Nursing Education Consortium (ELNEC) Critical Care conference, and this confirmed his calling to palliative care. He wants to return to school to obtain a master's degree to become an acute care APRN, with specialty training in palliative care. Alternatively, he is considering a bachelor of science in nursing (BSN) to doctor of nursing practice (DNP) program to develop the clinical leadership and quality improvement skills needed to influence his hospital system to improve end-of-life care for critically ill patients.

DEFINITION OF ADVANCED PRACTICE NURSING

Advanced practice registered nurses (APRNs) have played a pivotal role in palliative care over the past 20 years and will continue to shape the future of hospice and palliative care. Broadly defined and practice-focused, APRNs treat and diagnose illnesses, advise the public on health issues, manage chronic disease, and engage in continuous education to remain current in their knowledge of developments in the field. APRNs hold at least a master's degree, in addition to the initial nursing education and licensing required for all registered nurses (RNs). Based on the definition originally developed by the American Association of Colleges of Nursing (AACN), the term *"APRN"* refers to master's-prepared nurses who provide direct clinical care.[1]

ROADMAPS FOR EDUCATION

In the late 1990s, a national dialogue was ignited about the ability of the healthcare system to provide care to patients with life-threatening illness. In response to the dearth of end-of-life content in most nursing curricula at the time, combined with the realities of an aging population, the expense of unnecessarily prolonged dying driven by advanced technology, and public apprehension about suffering, the AACN, supported by the Robert Wood Johnson Foundation, assembled a panel of experts in 1997 to develop end-of-life competency statements.[2] This project, conducted in accordance with the mandate by the International Council of Nurses (ICN), detailed nurses' unique role in and responsibility for ensuring that individuals experience a peaceful death.[3] A round table of expert nurses and other healthcare professionals, on the premise that the precepts underlying hospice care are essential principles for all end-of-life care, developed an interdisciplinary approach to the educational preparation of nursing students for end-of-life practice. The panel developed 16 end-of-life competency statements to be included in multiple content areas, including health assessment, pharmacology, psychiatric–mental health nursing, nursing management courses, ethical/legal courses, cultural issues content, nursing research, and professional issues/healthcare settings.[2]

The *Clinical Practice Guidelines for Quality Palliative Care* were originally published in 2004 by the National Consensus Project for Quality Palliative Care (NCP).[4] The NCP started as a partnership of five national palliative care organizations: the American Academy of Hospice and Palliative Medicine (AAHPM), the Center to Advance Palliative Care (CAPC), the Hospice and Palliative Nurses Association

(HPNA), the Last Acts Partnership, and the National Hospice and Palliative Care Organization (NHPCO), later joined by the National Palliative Care Research Center and the National Association of Social Workers. The *Clinical Practice Guidelines* was the result of professional consensus in making recommendations about the development of palliative care programs by creating clinical practice guidelines that improve the quality of palliative care in the United States. The fourth edition of the *Clinical Practice Guidelines for Quality Palliative Care*, published in 2018, further delineates the original eight domains identified.[4] Domain 1, Guideline 1.1 states that the interdisciplinary team includes palliative care professionals with the appropriate patient population-specific education, credentialing, and experience and the skills to meet the physical, functional, psychological, social, cultural, and spiritual needs of both patient and family. Of particular importance is assembling a team, which includes chaplains, nurses, advanced practice providers (physician assistants and APRNs), pharmacists, physicians, and social workers, appropriately trained and, ideally, certified in hospice and palliative care, when such certification is available.[4]

Building on the work of the NCP, the National Quality Forum (NQF), a nonprofit public–private partnership, focused on improving the quality of healthcare through setting voluntary consensus standards, in 2006 developed *A National Framework and Preferred Practices for Palliative and Hospice Care Quality* (NQF Preferred Practices).[5] They incorporated the principles of the *Clinical Practice Guideline* domains into the framework, which were directly reflected in the preferred practices.

The NQF identified 38 preferred practices, including educational standards directly relatable to advanced practice education. NQF Preferred Practices 3, 4, and 5 directly addressed education.[5]

- *Preferred Practice 3.* Provide *continuing education* to all healthcare professionals on the domains of palliative care and hospice care.

- *Preferred Practice 4.* Provide *adequate training and clinical support* to assure that professional staff is confident in their ability to provide palliative care to patients.

- *Preferred Practice 5.* Hospice care and specialized palliative care professionals should be *appropriately trained, credentialed, and/or certified* in their area of expertise.

The NCP Clinical Guidelines recommend that Palliative care programs ensure appropriate levels of education for all palliative care professionals. "Advanced practice nurses, physicians, and rehabilitation therapists must have graduate degrees in their respective disciplines, with appropriate professional experience in hospice and palliative care."[4, p.6]

In 2010, the Institute of Medicine (IOM) published landmark recommendations on how to transform the nursing profession so that nurses can fully impact the nation's health. This document, entitled, *The Future of Nursing: Leading Change, Advancing Health*, was congruent with many palliative position statements already mentioned in this chapter

as it attempted to address the needs of an aging population, the growing number of people with chronic diseases, and the need for care coordination.[6] This report has influenced nursing education and practice for the past decade. Eight key recommendations were proposed, with two related to the promotion and elevation of nursing education[6]:

1. Nurses should practice to the full extent of their education and training.

2. Nurses should achieve higher levels of education and training through an improved education system that promotes seamless academic progression.

In response to the IOM report, the Robert Wood Johnson Foundation partnered with the American Association of Retired Persons (AARP) to launch a national campaign—the Future of Nursing: Campaign for Action—to advance the report's recommendations through the establishment of state-based coalitions. Preliminary data at 10 years after the report reveals significant improvements, such as a doubling of the number of practicing nurses with doctoral degrees and a significant expansion of the number of nurses permitted to practice at the full extent of their education and training.[7] The Campaign's formal progress report was originally postponed due to the COVID pandemic but has now been posted to support the release of the new *Future of Nursing 2020–2030 Charing A Path to Achieve Health Equity.*[8]

In 2021, the AACN amended *The Essentials: Core Competencies for Professional Nursing Education.* For all levels of nursing education: baccalaureate, masters, and doctoral.[9] The new essentials are competency-based and provide educational standards for nursing practice as defined within competencies for ten domains. competencies, and sub-competencies for advanced entry-level nursing practice.[9] Hospice, palliative, and supportive care features dominantly, as one of the four defined spheres of care.

> The competencies accompanying each domain are designed to be applicable across four spheres of care (disease prevention/promotion of health and wellbeing, chronic disease care, regenerative or restorative care, and hospice/palliative/supportive care), across the lifespan, and with diverse patient populations. While the domains and competencies are identical for both entry and advanced levels of education, the sub-competencies build from entry into professional nursing practice to advanced levels of knowledge and practice.[9, p.1]

PRIMARY PALLIATIVE CARE VERSUS SPECIALTY PALLIATIVE CARE

With the expansion of the field of palliative care, specialist workforce shortages have become apparent in all disciplines, including advanced practice nursing. There are not enough specialty-trained palliative care clinicians to meet the needs of all patients. As a solution, the concept of *primary palliative care* has evolved. Primary palliative care should be provided by all healthcare professionals and includes the management of chronic illness, basic symptom management, communication, and the appropriate completion of advance directives. Specialty palliative care is provided by professionals with more extensive training and certification in palliative care and is focused on patients and families with more complex needs and serious, advanced illness. It is hypothesized that a combination of generalist and specialist palliative care can meet the palliative care needs of our population in a more sustainable and cost-effective manner.[1]

All APRNs are educated to obtain the knowledge, skills, and competency to perform basic primary palliative nursing. However, additional graduate education and preparation is needed to promote practice at an advanced specialty level. More graduate programs are now including population-focused specialty palliative care education as either elective courses or as more extensive and formal specialty course programs.

PRIMARY PALLIATIVE REGISTERED NURSING PRACTICE

Since the essence of palliative care is embedded in all nursing practice, all nurses already practice primary palliative care. This is inherent in the definition of registered professional nursing as the alleviation of suffering through the diagnosis and treatment of human response to illness[10] and advocacy in the care of individuals, families, communities, and populations. By the nature of their role, all nurses provide physical and psychosocial symptom management. They also have the skills to assess and assist care-planning discussions and to identify spiritual issues and cultural concerns.

Many undergraduate baccalaureate programs offer specific courses in palliative care or incorporate elements of palliative nursing into required classes. After graduating from an accredited nursing program, RNs at the generalist level are required to pass the National Council Licensure Examination (NCLEX-RN), which includes palliative care content.[11] Funded by the Cambia Foundation, the AACN, in conjunction with End of Life Nursing Education Consortium (ELNEC), released the *Competencies and Recommendations for Education Undergraduate Nursing Students (CARES)* document to define palliative care competencies and an online associated curriculum. This work was revised in 2020 to address the needs of new graduate nurses as well.[12,13]

In 2017, the HPNA, in conjunction with the Hospice and Palliative Credentialing Center and the Hospice and Palliative Nurses Foundation, organized a Palliative Nursing Summit in Washington, DC, entitled *Palliative Care: Nurses Leading Change and Transforming Care.* The goal of this summit was to convene leaders from various nursing specialty organizations to develop a collaborative nursing agenda for primary palliative nursing. The work of the summit focused on three aspects of palliative nursing: communication/advance care planning, coordination/transitions of care, and pain and symptom management.[14]

ADVANCED PRACTICE PRIMARY PALLIATIVE NURSING

In 2018, the Cambia Foundation funded an initiative to develop competencies for primary palliative care for master's-prepared advanced practice nurses. ELNEC faculty developed and later revised a document entitled, "G-CARES: Primary Palliative Care Competencies for Masters and DNP Nursing Students".[15] These competencies align with the AACN *Essentials* and the fourth edition of the *NCP Guidelines for Quality Palliative Care.* The twelve primary palliative care competencies are expected of all graduate nursing students, including APRN, Clinical Nurse Leaders (CNL), nurses in education, administration, informatics, and public health, and DNP students who will be directly or indirectly providing primary palliative care for seriously ill patients and their families, from infants and children through geriatric populations and across the illness trajectory. These primary palliative competencies can be applied to graduate students who will be providing direct primary palliative care across any clinical, community, or technology-mediated (telehealth) setting.[15]

Generalist palliative care competencies are included in the competency statements listed by several nursing organizations.[16–18] The National Organization of Nurse Practitioner Faculty (NONPF) *Nurse Practitioner Core Competencies Content* identifies general core competencies in the realms of communication, cultural competence, ethics, and palliative and end-of-life care.[16] It is important to note that the NONPF competencies are inclusive of all advanced practice nursing specialties and populations, including pediatrics, family, acute care, psychiatric-mental health, and primary care.[19] Similarly, Midwifery Core Competencies include competencies in the realms of communication, collaboration, bioethics, psychosocial, and end-of-life care for the stillborn and family.[17] Clinical nurse specialist (CNS) competencies include relationship-building communication to promote a peaceful end-of-life and engage in difficult conversations, as well as advocacy of ethical principles and ethical conflict resolution of nurses and staff.[18] Table 2.1 outlines generalist-level advanced practice competencies that pertain to palliative care.

ADVANCED PRACTICE SPECIALTY PALLIATIVE NURSING

As described in *Palliative Nursing: Scope and Standards of Practice,*[20] there are two roles in advanced practice specialty palliative nursing practice. One advanced practice role is the graduate-level–prepared specialty nurse educated at the master's or doctoral level in nondirect care roles (e.g., education, research, administration). These nurses practice in a variety of settings such as academic medical centers, schools of nursing, specialty clinics, community settings, academic research or education settings, and various professional organizations. They promote educational programs in palliative care, palliative nursing research, and program development for diverse programs. Although advanced palliative nursing certification

GENERALIST-LEVEL PALLIATIVE CARE COMPETENCIES	NURSE PRACTITIONER (NONPF) ADULT-GERI ACUTE CARE NP ADULT-CARE PRIMARY CARE NP FAMILY NP PEDIATRIC NP NEONATAL NP PSYCHIATRIC MENTAL HEALTH NP	MIDWIFERY (ACNM)	CLINICAL NURSE SPECIALIST (NACNS)
Communication	Leadership competencies • Communicates practice knowledge effectively, both orally and in writing	Hallmarks of midwifery • Skillful communication, guidance, and counseling • Collaboration with other members of the interprofessional healthcare team	Direct care • Uses relationship-building communication to promote health and wellness, healing, self-care, and peaceful end-of-life • Uses advanced communication skills in complex situations and difficult conversations
Ethics	Ethics competencies • Integrates ethical principles in decision-making. • Evaluates the ethical consequences of decisions • Applies ethically sound solutions to complex issues related to individuals, populations, and systems of care	Professional responsibilities • Broad understanding of the bioethics related to the care of women, newborns, and families	Nurses and nursing practice • Leads efforts to resolve ethical conflict and moral distress experienced by nurses and nursing staff. Organizations/Systems • Advocates for ethical principles in protecting the dignity, uniqueness, and safety of all
Cultural competency	Health delivery system competencies • Facilitates the development of healthcare systems that address the needs of culturally diverse populations, providers, and other stakeholders Independent practice competencies • Incorporates the patient's cultural and spiritual preferences, values, and beliefs into healthcare		
Symptom management and end-of-life care	Independent practice competencies • Provides the full spectrum of healthcare services to include health promotion, disease prevention, health protection, anticipatory guidance, counseling, disease management, palliative, and end-of-life care	Components of midwifery care of women • Measures to support psychosocial needs during labor and birth Components of midwifery care of the newborn • End-of-life care for stillbirth and conditions incompatible with life	

From National Organization of Nurse Practitioner Faculties[16]; American College of Nurse Midwives Board of Directors[17]; National Association of Clinical Nurse Specialists[18]; Population-Focused Competencies Task Force.[19]

is not available in these areas, generalist hospice and palliative certification is encouraged. Currently, appropriate examinations offered are for the RN, administrator, generalist pediatric nurse, and perinatal loss expert.[21]

The second, more common level of advanced palliative nursing practice is that of the APRN, a nurse educated at the master's level or above and practicing within one of the four roles defined by the 2008 *Consensus Model for APRN Regulation: Licensure, Accreditation, Certification, and Education (LACE)* document developed by the APRN Consensus Work Group & National Council of State Boards

of Nursing APRN Advisory Committee.[22] According to this document, the APRN is a RN educated at the master's, post-master's, or doctoral level in one of four roles: a CNS, nurse practitioner (NP), certified nurse midwife (CNM), or certified RN anesthetist (CRNA). National certification is required to delineate basic advanced practice competency at the population level. Specialty practice (such as palliative care or oncology) allows depth in one's practice within the established population foci.[22] CRNAs and CNMs working in palliative care may practice in areas like pain management or perinatal palliative care. Most hospice and palliative specialty

APRNs are CNSs and/or NPs. The national certification for palliative care advanced practice nursing is offered for specialty certification on top of basic population certification.[21]

SCOPE AND COMPETENCIES OF THE SPECIALIST PALLIATIVE APRN

The specialty palliative APRN role was first identified 20 years ago when nursing leaders from academia, clinical practice, and research held a national leadership meeting to discuss the vital role of APRN in palliative care (see Chapter 1). While palliative care is most often delivered by multidisciplinary teams, APRNs often lead these teams and are the glue that holds them together to provide optimal care.[23]

The skills required for advanced practice in palliative nursing have been defined by the professional organization that represents this discipline. The American Nurses Association (ANA) and the HPNA have defined standards for practice in the document *Palliative Nursing: Scope and Standards of Practice*, which includes standards specific to advanced nursing practice.[20] In the 2021 sixth edition, the document is accompanied by a more specific delineation of competencies in the HPNA publication entitled *Competencies for the Palliative and Hospice APRN*.[24] This document describes advanced core competencies that represent the knowledge, skills, and attitudes advanced practice hospice and palliative care nurses demonstrate when providing evidence-based care to patients and families experiencing life-limiting, progressive illness. This care encompasses the physical, psychosocial, emotional, and spiritual realms. Thus, graduate education must include these competency domains. Box 2.1 lists the basic areas of palliative APRN competency as defined by the HPNA.[24]

DEFICITS IN NURSING EDUCATION

The topics of palliative and end-of-life care have been historically neglected within both medical and nursing education.[25] In a landmark study of nursing textbooks, Dr. Betty Ferrell and colleagues[26] first documented these deficits, finding that only 2% of nursing textbooks contained any reference to end-of-life care. Ten years later, deficits still remained. Shea

---

Box 2.1 PALLIATIVE NURSING: SCOPE AND STANDARDS OF PRACTICE DEFINED AREAS OF SPECIALTY PALLIATIVE APRN EXPERTISE

Clinical Judgment
  Within palliative care, the palliative nurse demonstrates clinical judgment, clinical reasoning, critical thinking, and decision-making surrounding palliative nursing, integrating global knowledge of multidimensional needs of individuals with serious illness and their families using the nursing process.
Advocacy and Moral Agency
  The palliative nurse integrates knowledge, attitudes, behaviors, and skills that are consistent with nursing professional standards, nursing codes of ethics, and scope of practice into their palliative nursing practice. This includes advocating for human rights of all individuals, with the goal of addressing and reducing health disparities, inequities, racism, and discrimination of people of color, LGTBQ+ individuals, and other marginalized groups.
Caring Practices
  The palliative nurse integrates caring practices to create a compassionate, supportive, and therapeutic environment for individuals with serious illness, families, and staff, including vigilance, engagement, and responsiveness.
Collaboration
  The palliative nurse collaboratively engages with individuals with serious illness, their families, and healthcare providers in a way that promotes each person's contributions toward achieving optimal yet realistic individual and family goals.
Systems Thinking
  The palliative nurse identifies and utilizes the evidence and body of knowledge for palliative care delivery and clinical practice, as well as the tools to manage the environmental and system resources for the individual with serious illness, their family, and staff within a healthcare system and a community.
Response to Diversity
  The palliative nurse has the cultural sensitivity to recognize, appreciate, and incorporate the cultural needs and preferences of individuals with serious illness into the provision of care. Assessment includes but is not limited to cultural identity, spiritual beliefs, sexual orientation, gender identity, gender expression, ethnic identity, socioeconomic status, age, educational level, and values.
Facilitation of Learning
  The palliative nurse facilitates learning for individuals with serious illness, their families, nurse colleagues, other members of the healthcare team, and the community.
Clinical Inquiry
  The palliative nurse utilizes the ongoing process of questioning and evaluating palliative practice and providing informed practice based on the established palliative care research evidence and related information.

From Dahlin.[24]

and colleagues examined knowledge about end-of-life care of experienced nurses returning for graduate study and found that, for the most part, graduate students had no previous palliative care education (86.7%) and linked palliative care solely with end-of-life care.[27] To address this gap, the ELNEC-APRN curriculum was developed to promote optimal practice in 2013.[28] In 2018, the results of the first known national survey specific to APRNs practicing in hospice and palliative care was published, revealing that 60% still had no palliative care content in their graduate programs, and the majority of specialty APRNs received training through continued education.[29]

CHANGES IN APRN EDUCATION: THE LACE MODEL

As described earlier, major changes in the education and licensing of advanced practice nurses came about with the proposal of the LACE model, a uniform model of regulation of APRNs across the states.[22] The model established foundational requirements for educational tracks leading to APRN licensure. This model recategorizes APRNs, mandating that they have education and certification within a population focus. The consensus model specifies four advanced practice registered nursing roles which fall within at least one of six population-based foci: family/individual across the lifespan, adult-gerontology, pediatric, neonatal, women's health/gender related, or psychiatric/mental health). After extensive national dialogue, the decision was made to define the adult population as "adult-gerontology" in order to increase the number of APRNs prepared to care for the growing older population.[22] This move has had a profound impact on the education of APRNs in that all adult programs now have a melded adult-gerontology focus. Increasing geriatric curriculum in all adult programs will, it is hoped, result in increased palliative care content as well.

CURRENT EDUCATIONAL MODELS: GRADUATE EDUCATION IN SPECIALTY PALLIATIVE CARE

As the specialty of palliative care has evolved over the past 20 years, so, too, have the educational models that form the basis of specialty advanced practice palliative nursing education. In 1998, the Breen School of Nursing at Ursuline College in Ohio offered the first master of science in nursing (MSN) program for the preparation of palliative CNSs. The same year, a program specifically designed to prepare palliative NPs was established at New York University. Both pioneering APRN programs included basic master's-level essential coursework, with clinical practice.[25]

Since these original programs were offered, several different models have been developed to integrate specialist palliative nurse education and clinical practice into master's programs. Framed as minors, certifications, and subspecialties, university programs have delivered content in a variety of formats ranging from single-course didactic elective classes to extensive clinical and classroom-based specialty tracks. Interprofessional master's programs with no clinical component have also been developed. Currently, there is a lack of consistency and standardization among programs, although some resources exist to assist with curriculum development. As the specialty palliative nursing organization, the HPNA developed both scope and standards and competencies for advanced practice. In addition, the HPNA established guidelines for clinical education entitled *Standards for Clinical Education*.[30] There has been recent work under way to develop consensus guidelines for graduate specialty palliative nursing education, and guidance is eagerly anticipated by many academic educators and administrators.[31]

With the expanding need for palliative APRNs, several universities have developed post-master's certificate programs. Designed for practicing APRNs who wish to develop a new area of expertise, these programs are increasingly popular among working advanced practice nurses wanting to move into palliative care. A variety of formats exist, from purely didactic online programs to 12-credit academic programs with up to 500 clinical practicum hours. Some programs are merged with DNP degree programs.

DOCTORAL EDUCATION IN PALLIATIVE CARE: PHD, DNS, DNSC, AND DNP

Doctoral education for the palliative care nurse provides the opportunity to contribute to the state of knowledge in the field. PhD, DNS, and DNSc programs in nursing provide the tools for nurses to design, conduct, analyze, and report theoretical and clinical research related to the care of those with advanced, progressive illness, while the DNP is a clinically based doctoral degree designed to translate evidence into practice and effect systems change.[32,33] Table 2.2 outlines the fundamental characteristics of PhD, DNS, DNSc and DNP programs of study.[32,33]

THE PALLIATIVE NURSE PREPARED AS PHD, DNS, OR DNSC

There is an urgent need for PhD-, DNS-, and DNSc-prepared nurses committed to increasing the body of knowledge within palliative nursing. *The Hospice and Palliative Nurses Associations (HPNA) 2019–2022 Research Agenda* highlights the need to integrate evidence into practice and guides nurse researchers in prioritizing research studies.[34] The *HPNA Research Agenda* emphasizes the need for well-designed studies to provide the necessary evidence-based foundation for optimal care of patients and their families along the full trajectory of serious illness. Within the framework of the eight NCP domains discussed earlier in this chapter, five priority gaps in palliative knowledge were identified by HPNA members emphasizing (1) Domain 1: Structure and Processes of Care, (2) Domain 2: Physical Aspects of Care, and (3) Domain 4: Social Aspects of Care.[5] In spring of 2018, the HPNA Research Special Interest

Table 2.2 PhD, DNS, DNSc, AND DNP PROGRAMS

	PHD, DNS, DNSC	DNP
Focus	Nursing research	Nursing practice
Degree Objectives	To prepare nurse scientists to develop new knowledge for the science and practice of nursing. Graduates will lead interdisciplinary research teams, design and conduct research studies, and disseminate knowledge for nursing and related disciplines.	To create nursing leaders in interdisciplinary healthcare teams by providing students with the tools and skills necessary to translate evidence gained through nursing research into practice, improve systems of care, and measure outcomes of patient groups, populations and communities
Curriculum Focus	Emphasis on research methodology, theory and meta-theory. Cognates, courses in other disciplines that complement nursing science, are required. They provide knowledge of basic and social sciences that is relevant to the student's research focus.	Emphasis on translation of research to clinical practice. Specialized emphasis or tracks of practice: • Direct care of individual patients • Care of patient populations • Practice that supports patient care
Point of Entry	BSN or MSN (or related master's degree)	BSN or master's in advanced practice nursing
Dissertation	Dissertation, including a dissertation defense, is required.	Dissertation requirements differ and must be grounded in clinical practice. They vary greatly and may include: • No dissertation • Thesis • Capstone project
Clinical Requirements	Field research requirements vary.	Clinical practicum/residency requirements vary.
Employment Opportunities	Nurse scientist, nursing faculty	Healthcare administration, clinical nurse faculty

Adapted from Edwards N, Coddington J, Erler C, Kirkpatrick J. 2018[32]; American Association of Colleges of Nursing. DNP Education. 2020.[33]

Group (SIG) members met to generate a list of research area gaps.[34] Subsequently, the Research Advisory Council (RAC) members and other identified experts reached consensus on five research priorities: (1) pediatric hospice and palliative nursing research; (2) family caregiving; (3) interprofessional education and collaborative practice (IPECP); (4) Big Data science, precision health, and nursing informatics; and (5) implementation science.[34] In this document, the HPNA also strongly recommended an interdisciplinary research team approach, which PhD-prepared nurses are uniquely positioned to lead because they are among the frontrunners in developing interprofessional education models embodying the teamwork competency.

The HPNA is not alone in recognizing the dearth of research in end-of-life care and the need for evidence-based practice development. The AAHPM partnered with the HPNA Research Advisory Group on an initiative called *Measuring What Matters*.[35] The purpose of the initiative is to provide measures for palliative care programs to use in program improvement, which would be a companion to the NCP guidelines previously discussed.

The science of palliative care has been targeted as a priority area for the National Institute of Nursing Research (NINR). In 2011, the NINR, the lead National Institutes of Health (NIH) funder of palliative care, conducted a State-of-the-Science Conference on Improving End-of-Life Care and affirmed its commitment to funding and supporting research

in palliative care.[36] The 2016 NINR Strategic Plan identified two palliative care research foci, *Symptom Science: Promoting Personalized Health Strategies* and *End-of-Life and Palliative Care: The Science of Compassion* (NINR, 2016). The NINR Strategic Plan is due to be updated in 2021. At time of publication, several major funding opportunities for palliative nursing were open. Table 2.3 provides examples of funding opportunities for nurse researchers in palliative care.[37]

THE DNP-PREPARED PALLIATIVE NURSE

The DNP is a terminal degree for nurses interested in a clinically focused, rather than research-based, doctorate. The development of this degree emerged from the need for highly educated, expert clinicians who could assume clinical leadership roles in shaping policy, developing clinical education and quality initiatives, and translating evidence at the point of patient contact.

There are currently two entry points for DNP education. The first is the post-bachelor's (BSN to DNP) program that integrates the preparation of APRNs within the roles and population foci described earlier. The other option is the post-master's DNP, for the master's-prepared APRN who is already practicing. Palliative education can be integrated into either option. Students in the BSN-to-DNP program can add the specialty to their population focus, and post-master's students can gain specialized knowledge while fulfilling the requirements for the doctoral degree.

Table 2.3 NATIONAL INSTITUTE OF NURSING RESEARCH (NINR) FUNDING OPPORTUNITIES FOR PALLIATIVE CARE RESEARCH

FUNDING OPPORTUNITY	TYPE OF GRANT*
End-of-life and palliative needs of adolescents and young adults with serious illnesses	R01, R21
End-of-life and palliative care health literacy: Improving outcomes in serious, advanced illness	R01
Advancing the science of geriatric palliative care	R01, R03, R21
End-of-life and palliative care approaches to advanced signs and symptoms	R01, R21

* Definition of grant types

R01: National Institute of Health (NIH)'s most commonly used grant program, used to support a discrete, specified, circumscribed research project. No specific dollar amount. Usually granted for 3–5 years.

R03: NIH Small grant program. Provides limited funding: Up to $50,000 for up to 2 years. Provides limited funding for a variety of types of projects, including pilot or feasibility studies, collection of preliminary data, secondary analysis of existing data, small self-contained research projects, development of new technology.

R21: Encourages new, exploratory, and developmental research projects by providing support for the early stages of project development. Sometimes used for pilot and feasibility studies. Up to $275,000 for up to 2 years. No preliminary data are generally required.

From National Institute for Nursing Research. Funding Opportunities. 2020.[37]

The essential competencies of the DNP relate directly to the role of the palliative APRN, who often assumes systems-based responsibilities such as patient and professional education, quality improvement, and team leadership.[38] The DNP program requires a capstone project that demonstrates achievement of the DNP graduate's clinical competencies, emphasizes the translation of evidence into practice, and often provides the clinical scholarship leading to nursing policy change.[33]

Integrating palliative care content into master's and doctoral programs has been a challenge due to the high credit requirements of many programs. Lack of faculty expertise in palliative care has also been a barrier. The HPNA has produced the third edition of *Core Curriculum for the Hospice and Palliative Advanced Practice Registered Nurse.*[39]

The ELNEC developed several curricula in response to palliative care knowledge deficits among various levels of graduate faculty. For instance, funding from the National Cancer Institute promoted the development of an ELNEC Graduate Faculty Curriculum, which provided end-of-life train-the-trainer education to graduate nursing faculty. Over the 5 years of the ELNEC Graduate Curriculum project, 300 graduate nursing faculty members, representing 63% of the existing graduate schools of nursing, attended. Outcome data showed that thousands of graduate students have since been educated in this content.[40]

With a grant from the National Cancer Institute, ELNEC also developed a program entitled *Integrating Palliative Oncology Care Into Doctor of Nursing Practice (DNP) Education and Clinical Practice.*[41] The grant offered a national workshop to DNP nursing faculty and DNP clinical practitioners and covered information on establishing more formal palliative care coursework and integrating palliative care into core courses, clinical experiences, and DNP capstone projects.

There are a growing number of postgraduate clinical nursing fellowships available for APRNs. Most programs are sponsored by academic medical centers, and some use the fellowships as workforce development within their institutions, rather than an as opportunity for APRNs to provide leadership in education and program development on a broader level. These programs are usually 1-year postgraduate clinical fellowships for NPs, often offered alongside medical fellowships in major institutions where palliative care is well developed. However, a few programs have been developed for midcareer APRNs. Barriers for APRN fellowship program development include the variation of state licensing requirements, low salaries, and inability to temporarily leave other positions. Currently, work is under way to define consistent standards for palliative APRN fellowships.[42]

CONTINUING EDUCATION FOR THE APRN

Along with formal academic programs, professional continuing education in palliative nursing has flourished over recent years. The most significant and far-reaching continuing education initiative has been the national and international ELNEC program, previously mentioned. ELNEC began in 2000 and continues today to educate nursing faculty, clinical nurses, researchers, and administrators in palliative care, including specialty content for those teaching pediatrics, oncology, critical care, geriatrics, and veterans' care (visit https://www.aacnnursing.org/ELNEC). To date, more than 1 million nurses and other members of the interprofessional healthcare team have attended one of hundreds of national or international train-the-trainer courses held in every state across America and in more than 100 countries. The ELNEC curriculum also has been translated into 11 languages to further its international reach.[43]

The ANA and HPNA *Call to Action—Nurses Lead and Transform Palliative Care* states that all nurses should receive ELNEC training as a minimum.[44] To target the education needs of the APRN, a 2-day ELNEC APRN curriculum is offered. Recognizing both the clinical and program development needs of APRNs, the curriculum includes the following clinical and program development modules: Overview, Pain Management, Symptom Management, Communication, Final Hours, Business & Finance, Quality Measurement, Education, and Leadership. The program offers breakout sessions for communication and palliative care program development important for both the generalist and specialist palliative APRN. In addition, there are tracks for both adult and pediatric APRNs.[45] To address the interest in and need for detailed communication skills training, an ELNEC Communication course was also recently developed.[46] Participants are provided with diverse content that can be incorporated into various coursework within the specialist and graduate curriculum, so this course is attractive to nursing faculty as well.

For graduate-prepared APRNs who maintain a generalist practice outside of the clinical specialty realm, there is the ELNEC Core Curriculum. This content is divided into eight modules: Nursing Care at the End of Life; Pain Management; Symptom Management; Ethical/Legal Issues; Cultural Considerations in End-of-Life Care; Communication; Loss, Grief, Bereavement; and Preparation for and Care at the Time of Death. Table 2.4 details the curricular topics of the ELNEC Core, ELNEC APRN for adults and pediatrics, and ELNEC DNP courses.

A plethora of other continuing education programs are available for APRNs interested in developing or expanding their palliative care skill set. There are various conferences, such as the annual assembly co-organized by AAHPM and HPNA and the annual Clinical Practice Forum organized by HPNA. Nursing specialty organizations, such as the American Association of Critical Care Nurses (ACCN), the Oncology Nursing Society (ONS), and the Gerontological Advanced Practice Nursing Association (GAPNA) offer palliative care content at their annual conferences. Other interprofessional clinical conferences include those organized by the Center to Advance Palliative Care, the National Hospice and Palliative Care Organization, and the American Society of Clinical Oncology. Several academic and clinical settings offer brief specialized immersion courses, including the HPNA/Cambia week-long externships for experienced APRNs new to palliative care.[47] The Center to Advance Palliative Care, the City of Hope Pain and Palliative Care Resource Center, and the Palliative Care Network of Wisconsin are examples of extensive multifaceted repositories for practice and educational resources. Table 2.5 provides a sample of available palliative care educational resources for APRNs interested in continuing educational opportunities. A basic internet search will uncover a plethora of programs. It is especially important to note that, during the COVID pandemic, many opportunities were offered free of charge.

Table 2.4 END-OF-LIFE NURSING EDUCATION CONSORTIUM (ELNEC) CURRICULA

ELNEC CORE[43]	ELNEC APRN[45]	ELNEC APRN PEDS[45]	INCORPORATING PALLIATIVE CARE INTO DNP CURRICULUM[41]
Introduction to Palliative Care	Overview of Palliative Care	Overview of Palliative Care	Overview: Palliative Care; Update on Cancer Care
Pain Management in Palliative Care	Pain Management	Pain Management	Leading Teams in Pain and Symptom Management
Symptom Management in Palliative Care	Symptom Management	Symptom Management	Interprofessional Teams
Ethical Issues in Palliative Care	Communication	Communication	Enhancing Communication
Cultural Considerations in Palliative Care	Final Hours	Final Hours	Changing Institutional Culture
Communication in Palliative Care	Business and Finance	Loss Grief and Bereavement	Principles of Business, Finance, and Economics to Improve Palliative Oncology Care
Loss, Grief, and Bereavement	Quality Management	Improving Quality Care in Palliative Care	Principles of Regulation, Outcomes Measurement, Guidelines, and Quality Improvement to Improve Palliative Oncology Care
Final Hours of Life	Generalist vs Specialty Palliative Care	Issues Regarding Billing & Legislation	Incorporating Palliative Care into Core and Clinical Coursework
	Leadership	Neonatal/Perinatal Palliative Care	DNPs Leading Health Systems Change

From American Association of Colleges of Nursing[43]; Buller et al.[46]

Table 2.5 CONTINUING EDUCATION RESOURCES

ORGANIZATION	EDUCATIONAL OPPORTUNITIES	WEBSITE
American Academy of Hospice and Palliative Medicine (AAHPM)	Conferences Webinars Online CE course Publications Online newsletter Pediatric resources	www.aahpm.org
American Association of Critical Care Nurses (AACN)	Self-assessments E-learning Online resources and protocols	www.aacn.org
American Society of Pain Management Nurses (ASPMN)	Conferences Online education Books and products Webinars	www.aspmn.org
Center to Advance Palliative Care (CAPC)	Online resources Webinars Conferences	www.capc.org
Gerontological Advanced Practice Association (GAPNA)	CE courses Conferences Special interest group	www.GAPNA.org
Hartford Institute for Geriatric Nursing	Webinars Podcasts CE courses Competencies and guidelines	www.hign.org
Hospice and Palliative Nurses Association (HPNA)	Conferences Books and products E-learning courses	www.advancingexpertcare.org
National Hospice and Palliative Care Organization (NHPCO)	Webinars Conferences Online courses Pediatric resources Educational products	www.nhpco.org/education
Oncology Nursing Society (ONS)	Conferences CE courses Online resources and guidelines Books and products	www.ons.org
Palliative Care Network of Wisconsin (PCNOW)	*Palliative Care Fast Facts and Concepts* QI resources Patient resources	https://www.mypcnow.org/
Vital Talk	Video resources Conferences	www.vitaltalk.org

Note: Arranged alphabetically; membership may be required.

FUTURE DIRECTIONS IN APRN EDUCATION

As palliative care continues to rapidly expand, graduate, post-graduate, and continuing education programs will also grow, affording APRN educators the opportunity for innovation and creativity. Several trends in APRN education are emerging.

INTERPROFESSIONAL EDUCATION

Interprofessional education has become a mandate for the health sciences. Described as health professionals learning with and about each other in the educational and practice settings, interprofessional education is interactive, cooperative, and experiential.[49] Four basic competencies, as developed by a collaborative expert panel, are (1) communication of roles and responsibilities, (2) demonstration of values and ethics in collaborative practice, (3) negotiation of roles, and (4) interprofessional teamwork.[49] Given the holistic preparation and focus of advanced practice nursing, APRNs often play leading roles on interprofessional teams. Advanced practice nurse educators must work with faculty colleagues across disciplines to ensure that advanced practice nursing is well represented in interprofessional program planning, literature, and research for interprofessional practice.

MENTORSHIP

Mentorship is an important aspect of palliative nursing education. APRNs serve as mentors to nursing staff of all levels. APRNs frequently formally and informally mentor new practitioners in other fields, including medical students and residents, social workers, and other interdisciplinary team members. As palliative care programs continue to expand, experienced APRNs mentor both new graduates, experienced APRNs moving into palliative care, and nursing professionals at all levels. Nurses report that mentoring conversations improve their effectiveness in integral palliative skills, like communication.[50] Focused mentorship can help to develop critical thinking, expand evidence-based practice, and sustain resilience in APRNs.[51]

ONLINE AND LONG-DISTANCE EDUCATION

Online and long-distance educational programs have become the norm in many academic circles. Long-distance learning makes advanced education accessible to nurses in remote areas and provides a flexible platform for continuing education for nurses with varying responsibilities and work hours. However, this framework can create substantial challenges in teaching subjects that can be emotion-laden and necessitate interpersonal work.[52] Advanced practice palliative nursing education requires significant direct role-playing for communication training. Use of online video streaming is one answer to this need for interactive work, and the required transition to virtual education during the COVID pandemic has led to improving educational technology that will undoubtedly influence the continuing development of online palliative care education.

SIMULATION

Simulation, particularly in relation to teaching communication skills, has increasingly become a mainstay of palliative care education at both the generalist and specialist levels. Simulation is now a common component of most advanced practice and palliative nursing educational programs.[53] Table 2.6 shows examples of program-specific palliative and end-of-life simulation scenarios utilized at a large urban university.

Although there remains a paucity of research regarding the translation of palliative care simulation pedagogies to clinical competence, these exercises are subjectively well-received by students who appreciate the opportunity for practice.[53] The first randomized controlled trial of patient- and family-reported outcomes revealed disappointing results, but a subsequent randomized trial of a simulation-based multisession workshop to improve palliative care communication skills (Codetalk) resulted in an improvement in trainee's overall self-assessment of competence in communication skills ($P < .001$).[54] The intervention was also associated with an improvement in trainee self-assessments of three of the four skill-specific indicators: expressing empathy, discussing spiritual issues, and eliciting goals of care.[54] Another study employed an exploratory, pre- and post-test design with additional qualitative data to evaluate a pilot project, "TeamTalk," which adapted VitalTalk methodology for interprofessional learners to develop communication skills in palliative care.[54] Attitudes toward interprofessional collaboration improved from pre- to post-test, with no difference among the professional groups. Self-confidence for interprofessional communication improved in "eliciting the contributions of colleagues, including those from other disciplines" ($p < 0.001$) for all learners during Year 2; chaplains improved in the greatest number of areas (15/19), followed by nurses (7/19) and physicians (4/19).[54] Further rigorous outcome research is needed to ascertain the efficacy of this teaching strategy.

Table 2.6 EXAMPLES OF END-OF-LIFE SIMULATION SCENARIOS

Advanced practice population program	Simulation scenario
Family nurse practitioner Adult-gerontology primary care nurse practitioner	• Difficult communication: Advance directives, breaking bad news, requests for non-disclosure of patient information • Introducing palliative care • COVID-19: Stable and unstable adults (telehealth)
Adult-gerontology acute care nurse practitioner	• Leading family meetings • Withdrawal of life support • Advanced directives: End-stage renal disease
Pediatric nurse practitioner	Goals of care family meetings, breaking bad news, addressing opioid fears
Midwifery	Perinatal loss and bereavement: Stillborn
Psychiatric-mental health nurse practitioner	Grief and bereavement counseling

Developed by New York University Rory Meyers College of Nursing.

TELEHEALTH EDUCATION

The COVID-19 pandemic accelerated the use of telehealth technology in hospice and palliative settings, necessitating the rapid development of telehealth curricula in advanced practice nursing programs. (See Chapter 17, "The Palliative APRN in Telehealth".) Guidelines compliant with the Health Insurance Portability and Accountability Act (HIPAA) were liberalized by the Department of Health and Human Services, allowing for a variety of nonpublic-facing video communication tools to be utilized as telehealth platforms.[55] Successful utilization of telehealth intervention to support end-of-life care and family meetings has been reported; however, these cases highlight the need to increase training for frontline care staff and those in palliative APRN programs to achieve telehealth competency.[55,56]

In 2018, the NONPF published a position statement, *NONPF Supports Telehealth in Nurse Practitioner Education*, that suggests new strategies are needed to effectively address the national healthcare provider shortage, complexity of disease, aging of our population, and limited access to care. Included in the position paper were eight recommended NP competencies (see Box 2.2).[57] The shortage of palliative care specialist providers makes telehealth an attractive option for hospice and palliative care organizations, and the recent COVID pandemic made the intervention integral. Integration of telehealth curricula has been developing rapidly in both generalist and specialist palliative APRN education.

A CALL TO ACTION FOR PALLIATIVE CARE NURSE EDUCATORS

Since the mid-1990s, healthcare experts have called for improved palliative care for patients with serious illness, and major advances have been made in establishing palliative care as a recognized nursing and medical specialty. Yet much work remains to be done. There is growing evidence that palliative care in terminal illness can improve quality of life, reduce cost, and may prolong survival.[58,59] In September 2014, the IOM released a report, *Dying in America: Improving Quality and Honoring Individual Preferences Near the End of Life*, with a chapter dedicated to education in palliative care.[60] Progress has been made since the early descriptive studies about the deficits in care and the initial IOM report calling for sweeping changes in end-of-life care. But because advance care planning and patient-centered care have yet to be fully integrated into healthcare, many perceive that the recommendations of this report remain timely.

Healthcare reform has moved palliative care upstream and into the community, with a focus on establishing an operational definition of the seriously ill along with quality indicators for necessary changes needed within the health care system.[62] In 2017, a new call to action was proposed by the ANA and the HPNA, which summed up the role of nursing in the future of palliative care: that all patients, families, and communities experiencing serious illness should receive quality palliative care by the delivery of primary palliative nursing by every nurse in all settings.[44] These national mandates lead us to continue to develop both primary and specialty palliative care education for advanced practice nursing.

Recent changes in the structure of advanced nursing education (adaptation of the LACE model and rapid development of DNP programs) complicate educational efforts for specialized palliative care. There are currently not enough APRN programs with a palliative care focus to meet current workforce needs. However, these changes also present opportunities for innovative programs that can be integrated into generalist APRN as well as specialist educational efforts. Work is in progress to delineate content for graduate nursing programs specialty palliative APRN entry into practice.[31] Legislation introduced into Congress is evidence that policymakers are starting to realize the importance of palliative care education. The *Palliative Care Training Act of 2004* addressed the critical health workforce need by calling for funding for education centers to expand interdisciplinary training in palliative and hospice care.[63] The Act also funds advanced education nursing grants, academic career awards, and career incentive awards to support nurses and other healthcare providers who provide palliative and hospice care training. It did not pass on first rounds, but the bill was reintroduced in 2017 as the *Palliative Care Health Education and Training Act (PCHETA)*. It passed in the House of Representative in 2019 and made it to the final docket in 2020, but with COVID-19, it was dropped from bills for review in the Senate[64] (see Chapter 10, "The Palliative APRN in the Emergency Department").

Box 2.2 THE NATIONAL ORGANIZATION OF NURSE PRACTITIONER FACULTY (NONPF) SUGGESTED TELEHEALTH NURSE PRACTITIONER COMPETENCIES

1. Telehealth etiquette and professionalism while videoconferencing
2. Skills in using peripherals, such as otoscope, stethoscope and ophthalmoscope
3. An understanding of when telehealth should and should not be used
4. An understanding of privacy/protected health information (PHI) regulations
5. Proficiency in the use of synchronous and asynchronous telehealth technology
6. Knowledge of appropriate documentation and billing of telehealth technology
7. An ability to collaborate interprofessionally using telehealth technologies
8. Proficiency in taking a history, performing an appropriate physical exam, and generate differential diagnoses using telehealth

From National Organization of Nurse Practitioner Faculties.[57]

SUMMARY

The discipline of palliative care is expanding, and its professional knowledge base is growing. There is a growing awareness among the public, in the health professions, and among policymakers that palliative care education is integral to overall healthcare. The nursing profession has a mandate to educate its members through formal academic programs and continuing professional education to remain at the forefront of palliative care practice. The HPNA calls for nursing educators to take an active stance in promoting palliative care education for both specialist and generalist APRNs. Their position statement on the value of the APRN calls for nursing educators to become knowledgeable and expand the following areas:

- Continuing education to prepare and develop existing APRNs in palliative care competencies

- Integration of core palliative care competencies into programs for all APRN students, regardless of role or degree

- Provision of academic programs for specialized palliative care

- Provision of clinical mentoring in palliative care[65]

The current healthcare environment provides an exciting time to practice palliative nursing, and many opportunities exist for nurses to take a leadership role in developing and leading palliative care programs in all settings. By providing advanced education for specialized clinical experts and expanding the primary palliative care knowledge base for generalist APRNs, palliative care educators can ensure that nursing remains at the forefront of this essential and rewarding work.

REFERENCES

1. Wiencek C, Wolf A. The advanced practice registered nurse. In Ferrell B, Paice J, eds. *Oxford Textbook of Palliative Nursing. 5th ed.* New York: Oxford University Press; 2019: 809–816.
2. American Association of Colleges of Nursing. *Peaceful Death: Recommended Competencies and Curricular Guidelines for End-of-Life Nursing Care.* Washington, DC: American Association of Colleges of Nursing; 1997. https://eric.ed.gov/?id=ED453706
3. International Council of Nurses. *Basic Principles of Nursing Care.* Washington, DC: American Nurses Publishing; 1997.
4. National Consensus Project for Quality Palliative Care. *Clinical Practice Guidelines for Quality Palliative Care 2018.* Richmond, VA: National Coalition for Hospice and Palliative Care. https://www.nationalcoalitionhpc.org/wp-content/uploads/2018/10/NCHPC-NCPGuidelines_4thED_web_FINAL.pdf
5. National Quality Forum. *A National Framework and Preferred Practices for Palliative and Hospice Care Quality.* Washington, DC: National Quality Forum; 2006. https://www.qualityforum.org/Publications/2006/12/A_National_Framework_and_Preferred_Practices_for_Palliative_and_Hospice_Care_Quality.aspx
6. Institute of Medicine of the National Academies. *The Future of Nursing: Leading Change, Advancing Health.* Washington, DC: National Academies Press; 2011. https://pubmed.ncbi.nlm.nih.gov/24983041/
7. Campaign for Action. Dashboard Indicators. 2021. https://campaignforaction.org/resource/dashboard-indicators/
8. National Academies of Sciences, Engineering, and Medicine 2021. *The Future of Nursing 2020–2030: Charting a Path to Achieve Health Equity.* Washington, DC: The National Academies Press. https://doi.org/10.17226/25982
9. American Association of Colleges of Nursing. The Essentials: Core Competencies for Professional Nursing Education. 2021. https://www.aacnnursing.org/AACN-Essentials
10. New York State Nurses Association. *Scope of Practice.* Article 139, Nursing. New York: New York State Nurses Association. 2010. https://www.nysna.org/nursing-practice/practice-resources/scope-practice#.X3iiv2dKi00
11. National Council of State Boards of Nursing (NCBSN). *NCLEX-RN Examination. Test Plan for the National Council Licensure Examination for Registered Nurses.* 2019. https://www.ncsbn.org/2019_RN_TestPlan-English.pdf
12. Ferrell B, Malloy P, Mazanec P, Virani R. CARES: AACN's new competencies and recommendations for educating undergraduate nursing students to improve palliative care. *J Prof Nurs.* 2016;32:327–333. doi:10.1016/j.profnurs.2016.07.002
13. American Association of Colleges of Nursing. *ELNEC Undergraduate/New Graduate Curriculum.* 2021. https://www.aacnnursing.org/ELNEC/About/ELNEC-Curricula
14. Welsh S, Matzo M, Hultman T, Reifsnyder J. Palliative Nursing Summit: Nurses leading change and transforming care: Our journey to the summit. *J Hosp Palliat Nur.* 2018:20;6–14. doi:10.1097/NJH.0000000000000412
15. Lippe M, Davis A, Stock N, Mazanec P, Ferrell B. Updated palliative care competencies for entry-to-practice and advanced-level nursing students: New resources for nursing faculty. *Journal of Professional Nursing.* 2022;42:250-261. doi:10.1016/j.profnurs.2022.07.012
16. National Organization of Nurse Practitioner Faculties. Nurse Practitioner Core Competencies Content. 2017. https://cdn.ymaws.com/www.nonpf.org/resource/resmgr/competencies/2017_NPCoreComps_with_Curric.pdf#:~:text=Nurse%20Practitioner%20Core%20Competencies%20Content%20A%20delineation%20of,Anne%20Dumas%2C%20PhD%2C%20RN%2C%20FNP-BC%2C%20GNP-BC%2C%20FAANP%2C%20FAAN
17. American College of Nurse Midwives Board of Directors. Basic Competency Section, Division of Advancement of Midwifery. 2020. https://www.midwife.org/acnm/files/acnmlibrarydata/uploadfilename/000000000050/ACNMCoreCompetenciesMar2020_final.pdf
18. National Association of Clinical Nurse Specialists. Statement on Clinical Nurse Specialist Practice and Education. 2019. https://nacns.org/resources/practice-and-cns-role/cns-competencies/
19. Population-Focused Competencies Task Force. Population-Focused Nurse Practitioner Competencies: Family/Across the Lifespan, Neonatal, Acute Care Pediatric, Primary Care Pediatric, Psychiatric-Mental Health, & Women's Health/Gender-Related. 2013. https://cdn.ymaws.com/www.nonpf.org/resource/resmgr/competencies/populationfocusnpcomps2013.pdf
20. Dahlin C, Hospice and Palliative Nurses Association. *Palliative Nursing: Scope and Standards of Practice.* 6th ed. Pittsburgh, PA: Hospice and Palliative Nurses Association; 2021.
21. Hospice and Palliative Credentialing Center. About Certification. 2021. https://advancingexpertcare.org/HPCC/CertificationWeb/Certification_FAQ.aspx
22. National Council of State Boards of Nursing (NCBSN). National Council of State Boards of Nursing (NCBSN). The Consensus Model for APRN Regulation, Licensure Accreditation, Certification and Education. . 2022. http://www.ncsbn.org/nursing-regulation/practice/aprn/aprn-consensus.page
23. Dahlin C, Coyne P. The Palliative APRN Leader. *Ann Palliat Med.* 2019;8 Supp 1:1–9. doi:10.21037/apm.2018.06.03
24. Dahlin C. *Competencies for the Palliative and Hospice APRN.* 3rd edition. Pittsburgh, PA: Hospice and Palliative Nurses Association; 2021.

25. Malloy P, Davis A. Nursing education. In Ferrell BR, Paice JA eds. *Oxford Textbook of Palliative Nursing.* 5th ed. New York: Oxford University Press; 2019:844–854.

26. Ferrell BR, Virani R, Grant M. Analysis of end-of-life content in nursing textbooks. *Oncol Nurs Forum.* 1999;26:869–876. doi:10.1089/jpm.1999.2.161

27. Shea J, Grossman S, Wallace M, Lange J. Assessment of advanced practice palliative care nursing competencies in nurse practitioner students: Implications for the integration of ELNEC curricular modules. *J Nurs Educ.* 2010;49:183–188. doi:10.1089/jpm.1999.2.161

28. Dahlin CM, Coyne PJ, Paice J, Malloy P, Thaxton CA, Haskamp A. ELNEC-APRN: Meeting the needs of advanced practice nurses through education. *J Hosp Palliat Nurs.* 2017:19;261–265. doi:10.1097/NJH.0000000000000340

29. Pawlow P, Dahlin C, Doherty C, Ersek M. The hospice and palliative care advanced practice registered nurse workforce: Results of a national survey. *J Hosp Palliat Nurs.* 2018;20:349–357. doi:10.1097/NJH.0000000000000449

30. Hospice and Palliative Nurses Association. *Standards for Clinical Education.* 2nd ed. 2015. https://advancingexpertcare.org/HPNA/HPNAweb/Education/Standards_for_Clinical_Education.aspx, https://www.ncsbn.org/2019_RN_TestPlan-English.pdf

31. Dahlin C, Ersek M, Wholihan D, Wiencek C. Specialty palliative APRN practice through state-of-the-art graduate education: Report of the HPNA Graduate Faculty Council. *J Pain Sympt Manag.* 2019;57:445. doi:https://doi.org/10.1016/j.jpainsymman.2018.12.189

32. Edwards N, Coddington J, Erler C, Kirkpatrick J. The impact of the role of doctor of nursing practice nurses on healthcare and leadership. *Med Research Arch.* 2018;6:1–11. doi:https://doi.org/10.18103/mra.v6i4.1734

33. American Association of Colleges of Nursing. DNP Education. Washington, DC. 2021. https://www.aacnnursing.org/Nursing-Education-Programs/DNP-Education

34. Hospice and Palliative Nurses Association. Research Agenda: 2019–2022. *Pittsburgh, PA: HPNA.* https://journals.lww.com/jhpn/Fulltext/2019/08000/HPNA_2019_2022_Research_Agenda__Development_and.18.aspx

35. American Academy of Hospice and Palliative Medicine. *AAHPM & HPNA: Measuring What Matters.* Chicago, IL: AAHPM. http://aahpm.org/quality/measuring-what-matters

36. National Institute for Nursing Research. *The NINR Strategic Plan: Advancing Science, Improving Lives.* Bethesda, MD: National Institute for Nursing Research 2016. https://www.ninr.nih.gov/aboutninr/directors-message/directors-message-strategicplan-2016

37. National Institute for Nursing Research. Funding Opportunities. 2021. https://www.ninr.nih.gov/researchandfunding/fundingopportunities

38. American Association of Colleges of Nursing. *The Essentials of Doctoral Education for Advanced Nursing Practice.* Washington, DC: American Association of Colleges of Nursing; 2006. https://www.aacnnursing.org/Portals/42/Publications/DNPEssentials.pdf

39. Dahlin CM, Moreines Tycon L, Root M. *Core Curriculum for the Hospice and Palliative Advanced Practice Registered Nurse.* Pittsburgh, PA: Hospice and Palliative Nurses Association; 2020.

40. Paice JA, Ferrell BR, Virani R, Grant M, Malloy P, Rhome. Appraisal of the graduate End-of-Life Nursing Education Consortium (ELNEC) training program. *J Palliat Med.* 2006;9:353–360. doi:10.1089/jpm.2006.9.353

41. Fennimore L, Wholihan D, Breakwell S, Malloy P, Virani R, Ferrell B. Integrating palliative oncology care into doctor of nursing practice (DNP) education and clinical practice. *J Prof Nurs.* 2018;34:444–448. doi:10.1016/j.profnurs.2018.09.003

42. Dahlin C, Wholihan D, Johnstone-Petty M. Palliative APRN fellowship guidelines: A strategy for quality specialty practice: Report of the HPNA APRN Fellowship Council. *J Pain Sympt Manag.* 2019;57:363. doi:https://doi.org/10.1016/j.jpainsymman.2018.12.029

43. American Association of Colleges of Nursing. ELNEC. End-of-Life Nursing Education Consortium: Fact Sheet. 2021. https://www.aacnnursing.org/Portals/42/ELNEC/PDF/ELNEC-Fact-Sheet.pdf

44. American Nurses Association and Hospice and Palliative Nurses Association. *Call to Action: Nurses Lead and Transform Palliative Care.* Silver Spring, MD: American Nurses Association; 2017. http://www.nursingworld.org/CallforAction-NursesLeadTransformPalliativeCare

45. American Association of Colleges of Nursing. ELNEC Curricula. 2021. https://www.aacnnursing.org/ELNEC/About/ELNEC-Curricula

46. Buller H, Virani R, Malloy P, Paice J. End-of-Life Nursing Education Consortium (ELNEC) communication curriculum for nurses. *J Hosp Palliat Nurs.* 2019;21:E5–E12. doi:10.1097/NJH.0000000000000540

47. Gentry J, Dahlin C. The evaluation of a palliative care advanced practice nursing externship. *J Hosp Palliat Nurs.* 2020;22:172–179. doi:10.1097/NJH.0000000000000637

48. Goldsberry J. Advanced practice nurses leading the way: Interprofessional collaboration. *Nurse Educ Today.* 2018;65:1–3. doi:10.1016/j.nedt.2018.02.024

49. Interprofessional Education Collaborative (IPEC). *Core Competencies for Interprofessional Collaborative Practice.* Washington, DC: Interprofessional Education Collaborative. 2016. https://ipec.memberclicks.net/assets/2016-Update.pdf

50. Mazanec P, Aslakson RA, Bodurtha J, Smith T. Mentoring in palliative nursing. *J Hosp Palliat Nurs.* 2016;18:488–495. doi:10.1097/NJH.0000000000000297

51. Burgunder-Zdravkovski L, Guzman Y, Creech C, Price D, Filter M. Improving palliative care conversations through targeted education and mentorship. *J Hosp Palliat Nurs.* 2020;22:319–326. doi:10.1097/NJH.0000000000000663

52. Bishop C, Mazanec P, Bullington J, Craven H, Dunkerley M., Pritchett J, Coyne P. Online ELNEC: CORE curriculum for staff nurses: An education strategy to improve clinical practice. *J Hosp Palliat Nurs.* 2019;21:531–539. doi:10.1097/NJH.0000000000000593

53. Brown CE, Back AL, Ford DW, et al. Self-assessment scores improve after simulation-based palliative care communication skill workshops. *Am J Hosp Palliat Care.* 2018;35(1):45–51. doi:10.1177/1049909116681972

54. Donesky D, Anderson WG, Joseph D, et al., TeamTalk: Interprofessional team development and communication skills training. *J Palliat Med.* 2020;23(1):40–47. doi:10.1089/jpm.2019.0046

55. Calton B, Nauzley A, Fratkin M. Telemedicine in the time of coronavirus. *J Pain Symptom Manage.* 2020;60:e12–e14. doi:10.1016/j.jpainsymman.2020.03.019

56. Ritchey KC, Foy A, McArdel E, Gruenewald DA. Reinventing palliative care delivery in the era of COVID-19: How telemedicine can support end of life care. *Am J Hosp Palliat Med.* 2020;37:992–997. doi:10.1177/1049909120948235

57. National Organization of Nurse Practitioner Faculties. NONPF Supports Telehealth in Nurse Practitioner Education. 2018. https://cdn.ymaws.com/www.nonpf.org/resource/resmgr/2018_Slate/Telehealth_Paper_2018.pdf

58. Temel JS, Grear JA, Muzikansky MA, et al. Early palliative care for patients with metastatic non-small cell lung cancer. *N Engl J Med.* 2010;363:733–742. doi:10.1056/NEJMoa1000678

59. Prescott AT, Hull JG, Dionne-Odom JN, et al. The role of a palliative care intervention in moderating the relationship between depression and survival among individuals with advanced cancer. *Health Psychol.* 2017;36:1140–1146. doi:10.1037/hea0000544

60. Committee on Approaching Death: Addressing Key End of Life Issues; Institute of Medicine. *Dying in America: Improving*

Quality and Honoring Individual Preferences Near the End of Life. Washington, DC: National Academies Press; 2015 https://www.ncbi.nlm.nih.gov/books/NBK285681/

61. Kelley AS, Bollens-Lund E. Identifying the population with serious illness: The "denominator" challenge. *J Palliat Med.* 2017;21:S7–S16. doi:10.1089/jpm.2017.0548

62. Schneider EC, Abrams M, Shah A, Lewis C, Shah T. *Health Care in America: The Experience of People with Serious Illness.* New York, NY: Commonwealth Fund. 2018. https://www.commonwealthfund.org/sites/default/files/2018-10/Schneider_HealthCareinAmerica.pdf

63. Bulanda R. A step toward normalizing end of life care: Implications of the Palliative Care Health Education and Training Act (PCHETA). *Northern Illinois Univer Law Review.* 2019. https://commons.lib.niu.edu/bitstream/handle/10843/20260/39-2-Bulanda-330-358-PDFA.pdf?sequence=1&isAllowed=y

64. Sinclair S. Flex your policy muscles with the Palliative Care Health Education and Training Act. 2017. Center to Advance Palliative Care Blog Post. May 15, 2019. Available at https://www.capc.org/blog/palliative-pulse-palliative-pulse-june-2017-flex-advocacy-muscles-pcheta/

65. Hospice and Palliative Nurses Association. *Position Statement: Value of the APRN in Palliative Care.* Pittsburgh, PA: Hospice and Palliative Nurses Association; 2015. https://advancingexpertcare.org/position-statements/

3.

CREDENTIALING, CERTIFICATION, AND SCOPE OF PRACTICE ISSUES FOR THE PALLIATIVE APRN

Kerstin Lea Lappen, Matthew McGraw, and Kate Meyer

KEY POINTS

- The Consensus Model for APRN Regulation, Licensure, Accreditation, Certification, and Education (LACE), developed in 2008, provides guidance for states to adopt uniformity in the regulation of APRN roles and will have an ongoing impact on advanced palliative nursing practice, the curriculum for advanced practice nursing educational programs, and on the US healthcare system.

- Palliative advanced practice registered nurses (APRNs) must understand credentialing requirements to practice safely, legally, and to the fullest extent of their scope.

- Advanced specialty palliative nursing certification is a valuable endeavor to demonstrate the APRN's expertise and commitment to quality care and to the profession.

CASE STUDY: THE CLINICAL NURSE SPECIALIST

Denise earned her graduate degree in nursing in 2002, with a specialty focus as a medical-surgical clinical nurse specialist (CNS). However, her credential title changed in 2008 to CNS in adult health. Denise's work experience had always been in hospice and pain management. In addition to achieving her CNS certification for entry to practice, she became board certified as an advanced practice certified hospice and palliative nurse. She was hired to work as a consultant for a palliative care service in a large urban hospital. Denise is fortunate to live in a state that recognizes the CNS as an advanced practice registered nurse (APRN) who is able to bill for services and have prescriptive privileges. Her state's law allows APRNs to practice independently, without a collaborative practice or prescriptive agreement with a physician. Denise recently implemented a rural palliative telehealth service, and her employer is interested in expanding the program to neighboring states. Her CNS and nurse practitioner (NP) colleagues want to continue to practice to the full extent of their scope but worry about regulations in other states. As she begins researching how to roll out this initiative, her mentor commented that the project would be worthy for a Doctor of Nursing Practice project stating, "If you're going to do the work, you may as well take the credit."

INTRODUCTION

In 2002, Promoting Excellence in End-of-Life Care, a national program office of the Robert Wood Johnson Foundation, published *Advanced Practice Nurses Role in Palliative Care: A Position Statement from American Nurse Leaders*[1] to spark conversation among nursing leaders about how to improve the state of palliative advanced practice nursing, illustrate successful models of palliative advanced practice registered nursing practice, and promote the advanced practice nurse's role in providing palliative care. The final position statement called on leaders in the clinical professions, nursing educators, health service providers, healthcare payers, and public policy advocates to take the following actions:

- Continue to discuss the advanced practice registered nurse (APRN) role and opportunities and strategies to advance it in palliative care.

- Educate nursing faculty about palliative care to develop curriculum and competencies for both APRN students and existing APRNs with the goal being the integration of primary palliative care principles into nursing education and practice. Additionally, clinical tracks should be developed for APRN students who intend to specialize in palliative care.

- Work with payers of health services to recognize the specialty of palliative care and provide APRNs with adequate and consistent compensation that is commensurate with the APRN scope of practice, authority, and responsibility, regardless of practice setting or specialty.

- Call on the National Council of State Boards of Nursing (NCSBN) and individual state boards of nursing to work collaboratively to consistently recognize APRN scopes of practice and privileges regardless of specialty and subspecialty.

- Ask health systems and health service providers to develop or expand practice opportunities for APRNs in all settings that care for patients who may experience life-limiting illnesses.

- Hold APRNs practicing in the specialty of palliative care accountable for the documentation and dissemination of outcomes of practice experience and roles and for engaging in interdisciplinary research with an emphasis on translating findings into practice.

- Clarify the challenges that APRNs face in training and licensure, along with regulatory and reimbursement barriers.

It was felt that, with the development of registered nurse and advanced practice registered nurse certification examinations and the creation of undergraduate and graduate advanced practice programs in palliative care, palliative nursing would be on the road to being recognized as a specialty in all states.[1]

There has been substantial progress for the APRN in the two decades since the position statement was published in 2002. Four major initiatives have contributed to this growth in APRN practice. First, in 2008, the NCSBN and the Advanced Practice Nursing Consensus Work Group developed uniform APRN regulations that culminated in the publication of the *Consensus Model for APRN Regulation: Licensure, Accreditation, Certification & Education (The APRN Consensus Model)*.[2] NCSBN launched the Campaign for Consensus that continues to work toward states' adoption of the recommendations in the *APRN Consensus Model*. The goal was to have full implementation by 2015. As of early 2021, roughly half of the states and US territories have fully adopted and implemented legislation to support the *APRN Consensus Model* recommendations, with partial adoption by other states. Many palliative APRNs have been influenced by this work. The NCSBN website provides updated information about APRN practice in each state and territory.[3]

Second, in 2010, after a 2-year joint effort to assess the state of the nursing profession; the historical, cultural, regulatory, and policy barriers; and the future needs of the country, the Robert Wood Johnson Foundation and the Institute of Medicine (IOM) published the influential report *The Future of Nursing: Leading Change, Advancing Health*.[4] In addition to addressing challenges in the nursing education system, the blueprint outlined recommendations to remove legal barriers to APRN practice. To achieve this recommendation, the IOM specified directives for Congress, state legislatures, the Centers for Medicare and Medicaid Services (CMS), the Office of Personnel Management for Federal Employees, the Federal Trade Commission (FTC), and the Antitrust Division of the Department of Justice. It is a clear indication that those who influence public policy and cultural change, such as the IOM, recognized the critical role APRNs play in the healthcare landscape of the country. The document specifically instructed Congress to expand the Medicare program to include coverage of APRN services that are within the scope of practice under applicable state law, just as physician services are now covered. CMS required that hospitals that participate in the Medicare program remove barriers that limit clinical privileges and membership on medical staffs for APRNs, thus promoting wider access to palliative care.

The work started by the IOM did not stop there as the recommendations of the report were monitored over the decade. A new report was planned for 2020 which was delayed enabling the inclusion of emergent health issues influenced by the COVID-19 global pandemic and the exacerbation of social injustice and systemic racism. Through the convening of a diverse expert panel, The National Academies of Sciences, Engineering and Medicine examined how nursing profession would meet these demands. *The Future of Nursing 2020–2030 Charting a Path to Health Equity* was issued in May 2021 and it builds on the prior themes to have nurses be on the forefront of achieving health equity.[5]

Third, coming on the heels of the *Consensus Model* and the *Future of Nursing* report, the implementation of the 2010 Affordable Care Act brought about an overhaul in healthcare unprecedented since the creation of the Medicare and Medicaid programs in 1965. To meet the increased demand due to increased access to healthcare coverage, APRNs have filled the gap of healthcare providers. However, there is a palliative care workforce shortage, exacerbated by the COVID-19 pandemic. Palliative APRNs will need to practice to the full extent of their scope to support the needs of a cultural shift and a changing US demographic.

Finally, in late 2016, the Department of Veterans Affairs (VA) issued a final rule granting full practice authority to three of the four advanced-practice roles (NP, certified nurse midwife [CNM], and CNS).[6] Largely driven by desire to improve access to care, the VA has stated that the omission of certified registered nurse anesthetists (CRNAs) in the rule was based not on their competence but rather on a lack of issues related to access problems to anesthesiology. The intent of the rule allowed APRNs to practice to the full extent of their license without clinical supervision, thereby addressing the provider shortage which has historically resulted in delayed care for veterans and ultimately poor health outcomes.[7] Perhaps the most significant aspect of this rule is the declaration that removes the requirement for supervision or collaboration for those APRNs employed by the VA. This federal declaration supersedes state law, removing the barrier of variability by state. Palliative APRNs practice more consistently and to the full extent of their scope of practice. Moreover, more veterans have access to quality palliative care.

UNDERSTANDING THE *APRN CONSENSUS MODEL*: WHAT DOES IT MEAN AND WHY SHOULD ONE CARE?

The profession of advanced practice nursing has historically been a convoluted and complicated web of educational degrees, certifications, and regulations. Moreover, oversight occurs within multiple layers of hierarchies, including the CMS, state statutes and state boards of nursing, and individual institutional privileging and credentialing requirements. The number of APRNs continues to grow at a rapid rate, currently numbering 290,000 NPs[8] and 70,000 specialists[9] in the United States and its territories. Between 2010 and 2017, the number of NPs more than doubled. The forecasted annual growth of practitioners between 2016 and 2030 is greater among NPs (6.8%) than physicians (1.1%) and physician assistants (4.3%). The lack of uniformity and cohesion in the laws and regulations creates confusion for employers and consumers and barriers and inconsistencies in how and where APRNs may practice. Knowing that APRNs will represent a larger proportion of healthcare, there is an opportunity to increase state and federal representation and align laws and regulations.[7,10]

The *APRN Consensus Model* was created to guide all states and jurisdictions in implementing and overseeing the uniform licensure, accreditation, certification, education, and practice of APRNs.[2,11-14] The *APRN Consensus Model* is composed of seven major elements (Box 3.1). APRNs should understand their own state regulations regarding title, recognition, education, credentialing, licensing, and independence to practice. If the APRN were to change jobs or location of employment, would their scope of practice be more or less restricted? Indeed, could they practice at all? The following elements are addressed in the *APRN Consensus Model*; APRNs should review these within their setting:

- *Title*: The purpose of a title is to differentiate professions, provide clarity to the consumer, and ensure consistent recognition regardless of location of practice.[2,11] The *APRN Consensus Model* has designated "advanced practice registered nurse" as the agreed-upon title. One would think something as basic as a title would be straightforward, but, unfortunately, this is not the case. There is wide variability across the country in the use and legal recognition of "APRN." Other titles used include advanced practice nurse (APN), nurse specialist, and advanced registered nurse practitioner (ARNP).

- *APRN Roles and Recognition*: There are four defined APRN roles with specific designated titles.

  - Certified nurse practitioner (CNP)
  - Clinical nurse specialist (CNS)
  - Certified registered nurse anesthetist (CRNA)
  - Certified nurse midwife (CNM)

  CNPs and CNSs are most common in the field of hospice and palliative care and are currently the only roles eligible for advanced practice specialty hospice palliative nursing certification.

- *Role Recognition Adoptions*: States vary in recognizing all four APRN roles, which certainly affects the ability of an APRN to move easily across state lines and continue to practice. Several states do not recognize the CNS role and have placed the CNS in a "nurse practitioner" designation.

- *Licensure*: State boards of nursing vary regarding required certifications, registrations, and licenses for permission to practice. Many states allow the APRN to practice with only an RN license and additional APRN certifications. The *APRN Consensus Model* requires a separate APRN license in addition to the RN license. This additional licensure will ensure consistency in recognizing the APRN role from state to state and will give APRNs the flexibility to relocate for jobs and maintain their essential scope of practice.

- *Graduate or Postgraduate Education*: The *APRN Consensus Model* requires that the APRN be educated by a nationally accredited program of nursing, with a minimum of a master's degree. The educational program must include the three core courses: advanced physiology or pathophysiology, advanced health assessment, and advanced pharmacology, with clinical and didactic experiences.[2,11] The graduate nursing educational path changed with the adoption of the *APRN Consensus Model* in that all APRN students must be educated in one of six specific populations.[2]

The selection of population focus will dictate to what practice the APRN will be restricted. For example, a CNP whose education and clinical preparation was in women's health would not be able to practice in adult/gerontology without additional education and certification. In the evolution of graduate-level nursing, the emphasis pivoted from role preparation (administration and education) to specialized clinical knowledge and practice (advanced practice nursing). Other health-related fields, including pharmacy, dental surgery, medicine, physical therapy, and psychology have clinical doctorate-level training. In 2004, the American Association of Colleges of Nursing (AACN) proposed moving APRN education from the master's to the doctoral level, achieving parity with our colleagues in a terminal degree.[15] There are currently two tracks for the doctoral-prepared nurse: the research-focused Doctor of Philosophy (PhD) or Doctor of Nursing Sciences (DNS, or DNSc) and the practice-focused Doctor of Nursing Practice (DNP) (Box 3.2).

Box 3.1 SEVEN ELEMENTS OF THE APRN CONSENSUS MODEL

I. Title

II. APRN Roles and Recognition

III. Licensure

IV. Graduate or Postgraduate Education

V. Certification

VI. Independent Practice

VII. Full Prescriptive Authority

Box 3.2 TERMINAL DEGREES IN NURSING

Terminal degrees in nursing prepare nurses as experts in health administration, education, clinical research, and advanced clinical practice

Research-focused:

- Doctor of Philosophy (PhD)

- Doctor of Nursing Science (DNS or DNSc)

- Doctor of Education (EdD)

Practice-focused:

- Doctor of Nursing Practice (DNP)

The PhD, DNS, or DNSc in nursing has an accepted reputation for building the body of nursing knowledge through research. The DNP has come to address the need for enhanced nursing leadership, implementation of evidenced-based nursing practice, and broadening the educational experience of nursing faculty. It has been formalized that preparation at the practice doctorate (i.e., DNP with a clinical focus) includes advanced preparation in nursing practice based on nursing science and is at the highest level of nursing practice.[16] Furthermore, the AACN (2018) in its white paper, describes how the DNP curriculum prepares nurses to generate new knowledge through innovation of practice change, the translation of evidence, and the implementation of quality improvement processes in specific practice settings, systems, or with specific populations to improve health or health outcomes.[17]

Postgraduate programs in palliative care are gaining traction and include observerships, practicums, preceptorships, internships, externships, residencies, and fellowships.[18] Palliative APRN fellowships are typically 1-year programs offered in academic settings, often within a teaching hospital. A palliative care fellowship provides specialized clinical training and education in palliative care and may be in collaboration and conjunction with palliative medicine and social work fellowships. A palliative APRN fellowship program includes the orientation to and history of palliative nursing and nursing leadership, advanced education and lectures taught by interprofessional faculty, clinical experiences mentored by an APRN (who is ideally certified as an advanced certification hospice and palliative nurse [ACHPN]), and APRN role development supervised by an APRN. A fellowship program includes the completion of a palliative-focused project/case study, quality improvement project, or research study.[18]

- *Certification*: The *APRN Consensus Model* requires that all APRNs obtain certification to practice by passing a psychometrically sound and nationally accredited examination at the advanced practice nursing level that measures competency in the specific population of practice.[2,11] The organization providing the certification program must be nationally accredited by the American Board of Nursing Specialties or the National Commission for Certifying Agencies.[2] The APRN must also demonstrate ongoing competence to maintain certification. Though advanced palliative and hospice care is not one of the population foci in the *APRN Consensus Model*, APRNs who practice in this specialty are encouraged to seek specialty certification to demonstrate their commitment to the field and to the patients they serve.

- *Independent Practice*: The *APRN Consensus Model* lobbies for the APRN to practice to full stated scope without physician supervision. In many states, there has been legislation to promote this practice; however, it has been met with fierce resistance from the medical establishment. APRNs should be very familiar with the

CMS requirement to work in collaboration with a physician with medical direction and appropriate supervision (though this supervision does not need to be direct) as required by the law of the state in which the services are furnished.[19] As part of the credentialing and privileging process, many state legislatures and/or individual institutions require the APRN to have a collaborative practice and/or prescribing agreement with a supervising physician. The *APRN Consensus Model* accentuates a hallmark of APRN practice which is voluntary collaboration that emphasizes the interdependence and interreliance of healthcare professionals.[2,11] In the adoption of this element of practice without physician oversight, some states have specified a period of physician or APRN supervision of newly graduated APRNs to ensure a smooth transition with close mentoring and guidance.

- *Full Prescriptive Authority*: The ability of the APRN to prescribe pharmacologic and nonpharmacologic therapies without physician oversight and/or a written collaborative agreement is the element of the *APRN Consensus Model* that has been met with the most opposition, primarily from organized medical groups. This is despite evidence that APRN outcome measures are equivalent to those of other medical providers.[7,11,20] Full prescriptive authority is key to being able to provide care to populations with limited access to healthcare.

The NCSBN continues to track each state's progress toward adoption of the seven elements. APRNs can access the most accurate and up-to-date status of adoption of the Consensus Model by checking the website.[3]

- *Scope of Practice*: "The advanced practice hospice and palliative registered nurse responds to the individual, professional, and societal needs related to the experience of serious or life-threatening illness through the nursing process."[21] Through graduate-level education at the master's or doctorate level, APRNs differ from generalists by being able to synthesize complex data, develop and implement advanced care plans, and provide leadership in hospice and palliative nursing. Besides the clinical focus of the CNS and CNP, there are graduate-level prepared nurses who are APNs. In hospice and palliative care, they may function as leaders/administrators, educators, researchers, consultants, case managers, program developers, and policymakers.

- *The Political Landscape of Advanced Practice Registered Nursing*: APRNs have struggled with practice barriers imposed by restrictive legislation, often supported by the political influence of medical associations. These restrictions lack any evidence or data showing inadequacies or concerns about the safety and outcomes of practice by APRNs—in fact, there is much evidence to the contrary. Multiple studies have found either no difference or actual improvement in comparable patient outcomes between APRNs and physicians. Also, APRNs show substantial cost savings and cost avoidance in the provision of care.[22] The consistent conclusion from these studies is that patient outcomes of care provided by APRNs are similar in terms of safety, effectiveness, quality, and patient satisfaction—in some aspects, they are better than care provided by physicians alone. APRNs are also recognized for their inherent focus on collaborative practice.[7,20,22]

It is extremely significant that the FTC, which exists to monitor and prevent any unfair or deceptive acts or practices that would impair competition in the marketplace, including the healthcare industry, published a policy paper in March 2014 called *Policy Perspectives: Competition and the Regulation of Advanced Practice Nurses*.[23]

The paper supports the ability of APRNs to practice to the full extent of their scope without unnecessary, unjustified, and restrictive supervisory requirements and collaborative practice agreements with physicians. The paper states that "APRN scope of practice limitations should be narrowly tailored to address well-founded health and safety concerns, and should not be more restrictive than patient protection requires."[23] The FTC recognizes that the scope of practice of any healthcare provider should be consistent with each professional's education and training, licensure and certification, and experience and capabilities. Current legislative or institutional requirements for physician supervision of the APRN to practice independently are identified by the FTC as a concern because they give one group of healthcare professionals control over another, resulting in restricted access to the market and potentially denying healthcare consumers the benefits of greater competition.[23]

In the policy paper, the FTC identified several concerns about the present state of APRN scope of practice where unwieldy and unwarranted restrictions, under the guise of "consumer protection," are actually contributing to less competition and, thus, less protection, including:

- Less access to safe and effective care, especially in under-served areas and for populations that are experiencing, in particular, primary care provider shortages.

- Impaired development of innovative models of healthcare delivery to meet the needs of the healthcare consumers.

- Increased costs and less oversight of cost containment.

- Less focus on the importance of measuring quality outcomes, with subsequent serious health and safety consequences.

This report, along with the *APRN Campaign for Consensus* and the IOM *Future of Nursing* recommendations discussed previously, have positioned APRN practice in its strongest standing to date. It remains to be seen how legislators, policymakers, and administrators will heed and implement these recommendations. Palliative APRNs can influence and support further changes and improvements in being able to practice to the fullest extent of their scope by getting involved with their professional organizations, as well as staying informed about and engaged in practice issues critical to APRN professional health.

THE PROFESSIONAL LANDSCAPE OF ADVANCED PRACTICE REGISTERED NURSING

The scope and standards of APRN practice are defined by the national professional nursing organizations specific to the population focus for which they were educated. The APRN's clinical scope includes the tasks of performing advanced assessments; interpreting diagnostic studies; forming a differential diagnosis; prescribing pharmacologic and nonpharmacologic treatments and equipment; ordering additional diagnostic tests, consultants, and support services; and evaluating the response to treatment.[24]

APRNs are accountable to patients for the quality of the care they provide. They must be able to recognize the limits of their education, knowledge, and experience. They should know when to refer patients to other providers and practitioners for appropriate management when they are confronted by a situation that is outside their area of expertise. With this increased responsibility, no matter how long a nurse may have practiced as an RN, when they become an APRN, there is usually a period of transition and uncertainty. Many questions may arise about what is now within the scope of practice for the APRN, such as:

- Does the APRN role allow the APRN to prescribe, and, if so, are there any restrictions on what classes of medications may be prescribed?

- If the APRN was trained in the population of family practice, given that their education and training was not in the population focus of adult/gerontology, can they provide care to an older adult entering the end stage of a chronic illness?

- Is the APRN's knowledge base adequate to diagnose and treat conditions for which they are seeing a patient?

- What are the limitations on the services that a CNS or CNP employed by a hospice program can provide in light of CMS rules that dictate which medical providers may complete face-to-face assessments and recertification of terminal illness?

These and other questions may cause the hospice and palliative APRN some level of anxiety because the responsibilities and liabilities change with the increased scope of practice. The American Nurses Association (ANA), along with Hospice and Palliative Nurse Association (HPNA), are the primary sources for guidelines about the scope and standards of APRN practice.[24] Above all, practice must be safe, quality-focused, and evidence-based. In response to the dilemma of what is considered appropriate practice within accepted scope, ANA advises the APRN to first consider the published scope and standards of practice. Now in its fourth edition, *Nursing: Scope and Standards of Practice*, published in 2021, includes specific information about the scope of the APRN.

Second, the APRN should determine the current state laws and regulations that dictate his or her practice limitations. In addition to the NCSBN website, each state's board of nursing is the source of up-to-date and pertinent legislation that governs the practice of APRNs in the jurisdiction where they work.

Third, APRNs should review the institutional policies and procedures that apply to their practice. Although CMS and state regulations provide the "outer limits" of APRN scope of practice, APRNs may find their practice further limited by the interpretation and application of those regulations in individual institutions/facilities or health systems. For instance, CMS may allow a CNS to prescribe, but the hospital where a CNS is employed may have very stringent collaborative agreement requirements or restrictions that limit the CNS's ability to prescribe medications. Although the professional credentialing process at a facility or institution may choose to be more restrictive, a motivated and informed cohort of APRNs can change practice at the ground level so that local rules and regulations mirror the rules and regulations of the larger governing body.

Finally, the APRN should do an objective review of their skills and expertise in a process of self-determination, taking into account the skills and expertise of other members of the healthcare team and available consultants. The prudent APRN should also consider risk management and potential liability issues in particular situations and consider consulting with the institution's risk management or legal department or the malpractice insurer for support and clarification regarding a scope-of-practice question. There are many good resources available that offer guidance to the APRN wanting to gain a deeper understanding of legal issues, including *Law and Ethics in Advanced Practice Nursing*.[25]

The APRN who practices in hospice and palliative care will find further information and guidance in the following resources specific to the specialty of palliative nursing:

- The Hospice and Palliative Nurses Association, *Palliative Nursing: Scope and Standards of Practice* (2021). A necessary resource for both APRNs and RNs, this edition discusses in detail what is expected of all hospice and palliative RNs and APNs. Practice accountabilities are divided into 16 standards with accompanying competencies, with additional competencies specified for APRNs. These standards provide the framework for guiding and evaluating the nurse's practice, along with behaviors and outcomes that would demonstrate whether he or she is meeting the minimal level of compliance with the standard.[21]

- Hospice and Palliative Nurses Association, *Competencies for the Palliative and Hospice Advanced Practice Registered Nurse* (3rd edition, 2021). This resource describes the explicit intellectual, interpersonal, technical, and moral competencies that are outcome-specific, measurable, and

considered necessary for quality palliative nursing.[26] It includes the following core characteristics applicable to the APRN, which are further delineated by advanced core behaviors based on the American Association of Critical Care Nurses *Synergy Model*[27]:

- Clinical judgment
- Advocacy and moral agency
- Caring practices
- Collaboration
- Systems thinking
- Response to diversity
- Facilitation of learning
- Clinical inquiry

- Hospice and Palliative Nurses Association, *The Core Curriculum for the Hospice and Palliative Advanced Practice Registered Nurse* (2020). This book reflects the current evidence-based knowledge in advanced hospice and palliative nursing practice. The Core Curriculum provides a foundational work for the APRN and includes sections on role and practice concerns, management of common symptoms, psychosocial and spiritual aspects of care, and specific pathophysiology and disease-specific management. There is also information on vulnerable and special populations and an appendix with many references and tools for practice.[28]

- The National Consensus Project for Quality Palliative Care (NCP), *Clinical Practice Guidelines* (4th edition, 2018). This collaborative effort of ten national palliative care organizations, including the HPNA, published a set of guidelines and recommendations for high-quality palliative care in eight domains of practice (Box 3.3).[29] Currently in its fourth edition, this updated publication builds on the work and developments that have occurred in hospice and palliative care since earlier guidelines were published in 2004, 2009, and 2013, with a focus on improving access to quality palliative care for all those with serious illness.

Box 3.3 **NATIONAL CONSENSUS PROJECT FOR QUALITY PALLIATIVE CARE,** *CLINICAL PRACTICE GUIDELINES* **EIGHT DOMAINS OF CARE**

   I. Structure and Processes of Care

  II. Physical Aspects of Care

 III. Psychological and Psychiatric Aspects of Care

 IV. Social Aspects of Care

  V. Spiritual, Religious, and Existential Aspects of Care

 VI. Cultural Aspects of Care

VII. Care of the Patient Nearing End of Life

VIII. Ethical and Legal Aspects of Care

- American Association of Colleges of Nursing and City of Hope, *End-of-Life Nursing Education Consortium* (ELNEC). This educational initiative was founded in 2000, by Dr. Betty Ferrell and colleagues, to develop educational tools for undergraduate nursing faculty to ensure that topics in palliative care were taught as part of the nursing curriculum. Various versions of the curriculum have been developed for nurses in general practice and for special populations, such as veterans, pediatrics, geriatrics, and critical care units. ELNEC offers a course that addresses the unique needs of APRNs who are developing, leading, joining, or participating in a hospice and/or palliative care program or are incorporating palliative care into their current APRN role.[30]

CREDENTIALING

The terms "credentialing," "accreditation," "licensure," and "certification" are often misunderstood and thus are frequently used interchangeably and incorrectly. In a general sense, "credentialing" is an umbrella term that refers to several different processes overseen by a number of regulatory bodies (Box 3.4), such as licensure, certification, accreditation, recognition, and registration.[31]

Licensure involves a mandatory process by which a government agency grants time-limited legal status and permission for a person to engage in the practice of a profession in the public domain. Licensure signifies the provider has met minimal standards of competence, typically by passing a psychometrically sound examination. A license grants permission to use a particular title and provides protection of that title. It also defines a scope of practice for the profession. Licensure ultimately serves to protect the consumer and the public health, safety, and welfare. To this end, the individual state boards of nursing must have processes in place for anyone to file a complaint against a nurse whom they believe has acted in violation of nursing rules and the defined scope of practice. For instance, a consumer who has suffered harm from incompetent prescribing practices of an APRN could file a complaint with the board of nursing. The complaint would be investigated to determine if the APRN acted in an illegal or incompetent manner. If found to be at fault, discipline for the APRN would likely include restrictions or even suspension of the professional license and thus the ability to practice.

Credentialing differs from licensure in that a credential it is a designation issued by a nongovernmental agency or association that the public can look to for assurance that an individual provider has achieved specific standards of competence that have been defined and promoted by the profession. APRNs may be familiar with the credentials granted by the American Nurses Credentialing Center or the American Academy of Nurse Practitioners after passing an accredited certification exam. There are different kinds of credentialing applicable to the APRN, and these are important to understand and differentiate.

"Entry to practice" credentialing is the "end product" of an educational program, achieved after graduation and the successful completion of a psychometrically sound examination from an accredited certification organization in the area of practice the provider was educated in. Successful completion of the exam provides the APRN with the required certification to obtain licensure to practice according to state statute and grants the legal right to use a specific title.

"Professional" credentialing is the process by which safe, high-quality, and competent care by APRNs (and other providers) is determined and verified by the facility or institution in which the APRN will be working. The Joint Commission requires that institutions have a systematic process to evaluate the provider who is applying for privileges.

The credentialing application is extensive and typically includes the elements listed here. APRNs should begin keeping a portfolio immediately after graduation that contains these documents for quick reference for any questions and future recredentialing processes[31]:

- Education, including proof of graduation and degree

- Previous work history

- Current licenses and certifications, National Provider Identifier (NPI) number, Drug Enforcement Administration (DEA) registration number, and a state registration for controlled substances

- Professional memberships

- Continuing education and competency assessments

- Collaborative practice and prescriptive agreements, if required

- Immunization status

- Any past or current disciplinary actions or suspensions from pertinent boards of practice

- Any past or current legal proceedings, both personal and professional

- Any physical, mental health, or chemical dependency issues that could affect one's ability to practice safely and competently

- References from peers and a current resume.

Box 3.4 **HEALTHCARE REGULATORY BODIES**

- Federal and state law, including the Centers for Medicare and Medicaid Services (CMS) laws

- State boards of nursing

- Healthcare Quality Organizations—The Joint Commission (TJC), DNV-GL, Community Health Accreditation Partner (CHAP), Accreditation Commission for Heath Care (ACHC)

- Hospital and facility provider bylaws and policies

- National certification associations and programs

- Professional organization statements

A credentialing committee at the institution reviews the application and, if approved, the APRN is granted privileges to practice. Clinical privileges are delineated to clarify specific sites where the APRN is able to practice and which practices and procedures the provider is allowed to provide, including prescriptive privileges. Clinical practice is often guided by, or in some cases is required to be based on, written guidelines and evidence-based protocols. There are many guidelines and evidence-based protocols in existence, so the APRN need not create something new. Rather, the APRN can adapt these to their setting. Depending on the specific practices and procedures the provider is requesting permission to perform, the committee may also require evidence of demonstrated competence.

Upon initial credentialing and privileging, APRNs can expect there to be a specified period of time in which their practice is closely monitored and evaluated by direct peer feedback and/or medical record review. Reappointments typically occur every 2 years, and the APRN must provide evidence of continued competency.

Payer credentialing involves the application for authorization to bill for reimbursement through Medicare, Medicaid, and other for-profit and nonprofit insurance carriers. The paperwork for credentialing varies widely by payer, but all processes begin by obtaining an NPI number, which recognizes the APRN as a unique healthcare provider under the Health Insurance Portability and Accountability Act (HIPAA) of 1996 guidelines and as one who maintains certifications and licensure.

THE VALUE AND PROCESS OF SPECIALTY CERTIFICATION

In most states, the CNP or CNS must obtain certification from a national, accredited certification organization after graduation from a master's or doctoral program in nursing in order to practice. Certification serves as a form of regulation by the state boards of nursing in recognizing a minimal level of competence. Certification is also now required for reimbursement for services through CMS, and as discussed previously, is required for practice, professional, and payer credentialing.

Specialty certification as an ACHPN is available through the Hospice and Palliative Credentialing Center (HPCC). It is voluntary for the individual APRN, but many employers require the additional specialty certification at the time of hire or require the nurse to obtain it within a specified time frame. The APRN is reminded, however, that the *APRN Consensus Model* now requires that the graduate student education program be focused on one of the six specific populations discussed earlier, with successful completion of the corresponding certification exam for entry to practice. In most states, hospice and palliative care is considered a "specialty" and the ACHPN examination is not accepted for entry to practice. The APRN should check with the individual state board of nursing and CMS to determine requirements for licensure and billing.

Some hospice and palliative APRNs wonder why they should work toward specialty certification in advanced hospice and palliative care when it might not be required. After all, it is an additional expense that may or may not be reimbursed by one's employer, and it is stressful and time-consuming to sit for an exam. But there are actually many benefits to obtaining certification in the specialty one practices in, and these perceived and actual values have been described in a study conducted by the American Board of Nursing Specialties.[32] They include:

- An expanded and deeper knowledge base. The exercise of studying for the exam actually contributes to learning new information about the specialty.

- A commitment to professional growth, enhanced feelings of personal accomplishment, professional satisfaction, and increased empowerment and confidence in the role.

- Enhanced credibility and respect of coworkers; being seen as a staff resource.

- The standard of practice is raised throughout the profession, which in the long run serves to improve patient care outcomes and safety.

- Employers have found that specialty-certified nurses are desirable employees because certification reflects dedication to their profession and to providing the most relevant, evidence-based, and cutting-edge care to patients and their families.

- Financial benefits and professional growth. In addition to possible bonuses and salary increases, APRNs with specialty certification are often viewed as more competent and able to take on more responsibility, which can lead to career advancement and opportunities.

- Managers and employers have found that certified nurses help ensure a highly trained, progressive team, which elevates the perception of the medical facility or program. Hospitals applying for or renewing American Nurses Credentialing Center Magnet status or programs seeking The Joint Commission for specialty certification in palliative care must have a greater percentage of certified providers.[32]

SPECIFICS AND PROCESS OF ATTAINING THE ACHPN

Initial certification as an ACHPN is attained by passing a psychometrically sound, computer-based examination. The content of the examination has been developed from a national job analysis survey that identified the activities performed by hospice and palliative APRNs. A task force of experienced hospice and palliative APRNs determined from the job analysis the activities and knowledge critical to the practice of the hospice and palliative APRN. These are specified in the Detailed Content Outline in the ACHPN Candidate

Handbook.[33] The content outline can be used to guide self-assessment and a study plan for the exam.

Although there is not a test question pertaining to each topic on the content outline, every question on the exam can be linked back to the outline. The questions are written by experienced APRNs in the field and are scrutinized by members of the HPCC APRN Exam Development Committee, with the guidance of a statistician from the professional testing agency that assists in the development, administration, scoring, and analysis of the certification examination.

RECERTIFICATION

HPCC certification must be renewed every 4 years through the Hospice and Palliative Accrual for Recertification process. It is the expectation that the APRN has continued to develop professionally with experience and exposure to new knowledge over that 4-year period. Continuing education and professional activities, along with a minimum number of practice hours, are the main requirements for certification renewal. Professional activities are converted to points, with a requirement to accrue an established minimum number of points in the 4-year period. Professional activities the APRN can complete for recertification include[33]:

- Continuing nursing education
- Continuing medical education
- Academic education
- Professional publications
- Professional presentations
- Item writer workshop participation
- Self-assessment examination completion
- Professional volunteer activities related to hospice and palliative care
- Clinical mentoring/preceptorship of graduate nursing students

In support of the goal of encouraging continued competence in practice, a situational judgment exercise is also required for recertification. This is an open-book, online exercise that uses real-life, case-based scenarios to test the candidate's critical reasoning and clinical application beyond the level of the initial certification exam. As candidates are led through the scenario, they are asked to make decisions about what pertinent information to gather to guide decisions about the care and treatment of the patient and family. The cases involve more than just clinical decision-making; they also address professional judgment, patient education, communication, ethics, and collaborative practice issues. Points are accrued toward recertification based on the score achieved.

To accomplish recertification efficiently, the APRN should organize activities, dates, and documentation during the 4-year accrual period. As most APRNs need to gather this information to recertify for their primary practice certification, relicensure, and credentialing, it should not require significant extra work. Although online documentation makes recordkeeping easier and more efficient, it is still important for the APRN to keep copies of continuing education certificates of attendance and documentation to support other professional development activities. It is much better to acquaint oneself with the recertification requirements soon after initial certification rather than waiting for the deadline to be looming and discover that meeting the recertification requirements will be more challenging than anticipated.

Certification and recertification in advanced hospice and palliative care demonstrate professional commitment and mastery of the field. While they are not necessarily required to practice in the field, they speak to the APRN's professional commitment and dedication to the specialty.

CASE STUDY: THE CLINICAL NURSE SPECIALIST (CONTINUED)

Denise educated herself about the variations in APRN scope of practice in the states she planned to deploy the CNS and NP team members to implement a rural palliative telehealth service. The project synced with graduate coursework in a DNP program, which led to national presentations and recognition for her innovation in palliative care. Denise was later invited to work on political advocacy projects exploring the variability of APRN practice across regions. What started as a program-level growth project morphed into a career-changing endeavor exploring the system-level variability in APRN practice.

SUMMARY

The landscape of our healthcare system is constantly changing, and APRNs will need to rise to the challenge to provide high-quality, efficient, cost-effective, and accessible care. The hospice and palliative APRN will increasingly be called upon to meet the needs of an aging population. To practice safely, legally, and to the fullest extent of their scope, APRNs must have a working knowledge of the sometimes confusing world of credentialing, privileging, certification, and licensure. APRNs must understand potential changes to their own practice regarding the implementation of the NCSBN *APRN Consensus Model* and the lifting of current restrictions to independent practice. APRNs practicing in the specialty of hospice and palliative care may best demonstrate their expertise and ongoing competence, in addition to professionalism, by achieving advanced certification in hospice and palliative care.

REFERENCES

1. Promoting Excellence in End-of-Life-Care. *Advanced Practice Nurses Role in Palliative Care: A Position Statement from American Nurse Leaders.* Missoula, MT: Promoting Excellence in End-of-Life Care

(a project of the Robert Wood Johnson Foundation); 2002. http://www.mywhatever.com/cifwriter/content/41/pe3673.html

2. National Council of State Boards of Nursing. *APRN Consensus Model: The Consensus Model for APRN Regulation, Licensure, Accreditation, Certification and Education.* Chicago, IL: National Council of State Boards of Nursing. 2008. https://ncsbn.org/aprn-consensus.htm

3. National Council of State Boards of Nursing. APRN Consensus Model Implementation Status. 2019. https://ncsbn.org/APRN_Consensus_Grid_Apr2019.pdf

4. Institute of Medicine. *The Future of Nursing: Leading Change, Advancing Health.* Washington, DC: The National Academies Press; 2011. doi:10.17226/12956. https://pubmed.ncbi.nlm.nih.gov/24983041/

5. National Academies of Sciences, Engineering, and Medicine 2021. *The Future of Nursing 2020–2030: Charting a Path to Achieve Health Equity.* Washington, DC: The National Academies Press. https://doi.org/10.17226/25982.

6. US Department of Veterans Affairs. Office of Public and Intergovernmental Affairs. (2016, December 14). VA grants full practice authority to advanced practice registered nurses [press release]. https://www.va.gov/opa/pressrel/pressrelease.cfm?id=2847

7. Fauteux, N, Brand, R, Fink J, Frelick M, Werrlein, D. The case for removing barriers to APRN practice. Robert Wood Johnson Foundation. *Charting Nursing's Future.* 2017;30:1–10. https://www.rwjf.org/en/library/research/2017/03/the-case-for-removing-barriers-to-aprn-practice.html

8. American Association of Nurse Practitioners. NP Fact Sheet. Austin, TX: AANP. Updated May. 2021. https://www.aanp.org/about/all-about-nps/np-fact-sheet

9. ExploreHealthCareers.org. Clinical Nurse Specialist. 2021. https://explorehealthcareers.org/career/nursing/clinical-nurse-specialist/

10. Auerbach DI, Buerhaus PI, Staiger DO. Implications of the rapid growth of the nurse practitioner workforce in the U.S. *Health Aff.* 2020;39(2): 273–279. doi:10.1377/hlthaff.2019.00686

11. Cahill M, Alexander M, Gross L. The 2014 NCSBN Consensus Report on APRN Regulation. *J Nurs Regul.* 2014;4(4): 5–12. doi:10.1016/S2155-8256(15)30111-3

12. Doherty CL, Pawlow P, Becker D. The consensus model: What current and future NPs need to know. *American Nurse Today.* 2018;13(1),65–67. https://www.myamericannurse.com/consensus-model-nps/

13. National Council of State Boards of Nursing. APRN Consensus Model Frequently-Asked Questions. Chicago, IL: NCSBN. August 19, 2010. https://ncsbn.org/APRN_Consensus_Model_FAQs_August_19_2010.pdf

14. Mack R. Increasing access to health care by implementing a consensus model for advanced practice registered nurse practice. *J Nurs Pract.* 2018;14(5):419–424. doi:10.1016/J.NURPRA.2018.02.008

15. American Association of Colleges of Nursing. *AACN Position Statement on the Practice Doctorate in Nursing.* Washington, DC: AACN; 2004. https://www.aacnnursing.org/DNP/Position-Statement

16. American Association of Colleges of Nursing. *The Essentials of Doctoral Education for Advanced Nursing Practice.* Washington, DC: AACN; 2006. https://www.aacnnursing.org/Portals/42/Publications/DNPEssentials.pdf

17. American Association of Colleges of Nursing. *Defining Scholarship for Academic Nursing Task Force Consensus Position Statement.* Washington, DC: AACN; March 26, 2018. https://www.aacnnursing.org/News-Information/Position-Statements-White-Papers/Defining-Scholarship-Nursing

18. Hospice and Palliative Nurses Association. Palliative care APRN fellowships. 2021. https://advancingexpertcare.org/aprn-fellowship

19. Department of Health and Human Services Centers for Medicare and Medicaid Services. Medicare Learning Network. Medicare Information for Advanced Practice Registered Nurses, Anesthesiologist Assistants, and Physician Assistants. Baltimore, MD. April 2020. https://www.cms.gov/Outreach-and-Education/Medicare-Learning-Network-MLN/MLNProducts/Downloads/Medicare-Information-for-APRNs-AAs-PAs-Booklet-ICN-901623.pdf

20. Kurtzman ET, Barnow BS, Johnson JE, Simmens SJ, Infeld DL, Mullan F. Does the regulatory environment affect nurse practitioners' patterns of practice or quality of care in health centers? *Health Serv Res.* 2017;52(12):437–458. doi:10.1111/1475-6773.12643

21. Dahlin C. *Palliative Nursing: Scope and Standards of Practice.* 6th ed. Pittsburgh, PA: Hospice and Palliative Nurses Association; 2021.

22. Dubree M, Jones P, Kapu A, Parmley CL. APRN practice: Challenges, empowerment, and outcomes. *Nurse Leader.* 2015;13(2):43–49. doi:10.1016/j.mnl.2015.01.007

23. Gilman DJ, Koslov TI. *Policy Perspectives: Competition and the Regulation of Advanced Practice Nurses.* Federal Trade Commission; 2014. https://www.ftc.gov/system/files/documents/reports/policy-perspectives-competition-regulation-advanced-practice-nurses/140307aprnpolicypaper.pdf

24. American Nurses Association. *Nursing: Scope and Standards of Practice.* 4th ed. Silver Spring, MD: ANA/Nursebooks.org; 2021.

25. Kjervik D, Brous EA. *Law and Ethics in Advanced Practice Nursing.* New York: Springer; 2010.

26. Dahlin C. *Competencies for the Palliative and Hospice APRN.* 3rd ed. Pittsburgh, PA: Hospice and Palliative Nurses Association; 2021.

27. American Association of Critical Care Nurses. *AACN Synergy Model for Patient Care.* 2nd ed. 2018. https://www.aacn.org/nursing-excellence/aacn-standards/synergy-model

28. Dahlin C, Morienes LT, Root M, eds. *Core Curriculum for the Hospice and Palliative Advanced Practice Registered Nurse.* 3rd ed. Pittsburgh, PA: Hospice and Palliative Nurses Association; 2020.

29. National Consensus Project for Quality Palliative Care. *Clinical Practice Guidelines for Quality Palliative Care,* 4th ed. Richmond, VA: National Coalition for Hospice and Palliative Care; 2018. https://www.nationalcoalitionhpc.org/ncp

30. American Association of Colleges of Nursing. ELNEC website. 2021. http://www.aacn.nche.edu/elnec

31. Smolenski MC, Gagan MJ. Credentialing, certification, and competence: Issues for new and seasoned nurse practitioners. *J Am Acad Nurse Pract.* 2005;17(6):201–204. doi:10.1111/j.1041-2972.2005.00033.x

32. American Board of Nursing Specialties. *Specialty Nursing Certification: Nurses' Perceptions, Values and Behaviors.* Birmingham, AL: ABNS; 2006. https://www.nursingcertification.org/resources/documents/research/white_paper_final_12_12_06.pdf

33. Hospice and Palliative Credentialing Center. ACHPN® Candidate Handbook. August 2021. https://advancingexpertcare.org/HPNA/Certification/Credentials/APRN_ACHPN/HPCC/CertificationWeb/ACHPN.aspx?hkey=fe8a39d4-bbe7-4acf-83c2-a13d29670579

SECTION II

PALLIATIVE APRN ROLES

4.

THE PALLIATIVE APRN IN ADMINISTRATION

Karen Mulvihill

KEY POINTS

- Graduate and doctoral programs do not provide the skills necessary to lead.

- The advanced practice registered nurse (APRN) interested in leadership roles need to seek out education in leadership and opportunities to lead.

- The APRN should seek out and utilize existing resources to develop their leadership skills.

- Conflict and change management are important skills in leading interdisciplinary teams.

CASE STUDY: LEADERSHIP

Cheryl is a new director for an inpatient palliative care team at a moderate-sized teaching hospital. One of her first tasks in the new role is to do the annual performance reviews for the 15 employees who report to her. She does not know where to begin and feels like an imposter in this role. Cheryl feels uncomfortable providing constructive feedback to her employees because she has never had to do that before. Although she is grateful for the chance to advance her career and experience, she wonders how she got into the role, given her lack of leadership experience.

INTRODUCTION

Florence Nightingale was the first nurse to recognize the need to formalize nursing as a practice, and she led the way for all nurses to ask, "How can I do more?" She was the first to identify the role of hygiene and sanitation in illness, thus becoming the first epidemiologist. She was the original nurse leader. Nursing roles have developed and expanded over time, placing more nurses in leadership positions. Advanced practice registered nurse (APRNs) are in a prime position to lead at local, regional, state, national, and global levels. Administration leadership roles may include myriad tasks such as developing programs, hiring and managing staff, creating strategic plans, education planning, quality improvement initiatives, and leading policy initiatives. The first step in being a leader is understanding leadership concepts and developing the necessary skills to be an effective leader.

Leadership is a core competency at all levels of nursing education and practice. The American Nurses Association (ANA) *Nursing Scope and Standards of Practice* and the Hospice and Palliative Nurses Association (HPNA) *Palliative Nursing: Scope and Standards* identifies leadership as a standard of professional performance for both registered nurses (RN) and graduate-level prepared registered nurses (Boxes 4.1 and 4.2).[1,2] The standard set the expectation for nurses to assume leadership roles at all levels. The *Nursing Scope and Standards of Practice* and the *Palliative Nursing: Scope and Standards* include ethical practice, accountability, communication, and moving the profession forward. The graduate-level competencies and advanced focus on decision-making, interprofessional teams, promoting policy, and role development through expert practice and mentoring.[1,2]

The ANA sets practice for all nurses at both the RN and APRN levels of practice. The ANA *Nursing Scope and Standards of Practice* set the stage for guidelines for education, clinical practice, advocacy, administration, and research in nursing professions. The competencies focus on enhancing the effectiveness of the interdisciplinary team and outcomes through quality initiatives and research, promoting role development of advanced practice palliative nurses, modeling expertise, and mentoring (Box 4.2).[1]

In 2010, the *Patient Protection and Affordable Care Act (ACA)* was passed and was important for healthcare reform. Subsequent to this legislation, the Institute of Medicine (IOM) and the Robert Wood Johnson Foundation (RWJF) collaborated on *The Future of Nursing: Leading, Change, Advancing Health.*[3] The committee focused their charge on the role of nursing in the context of the entire workforce, expanding nursing faculty to meet the healthcare demand for an increased nursing workforce, developing innovative solutions for healthcare delivery and staffing, and retaining nurses in all settings. A key message in the report is grounded in nurses being full partners in redesigning the healthcare system. Specifically, the overall message of the report is that in order to transform our healthcare system, the nursing profession must develop competent leaders to collaborate with other healthcare professionals and use their knowledge to identify innovative models of quality care and healthcare delivery.[3] Being a full partner involves "identifying problem areas of waste, devising and implementing a plan for improvement, tracking improvement over time, and making necessary adjustments to realize established goal."[3 (pp. 8)]

In 2017, the ANA and HPNA collaborated to create the *Call for Action: Nurses Lead and Transform Palliative Care.*[4] The document calls nurses to lead in practice, education, administration, policy, and research.[4] As a leader, palliative APRNs

Box 4.1 ANA SCOPE AND STANDARDS-STANDARD 12: LEADERSHIP

The registered nurse:

- Retains accountability for delegated nursing care.

- Promotes effective relationships (relational coordination) to achieve quality outcomes and a culture of safety.

- Engages in an interprofessional environment that promotes respect, trust, and integrity.

- Embraces practice innovations and role performance to achieve life-long personal and professional goals.

- Communicates to manage change and address conflict.

- Mentors colleagues and others to enhance their knowledge, skills, and abilities.

- Participates in professional activities and organizations for professional growth and influence.

- Advocates for all aspects of human and environmental health in practice and policy.

Additional Competencies for the Graduate-Level Prepared Registered Nurse, Including the APRN

In addition to the competencies of the registered nurse, the graduate-level prepared registered nurse including the APRN:

- Engages in decision-making bodies to implement an effective interprofessional environment that improves healthcare consumer outcomes and satisfaction.

- Interprets advanced practice nursing roles for policy makers and healthcare consumers.

- Models expert nursing practices to interprofessional team members and healthcare consumers.

- Mentors colleagues in their professional growth and participation in succession planning.

Adapted from American Nurses Association.[1]

have a role in promoting specialty palliative nursing. They ensure staff having training in primary palliative care, facilitate specialty palliative care training, foster specialty palliative nursing certification, create and implement palliative care nurse residency and fellowship programs, and seek funding for programs. Palliative APRN administrators are positioned to facilitate workforce strategies to explore and implement innovative models of care to address cultural diversity and staffing challenges as well as initiatives for equitable access to quality palliative care.[4]

The American Association of Colleges of Nursing (AACN) has recently updated *The Essentials: Core Competencies for Professional Nursing Education.*[5] The document provides core competencies across all levels of nursing education with specific subcompetencies for advanced nursing practice. The competencies are divided into domains and competencies which represent the four spheres of care: disease prevention, promotion of health and well-being, chronic disease care, regenerative or restorative care, and hospice, palliative, and supportive care.[5] In addition to the updated *Essentials*, the AACN has provided specific guidance for masters' and doctoral programs, requiring leadership to be part of the APRN's education. AACN Essential II *Organizational and Systems Leadership*[6] states "that organizational and systems leadership are critical to the promotion of high quality and safe patient care. Leadership skills are needed that emphasize ethical and critical decision-making, effective working relationships, and a systems-perspective."[5 (pp. 4)]

To be effective, palliative APRNs must rely on their graduate education. Whether master's-prepared or doctorally prepared, leadership has been part of the APRN's education as outlined by the American Association of Colleges of Nursing (AACN). The AACN *Essentials of Master's Education* states that graduates must be prepared "to lead change to improve quality outcomes, advance the culture of excellence through lifelong learning, build and lead interprofessional teams, integrate care across the healthcare system, design innovative nursing practice and translate evidence into practice."[6 (pp. 3-4)]

The AACN *The Essentials of Doctoral Education for Advanced Practice Nursing* states that "enhanced leadership skills to strengthen practice and health care delivery" as a program benefit.[7 (pp. 5)] The essential for organization and systems leadership focuses on health disparities, policy development, quality improvement at both practice and policy levels, and "principles of economics and finance to redesign effective and realistic care delivery strategies."[7 (pp. 10)]

In a *US News & World Report* review of the top five graduate nurse practitioner and clinical nurse specialist programs, all of the top five programs had a basic leadership class as part of the standard curriculum across all advanced practice programs.[8,9] Upon review of the graduate nursing curriculum at those top five schools, graduate programs only include one class focused on leadership competencies, with doctoral programs providing greater emphasis on leadership development.[10-14] Further review revealed that the top five doctor of nursing practice programs had at least one leadership-focused class across their advanced practice programs.[10-14] However, a single class on leadership is not enough to provide the graduate nurse with the leadership competencies needed to move into leadership roles.

The palliative registered nurse:

- Contributes to the establishment of an environment that supports and maintains respect, trust, and dignity.

- Encourages innovation in palliative nursing practice and role performance to attain personal and professional objectives, goals, and vision.

- Communicates to manage change and address conflict within palliative care delivery.

- Mentors colleagues for the advancement of palliative nursing practice and the nursing profession to enhance safe, quality, and equitable palliative care.

- Retains accountability for delegated care.

- Contributes to the evolution of the specialty of palliative nursing through participation in professional organizations.

- Influences local, regional, national, and international policies to promote health and access to quality palliative care.

- Influences decision-making bodies to improve the professional practice environment and outcomes for individuals with serious illness.

- Leads palliative care teams across settings to create new models of palliative care delivery.

Additional Competencies for the Graduate-Level Prepared Palliative Registered Nurse and the Palliative Advanced Practice Registered Nurse

The graduate-level prepared palliative registered nurse or the palliative APRN:

- Enhances the effectiveness of the palliative interdisciplinary team and outcomes through quality initiatives and research.

- Promotes advanced palliative practice nursing and role development by interpreting its role for the palliative interdisciplinary team, health colleagues, the public, and policymakers.

- Models expert advanced palliative nursing practice to the palliative interdisciplinary team, interprofessional colleagues, and other individuals.

- Mentors colleagues in the acquisition of clinical knowledge, skills, abilities, and management of individuals with serious illness.

Adapted from Dahlin.[2]

Although graduate nursing education contains leadership competencies, APRNs need further leadership skills. One option is to study leadership in an academic program with a focus on leadership. There are several master's programs focused on clinical leadership, nursing administration, and nurse executives. There are also clinical doctorate and research doctorate programs with a focus on leadership, including executive leadership, clinical leadership, and health system executive tracks. Other options include accelerated leadership programs specifically for nurses or business leadership programs for health professionals.

Huston identified essential competencies to prepare nurses for leadership (Box 4.4).[15] The aim is for nursing programs and healthcare organizations to integrate these competencies into their programs for developing future leaders. The focus on a global vision of nursing and systems thinking.

LEADERSHIP COMPETENCIES

The first step in developing nurse leaders is to have a set of core competencies for nurse leaders. The ANA is the primary resource and voice for the millions of nurses across the

Box 4.3 AMERICAN NURSES ASSOCIATION LEADERSHIP COMPETENCIES

- Collaboration

- Education

- Environmental health

- Ethics

- Evidence-based practice and research

- Leadership

- Professional practice evaluation

- Quality of practice

- Resource utilization

Adapted from American Nurses Association.[16]

country. It provides guidance and education in all areas of nursing practice, certification, accreditation, research, and advocacy. The ANA Leadership identified 10 competencies for nurse leaders based on the ANA Competency Model, which pulls together the *Nursing Scope and Standards of Practice*, the *Code of Ethics for Nursing*, and *Nursing's Social Policy* Statement (Box 4.3).[16] The model follows the ANA's *Model of Professional Practice*, which focuses on quality, safety, and evidence, with self-determination being the main focus of leadership. The ANA has developed a curriculum on leadership using evidence-based practice and a multidisciplinary approach to develop the nurse expert as they move into leadership roles.[16] The important message is that the nursing leader leads themselves, leads others, and leads organizations.

Core competencies in leadership have also been established by advanced practice nursing professional organizations. The National Association of Clinical Nurse Specialist (NACNS) produced *Systems Leadership Competency*, which states that the clinical nurse specialist (CNS) should "manage change and empower others to influence clinical practice and political processes both within and across systems."[17 (pp. 20)] Other leadership competencies for the CNS role include organization and systems leadership, healthcare business and finance, and professional development of healthcare team members, as well as continuing education, role-modeling, mentorship, coaching, and preceptorship.[17] The National Organization of Nurse Practitioner Faculty (NONPF) established leadership as part of its core competencies as well. The core competencies include initiating and guiding change, fostering collaboration with stakeholders, using critical and reflective thinking, advocating for better access and quality of care, advancing practice, expert communication, and participation in professional organizations.[18]

PALLIATIVE NURSING LEADERSHIP

The HPNA focuses on leadership within the specialty of palliative nursing. Advancing Expert Care, comprised of HPNA, the Hospice and Palliative Credentialing Center (HPCC), and the Hospice and Palliative Nurses Foundation (HPNF) published the *Palliative Nursing Leadership Position Statement*, which states that[19]:

- Palliative nursing leadership is transformative, leading to improved care of patients with advanced serious illnesses and influencing the values of care across all healthcare delivery settings.

- Palliative nursing leadership should be encouraged, developed, and recognized at all levels and in all aspects of palliative nursing, including clinical practice, management and administration, education, research, and policy.

- Palliative nursing leadership is advanced by palliative nurse involvement with national healthcare initiatives, collaboration with other nursing specialties, and engagement of other healthcare professionals to enhance quality palliative care.

The position statement supports transformational leadership within palliative nursing and has identified the skills of self-assessment, listening, feedback, orchestration of interprofessional care, and negotiation as valuable in building integrity is palliative nursing.[19] These skills are developed through education, collaborative practice, practice expertise, and self-awareness. The HPNA is training future nurses leaders within their Leadership Development program. The goal of the program "is to support nurses who wish to enhance their leadership skills, and to advance nurses into national leadership roles to serve as change agents to influence the future of palliative nursing practice and policies."[20]

The National Hospice and Palliative Care Organization (NHPCO) has a leadership and management conference to support leaders.[21] The Center to Advance Palliative Care (CAPC) has Palliative Care Leadership Centers (PCLCs) where new program leaders can work in an organization similar to their own to learn from expert leaders.[22] These PCLCs are a good resource for new programs and provide mentors to help nurses along the journey of program development.[22] The American Academy of Hospice and Palliative Medicine has a leadership development page with resources for new and experienced leaders.[23] These serve as resources to advance leadership skills for the APRN.

In summary, leadership education within graduate programs is often not enough to prepare the APRN to take on leadership roles. Therefore, the palliative APRN must pursue other resources to attain the competencies listed in (Box 4.4). The ANA, HPNA, and other palliative care organizations are prioritizing future palliative care leaders and offering further skill development through education, training, and resources such as position statements, competencies, and leadership mentorships.

PALLIATIVE APRN LEADERSHIP: FROM BEDSIDE TO BOARDROOM

The move from clinical practice to leadership is often fraught with challenges. Leadership positions in healthcare are often patriarchal, with male physicians occupying leadership roles. APRNs may be emotionally attached to their role as a "nurse" and find it difficult to move from a subordinate role into one of leadership.[24] Palliative APRNs need to shift their thinking to overcome this expectation and see leadership as part of their role as well. Palliative APRN leaders must seek opportunities to be on committees and boards for their organizations and professional associations. Through these experiences, they gain leadership skills and experience and have a place to practice these skills. These will serve them in their administrative roles.

One leadership challenge is maintaining a clinical practice while developing leadership skills and competencies. The APRN may not be given the nonacademic time to serve in these roles and may need to pursue education and leadership activities on their own time. Leadership activities may include participating in local and national organizations and serving on boards that allow them ways to expand their roles outside of their clinical practice.

Box 4.4 ESSENTIAL COMPETENCIES FOR APRN LEADERS

1. A global perspective or mindset regarding healthcare and professional nursing issues.

2. Technology skills that facilitate mobility and portability of relationships, interactions, and operational processes.

3. Expert decision-making skills rooted in empirical science.

4. The ability to create organization cultures that permeate quality healthcare and patient/worker safety.

5. Understanding and appropriately intervening in political processes.

6. Highly developed collaborative and team-building skills.

7. The ability to balance authenticity and performance expectations.

8. The ability to envision and proactively adapt to a healthcare system characterized by rapid change and chaos.

Adapted from Huston.[15]

Finding palliative APRN leader role models may be a challenge. Many healthcare organizations are physician-led. Therefore, it may be difficult to identify nurse role models and mentors to develop leadership competencies. It may be even more difficult to find mentors willing to support the APRN's move into an actual leadership position. Mentors may take many forms, from registered nurses to physician colleagues. According to Johnson, "Role models help create a positive work culture where all staff feel the impact of their efforts. They inspire trust, have a higher rate of job satisfaction, and help others to have the same."[25 (p. 289)] Role models from within the healthcare system and organizations are necessary to move palliative APRNs into roles outside clinical practices.[26]

Volunteering to serve on a board is a great place to start, but the first experience can be stressful. The ANA prioritized supporting nurses to sit on board by establishing the *Nurses on Boards Coalition*. This coalition offers both help in identifying boards that are looking for nurses and resources to encourage nurses to ensure their voices are heard.[27] Professional organizations, local chapters, organizational committees, and other committees provide opportunities for palliative APRNs to be part of a board.

A visible form of leadership occurs at organizational and department meetings. Meetings are essential vehicle to provide and glean information and keep a team together. Efficient and effective meetings are important for moral and action. Leading meetings is skill that many healthcare clinicians learn by example, rather than in any of their education and training. Being a committee or board member provides experience and promotes confidence and skill at leading meetings. Key strategies to successful meetings will help the APRN leader be more effective (Box 4.5).[28]

LEADERSHIP IN CLINICAL SETTINGS

Since the 1990s, APRNs have been leaders in palliative care in both program development and clinical care. The leadership role varies with location of practice. At a systems level, the palliative APRN leader develops a shared vision "to change the status quo of current care delivery to patients with advanced illnesses in the areas of effectiveness, efficiency, and timeliness, achieved through evidence-based palliative nursing practices."[29 (pp. 4)] The palliative APRN needs to advocate for advancement into leadership positions. With all the resources available to lead, now is the time for APRNs to take this important step. Here are some questions to consider when seeking leadership roles.

Who are the advocates, partners, and cheerleaders of your program?

How can your program get the most visibility?

Is the palliative APRN embedded in oncology leading the palliative care initiative?

Have you been successful in palliative care screening and automatic referral within the hospitalist service?

All these potential questions can be answered through communication, education, and consistency, using what your team provides and in your working environment.

At the academic medical setting, APRNs may find themselves starting palliative care programs with a physician partner and then leading those programs as director. The APRN may develop and lead palliative care fellowship programs for both nursing and medicine. The palliative APRN is in a prime position to advocate for incorporating the appropriate palliative care curriculum into healthcare academic programs that have educational agreements with an academic center. They may develop and lead palliative care education initiatives for medical schools, schools of nursing, schools of social work, and spiritual care programs to name a few. This may include preceptorships, practicums, rotations, or orientation to the specialty.[2] The academic center also provides a robust opportunity to lead a truly interdisciplinary team and educate about palliative care.

Box 4.5 PLANNING A SUCCESSFUL MEETING

- The agenda should be well-planned and published in advance.

- The committee should ideally create a charter for itself so that its intent and link to the larger organization are clear.

- Ground rules should be established early on.

- Meetings should start and end on time.

- Each meeting should have a stated purpose.

- Participants should come to the committee with their assignments complete and ready to participate fully in the work of the group.

- Opposing viewpoints should be welcomed and respected.

- The group should remain focused.

- Meaningful reports should be generated summarizing the committee's work.

- Time spent in committee meetings and in the accomplishment of committee tasks should further the goals of the organization.

Adapted from Rundio et al.[28]

In community hospitals, the palliative APRN may be the only palliative care provider or may have a very small team. The palliative APRN leader will need to collaborate with all departments and work together to ensure quality care for patients and their families. Policy development and education will be a key role and a chance to foster collaboration. Additionally, the leadership role may expand beyond palliative care and include oversight of other smaller departments. Thus, there may be fewer people to do more work. Physician partners may only be part-time, resulting in the need to balance clinical work with a leadership role.

The community care setting is a growing area for palliative APRNs. Both clinical leadership and administrative leadership are essential for program development in office practices and clinics. This may include primary care practices and specialty clinics such as cancer care, heart failure clinics, and pulmonary clinics. The palliative APRN will need to use leadership skills to conduct a needs assessment and develop a strategic plan for program development and expansion. They will need clinical leadership to build relationships with providers and ensure expert communication with the care team, patient, and family.

In rural areas, the palliative APRN may have their own business because some states allow independent practice. The translates into the APRN being a clinical leader, an administrative leader of their practice, and a community leader in promoting an understanding of palliative care. The opportunity to be the "face of palliative care" necessitates APRN leadership skills of needs assessment, project management, and influence local and state policy.

With the aging of the population, long-term care is a growing place of leadership for palliative APRNs. Skilled facilities, such as chronic care/rehabilitation hospitals, skilled nursing facilities, long-term care, and assisted living facilities, provide opportunities to develop palliative care initiatives across the continuum of care. Several models highlight how APRNs

are leading the way in these settings. Insurers may offer the services of palliative APRNs to assess and manage patients with serious illness. A large inpatient service may expand its consultative services into long-term facilities. This may be a palliative APRN who rounds with facility staff, participates in care meetings, and establishes palliative care policies and standards for the facilities. Home health and hospice agencies may also employ APRNs to provide quality palliative care services within long-term care facilities.

LEADERSHIP THEORIES AND STYLE

Over the years, different leadership theories and styles have developed (Box 4.6). Having an understanding of one's style is critical to effective and compassionate leaderships. It is also important that a good leader adapt their style based on the climate of their team. During times of crisis, the leader may need to be authoritarian to get through disasters and emergencies. In a transition, the leader may need to be flexible. *Transactional leadership* is derived from the principles of social-exchange theory. Interactions between a leader and employee are meant to achieve balance.[30] *Transformational leadership* is a model that is often used by nurse leaders. The transformational leader inspires others to understand why change is necessary and to see the vision for the future.[30] Another type of leadership is *connective leadership*. Connective leadership depends on bringing employees together and uses collaboration, cooperation, collegiality, and coordination to lead. *Shared leadership* recognized the leaders in everyone, both formal and informal leaders. Shared governance and self-directed teams are examples of shared leadership.[31] Finally, there is the *servant leader*. The servant leader puts the needs of others before their own and inspires others to do the same.[31] *Adaptive leadership* has become important and was even more so during the COVID-19 pandemic, when teams had to be flexible to meet increasing challenges.

- Coaching: Focused on developing staff

- Visionary: Have a clear vision of where the program should be and how to get there

- Servant: Believe in people first

- Autocratic: The leader makes all the decisions on their own

- Laissez-faire: Hands-off leadership

- Bureaucratic: Based on rules

- Democratic: Decisions are shared

- Pacesetter: Very high standards and goals to get things done

- Transformational: Leaders inspire others to produce change

- Transactional: Punishments and incentives are used to motivate staff

Adapted from Campbell.[29]

Transformational leadership is an appropriate model in palliative care.[30] Palliative APRNs are inherently transformational leaders by nature, being able to translate vision into reality, utilize effective communication skills, sustain a commitment to others, and always think bigger. Transformational leaders are continuous learners themselves while supporting the role development of their team members. They create safe and supportive environments and, through their own development, serve as role models. The transformational leader encourages the team through empowerment to identify issues, set goals, and resolve problems as they arise.[30] These characteristics are common of well-functioning teams, and a team is the heart of palliative care. There are four domains in transformational leadership: idealized leadership, inspired motivation, intellectual stimulation, and individualized consideration.[30]

Communication is an essential aspect of leadership. There are three types of communication that leaders use in managing teams: upward, downward, and lateral or diagonal. *Upward communication* comes from your employees to the leader. *Downward communication* flows from the leader to the employees and is used to direct and inform them. Downward communication can appear authoritative and, depending on the content, may not be perceived as in the way that is meant. An example may be a staff meeting where the leader is giving organizational updates, or it could be having a difficult conversation with an employee. *Lateral* or *diagonal communication* may be used across groups and departments, often when there are projects or committees involving different departments. Lateral communication can also be a "give and take" conversation where the leader is at the same level as the employee. Being an expert communicator is a skill that all leaders must master, but it is especially true in palliative care.

Emotional intelligence also enhances leadership. There are four key competences to lead with good emotional

intelligence: self-awareness, self-management, social awareness, and relationship management.[31] *Self-awareness* includes understanding your own emotions and understanding your strengths and weaknesses. *Self-management* is about keeping your emotions in check and being transparent and positive in all you do. Empathy and organizational awareness fall under *social awareness*. The most important competence is *relationship management*. Competence in emotional intelligence is reflected in being a visionary and being able to influence others.

Traits that are necessary to be an effective leader are the ability to build relationships and develop trust, think critically, utilize effective communication skills, be accountable for actions, provide constructive feedback, perform self-assessment, and be skilled at conflict negotiations.[32] The true goal of the palliative APRN leader is to focus on ways to improve the quality of care for the seriously ill, which can be achieved by leading teams, motivating others, and changing behaviors to work collaboratively.[32]

THE PROGRAM LEADER IN PALLIATIVE CARE

To lead a quality palliative care program, the program should be focused on the National Consensus Project for Quality Palliative Care *Clinical Practice Guidelines for Quality Palliative Care* (NCP). The NCP *Clinical Practice Guidelines* Domain 1: Structure and Process focuses on the organizational framework of your program, including interdisciplinary team (IDT) composition and the delivery of care and services in your program.[33] The frequency and function of the IDT and ensuring that the IDT is properly trained and continues to learn encourages certification and continued competence. The APRN leader needs to ensure appropriate policies and procedures are in place based on the healthcare setting.

The APRN leader promotes effective communication across the continuum of care to continually assess and reassess communications to ensure quality care. Leading staff may be the most difficult task the leader has to face. All team members are unique, with unique needs and styles. An effective leader must embrace each person's unique abilities and what they contribute to the team.

TEAM HEALTH AND WELLNESS

Palliative care professionals meet patients and families with serious illness during difficult times. The work involves continual grief and loss and is difficult on the interdisciplinary team. The NCP *Clinical Practice Guidelines* Domains 1.7 and 1.8 are focused on caring for the IDT.[33] Well-being and health is a priority for all palliative care teams. Both the leader and the team are responsible for team wellness. Getting to know the team members will help one's understanding of what matter most to them in developing a team and individual wellness plan. This should be a part of the team's strategic plan, and the palliative leader must recognize the emotional impact that palliative care has on the team.

The Institute of Health Improvement (IHI) published a white paper, *A Framework for Improving Joy in Work*, to address clinician burnout. The white paper describes burnout as an epidemic, and this is especially true in the field of palliative care.[34] The IHI identifies four steps to help employees restore and foster joy in their work, with each step serving as a foundation for the next. Step One is to ask staff "What matters to you?,"[34] a frequent question that palliative care clinicians ask their patients. Step Two is that the APRN leader must then seek out barriers to employees finding joy in their work. Step Three takes place is on a systems level, in which there needs to be a commitment to joy at work at all levels in the organization. Finally, Step Four is the quality improvement process of testing approaches and evaluating outcomes of the approach that is chosen for organizational implementation.

The National Academy of Sciences, Engineering, and Medicine published *Taking Action Against Clinician Burnout* to promote professional well-being by highlighting clinician burnout, improving understanding of challenges to clinician well-being, and advancing evidence-based solutions to take better care of the caregiver.[35] The Academy recommends the following step-wise approach to promote well-being:

Goal 1: Create positive work environments.

Goal 2: Create positive learning environments.

Goal 3: Reduce administrative burdens.

Goal 4: Enable technology.

Goal 5: Provide support to clinicians and learners.

Goal 6: Invest in research.

The CAPC published *Strategies for Maximizing the Health/Function of Palliative Care Teams* to guide development processes to promote team health.[36] Maintaining a health team takes time and deliberate attention and is the responsibility of all team members. The leader needs to pay close attention to team health and address issues early on. The CAPC monograph provides resources that range from assessing team health to implementing interventions to get the team back on track. It is important for teams to take time together to debrief difficult cases and grieve the losses they face on a regular basis. Staff should be aware of staff support groups and employee assistance programs to help cope with the stress and emotions of their daily work. Chaplain partners can provide regular debriefings during IDT meetings and other self-care activities. Other considerations include regular meetings focused on self-care activities such as meditation, coloring, or journaling. Yearly IDT retreats, which take place outside of the office, are a great way to build teams and to get to know each other better.

The APRN leader should structure such programs in a way that allows for some flexibility with schedules and values employees' time off. Creating a wellness policy is a way to show that self-care is a priority. Have each team member create an individualized self-care plan and include it as part of their yearly development goals. A team lunch is a great opportunity to educate about self-care and provide time to complete care plans. When mid-year and annual reviews occur, be sure to ask how team members have been managing their self-care and if they are meeting the goals they set for themselves. They do not need to share their care plan, but discussion at review demonstrates its importance. Finally, be sure to ask if there is anything that you, as their leader, can do to help them reach their goals and then actually work out a plan to achieve that.

During the crisis levels of COVID-19 pandemic, palliative care teams faced role changes and increased patient volume. Increased volumes put teams at higher risk of compassion fatigue and burnout. Also unique to the pandemic was the new anxiety and stress of providers getting sick themselves and bringing infection home to their families and others.[37] Palliative care teams had to use innovative ways to stay in touch with other team members, other teams, patients, and families.

In summary, team wellness is an essential aspect of leadership. Compassionate leadership and organizational support are needed to ensure healthy teams. The key to a successful team lies in empowering your team to make decisions, stick to agreed-on consultation requirements to ensure consistency in the referral process, and be very clear on the rules of engagement. Role-modeling and ensuring team wellness ensures program sustainability.

STAFF RECRUITMENT AND RETENTION

Hiring new employees can be challenging in palliative care. Not everyone has the ability to work in palliative care. New hires are costly to orient, onboard and train, so hiring the wrong candidate can be financially draining. The APRN leader is looking for a team member who has the required skill set for palliative care and who is a good fit with the team culture. Consider internal candidates for positions to help decrease onboarding and training costs.

Recruitment is usually done through human resources departments. Resources to make the recruiting process successful include: advertisement and social media networking, conferences and trade shows, employee personal networks, healthcare industry contacts and professional organization, organization websites, and being listed as an employer of choice.[38] However, now more than ever, it is important to consider workforce diversity. Does your team diversity match the diversity of the patients you serve? If not, why, and what is your plan for recruiting diverse team members?

To be successful and transparent, including your team in the interview process is a proven strategy. It also demonstrates that their opinions are valued. The first step in the hiring process is ensuring a clear and concise job description. Is the position appropriate for new graduate nurses or are you looking for experienced nurses?

When interviewing candidates, be sure to ask about their 1- and 5-year plans. Where do they see themselves in 1 year? In 5 years? Does their answer fit in with the goals of your program? Ask about how they resolve conflict and for examples of a time when they had to advocate for a patient. A strong candidate will be able to negotiate patient goals with care teams. Also, be sure to ask why they want to be part of the team, and, if new to palliative care, why they are interested in the field now. The decision to hire a new graduate or experienced candidate must take into consideration the team's bandwidth for orientation and training resources as well as the practice environment. A new graduate may have more support within an inpatient team rather than in a community program.

Employee retention is vital to a successful program. As the leader, it is your responsibility to support employees so they can develop meaningful careers that they are proud of. Onboarding a new employees should include the mission and vision of the program and the broader organization, if appropriate. Performance expectations and goals need to be clearly identified for each employee. It is important to include employee developmental goals as well as performance goals. How the employee's performance is measured should be clearly identified upon hiring. Employee satisfaction is key to retention and healthy teams. Employee satisfaction can be defined as "the terminology used to describe whether employees are happy and content and fulfilling their desires and needs at work. . . . [It] is a factor in employee motivation, employee goal achievement, and positive employee morale in the workplace."[38] Heathsfield Important strategies for retaining employees are effective communication, workplace diversity, hiring of skilled employees, and having a training and development plan for employees.[38]

Frequent turnover is a sign of issues within the team. Turnover can negatively affect team morale and patient satisfaction, not to mention quality of care. The APRN leader must conduct a deep dive with team to determine the reasons for turnover. Given the diversity of teams, this can be especially challenging for the APRN palliative leader.[36]

GIVING FEEDBACK

Performance appraisals are a foundational aspect of leadership. The APRN leader should provide the employee with feedback on their performance and planning for future goals. Provide objective appraisals that focus on their positive performance for the year; this is not the time for addressing poor performance or behavior. There should be no surprises at an annual performance review, which means frequent updates and touchpoints with employees throughout the year.

While there are many models to assist with providing feedback, the Plus/Delta model is easy to remember and follow.[39] The Plus/Delta model is a well-known way of providing feedback in a constructive, positive way and is very useful in the palliative care setting. The Plus-Delta model is great for individual and team evaluations and feedback. The Plus looks at the positive aspects: what went well. The Delta identifies what could be done better, improved, or changed. It takes the

negative and turns it into an opportunity to learn about ways to improve.[39]

CONFLICT MANAGEMENT

Conflict management is also an essential aspect of leadership when addressing employee behaviors. Moreover, it requires the leader to be objective and nonjudgmental. When addressing a behavior that is not aligned with expectations, it is important to address the behavior not the person[40] (Figure 4.1). First, assess the situation and identify the behavior. Was it a policy breach? Was the employee aware that a policy exists? Was it a misconception or a personality conflict? Address the behavior clearly and concisely without judgment. The next step is to be clear about your expectation and how the behavior goes against that expectation. Then stop and listen to the employee's response. Determine if there is "will" or "skill" involved. If it is skill, then the solution may be a policy review or retraining. If it is "will," it may be more challenging and implies a personality issue which may not be easily resolved. It is important to stop once consequences are given and move on. End the conversation when compliance is reached. Again, clear and concise is key. Do not prolong the conversation. If progress is not being made, consult with human resource partners for further guidance.[40]

An example of inappropriate behavior occurs when the leader witnesses an employee using their cellphone on the floor when there is a clear policy prohibiting cellphone use. The leader approaches the employee and states "I saw you were on your cellphone on the nursing unit. We have a policy prohibiting cellphone use on the units. Were you aware of the policy?" If the employee states they were not aware of the policy, then you can direct them to the policy for clarification. If they are already aware of the policy but still used the cellphone, the response may be that if they continue to use the cellphone on the unit, they will be written up. Then the employee should respond with "OK" and "Thank you, I won't do it again," in which case you can move on. If they start with excuses and other comments, reiterate the consequences of cellphone use and end the conversation. If conflict continues, human resource involvement may be necessary.

There are many different types of conflict, and conflict is inevitable. The goal of conflict management is to maintain a sense of equilibrium. Not all conflict is bad, and it can be used to stimulate growth and coping behavior.[40] Conflict may be intrapersonal (within oneself), interpersonal (between the self and another person), intragroup (among members of a particular group), or intergroup (among members of two or more groups).[40] The goal of conflict resolution is to reach a "win-win" for both parties. Strategies for conflict resolution include focusing on goals, not personalities; meeting the needs of both parties equally, if at all possible; and building consensus. Common conflict resolution strategies include compromise, competing, cooperating, smoothing, avoiding, and collaborating.[40] *Compromising* is a positive solution while avoiding is a negative solution. Conflict will not be resolved if avoided. *Compromise, cooperating,* and *collaborating* will help resolve conflict and move forward.

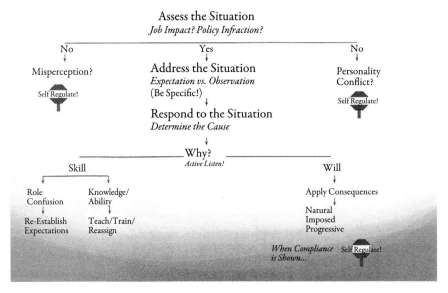

Assess the Situation
Job Impact? Policy Infraction?

No — Yes — No

Misperception? — **Address the Situation** — Personality Conflict?
Expectation vs. Observation
(Be Specific!)

Self Regulate! — **Respond to the Situation** — Self Regulate!
Determine the Cause

—————— Why? ——————
Active Listen!

Skill — Will

Role Confusion — Knowledge/Ability — Apply Consequences

Re-Establish Expectations — Teach/Train/Reassign — Natural Imposed Progressive

When Compliance is Shown... — Self Regulate!

Figure 4.1 Professional performance model.[40]

In summary, it is important to face conflict head on and not avoid it. Practicing the conversation before addressing it will help the leader be more prepared. Be concise and to the point. There is no need to drag on or entertain ongoing arguing by the employee. Use your human resources if the situation does not go as planned.

STRATEGIC PLANNING AND PROGRAM DEVELOPMENT FOR PALLIATIVE CARE NURSE LEADERS

The NCP *Clinical Practice Guidelines* Domain 1: Structure and Process has specific preferred practices to help guide strategic planning and program development (Box 4.7).[33] It is important to do a thorough needs assessment for the project and identify champions to lead and encourage buy-in to the project.

NEEDS ASSESSMENT

The first step in creating a strategic plan for program development is to conduct a thorough needs assessment. The needs assessment will help to focus areas of development and set goals and priorities. Currently available resources will be identified, and, when conducted correctly, the assessment will identify champions from the organization that will help push the plan forward. By interviewing stakeholders for their input, champions can be identified and a leadership team for the project can be created who will drive the strategic plan and program development.[42]

The CAPC has resources and tools to assist in completing a proper needs assessment.[42] An example of a tool can be found for both inpatient programs and community programs at www.CAPC.org. The community needs assessment identifies four steps to a thorough needs assessment: self-assessment, stakeholder input, data analysis, and conclusions and next steps.[42]

Box 4.7 NCP *CLINICAL PRACTICE GUIDELINES*

Domain 1-Structure and Processes 1.10

1.10.1   A community needs assessment is conducted to identify populations in need of palliative care, determine if demand and resources are sufficient to support a sustainable palliative care program model, design services specific to the target population(s), and identify partners.

1.10.2   Based on the needs assessment, a business plan with anticipated revenue and expenses is developed to ensure continuity of service to patients and families.

1.10.3   When launching a new program, key performance metrics are agreed on in advance to define when a program is meeting its goals.

1.10.4   The IDT develops strategic plans to prepare for changes in the target population and market forces, as well as other opportunities or threats that may affect the sustainability and growth of the program

Adapted from National Consensus Project for Quality Palliative Care.[33]

Once the needs assessment is complete, the leader can use those results to create a strategic plan. *Strategic planning* may include program development, expanding your current program, or starting an inpatient palliative care unit. The plan allows for the setting of long-term objectives, creating a timeline for activities, and setting priorities for the program.

An important step in creating a strategic plan is assessment of your current status. Determining the strengths, weaknesses, opportunities, and threats using a SWOT analysis model will help the leader stay focused. The *SWOT analysis* will help the leader determine what they are doing well, what needs to improve, what the opportunities are, and what the barriers or threats to the project will be.

Goal setting is the next step. What are the goals for the project? What is the vision? It is important to align the values of the project with the values of the bigger organization to ensure buy-in from other leaders within the organization. Prioritizing goals and determining which steps need to happen first will allow for a greater chance at success. A clear plan for evaluation of the project is important to keep the project on track. What are the measures of success and the overall outcome being sought? Establishing how the project will be evaluated is important from day one of the project.[42]

The next step is *program development*, and this is where the work really starts. The strategic plan is broken down even farther and specific tasks are assigned to the appropriate person in order to start moving the project forward. These tasks will include timelines, budgets, objectives, marketing, and data gathering. The CAPC has resources available to help the leader in palliative care be successful.[42]

TEAM BUILDING

The interdisciplinary team is the heart of palliative care. In a sentinel article by Tuckman, in 1965, he identified the five states of team development as forming, norming, storming, performing, and adjourning.[43] *Forming* occurs as team members get to know each other and learn how best to communicate. Roles and responsibilities are established, as well as group rules of engagement. In *norming*, the team begins to function together, and they find their normal place in the group. In the *storming* state, conflict arises and needs to be dealt with to ensure the team's performance is meeting expectations. *Performing* occurs when the team develops a rhythm and process to working collaboratively and effectively. *Adjourning* does not happen with long-term teams, but can be modified to apply when a member leaves the team. When a member of the team resigns, the other team members should take the opportunity to get feedback from their co-worker on what they did well and what could have been done differently. This is a good opportunity to practice using a feedback model.

CHANGE MANAGEMENT

Change is an inevitable aspect of life. It may be difficult or easy. APRN leaders are at the forefront of change in palliative care. Implementing palliative care services requires a culture shift from thinking of palliative care as hospice to its integration at the onset of a serious illness. Change for the palliative APRN leader can range from culture change, role change, and department change, to changes in team members and dynamics. The role of the palliative APRN leader in change can be difficult. The Kurt Lewin Change Model is well-known and laid the groundwork for other theories on change management.[44] Lewin's Change Model identifies three steps to change: unfreezing, movement, and refreezing.[44,45] The transformational leader model type is more conducive to change in that it is a collaborative model that ensures employee involvement in decision-making during the process. Transparency in the unfreezing phase of change is crucial and will increase trust and decrease resistance to the change. Involving employees in the "movement" phase is key to employee satisfaction. Checking in with them frequently and adjusting the process in real time will help with achieving, implementing, and "refreezing" the new process.[44,45]

QUALITY MANAGEMENT PLAN

As a leader in palliative care, it is important to develop a means of continually evaluating a program in meaningful ways and then analyzing that data to identify areas for improvement. The NCP *Clinical Practice Guidelines* Palliative Care Domain 1: Structure and Process identifies data analysis, and having a continuous quality improvement (CQI) initiative is essential in a quality palliative care program (Box 4.8).[33] It is the program leader's responsibility to pull this together and present the analyzed data in a constructive way. Utilize the IDT to determine where there is need for improvement and to establish the plan using CAPC data collection recommendations.[46]

The Joint Commission (TJC) Standards for Palliative Care Programs[47] currently include a pain screen within 24 hours, a comprehensive pain assessment, dyspnea screen, documentation of goals of care conversation, and a plan of care that can travel with patients across settings. These are solid measures for new palliative care programs.

The Palliative Care Quality Collaboration (PCQC) is a national database which allows programs to benchmark against other programs and can help with goal setting in your palliative care program.[48] Examples of some national measures are days from hospital admission to consult, length of stay on the palliative care program, and number of consults per hospital admissions. Utilizing the plan–do–check–act (PDCA) cycle assists with successful improvement in your processes.

RISK MANAGEMENT

Risk management is inherent in palliative care. Palliative care programs should have a way to address complaints. Inpatient issues that may arise include clarification of advance directive documents, conservatorship, medication errors, and other legal issues. In outpatient programs, common risk issues arise around opioid contracts and prescribing and compliance.

Box 4.8 NCP *CLINICAL PRACTICE GUIDELINES*

Domain 1-Structure and Processes 1.9

1.9.1 The program measures and improves quality by systematically collecting and analyzing data on care processes and outcomes specific to the patient population and organization's capacity, setting improvement targets, and planning and implementing change. This cycle is repeated in an iterative and ongoing fashion until it achieves sustained improvement.

1.9.2 The interdisciplinary team (IDT) considers the six domains of healthcare quality as defined in 2001 by the Institute of Medicine (safe, effective, patient-centered, timely, efficient and equitable) in the design of its continuous quality improvement (CQI) program.

1.9.3 The IDT identifies care coordination measures and integrates these into CQI initiatives.

1.9.4 To the extent possible, the IDT uses assessment instruments, quality measures, and experience of care surveys that are validated, clinically relevant, and cross-cutting across settings or populations.

1.9.5 Patients, families, clinicians, and other partners participate in the evaluation of the IDT.

1.9.6 The IDT participates in quality reporting and accountability programs, as required or necessary to maintain licensure or accreditation

Adapted from National Consensus Project for Quality Palliative Care.[33]

Inpatient programs may utilize their organizational risk management departments to help clarify legal issues that may arise. Community programs face some of the same issues as well as new ones, such as patient safety in the home setting, caregiver strain, and compliance with medication regimens. Opioid contracting is especially important due to increased risk of diversion in the community setting. Long-term care (LTC) facilities may have their own risk management programs. Some of the issues faced in LTC may include dietary requirements, difficulty negotiating appropriate patient-centered care plans, issues with reaching family members or conservators, and following through with end-of-life care plans. It is important to understand the risks and advocate for patients who otherwise may not have a voice.

The risk management department is very helpful in ensuring proper documentation when patients are not following the contract. These patients may need to discontinue opioids or even be discharged from the practice while maintaining the providers' obligation to the patient. Risk management can help with policy creation and keep you up to date on laws in your state. It is important to develop a relationship with your risk management department to maintain compliance and ensure that you and your team are practicing within the laws of your state. Ethics committees and consults can also be helpful in resolving conflicts that involve patient safety, autonomy, and social justice.

COMPLIANCE WITH CERTIFYING AGENCIES

There are a few different means to reaching the specialty palliative care program designation. All organizations offering this designation recognize excellence in palliative care services and validate compliance with NCP guidelines, CQI, and that the program provides family-centered care. TJC is a global leader for healthcare accreditation and offers disease-specific certifications. Their designation offers Palliative Care Certification for hospital and community programs under home health and hospice.[47] The Community Health Accreditation Partners (CHAP) offers specially palliative care certification to community programs. Valid for 3 years, CHAP is progressive in offering the designation to palliative care programs at physician offices, assisted living facilities, skilled nursing facilities, and home health agencies as well as to independent providers of palliative care.[49] The Accreditation Commission for Health Care (ACHC) has a distinction for home health agencies and private duty agencies for palliative care that are focused on family-centered care and quality of life throughout the continuum of care and that address all realms of the patient and family based on the NCP guidelines.[50] They are developing a certification program as well. DNV is a certifying body for inpatient programs and recognizes excellence in palliative care treatment and delivery.[51] Its requirements provide a "framework that assists organizations in the development and implementation of processes and systems which improve operational effectiveness and enhance positive health outcomes to improve the palliative care patient's quality of life."[51]

SUMMARY

With the changing landscape of healthcare, palliative APRNs are leading programs across settings and populations.[52] The expertise and experience of palliative APRNs provides them with the foundation of a compassionate and effective leader to lead and develop interprofessional team members.[52,33] There are resources to help palliative APRNs expand their knowledge and skills as leaders, allowing them to use knowledge and expertise to move the field of palliative care forward in new and innovative ways (Box 4.9). Palliative APRNs should embrace stepping outside their comfort zone of clinical work and bravely take on roles in leadership.

Box 4.9 PALLIATIVE NURSING LEADERSHIP RESOURCES

Nursing Organizations

- American Association of Colleges of Nursing

  o Leadership Development
    https://www.aacnnursing.org/Resources-for-Deans/Leadership-Development

- American Association of Critical Care Nurses—Leadership resources

- American Nurses Association

  o Nursing Leadership and Excellence

    https://www.nursingworld.org/continuing-education/ce-subcategories/leadership/

  o ANA Leadership Institute Competency Model

    https://www.nursingworld.org/~4a0a2e/globalassets/docs/ce/177626-ana-leadership-booklet-new-final.pdf

- American Organization for Nursing Leadership

- National League for Nursing—Leadership Institute

  o Nursing Leadership Network – NLN Leadership Institute – LEAD and SIMULATION

    http://www.nln.org/professional-development-programs/leadership-programs

- Hospice and Palliative Nurses Association—Leadership Resources

- Oncology Nursing Society—Leadership Competencies

- Sigma Theta Tau

  o Nurse Leadership Academy for Practice

    https://www.sigmanursing.org/learn-grow/sigma-academies/nurse-leadership-academy-for-practice

  o New Academic Leadership Academy

    https://www.sigmanursing.org/learn-grow/sigma-academies/new-academic-leadership-academy

  o Experienced Academic Leadership Academy

    https://www.sigmanursing.org/learn-grow/sigma-academies/experienced-academic-leadership-academy

- Foundation Supported Toolkits

  o AARP Foundation and Robert Wood Johnson Foundation

    - Campaign for Action: Promoting Nursing Leadership Tool Kit

      http://campaignforaction.org/resources/#p=1

    - Wisconsin Center for Nursing–A Leadership Toolkit: Leadership Resources for Nurses

      https://campaignforaction.org/wp-content/uploads/2015/08/Leadership-Toolkit-WI.pdf

- National Palliative Care Organizations

  o Center to Advance Palliative Care—Leadership Skills

  o National Hospice and Palliative Care Organization

Academic Programs for Leadership Development

- Executive Leadership Certificate Programs

  o Wharton School of Business–Nurse Leaders Program

  o Cornell–Healthcare Leadership

  o Duke University–Nursing and Health Care Leadership

(continued)

Box 4.9 Continued

- Schools of Nursing

  o MSN in Nursing Leadership and Administration

- Duke University–Nursing and Health Care Leadership

- George Washington University–MSN Nursing Leadership and Management

  o Certificate Programs

- Duke CE–Nursing leadership

- Drexel–Nursing Leadership in Health Systems

- Seton Hall–Health Care Administration

- Stoneybrook–MSN Nursing Leadership

REFERENCES

1. American Nurses Association. *Nursing: Scope and Standards of Practice*. 3rd ed. Silver Springs, MD: American Nurses Association; 2015.
2. Dahlin C. *Palliative Nursing: Scope and Standards of Practice*. 6th ed. Pittsburgh, PA: Hospice and Palliative Nurses Association; 2021.
3. Institute of Medicine. *The Future of Nursing: Leading Change, Advancing Health*. Washington, DC: National Academies Press; 2010. https://www.nap.edu/read/12956/chapter/1
4. American Nurses Association and Hospice and Palliative Nurses Association. Call for action: Nurses lead and transform palliative care. Silver Spring, MD: ANA. March 13, 2017. https://www.nursingworld.org/~497158/globalassets/practiceandpolicy/healthpolicy/palliativecareprofessionalissuespanelcallforaction.pdf
5. American Association of Colleges of Nursing. The Essentials: Core competencies for professional nursing education. April 7, 2021. Washington, DC: AACN. https://www.aacnnursing.org/Portals/42/AcademicNursing/pdf/Essentials-Final-Draft-2-18-21.pdf
6. American Association of Colleges of Nursing. The essentials of master's education in nursing. 2011. Washington, DC: AACN. https://www.aacnnursing.org/portals/42/publications/mastersessentials11.pdf
7. American Association of Colleges of Nursing. Essentials of doctoral education for advanced nursing practice. 2006. Washington, DC: AACN. https://www.aacnnursing.org/DNP/DNP-Essentials
8. US News and World Report. Education. 2021 best nursing schools: Master's. https://www.usnews.com/best-graduate-schools/top-nursing-schools/nur-rankings
9. US New and World Report. 2021 Education. best nursing schools: Doctorate of nursing. https://www.usnews.com/best-graduate-schools/top-nursing-schools/dnp-rankings
10. The Ohio State University College of Nursing. Psychiatric mental health nurse practitioner. 2021. https://nursing.osu.edu/academics/graduate-specializations/psychiatric-mental-health-nurse-practitioner
11. University of California at San Francisco. Family nurse practitioner curriculum. July 15, 2019. https://nursing.ucsf.edu/sites/nursing.ucsf.edu/files/inline-files/SampleMSFNPCurriculum_7-15-19.pdf
12. Duke School of Nursing. MSN curriculum requirements AGNP acute care. August 28, 2014. https://nursing.duke.edu/sites/default/files/documents/etc/duson_msn_curriculum_requirements_agnp_acute_care.pdf
13. University of North Carolina School of Nursing. AGPCNP suggested plan of study UNC School of Nursing. 2021. https://nursing.unc.edu/academic-programs/msn/advanced-practice-areas/agpcnp-suggested-plan-of-study/
14. Vanderbilt School of Nursing. Curriculum adult-gerontology acute care nurse practitioner (AGACNP) MSN. 2020. https://nursing.vanderbilt.edu/msn/agacnp/agacnp_curriculum.php
15. Huston C. Preparing nurse leaders for 2020. *J Nurs Manag.* 2008;16(8):905–911. doi:10.1111/j.1365-2834.2008.00942.x
16. American Nurses Association. Nursing leadership and excellence: competency model 2018. 2018. https://www.nursingworld.org/~4a0a2e/globalassets/docs/ce/177626-ana-leadership-booklet-new-final.pdf
17. National Association of Clinical Nurse Specialists. Statement on CNS practice and education 3rd ed. 2019. https://nacns.org/professional-resources/practice-and-cns-role/cns-competencies/
18. National Organization of Nurse Practitioner Faculty. Nurse practitioner core competencies content: A delineation of suggested content specific to the NP core competencies 2017. NP Core Competencies Content Work Group. 2017. https://cdn.ymaws.com/www.nonpf.org/resource/resmgr/competencies/2017_NPCoreComps_with_Curric.pdf
19. The Hospice and Palliative Nurses Association. Position statement: Palliative nursing leadership. October 2014. https://advancingexpertcare.org/position-statements
20. The Hospice and Palliative Nurses Association. HPNA Year of Leadership. 2021. https://advancingexpertcare.org/HPNAweb/Education/Year_of_Leadership.aspx
21. National Hospice and Palliative Care Organization. Conferences. 2020. https://www.nhpco.org/education/nhpco-conferences
22. Center to Advance Palliative Care. Palliative care leadership centers. Locations and Training Dates. 2021. https://www.capc.org/palliative-care-leadership-centers/palliative-care-training-locations/
23. American Academy of Hospice and Palliative Medicine. Leadership development. 2021. http://aahpm.org/career/leadership
24. Anderson C. Exploring the role of advanced nurse practitioners in leadership. *Nurs Stand.* 2018;33(2):29–33. doi:10.7748/ns.2018.e11044
25. Johnson JA. Nursing professional development specialists as role models. *J Nurses Prof Dev.* 2015;31(5):297–299. doi:10.1097/NND.0000000000000202
26. Elliott N, Begley C, Sheaf G, Higgins A. Barriers and enablers to advanced practitioners' ability to enact their leadership role: A scoping review. *Int J Nurs Stud.* 2016;60(2016):24–45. doi:10.1016/j.ijnurstu.2016.03.001
27. Nurses on Boards Coalition. About our story. 2021. https://www.nursesonboardscoalition.org/about/
28. Rundio A, Wilson, V Meloy F. *Nurse Executive.* 3rd ed. Silver Springs, MD: ANA Enterprise; 2016.
29. Campbell M. 10 Proven types of leadership styles: What's the one for you. October 13, 2019. https://www.growthtactics.net/10-common-types-of-leadership-styles/

30. Pearson MM. Transformational leadership principles and tactics for the nurse executive to shift nursing culture. *J Nurs Adm.* 2020;50(3):142–151. doi:10.1097/NNA.0000000000000858

31. Goleman D, Boyatzis R, McKee A. *Primal Leadership: Learning to Lead with Emotional Intelligence.* Boston: Harvard Business School Press; 2002: 39.

32. Dahlin C, Coyne P, Goldberg J, Vaughan L. Palliative care leadership. *J Palliat Care.* 2019;34(1):21–28. doi:10.1177/0825859718791427

33. National Consensus Project for Quality Palliative Care. *Clinical Practice Guidelines for Quality Palliative Care.* 4th ed. Richmond, VA; National Coalition for Hospice and Palliative Care; 2018. https://www.nationalcoalitionhpc.org/ncp/

34. Institute for Healthcare Improvement; Perlo J, Balik B, Swensen S, Kabcenell A, Landsman J, Feeley D. *IHI Framework for Improving Joy in Work.* IHI White Paper. Cambridge, MA: Institute for Healthcare Improvement; 2017. http://www.ihi.org/resources/Pages/IHIWhitePapers/Framework-Improving-Joy-in-Work.aspx

35. National Academies of Sciences, Engineering, and Medicine. *Taking Action Against Clinician Burnout: A Systems Approach to Professional Well-Being.* Washington, DC: National Academies Press; 2019. https://doi.org/10.17226/25521

36. Atillio T, Dahlin C, Remke, S, Tucker R, Weissman D. Strategies for maximizing the health/function of palliative care teams. Center to Advance Palliative Care. 2016. https://www.capc.org/training/improving-team-performance/

37. Mills J, Ramachenderan J, Chapman M, Greenland R, Agar M. Prioritizing workforce wellbeing and resilience: What COVID-19 is reminding us about self-care and staff support. *Palliat Med.* 2020;34(9):1137–1139. doi:10.1177/0269216320947966

38. Heathfield SM. Employee satisfaction: Make employees satisfaction surveys successful. The Balance Careers. Updated October 31, 2020. https://www.thebalance.com/employee-satisfaction-1918014

39. Helminski L, Koberna S. Total quality in instruction: A systems approach. In: Roberts HV, ed. *Academic Initiatives in Total Quality for Higher Education.* Milwaukee, WI: ASQC Quality Press; 1995: 322.

40. Albright RR. Professional performance model. Presented at Nuvance Health Leadership seminar. October 18, 2019. Danbury, CT.

41. Center to Advance Palliative Care. Designing a hospital inpatient palliative care program. June 22, 2020. https://www.capc.org/toolkits/starting-the-program/designing-an-inpatient-palliative-care-program/

42. Center to Advance Palliative Care. Needs assessment: Ensuring successful community-based palliative care. 2015. https://www.capc.org/operational-courses/community-palliative-care-program-design/needs-assessment-ensuring-successful-community-based-palliative-care/

43. Tuckman BW. Developmental sequence in small groups. *Psych Bull.* 1965;63(6):384–399. doi:10.1037/h0022100.

44. Lewin K. *Field Theory in Social Science.* New York: Harper & Row; 1947.

45. Hussain ST, Lei S, Akram T, Haider MJ, Hussain SH, Ali M. Kurt Lewin's change model: A critical review of the role of leadership and employee involvement in organizational change. *J Innov Knowl.* 2018;3(3):123–127. doi:10.1016/j.jik.2016.07.002

46. CAPC. Recommended Program Measures and CAPC Measurement Toolkit. CAPC.org. Last updated June 22, 2020. https://www.capc.org/toolkits/measurement-best-practices/

47. The Joint Commission. Palliative care certification. 2021. https://www.jointcommission.org/accreditation-and-certification/certification/certifications-by-setting/hospital-certifications/palliative-care-certification/

48. Palliative Care Quality Collaborative. Home page. 2021. https://www.palliativequality.org/

49. Community Health Accreditation Partners. Palliative care certification. 2019. https://chapinc.org/palliative-certification/

50. Accreditation Commission for Health Care. Home health distinction in palliative care. 2017. https://cc.achc.org

51. DNV Healthcare. DNV GL Healthcare's palliative care program certification. 2018. https://www.dnvgl.us/assurance/healthcare/PalliativeCare.html

52. Dahlin C, Coyne P. The palliative APRN leader. *Ann Palliat Med.* 2019;8(Suppl 1):S30–S38. doi:10.21037/apm.2018.06.03

5.

THE PALLIATIVE APRN IN NURSING EDUCATION

Carrie L. Cormack and Kathleen O. Lindell

KEY POINTS

- Palliative advanced practice registered nurses (APRNs) have the expertise and background to lead and implement palliative nursing education across all levels to meet the current needs of individuals with serious illness and facing end of life.

- Primary palliative care skills and knowledge are essential for all nurses at any level to help meet the needs of the increasing acuity and complexity of healthcare.

- The American Association of Colleges of Nursing (AACN) and End of Life Nursing Education Consortium (ELNEC) primary palliative care competencies provide a framework for undergraduate and graduate nursing programs to prepare students to care for individuals with serious illness and their families.

- Specialty graduate palliative care programs are necessary to help meet the urgent need for providers with advanced specialty skills in palliative care.

- Competencies for the hospice and palliative APRN guide the education of specialty advanced palliative nursing practice.

---

the critical knowledge required to provide primary palliative care in their chosen healthcare settings and positively impact the lives of patients and families facing serious illness and end of life.

In addition to preparing all students in primary palliative care, the palliative care faculty developed and launched a post-MSN-to-DNP in palliative care track specialty designed specifically for the working APRN interested in gaining deeper experience and focus on the needs of individuals with serious illness and their families. This was achieved with the assistance of an outside palliative APRN consultant to assist with the development and implementation of curriculum changes as well as the design of the new program. The current level of faculty expertise in palliative care was assessed by the consultant, and a faculty workshop for training in the new program was offered. Under the APRN leadership, all faculty at the college of nursing are now required to complete mandatory End of Life Nursing Education Consortium (ELNEC) training in addition to participation in palliative care workshops and conferences. Due to Caroline's initiative and the comprehensive approach to support specialty APRN faculty, the college has led the integration of palliative care across academic nursing programs, promoted specialty practice, and contributed to the needs of the workforce.

CASE STUDY: THE PALLIATIVE APRN EDUCATOR

Advanced practice registered nurses (APRNs) play an important role in the delivery of palliative care and palliative care education. Caroline is a Doctor of Nursing Practice (DNP) faculty member at a prominent college of nursing. She has worked with the dean and other members of the leadership team to ensure a commitment to prioritize palliative care across all educational programs, in practice, scholarship, and research, with the downstream effect being promoting and improving quality of life for individuals with serious illness and their families. The college supported both the education and training of specialty palliative APRN faculty as well as their sitting for the specialty palliative care certification examination. These specialty palliative APRNs have led significant curriculum changes, including the incorporation of primary palliative care across all programs (registered nurse-bachelor of science in nursing [RN-BSN], accelerated bachelor of science in nursing [ABSN], master of science in nursing [MSN]/DNP, and doctoral degrees [doctor of philosophy PhD, doctor of nursing science [DNS]]). By doing this they ensure that all nursing students graduating from the nursing programs are equipped with

---

INTRODUCTION

The National Hospice and Palliative Care Organization (NHPCO) defines palliative care as "patient and family-centered care that optimizes quality of life by anticipating, preventing, and treating suffering. Palliative care throughout the continuum of illness involves addressing physical, intellectual, emotional, social, and spiritual needs and to facilitate patient autonomy, access to information, and choice."[1]

Palliative advanced practice registered nurses (APRNs) fill an important gap in access to evidence-based, high-quality care. With a background to provide holistic, person-centered care and advocate and seek patient goals of care,[2,3] care provided by an APRN correlates perfectly with palliative care.[4] APRNs have emerged as leaders in palliative care over the past several years. Leadership from APRNs in palliative care includes the domains of clinical care, advocacy and policy, research, administration and management, and education.[5] The APRN as educator has a significant role in shaping the future generation of APRNs and specialty practice APRNs. These APRN educators must use their expertise to facilitate education in primary and specialty palliative skills and clinical practice, and they must use leadership skills to shape change in nursing curriculum within schools of nursing. They may also shape change in nursing professional development with educational and clinical programs.

Nursing programs, especially those led by palliative APRNs as educators, must step up to the task of promoting palliative care education for both generalist and specialty nursing care. In order for nursing to remain at the forefront of this important work, palliative APRN educators must lead the way to properly prepare nurse graduates at all levels of education, within both academic and preparatory programs, to provide high-quality care to individuals with serious illness and their families.

Chapters 1 and 2 of this textbook discuss other aspects of the APRN role in education, including serving as mentors to other nurses and interprofessional colleagues and participating in palliative care research. This chapter focuses on the roles and opportunities for the palliative APRN in education, specifically for those teaching palliative care content and leading program development and implementation.

PALLIATIVE APRN EDUCATION

FACULTY

The Institute of Medicine's 2014 report, *Dying in America*, expressed the need for more professional palliative care education.[6] This includes both primary palliative care and specialty palliative care. For nursing programs seeking to follow these recommendations, acquiring nursing faculty who are practicing at a high level of expertise in palliative care is essential.

APRNs with experience and expertise in palliative care are in a desirable position to serve as faculty and teach palliative care content across all levels of nursing students. This includes associate's, bachelor's, master's, and doctoral programs.

In addition to having palliative care experience and training, there are several considerations APRNs should make when seeking to transition from bedside patient care to academia. It is important for APRNs to thoroughly research the expectations of the academic institution, including education requirements and expectations,[7] well in advance of this transition. Taking time to fully consider the role change and its impact may help ease any strain associated with this change. Seeking and establishing a formal mentor in the process can also be helpful. APRNs with specialty palliative certification or advanced certification in hospice and palliative nursing (ACHPNs) are especially fit for a faculty role because certification is evidence of expertise in the area of palliative and hospice care. Palliative nursing certification is achieved through the Hospice and Palliative Credentialing Center (HPCC)[8] (see Chapter 3).

Palliative APRNs are well-situated to articulate the current needs of patients facing serious illness and end of life and to identify areas on which nursing education should focus.[9] Palliative APRN nursing faculty are in a unique position to fill this gap and improve the quality of life for patients and families by educating students in palliative care.[10] Furthermore, palliative APRN faculty have the expertise and background to lead and implement curriculum and program changes while addressing potential barriers and overall impact.

PRIMARY PALLIATIVE NURSING EDUCATION

In 2017, the *Call to Action: Nurses Lead & Transform Palliative Care*, a collaboration between by the American Nurses Association (ANA) and the Hospice and Palliative Nurses Association (HPNA), was published.[11] This document includes recommendations for *all* nurses caring for patients with serious illness and their families to be prepared in primary palliative care. This foundational palliative care knowledge and skills are the care provided by non-palliative care specialty nurses to patients with serious or life-threatening illness.[12,13]

Primary palliative nursing education involves teaching skills such as common pain and symptom assessment and management and role modeling communication techniques such as goals of care, advance directives, and providing information about resources available to patients and families in need.[13] Because of the increasing acuity and complexity of patient care, providing this education is urgent and necessary across all levels of nursing programs. At time of graduation, new graduates should be expected to be competent in caring for patients who are seriously ill and their families, which further emphasizes the need for this content to be embedded into nursing programs.[10]

COMPETENCIES

To provide a framework for APRN nursing faculty to teach primary palliative care content, the AACN partnered with the ELNEC and released undergraduate and graduate primary palliative care competencies.[14,15] By embedding these competencies into nursing programs, APRN faculty will ensure that students are prepared to provide high-quality care for individuals with serious illness and their families from time of diagnosis through the trajectory of a disease or illness. These competencies give faculty a road map and establish goals as they plan and develop the palliative care content.

For undergraduate programs, the document *CARES: Competencies and Recommendations for Educating Undergraduate Nursing Students: Preparing Nurses to Care for the Seriously Ill and Their Families*[10,14] outlines the 17 competencies that all undergraduate nursing students should achieve by the time of graduation. The document reiterates the importance of each competency and provides recommendations for how to incorporate them into nursing courses and explanations of how they align with the AACN *Essentials of Baccalaureate Education*,[16] which is essential for accreditation purposes.[10]

At the graduate level, palliative nursing faculty also have primary palliative care competencies to help guide this work. *Graduate Competencies and Recommendations for Educating Nursing Students* (G-CARES)[15] was developed on the foundation of the CARES[14] document for master's and DNP nursing students. These competencies prepare graduates to "lead clinical practice, healthcare systems, quality improvement, and academic changes needed to advance the access of primary palliative care to all patients with serious illness."[15(p. 4)] Graduate-level competencies are further broken down into two categories, one for all graduate nursing students and the other for those who will be providing direct primary palliative care to patients and families. Because the undergraduate competencies are aligned with the nursing essentials, the graduate competencies are also aligned with the *AACN Master's Essentials* and *DNP Essentials*.[15] These competencies, at both the undergraduate and graduate levels, have marked a significant change in the way palliative care is taught in nursing programs.[10]

In addition to the previously mentioned *Essentials* aligned with baccalaureate, master's, and DNP education,[15,16] in April 2021, the AACN released, *The Essentials: Core Competencies for Professional Education*, to provide a framework for nursing across the discipline.[17] This document introduces 10 domains and competencies that highlight the uniqueness of the nursing profession. The AACN has recognized that one of the competencies across the 10 domains is the importance of hospice, palliative, and supportive care and has listed this as one of the areas of focus. This document will support APRN nursing faculty to teach palliative care content and expanding programs in this area and will assist faculty with "bridge(ing) the gap between education and practice."[17(p. 1)] The concepts of compassionate care and ethics are woven throughout, highlighting the importance of these essential aspects of nursing practice.

INTEGRATING PRIMARY PALLIATIVE CARE INTO NURSING CURRICULUMS

APRN faculty should utilize available resources for embedding primary palliative care into existing programs. The CARES[14] and G-CARES[15] documents have appendices that specifically outline for faculty how the competencies are linked to palliative care content.[10,15] Relying on these tools ensures that the approach is standardized for all students. Once the competencies are established, there are several options for offering palliative care content. Consideration must be given to the flexibility of the whole nursing curriculum and whether there is space for new content. The integration of content into the curricula may be achieved by two approaches. Specific courses in palliative care may be developed anew and implemented, or palliative care content may be embedded into existing courses.

Determining how palliative care content will be integrated into programs must be carefully considered by APRN faculty and nursing program leaders. One option is to offer a separate course or unit in palliative care, which may be offered to all students or as an elective. This is appealing for nursing students with a passion for palliative care or seeking to enhance their current knowledge of and preparedness for caring for patients with serious illness. The second option for programs is to take a more integrated approach to embed palliative care

content throughout the existing curriculum. Implementing this approach to learning has allowed for palliative care concepts to be introduced, reiterated, and reinforced continually until the desired competencies are attained.[18] Either approach should include both didactic and clinical opportunities when possible.[19]

In an effort to support faculty to teach palliative care content, ELNEC[20] has developed online curriculums in primary palliative care specifically for nursing students. Utilizing these curriculums are one option for nursing faculty seeking to integrate this content. The content of these curricula is based on the ELNEC-Core curriculum, originally released in 2001, which was developed to guide palliative care education for nurses.[21] These online curricula specifically meet the undergraduate and graduate competencies for primary palliative nursing and include recommendations for achieving these competencies.[14,15] A benefit for faculty using this program is that there is no need to create similar type modules or courses for their students. Offered through Relias Learning Academy,[22] access to the curricula may be purchased individually at a minimal fee per student or in a bundle by nursing programs. Each curriculum is comprised of six modules, each designed to take students approximately 1–1.5 hours to complete. Included within each module are learning activity sessions, case studies, video vignettes, and certification board–like type questions.[10,15]

The format of incorporating these online ELNEC curricula into existing programs should be individualized based on nursing program structure. As noted earlier, this content may be embedded into existing courses within a program or offered as separate electives. Faculty options for offering the online ELNEC curriculum modules include

- *Option 1*: Offer the online modules as stand-alone, self-paced assignments, where students are given a final due date for completion. This format gives students the autonomy to work at their own pace and can be ideal, especially for the adult learner or within an online program. This is also a likely more practical method for the graduate student who may be more accustomed to self-study exercises as well as the sensitive content explored in the palliative care modules.
- Table 5.1 is an example of the ELNEC Graduate Modules offered in an accredited online DNP program. Within this example, the ELNEC Modules are offered during the last semesters of the DNP program (semesters 5/6) during the residency course. This placement was a deliberate faculty decision due to the higher level of thinking and decision-making required for some palliative care concepts. Students nearer to graduation have completed four semesters of clinical experience and are functioning at the level of a master's-prepared nurse. A lecture is given to all DNP students by a palliative APRN in the semester prior to opening the modules; this lecture reviews the foundations of palliative care as well as some advanced techniques in primary palliative care appropriate for APRN-level learning.

Table 5.1 EXAMPLE OF PRIMARY CARE PALLIATIVE EDUCATION EMBEDDED INTO A DOCTOR OF NURSING PRACTICE (DNP) PROGRAM

DNP COURSE	ELNEC GRADUATE MODULE	SUPPLEMENTAL ACTIVITIES
Semester 4		
Advanced Care Management 2 (clinical course #2)	—	Guest lecturer/content expert "Advanced Palliative Care Techniques" including Loss and Bereavement exercise,[23] case studies, and video vignettes
Semester 5		
Residency I	Module 1: Introduction to Palliative Care Module 2: Communication in Palliative Care Module 3: Pain Management in Palliative Care	Ongoing consultation available by lead palliative care faculty Specialty clinical opportunities available
Semester 6 (Final Semester in Program)		
Residency II	Module 4: Symptom Management in Palliative Care Module 5: Final Hours of Life Module 6: APN Leadership in Serious Illness	Ongoing consultation available by lead palliative care faculty Specialty clinical opportunities available

- *Option 2*: The modules can be offered in more traditional face-to-face learning platforms, in-person or virtually, where an instructor uses PowerPoint presentations to teach each module to a group of students. While this may be more time-consuming, it allows students the opportunity to digest and reflect on the content, interact, ask questions, and collaborate with faculty and other experts in real time. Palliative care content can be emotionally challenging for some students. Having an opportunity to debrief with faculty and others may be beneficial.[23,24,25]

- *Option 3*: Faculty may choose to offer these modules in a hybrid platform. This may include assigning a module to be completed independently and follow-up with interactive group discussion. The format of this session varies from Q&A opportunities, expert guest lectures, interactive group discussions, activities such as grief and bereavement exercises, and case studies.

  See Table 5.2 for an example of this hybrid approach where the ELNEC Undergraduate Curriculum is embedded into an existing ABSN degree program along with supplemental activities following the completion of each module. Credit is given toward each semester grade for completion of each module.

- *Option 4*: The ELNEC modules may be offered as an in-person ELNEC course, held over 1–2 days, that student may take on their own timeline but that is required for graduation. This could include core, geriatric, pediatric APRN or critical care and may be offered independently within a school of nursing or in collaboration with a healthcare organization. The challenge is that many students may wait to do this at the end of their education and regret that they did not have the information earlier.

Having the options and flexibility of palliative care integration gives faculty autonomy with the program structure and design and supports the unique needs of each individual nursing program. For both undergraduate and graduate students, a certificate of completion of ELNEC training is available at the end of the program for students' curriculum vitae and portfolio to demonstrate this training to future employers.

Programs that choose not to utilize the online ELNEC Undergraduate and Graduate Curricula, should still access and use the faculty resources available through AACN ELNEC resources, including curriculum guidelines, modules, and a section designated for professional development (https://www.aacnnursing.org/ELNEC/Resources). APRN faculty who have undergone ELNEC training may elect to offer separate ELNEC modules such as communication or pain and symptom management, aligning them with existing coursework. These programs may rely more heavily on the expertise of the experienced APRN faculty teaching in the programs than when embedding palliative care content. Panel discussions with interdisciplinary team (IDT) members or content experts can be helpful for students as well as offering clinical opportunities with members of a palliative care team.

DEVELOPING SPECIALTY PALLIATIVE NURSING GRADUATE PROGRAMS

Specialty palliative nursing at the advanced practice level is distinguished from primary palliative nursing. At this level, APRNs have advanced skills, knowledge, communication techniques, and clinical judgment to care for individuals with serious illness and their families.[11,26] The world, especially the United States, is facing an increased incidence of serious illness, aging demographics, and advancing healthcare technologies; the need for providers with advanced specialty skills in palliative care is urgent. Specialty palliative APRNs (postgraduate certificate or post-MSN-to-DNP degree) with expert palliative care knowledge and skills are essential to meet this demand.[27,28]

Table 5.2 EXAMPLE OF PRIMARY CARE PALLIATIVE EDUCATION EMBEDDED INTO AN ACCELERATED BACHELOR OF SCIENCE IN NURSING (ABSN) PROGRAM

BSN COURSE	ELNEC UNDERGRADUATE MODULE	SUPPLEMENTAL ACTIVITY
Semester 1		
Foundations & Gerontologic Nursing	Module 1: Introduction to Palliative Nursing	Question/Answer session with guest lecturer/ content expert Simulation part 1
Semester 2		
Psychiatric and Mental Health Nursing	Module 2: Communication in Palliative Care	Question/Answer session with guest lecturer/ content expert; Simulation part 2
Medical Surgical Nursing I	Module 3: Pain Management in Palliative Care Module 4: Symptom Management in Palliative Care	Question/Answer session with guest lecturer/ content expert
Semester 3		
Population-Focused Nursing	Module 5: Loss, Grief, and Bereavement	Question/Answer session with guest lecturer/ content expert; Loss/grief/bereavement exercise[23]; Allow palliative care clinical group to share their clinical experiences with the class
Nursing Care with Children and Their Families	Module 6: Final Hours of Life	Question/Answer session with guest lecturer/ content expert. Have a hospice nurse come in and talk about applicable clinical experience

In addition to providing all nurses with a foundational knowledge of primary palliative care skills, nursing programs also have a responsibility to prepare more specialty palliative APRNs. Until recently, however, there has been a lack of consistency or models for graduate programs to follow when creating or providing this content. In 2015, a graduate faculty workgroup was formed with the goal of achieving consensus on the preparation of APRNs to practice specialized palliative care.[29] The faculty workgroup was comprised of graduate nursing faculty members from around the country involved with the education of nurses and led by Constance Dahlin, Clareen Wiencek, and Dorothy Wholihan, all of whom hold advanced degrees in nursing science. This section of the chapter will articulate the standards developed by the workgroup and later refined by additional APRN faculty experts for entry into specialty palliative APRN practice and serve as a guidebook for nursing programs seeking to prepare entry-level APRNs to practice specialized palliative care.

The standards for APRN entry into specialty palliative care practice include roles and expectations for both clinical nurse specialists (CNS) and nurse practitioners (NP). They were created with the acknowledgment that there are different models for specialty palliative care graduate nursing programs (i.e., postgraduate certificates, MSN/DNP programs, minor in palliative care). Program structure also varies from face-to-face, online, to hybrid. The goal when developing these standards was to set in place essential components applicable to any graduate nursing program regardless of format or structure.

EXISTING PROFESSIONAL AND REGULATORY STANDARDS

Nursing programs seeking to prepare APRNs to practice in specialty palliative care must be familiar with the recommendations and standards used to guide both palliative nursing and APRN practice. See Table 5.3 for a list of foundational documents used by the faculty workgroup and recommended for integration. The table also lists the relevance of each resource. As new curriculum is developed, APRN faculty should utilize these as well as accreditation documents to ensure that content maintains best practice and quality standards. When developing new programs in specialty palliative care, nursing faculty and leaders must follow all state and accrediting organization guidelines.

ORGANIZING FRAMEWORK: THE SYNERGY MODEL

The graduate faculty workgroup chose to use the AACN *Synergy Model*[30] as an organizing framework for the development of the standards. This model stems from the understanding that patient and family needs are similar across all health conditions and illness trajectories. These needs are what shape a nurse's practice and helps define nursing characteristics and competences. This model is the basis of *Palliative Nursing Scope and Standards*[26] and is comprised of eight domains including Clinical Judgement, Advocacy and Moral Agency, Caring Practices, Collaboration, Systems Thinking,

Table 5.3 RESOURCES FOR GRADUATE SPECIALTY PALLIATIVE CARE CONTENT INTEGRATION

RESOURCES FOR INTEGRATION	RELEVANCE
American Association of Colleges of Nursing (AACN) and City of Hope *End-of-Life Nursing Education Consortium (ELNEC) APRN Curriculum*[31]	The ELNEC project is a national and international education initiative to improve palliative care. ELNEC is a partnership between the AACN, in Washington, DC, and the City of Hope, Duarte, CA. The project provides undergraduate and graduate nursing faculty, continuing education providers, staff development educators, specialty nurses in pediatrics, oncology, critical care, and geriatrics, and other nurses with palliative care training.
AACN *Graduate Competencies and Recommendations for Educating Nursing Students (G-CARES)*[15]	The G-CARES document builds on the American Association of Colleges of Nursing (AACN) *Competencies and Recommendations for Educating Undergraduate Nursing Students* (CARES) document. CARES identifies the 17 essential competencies undergraduate nursing students need to have completed by the end of their pre-licensure education.
AACN *Competencies and Recommendations for Educating Undergraduate Nursing Students to Improve Palliative Care* (CARES)[14]	This is a set of competencies and recommendations that will guide the education of future nurses on providing quality end-of-life care.
AACN *Doctoral Education for Advanced Nursing Practice*[32]	Outlines the necessary curriculum content and expected competencies of graduates from baccalaureate, master's, and Doctor of Nursing Practice programs, as well as the clinical support needed for the full spectrum of academic nursing.
AACN *Synergy Model*[30]	The AACN *Synergy Model* 2nd ed. for Patient Care is a conceptual framework that aligns patient needs with nurse competencies. The central idea of the model is that a patient's needs drive the nurse competencies required for patient care. When nurse competencies stem from patient needs, and the characteristics of the nurse and patient match, synergy occurs. This synergy enables optimal outcomes. The model identifies eight patient characteristics and eight nurse competencies.
American Nurses Association (ANA) *Code of Ethics for Nurses with Interpretive Statements*[33]	This is a guide for all nurses regarding the professional responsibilities consistent with the quality in nursing care and the ethical obligations of the profession.
ANA/HPNA *Call to Action: Nurses Lead and Transform Palliative Care*[11]	The call for action, which has been approved by members of the ANA and HPNA Boards of Directors, outlines 12 key recommendations that indicate the steps necessary to achieve quality primary palliative nursing, regardless of setting.
ANA *Nursing: Scope and Standards*[34]	Provides detailed and practical discussion of the competent level of nursing practice and professional performance. Outlines key aspects of nursing's professional role and practice for any level, setting, population focus, or specialty.
Center to Advance Palliative Care (CAPC)[35]	This is a national organization dedicated to increasing the availability of quality palliative care services for people facing serious illness. As the leading resource for palliative care development and growth, CAPC provides healthcare professionals with the training, tools and technical assistance necessary to start and sustain successful palliative care programs in hospitals and other healthcare settings.
Hospice and Palliative Nurses Association (HPNA) *Competencies for the Palliative and Hospice APRN*[36]	Describes the explicit intellectual, interpersonal, technical, and moral competencies necessary for specialty quality advanced palliative nursing practice. Advanced practice is inclusive of APRNs and graduate-prepared nurses with doctoral education. Competencies are outcome-specific and measurable.
HPNA *Palliative Nursing: Scope and Standards of Practice*[26]	Provides information that encompasses hospice and palliative nursing. Provides essential guidance in the form of standards and competencies for all levels of practice for palliative nursing.
National Consensus Project for Quality Palliative Care *Clinical Practice Guidelines*, 4th ed.[12]	This 4th edition creates a blueprint for excellence by establishing a comprehensive foundation for gold-standard palliative care for all people living with serious illness, regardless of their diagnosis, prognosis, age, or setting.
National Council of State Boards of Nursing (NCSBN)[37]	The organization through which nursing regulatory bodies act and counsel on matters affecting public health, safety and welfare. This includes but is not limited to nursing licensure examinations.

Response to Diversity, Facilitation of Learning, and Clinical Inquiry.[30] In creating the standards for specialty palliative graduate nursing education, each of the eight content areas was explored and aligned with competencies from the *HPNA Competencies for the Palliative and Hospice APRN*.[36] In addition, essential content for program implementation was identified, including resources to guide curricula development and for faculty to gain expertise. Box 5.1 lists the *Palliative and Hospice APRN Competencies* aligned with each domain. The following section outlines the essential content necessary for graduate faculty to incorporate into a specialty care program as well as supporting resources.

Clinical Judgment

Faculty must ensure that students are prepared to practice diagnostic reasoning, clinical decision-making, and effective communication techniques with patients and families (Box 5.2). This competency encompasses a vast array of APRN skills including clinical judgment, clinical reasoning, and decision-making at an advanced level of practice. In addition, they must be knowledgeable about illness trajectories across all setting and various specialties, including anticipatory guidance. Comprehensive palliative physical assessment skills and incorporation of these skills and tools per the *NCP Clinical Practice Guidelines*[12] are essential and should be assessed for competency throughout the program. This may be done through the use of standardized patients or in clinical settings with expert preceptors.

Specialty palliative APRNs nurses must fully manage and support patients and families nearing end of life. This may include coordination of care as well as palliative pharmacological and nonpharmacological options to address pain and symptoms associated with advanced illness. Competent history-taking and assessment skills, knowledge of common complications, considerations of opioid use and misuse, and socioeconomic factors are essential. APRNs should be comfortable documenting and revising the plan of care for

---

Box 5.1 PALLIATIVE APRN COMPETENCIES ALIGNED WITH *SYNERGY MODEL* DOMAINS

Clinical Judgment
  The palliative APRN demonstrates advanced clinical judgment, clinical reasoning, and decision-making as appropriate to advanced practice nursing, based on expert knowledge and skill in the assessment (history, current concerns, and physical examination), diagnosis, planning, and management of complex human responses, and the integration of global knowledge of the multidimensional care needs of individuals with serious illness and their families.

Advocacy and Moral Agency
  The palliative APRN integrates knowledge, attitudes, behaviors, and skills that are consistent with and assumes responsibility for advanced practice nursing professional standards, nursing codes of ethics, and advanced practice scope of practice within their care delivery. The palliative APRN serves as a moral agent to identify and resolve moral and ethical concerns, including advocating for human rights of all individuals with the goal of addressing and reducing health disparities, inequities, racism, and discrimination.

Caring Practices
  The palliative APRN integrates advanced caring practices to create a compassionate, supportive, and therapeutic environment for individuals with serious illness (perinates, neonates, children, adolescents, young adults, and older adults) and their families with the aim of promoting comfort, healing, and preventing unnecessary suffering. This is accomplished by, but is not limited to, vigilance, engagement, and responsiveness to themselves, individuals, families, and other healthcare providers.

Collaboration
  The palliative APRN collaboratively engages with individuals with serious illness, their families, and healthcare providers in the provision of palliative care, with the focus on patient-centered and family-focused care in a way that promotes each person's contributions toward achieving optimal yet realistic individual and family goals.

Systems Thinking
  The palliative APRN identifies and utilizes the evidence and body of knowledge for palliative care delivery and advanced clinical practice, as well as the tools to proactively manage the environmental and system resources for the individual with serious illness, their family, and staff within a health organization, a care system, and a community.

Response to Diversity
  The palliative APRN has the cultural sensitivity to recognize, appreciate, and incorporate the differing cultural needs of individuals with serious illness into the provision of care, which may include but is not limited to cultural differences, spiritual beliefs, sexual orientation, gender identity, gender expression, race, ethnicity, lifestyle, socioeconomic status, age, and values.

Facilitation of Learning
  The palliative APRN provides and facilitates learning for individuals with serious illness, their families, nurse colleagues, other members of the healthcare team, and the community in formats appropriate to the environment (i.e., virtual, in-person, or hybrid models).

Clinical Inquiry
  The palliative APRN continually questions and evaluates advanced palliative nursing practice and palliative care and provides informed practice based on the established palliative care research evidence and related information. In addition, the palliative and hospice APRN uses research to promote improved outcomes for individuals with serious illness and the community.

individuals with serious illness and their families based on evolving needs and preferences and complex, competing, and shifting priorities in goals of care.

Advocacy and Moral Agency

Advocacy is intertwined with ethical principles and ethical theories and is an essential component in graduate nursing education and should include defining and identifying ethical conflicts and moral distress associated with families, patients, and staff and developing interventions to address these (Box 5.3). Goals of care conversations with families also fall under this umbrella including how to identify, document, and follow through on patients wishes and preferences for care including advance care planning. Faculty should model strategies to help patients and families weigh the pros and cons of aggressive life-prolonging or life-saving treatment and how these align with their goals of care. This may be best accomplished through the use of role-play and case studies. Faculty should ensure that students are practicing in accordance with the professional standards of the current versions of the ANA *Nursing: Scope and Standards of Practice* and HPNA's *Palliative Nursing: Scope and Standards of Practice* as well as the ANA *Code of Ethics for Nurses* and HPNA's *Code of Ethical Conduct*, which articulate the moral foundation of palliative and hospice advanced practice nursing. Students should also incorporate into their practice all appropriate federal laws, regulations, and standards from the Centers for Medicare and Medicaid Services (CMS) and state statutes, regulations, and laws as well as currently accepted professional standards of advanced practice nursing.

Caring Practices

Palliative APRN faculty must teach and role-model compassionate caring and patient- and family-centered care (Box 5.4). Theoretical models of caring are essential to nursing practice and even more significant when caring for individuals with serious illness and at end of life. The APRN in education must value the role of compassion and kindness and exhibit these traits in all aspects of their interactions, including with students, colleagues, and patients and families. Demonstration of compassion and respect for the inherent dignity, worth, and unique attributes of all people is essential. Self-care, caregiver burden, and compassion fatigue, as well as moral distress

and building resilience, are important content areas in this domain.

Collaboration

APRNs must be full partners with interprofessional team members,[38] especially when caring for individuals with serious illness (Box 5.5). To support an IDT team process, APRNs must be able to identify complementary areas of expertise as well as overlapping areas of expertise among disciplines and how this contributes to the care being provided to the patient and family. Demonstrating this teamwork will establish a climate of trust, respect, and partnership between individuals and families with serious illness and IDT members in the provision of specialty palliative care. Team communication skills and opportunities to work with or shadow palliative care IDT members in a clinical setting would be beneficial to the students. The Cambia Health Foundation Sojourns Scholars

Program has implemented a wide range of projects to advance leadership in palliative care.[39]

Systems Thinking

Systems thinking includes concepts such as system theories, healthcare finances, and policy work (Box 5.6). These topics are often covered in courses throughout an MSN/DNP program. Faculty must ensure that students focus on palliative care in relation to these consent areas. The students should examine the application of program cost-effectiveness measures, metrics, and marketing, as well as measures for quality improvement and accountability. Working with team members in various healthcare delivery settings, systems, and as part of interprofessional teams will allow students to get a behind the scenes experience of some of the access, barrier, cost, efficacy, and quality issues that present when making palliative care decisions with patients and families.

Response to Diversity

Nurse educators are responsible for instilling the importance of culturally respectful care from the start of a student's educational journey. Students much learn to recognize and appreciate the cultural needs of individuals with serious illness and their families, which may include but are not limited to cultural differences, spiritual beliefs, sexual orientation, gender identity, gender expression, race, ethnicity, socioeconomic status, age, and values. Self-reflection on one's own values, beliefs, and perspectives and how this may impact the delivery of culturally sensitive care should be discussed and incorporated into all aspects of a program. Spiritual and religious influences on illness, grief, and bereavement should be explored and understood, including the cultural aspects of palliative care. An important aspect of this is introducing students to health disparities and social injustices within palliative care and how this may be approached and resolved. Chapter 35, "Culturally Respectful Palliative Care," further outlines the importance of care and may provide tools helpful for faculty embedding this content into their curriculums.

Facilitation of Learning

Knowledge about and involvement with existing professional associations and standards will be essential for graduate students to provide palliative care education to others in their role as palliative APRNs (Box 5.8). This includes not only patients and families, but other healthcare professionals and community members. As discussed earlier, ELNEC Modules and resources[20,22] were specifically designed to advance palliative care education and should be introduced to students as a resource early in their program. Other associations such as the HPNA,[40] the Center to Advance Palliative Care (CAPC),[35] and the NHPCO[1] should be explored for their valuable patient, family, and provider resources, including educational materials and toolboxes.

Box 5.7 RESOURCES FOR CURRICULAR DEVELOPMENT: RESPONSE TO DIVERSITY

American Association of Colleges of Nursing. *ELNEC APRN Curriculum: Overview Module.* 2021. https://www.aacnnursing.org/ELNEC/About/ELNEC-Curricula

Beaune L, Morinis J, Rapoport A, et al. Paediatric palliative care and the social determinants of health: Mitigating the impact of urban poverty on children with life-limiting illnesses. *Paediatr Child Health.* 2013;18(4):181–183.

Kirby E, Lwin Z, Kenny K, Broom A, Birman H, Good P. "It doesn't exist . . . ": Negotiating palliative care from a culturally and linguistically diverse patient and caregiver perspective. *BMC Palliat Care* 2018;17(1):90.

Koroukian SM, Schiltz NK, Warner DF, et al. Social determinants, multimorbidity, and patterns of end-of-life care in older adults dying from cancer. *J Geriatr Oncol.* 2016;8(2):117–124.

National Academy of Medicine. The Future of Nursing 2020–2030. Charting a Path to Achieve Health Equity. Washington, DC: National Academies Press; 2021. https://nam.edu/publications/the-future-of-nursing-2020-2030/.

Phillips JM, Malone B. Increasing racial/ethnic diversity in nursing to reduce health disparities and achieve health equity. *Public Health Rep.* 2014;129(Suppl 2):45–50.

Washington H. *Medical Apartheid: The Dark History of Medical Experimentation on Black Americans from Colonial Times to the Present.* New York: Penguin Random House; 2008.

Wicks Newsome M, Alejandro J, Bertrand D, Boyd C, Coleman C, Haozous E, Meade C, Meek P. Achieving advance care planning in diverse and underserved populations. *Nurs Outlook.* 2019;66(3):311–315.

Clinical Inquiry

Graduate nursing programs will prepare APRNs to evaluate evidence related to clinical practice in palliative care using standardized approaches related to the domains of the NCP *Clinical Practice Guidelines*[12] (including pain and symptom management, grief and bereavement, and spiritual care). Quality improvement principles and methods to promote change in nursing practice related to palliative care should be emphasized and modeled.

Evaluation of Content Areas

When integrating primary palliative care content into existing nursing curriculums or developing specialty palliative care programs, faculty should utilize a combination of innovative teaching modalities. These may include but are not limited to the following:

- Journaling
- Self-reflection
- Written assignment (e.g., resolution of ethical cases)
- Problem-based learning
- Simulation (high- and low-fidelity; using standardized patients)
- Case studies
- Content expert lectures
- Panel discussions (IDT)
- Group discussions
- Role-plays
- Interviews
- Book club review and/or movie reviews

- Graded case presentation or case studies
- Readings, podcasts, videos
- Clinical rotations
- Examinations (e.g., multiple-choice, short-answer, case-based questions)

In addition to the listed teaching modalities, faculty and program leaders must evaluate the outcomes of the palliative care programs and initiatives. This may be done through

- Course summaries
- Student academic outcomes (e.g., grade point averages, certification pass rate, oral or practical evaluation)
- Preceptor evaluations of student clinical work
- Student evaluations of program
- Student clinical outcomes
- Clinical preceptor and site evaluations
- Electronic student record of patient encounters for number and type of palliative care encounters and care provided
- Program outcome metrics
- Tracking admissions, attrition, certification pass rates, transcripts, etc.

Clinical Experiences

The HPNA *Standards for Clinical Education* (2nd ed.)[19] should be used by faculty when incorporating clinical opportunities into nursing programs. These standards outline types of clinical experiences, including those for the RN and those for the APRN. The standards also review criteria for suitable preceptors, curriculum needs, and evaluation requirements.

Practicum specialty hours should be included, at the minimum with graduate specialty palliative care programs but may also be considered for undergraduate and graduate students as optional experiences for students seeking to gain additional expertise. Supervised practicum experiences are essential to the development of specialist graduate-level skills. Students should be exposed to both palliative and hospice care to assure competency in complex pain and symptom management, communication, and conflict resolution across the lifespan, and in various clinical settings.

Advanced certification in hospice and palliative nursing by the HPCC, requires didactic and clinical hours, including functioning as a CNS or NP with hospice and palliative advanced nursing practice of 500 hours in the most recent 12 months or 1,000 hours in the most recent 24 months prior to applying for the exam.[8] Programs may consider meeting the requirements for sitting for certification by the end of their programs.

BARRIERS

Literature is abundant on the barriers that exist to integrating palliative care for individuals with serious illness and their families.[41] Among these barriers, a recurrent theme is the lack of and need for more education and training, including preparing specialty trained providers in palliative care.[6,11] Other barriers include time to attend such education, financial support, and space within nursing program curricula. This chapter has outlined solutions for APRN faculty to meet this need and incorporate elements of palliative care into existing and new nursing program curricula. Unfortunately, nursing programs and educators also face barriers when answering this call to action.

Despite having the support of the recommendations and guidelines published by organizations such as the National Academy of Medicine (formerly the Institute of Medicine),[6] the ANA, and the HPNA[11] to advance palliative care education, faculty should anticipate challenges in developing and rolling out this content. The first step for faculty should be obtaining organizational buy-in. Palliative care education should be a prioritized part of the organizational strategic plan if programs are to be successful when changing curricula. Communication with senior leadership and focusing on the known benefits of palliative care practice, including improving pain and symptoms, enhancing quality of life, reducing caregiver stress and burdens, and decreasing hospital costs and lengths of stay.

Expert APRN faculty should be prepared to provide education to those who may not be as familiar with the guidelines, recommendations, and benefits of increasing palliative care education. This includes not only senior leadership but also faculty who will be supporting students throughout their program. In the case study, an interactive faculty workshop was developed and implemented, faculty were mandated to complete the online ELNEC modules, and periodic "lunch and learn" mini conferences were offered on palliative care topics. When palliative care education is named a priority in strategic planning, it opens the door for advancement in this area.

Another barrier in implementing new content may exist because of already crowded curricula. A comprehensive review of courses should be completed to identify outdated content that may be removed from the curriculum to make necessary room for palliative care material. Additionally, curriculum change comes with a price tag. As with many new initiatives, finances are another barrier that faculty may face when incorporating palliative care into nursing programs. Financial impacts extenuate the importance of leadership and stakeholder buy-in. Expenses may include faculty time, marketing, access to the online ELNEC curriculum, expert consultative fees, professional development, and additional training necessary for faculty. APRN faculty should work with leadership to secure funding through grants, philanthropy, and allocations in the budget for palliative care initiatives.

Last, securing appropriate clinical sites with trained preceptors may be a barrier for programs wanting to offer students hands-on practical experience with patients and families in palliative care. Securing community partners will be essential early on in program development, and this will include specialty palliative care providers as well as IDT members. Offering students opportunities to engage with individuals with serious illness across the lifespan is optimal and may require travel, especially for those living in rural areas. Faculty should consider hospital-based care, community or outpatient care, residential facilities, and home-based palliative and hospice organizations.

SUMMARY

It is generally recognized that there is a need to increase palliative education across all levels of nursing programs in order to meet the demands associated with individuals with serious illness. Experienced APRNs in the field of palliative care should consider this an opportunity to take a leadership role in educating future nurses and advanced practice nurses in palliative care. Palliative care education is vital to answering the call to increase both primary and specialty palliative care access for individuals with serious illness and their families. Palliative APRN educators should use the resources available in addition to their experience and expertise to obtain leadership buy-in, develop and design curricula, implement curriculum changes, and support students and other faculty throughout the process. Based on their competence, expertise, and professionalism, palliative APRN educators are in a unique position to overcome existing barriers and truly make an impact on the lives of patients and families.

REFERENCES

1. National Hospice and Palliative Care Organization. Explanation of palliative care. October 2021. https://www.nhpco.org/palliative-care-overview/explanation-of-palliative-care/
2. American Association of Colleges of Nursing. Common advanced practice registered nurse doctoral-level competencies. Washington, DC, AACN. October 2017. http://www.aacnnursing.org/Portals/42/AcademicNursing/pdf/Common-APRN-Doctoral-Competencies.pdf
3. American Association of Nurse Practitioners. Scope of practice for nurse practitioners. Austin, TX; AANP. Revised 2019. Austin, Tx. https://www.aanp.org/advocacy/advocacy-resource/position-statements/scope-of-practice-for-nurse-practitioners
4. Fennimore L, Wholihan D, Breakwell S, Malloy P, Virani R, Ferrell B. A framework for integrating oncology palliative care in doctor of nursing practice (DNP) education. *J Prof Nurs*. 2018;34(6):444–448. doi:10.1016/j.profnurs.2018.09.003
5. Dahlin C, Coyne P. The palliative APRN leader. *Ann Palliat Med*. 2019;8(Suppl 1):S30–S38. doi:10.21037/apm.2018.06.03
6. Institute of Medicine. *Dying in America: Improving Quality and Honoring Individual Preferences Near the End of Life*. Washington, DC: National Academies Press; 2015. https://www.nap.edu/catalog/18748/dying-in-america-improving-quality-and-honoring-individual-preferences-near
7. American Association of Colleges of Nursing. Transitioning from clinical nursing to nursing faculty. Washington, DC, AACN. 2014. https://www.aacnnursing.org/Teaching-Resources/Tool-Kits/Transitioning-Clinical-Faculty
8. Hospice and Palliative Credentialing Center. Advanced Certified Hospice and Palliative Nurse. 2021. https://advancingexpertcare.org/HPNA/HPCC/CertificationWeb/ACHPN.aspx
9. Schneider E, Abrams M, Shah A, Lewis C, Shah T. *Health Care in America: The Experience of People with Serious Illness*. New York, NY: Commonwealth Fund; October, 2018. https://www.commonwealthfund.org/sites/default/files/2018-10/Schneider_HealthCareinAmerica.pdf
10. Ferrell B, Malloy P, Mazanec P, Virani R. CARES: AACN's new competencies and recommendations for educating undergraduate nursing students to improve palliative care. *J Prof Nurs*. 2016;32(5):327–333. doi:10.1016/j.profnurs.2016.07.002
11. American Nurses Association, Hospice and Palliative Nurses Association. *Call for Action: Nurses Lead and Transform Palliative Care*. Silver Spring, MD: American Nurses Association; March, 2017. https://www.nursingworld.org/~497158/globalassets/practiceandpolicy/health-policy/palliativecareprofessionalissuespanel-callforaction.pdf
12. National Consensus Project for Quality Palliative Care. *Clinical Practice Guidelines*, 4th ed. Richmond, VA: National Coalition of Hospice and Palliative Care; 2018. https://www.nationalcoalitionhpc.org/ncp/
13. Dahlin C. Palliative care: Delivering comprehensive oncology nursing care. *Semin Oncol Nurs*. 2015;31(4):327–337. doi:10.1016/j.soncn.2015.08.008
14. American Association of Colleges of Nursing. CARES: Competencies and recommendations for educating undergraduate nursing students: Preparing nurses to care for the seriously ill and their families. Washington, DC, AACN. 2016. https://www.aacnnursing.org/Portals/42/ELNEC/PDF/New-Palliative-Care-Competencies.pdf
15. American Association of Colleges of Nursing, End of Life Nursing Education Consortium. G-Cares competencies in primary palliative

care for graduate nursing students in master's and DNP programs. Washington, DC, AACN. 2019. https://www.aacnnursing.org/Portals/42/ELNEC/PDF/Graduate-CARES.pdf

16. American Association of Colleges of Nursing. The essentials of baccalaureate education for professional nursing practice. Washington, DC, AACN. 2008. https://www.aacnnursing.org/Education-Resources/Tool-Kits/Baccalaureate-Essentials-Tool-Kit

17. American Association of Colleges of Nursing. Essentials: Core competencies for professional nursing education. Washington, DC, AACN. 2021. https://www.aacnnursing.org/AACN-Essentials

18. Ramjan JM, Costa CM, Hickman LD, Kearns M, Phillips JL. Integrating palliative care content into a new undergraduate nursing curriculum: The University of Notre Dame, Australia-Sydney experience. *Collegian (Royal College of Nursing, Australia)*. 2010;17(2):85–91. doi:10.1016/j.colegn.2010.04.009

19. Hospice and Palliative Nurses Association. *HPNA Standards for Clinical Education of Hospice and Palliative Nurses*. 2nd ed. Pittsburgh, PA: Hospice and Palliative Nurses Association; 2015. https://advancingexpertcare.org/HPNA/HPNAweb/Education/Standards_for_Clinical_Education.aspx

20. American Association of Colleges of Nursing. End of Life Nursing Education Consortium (ELNEC). About ELNEC. September 2021. http://www.aacnnursing.org/elnec

21. American Association of Colleges of Nursing. ELNEC fact sheet. August, 2021. https://www.aacnnursing.org/Portals/42/ELNEC/PDF/ELNEC-Fact-Sheet.pdf

22. ELNEC Academy. Relias Learning, ELNEC Academy. September, 2021. https://elnec.academy.reliaslearning.com/

23. Ebberts, M. A grief and bereavement exercise for small groups based on Peak R, Wooldridge J. Hospice of Marin. https://5y1.org/document/death-and-dying-educational-pdf.html

24. Gallagher O, Saunders R, Tambree K, Alliex S, Monterosso L, Naglazas Y. Nursing student experiences of death and dying during a palliative care clinical placement: Teaching and learning implications. Teaching and Learning Forum 2014: Transformative, Innovative and Engaging. 2014. University of Notre Dame, Australia. https://core.ac.uk/download/pdf/61303912.pdf

25. Bishop CT, Mazanec P, Bullington J, et al. Online end-of-life nursing education consortium core curriculum for staff nurses: An education strategy to improve clinical practice. *J Hosp Palliat Nurs*. 2019;21(6):531–539. doi:10.1097/NJH.0000000000000593

26. Dahlin C. *Palliative Nursing: Scope and Standards of Practice*. 6th ed. Pittsburgh, PA: Hospice and Palliative Nurses Association; 2021.

27. Lupu D, Quigley L, Mehfoud N, Salsberg ES. The growing demand for hospice and palliative medicine physicians: Will the supply keep up? *J Pain Symptom Manage*. 2018;55(4):1216–1223.

28. Meier DE, Back AL, Berman A, Block SD, Corrigan JM, Morrison RS. A national strategy for palliative care. *Health Aff (Millwood)*. 2017;36(7):1265–1273. doi:10.1377/hlthaff.2017.0164

29. Dahlin C, Ersek M, Wholihan D, Wiencek C. Palliative APRN fellowship guidelines: A strategy for quality specialty practice: Report of the HPNA Graduate Faculty Council (SA509). Abstract for the Annual Assembly. *J Pain Symptom Manage*. 2019;57(2):445.

30. American Association of Critical Care Nurses. *Synergy model for patient care*. 2nd ed. Aliso Viejo, CA. 2018. https://www.aacn.org/nursing-excellence/aacn-standards/synergy-model

31. American Association of Colleges of Nursing. ELNEC-APRN. September, 2021. https://www.aacnnursing.org/ELNEC/About/ELNEC-Curricula

32. American Association of Colleges of Nursing. Essentials of doctoral education for advanced nursing practice. Washington, DC. 2006. www.aacnnursing.org/Portals/42/Publications/DNPEssentials.pdf

33. American Nurses Association. *Code of Ethics for Nurses with Interpretive Statements*. 3rd ed. Silver Spring, MD: Nursesbooks.org; 2015.

34. American Nurses Association. *Nursing Scope and Standards of Practice*, 4th ed. Silver Spring, MD: Nursesbooks.org; 2021.

35. Center to Advance Palliative Care (CAPC). Home page. October 2021. https://www.capc.org/

36. Dahlin C. *Competencies for Palliative and Hospice APRN*. 3rd ed. Pittsburgh, PA: Hospice and Palliative Nurses Association; 2021.

37. National Council of State Boards of Nursing (NCSBN). History of the APRN. October 2021. https://www.ncsbn.org/737.htm.

38. Dahlin C, Coyne P. History of the advanced practice role in palliative nursing. In Dahlin C, Coyne P, Ferrell B, eds. *Advanced Practice Palliative Nursing*. New York: Oxford University Press; 2016:3–12.

39. Dahlin C, Sanders J, Calton B, et al. The Cambia Sojourns Scholars Leadership Program: Projects and reflections on leadership in palliative care. *J Palliat Med*. 2019;22(7):823–829. doi:10.1089/jpm.2018.0523

40. Hospice and Palliative Nurses Association. Home Page. 2021. https://advancingexpertcare.org/

41. Aldridge MD, Hasselaar J, Garralda E, et al. Education, implementation, and policy barriers to greater integration of palliative care: A literature review. *Palliat Med*. 2016;30(3):224–239. doi:10.1177/0269216315606645

6.

THE PALLIATIVE APRN IN POLICY AND PAYMENT MODELS

Marian Grant

KEY POINTS

- Palliative care achieves all the key objectives of health reform and recent health policy revisions.

- Recent federal legislation and regulation is improving access to palliative care services.

- Healthcare payment is shifting toward paying for outcomes and value and palliative care can contribute to achieving those goals.

- New payment models could also increase access to palliative care services.

- Health policy and payment policy affect patient care and access to care, what palliative APRNs can do clinically, and what they can be reimbursed for.

- Advanced practice registered nurses (APRNs) can play a significant role in the development of policy and payment.

CASE STUDY 1: PALLIATIVE CARE REIMBURSEMENT

Shanice is a nurse practitioner (NP) who is a new member of an inner-city hospital's palliative care team. She really likes the people she works with, but she has been struck by the fact that the team seems more heavily staffed with physicians and NPs than with nurses, social workers, or even a chaplain. She knows from her previous hospice experience that the most holistic care is delivered by a fully interdisciplinary team. When she questioned the team about the interdisciplinary mix, her teammates answered that the hospital only wants billable providers on the team. This was a new concept to her because, when she worked in hospice, billing for her services did not come up. She also loved working in the home setting and was hoping that this might be an option on this new palliative care team, but now it seems that the hospital cannot afford to start a home-based palliative care program since there is not adequate payment for such a program.

Fortunately, one of the other palliative NPs on the team has become very involved in federal and state policy efforts and has been able to answer Shanice's questions and show her how policy shapes their team's makeup and responsibilities. This NP suggested that Shanice learn more about policy, and this chapter will cover some of the key things she has learned.

INTRODUCTION

Most palliative advanced practice registered nurses (APRNs) know it is important to be knowledgeable and current on palliative clinical practice. What some palliative APRNs do not realize, however, is the value of being aware of ongoing health policy and payment models. This knowledge is important because clinical practice in the United States is regulated. The care patients can receive, including access to palliative care, along with what APRNs can do and be reimbursed for, all depend on health policy and payment regulations (see Appendix I for information on reimbursement).

This chapter provides an overview on health policy and payment and how they relate to patient care, palliative care delivery, and APRN practice. To illustrate core concepts, two case studies are threaded throughout the chapter.

HEALTHCARE IN THE UNITED STATES

In 2018, US healthcare spending was $3.6 trillion or $11,172 per person. As a share of the nation's Gross Domestic Product (GDP), this health spending accounted for 17.7%.[1] That makes healthcare a major sector of the US economy and larger than manufacturing.

Healthcare has therefore become an important national issue given its size and role in the economy. However, although the United States leads the world in health technology and innovation, it lags on other important health aspects.

- The United States spends nearly twice as much other developed countries on healthcare, paradoxically having the lowest life expectancy and the highest suicide rates among the 11 other developed nations.

- The United States has the highest chronic disease burden, with an obesity rate that is two times higher than other developed countries.

- Compared to peer nations, the United States has among the highest number of hospitalizations from preventable causes and the highest rate of avoidable deaths.[2]

It is estimated that the care for only 5% of the US population represents close to 50% of total healthcare spending.[3] Healthcare in the United States is not only expensive for the government or insurance companies paying for it, but also for patients and their families. Specifically, as the costs of health insurance and medications have increased, so have deductibles, copays, and out-of-pocket expenses. It is estimated that these expenses cost the average American household $5,000 per year, twice the amount from 1984.[4] Approximately 60% of health insurance in this country is employment-based, and being unemployed unfortunately often goes hand in hand with being uninsured.[5] These issues, along with problems of health coverage and access in the United States became magnified during the COVID-19 pandemic.[6] The pandemic highlighted lack of access to care, higher morbidity and mortality among minority and vulnerable populations, and lack of systems to provide good care in the home, thereby revealing many of the underlying problems with the US healthcare system.[6] The US health system is really not a system; rather it is inefficient, uncoordinated, and many Americans are under- or uninsured. Moreover, systemic racism and inequity continue to result in health disparities for minority communities that cause shorter life spans and higher morbidity.[7]

HEALTHCARE REFORM

It is therefore not surprising that the US healthcare system has been undergoing reform for some time. Much of that reform has been driven by what is called "the triple aim." This is the goal of concurrently

- Improving the patient experience of care (including quality and satisfaction);

- Improving the health of populations; and

- Reducing the per capita cost of healthcare.[8]

These goals may sound familiar, but they are not obvious partners. Trying to improve something while at the same reducing costs can be challenging. Nonetheless, doing all three together has been the goal of many federal and state health policy changes. More recently, there has been talk of adding a fourth aim: "the quadruple aim." Possible additions include improving clinician satisfaction, pursuing health equity, and other priorities.[9] However, from a policy perspective, the original triple aim continues to be the most consistent goal even if it has yet to be fully realized.

Another factor in healthcare reform is the aging of the American population. The 73 million "baby boomers," those born between 1946 and 1964, will all be older than 65 in 2030.[10] At that point, they and others over age 65 will represent 20% of the population, or one in five Americans.[10] Since the number of chronic conditions increases with age, almost half of all people aged 45–64 and 80% of those 65 and over have multiple chronic conditions.[11] This means that older people will represent increasingly more of the patients in the US health system. The aging of the population has been anticipated for a long time. However, recent developments, like the COVID-19 pandemic and its higher mortality in nursing homes,[12] have demonstrated that our health system is not ready to provide safe and appropriate care for older patients[13] and that further reform is still needed.

PALLIATIVE CARE AND HEALTHCARE REFORM

Fortunately, palliative care is a solution to many of healthcare's current problems. First, it can deliver all three of the triple aims.[14] It can improve the quality and satisfaction of an individual's care by addressing their specific needs and providing support. Then, it can improve the health of the seriously ill population by, again, addressing physical symptoms, emotional and social issues, and providing support. Finally, it typically does this at equal or less cost than care without palliative care.[15] This is achieved primarily due to the goals of care conversations palliative care teams have with patients. Those conversations focus on what matters most to the individual; then the treatment plan is developed to deliver on those personal goals. In many cases, once people are more aware of their health situation and prognosis and have been given the full range of treatment options, including less aggressive ones, they often choose a less aggressive approach, which saves money for them and those paying for their care.[16] Even when people choose to continue pursuing all aggressive care, palliative care does not end up costing more because palliative care combined with aggressive care usually results in less hospitalizations or readmissions by better anticipating and managing health crises.[16] It is because of this financial consideration that many hospitals have palliative care programs to both improve patient care and control healthcare costs. Shanice has heard her team talk about these benefits being why her team was able to add new staff recently.

Palliative care is appropriate for aging individuals, especially those with multiple chronic illnesses, as its focus on improving or maintaining quality of life. Shanice sees not only how her patients individually benefit from the palliative care services she and her team deliver, but she is also becoming aware of her team's success, and her hospital's interest, in reducing readmissions, intensive care unit (ICU) length of stay, and mortality—in the latter case by increasing hospice referrals—all of which palliative care has been shown to help achieve.[17]

HEALTH POLICY

According to the World Health Organization (WHO) health policy refers to

Decisions, plans, and actions that are undertaken to achieve specific healthcare goals within a society. An explicit health policy can achieve several things: it defines a vision for the future which in turn helps to establish targets and points of reference for the short and medium term. It outlines priorities and the expected roles of different groups; and it builds consensus and informs people.[18]

Health policy can be formed at the institutional, local, state, or federal level and involves multiple stakeholders from citizens, patients, clinicians, healthcare providers and systems, government officials, policy experts, and professional and advocacy organizations, to name just a few. Their combined effort leads to health policy in the United States The following content explains key federal policy components.

LEGISLATION

In the United States, governmental health policy is achieved via two mechanisms. The first is legislative action through new laws. The second is regulatory action through the interpretation and implementation of those laws. *The Affordable Care Act* (ACA), also known as Obamacare, was a law passed in 2009.[19] Its provisions were then translated into regulations to provide the specifics on, for instance, how children receiving hospice could also receive concurrent curative care[20] (see Figure 6.1).

In terms of federal legislation, palliative care currently enjoys strong support in Congress in both the House and Senate and among both Republicans and Democrats. That is because members of Congress and their staff often have personal experience with serious illness that drives their interest in improving care. Some members of Congress are also nurses and physicians who likely better appreciate the benefits of palliative care.[21] Nonetheless, it can take several sessions of Congress to get a bill passed. This has been the case with the *Palliative Care and Hospice Education and Training Act* (PCHETA), a bill to increase the funding for training physicians, nurses, and other team members, which has been introduced repeatedly since 2012[22] and which has only ever passed in the House. See Box 6.1 for details on PCHETA.

Shanice has started advocating for PCHETA by responding to her nursing association's requests that she contact her elected federal officials to get them to support this and other important bills. She has also learned that members of Congress are interested in hearing both from their constituents and nurses, since nurses represent the largest healthcare workforce[23] and have been consistently rated the profession with the highest levels of honesty and ethics by the public since 2002.[24] Constituents who are also nurses are, therefore, likely to get a welcome response from their elected officials' offices.

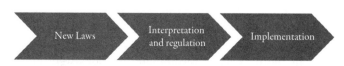

Figure 6.1 Government health policy.

REGULATION

As noted, regulations are the other way health policy is implemented. While the wording for enacted laws is set in statute, the regulations for those laws must be interpreted from that wording and, in the case of some laws, periodically updated. The federal regulatory process includes a mandatory 60-day period for the public to comment on any proposed regulations, which is an opportunity to both educate and advocate for palliative care with the various regulatory agencies. Every year, the Centers for Medicare and Medicaid Services (CMS) update regulations for major aspects of healthcare such as hospital, hospice, nursing home, home health, and the Medicare drug (Part D) programs. These updated regulations dictate what and how healthcare providers like APRNs and physicians will be paid. Major palliative care organizations monitor federal regulations and advocate to include palliative care in programs for those with serious illness wherever possible.[25] They also monitor regulations to advocate that activities like advance care planning be included or required in as many federal programs as possible. For instance, after advocacy from the field, CMS introduced new billing codes for advance care planning in 2016, and nurse practitioners are among the healthcare providers who are eligible for reimbursement for having these conversations using these codes.[26]

MEDICARE ADVANTAGE SUPPLEMENTAL BENEFITS

Getting bills passed in Congress has become increasingly difficult due to increased partisanship, although regulatory opportunities in general, as well as for palliative care

Box 6.2 MEDICARE ADVANTAGE (MA) KEY DETAILS

- Available to Medicare beneficiaries as an alternate to traditional Medicare

- Provided via commercial health insurance plans

- Has become increasingly popular among those beneficiaries as it often provides additional benefits like dental, vision, and hearing services, things unfortunately not yet covered by traditional Medicare

Source: US Department of Centers for Medicare and Medicaid Services.[68]

specifically, have increased over the past few years. This likely reflects the government's recognition of the needs of those living with serious illness[27] and the aging of the population. Some serious illness examples include allowing Medicare Advantage (MA) health insurance plans to offer additional services, such as home-based palliative care, to those with serious illness.[28] See Box 6.2 for more on MA.

Shanice read recently that the head of the big MA organization in her state is interested in offering home-based palliative care, and her team has discussed whether that might be an opportunity for them to pilot such a program with that MA plan.

TELEHEALTH

Another federal policy opportunity has been increasing flexibility for healthcare programs to be in touch with patients via telehealth. Historically, telehealth was limited to only patients in rural areas and required these patients to go to a designated healthcare facility to interact with providers elsewhere.[29] The COVID-19 pandemic resulted in some CMS waivers that allowed providers to contact patients at home in any geographic area, even using the telephone if the patient did not have a device that allowed video interaction. Shanice and her team were able to check on patients at home via telephone during the pandemic and found it surprisingly effective. Another hospital in her city has a palliative care discharge program where patients are given tablet devices to follow-up with the team virtually after discharge.[30] Many of these patients are elderly and have limited transportation options, and the team at the hospital has found telehealth with them surprisingly effective. Because of these types of experiences, the use of telehealth surged in 2020 during the pandemic and both providers and patients found it helpful. The federal government has subsequently started making some of these changes permanent, including home visits for the evaluation and management of a patient where the law allows telehealth services in the patient's home and certain types of visits for patients with cognitive impairments via new legislation and regulations.[31] (See Box 6.3 and Chapter 17, "The Palliative APRN in Telehealth.")

Box 6.3 EXAMPLES OF CMS TELEHEALTH WAIVERS THAT BECAME PERMANENT

Contacting patient at home via telehealth in states where allowed

Contacting patient with cognitive impairment via telehealth

SOCIAL DETERMINANTS OF HEALTH

CMS is also interested in assessing and modifying payment in Medicare programs for those beneficiaries with social risk factors such as income, geographic location, education level, etc. It is estimated that these "social determinants of health" contribute up to 80% of health outcomes,[32] and they are particularly important for those with serious illness as many with social risk factors have poorer outcomes and they and their families would benefit from additional services, including palliative care (see Chapter 20, "Health Disparities"). Shanice's care of people with lower-income, living near her city hospital, makes her very aware of social determinants of health and health disparities. A church in her neighborhood is developing a program to support family caregivers, for instance, and asked her to talk to their health committee about palliative care.

PAYMENT MODELS

Payment is a major focus area for health policy reform because it so strongly impacts care delivery. In many cases, you can change clinical practice by changing what is and is not paid for.

CASE STUDY 2: PRACTICE AUTHORITY

Derrick is a CNS who has now also joined the palliative care team Shanice works on. His previous experience was at the cancer center affiliated with their hospital, but he was interested in developing his palliative care skills and has been glad to join the palliative care team. In regard to policy, he has already been involved with some issues as state regulations limit his CNS scope of practice. This has been frustrating for him because he previously worked in a state where CNSs had full practice authority. His state CNS association has been lobbying for legislation to expand scope of practice, and he ended up on that association's policy committee and is knowledgeable about this issue and process.

FEE FOR SERVICE

Historically in the United States, healthcare providers have been paid on a fee-for-service (FFS) basis.[33] This means that each procedure or intervention has an agreed-upon fee attached to it. While this system sounds simple and made sense in the days when medical interventions were more limited, over time there has been the realization that it can inadvertently encourage healthcare providers to do more interventions or tests than needed since that can help boost income. An additional problem with an FFS model was highlighted when patients stopped seeing their providers or coming into the hospital during the COVID-19 pandemic in 2020.[34] Since visits, procedures, and testing were all reduced by infection concerns from the pandemic, FFS revenue to clinical practices and hospitals was reduced as well. It was estimated that this could be a loss of revenue of $15 billion to the primary care system alone.[35] Shifting to telehealth helped mitigate some of that patient contact and revenue loss, but healthcare organizations were significantly affected even though patients with serious illness were still ill and in need of care. Almost overnight, shifting from an FFS model became even more urgent.

Another consequence of an FFS model is that it focuses healthcare delivery on those interventions or providers that can be reimbursed. This has led palliative care programs to have proportionately more billable providers, such as physicians, APRNs, and physician assistants, versus nonbillable clinicians such as nurses, social workers, or chaplains. It also encourages those billable providers to focus on billable activities, such as medical interventions, rather than on nonbillable ones, such as providing spiritual or family support. This is why Shanice and Derrick's palliative care team is configured in the way that it is, with more physicians and APRNs and fewer of the other disciplines, which is unfortunate because it means the reality of payment often overrides the goal of interdisciplinary palliative care.

The FFS model has also made providing a home-based palliative care program too costly for a hospital since the reimbursement of only the billable providers for mostly medical services is not enough to cover the additional costs of nonbillable staff and their time and travel to peoples' homes. FFS is not just an issue for palliative care. The FFS payment structure encourages all healthcare providers to focus more on medical interventions than psychosocial ones that, while possibly needed, are not reimbursable. The result is a health system more focused on interventions than health. Of note, hospice care is not per FFS intervention or provider-based but is a daily amount per patient basis or per diem.[36] It is therefore required to have interdisciplinary teams because the payment for those services is bundled across the team.

VALUE-BASED PAYMENT

For these reasons, there is now a steady shift from paying providers on an FFS basis to paying them for *value* or *outcomes*.[37] The premise of this shift to value-based payment (VBP) is to promote and reward/pay for activities that increase quality or improve patient outcomes. At present, 30% of Medicare payments are value-based, and the federal government has the goal of eventually getting to 100% by 2025 (see Table 6.1).

MERIT-BASED INCENTIVE PAYMENT SYSTEM

A law in 2015, the *Medicare Access and CHIP Reauthorization Act* (MACRA),[38] established the Quality Payment Program, of which the most significant element is the Merit-Based Incentive Payment System or MIPS. MIPS is a VBP designed to tie payments to quality and cost-efficient care, drive improvement in care processes and health outcomes, increase the use of healthcare information, and reduce the cost of care. Most healthcare providers, including APRNs, likely participate in this program, which has four components.

- *Quality*: Practices pick six quality measures from a set list to report and have their performance measured on. In 2020, this category was weighted at 45%.

- *Promoting interoperability*: Practices have an incentive to share information with other clinicians or patients via information technology to improve and coordinate care. This used to be called "meaningful use." In 2020, this category was weighted at 25%.

- *Improvement activities*: This assesses how practices improve care processes, enhance patient engagement in care, and increase access to care. Practices can choose from a list of activities appropriate to them such as enhancing care coordination, patient and clinician shared decision-making, and expansion of practice access. In 2020, this category was weighted at 15%.

- *Cost*: The cost of the care provided is calculated by CMS based on the practice or provider's Medicare claims. MIPS uses cost measures to gauge the total cost of care during the year or during a hospital stay. In 2020, this category was weighted at 15%.[39]

Table 6.1 PERCENTAGE OF US HEALTHCARE PAYMENTS TIED TO QUALITY AND VALUE

YEAR	MEDICAID	COMMERCIAL	MEDICARE ADVANTAGE	TRADITIONAL MEDICARE
2020	15%	15%	30%	30%
2022	25%	25%	50%	50%
2025	50%	50%	100%	100%

Source: Healthcare Payment Learning & Action Network.[69]

The way MIPS works is that practices are scored each calendar year on their weighted performance across these four areas. Payment to the practice can be increased by up to 9% for exceptional performance across these areas. The weighting of the cost area has steadily increased since the program was launched in 2017 and is scheduled to go up to 30% in 2022, while the quality area will go down to 30% at that time.

Interestingly, palliative care can help practices improve their MIPS score and, therefore increase payment, by improving their patients' care, their care coordination, and reducing unwanted or unnecessary costs. This gives practices a financial incentive to include palliative care in addition to usual care. Derrick's contacts have resulted in an oncology practice in their area expressing interest in piloting palliative care to some of their clinic patients. While this is primarily because the evidence increasingly shows that patients with cancer tolerate their treatments better and have better outcomes by adding palliative care to usual oncology care,[40] it does not hurt that palliative care could also help this oncology practice have higher MIPS scores and, therefore, payment.

ACCOUNTABLE CARE ORGANIZATIONS

An additional VBP arrangement is accountable care organizations (ACOs). ACOs were established in the ACA[41] and are an example of lesser known aspects of that law that sought to simultaneously improve quality and reduce healthcare costs. ACOs are groups of doctors, hospitals, and other healthcare providers who come together voluntarily to give coordinated high-quality care to their Medicare patients.[41] The goal of coordinated care is to ensure that patients get the right care at the right time while avoiding unnecessary duplication of services and preventing medical errors. When an ACO succeeds in both delivering high-quality care and spending healthcare dollars more wisely, the ACO will share in the savings it achieves for the Medicare program.[42] The payment concept behind ACOs is that of encouraging savings versus usual care. ACOs can either get a share of those savings, which is called *one-sided risk* since there is only the chance for higher payment, or they can participate in *two-sided risk*, where their share of any savings can be higher, but they can also be penalized if there are no savings. The number of ACOs has been somewhat stable due to the challenges of delivering savings year after year.[43] Again, this arrangement is

also an opportunity to incorporate aspects of palliative care into the care that ACOs deliver,[44] since, as noted earlier this chapter, palliative care can improve quality while potentially reducing costs. The health system that Shanice and Derrick's hospital is a part of has an ACO for its outpatient clinics and that ACO has also been talking to their palliative care team about ways to work together.

ALTERNATE PAYMENT MODELS

A final VBP option is that of alternate payment models (APMs) or care model demonstrations. Here, the federal government develops and offers new clinical models that seek to change care delivery by changing how that care is paid for. The ACA established a new department in CMS, that of the Innovation Center (CMMI).[45] CMMI is tasked with testing new care models with the goal of delivering care at comparable or lower cost to traditional Medicare programs. Subsequently, MACRA established a new process that allowed providers to submit their own alternate payment models to a committee called the Physician-Focused Payment Model Technical Advisory Committee (PTAC).[27] (Many nurses are dissatisfied with the name of this committee.) Practices participating in a PTAC-supported advanced APM are released from having to participate in the more complicated MIPS program and also receive a 5% lump sum bonus each year.[46] Because serious illness affects both quality of life for patients and the cost of their care, there have been several APMs for this population since CMMI was created in 2009. Two that were approved by PTAC were models developed by the American Academy of Hospice and Palliative Medicine (AAHPM) and the Coalition to Transform Advanced Care (C-TAC).[47] However, while the committee approved these models, they were not subsequently picked up for testing by CMMI. See Table 6.2 for a review of value-based models. Other CMMI models for serious illness are described below.

Medicare Care Choices Model

The Medicare Care Choices Model (MCCM) was an attempt to revise the Medicare Hospice Benefit (MHB). As many people likely know, the MHB currently requires patients to forego curative treatment when they enroll in hospice.[36] This limitation made sense in the early 1980s, when the MHB was

Table 6.2 VALUE-BASED MODELS

NAME	MERIT-BASED INCENTIVE PAYMENT SYSTEM (MIPS)	ACCOUNTABLE CARE ORGANIZATIONS (ACOs)	ALTERNATE PAYMENT MODELS (APMs)
Goal	Payment for quality and cost efficient care	Coordinated high-quality care to their Medicare patients	New clinical models that change care delivery by changing how that care is paid for
Strategy	Achieved by driving improvement in care processes and health outcomes, increasing the use of healthcare information, and reducing the cost of care	Achieved by ensuring that patients get the right care at the right time, while avoiding unnecessary duplication of services and preventing medical errors	Physician-Focused Payment Model Technical Advisory Committee (PTAC) released from having to participate in the more complicated MIPS program and also receive a 5% lump sum bonus each year

established mainly for cancer patients for whom there were not many treatment options. However, it has become increasingly problematic since then as more curative and palliative treatments are available. Shanice is all too aware of the MHB's limitations from her work as a hospice NP, where many of her patients delayed selecting hospice until the last days of life as they sought curative treatment instead.[48] CMS is also aware of these issues but is restricted from changing the MHB without evidence that any such changes would be cost-neutral or cheaper.

The MCCM was a way to test concurrent hospice and curative care as a 5-year model that launched in 2016, with the goal of allowing patients who met specific criteria to receive some hospice services in addition to curative treatment.[49] Instead of being paid their usual daily rate, participating MCCM hospices were paid $400 for per patient per month. For that fee, they were to provide symptom management and other support. The enrollment criteria limited eligible patients to having only four types of illnesses: advanced cancer, chronic obstructive pulmonary disease (COPD), congestive heart failure, or human immunodeficiency virus/acquired immunodeficiency syndrome (HIV/AIDS), and there were also limits on their Medicare insurance status.[49] The latter limits were loosened in 2017, when not enough patients were enrolled.[50] In 2020, CMS announced that they will extend the model by another year[50] and may further revise the elements of the model to make it available to more patients and to pay hospices more to participate. Shanice's former hospice was an MCCM participant, and she knew firsthand how challenging it was to provide appropriate care to those patients given the low monthly payments. Nonetheless, her hospice found that enough of their MCCM patients opted for full hospice sooner in their illness and therefore had longer lengths of stay with her hospice at the higher hospice daily rate. Derrick was also used to referring his former cancer patients to this MCCM program and is now grateful that this hospice offers MCCM as a way for their discharged palliative care patients not yet ready to choose full hospice to get some aspects of hospice care at home.

Primary Care First Model

A new CMMI model for serious illness will start in 2021. It is called the Primary Care First model and is intended to improve care and care coordination for those patients lacking a primary care provider. Even though the focus is primary care, this model has an option for primary care practices to enroll patients with serious illness and work with palliative care programs and/or hospices to help provide more supportive care to these patients. Again, payment is limited, and participating programs will have to be efficient in their care delivery.[50] Another related model, Direct Contracting, will let ACOs taking care of large groups of patients (5,000 or more) allow those patients to have concurrent hospice and curative care as appropriate.[51] Derrick and Shanice have heard the MCCM hospice in their area is interested in applying for the Serious Illness part of the new primary model since the hospice has learned how to optimize operations through its MCCM experience. And their health system's ACO is exploring the Direct Contracting option. The latter could be a way to fund the home-based palliative care program their team hopes for.

Medicare Advantage Value-Based Insurance Design Model

A final new model that has opportunities to improve access to care for serious illness is the Medicare Advantage Value-Based Insurance Design Model (MAV-BID).[52] This is scheduled to start in 2021 and will allow MA plans to offer hospice. Currently, any patient in an MA plan who chooses hospice has to withdraw from that plan and their providers, go into traditional Medicare, and get hospice via the MHB there. This transition was not always smooth for patients, and some were reluctant to leave their previous MA network providers. Hospices, however, have been concerned that private insurance companies, who are the organizations that provide MA, may choose to do hospice on their own and not work with existing hospices in their areas. However, those MA plans that do work with existing hospices will be able to be flexible about when patients can enroll in hospice and can let them also have concurrent curative care. This could allow patients with serious illness enrolled in MA to get home-based palliative care as they transition into hospice care. Derrick and Shanice are guessing that the large MA plan in their state will likely want to participate in this VBID model and that this may give their patients who have MA an additional care option. See Table 6.3 for a comparison of CMMI models.

Table 6.3 CMS INNOVATION CENTER (CMMI) MODELS

MODEL	MEDICARE CARE CHOICES MODEL (MCCM)	PRIMARY CARE FIRST (PCF) MODEL	MEDICARE ADVANTAGE VALUE-BASED INSURANCE DESIGN MODEL (MAV-BID)
Year initiated and purpose	2016 launch for a 5-year test of concurrent hospice and curative care, now expanded through 2021	2021 launch to improve care and care coordination for those patients lacking a primary care provider.	2021 launch to allow MA plans to offer hospice
Goal	Allowing patients who met specific criteria to receive some hospice services in addition to curative treatment[49]	An option for primary care practices to enroll patients with serious illness and work with palliative care programs and/or hospices to help provide more supportive care to these patients	Goal of continuity of care, smoother transition of care

Health Insurance Company Models

In a good example of the benefits of a health system with public and private components, Aetna, a national health insurer, launched the Aetna Compassionate Care Program (ACCP) in 2004, targeting members diagnosed with an advanced illness with a view to increase access to palliative care and hospice services. This programs continues to this day and has reported encouraging outcomes, such as 79% of members choosing hospice versus 59% of members not in the program and having improved quality of life while saving money in less aggressive treatment at the end of life.[53] More large health insurance plans have explored offering similar palliative care benefits or hiring community-based palliative care providers like Aspire,[54] Optum,[55] Resolution Care,[56] and Landmark[57] to provide these benefits to their members.

STATE POLICY

So far, this chapter has focused on federal policy and payment, but there are also encouraging developments for palliative care at the state level. Perhaps the most important is a 2018 California law that required all of the state's managed Medicaid programs to offer home-based palliative care to patients with advanced illness.[58] Because this was a statewide requirement, there was suddenly the need to set up home-based palliative care programs to provide these services in all 58 counties of California. Innovative programs sprang up, some using telehealth to reach patients in the most rural parts of the state.[56] These programs are young and working hard to overcome logistical barriers, such as identifying appropriate patients, seeing them quickly and regularly, and doing so on a cost-efficient basis. But the law and the home-based palliative care infrastructure it is building are of interest, and other states are now considering similar legislation as well.[59]

Other states are also using legislation to set up palliative care councils to study opportunities for serious illness care and to begin to develop the infrastructure to deliver it.[60] New York passed laws requiring hospitals and other providers to tell patients of the existence of palliative care,[61] but this law did not include money to pay for implementing that requirement. Maryland passed a law in 2013, requiring all hospitals with more than 50 beds to provide basic aspects of palliative care,[62] although it is unclear if this has really improved access to palliative care there.[63] Other states have various additional bills which suggest a growing local interest in palliative care.[59] Derrick was part of an effort to lobby state legislators to consider a palliative care council bill in their state. He's also participated in his state's annual "Nurses Day," where nurses visit the state capitol to advocate for legislation they support. (He also met with state legislators to educate them about the benefits of expanding CNS scope of practice.)

Finally, local health insurance companies and other payers are setting up home- or community-based palliative care programs on their own as well. These are similar to the federal models but involve local health plans working with a palliative care program to identify patients who could benefit from these services and then help them access this care.[64] Insurance companies have the incentive to both improve the quality of their care and to reduce costs, and, once again, palliative care can help do this for people with serious illness. Derrick learned of Blue Shield of California's home-based palliative care program at a national palliative care conference[65] and is hoping that their program could explore the same with the large insurance company in their area.

CASE STUDY: PRACTICE AUTHORITY (CONCLUSION)

After a smooth transition to the palliative care team, Derrick was able to help Shanice develop a better understanding of the importance of health policy to the care they deliver and that their patients and their families need. Both have seen how clinicians, APRNs in particular, need to be involved with policy developments since many of the care and payment models assume APRN participation. In the process, Derrick has started to become a policy expert in his own right and is becoming recognized for that expertise in nursing. Both he and Shanice have learned the truth to the policy saying: Be at the table or on the menu.[66] But, most important, they have learned how to use policy to improve the access and quality of the care that their patients and their families get—which has made them even more effective palliative APRNs.

SUMMARY

This chapter has discussed how health policy and payment policy affect the care of those with serious illness, particularly in regard to access to palliative care. It has used case studies of two APRNs, an NP and a CNS, to show the implications of policy on APRN practice. Palliative care has been shown to meet the triple aim of health reform by improving the quality of care and the health of the serious illness population and showing how unnecessary and unwanted treatments, and their resulting costs, can be reduced. Palliative care's contribution to value-based payment has also been shared. The chapter has reviewed some key legislative and regulatory developments that are encouraging for those living with serious illness and their access to palliative care services. Several encouraging alternate payment models and demonstrations will launch in the next few years that could further improve access and care for those with serious illness. Finally, the case study examples of the two APRNs show how palliative APRNs can become involved with policy and contribute to this important area.

REFERENCES

1. Hartman M, Martin AB, Benson J, Catlin A. The National Health Expenditure Accounts Team. National healthcare spending in 2018: Growth driven by accelerations in Medicare and private insurance spending: *Health Aff (Millwood)*. 2020;39(1):8–17. doi:10.1377/hlthaff.2019.01451

2. Tikkanen T, Abrams M. US healthcare from a global perspective, 2019: Issue Briefs, January 20, 2020. Higher spending, worse outcomes? New York, NY: Commonwealth Fund. https://www.commonwealthfund.org/publications/issue-briefs/2020/jan/us-health-care-global-perspective-2019

3. Institute of Medicine. *Dying in America: Improving Quality and Honoring Individual Preferences Near the End of Life.* Washington, DC: National Academies Press; 2014. https://www.nap.edu/catalog/18748/dying-in-america-improving-quality-and-honoring-individual-preferences-near

4. Leonhardt M. Americans now spend twice as much on healthcare as they did in the 1980s. CNBC. October 9, 2019. https://www.cnbc.com/2019/10/09/americans-spend-twice-as-much-on-health-care-today-as-in-the-1980s.html

5. Dougherty C. The massive impact of COVID-19 on US healthcare. BRINK–News and Insights on Global Risk. July 13, 2020. https://www.brinknews.com/the-massive-impact-of-covid-19-on-us-health-care/

6. Seervai S. Blog. Coronavirus reveals flaws in the US health system. New York, NY; Commonwealth Fund. March 6, 2020. https://doi.org/10.26099/fmdc-jp90

7. National Academies of Sciences, Engineering, and Medicine; Health and Medicine Division; Board on Population Health and Public Health Practice; Committee on Community-Based Solutions to Promote Health Equity in the United States; Baciu A, Negussie Y, Geller A, et al., editors. Communities in Action: Pathways to Health Equity. Washington (DC): National Academies Press (US); 2017 Jan 11. 2, The State of Health Disparities in the United States. https://www.ncbi.nlm.nih.gov/books/NBK425844/

8. Institute for Healthcare Improvement. Initiatives. IHI triple aim initiative. Boston, MA. 2021. http://www.ihi.org:80/Engage/Initiatives/TripleAim/Pages/default.aspx

9. Feeley D. The triple aim or the quadruple aim? Four points to help set your strategy. Line of Sight. Institute of Health Improvement Blog. November 28, 2017. Available at http://www.ihi.org/communities/blogs/the-triple-aim-or-the-quadruple-aim-four-points-to-help-set-your-strategy

10. United States Census Bureau. By 2030, All Baby Boomers will be age 65 or older. United States Census Bureau. Washington, DC. December 10, 2019. https://www.census.gov/library/stories/2019/12/by-2030-all-baby-boomers-will-be-age-65-or-older.html

11. Home Care, Hospice and Palliative Care Alliance of New Hampshire. CMS provides guidance on medicare advantage supplemental benefits. Manchester, NH. May 3, 2018. https://homecarenh.org/wp-content/uploads/2018/05/cms-provides-guidance-on-medicare-advantage-supplemental-benefits/

12. Gregg G, Roy A. Nursing homes & assisted living facilities account for 45% of COVID-19 deaths. FREOPP.org. May 7, 2020. https://freopp.org/the-covid-19-nursing-home-crisis-by-the-numbers-3a47433c3f70

13. LaFave S. The impact of COVID-19 on older adults. The Hub. Johns Hopkins University. May 5, 2020. https://hub.jhu.edu/2020/05/05/impact-of-covid-19-on-the-elderly/

14. Meier DE, Back AL, Berman A, Block SD, Corrigan JM, Morrison RS. A national strategy for palliative care. *Health Aff.* 2017;36(7):1265–1273. doi:10.1377/hlthaff.2017.0164

15. Lustbader D, Mudra M, Romano C, et al. The impact of a home-based palliative care program in an accountable care organization. *J Palliat Med.* 2017;20(1):23–28. doi:10.1089/jpm.2016.0265

16. May P, Garrido MM, Cassel JB, et al. Palliative care teams' cost-saving effect is larger for cancer patients with higher numbers of comorbidities. *Health Aff.* 2016;35(1):44–53. doi:10.1377/hlthaff.2015.0752

17. Elnadry J. Home-based palliative care reduces hospital readmissions (S735). *J Pain Symptom Manage.* 2017;53(2):428–429. doi:10.1016/j.jpainsymman.2016.12.245

18. World Health Organization. Health system governance. Geneva, Switzerland. 2021. https://www.who.int/topics/health_policy/en/

19. HealthCare.gov. Affordable Care Act (ACA). Washington, DC. 2021. https://www.healthcare.gov/glossary/affordable-care-act/

20. Mary Labyak Institute for Innovation. Pediatric concurrent care. Alexandria, VA; National Hospice and Palliative Care Organization; 2012. https://www.uclahealth.org/Palliative-Care/Workfiles/Pediatric-Concurrent-Care.pdf

21. Warner. Warner, Isakson, Blumenauer & Roe introduce bipartisan legislation to enhance planning options for patients with advanced illnesses. US Representative Phil Roe. June 12, 2017. https://www.warner.senate.gov/public/index.cfm/2017/6/warner-isakson-blumenauer-roe-introduce-bipartisan-legislation-to-enhance-planning-options-for-patients-with-advanced-illnesses

22. Ramthum S, Kocinski J. PCHETA. AAHPM Quarterly. Winter 2020. 16 Feature | AAHPM. http://aahpm.org/quarterly/winter-16-feature

23. American Association of Colleges of Nursing. Nursing fact sheet. Updated April 1, 2019. https://www.aacnnursing.org/News-Information/Fact-Sheets/Nursing-Fact-Sheet

24. Reinhart RJ. Nurses continue to rate highest in honesty, ethics. Gallup.com. January 6, 2020. https://news.gallup.com/poll/274673/nurses-continue-rate-highest-honesty-ethics.aspx

25. Coalition to Transform Advanced Care. Regulatory work. 2021. https://www.thectac.org/regulatory/

26. CMS. Frequently asked questions about billing the physician fee schedule for advance care planning services. July 14, 2016. https://www.cms.gov/medicare/medicare-fee-for-service-payment/physicianfeesched/downloads/faq-advance-care-planning.pdf

27. US Department of Health and Human Services. ASPE—Office of the Assistant Secretary for Planning and Evaluation. Physician-focused payment model technical advisory committee (PTAC). February 17, 2016. Updated June 22, 2020. https://aspe.hhs.gov/ptac-physician-focused-payment-model-technical-advisory-committee

28. US Department of Health and Human Services. Centers for Medicare and Medicaid Services. Medicare Drug & Health Plan Contract Administration Group. Reinterpretation of "primarily health related" for supplemental benefits. April 17, 2018. https://www.nahc.org/wp-content/uploads/2018/05/HPMS-Memo-Primarily-Health-Related-4-27-18.pdf

29. Center for Connected Health Policy. Introduction to Telehealth Policy. 2021. https://www.cchpca.org/telehealth-policy/telehealth-and-medicare

30. Costantino R, Gressler L, Rothwell C, Groninger H, Kearney C, Walker K. Examining the effects of palliative telehealth connecting hospital to home (Patch) program on quality of life. *J Pain Symptom Manage.* 2018;56(6):e104. doi:10.1016/j.jpainsymman.2018.10.350

31. Access to Telehealth. President Donald J. Trump is expanding access to telehealth services and ensuring continued access to healthcare for rural Americans. White House Archives. August 3, 2020. https://trumpwhitehouse.archives.gov/briefings-statements/president-donald-j-trump-expanding-access-telehealth-services-ensuring-continued-access-healthcare-rural-americans/

32. Magnan S. Social determinants of health 101 for healthcare: Five plus five. *NAM Perspect.* October 9, 2017. doi:10.31478/201710c

33. Healthinsurance.org What is fee-for-service? June 5, 2017. https://www.healthinsurance.org/glossary/fee-for-service/

34. Mehrotra A, Chernew M, Linetsky D, Hatch H, Cutler D. The impact of the COVID-19 pandemic on outpatient visits: A rebound emerges. May 19, 2020. New York, NY: Commonwealth Fund. https://www.commonwealthfund.org/publications/2020/apr/impact-covid-19-outpatient-visits

35. Basu S, Phillips RS, Phillips R, Peterson LE, Landon BE. Primary care practice finances in the United States amid the COVID-19 pandemic. *Health Aff* (Millwood). 2020;30(9):1605–1614. doi:10.1377/hlthaff.2020.00794

36. US Department of Centers for Medicare and Medicaid Services. Medicare.gov Hospice care coverage. 2021. https://www.medicare.gov/coverage/hospice-care

37. US Department of Centers for Medicare and Medicaid Services. What are the Value Based Programs? CMS.gov. 2021. Page Last Modified: 01/06/2020. https://www.cms.gov/Medicare/Quality-Initiatives-Patient-Assessment-Instruments/Value-Based-Programs/Value-Based-Programs

38. US Department of Centers for Medicare and Medicaid Services. MACRA. CMS.gov. Page Last Modified: 11/18/2019. https://www.cms.gov/Medicare/Quality-Initiatives-Patient-Assessment-Instruments/Value-Based-Programs/MACRA-MIPS-and-APMs/MACRA-MIPS-and-APMs

39. U.S. Centers for Medicare and Medicaid Services. Quality Payment Program. Participation Options Overview. MIPS. 2021. https://qpp.cms.gov/mips/overview

40. Haun MW, Estel S, Rücker G, et al. Early palliative care for adults with advanced cancer. *Cochrane Database Syst Rev.* 2017;6(6):CD011129. doi:10.1002/14651858.CD011129.pub2

41. Gold J. Accountable care organizations, explained. Kaiser Health News. September 14, 2015. https://khn.org/news/aco-accountable-care-organization-faq/

42. US Department of Centers for Medicare and Medicaid Services. Accountable care organizations (ACOs). CMS.gov. Page Last Modified: 03/04/2021. https://www.cms.gov/Medicare/Medicare-Fee-for-Service-Payment/ACO

43. Muhlestein D, Bleser W, Saunder R, Richards R, Singletary E, McClellan M. Spread of ACOs and value-based payment models in 2019: Gauging the impact of pathways to success. Health Affairs Blog. October 21, 2019. Available at https://www.healthaffairs.org/do/10.1377/hblog20191020.962600/full/

44. Center to Advance Palliative Care. Strategies for health systems, health plans, and ACOs. 2021. New York, NY: CAPC. https://www.capc.org/strategies/

45. Kaiser Family Foundation. "What is CMMI?" and 11 other FAQs about the CMS Innovation Center. February 27, 2018. https://www.kff.org/medicare/fact-sheet/what-is-cmmi-and-11-other-faqs-about-the-cms-innovation-center/

46. Doolittle D. Get details about your 5% medicare bonus. Texas Medical Association. Updated November 5, 2019. https://www.texmed.org/Template.aspx?id=51937

47. Coalition to Transform Advanced Care. HHS panel advances C-TAC and AAHPM's payment models. Coalition to Transform Advance Care. C-TAC News. Published March 26, 2018. Available at https://www.thectac.org/2018/03/hhs-panel-advances-c-tac-and-aahpms-payment-model-proposal/

48. National Hospice and Palliative Care Organization. *NHPCO hospice facts & figures 2020 edition.* Alexandria, VA: NHPCO. August 20, 2020. https://www.nhpco.org/wp-content/uploads/NHPCO-Facts-Figures-2020-edition.pdf

49. US Department of Centers for Medicare and Medicaid Services. Medicare Care Choices Model (MCCM): The first two years. December 11, 2017. CMS.gov. https://www.cms.gov/newsroom/fact-sheets/medicare-care-choices-model-mccm-first-two-years

50. Sinclair S, Silvers A. Payment and program financing. FAQs on the new seriously ill population alternative payment model option. Center to Advance Palliative Care Blog, November 1, 2019. Available at https://www.capc.org/blog/faqs-new-seriously-ill-population-sip-alternative-payment-model-option/

51. US Department of Centers for Medicare and Medicaid Services. Direct contracting. CMSgov. April 22, 2019. https://www.cms.gov/newsroom/fact-sheets/direct-contracting

52. US Department of Centers for Medicare and Medicaid Services. Medicare Advantage value-based insurance design model. CMS.gov Last updated on: 08/17/2021. https://innovation.cms.gov/innovation-models/vbid

53. Baquet-Simpson A, Spettell CM, Freeman AN, et al. Aetna's compassionate care program: Sustained value for our members with advanced illness. *J Palliat Med.* 2019;22(11):1324–1330. doi:10.1089/jpm.2018.0359

54. Aspire Health. Home page. 2021. http://aspirehealthcare.com/

55. Optum care. Home page. 2021. Home page. https://www.optum-care.com

56. Resolution Care Network. Home page. 2021. https://www.resolutioncare.com/

57. Landmark. House calls conversations: Palliative care. May 15, 2019. https://www.landmarkhealth.org/palliative-care/

58. Department of Healthcare Services. Palliative care and SB 1004. CA.gov. Last modified date: 3/23/2021. https://www.dhcs.ca.gov/provgovpart/Pages/Palliative-Care-and-SB-1004.aspx

59. National Academy for State Healthcare Policy. State strategies to build and support palliative care. Last updated August 23, 2021. https://www.nashp.org/state-strategies-to-address-palliative-care/

60. Sinclair S. A new foundation for state palliative care policy activity. Center to Advance Palliative Care Blog. Updated April 30, 2019. Available at https://www.capc.org/blog/new-foundation-state-palliative-care-policy-activity/

61. New York State Department of Health. Palliative Care Access Act (PHL Section 2997-d): Palliative care requirements for hospitals, nursing homes, home care and assisted living residences (enhanced and special needs). Revised: August 2011. https://www.health.ny.gov/professionals/patients/patient_rights/palliative_care/phl_2997_d_memo.htm

62. Lacasse L. Palliative care legislation signed in Maryland. American Cancer Society Cancer Action Network. Cancer CANdor Blog. May 7, 2013. Available at https://www.fightcancer.org/cancer-candor/palliative-care-legislation-signed-maryland

63. Gibbs KD, Mahon MM, Truss M, Eyring K. An assessment of hospital-based palliative care in Maryland: Infrastructure, barriers, and opportunities. *J Pain Symptom Manage.* 2015;49(6):1102–1108. doi:10.1016/j.jpainsymman.2014.12.004

64. BlueCross Blue Shield. Blue Shield of California expands palliative care program, offers home-based care statewide. March 15, 2018. https://www.bcbs.com/press-releases/blue-shield-of-california-expands-palliative-care-program-offers-home-based-care

65. Vallene, K. A health plan's approach to providing palliative care everywhere. CAPC National Seminar 2018. Poster Session: Collaborative Models. https://www.capc.org/seminar/poster-sessions/a-health-plans-approach-to-providing-palliative-care-everywhere/

66. Murray P. If you're not at the table, you're on the menu. Medium. May 23, 2017. https://medium.com/@PattyMurray/if-youre-not-at-the-table-you-re-on-the-menu-932c0f76550a

67. Congress.gov. H.R.647—116th Congress (2019–2020): Palliative Care and Hospice Education and Training Act. October 29, 2019. https://www.congress.gov/bill/116th-congress/house-bill/647

68. US Department of Centers for Medicare and Medicaid Services. Medicare Advantage Plans cover all Medicare services. Medicare.gov. 2021. https://www.medicare.gov/what-medicare-covers/what-medicare-health-plans-cover/medicare-advantage-plans-cover-all-medicare-services

69. Healthcare Payment Learning and Action Network. What is the Healthcare Payment Learning & Action Network? Last updated on: 06/21/2021. https://hcp-lan.org

7.

THE PALLIATIVE APRN IN RESEARCH AND EVIDENCE-BASED PRACTICE

Janice Linton and Joan G. Carpenter

KEY POINTS

- Research is a systematic investigation that contributes to generalizable knowledge.

- Advanced practice registered nurses (APRNs) evaluate and apply research evidence in quality improvement projects and evidence-based practice.

- Evidence-based practice embodies the "quadruple aim" of improved patient outcomes, with high-quality care, at better cost, delivered by empowered clinicians.

CASE STUDY: FRAMING A RESEARCH QUESTION

A palliative advanced practice registered nurse (APRN) in the post-acute nursing home care setting noticed that many of his patients experience high levels of anxiety and insomnia after admission. Their medical diagnoses and comorbidities varied, but one commonality is that all had cognitive impairment and had been recently discharged from a hospital setting. He knew that changes in care setting can exacerbate confusion, but he also recognized that a change in care setting may disrupt the therapeutic interventions that were started and stabilized in the hospital. While he has managed their anxiety and insomnia with medications and improved their comfort, he began to consider how he might research this clinical problem and develop non-drug therapies to manage it.

INTRODUCTION

The advanced practice registered nurse (APRN) in research is uniquely situated to generate new evidence that is meaningful to advance hospice and palliative care science.[1] Through their holistic approach to patients with serious illness and care partners, palliative APRNs evaluate and apply research evidence in quality improvement (QI) projects and evidence-based practice (EBP).[2] However, some APRNs may be unsure how to integrate these activities into their busy clinical practice. Furthermore, APRNs may have had limited exposure to research and QI in their education and training. The purpose of this chapter is to explore and expand the role of the APRN in research, QI, and EBP activities with a focus on hospice and palliative care.

DEFINING RESEARCH

"RESEARCH" AND "NOT RESEARCH"

According to the Code of Federal Regulations that govern the conduct of research, 45 CFR 46.102,[3] research is "a systematic investigation including research development, testing and evaluation, designed to develop or contribute to generalizable knowledge." Therefore, a project is research if it uses a commonly accepted scientific method and its results will be applied to the wider population that the study sample represents. In contrast, a project that includes an arbitrary collection of information without wide generalizability is not considered research.

The interpretation of the term "systematic investigation" depends on the scientific method—that is, the organized approach to gathering information. It is possible for research to be systematic without reflecting the process of the traditional scientific method (e.g., hypothesis testing using controlled experiments). For example, a palliative APRN may conduct interviews and observe the actions of nurses in an inpatient hospice unit caring for individuals with dyspnea. In this example, there may not be a hypothesis prior to data collection about how the nurses will respond to and treat dyspnea; however, data collection is purposeful in the selection of participants, decisions about actions to record, and interview questions to ask (e.g., data collection). To help clarify this, the Office of Human Research Protections (commonly referred to as OHRP) offers guidance of the systematic process of research as, "observations are obtained under clearly specified, and, where possible, controlled conditions that can be measured and evaluated."[4]

SYSTEMATIC INQUIRY

Systematic investigation involves the collection and use of data. To conduct an investigation, the palliative APRN develops a study plan. This includes several steps that begin with a statement of the problem and its significance and

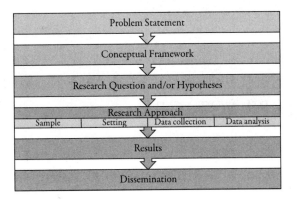

```
┌─────────────────────────────────────────────────────┐
│                 Problem Statement                     │
├─────────────────────────────────────────────────────┤
│                        ▽                              │
│                Conceptual Framework                   │
├─────────────────────────────────────────────────────┤
│                        ▽                              │
│         Research Question and/or Hypotheses           │
├─────────────────────────────────────────────────────┤
│                        ▽                              │
│                  Research Approach                    │
├──────────┬──────────┬──────────────┬─────────────────┤
│  Sample  │ Setting  │ Data collection│  Data analysis │
├──────────┴──────────┴──────────────┴─────────────────┤
│                      Results                          │
├─────────────────────────────────────────────────────┤
│                        ▽                              │
│                   Dissemination                       │
└─────────────────────────────────────────────────────┘
```

Figure 7.1 Framework for a Study Plan

end with a dissemination strategy. In between, the palliative APRN considers several key elements: a conceptual framework that organizes the research variables, the research question to be answered by the study, and, if needed, a list of hypotheses to be tested. An essential element is a depiction of the research approach—a description of the potential participants, the setting where the study will take place, and the process of data collection and analysis. It is important also to remember that beyond just reporting research results to the study team, the APRN should create a plan to widely disseminate systematic inquiry. This may involve presentations at peer-reviewed, professional conferences and local opportunities to present the research within the community or the organization where it was conducted, as well as articles in journals. Including the study site in the dissemination plan is recommended because study sites often state that they don't hear back from the team that conducted research in their settings. The framework in Box 7.1 presents a structured way of thinking through a study plan.

DATA AS EVIDENCE

Data are plain facts. When data are collected, processed, organized, structured, or presented in a given context to be useful, they are called *evidence*. Pieces of evidence can be used in an analysis of a problem, such as the diagnosis and treatment of a health condition. Research data can be quantitative or qualitative information that is collected, observed, or created for purposes of analysis to produce original research results. Table 7.1 provides common data definitions and related phrases.

It's important to remember that, more often than not, the plural form of data should be used. For example, "*these data* support previous findings" and "*the data* challenge current practice." Research data are generated for different purposes and through different processes and may be grouped into different categories. Each category of research may require a different type of data management plan. Two commonly accepted approaches to conducting research and collecting data are through qualitative and quantitative research methods.

QUALITATIVE RESEARCH

Qualitative data are narrative or subjective and often describe attitudes, beliefs, and feelings. They are not arrived at by statistical or other quantitative techniques. Rather, the goal is to understand behavior in a natural setting and the perspective of research participants within the context of their everyday life. Qualitative research is inductive, rather than deductive. Common methods palliative APRNs may use for qualitative inquiry include interviewing, ethnography, participant observation, and focus groups. APRNs may conduct primary data collection or analyze previously collected data (e.g., secondary data analysis).

An example of qualitative research is the study by Lim et al.[5] They provide several examples of ways to apply qualitative inquiry in a previously conducted clinical trial testing a palliative care intervention. First, the team analyzed clinician documentation in medical records to describe the different components of a palliative care intervention. Second, they conducted focus groups and interviews to explore clinicians' perspectives on the results from the first study and validate their findings. Last, they performed an analysis of patient–clinician palliative care intervention audio recordings to endorse the findings from the first two studies. Applying qualitative inquiry in this way, the investigators were able to provide a deeper understanding of different components of the palliative care intervention.

Because of the subjective nature of qualitative research, it is important for investigators to maintain objectivity, avoid bias, and ensure trustworthiness when conducting qualitative inquiry. Credibility, dependability, and transferability are three concepts that strengthen trustworthiness. To achieve credibility, a researcher and their team members keep active documentation about the process. They write field notes describing events during data collection, keep a study diary that includes reflections during data collection and analysis, and conduct regular debriefing sessions. Debriefing and reflexive dialogue through discussion of beliefs, values, and assumptions help to prevent imposing preexisting views on data and diminish bias.[6] An audit trail that contains detailed analytic memos made during data analysis contributes to dependability. In addition, when two or more data sources are employed, the investigator can use triangulation to develop a comprehensive understanding of the data and ensure dependability.[7] Transferability, or how results from qualitative inquiry can be applied to other contexts, can be strengthened with the use of an audit trail, field notes, and memos. Researchers often refer to "think description" as a way for others to determine to what extent the study findings transfer to other people and settings, or another context.[8]

QUANTITATIVE RESEARCH

The main purpose of quantitative research is to use numerical data to describe a situation or event, explain a relationship, or determine causality between independent (intervention) and dependent (outcome) variables.[9] Quantitative data are

Table 7.1 DATA DEFINITIONS AND RELATED PHRASES

Categorical data	Categorical data are qualitative and suited to classification into categories. Further divisible into nominal (names), ordinal (levels of quality, development), and dichotomized (mutually exclusive).
Continuous data	Data that have an infinite number of possible values.
Database	An organized collection of data. A medical database is all the information that exists in the practice at any time.
Data adjustment	For useful results, data often need to be modified before analysis (e.g., for age, sex, or difficulty or number of attempts).
Data aggregation	A collection of protected health information used to conduct data analysis relating to the healthcare operations of the entity.
Data analysis	Submission of data to statistical analysis; includes sorting into categories and determining relationships between variables.
Data capture	A mechanism for collecting specified segments or categories of data from a stream of automatically recorded data, some of which may be irrelevant for the specific purpose.
Data processing	The collection of data, processing of the data to obtain usable information, and communication of this usable information.
Observational data	Data captured in real time, usually irreplaceable (e.g., sensor data, survey data, sample data, neurological images).
Ordinal data	A type of data containing limited categories with a ranking from the lowest to the highest (e.g., none, mild, moderate, severe). Subjects placed in order from high to low. For instance, an employer might rank applicants for a job on their professional experience, giving a rank of 1 to the subject who has the least experience, 2 to the next highest, and so on. This rank does not tell us by how much subjects differ.
Pre-existing data	Data that were in existence before the commencement of a study. Of limited value unless they are exactly the data required, they have been collected adequately, and a group of pre-existing controls with their corresponding data can be identified.
Prevalence data	Disease occurrences are recorded against the size of the population at risk at the time.
Ratio-level data	A higher level of data than the interval level because the ratio has an absolute zero point that we know how to measure. Thus, weight is an example of the ratio scale because it has an absolute zero that we can measure.
Raw data	Data as they are collected, before any calculation, ordering, etc., has been done.

Adapted from The Free Dictionary website (http://medicaldictionary.thefreedictionary.com/data).

measurable; data are collected, analyzed, and expressed in statistical form with numbers using descriptive and inferential statistics. Descriptive statistics can be used to answer questions that explore situations. For example, a palliative APRN may ask, "What is the length of stay in the hospital for patients after a palliative care consultation?" Inferential statistics elucidate the relationships among study variables and are often more complex than descriptive studies: "Are patients who receive a palliative care consultation more or less likely to be discharged home from the hospital on hospice care?" Studies that aim to predict and control or manipulate variables in experimental or quasi-experimental study designs rely on inferential statistics.

Well-conducted quantitative research studies depend on the extent to which an APRN enhances the quality of a study. Measurement of validity and reliability are important concepts to support rigor in quantitative studies.[10] Internal validity means that a test or instrument used in a study is precise in measuring what it is supposed to. External validity is also known as *generalizability*—the likelihood that findings will apply to a larger population than the study sample. Reliability implies consistency; that is, that the research methods produce the same results on the same object of measurement in the same setting over a number of repeated observations. To ensure validity and reliability, the palliative APRN should make sure that the research design is appropriate for the question to be answered and that the research is conducted carefully by a highly qualified team.

MIXED METHODS

Using both quantitative and qualitative data, mixed-method research integrates them and draws interpretations based on both sets of data to understand a research question. Combining the data, the researcher uses the strength of each approach in one method to better understand a phenomenon that quantitative or qualitative data may not explain individually. The key ingredient in this method is the *integration* of the two data sources, not just the gathering of quantitative and qualitative data. According to Creswell,[11] three mixed-method designs include convergent, explanatory sequential, and exploratory sequential. *Convergent designs* collect both quantitative and qualitative data at the same time; researchers analyze the data together. In an *explanatory sequential design*, investigators use quantitative methods and then qualitative methods to explain the quantitative results. In an *exploratory sequential design*, qualitative methods are used to explore a problem. The results are then used to build a quantitative phase of the project.

QUALITY IMPROVEMENT

QI is intended to improve a known gap in performance (e.g., standard) at a specific clinical site for an immediate effect to those involved. The purpose of QI is to apply what is already known (e.g., evidence) in local practice; its intent is to improve care in a specific setting. It is distinct from research: research methods are designed to add new, generalizable knowledge to

what was previously known. In QI, APRNs may see observable results over time with direct benefit to those people directly involved. QI approaches may include qualitative, quantitative, or mixed methods. Furthermore, a project may be both QI and research. Palliative APRNs need to make sure they have the appropriate level of regulatory and organizational oversight for a project. Institutional Review Boards (IRBs) review and monitor human subject research and provide insight on whether a project qualifies as research or QI. Table 7.2 lists organizational research resources for palliative APRNs, and many of these resources also can be used to inform QI projects.

CASE STUDY: FRAMING A RESEARCH QUESTION (CONTINUED)

The palliative APRN met with one of his colleagues to discuss the anxiety and insomnia he has observed in his post-acute care patients. His colleague introduced him to a PhD-prepared nurse investigator with a funded research program studying persons

Table 7.2 ORGANIZATIONAL RESEARCH RESOURCES FOR PALLIATIVE APRNS

ORGANIZATION	DESCRIPTION	WEBSITE	UNIQUE ASPECTS
Hospice and Palliative Nurses Association (HPNA)	HPNA is the national professional organization that represents the specialty of palliative nursing. Research is one of five pillars of excellence.	https://advancingexpertcare.org/HPNA/Default.aspx	Opportunities for grant funding through the foundation and networking through the research special interest group Supports training and development for early-career APRN investigators through the research scholars program and the emerging research scholars special interest group Research agenda offers foci for increasing practice evidence Research advisory council
American Academy of Nurse Practitioners (AANP) Network for Research	The AANP Network for Research (AANPNR) is an online community for AANP members interested in research. It is a web-based platform to share resources and ideas with other NPs as well as a monthly newsletter with information on funding opportunities, upcoming conferences, research updates.	https://www.aanp.org/about/research-opportunities/aanp-network-for-research-aanpnr	Offers a variety of methods to collect high-quality data through surveys Researchers may also submit a set of tailored questions through AANP's annual surveys Unique access to the NP workforce
National Institute of Nursing Research (NINR) of the National Institutes of Health (NIH)	NINR supports and conducts clinical and basic research and research training on health and illness that develops the scientific basis for clinical practice.	https://www.ninr.nih.gov/ https://www.ninr.nih.gov/researchandfunding/desp/oepcr	The lead NIH institute on end-of-life and palliative care research and training.
Palliative Care Research Cooperative	The PCRC is an interdisciplinary research community committed to advancing rigorous palliative care science and improving care for people with serious illness.	https://palliativecareresearch.org	Develops efficient palliative care research capacity nationally Infrastructure Supports the conduct, analysis, and dissemination of high-quality research in palliative care Trains and mentors new, existing, and future clinician-scientists committed to advancing palliative care research

living with mild cognitive impairment and dementia and their family care partners. They quickly reviewed and discussed the existing literature that describes this problem and realized there was very little evidence to guide practice. At that point, they wanted to design a project but could not decide if it should be research or QI.

- What do you think are the best next steps?

- What method do you think would help them come to a better understanding of his clinical phenomenon?

- What are the strengths and benefits of each of the approaches just described?

- What challenges might they face?

APPLYING RESEARCH EVIDENCE

Evidence comes from research, quality improvement projects, consensus statements, guidelines, expert opinions, practice and experience, and patient values. Delivering evidence-based care to improve patient outcomes and clinical practice is the role of palliative APRNs. APRNs may recall that, for decades, the protocol to maintain the patency of intravenous catheters was flushing every 8 hours with a heparin solution. Flushing intravenous catheters with heparin presented risks such as heparin-induced thrombocytopenia.[12] Research later supported that normal saline is effective in reducing catheter occlusion.[13] Normal saline solution flush is now a part of the current practice to maintain the patency of intravenous access. Protocols and practice are no longer driven by "the way we have always done things" but by high-quality, EBP.

EVIDENCE-BASED PRACTICE

EBP is a structured problem-solving approach for health-related issues using the triad of best research (external evidence), clinical expertise (internal evidence), and patient preferences and values to support clinical decision-making for best outcomes (Figure 7.2).[14] EBP embodies the Quadruple Aim[15] of improved patient outcomes, with high-quality care, at better cost, delivered by empowered clinicians. Individuals are living longer, but many endure chronic and life-threatening illnesses. When hospitalized, these individuals facing life-threatening illnesses require interdisciplinary collaboration between intensivists, oncologists, and palliative care teams. Palliative APRNs engage in goals-of-care conversations with patients and families and use best evidence to support patient preferences and values. Palliative APRNs, empowered to engage in EBP, follow a seven-step systematic approach beginning with a deep sense of inquiry.

CASE STUDY: EVIDENCE-BASED PRACTICE

Mr. B, was a 75-year-old man who presented to the hospital for respiratory distress secondary to congestive heart failure exacerbation. He was in respiratory failure requiring ventilator support. His hospital course included recurrent pulmonary effusions,

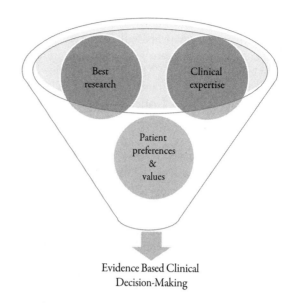

Figure 7.2 Evidence-based practice elements.

despite ongoing diuretic therapy, and therapeutic thoracentesis. Lab results were significant for acute renal failure and hypoalbuminemia. Mr. B was extubated once during the hospitalization, but required reintubation in less than 24 hours. Documentation from specialists reflects Stage IV heart failure and cardio-renal syndrome requiring inotropic support. Mr. B was alert and engaged in his care, but when ventilator rates decreased, he became anxious and tachypneic.

A palliative APRN was consulted for a goals-of-care consultation. During the initial visit with Mr. and Mrs. B, the APRN discussed symptoms needs, illness understanding, treatment and treatment options. Mr. B's goals were control of his breathlessness and anxiety especially with ventilator changes. He knew his condition was serious but was hopeful to be breathing on his own in a couple of days. He was not interested in dialysis or ventricular assist devices. The APRN supported hope for this but expressed concern about his end-stage heart condition and failing kidneys. Mr. B agreed to a time-limited trial of low-dose extended-release morphine administered as disintegrating capsule pellets for shortness of breath and an anxiolytic timed prior to ventilator weaning. During the follow-up encounter, they discussed additional preferences for care and values. Due to increasing fatigue, the ICU team considered a tracheostomy and feeding tube.

A family meeting was held with Mr. B, Mrs. B, and the palliative care and ICU teams. The result was acknowledgment of the patient's terminal heart condition. Goals of care shifted to optimizing comfort and quality and a do-not-resuscitate code status. There was discussion of ventilator discontinuation because Mr. B stated that he did not want a prolonged withdrawal, in which the protocol was decreasing the delivered breaths from the ventilator by two every 15–30 minutes. However, the process was not evidence-based.

EVIDENCE-BASED PRACTICE

More than a decade ago, the National Academy of Medicine (NAM) set forth a goal that, by 2020, the best evidence will drive and support 90% of clinical decision-making. According to the NAM's vision, patients will receive current, timely, accurate, and appropriate care with clinical decision-making grounded in EBP.[16] Palliative APRNs must be knowledgeable about the seven steps[14] of EBP and apply this stepwise approach to meet the goal of improved patient outcome, improved clinician practice, and improve organizational outcomes.

SEVEN STEPS OF EBP

1. Cultivate a spirit of inquiry with the EBP culture and environment.

2. Ask the burning clinical question in a population, intervention, comparison, outcome, time (PICOT) format.

3. Search for and collect the most relevant best evidence.

4. Critically appraise the evidence (i.e., rapid, critical appraisal, evaluation, synthesis, and recommendations).

5. Integrate the best evidence with one's clinical expertise and patient preferences and values in making a practice decision change.

6. Evaluate outcomes of the practice decision or change based on evidence.

7. Disseminate the outcomes of the EBP decision or change.[14]

As leaders, innovators, and healthcare systems thinkers, palliative APRNs must consistently question approaches to clinical practice and organizational norms. Organizational culture and environment must embrace a spirit of inquiry. The Hospice and Palliative Nurses Association (HPNA) *Position Statement on Evidence-Based Practice* recommends that healthcare employers of hospice and palliative nurses have the infrastructure to support EBP.[17] Is the clinical practice of terminal weaning for a Stage IV heart failure patient, whose preference and values are to de-escalate nonbeneficial interventions such as mechanical support, current, timely, and appropriate?

Clinical questions rooted in the spirit of inquiry are formulated as a PICO (population, intervention, comparison, outcome) or PICOT (population, intervention, comparison, outcome, time) question. For the patient in the preceding case study, a well-formulated PICOT would be stated as follows:

> In patients who are terminally ill and on a ventilator, whose preference is comfort-focused care (population), how does a compassionate extubation protocol (intervention) compared to terminal weaning protocol (comparison) impact the time of death during a 12-hour period (time)?

Not all clinical problems are intervention-focused, and the (I) can be driven by an issue of interest or a meaning type question. A meaning type clinical question would be stated

How do families (P) with terminally ill loved ones undergoing terminal weaning (I) perceive the suffering of the patient (O) during the 2-hour weaning process (T)?

Clinical questions in a PICOT format drive the literature search and allow the APRN to move through Step Two of collecting the most relevant and best evidence.[14] The best evidence to drive intervention= or treatment-based decisions is systematic reviews or meta-analysis of randomized controlled trials (RCTs). Palliative APRNs have formalized education and experience with EBP and literature search methods.[18] Finding information from reliable sources is pivotal to identifying the best evidence. Professional online databases or search engines such as the Cumulative Index to Nursing and Allied Health Literature (CINAHL), Cochrane Database of Systematic Reviews, MEDLINE, Ovid, and PubMed are appropriate sites that publish peer-reviewed articles. Clinical practice guidelines (CPGs) are robust, systematic evidence-based recommendations that help APRNs in clinical decision-making to optimize the care of a specific population.[19] The Agency for Healthcare Research and Quality is a reliable repository for CPGs. Government sites such as the Center for Disease Control and Prevention and the US Department of Health and Human Services are other sources for peer-reviewed clinical information.

CRITICAL APPRAISAL OF THE EVIDENCE

Critical appraisal of the evidence allows the APRN to evaluate research studies collected from literature searches and examine keys factors such as validity, reliability, and applicability.

- *Are the results of the study valid (Validity)?* Did the researcher use the best methods possible to measure key concepts in the study adequately? Is a questionnaire on nurses' perception of patient suffering during discontinuation of life-sustaining therapy truly measuring perception of patient suffering or measuring the nurse's discomfort with the end-of-life practices?

- *What are the results (Reliability)?* Did the researcher get a consistent answer when using the same instrument of measure more than once? When assessing symptom burden in a group of oncology patients receiving palliative care compared to patients receiving usual oncology care, does the Edmonton Symptom Assessment System (ESAS) tool measure patient-reported pain, fatigue, nausea, depression, anxiety, drowsiness, shortness of breath, appetite, well-being, and sleep when used?[20]

- *Will the results help me deliver care to my patient (Applicability)?* Are the participants in the study similar to the patients seen in the ARPN's practice? If the intervention in the study aligns with patient preferences, will the benefits outweigh the risks and be feasible to apply in the practice setting? If a systemic review provided evidence to support compassionate extubation in ICU patients with brainstem infarctions, would a similar discontinuation of life support method apply to patients with similar neurologic events receiving palliative care services?

INTEGRATING THE EVIDENCE WITH CLINICAL EXPERTISE AND PATIENT PREFERENCES

Combining (a) critical appraisal and synthesis of the best evidence, (b) APRN clinical expertise, and (c) patient preferences is the next step in the EBP process. Clinical expertise is a culmination of the palliative APRN's education, training, clinical reasoning, clinical skills, and experience caring for a particular population. The centrality of patient preferences is pivotal to clinical decision-making. The assessment of a patient living with lung cancer revealed recurrent hospital admissions for anxiety and shortness of breath. During the patient encounter, the palliative APRN discussed multiple EBP, clinical experience, and benefits of extended-release morphine for dyspnea. Although compelling evidence supported morphine for symptom relief, the patient had reservations about the medication, and a shared decision was made to support the patient's preference and explore other treatment options.

EVALUATING THE OUTCOME OF PRACTICE CHANGE

Did the EBP change affect patient outcomes and yield similar results, as outlined in the literature? The palliative APRN must determine the clinical significance of the practice change on a micro and a macro level. Breathlessness, a common symptom in patients living with lung cancer, is challenging to manage in the outpatient setting. The usual care for breathlessness is pharmacologic administration of opioids and benzodiazepines. Evidence from a nurse-driven home-based program for managing breathlessness in cancer patients revealed that an educational program involving in-home pulmonary rehabilitation improved the level of breathlessness experience the participants.[21] When evaluating outcomes of practice change, the palliative APRN implementing the in-home pulmonary rehabilitation for persons living with lung cancer anticipates the outcome of symptom control of dyspnea—the impact of EBP on a micro level. With effective practice change based on evidence, patients living with lung cancer can be managed through in-home pulmonary rehabilitation, ultimately reducing emergency department utilization and hospital readmissions—the impact of EBP on a macro level.

DISSEMINATING THE OUTCOMES OF THE EBP CHANGE

The *Essentials of a Master's Prepared Nurse* set forth by the American Association of Colleges of Nursing includes

Translating and Integrating Scholarship into Practice. This essential recognizes that the APRN functions as an agent of change and disseminates best practice results.[22] The final step in the EBP process is disseminating the outcomes. Palliative APRNs are leaders who improve healthcare processes and outcomes. Too often, significant EBP change is not shared with other healthcare providers, thus limiting the benefits for other patients. Dissemination of the outcomes can be at the clinical practice site through collegial "lunch and learns." Palliative APRNs must broaden their sphere beyond individual patient care and influence practice change by sharing clinical outcomes at local, state, and national conferences and through peer-reviewed publications. There is rigor to disseminating the outcomes, but there is a tremendous value for the patient, provider, and healthcare system. Palliative APRNs garner and disseminate best evidence through local and national palliative care organizations such as the HPNA, the Center to Advance Palliative Care (CAPC), and the End of Life Nursing Education Consortium (ELNEC) but also through other appropriate professional nursing organizations such as the American Association of Critical Care Nurses, the Oncology Nursing Society, and the like. EBP to support high-quality palliative care is also disseminated in palliative peer-reviewed journals such as the *Journal of Hospice and Palliative Nursing*, the *Journal of Pain and Symptom Management*, and the *Journal of Palliative Medicine*.

EVIDENCE-BASED COMPETENCIES FOR THE PALLIATIVE APRN

EBP is a widely used concept among healthcare providers, but APRNs report lacking the skills and competencies to effectively implement EBP.[23] The American Nurses Association (ANA) defines competency as "an expected level of performance that integrates knowledge, skills, abilities, and judgment, based on established scientific knowledge and expectations for nursing practice."[24] Inadequate preparation at the academic level, the traditional pattern of healthcare delivery (e.g., "we have always done it this way"), and lack of organizational support impact APRNs' ability to consistently implement EBP.[23] Melnyk et al. developed an EBP competencies model with 24 elements for RNs and APRNs (Table 7.3).

While APRNs do not report high levels of competency in the any of the EBP competencies elements, they feel the most competent in questioning clinical practice to improve quality of care but least competent in leading transdisciplinary teams.[23] Studies support that structured education through academic–practice partnerships and principles of EBP readiness have been effective in enhancing knowledge and confidence in evidenced-based practice design and implementation.[25,26] Advancing the NAM's vision of clinical decision-making grounded in EBP[16] requires organizational culture and infrastructure for practice change sustainability of best processes. Organizations must foster and support APRNs in clinical inquiry, have clear EBP implementation processes, and develop competent EBP mentors to maintain the culture of best practice.

Table 7.3 EBP COMPETENCIES

Evidence-based practice competencies

EBP competencies for registered nurses (RNs)	EBP competencies for APRNs All competencies for professional registered nurses with the following additional competencies
1. Questions clinical practices for the purpose of improving the quality of care	14. Systematically conducts an exhaustive search for external evidence[a] to answer clinical questions
2. Describes clinical problems using internal evidence	15. Critically appraises relevant pre-appraised evidence (i.e., clinical guidelines, summaries, synopses, syntheses of relevant external evidence) and primary studies, including evaluation and synthesis
3. Participates in the formulation of clinical questions using PICOT format.	16. Integrates a body of external evidence from nursing and related fields with internal evidence[b] in making decisions about patient care
4. Searches for external evidence to answer focused clinical questions	17. Leads transdisciplinary teams in applying synthesized evidence to initiate clinical decisions and practice changes to improve the health of individuals, groups, and populations
5. Participates in critical appraisal of preappraised evidence	18. Generates internal evidence through outcomes management and EBP implementation projects for the purpose of integrating best practices
6. Participates in the critical appraisal of published research studies to determine their strength and applicability to clinical practice	19. Measures processes and outcomes of evidence-based clinical decisions
7. Participates in the evaluation and synthesis of a body of evidence gathered to determine its strength and applicability to clinical practice	20. Formulates evidence-based policies and procedures
8. Collects practice data (e.g., individual patient data, quality improvement data) systematically as internal evidence for clinical decision-making in the care of individuals, groups, and populations.	21. Participates in the generation of external evidence with other healthcare professionals
9. Integrates evidence gathered from external and internal sources in order to plan evidence-based practice changes	22. Mentors others in evidence-based decision-making and the EBP process
10. Implements practice changes based on evidence and clinical expertise and patient preferences to improve care processes and patient outcomes	23. Implements strategies to sustain an EBP culture
11. Evaluates outcomes of evidence-based decisions and practice changes for individuals, groups, and populations to determine best practices	24. Communicates best evidence to individuals, groups, colleagues, and policymakers
12. Disseminates best practices supported by evidence to improve quality of care and patient outcomes	
13. Participates in strategies to sustain an evidence-based practice culture	

[a] External evidence is evidence generated outside a clinical setting such as from systematic reviews, randomized controlled trials and practice guidelines.

[b] Internal evidence is evidence generated internally within a clinical setting, such as patient assessment data, outcomes management, and quality improvement data.

From Melnyk et al.[23]

IMPLEMENTING EBP

How we evolve from the "way we have always done things" to implementing EBP requires structural change. Leading organizations such as the National Academy of Medicine, the Agency for Healthcare Research and Quality, the American Association of Colleges of Nursing, and the US Preventative Services Task Force mandate EBP implementation, but barriers prohibit adoption among all healthcare providers.[27] The path from clinical inquiry to practice change for best patient outcomes can be met with layers of administrative decisions, financial constraints, stakeholder influences, decision-making biases, time and training constraints, and attitude about EBP. Several models have been developed to implement EBP. There are differences in the application of the models but the commonalities include practice problem, change agents, high-quality research, implementation and evaluation of practice change, and infrastructure to sustain practice change. The following is a list of models to guide EBP implementation:

- The Iowa Model of Evidence-based Practice to promote quality care[28]

- John Hopkins Nursing Evidence-Based Practice Model[29]

- Stetler Model of Evidence-Based Practice[30]

- Model for Evidence-Based Practice Change[31]

- Advancing Research and Clinical Practice Through Close Collaboration (ARCC)[32]

- Promoting Action on Research Implementation in Health Services (PARIHS) Framework[33]

- The Clinical Scholar Model[34]

- The Stevens Star Model of Knowledge Translation[14]

Palliative APRNs are experts in comprehensive management for patients living with serious illnesses. There is a deliberate focus on patient preferences during palliative encounters. The palliative APRN serves as an EBP mentor for critical care teams involved in goal-directed therapy for patients wanting to defer nonbeneficial intervention and optimize quality of life. EBP mentors are knowledgeable catalyst for EBP change.[35] As EBP mentors, palliative APRNs are aware that each EBP model has emphasis, strategies, and phases for implementation.

The Iowa Model of Evidence-Based Practice to promote quality care guides clinicians in decision-making about patient-related or organizational-focused issues.[28] The model outlines a multiphase strategic change process with feedback loops for ongoing improvement in quality of care. The initial phase or trigger begins with the clinicians' awareness of a problem-focused or knowledge-focused opportunity. Organizational problem-focused triggers include clinical issues, benchmark data comparison, and process improvement data. Knowledge-focused triggers include publication of research and change in protocols based on guidelines.[28] Utilizing the Iowa Model of Evidence-Based Practice to promote quality care as a framework (Figure 7.3) the palliative APRN can implement EBP to support the clinical inquiry "In terminally ill mechanically ventilated patients whose preference is comfort-focused care (population), how does a compassionate extubation protocol (intervention) compared to terminal wean protocol (comparison) impact the time of death during a 12-hour period (time)?" The stepwise approach described next provides an example of the Iowa EBP Model.[28]

Step 1: Identifying triggering issues and opportunities. Terminal weaning versus compassionate extubation from nonbeneficial ventilator support is an element of care where palliative APRNs and the critical care teams collaborate. *Terminal weaning* is defined as the incremental decrease in ventilator assistance, such as oxygen supply, respiratory rate, positive expiratory pressure support, or tidal volume, before removal of the endotracheal tube. *Compassionate extubation* is defined as removal of invasive mechanical ventilatory support, specifically the endotracheal tube, with no decrease in ventilator support. Palliative APRNs support patients, families, and bedside nurses through difficult medical decisions. Critical care nurses often express moral distress when caring for patients who endure a prolonged ventilator discontinuation weaning protocol but whose treatment preferences include comfort-focused care and removal from machines. These nurses see the duration for terminal weaning according to protocol as prolonging suffering for patients and families. Others express moral issues of hastening of the dying process during a compassionate extubation process. The example of the clinical question proposed presents a problem-focused trigger.

Step 2: Identifying the purpose of the clinical question and the priority for the organization. The palliative APRNs collaborates with the direct care nurses to determine if the current organization's withdrawal protocol aligns with current practice and patient preferences.[28] The organization values high-quality patient- and family-centered care. Honoring patient's treatment preferences is a key performance indicator and metric for the critical care physicians and team.

Step 3: Forming a team of stakeholders, conducting a literature search, and critically appraising the evidence for reliability, validity and application in current practice. The ARREVE observational study on terminal weaning or immediate extubation for withdrawal of support in critically ill patients reported no difference in ICU time of death after the initiation of terminal weaning and compassionate extubation.[36] Emerging themes from a qualitative study on the ICU team's perception of compassionate extubation and terminal weaning indicated that compassionate extubation eliminated medicalization of the dying process, reduced ambiguity of the dying process, and provided greater patient comfort. Themes for provider's preferences for terminal weaning included time for the patient to adapt to symptom management medications, better patient comfort, and optimizing any possibility of survival.[37] APRNs are scholarly experts in assessing the quality of both studies.

Leading the EBP initiative, the palliative APRN along with the palliative care team collaborates with the critical care physician champion, critical care medical residents, clinical nurse specialists, direct care registered nurses, nurse managers, pharmacists, respiratory therapists, and a patient-family champion. When the team has determined that there is supportive evidence for safe practice change, adequate resources are available, and administrative buy-in is established, they proceed to define, design, and pilot the practice change.

Step 4: Defining, designing, and piloting the practice change. The palliative APRN role is to increase the ICU team's awareness of terminal weaning and compassionate extubation processes. The APRN develops a compassionate extubation protocol with the ICU physician team to pilot in 10-bed unit. The team will standardize the implementation process, including material for the nurses and respiratory therapists. The team will determine and announce a pilot date

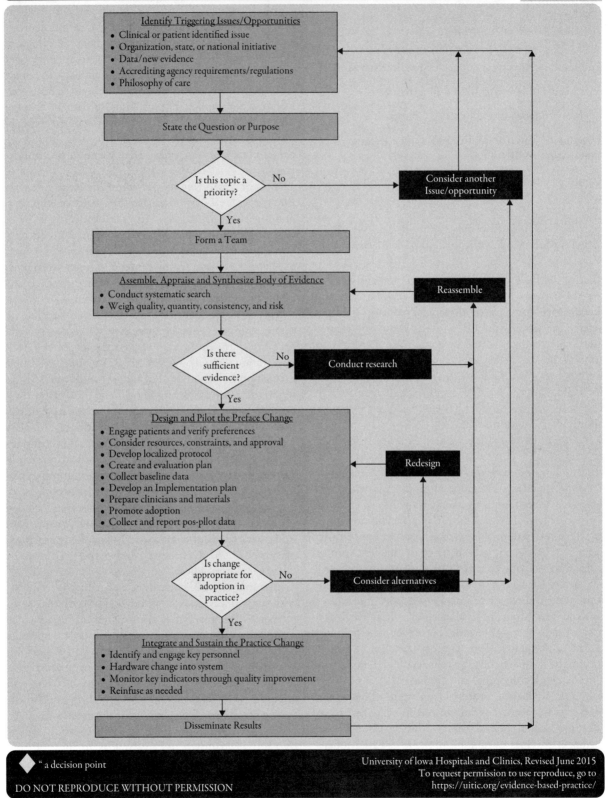

The Iowa Model Revised: Evidence-Based Practice to Promote Excellence in Health Care

Identify Triggering Issues/Opportunities
- Clinical or patient identified issue
- Organization, state, or national initiative
- Data/new evidence
- Accrediting agency requirements/regulations
- Philosophy of care

State the Question or Purpose

Is this topic a priority?

No → Consider another Issue/opportunity

Yes

Form a Team

Assemble, Appraise and Synthesize Body of Evidence
- Conduct systematic search
- Weigh quality, quantity, consistency, and risk

Reassemble

Is there sufficient evidence?

No → Conduct research

Yes

Design and Pilot the Preface Change
- Engage patients and verify preferences
- Consider resources, constraints, and approval
- Develop localized protocol
- Create and evaluation plan
- Collect baseline data
- Develop an Implementation plan
- Prepare clinicians and materials
- Promote adoption
- Collect and report pos-pllot data

Redesign

Is change appropriate for adoption in practice?

No → Consider alternatives

Yes

Integrate and Sustain the Practice Change
- Identify and engage key personnel
- Hardware change into system
- Monitor key indicators through quality improvement
- Reinfuse as needed

Disseminate Results

◆ " a decision point

DO NOT REPRODUCE WITHOUT PERMISSION

University of Iowa Hospitals and Clinics, Revised June 2015
To request permission to use reproduce, go to
https://uitic.org/evidence-based-practice/

Figure 7.3 The Iowa model revised: Evidence-based practice to promote excellence in health care.

Used with permission from Iowa Model, Buckwalter KC, Cullen L, et al. Iowa Model of Evidence-Based Practice: Revisions and validation. *Worldviews Evid Based Nurs* 2017;14(3):175–182. doi:10.1111/wvn.12223.28

and duration of the pilot. During the goals-of-care conversation with patients and families opting for comfort-focused care, the APRN will engage in a discussion of preferences for withdrawal of mechanical ventilator and, in conjunction with the critical care physician champion, identify candidates for terminal weaning and compassionate extubation. The APRN evaluates outcomes and modifies steps as needed. Post-pilot data are collected and reported to the team and practice change is adopted across all critical care units.

Step 5: Integrating and sustaining the practice change. After the reviewing the post-pilot data, the palliative APRN re-engages stakeholders along with the senior administrative team to hardwire system-level practice change. One of the EBP competencies of the APRN is implementing strategies to sustain an EBP culture.[23] A plan for sustainability of EBP

Box 7.1 RESEARCH, QUALITY IMPROVEMENT, AND EVIDENCE-BASED PRACTICE PRIORITIES FOR PALLIATIVE APRNS

2019 HPNA Research Agenda[39]

1. Pediatric hospice and palliative nursing research
2. Family caregiving
3. Interprofessional education and collaborative practice
4. Big Data science, precision health, and nursing informatics
5. Implementation science

2017 ANA and HPNA Call for Action: Nurses Lead and Transform Palliative Care[40]

1. Conduct systematic examinations of the current palliative nursing workforce, including those practicing primary palliative nursing, frontline nursing staff, and palliative nurse specialists
2. Clarify the scope of primary and specialty palliative nursing practice
3. Identify effective approaches to standardize palliative nursing education and evaluate its impact on the competencies of nurses practicing primary palliative nursing and, ultimately, its impact on patient and family outcomes
4. Examine the complex interplay of individual and environmental factors that can contribute to compassion fatigue and burnout of nurses and other palliative workforce members

2016 National Institute of Nursing Research Strategic Plan: Advancing Science, Improving Lives[41]

1. Symptom Science: Promoting personalized health strategies
2. Self-Management: Improving quality of life for individuals with chronic illness
3. End-of-Life and Palliative Care: The science of compassion

2015 Institute of Medicine Dying in America: Improving Quality and Honoring Individual Preferences Near the End of Life[42]

1. Delivery of person-centered, family-oriented care
2. Clinician–patient communication and advance care planning
3. Professional education and development
4. Policies and payment systems
5. Public education and engagement

---

includes competency-based education, EBP mentors, steering committee researchers, and EBP champions.[38]

Step 6: Disseminating the results. The palliative APRN disseminates the results to the critical care nursing team. The APRN will share patient, family, and staff satisfaction results with the senior leadership team at organizational reviews. On a larger scale, the APRN will present at local and nation conferences through podium or poster presentations. Finally, to expand the body of knowledge, the APRN will publish the results in palliative and critical care journals.

FUTURE WORK AND PRIORITIES

As healthcare clinicians, APRNs conduct projects that involve nursing issues and outcomes of care, including patient and family satisfaction with care. APRNs have the potential opportunity to serve as investigators of research projects and study team members, as well as translate their findings into practice. In public education and engagement, the ANA in collaboration with the HPNA published the 2017 *Call for Action: Nurses Lead and Transform Palliative Care.* The purpose of the document was to urge nurses to lead the growth of palliative care in several areas, including research. In this document, gaps in evidence and recommendations were identified. Box 7.1 lists additional organizational research, QI, and EBP priorities for palliative APRNs.

SUMMARY

Palliative APRNs in all settings are expected to be knowledgeable about research, QI, and EBP practices. Opportunities to generate knowledge and translate evidence into practice abound. Understanding the approach and type of data needed to inform these opportunities is an essential element of APRN practice. As healthcare leaders, APRNs directly impact patient outcomes. Best outcomes are driven by EBP. Palliative APRNs must be equipped with research knowledge and EBP implementation processes to guide future practitioners and advance both palliative nursing and palliative care. There are barriers to conducting research and translating the evidence from research to practice but the benefits of research and EBP have been supported for decades. A coalition of research and EBP mentors is necessary for sustainable best practice.

REFERENCES

1. Powers J. Increasing capacity for nursing research in magnet-designated organizations to promote nursing research. *Appl Nurs Res.* 2020;55:151286. doi:10.1016/j.apnr.2020.151286
2. Falkenberg-Olson AC. Research translation and the evolving PhD and DNP practice roles: A collaborative call for nurse practitioners. *J Am Assoc Nurse Pract.* 2019;31(8):447–453. doi:10.1097/JXX.0000000000000266
3. US Department of Health and Human Services. Office for Human Research Protections. Protection of Human Subjects, 46 C.F.R. §46.102. Electronic Code of Federal Regulations. July 28, 2018. https://www.ecfr.gov/cgi-bin/retrieveECFR?gp=&SID=83cd09e1c0f5c6937cd9d7513160fc3f&pitd=20180719&n=pt45.1.46&r=PART&ty=HTML

4. US Department of Health and Human Services. The Office of Research Integrity. Basic research concepts: Additional sections. Glossary of terms. 2021. https://ori.hhs.gov/basic-research-concepts-additional-sections

5. Lim CT, Tadmor A, Fujisawa D, et al. Qualitative research in palliative care: Applications to clinical trials work. *J Palliat Med.* 2017;20(8):857–861. doi:10.1089/jpm.2017.0061

6. Creswell JW, Poth CN. *Qualitative Inquiry and Research Design: Choosing Among Five Approaches.* 4th ed. Thousand Oaks, CA: Sage; 2018:253–286.

7. Carter N, Bryant-Lukosius D, DiCenso A, Blythe J, Neville AJ. The use of triangulation in qualitative research. *Oncol Nurs Forum.* 2014;41(5):545–547. doi:10.1188/14.ONF.545-547

8. Korstjens I, Moser A. Series: Practical guidance to qualitative research. Part 4: Trustworthiness and publishing. *Eur J Gen Pract.* 2018;24(1):120–124. doi:10.1080/13814788.2017.1375092

9. Rutberg S, Bouikidis CD. Focusing on the fundamentals: A simplistic differentiation between qualitative and quantitative research. *Nephrol Nurs J.* 2018;45(2):209–212.

10. Heale R, Twycross A. Validity and reliability in quantitative studies. *Evid Based Nurs.* 2015;18(3):66–67. doi:10.1136/eb-2015-102129

11. Creswell JW. *A Concise Introduction to Mixed Methods Research.* Thousand Oaks, CA: Sage Publications; 2015.

12. Mitchell MD, Anderson BJ, Williams K, Umscheid CA. Heparin flushing and other interventions to maintain patency of central venous catheters: A systematic review. *J Adv Nurs.* 2009;65(10):2007–2021. doi:10.1111/j.1365-2648.2009.05103.x

13. Zhong L, Wang HL, Xu B, et al. Normal saline versus heparin for patency of central venous catheters in adult patients: A systematic review and meta-analysis. *Crit Care.* 2017;21(1):5. doi:10.1186/s13054-016-1585-x

14. Melnyk BM, Fineout-Overholt E. *Evidence-Based Practice in Nursing & Healthcare: A Guide to Best Practice.* 4th Philadelphia: Wolters Kluwer; 2019.

15. Feeley D. The triple aim or the quadruple aim? Four points to help set your strategy. Institute for Healthcare Improvement Blog. November 26, 2017. Available at http://www.ihi.org/communities/blogs/the-triple-aim-or-the-quadruple-aim-four-points-to-help-set-your-strategy

16. Institute of Medicine Roundtable on Evidence-Based Medicine. *Leadership Commitments to Improve Value in Healthcare: Finding Common Ground: Workshop Summary.* Washington, DC: National Academies Press; 2009. https://www.nap.edu/catalog/11982/leadership-commitments-to-improve-value-in-health-care-finding-common

17. Hospice and Palliative Nurses Association. HPNA position statement: Evidence-based practice. Pittsburgh, PA: HPNA. 2016. https://advancingexpertcare.org/position-statements

18. Fencl JL, Matthews C. Translating evidence into practice: How advanced practice RNs can guide nurses in challenging established practice to arrive at best practice. *AORN J.* 2017;106(5):378–392. doi:10.1016/j.aorn.2017.09.002

19. Institute of Medicine (US) Committee on Standards for Developing Trustworthy Clinical Practice Guidelines. *Clinical Practice Guidelines We Can Trust.* Washington, DC: National Academies Press; 2011. https://www.nap.edu/read/13058/chapter/1

20. Hui D, Bruera E. The Edmonton Symptom Assessment System 25 years later: Past, present, and future developments. *J Pain Symptom Manage.* 2017;53(3):630–643. doi:10.1016/j.jpainsymman.2016.10.370

21. Choratas A, Papastavrou E, Charalambous A, Kouta C. Developing and assessing the effectiveness of a nurse-led home-based educational programme for managing breathlessness in lung cancer patients: A feasibility study. *Front Oncol.* 2020;10:1366. doi:10.3389/fonc.2020.01366

22. American Association of Colleges of Nursing. The essentials of master's education in nursing. Washington, DC; AACN. 2011. https://www.aacnnursing.org/Portals/42/Publications/MastersEssentials11.pdf

23. Melnyk BM, Gallagher-Ford L, Zellefrow C, et al. The first U.S. study on nurses' evidence-based practice competencies indicates major deficits that threaten healthcare quality, safety, and patient outcomes. *Worldviews Evid Based Nurs.* 2018;15(1):16–25. doi:10.1111/wvn.12269

24. American Nurses Association. *Nursing Scope and Standards of Practice.* 4th ed. Silver Spring, MD; Nursingworld.org: ANA; 2021.

25. Harbman P, Bryant-Lukosius D, Martin-Misener R, et al. Partners in research: Building academic-practice partnerships to educate and mentor advanced practice nurses. *J Eval Clin Pract.* 2017;23(2):382–390. doi:10.1111/jep.12630

26. Saunders H, Vehvilainen-Julkunen K, Stevens KR. Effectiveness of an education intervention to strengthen nurses' readiness for evidence-based practice: A single-blind randomized controlled study. *Appl Nurs Res.* 2016;31:175–185. doi:10.1016/j.apnr.2016.03.004

27. Mayden KD. Evidence-based oncology practice: Competencies for improved patient outcomes. *J Adv Pract Oncol.* 2019;10(1):84–87. Epub 2019 Jan 1. PMID: 31308991.

28. Iowa Model C, Buckwalter KC, Cullen L, et al. Iowa Model of Evidence-Based Practice: Revisions and validation. *Worldviews Evid Based Nurs.* 2017;14(3):175–182. doi:10.1111/wvn.12223

29. Dang D, Dearholt S, Sigma Theta Tau International, Johns Hopkins University School of Nursing. *Johns Hopkins Nursing Evidence-Based Practice: Model and Guidelines.* 3rd ed. Indianapolis, IN: Sigma Theta Tau International; 2018.

30. Stetler CB. Updating the Stetler Model of research utilization to facilitate evidence-based practice. *Nurs Outlook.* 2001;49(6):272–279. doi:10.1067/mno.2001.120517

31. Rosswurm MA, Larrabee JH. A model for change to evidence-based practice. *Image J Nurs Sch.* 1999;31(4):317–322. doi:10.1111/j.1547-5069.1999.tb00510.x

32. Melnyk BM, Fineout-Overholt E, Giggleman M, Choy K. A test of the ARCC(c) model improves implementation of evidence-based practice, healthcare culture, and patient outcomes. *Worldviews Evid Based Nurs.* 2017;14(1):5–9. doi:10.1111/wvn.12188

33. Kitson A, Harvey G, McCormack B. Enabling the implementation of evidence based practice: A conceptual framework. *Qual Health Care.* 1998;7(3):149–158. doi:10.1136/qshc.7.3.149

34. Honess C, Gallant P, Keane K. The clinical scholar model: Evidence-based practice at the bedside. *Nurs Clin North Am.* 2009;44(1):117–130, xii. doi:10.1016/j.cnur.2008.10.004

35. Spiva L, Hart PL, Patrick S, Waggoner J, Jackson C, Threatt JL. Effectiveness of an evidence-based practice nurse mentor training program. *Worldviews Evid Based Nurs.* 2017;14(3):183–191. doi:10.1111/wvn.12219

36. Robert R, Le Gouge A, Kentish-Barnes N, et al. Terminal weaning or immediate extubation for withdrawing mechanical ventilation in critically ill patients (the ARREVE observational study). *Intensive Care Med.* 2017;43(12):1793–1807. doi:10.1007/s00134-017-4891-0

37. Cottereau A, Robert R, le Gouge A, et al. ICU physicians' and nurses' perceptions of terminal extubation and terminal weaning: A self-questionnaire study. *Intensive Care Med.* 2016;42(8):1248–1257. doi:10.1007/s00134-016-4373-9

38. Fisher C, Cusack G, Cox K, Feigenbaum K, Wallen GR. Developing competency to sustain evidence-based practice. *J Nurs Adm.* 2016;46(11):581–585. doi:10.1097/NNA.0000000000000408

39. Romo RD, Carpenter JG, Buck H, et al. HPNA 2019-2022 Research agenda: Development and rationale. *J Hosp Palliat Nurs.* 2019;21(4):E17–e23. doi:10.1097/NJH.0000000000000580

40. American Nurses Association, Hospice and Palliative Nurses Association. Call for action: Nurses lead and transform palliative care. Silver Spring, MD: American Nurses Association; 2017. https://www.nursingworld.org/~497158/globalassets/practiceandpolicy/health-policy/palliativecareprofessionalissuespanelcallforaction.pdf

41. National Institute of Nursing Research. The NINR strategic plan: Advancing science, improving lives, a vision for nursing science. Bethesda, MD: NINR. 2016. https://www.ninr.nih.gov/sites/files/docs/NINR_StratPlan2016_reduced.pdf

42. Institute of Medicine. *Dying in America: Improving Quality and Honoring Individual Preferences Near the End of Life.* Washington, DC: National Academies Press; 2015. https://www.nap.edu/catalog/18748/dying-in-america-improving-quality-and-honoring-individual-preferences-near

SECTION III

CLINICAL SETTINGS
OF PALLIATIVE APRNS

8.

THE PALLIATIVE APRN IN THE MEDICAL, SURGICAL, AND GERIATRICS PATIENT CARE UNIT

Phyllis B. Whitehead and Carolyn White

KEY POINTS

- More than 50% of all deaths occur in the acute care setting, where the focus is on active, curative treatment, not on managing symptoms and establishing realistic goals of care.

- Palliative advanced practice registered nurses (APRNs) are uniquely qualified to care for seriously ill patients by providing comprehensive, effective, compassionate, and cost-effective care that improves end-of-life care in acute care settings.

- Palliative APRNs orchestrate interdisciplinary care plans focused on alleviating suffering and promoting healing to enhance the quality of life for seriously ill patients and their loved ones.

CASE STUDY 1: EMERGENCY DEPARTMENT PALLIATIVE CARE

Paul was a 78-year-old Black American man who had been on hospice care at home for the preceding 3 weeks. His past medical history included dementia (diagnosed in 2015), hypertension, chronic kidney disease Stage 3 (glomerular filtration rate 30–59 mL/min), coronary artery disease, chronic diastolic heart failure, and squamous cell skin cancer of the right ear, right face, and right hand, untreated per his family's request. Paul's past medical history also included benign prostatic hypertrophy with urinary obstruction, chronic solar dermatitis, osteoarthritis, acute-on-chronic renal failure, and colon cancer (diagnosed in 2010). Paul's past surgical history included colectomy (2010) and exploratory abdominal laparotomy (2015). His medications included amlodipine, metoprolol, lisinopril, topical Metronidazole as needed for wound odor control, and oxycodone as needed for pain.

Paul presented to the emergency department with increased confusion and falls. His daughter, Nancy, reported Paul had been more confused and eating and drinking less for the past week. She also stated that his falls had increased. His review of systems revealed no fever, chest pain, or shortness of breath. According to Nancy, Paul had been having more difficulty swallowing his medications over the past few weeks. Nancy shared that Paul is a retired veteran.

Nancy also reported several episodes of bleeding from Paul's skin cancer lesions, which was a great concern to her. She also described how the hospice registered nurse came out to help with the wound care and medication management. She and the hospice nurses performed local wound care several times a week, mainly to contain the drainage and bleeding. However, Nancy wished no further diagnostic studies regarding the skin cancer and stated, "I don't want to put him through any additional distress of unnecessary treatments and interventions." She wanted the admitting physician to investigate for any easily treatable causes of Paul's confusion and agitation.

Nancy had been caring for her father for the past 8 years, first at his home and then at her home. He had been living with her for the past 3 years. His wife and siblings were deceased. Nancy was married with two adult children and four adult grandchildren. She was solely responsible for Paul's care and shared that her husband had expressed frustration that she was spending all of her time with Paul. She was considering nursing home placement as she was not sure she could care for him any longer. Overall, Paul was declining, with a very poor appetite, weight loss (20 pounds over the past 8 weeks), weakness and fatigue, and increased confusion, agitation, and falls.

Based on the conversation with Nancy and the review of the diagnostics and laboratory values (creatinine 1.83 mg/dL and estimated glomerular filtration rate 29 mL/min/1.73 m²; see Table 8.2), a palliative care consult was ordered for Paul to discuss goals of care, as well as his pain and symptoms. A family meeting was scheduled, and the palliative APRN Stacey reviewed the role of palliative care in Paul's care. Stacey asked Nancy to share her understanding of Paul's condition. After listening to Nancy's understanding of Paul's condition, she explained that a stroke, cerebral bleed, and infection had all been ruled out as sources of his encephalopathy. Stacey clarified that the confusion, agitation, and decline were related to Paul's dementia and that his other underlying heart and kidney diseases were not reversible.

INTRODUCTION

Patients who are seriously ill and hospitalized represent a specialized patient population that greatly benefit from the expanded skills and knowledge of palliative APRNs.[1,2] These patients and their loved ones have unique needs that are often unaddressed in a busy healthcare system.[3,4] By the year 2030, almost one in five adults will be over the age of 65 years and have at least one chronic illness.[5,6,7] The year 2030 marks an important demographic turning point in US history according to the US Census Bureau's 2017 National Population

99

Table 8.1 STAGES OF DEMENTIA

STAGE	IMPAIRMENT LEVEL
1	No impairment
2	Very mild decline: Unnoticeable memory lapses
3	Mild decline: Noticeable memory and concentration problems; losing items
4	Moderate decline: Forgetfulness of events; difficulty performing tasks
5	Moderate to severe decline: Gaps in memory, thinking; needs help with activities of daily living
6	Severe decline: Loss of awareness of recent experiences; remembers own name but has difficulty with others
7	Very severe decline: Total care; swallowing impaired; hospice eligible

Adapted from Ernecoff et al.[5]; Schoenherr et al.[2]; and Kyeremanteng et al.[6]

Projections. By 2030, all baby boomers will be older than age 65. This will expand the size of the older population so that 1 in every 5 residents will be of retirement age.[1]

By 2060, the United States is projected to grow by 79 million (previously 78 million) people, from about 326 million today to 404 million. The population is projected to cross the 400-million threshold in 2058. In coming years, the rate at which the US population grows is expected to slow down. The population is projected to grow by an average of 2.3 million people per year until 2030. But that number is expected to decline to an average of 1.9 million (previously 1.8 million) per year between 2030 and 2040, and continue falling to 1.6 million (previously 1.5 million) per year from 2040 to 2060.[1]

Often, patients with chronic illness have uncertain prognoses and poorly predictable disease trajectories resulting in numerous emergency department visits and hospital admissions. Hospitals have become places where patients go for "state-of-the-art" diagnostic and therapeutic interventions, procedures, complex surgeries, and powerful medications to support life at all costs. The modern acute care setting is overwhelmingly complicated and difficult to navigate for patients and their families, with countless specialists; it is often described as a "conveyer belt" approach to care.[2] Specialization of care may result in a sole focus on incremental improvement of a specific organ. This emphasis does not take into account "the big picture" of the patient's overall clinical condition or the way that specific organ interactions affect the disease process.[2] The prevalence of hospital-based palliative care services has increased by 26% during the past decade; 67% of all hospitals and greater than 90% of hospitals with more than 300 beds currently offer palliative care services.[2] Additional barriers that interfere with providing effective end-of-life care in acute care settings include (1) poor communication among clinicians, patients, and caregivers; (2) a focus on life prolongation and technology; and (3) unrealistic expectations on the part of patients and their loved ones.[3] To address these challenges, inpatient specialty palliative care programs have grown dramatically over the past decade. APRNs have become an integral part of these growing programs and are well-prepared to care for complex acutely ill patients.[2,3,4] APRNs may serve as the patient's attending provider or as a pain or palliative consultant. Their numerous acute care roles include (1) direct clinical care, (2) expert coaching and guidance to colleagues, (3) ethical decision-making skills, (4) collaboration, (5) clinical and professional leadership, (6) research skills, (7) consultation, and (8) education.[3,4,5]

Today, medical-surgical patients are sicker, with many comorbid conditions. One of the most challenging barriers in acute care settings is the lack of communication and coordination of patient care.[3] APRNs are well-positioned to address this barrier. For example, while making rounds on their patients, APRNs can model effective communication with the patient and family, nursing staff, and medical teams. APRNs can address pain and symptom management of patients while coaching and mentoring their colleagues on the most current evidence-based standards of care. Furthermore, APRNs can identify seriously ill patients earlier in their disease trajectory who would benefit from aggressive pain and symptom management as well as goals-of-care discussions that otherwise may go unaddressed.[2,4,6]

An illustration of this holistic approach to patient care is the unitary-caring praxis conceptual model for the palliative APRN embedded within the eight domains of the NCP Clinical Practice Guidelines (Figure 8.1).[7] The use of a model guided by nursing theory can enhance the care of seriously ill patients while promoting spiritual and emotional healing when physical healing may not be possible. A theoretical framework resembling the unitary-caring praxis provides guidance for the APRN in caring for seriously ill patients by translating the national guidelines into a comprehensive but practical approach to palliative care.

CHRONIC KIDNEY DISEASE

END-STAGE RENAL DISEASE

With the growing elderly population, the number of patients with acute kidney injury, Stage 4 and 5 chronic kidney disease, or end-stage renal disease (ESRD) and other comorbidities is increasing.[8] Mortality among ESRD patients is 10 to 100 times greater than in the general population when matched for age and gender. Many patients are older and have multiple comorbidities that add to their overall illness situation. The associated mortality is high even when the patients are on hemodialysis, about 20% annually. A review shows that for elderly patients starting dialysis (undifferentiated), 1-year survival is about 73% and 5-year survival is about 35%.[9,10] The cost associated with ESRD is staggering, with hemodialysis costing $89,000 per patient annually and amounting to $42 billion in the United States.[11] Only 1% of the Medicare population has ESRD, but it accounts for up to 7% of the annual budget.[11]

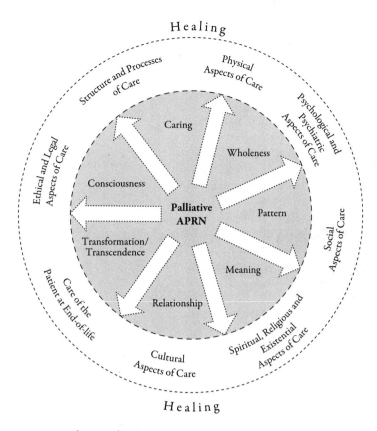

Figure 8.1 Palliative APRN unitary-caring praxis framework.
From Reed SM. A Unitary-Caring Conceptual Model for advanced practice nursing in palliative care. *Holist Nurs Pract.* 2010;24(1):23–34. Reprinted with permission from Wolters Kluwer Health, Inc.[7]

In 2000, the American Society of Nephrology and Renal Physicians Association published the first clinical practice guideline encouraging palliative care for ESRD patients. It was revised in 2010 to include information on an integrated prognostic model predicting the mortality of hemodialysis patients (available at http://touchcalc.com/calculators/sq).[12]

Patients with kidney disease face limited survival compared with the general population. Although mortality trends have improved, the median survival for those on maintenance dialysis is about 4–5 years. Despite this poor survival, hemodialysis continues to be offered in terms of longevity versus quality of life, especially at end of life. Patients on hemodialysis experience more hospital stays including more intensive care days, higher death risk while hospitalized, and less use of hospice as compared to those with advanced cancer or heart failure.[8]

It is clear that patients, loved ones, and hospitals need to be prepared to have end-of-life conversations, ideally before dialysis is initiated but most certainly when patients are functionally and physically declining despite dialysis. APRNs need to feel comfortable having the discussion with patients and their families regarding whether dialysis may offer a better quality and quantity of life compared to conservative management of symptoms.[2,13–16] For example, patients older than 80 years who start dialysis experience a significant loss of functionality within the first 6 months of treatment, requiring caregiver support or placement in a nursing home.[8] Unfortunately, randomized clinical trials evaluating the benefits of dialysis for older adults are lacking.[8,15–17]

Paramount is the collaboration between the hospital's nephrologists and the dialysis nurses to implement the American Society of Nephrology and Renal Physicians Association's published clinical practice guidelines for palliative care counseling and symptom management. Early palliative care involvement and integration into routine ESRD management are preferred for creating trusting relationships with patients and their loved ones. Several instruments have been developed by Cohen and colleagues—the Dialysis Discontinuation Quality of Dying (DDQOD) and the Dialysis Quality of Dying Apgar (QODA)—which help distinguish between good and bad deaths for dialysis patients and may assist with end-of-life discussions.[12,18] In 2018, the National Institute for Health and Care Excellence (NICE) published a guideline on conservative care of patients with chronic kidney disease.[18] The guideline recommends starting counseling at least 1 year before any therapy may be needed. It further suggests that ESRD management be based on individual factors such as frailty, cognition, other comorbidities, and patient preference.[2]

Palliative care renal literature and guidelines suggest that the elements of good end-of-life care for ESRD patients include (1) advance care planning for agreed level of care and preferred place of care; (2) appropriate transition from life-sustaining to comfort care, including potential discontinuation of dialysis; (3) ongoing dialogues with patients and caregivers regarding prognosis and treatment options; and (4) aggressive symptom management throughout disease progression.[19,20]

Physical assessment includes (1) skin turgor and color changes (i.e., gray-bronze color); (2) oliguria or anuria; (3) edema and/or ascites; (4) jugular vein distention; (5) fluid accumulation in the lungs; (6) blood pressure and orthostatic changes; (7) fluid retention resulting in weight gain; (8) hypocalcemia; (9) dry, flaky skin; (10) ammonia-smelling breath; (11) tremors/seizures; (12) easy bruising; and (13) signs of anemia.[1] Routine laboratory tests should be ordered, including blood urea nitrogen (BUN), creatinine, hemoglobin, hematocrit, calcium, phosphorus, sodium, and potassium. Other diagnostic testing may involve imaging (computed tomography [CT] or magnetic resonance imaging [MRI]), renal arteriograms, and kidney, ureters, and bladder (KUB) radiographs.[2,11,19] The APRN should assess for common symptoms such as nausea and vomiting, anxiety, depression, constipation, diarrhea, pruritus, pain, fatigue, and anorexia. Morphine should be avoided; fentanyl, methadone, and oxycodone are preferred in the treatment of pain.[11,19–21]

All reversible causes should be eliminated, especially in the treatment of acute renal failure. For ESRD, dialysis discussions should cover lifestyle changes, dietary restrictions, symptom management, potential complications, transplant option, and whether dialysis will continue until the patient dies or under what circumstances dialysis will be discontinued.[19–21] Once a decision is made to stop dialysis, all nonessential medications must be stopped to avoid toxicities and to stop or at least minimize fluid volume. Patient and family education must be provided on what to expect, especially alleviating the fear of "drowning in fluids" that accompanies stopping dialysis. The patient's diet should be liberalized so he or she can enjoy foods and beverages that have been restricted. The patient who has stopped dialysis has a prognosis usually measured in days to a few weeks. The APRN should review disposition planning options with the patient and family, including home with hospice, long-term care facility with hospice, or a residential hospice facility, and provide guidance in this decision.[11,15,21–23]

Hole et al. suggests a model of supportive care for integrated kidney care where patients are guided from aggressive treatments to conservative and supportive interventions based upon their trajectory and prognosis.[22] This model of supportive care examines how APRNs can make a distinct shift to a purely supportive approach including withdrawal of dialysis. Supportive care should be available to all patients with advanced chronic kidney disease.[22]

DEMENTIA

Dementia is a common diagnosis on medical, surgical, and geriatric units. Frequently, families do not understand that dementia is a life-limiting condition.[2] APRNs are uniquely positioned to initiate conversations to help families understand the disease trajectory for dementia patients. The incidence of dementia is growing, and by 2050 the number is expected to rise to 135 million.[24] Worldwide, 50 million individuals are living with dementia, and this number is predicted to double

Table 8.2 STAGES OF CHRONIC KIDNEY DISEASE

STAGE	GLOMERULAR FILTRATION RATE (GFR)	STATUS
1	>90	Normal kidney function
2	60–89	Declining GFR with comorbidities
3	30–59	Decline, incidence of anemia, malnutrition, poor quality of life, consider palliative care consult
4	15–29	Pre-dialysis, preparation for dialysis
5	<15	Renal replacement therapy, kidney transplant, or hospice care

Adapted from Axelson et al.[9] and Forzley et al.[11]

over the next 20 years.[24] Dementia, specifically Alzheimer's disease, is the fifth leading cause of death and accounts for 80% of the cases.[24] More than 5 million Americans live with dementia, with more than 1 million of those at late to end stage. This results in out of pocket expenses of $66,000 in the last year of life and societal costs exceeding $250 billion in 2018 and expected to double by 2030.[3,5] Dementia is a progressive, incurable condition that causes limitations in life and should be recognized as a life-limiting condition.[3,24,25]

Dementia can have many causes, such as Alzheimer's disease, vascular dementia, advanced Parkinson's or Huntington's disease, Lewy body disease, and excessive or chronic alcohol use.[3,24,25] Impairments in mental and physical functioning, such as memory loss, language impairment, personality changes, dysphagia, and inability to perform activities of daily living, characterize the condition.[3,24,25] There are seven stages of dementia (Table 8.1). The APRN should be familiar with these stages in order to help clinicians and families understand the role of palliative and hospice care for patients and their loved ones.

One challenge for the acute care APRN is the difficulty of identifying dementia as a life-limiting illness and the importance of getting a palliative care consult for the patient. Evidence shows that patients with end-stage dementia are less likely to be referred to palliative care than other non-oncological end-stage disease patients (9% vs. 25%), and dementia patients are likely to be prescribed fewer palliative medications (28% vs. 51%).[25,28] Only 27% of US nursing homes report any type of palliative or end-of-life care, despite 85% of large hospitals reporting specialty palliative care services.[25] Infections, hip fracture, and nutritional decline are common reasons for hospitalizations and signal worsened prognosis of a mortality risk of 20–50% within the next 6 months.[3,25] Caregivers' burden can be worsened when periods of stability are interrupted by acute exacerbations—in contrast to the more predictable decline in patients with advanced cancer.[3] Advance care planning and goal setting should be initiated early in the disease process, while the patient can provide guidance to loved ones. Due to the progression of dementia, it can be challenging for family and clinicians to know when to initiate palliation as a goal.[3,28]

The use of functionality and cognition scales, such as the Minimum Data Set 2 (MDS-2) or the Functional Assessment Staging (FAST) instruments, can be helpful in quantifying the stage and identifying appropriate palliative and/or hospice patients.[3,5] Both pain (39%) and dyspnea (46%) are common symptoms at end-of-life for many dementia patients.[3,5,28] They should be aggressively treated on a first-line basis with an opioid, such as morphine. Patients with dementia receive less analgesia than patients who are cognitively intact. They often cannot express themselves verbally and hence receive suboptimal palliative care.[28] The APRN should integrate the use of behavioral pain assessment tools, such as the Pain Assessment in Advanced Dementia Scale (PAINAD).[28,29] The American Society of Pain Management Nursing's *Position Statement on Pain Assessment in Patients Unable to Self-Report* recommends using patient self-report of pain if possible, review of known pain etiologies from the medical history, observation of pain-related behaviors, and family or proxy reports to assess for pain in the dementia patient.[3,5,28,29] Agitation may affect up to half of end-stage dementia patients, necessitating a calm environment and the treatment of reversible causes, such as pain, dyspnea, and constipation.[3] The APRN should assess for cognitive changes, including delirium. Tools such as the Mini-Mental State Examination (MMSE), the Short Portable Mental Status Questionnaire (SPMSQ), the Delirium Observation Screening Scale, and the Confusion Assessment Method (CAM) can be used to screen for cognitive changes and delirium to enhance symptom management.[3,5]

Infections, such as pneumonia from aspiration, urinary tract infections, or pressure ulcers from lack of mobility are a natural part of the disease progression.[3,25] The APRN must discuss with caregivers the role of antibiotics in the context of a life-prolonging intervention, especially in the late stages of the disease. Antibiotics are not benign and can cause complications, such as *Clostridium difficile* infection, so an early dialogue is warranted about the use of oral and/or intravenous antibiotics based on the patient's goals of care.[3,25]

Due to the prevalence of dysphagia (93%),[3,24,25,28] malnutrition and dehydration are common. Conversations on the use of medically administered hydration and nutrition should start early and continue as the disease progresses. There are many resources, such as the video from the University of North Carolina School of Medicine Palliative Care Resources on feeding options (http://www.med.unc.edu/pcare/resources/feedingoptions), to provide patients and their loved ones with accurate information on the benefits and risks of medically administered nutrition versus careful hand feeding so the patient and/or caregivers can make informed decisions. A speech-language pathologist referral should be considered to determine the safest oral intake/diet recommendations for the patient.

Frequently, loved ones ask how we can allow the patient to "starve to death."[3,5,30] A candid discussion on the natural dying process for a dementia patient is imperative. Using a careful selection of words, such as "fasting," and explaining that this process is not uncomfortable can be helpful for caregivers. Comparing the fasting state to a time when the loved one has been ill and did not have a desire to eat may also be helpful.[30] It is important to emphasize that the patient will be offered comfort foods and/or sips of beverages, despite the risk of aspiration, along with frequent oral care.[30] Providing the information and allowing loved ones time to process it while providing empathy are essential APRN skills.

HIP FRACTURES

Elderly patients hospitalized for hip fractures are common on medical-surgical units. As the population ages, the number of hip fractures are estimated to rise by 11.9% by 2030.[31–34] More than 250,000 older adults sustain hip fractures annually in the United States, and, by 2030, this number is expected to rise to 260,000.[35] Most hip fractures are treated surgically with only about 10% treated nonoperatively.[31,36] APRNs need to be familiar with the care of these patients, including pain and symptom management as well as the importance of initiating an early goals-of-care discussion with the patient (if possible) and family.[32,37] Although one may not consider consulting palliative care for a hip fracture alone, it may be appropriate if the patient has multiple comorbidities (e.g., heart failure, dementia, chronic pulmonary and kidney disease) and is frail even at baseline. Patients with hip fractures have significant comorbidities and have a 1-year mortality rate of approximately 30%.[32,34,36,38,39] Hip fractures in a patient older than 65 years old should trigger a palliative care consult.[34–36,38,39]

Having a goals-of-care conversation with the patient and family can align the patient's priorities of care (cure vs. quality of life) while ensuring that both surgical and conservative intervention options are fully discussed, including the benefits and risks (mortality) of each.[35–37,40] Many times the patient's main priority is to ambulate again, so surgery may be the better option if, realistically, rehabilitation is possible. It is important for patients and their loved ones to understand that pain and symptom management can be achieved via medical management.

In Case Study 1, although Paul did not sustain a fracture, he was at high risk because of his frequent falls. Hip fractures increase after the age of 60, and then exponentially after the age of 80.[35–37,40] Approximately 30% of community-dwelling senior citizens age 65 and up fall annually, with higher numbers in institutions.[38,39] Hip fractures are disabling and a major cause of morbidity and mortality in elderly individuals.[34–36] Common risk factors for falls include (1) cognitive dysfunction; (2) bowel/bladder incontinence; (3) medications, such as opioids, sedatives, and diuretics; (4) impaired balance; (5) environmental hazards, such as throw rugs and slippery floors; (6) pets; and (7) weakness.[32,34,36,38,39]

CASE STUDY 1: EMERGENCY DEPARTMENT PALLIATIVE CARE (CONTINUED)

Nancy said she knew Paul's prognosis was limited since he had been enrolled in hospice for the past 3 weeks. She wanted to focus on comfort/quality of life and did not want to pursue life-sustaining interventions or procedures, including resuscitation, dialysis, and mechanical ventilation. However, when Paul fell, Nancy did not notify Paul's hospice before calling 911 for assistance and instead revoked Paul's hospice benefit and came to the hospital for evaluation.

Stacey recommended transferring Paul to the hospital's palliative care unit for symptom management while a disposition plan was established. Since the focus was on comfort and no surgical intervention, a wound care consult was placed. The purpose was to create a plan to manage odor and drainage of the large fungating and necrotic lesions on Paul's face and hand.

Nancy said she could not continue to care for Paul at her home. Stacey reviewed disposition options with her, including long-term care with hospice versus skilled nursing care. Unfortunately, there were no local residential hospice facilities in Nancy's community. Stacey consulted the palliative care social worker to assist Nancy in disposition planning. In the meantime, Paul was transferred to the palliative care unit (PCU).

The PCU APRN observed Paul cry out in pain upon positioning, and per the nursing staff, wound dressing changes were reported to be very painful for Paul. Stacey changed Paul's medications since he had dysphagia. She scheduled oral oxycodone (20:1 concentrate) 10 mg for pain every 4 hours and 30 minutes prior to dressing changes to address his pain.

Stacey and the nursing staff also identified a potential source of Paul's distress related to his past military service. Stacey explored with Nancy about Paul's service and if he had shared his experiences. Knowing that Paul's military service may be contributing to Paul's agitation, Stacey reached out to the PCU's chaplain and social worker to integrate strategies into Paul's care plan.

Over the next 72 hours, Paul continued to decline. He was unable to eat or drink. Stacey discussed medically administered hydration and nutrition with Nancy, who shared that Paul never wanted a feeding tube. Nancy stated that she knew Paul was dying and that even though he was 78 years old, it was hard to lose her father. Stacey encouraged Nancy to speak with the hospital chaplain or the palliative care bereavement counselor. Nancy expressed appreciation for the additional support and met with each of them.

The nursing staff and the PCU APRN closely assessed Paul for any signs of pain and agitation as well as the effectiveness of his medications. They documented that Paul's pain was better controlled with the scheduled oxycodone but required dose titration over the next day. Stacey and the palliative care team (physician, nurses, social worker, counselor, chaplain, and pharmacist) made rounds daily and collaborated to provide intensive psychosocial and spiritual care to Paul and Nancy. Paul died peacefully 4 days after he came to the PCU. Nancy expressed deep appreciation for the care Paul received.

PALLIATIVE CARE AND ONCOLOGY

The Institute of Medicine (IOM) and the American Society for Clinical Oncology (ASCO) continue to recommend early palliative care interventions in order to provide high-quality cancer care.[1,25,41] ASCO has recommended full integration of palliative care as part of comprehensive cancer care in the United States by 2020.[1,41–44] There is clear evidence that cancer patients experience better outcomes with palliative care including less pain, dyspnea, and depression; better quality of life; similar if not improved survival; and reduced costs.[1,6,25,42,43,45] Unfortunately, fewer than 50% of patients with advanced cancer have palliative care consultation, and only one-third have goals-of-care discussions.[6,25,42,43,45] To address the gap in care of the cancer patient, it is essential that palliative APRNs step up to ensure quality care of these patients' needs.[25] Palliative APRNs are uniquely positioned to manage challenging pain and symptoms while promoting goals-of-care dialogues.

Lung cancer has the highest morbidity and mortality, of which 80% are non-small cell lung cancers (NSCLC).[47] In recent years, a new cancer treatment called immunotherapy has emerged. Immunotherapy offers a novel way to target cancer cells by engaging the body's own immune system.[46,47] Clinicians, patients, and their families are pursuing these treatments, even for those who may be at risk for low response rates and significant toxicities, such as those patients with low performance status and multiple comorbidities. Clinicians, both oncology and palliative, bear the challenge and responsibility of providing realistic and balanced information about the risks and benefits of these new immunotherapy agents.[48–50]

The APRN should understand that the typical side effects of chemotherapy, such as hair loss and blood cell abnormalities, are not prevalent with immunotherapy. These immunotherapy agents do, however, have side-effect profiles that include severe fatigue, diarrhea/colitis, pneumonitis, rash/pruritus, transaminitis, hypo- or hyper-thyroidism, diabetes, and adrenal insufficiency.[41,50] More commonly, skin side effects are often noticed initially, followed by colitis/diarrhea. Skin manifestations can occur in up to 40% of melanoma patients receiving immunotherapy.[51] These can include rash, pruritus, vitiligo, lichenoid dermatitis psoriasis, or oral mucosal inflammation.[50] Severe colitis occurs in fewer than 10% and can lead to increased risk of peritonitis and bowel perforation. Endocrine side effects also occur in approximately 10% of patients, and treatment should be targeted at replacing the affected hormone, treatment that is likely needed for life. Rarer side effects of immunotherapy can include episcleritis, uveitis, pancreatitis, neuropathies, nephritis, and cardiomyopathies.[50]

Typically, most immunotherapy toxicities have a relatively predictable time course. Skin toxicities or reactions present the earliest, sometimes only 2–3 weeks after initiation. More severe organ toxicities, such as colitis, hepatitis, and pneumonitis, appear between 5 and 12 weeks after initiation. Endocrine toxicities that affect the thyroid and adrenals often present from 8 to 14 weeks after initiation. Knowing these timelines can help clinicians plan for and prepare patients and involve the palliative care team when these side effects occur and even before they occur.[48,50] Of note, glucocorticoids should be considered in the treatment of some side effects of immunotherapy agents. Because glucocorticoids counteract the same immune system activated by immunotherapies, some clinicians may incorrectly believe that these steroids are contraindicated, fearing they may reduce the efficacy of the immunotherapy. This has not been proved by research, and often the glucocorticoid is a necessary life-saving intervention. In fact, most clinical trials of immunotherapies allow for glucocorticoid use up to a dose of oral prednisone 10 mg daily or its equivalent.[48,50] In some cases, low-dose glucocorticoids may be the only way a patient can continue with immunotherapy. Given their promise of potential durable remissions, the use of these immunotherapy agents will only grow. It is incumbent upon palliative APRNs to be aware of these new therapies, as well as their risks and benefits.

CASE STUDY 2: GOALS-OF-CARE DISCUSSIONS

Judy was a 26-year-old unmarried Latino woman who had been diagnosed with Stage IV non-small cell lung cancer (NSCLC) 6 months earlier. She was admitted over the weekend with intractable pain and dyspnea. The palliative APRN, Brook, met her on Monday morning rounds.

On reviewing her medical records, Brook observed that Judy presented with Stage IV disease with metastases to the brain and bones. She had undergone three cycles of cisplatin, vinblastine, and DTIC (CVD), but recent scans revealed widespread progressive disease. Judy rated her pain at 7/10 on patient-controlled analgesia (PCA) with morphine at a basal rate of 2 mg per hour, with a 2 mg bolus every 15 minutes as needed. Oxygen saturation was 94% on 2 liters of oxygen, but Judy complained of dyspnea.

Brook focused on establishing a bond with Judy and her parents, Ben and Jill, and worked to improve her symptoms. With Judy's permission, her parents stayed in the room during the initial assessment. She was "desperate" to be more comfortable but also wanted to be able to think and function coherently. Brook made it clear to Judy that she could be more comfortable, but it was going to take some adjustment in her current medications. The benefits of morphine were discussed—both for her pain and her breathing. Judy reported that she was tolerating the morphine fine, except for its constipating side effects. Judy was assured that the constipation could be countered with a good bowel regimen. Work began on improving her pain control. Brook reviewed the number of breakthrough doses Judy had attempted since her admission and adjusted her morphine dosage up to 3 mg/hr and gave her a 3 mg bolus every 20 minutes. Simultaneously, her bowel regimen was increased to include stool softeners and laxatives. An as-needed antiemetic was prescribed, as Judy had nausea with severe pain. Brook informed Judy that the first few days of titration might make her more sedated than she wanted, but she would adjust to the sedative effects to some degree over time and that Judy had been sleep-deprived due to her pain and dyspnea. Brook reinforced the principle of patient-controlled analgesia: that she was in control of how much she needed or wanted, and efforts to balance

her pain control with the level of sedation would be undertaken moving forward.

The next focus was her dyspnea. While the morphine would help with this, her chest x-ray from the preceding day revealed a large left pleural effusion and moderate right pleural effusion. Brook consulted with the oncologist to ask if he would consider tapping the effusions to improve her respiratory status. When he said yes, Brook made arrangements with the interventional radiology department to perform bilateral pleural taps later in the day or on Tuesday morning at the latest.

As the Brook left the room with them, Ben and Jill shared that Judy was the second of three daughters in their family. She was the first person in their family to go to college and then on to graduate school and had recently moved out of state to begin her career. Shortly after her move, Judy was diagnosed with NSCLC and elected to return to her parent's home to begin treatment. In her parent's words, she was the "golden child." Their home was a 1-hour drive away from the hospital. Their older daughter (28) lived out of state; their younger daughter (23) lived nearby but was finding being with her sister at this time very difficult. They shared that they were very aware of the gravity of their daughter's illness but were not prepared for what was ahead. Brook reassured them there were resources to help them feel better prepared. They agreed to meet with the social worker and confirmed that a chaplain would also be helpful for them. Brook discussed the plan and conversations with the nurse caring for Judy. The RN had already had a brief conversation with Judy's parents and agreed to reinforce the plan of care for the day and ensure that both the social worker and the chaplain visited.

On Tuesday, Judy's pain control was markedly improved, with a self-reported level of 2/10. Oxygen saturation was 99% after the pleural taps, and she did not feel she needed the oxygen all the time, A plan was made to meet to discuss next steps. With Judy's permission, Ben and Jill were included in the conversation. It was a difficult conversation. Judy and her parents were advised that the cancer had progressed in her bones and brain, which meant that the treatment she had received was not working. The oncologist reviewed other treatment options including immunotherapy, anticipated side effects, and the likelihood of the treatment extending her life. Judy shared that she wanted to try the immunotherapy, and her parents agreed that she would go home with the goal of starting the immunotherapy over the next week once the oncologist obtained approval for the medication. Brook converted her morphine from IV to oral in anticipation of discharge and made sure Judy had a good bowel regimen to prevent constipation. Brook reviewed the potential complications and provided follow-up instructions including a follow-up outpatient palliative care appointment.

Brook was on call for the palliative care service when she was consulted a few weeks later that Judy was admitted back to the oncology unit for renal failure related to her immunotherapy. Unfortunately, Judy had been unable to keep the palliative care outpatient appointment due to her fatigue. Brook was consulted now for symptom management and goals-of-care conversations. Understanding that Judy's renal function was poor, Brook transitioned Judy from oral morphine to a hydromorphone PCA. Brook met with Judy and her parents once Judy was more comfortable and settled into her oncology room. Judy shared that she was so tired and now ready to focus on her comfort and being at home. She wanted to go home to be with her family and dog. In collaboration with the case manager, a plan was begun to discharge her home with hospice.

By Thursday, planning was complete. All the home hospice equipment had been delivered to Judy's house. Her hospital bed was in the family room that looked out over the ocean; there was an adjacent bathroom. Although Judy was not wearing the oxygen all the time, it had been delivered and set up, anticipating that she would need it in the future. The hospice agency had visited with Judy's parents and her sister. The hospice nurse and social worker on their team would meet with them frequently, initially, to help them better understand what to expect as Judy's disease progressed. Ben and Jill contacted their pastor and advised him they were coming home with Judy, and he told him he would visit them as often as they needed him. Judy was discharged to home hospice on Thursday afternoon. Two weeks later, Judy died comfortably in her home, surrounded by her family and with her dog by her side.

Bereavement follow-up revealed that Judy's family felt supported during the transitional care process. As difficult as it was for them to have her decide to stop treatment, they saw her make a decision that she felt was best for her. Although she stopped treatment, Judy was actively engaged in managing her symptoms so she could continue to enjoy her life until the very end.

SURROGATE OR PROXY DECISION-MAKING

Because seriously ill patients like Judy often lose their decision-making capacity, the APRN may have to rely on loved ones to advocate for the patient's wishes.[11,25,40] State laws vary in the extent to which they authorize proxy decision-making; they also differ as to which family members have priority in the decision-making. Thus, the APRN should be familiar with the state's surrogate decision-making laws and regulations. The acute care APRN should initiate family meetings early during the hospital stay so that priorities of care can be established.

During the family meeting, the APRN needs to provide an accurate summary of the medical care to date, all of the medical treatment options being considered, and the potential outcomes, including prognosis. The APRN should summarize what the medical teams are recommending as the best care option(s) while focusing on the patient's preferences and values. For example, "In light of what we have talked about so far, what do you think Judy would want to do?"[40] The goals of the meeting are to minimize the surrogate decision-maker's burden of responsibility and remain focused on the patient's—not the decision-maker's—wishes.[11,25,40]

Whether the APRN is serving as the patient's attending or as a consultant, there is an expanding palliative care role in the acute care setting.[15] APRNs are defining hospitals' end-of-life policies and procedures as well as creating triggers for appropriate palliative care consults. APRNs provide optimal

symptom management, maximize patient and family function throughout treatment, and ensure seamless transitions to end-of-life care when cancer treatment is no longer possible or desirable.[15,40,51] With the majority of deaths occurring in

Table 8.3 INPATIENT APRN ELEMENTS AND ASSESSMENT

ELEMENTS	ASSESSMENT
Patient assessment	System review • Cardiac • Pulmonary • Renal • Neurological • Skin • Endocrine • Hepatic
Values and beliefs to facilitate advance care planning	• Goals-of-care conversations • AMD/DNR/POST/POLST/MOST completion[a] • Family meetings • Cultural assessment • Therapeutic presence
Communication and education to staff	• Inpatient nursing staff collaboration • Medical and surgical teams coordination • Case management/disposition planning • Delivery of serious news • Conflict management • Prognostication • Facilitation of interprofessional teams
Management of symptoms and procedures	• Pain • SOB • Constipation • Anxiety • Nausea • Bowel obstructions • Interventional radiology (i.e., venting gastrostomy tubes and drainage system catheter placements) • Paracentesis • Thoracentesis • Diagnostics, testing, laboratory • Placements of port-a-catheters and peripheral intravenous catheters • Opioid therapy • Nonopioid and nonpharmacological interventions • Dialysis • Medically administered hydration and nutrition management
Consultation	• Social work/counseling • Chaplaincy • Physical therapy/occupational therapy/speech language pathology • Wound team • Nutrition • Reiki • Pet therapy • Music therapy

[a] AMD, advance medical directive; DNR, do-not-resuscitate order; POST, physician orders for scope of treatment; POLST, physician orders for life-sustaining treatment; MOST, medical orders for scope of treatment.

acute care settings, where the focus of care is on active, curative treatment and not on managing symptoms or establishing realistic goals of care, palliative APRNs must be able to advocate for seriously ill patients and their loved ones.[41,52] Patients need APRNs who are skilled in the science of palliative medicine as well as in the art of holistic healing. With the ever-changing healthcare environment, palliative APRNs are essential in providing specialized interventions to meet the diverse needs of acute care patients (Table 8.3).

SUMMARY

This chapter discusses the specialized role of the palliative APRN in the ever-changing acute care environment. More than 50% of all deaths occur in medical, surgical, and oncology units where the focus is on active, curative treatment, not on managing symptoms and establishing realistic goals of care. Palliative APRNs are uniquely qualified to care for seriously ill patients by providing comprehensive, effective, compassionate, and cost-effective care that improves end-of-life care in acute care settings. Care must be focused on patients with common conditions including end-stage renal disease, dementia, hip fractures, and oncological conditions and their associated sequelae.

REFERENCES

1. May P, Normand C, Cassell JB, et al. Economics of palliative care for hospitalized adults with serious illness: A meta-analysis. *JAMA Intern Med.* 2018;178(6):820–829. doi:10.1001/jamainternmed.2018.0750
2. Schoenherr LA, Bischoff KE, Marks AK, O'Riordan DL, Pantilat SZ. Trends in hospital-based specialty palliative care in the United States from 2013 to 2017. *JAMA Netw Open.* 2019;2(12):e1917043. Published 2019 Dec 2. doi:10.1001/jamanetworkopen.2019.17043
3. Ernecoff NC, Zimmerman S, Mitchell SL, et al. Concordance between goals of care and treatment decisions for person with dementia. *J Palliat Med.* 2018;21(10):1442–1447. doi:10.1089/jpm.2018.0103
4. van Dusseldorp L, Groot M, Adriaansen M, van Vught A, Vissers K, Peters J. What does the nurse practitioner mean to you? A patient-oriented qualitative study in oncological/palliative care. *J Clin Nurs.* 2019(3-4);28:589–602. doi:10.1111/jocn.14653
5. Ernecoff NC, Lin FC, Wessell KL, Hanson LC. Quality of life with late-stage dementia: Exploring opportunities to intervene. *J Am Geriatr Soc.* 2019(6);67:1189–1196. doi:10.1111/jgs.15794
6. Kyeremanteng K, Ismail A, Wan C, Thavorn K, D'Egidio G. Outcomes and cost of patients with terminal cancer admitted to acute care in the final 2 weeks of life: A retrospective chart review. *Am J Hosp Palliat Med.* 2019;36(11):1020–1025. doi:10.1177/1049909119843285
7. Reed SM. A Unitary-Caring Conceptual Model for advanced practice nursing in palliative care. *Holist Nurs Pract.* 2010;24(1):23–34. doi:10.1097/HNP.0b013e3181c8e4c7
8. Lam DY, Scherer JS, Brown M, Grubbs V, Schell JO. A conceptual framework of palliative care across the continuum of advanced kidney disease. *Clin J Am Soc Nephrol.* 2019;14(4):635–641. doi:10.2215/CJN.09330818
9. Axelsson L, Alvariza A, Lindberg J, et al. Unmet palliative care needs among patients with end-stage kidney disease: A national registry study about the last week of life. *J Pain Symptom Manage.* 2018;55(2):236–244. doi:10.1016/j.jpainsymman.2017.09.015
10. Forzley B, Er L, Chiu HHL, et al. External validation and clinical utility of a prediction model for 6-month mortality in patients undergoing hemodialysis for end-stage disease. *Palliat Med.* 2018;32(2):395–403. doi:10.1177/0269216317720832
11. Mechler K, Liantonio J. Palliative care approach to chronic diseases: End stages of heart failure, chronic obstructive pulmonary disease, liver failure and renal failure. *Prim Care—Clin Off Pract.* 2019;46(3):415–432. doi:10.1016/j.pop.2019.05.008
12. Cohen L, Ruthazer R, Moss AH, Germain M. Predicting six month mortality for patient on maintenance hemodialysis. *Clin J Am Soc Nephrol.* 2010;5(1):72–79. doi:10.2215/CJN.03860609
13. Sellars M, Morton R, Clayton J, et al. Case-control study of end-of-life treatment preferences and costs following advance care planning for adults with end-stage kidney disease. *Nephrology (Carlton).* 2019;24(2):148–154. doi:10.1111/nep.13230
14. Sellars M, Clayton JM, Detering KM, Tong A, Power D, Morton RL. Cost and outcomes of advance care planning and end-of-life care for older adults with end-stage kidney disease: A person centred decision analysis. *PLoS One.* 2019;14(5):1–11, e0217787. Published 2019 May 31. doi:10.1371/journal.pone.0217787
15. Buonocore D, Wiegand DL. Palliative care for advanced practice nurses. *Am Assoc Crit Care Nurses Adv Crit Care.* 2015;28(2):108–109. doi:10.1097/NCI.0000000000000087
16. Ernecoff NC, Wessell KL, Hanson LC, et al. Does receipt of recommended elements of palliative care precede in-hospital death or hospice referral? *J Pain Symptom Manage.* 2020;59(4):778–786. doi:10.1016/j.jpainsymman.2019.11.011
17. Scott IA, Rajakaruna N, Shah D, Miller L, Reymond E, Daly M. Normalising advance care planning in a general medicine service of a tertiary hospital: An exploratory study. *Aust Heal Rev.* 2015;40(4):391–398. doi:10.1071/AH15068
18. Burns RB, Waikar SS, Wachterman MW, Kanjee Z. Management options for an older adult with advanced chronic disease and dementia. *Ann Intern Med.* 2020;173(3):217–225. doi:10.7326/M20-2640
19. O'Halloran P, Noble H, Norwood K, et al. Advance care planning with patients who have end-stage kidney disease: A systematic realist review. *J Pain Symptom Manage.* 2018;56(5):795–807. e18. doi:10.1016/j.jpainsymman.2018.07.008
20. Raghavan D, Holley JL. Conservative care of the elderly CKD patient: A practical guide. *Adv Chronic Kidney Dis.* 2016;23(1):51–56. doi:10.1053/j.ackd.2015.08.003
21. Bansal AD, Leonberg-Yoo A, Schell JO, Scherer JS, Jones CA. Ten tips nephrologists wish the palliative care team knew about caring for patients with kidney disease. *J Palliat Med.* 2018;21(4):546–551. doi:10.1089/jpm.2018.0087
22. Hole B, Hemmelgarn B, Brown E, et al. Supportive care for end-kidney disease: An integral part of kidney services across a range of income settings around the world. *Kidney Int Suppl.* 2020;10(1):e86–e94. doi:10.1016/j.kisu.2019.11.008
23. Hickish D, Roberts D. The nurse-led model of hospice care. *Int J Palliat Nurs.* 2019;25(3):143–149. doi:10.12968/ijpn.2019.25.3.143
24. Watt AD, Jenkins NL, McColl G, Collins S, Desmond PM. Ethical issues in the treatment of late-stage Alzheimer's Disease. *J Alzheimer's Dis.* 2019;68(4):1311–1316. doi:10.3233/JAD-180865
25. Hanson LC, Collichio F, Bernard SA, et al. Integrating palliative oncology care for patients with advanced cancer: A quality improvement intervention. *J Palliat Med.* 2017;20(12):1366–1371. doi:10.1089/jpm.2017.0100
26. Goebel JR, Ferolito M, Gorman N. Pain screening in the older adult with delirium. *Pain Manag Nurs.* 2019;20(6):519–525. doi:10.1016/j.pmn.2019.07.003
27. Herr K, Coyne PJ, Ely E, Gélinas C, Manworren RCB. Pain assessment in the patient unable to self-report: Clinical practice recommendations in support of the ASPMN 2019 position statement. *Pain Manag Nurs.* 2019;20(5):404–417. doi:10.1016/j.pmn.2019.07.005
28. Hum A, Tay RY, Wong YKY, et al. Advanced dementia: An integrated homecare programme. *BMJ Support Palliat Care.* 2020;10(4):e40. doi:10.1136/bmjspcare-2019-001798

29. Herr K, Coyne PJ, Ely E, Gélinas C, Manworren RCB. ASPMN 2019 position statement: Pain assessment in the patient unable to self-report. *Pain Manag Nurs.* 2019;20(5):402–403. doi:10.1016/j.pmn.2019.07.007

30. Greenfield SM, Gil E, Agmon M. A bridge to cross: Tube feeding and the barriers to implementation of palliative care for the advanced dementia patient. [published online ahead of print, 2020 Jul 31]. *J Clin Nurs.* 2020;10.1111/jocn.15437. doi:10.1111/jocn.15437

31. Sullivan NM, Blake LE, George M, Mears SC. Palliative care in the hip fracture patient. *Geriatr Orthop Surg Rehabil.* 2019;10:1–7. doi:10.1177/2151459319849801

32. Berry L, Castellani R, Stuart B. The branding of palliative care. *J Oncol Pract.* 2016;12(1):48–50. doi:10.1200/JOP.2015.008656

33. Scott J, Owen-Smith A, Tonkin-Crine S, et al. Decision-making for people with dementia and advanced kidney disease: A secondary qualitative analysis of interviews from the Conservative Kidney Management Assessment of Practice Patterns study. *BMJ Open.* 2018;8(11):e022385. Published 2018 Nov 12. doi:10.1136/bmjopen-2018-022385

34. Gleason LJ, Benton EA, Alvarez-Nebreda ML, Weaver MJ, Harris MB, Javedan H. FRAIL Questionnaire screening tool and short-term outcomes in geriatric fracture patients. *JAMDA.* 2017;18(12):1082–1086. doi:10.1016/j.jamda.2017.07.005

35. Ritchie CS, Kelley AS, Cenzer I, Smith AK, Wallhagen ML, Covinsky KE. High levels of geriatric palliative care needs in hip fracture patients before the hip fracture. *J Pain Symptom Manage.* 2016;52(4):533–538. doi:10.1016/j.jpainsymman.2016.07.003

36. Mehr DR, Tatum PE, Crist BD. Hip fractures in patients with advanced dementia: What treatment provides the best palliation? *JAMA Intern Med.* 2018;178(6):780–781. doi:10.1001/jamainternmed.2018.0822

37. Milte R, Crotty M, Miller MD, Whitehead C, Ratcliffe J. Quality of life in older adults following a hip fracture: An empirical comparison of the ICECAP-O and the EQ-5D-3 L instruments. *Health Qual Life Outcomes.* 2018;16(1):173. Published 2018 Sep 5. doi:10.1186/s12955-018-1005-9

38. Harries L, Moore A, Kendall C, Stringfellow TD, Davies A. Attitudes to palliative care in patients with neck-of-femur fracture: A multicenter survey. *Geriatr Orthop Surg Rehabil.* 2020;11:2151459320916931. Published 2020 Apr 16. doi:10.1177/2151459320916931

39. Joosse P, Loggers SAI, Van De Ree CLP, et al. The value of non-operative versus operative treatment of frail institutionalized elderly patients with a proximal femoral fracture in the shade of life (FRAIL-HIP): Protocol for a multicenter observational cohort study. *BMC Geriatr.* 2019;19(1):301. Published 2019 Nov 8. doi:10.1186/s12877-019-1324-7

40. Shaw M, Shaw J, Simon J. Listening to patients' own goals: A key to goals to care decisions in cardiac care. *Can J Cardiol.* 2020;36:1135–1138. doi:10.1016/j.cjca.2020.04.020

41. Shah N, Aiello J, Avigan DE, et al. The Society for Immunotherapy of Cancer consensus statement on immunotherapy for the treatment of multiple myeloma. *J Immunother Cancer.* 2020;8(2):1–15. doi:10.1136/jitc-2020-000734

42. McCorkle R, Jeon S, Ercolano E, et al. An advanced practice nurse coordinated multidisciplinary intervention for patients with late-stage cancer: A cluster randomized trial. *J Palliat Med.* 2015;18(11):962–969. doi:10.1089/jpm.2015.0113

43. Slama O, Pochop L, Sedo J, et al. Effects of early and systematic integration of specialist palliative care in patients with advanced cancer: Randomized controlled trial PALINT. *J Palliat Med.* 2020;23(12):1586–1593. doi:10.1089/jpm.2019.0697

44. Shippee ND, Shippee TP, Mobley PD, Fernstrom KM, Britt HR. Effect of a whole-person model of care on patient experience in patients with complex chronic illness in late life. *Am J Hosp Palliat Med.* 2018;35(1):104–109. doi:10.1177/1049909117690710

45. Zertuche-Maldonado T, Tellez-Villarreal R, Pascual A, et al. Palliative care needs in an acute internal medicine ward in Mexico. *J Palliat Med.* 2018;21(2):163–168. doi:10.1089/jpm.2017.0043

46. Dong J, Li B, Zhou Q, Huang D. Advances in evidence-based medicine for immunotherapy of non-small cell lung cancer. *J Evid Based Med.* 2018;11(4):278–287. doi:10.1111/jebm.12322

47. Bayer V, Amaya B, Banlewicz D, Callahan C, Marsh L, McCoy A. Cancer immunotherapy: An evidence-based overview and implications for practice. *Clin J Oncol Nurs.* 2017;21(2 Suppl):13–21. doi:10.1188/17.CJON.S2.13-21

48. Wong A, Billett A, Milne D. Balancing the hype with reality: What do patients with advanced melanoma consider when making the decision to have immunotherapy? *Oncologist.* 2019;24(11):e1190–e1196. doi:10.1634/theoncologist.2018-0820

49. Wiesenthal A, Patel S, LeBlanc T, Roeland E, Kamal AH. Top ten tips for palliative care clinicians caring for cancer patients receiving immunotherapies. *J Palliat Med.* 2018;21(5):694–699. doi:10.1089/jpm.2018.0107

50. Rapoport B, van Eeden R, Sibaud V, et al. Supportive care for patients undergoing immunotherapy. *Support Care Cancer.* 2017;25(10):3017–3030. doi:10.1007/s00520-017-3802-9

51. Gott M, Robinson J, Moeke-Maxwell T, et al. It was peaceful, it was beautiful: A qualitative study of family understandings of good end-of-life care in hospital for people dying in advanced age. *Palliat Med.* 2019;33(7):793–801. doi:10.1177/0269216319843026

9.

THE PALLIATIVE APRN IN THE INTENSIVE CARE SETTING

Clareen Wiencek

KEY POINTS

- Palliative care is now an expected component of high-quality care in the intensive care unit (ICU).

- The palliative advanced practice registered nurse (APRN) has the ideal skill set to influence clinical outcomes in the ICU.

- The palliative APRN needs to acquire knowledge about pain and symptom management, resuscitation outcomes, withdrawal and withholding of life-sustaining treatments, and quality improvement activities in the ICU.

CASE STUDY: ESTABLISHING TRUST

The palliative advanced practice registered nurse (APRN) responded to a consult for an 87-year-old female patient, Mrs. S, who had suffered a massive intracerebral hemorrhage. She had multiple comorbidities and had been living at home with her grandson, John, prior to the acute event. Mrs. S was minimally responsive, intubated and mechanically ventilated, and on vasopressor support. She was a full code as a default due to the absence of an advance directive. The APRN was consulted to help with goals of care and was informed that the patient's grandson was unreasonable and abrasive. After an examination of the patient, the palliative APRN met with the intensivist and John. She started the meeting by asking John what he understood about his grandmother's condition and what the doctors had told him, and affirmed John's obvious love and devotion for his grandmother. In addition, the APRN asked what a typical "good day" looked like for his grandmother and what activities gave her joy. During that meeting, she began to establish trust with John and began to de-escalate some of the aggressive behavior. The palliative APRN assured him that the ICU team was doing everything they could to support his grandmother and did not press for a change in code status during the first encounter. Over several days, trust continued to increase but the patient's condition did not improve. The team and John agreed that more aggressive intervention would be more harmful than helpful to his grandmother and agreed to a do-not-resuscitate (DNR) order. The palliative APRN helped John to consider his grandmother's quality of life and dignity and to begin to think about possibly discontinuing the ventilator rather than performing a tracheostomy and continued support in light of grave neurological outcomes. The palliative APRN made recommendations on how to manage the patient's agitation and

sedation while on the ventilator. Over one weekend, John contacted the APRN and told her that he was ready to discontinue the ventilator. He shared that his grandmother had come to him in a dream and asked that he let her go. The palliative APRN worked with the intensivist and bedside nurse to allow John time with his grandmother and then premedicated the patient prior to extubation and removal of the ventilator. Spiritual care provided presence and support prior to the actual procedure. Mrs. S died peacefully 4 hours later with her grandson at her side in the ICU. John expressed gratitude to the palliative APRN and ICU team for the compassionate care of his beloved grandmother. His memory of a good death was preserved through the skilled delivery of palliative care.

INTRODUCTION

The early intensive care units (ICUs) of the 1950s were opened to care for the sickest patients and to concentrate the knowledge and skills of the nurses and physicians who worked there. The aim was rescue and survival of the most critical patients in a more efficient and effective physical space.[1] This mission has not changed over the past 60 years, but technological and medical advances have transformed those early units into modern, high-tech centers within acute care hospitals. At first glance, palliative care may seem an incongruous fit for the ICU due to the fundamental difference between the ICU goals of cure and rescue and the palliative goals of quality of life and symptom management. However, after a decade of explosive growth in acute care–based palliative care programs and considerable expansion of the evidence base, palliative care in the ICU setting is no longer a novelty but an essential component of high-quality care.[2,3] Most critical care professional societies have issued position statements, protocols, or clinical practice guidelines that delineate the how and why of integrating palliative care in the care of the critically ill.[4–7] The Center to Advance Palliative Care (CAPC) launched the Improve Palliative Care in the ICU (IPAL-ICU) initiative in 2010, and it is an excellent resource for quality improvement (QI).[8] Given the ongoing shift in acceptance and viewpoints, the palliative advanced practice registered nurse (APRN) is ideally suited to deliver high-quality outcomes for critically ill patients and their families through the full integration of palliative care in the ICU setting, whether in the integrative or consultative role.[8]

All critically ill patients and their families have palliative care needs based on the definition found in the fourth edition of the National Consensus Project for Quality Palliative Care *Clinical Practice Guidelines* which states,

> Beneficial at any stage of a serious illness, palliative care is an interdisciplinary care delivery system designed to anticipate, prevent, and manage physical, psychological, social, and spiritual suffering to optimize quality of life for patients, their families and caregivers. Palliative care can be delivered in any care setting through the collaboration of many types of care providers. Through early integration into the care plan of seriously ill people, palliative care improves quality of life for both the patient and the family.[9(p. ii)]

This more expansive definition, broadening beyond just end-of-life care, has yet to be widely accepted in the ICU setting. However, all critically ill patients and their families have needs consistent with this definition: goal-oriented care that is aligned with their goals, preferences, and values; the management and relief of distressing symptoms related to the underlying critical illness and to the procedures and interventions inherent in that treatment; regular and effective communication between the critical care team and the patient and surrogate decision-makers, so common in the ICU setting; and deliberate planning for care transitions.[2]

The commonality of palliative needs in the critically ill and the palliative interventions to meet those needs can be driven by APRNs when they are allowed to practice to the full scope of their education, licensure, and certification. Full scope of practice was just one of the changes called for by the Institute of Medicine (IOM)'s 2010 report, *The Future of Nursing: Leading Change, Advancing Health*.[10] The palliative APRN, when practicing to full scope, can improve care for those patients who will survive the life-threatening episode and for those who will die in the ICU. Although palliative care is broader than just terminal care, death is common in the ICU: one in five Americans die in the ICU or during an ICU-related admission.[11]

The findings of the landmark Study to Understand Prognoses and Preferences for Outcomes and Risks of Treatments (SUPPORT)[12] and the 1997 IOM report *Approaching Death: Improving Care at the End of Life*[13] revealed that Americans do not die well. The SUPPORT investigators found that 50% of the more than 9,000 seriously ill patients enrolled in the study died with unrelieved pain and experienced an undesirable ICU admission in the last week prior to death.[13] Multiple studies since have reported limitations in the care of the critically ill. These discrepancies include unrelieved pain and other symptoms, inadequate communication and goal setting, divergence in goals of treatment, clinician burnout and moral distress, and inefficient resource utilization.[5,14] Since death is common in the ICU and usually occurs after a course of aggressive, life-sustaining interventions, experts assert that an ICU admission is actually a therapeutic trial, and, only when it fails do providers, patients, and families entertain a change in goals from survival at all costs

to palliation.[5] It is time to change that paradigm and fully integrate palliative care from time of admission. The palliative APRN can lead this transformation.

Although death remains common in the ICU setting, especially in medical units, the site of death is shifting. Teno and colleagues analyzed the care of Medicare beneficiaries in 2000, 2005, and 2009.[15] Between 1989 and 2007, home deaths increased from 15% to 24%. However, the rate of ICU use in the last month of life increased from 24.3% to 29.2% in 2009. It is commonly agreed that hospitals are not the preferred place of death, as patients strongly prefer to return home but only after the full trial of advanced, aggressive medical technologies such as those found in the ICU. As noted by Rothman, "in the mid-20th century death and dying was removed and rendered invisible once through hospitalization and again through the intimidating locked doors of the ICU."[1 (p. 2459)] The locked doors have opened for most ICUs, partially thanks to the efforts by the American Association of Critical Care Nurses (AACN) to promote open visitation,[16] and it is now time for palliative care to be fully present.

Palliative APRNs must take up the challenge presented by the life-saving technology in today's ICUs and the expanding evidence base that the critically ill and their families not only could benefit from palliative care but should also expect it. Also, the greater awareness that palliative care does have a place in the ICU has led prominent stakeholders to call for more systematic integration. These stakeholders include the Joint Commission, the Institute for Healthcare Improvement, the Critical Care Societies Collaborative, and the IOM. Toward the goal of optimizing the palliative APRN's impact in the ICU, this chapter focuses on five dimensions: pain and symptom management, communication, discontinuation of life-sustaining treatments, and resuscitation outcomes, and QI activities. Additionally, the impact of the 2020 coronavirus pandemic on how palliative care and critical care were and can be integrated during this global crisis and the provision of primary and secondary palliative care in the emergency department setting, as an entry into the ICU, will be addressed.

PAIN AND SYMPTOM MANAGEMENT

PAIN: PREVALENCE AND CLINICAL PRACTICE GUIDELINES

Pain is a common symptom in the critically ill. Despite more than 20 years of research and quantification of the pain experience, the incidence of significant pain is still 50% or higher in both medical and surgical ICU patients.[17–20] The seminal work by Puntillo[17] in 1990 was one of the first studies to describe the pain experience of critically ill patients, and the multicenter Thunder Project II provided strong evidence of the high incidence, up to 80%, of procedural pain in this population and the inadequate management and relief.[21] Such common procedures as turning, tracheal suctioning, line insertion, and dressing changes were found to be associated with significant levels of pain.[21] The stress response evoked by

Table 9.1 THE PADIS GUIDELINES FOR ADULT ICU PATIENTS: PAIN MANAGEMENT

RECOMMENDATION	STRENGTH	QUALITY OF EVIDENCE
Use an assessment-driven, protocol-based, stepwise approach for pain and sedation management in critically ill adults.	Conditional	Moderate
Use acetaminophen as an adjunct to an opioid to decrease pain intensity and opioid consumption for pain management in critically ill adults.	Conditional	Very low
Use low-dose ketamine (1–2 μg/kg/hr) as an adjunct to opioid therapy when seeking to reduce opioid consumption in postsurgical adults.	Conditional	Low
Use an opioid, at lowest effective dose, for procedural pain management in critically ill adults.	Conditional	Moderate
Use a neuropathic pain medication with opioids for neuropathic pain management in critically ill adults.	Conditional	Low
Do not routinely use IV lidocaine as an adjunct for pain management in critically ill adults.	Conditional	Low
Do not routinely use a COX-1 selective NSAID as an adjunct to opioid therapy for pain management in critically ill adults.	Conditional	Low
Suggest using music therapy or massage for pain management in critically ill adults.	Conditional	Low
Suggest offering relaxation techniques for procedural pain management in critically ill adults.	Conditional	Very low
Do not use local analgesia or nitrous oxide for pain management during chest tube removal in critically ill adults.	Conditional	Low

Adapted from Devlin et al.[22]

unrelieved pain in the critically ill can lead to impaired tissue perfusion, hyperglycemia, lipolysis, and impaired wound healing, thereby increasing not only patient discomfort but risk of prolonged morbidity.[20]

The evidence that most critically ill patients experience pain and that pain continues to be undermanaged led to the development of the *Clinical Practice Guidelines for the Management of Pain, Agitation and Delirium (PAD) in Adult Patients in the Intensive Care Unit* by the American College of Critical Care Medicine, the consultative body of the Society of Critical Care Medicine.[19] These 2013 guidelines were issued to define best practices for optimizing management of pain, agitation, and delirium in the critically ill; however, the authors report that only 60% of ICUs in the United States have implemented PAD guidelines, and compliance with such protocols remains low. These Guidelines were updated in 2018 to include immobility and sleep disruption, thus, they are now referred to as the *PADIS Guidelines*.[22]

There are several reasons behind the continued prevalence of suboptimal pain management in the critically ill. One of the main reasons is the conflict in goals between rescue and comfort.[18] Many ICU nurses and providers, especially those in training, may be concerned about and therefore reluctant to use medications such as opioids that could impact hemodynamic stability, threaten end-organ perfusion and function, or induce oversedation and respiratory depression.[18,22] Second, critical care practitioners may not have the experience or knowledge about the use of opioids and adjuvant

medications, including routes other than the parenteral route widely used in the ICU setting.[13,18] Third, there is a growing number of evidence-based management bundles and checklists used in the ICU setting that may complicate the delicate balance between treatment goals and quality of life for the patient.[18–20] Finally, the preponderance of nonverbal patients in the ICU limits the gold standard of patient self-report, resulting in the use of surrogate reports or interpretations and therefore potentially leading to a reluctance to administer pain medications in doses adequate for relief.[23] The palliative APRN practicing in the ICU must be aware of and accommodate to these realities of pain management, especially when in the consultative role. Table 9.1 lists the major recommendations from the 2018 *PADIS Guidelines* for pain management. The full document includes 37 recommendations noting the strength and quality of evidence. Chapter 43 provides a full discussion of pain management principles.

PAIN AND SPECIAL PATIENT POPULATIONS: NONVERBAL PATIENTS

The prevalence of critically ill patients unable to self-report pain is high due to a multitude of factors that include severity of illness, neurological dysfunction or injury, intentional sedation, metabolic disturbances, and vital organ dysfunction. This prevalence poses a challenge to optimal pain management for the palliative APRN. Since these patients cannot self-report, the APRN must use standardized scales and multiple measures on which to base assessment and management.[25] The palliative APRN should assess for behavioral signs of pain, such as grimacing, furrowed brow, restlessness, and delirium. Generally, vital signs as physiologic indicators are not sensitive for discriminating pain from other distressing triggers.[25] No single strategy will be sufficient, and the APRN must be aware that vital signs that are within normal ranges do not indicate an absence of pain.[25] In fact, the APRN should assume that pain is present for those on neuromuscular blockade and recommend appropriate analgesic therapy.[23]

Clinical practice guidelines call for a hierarchy of pain assessment techniques in the adult, nonverbal patient: self-report, ruling out potential causes of pain, observing patient behaviors, using surrogate reporting, and attempting an analgesic trial.[25] A therapeutic trial is indicated if a pathologic or procedural reason exists for pain. For mild to moderate pain, a non-opioid analgesic should be given initially; if the patient's behaviors improve, continue the regimen. If the pain-related behaviors do not improve, the APRN should order a trial dose of a short-acting opioid and observe the effect. If there is no change in behavioral indicators of pain, the dose should be increased by 25–50% and the nurse should observe the effect.[25]

The palliative APRN may use proxy reports of pain as a basis for management in the nonverbal patient. Proxy reports remain controversial; families often overestimate pain.[24] Even so, family members can provide valuable information, such as a history of chronic back pain, that can influence pain management outcomes.

Multiple scales are used to assess pain in the nonverbal adult population, but two scales are more commonly used and have sound psychometrics: the *Behavioral Pain Scale* (BPS) and the *Critical-Care Pain Observation Tool* (CPOT). These two scales are the most reliable and valid behavioral pain scales for assessing and monitoring pain in nonverbal medical, surgical, or trauma ICU patients and should be used at standardized intervals.[22,24,25]

PAIN AND SPECIAL PATIENT POPULATIONS: RENAL AND HEPATIC FAILURE

It is estimated that up to 25% of all ICU patients present with or develop acute renal failure, depending on the setting and the definition.[26] In addition to patients with acute renal failure, chronic kidney disease is prevalent in the ICU setting.

If opioids are used by the palliative APRN to manage pain in this population, certain medications must be avoided or used with caution. However, there is a lack of hard pharmacokinetic data that support specific treatment guidelines.[27] Meperidine, codeine, dextropropoxyphene (propoxyphene), and morphine should be avoided due to toxicity and/or the accumulation of active, nondialyzable metabolites.[27] Oxycodone and hydromorphone should be used with caution. Oxycodone undergoes hepatic metabolism, but 19% is excreted unchanged in the urine. Hydromorphone should be used prudently in patients who are not on dialysis due to the rapid accumulation of its active metabolite.[27] Fentanyl and

---

Box 9.1 GUIDELINES TO OPTIMIZE PAIN MANAGEMENT IN PATIENTS WITH HEPATIC FAILURE

1. Reduce long-term acetaminophen dosing to 2–3 g/day.

2. A one-time acetaminophen dose of 3–4 g/day may be safe.

3. Use reduced doses of non-steroidal anti-inflammatory drugs (NSAIDs) and opioids in patients with cirrhosis.

4. Avoid using NSAIDs in patients with compensated or decompensated cirrhosis due to the risk of inducing acute renal failure from prostaglandin inhibition.

5. Avoid using opioids in patients with a history of encephalopathy.

6. Avoid using codeine and meperidine at all times.

7. Decrease hydromorphone dose by 50% of normal dose and administer it at prolonged dosing intervals.

---

methadone are considered to be the safest opioids for patients in renal failure.[27]

The critically ill patient with hepatic failure also presents challenges in terms of optimal pain and symptom management. The greater the hepatic dysfunction, the greater the impairment in drug metabolism and removal.[28,29] The efficiency of drug removal by the liver depends on blood flow, plasma protein binding, and hepatic enzymes. Advanced liver dysfunction alters the effects of many medications as a result of changes in pharmacokinetics, abnormal accumulation of the free drug in plasma, and end-organ response. The palliative APRN should be aware that the majority of pain medications are largely metabolized by the liver and that opioid clearance is reduced and drug bioavailability increased in hepatic failure. Fentanyl is the preferred opioid in this population.[30] Given the variability in response, the right dose and interval of any opioid are those tolerated by the patient. Dosing should be based on close and frequent assessment of the patient's response.[30] Box 9.1 provides guidelines on how to optimize pain management in patients with hepatic failure.[28–30]

SYMPTOM MANAGEMENT: AGITATION AND DELIRIUM

Agitation is common in critically ill patients.[22] The palliative APRN should assess for possible causes of agitation when developing the treatment plan, such as pain, delirium, hypoxemia, or withdrawal from alcohol or opioids. Strong evidence now exists that prolonged deep sedation is associated with adverse outcomes and that light sedation from which the patient can be aroused and can follow simple commands is preferred.[22] Indeed, most ICUs have established treatment protocols with this goal. Due to the growing evidence that benzodiazepine use is strongly correlated with delirium in the acutely ill patient, patterns of use are changing. Currently, the dominant medications used for sedation of the critically ill patient are midazolam and propofol (Diprivan), with decreasing use of lorazepam, rare use of diazepam and barbiturates, and growing use of dexmedetomidine (Precedex).[22]

The palliative APRN caring for patients in the ICU should be familiar with the pharmacokinetics and side effects of propofol and dexmedetomidine due to their common use in this setting. Propofol is an intravenous sedative that binds to multiple central nervous system receptors to block neural impulses. It has sedative, hypnotic, anxiolytic, antiemetic, and anticonvulsant properties. Propofol does not possess any analgesic properties, so analgesics must be coadministered. This drug causes dose-dependent respiratory depression and hypotension but has rapid redistribution and a short duration, making it an ideal adjuvant for mechanical ventilator–related sedation that allows for daily sedation interruption protocols.[22,23] Dexmedetomidine is a selective alpha-receptor agonist with sedative, analgesic or opioid-sparing, and sympatholytic properties that was approved in the United States more than 10 years ago for short-term sedation (<24 hours) at a maximum dose of 0.7 µg/kg/hour. Its pattern of sedation differs significantly from other sedatives as patients are more easily arousable, but its onset is also quick (in about 15 minutes). Dexmedetomidine produces minimal respiratory depression and therefore is the only sedative approved in the United States for administration in non-intubated patients. However, patients' ventilator and oxygenation status must still be closely monitored as the drug can cause loss of oropharyngeal muscle tone, putting the patient at risk of airway obstruction. The most common side effects of dexmedetomidine are hypotension and bradycardia. The opioid-sparing effects of this sedative may reduce opioid requirements in the critically ill patient.[22]

Agitation can be distressing for the critically ill patient, family members, and the team. Preferred agents in the ICU have changed over the past decade based on research, and strong evidence now supports the use of subjective sedation scales at regular intervals. The most valid and reliable sedation assessment tools for adult ICU patients are the *Richmond Agitation-Sedation Scale* (RASS) and the *Sedation-Agitation Scale* (SAS).[22] These two scales demonstrated a high degree of interrater reliability and had robust methodology and sampling method. Table 9.2 provides recommendations from the 2018 PADIS guidelines on managing agitation and delirium in ICU patients.

Delirium is also highly prevalent in critically ill patients, affecting up to 80% of mechanically ventilated patients.[22] Strong evidence now exists that even one episode of delirium is an independent predictor of adverse clinical outcomes, such as increased mortality, increased hospital length of stay, higher costs of care, and long-term cognitive impairment.[31,32] Delirium is a syndrome associated with a change or fluctuation in mental status, inattention, and either disorganized thinking or an altered level of consciousness.[22] Hypoactive delirium and hyperactive delirium exist, with hypoactive being more common, and ICU clinicians often underestimate its clinical presence.[22] Formerly referred to as "ICU psychosis," it is no longer considered a benign condition in the ICU or acute care setting.

The ideal treatment for delirium is prevention and the use of standardized screening. The palliative APRN should be familiar with the *Confusion Assessment Method for the ICU* (CAM-ICU) and the *Intensive Care Delirium Screening Checklist* (ICDSC), which are the most valid and reliable instruments for the screening and monitoring of delirium in ICU patients.[22] Moderate-quality evidence exists that routine monitoring for delirium is feasible and that monitoring compliance rates exceed 90%.[22] There is mixed or a lack of evidence that haloperidol is effective as a preventive measure.

Table 9.2 PADIS GUIDELINES FOR ADULT ICU PATIENTS: AGITATION AND DELIRIUM

RECOMMENDATION	STRENGTH	QUALITY OF EVIDENCE
Use light sedation vs deep sedation in critically ill, mechanically ventilated adults.	Conditional	Low
Use propofol over a benzodiazepine for sedation in mechanically ventilated adults after cardiac surgery.	Conditional	Low
Critically ill adults should be regularly assessed for delirium with a valid tool.	N/A	N/A
Sedation strategies using non-benzodiazepines (propofol or dexmedetomidine) should be used over benzodiazepines for sedation in mechanically ventilated adult ICU patients.	Conditional	Low
Suggest not using haloperidol, dexmedetomidine, or ketamine to prevent delirium in all critically ill adults.	Conditional	Very low to low
Suggest not routinely using haloperidol to treat delirium.	Conditional	Low
Use a multicomponent, nonpharmacologic intervention that is focused on but not limited to reducing modifiable risk factors for delirium, improving cognition, and optimizing sleep, mobility, hearing, and vision in critically ill adults.	Conditional	Low

Adapted from Devlin et al.[22]

SYMPTOM MANAGEMENT: DYSPNEA

Dyspnea is a prevalent symptom in the critically ill population.[33] Puntillo and other members of the IPAL-ICU Advisory Board conducted a comprehensive literature review related to palliation of pain, dyspnea, and thirst.[33] Optimal treatment for dyspnea was found to be identification and amelioration of the underlying condition, patient positioning, and, sometimes, supplemental oxygen. As for other symptoms, the use of a standardized symptom assessment scale is correlated with better outcomes. The *Respiratory Distress Observation Scale* is the only reported behavioral scale for assessment of dyspnea. A systematic review by Lorenz and colleagues focused on the management of dyspnea at end of life.[34] Strong evidence supported the use of beta-agonists and opioids in patients with chronic obstructive pulmonary disease, and weak evidence supported the use of opioids to relieve dyspnea in patients with cancer.

Several options are available for the treatment of dyspnea in patients at end of life. Systemic opioids, either oral or parenteral, are considered first-line medications. Opioid receptors are found in the respiratory centers of the brain and peripherally in the respiratory tract and lung tissue. Clinicians have suggested that nebulized opioids would result in less systemic absorption, leading to a safer clinical profile. However, robust trials and systematic reviews have found these to be no more effective than placebo.[35] Guidelines from the American College of Chest Physicians recommend the use of systemic opioids for relief of dyspnea.[36] A robust Cochrane Review concluded that evidence does not support the routine use of benzodiazepines in patients with dyspnea without coexisting anxiety.[37] However, the treatment of underlying conditions that exacerbate dyspnea, such as edema or inflammation, can provide benefit if glucocorticoids, bronchodilators, and diuretics are used.[35]

SYMPTOM MANAGEMENT: OTHER CONSIDERATIONS

Although pain, dyspnea, and thirst are three of the most distressing and prevalent symptoms reported by critically ill patients,[33] other distressing symptoms can occur. These include anxiety, depression, nausea and vomiting, and sleep disturbances. The appropriate chapters in this text provide full discussions, as these are not unique to the ICU. What *is* unique is the impact that the delicate balance between the ICU goals of rescue and hemodynamic stability and the palliative goals of comfort and quality of life has on treatment plans. The palliative APRN needs to be aware of the medications and alternate routes that can be used in the ICU for patients across the continuum of survival to end of life because barriers exist to medication administration and choice of agents.[35] The choice of pharmacologic agents to treat symptoms must be considered after clear goals of care are established between the patient/family, ICU team, and palliative team.

Although symptom management requires a multimodal approach, pharmacologic agents are often used by the palliative APRN to relieve general symptoms. The route of administration is predominantly intravenous, but if this route no longer exists, medications can be given by the buccal, sublingual, rectal, nebulized, or transdermal route. Liquid concentrates, sometimes referred to as *intensol* (i.e., lorazepam intensol), are up to 10 times more potent and can be given orally in very small volumes. These are considered high-alert medications by the Institute for Safe Medication Practices. Topical agents may be used with the intent of systemic absorption to control symptoms at end of life, but the APRN should be cautious about using compounded formulations because evidence is lacking to support efficacy. Frail or cachectic patients may have lower absorption and therefore inadequate symptom management due to low body fat stores. Transdermal fentanyl patches must be used with caution in this scenario or not at all. Rectal medications should be avoided in patients with thrombocytopenia, neutropenia, diarrhea, abdominal-perineal resection, and anorectal disease. Although many agents can be given by this route, patient comfort and choice must be considered. The subcutaneous route may be used as an alternate to the intravenous route but does result in slower drug absorption rates. These are limited to volumes of 1 mL or less, but continuous infusions can be administered if more than 1 mL is needed and have been shown to provide more stable symptom control. Limited evidence supports the use of nebulized morphine and fentanyl and these should not be used as a regular alternative to parenteral or oral formulations. Nebulized lidocaine has been shown to be effective for intractable cough at end of life.[35]

THE PALLIATIVE APRN'S ROLE IN COMMUNICATION

Skilled communication is at the core of effective palliative care integration across all settings and is especially critical in the ICU. The transition from goals of rescue and cure to goals of comfort—or mixed goals combining elements of intensive care and palliative care—can be a turbulent time for patients, families, and the ICU team. The palliative APRN is ideally equipped with communication skills to help all stakeholders navigate this transition. As mentioned earlier in this chapter, the ICU setting is unique due to the delicate balance—and the potential divide—between ICU goals of rescue and the palliative goals of comfort and optimal quality of life. The ICU is the epitome of the technological imperative, so for a patient or family to request, or a consultant to suggest, the discontinuation or withholding of such technology can be a source of conflict unless grounded in expert listening and communication skills. Communication between ICU clinicians and families has been described as a delicate dance with many complex issues embedded in the relationship.[38] Skill is needed to deal with that complexity (see Chapter 32 "Advance Care Planning" and Chapter 33 "Family Meetings").

Regular communication between critically ill patients and their families and the ICU team is now considered an essential component of high-quality care.[2,5,39] Many studies have shown the value of proactive, structured clinician–family communication in the ICU on the establishment of goals of care. These same studies have demonstrated a positive impact on family members' psychological well-being, consensus among surrogate decision-makers and the ICU team, and utilization of ICU resources.[2,39–43] Yet regular meetings between families and ICU clinicians, as the standard of care, remain the exception and not the rule in many ICUs.[2]

The fact that practice is lagging behind evidence in this case may be due to the high incidence of surrogate decision-makers in the ICU. It is estimated that as many as 95% of critically ill patients lack decision-making capacity, requiring families to step forward to make often-difficult treatment decisions.[5] Prognostic uncertainty also exists, although at least one study reported that 87% of surrogate decision-makers preferred that physicians discuss an uncertain prognosis, as they consider this uncertainty to be an unavoidable feature of critical illness.[44]

The palliative APRN can use specific, evidence-based approaches to facilitate communication and goal setting in the ICU and remove the obstacles to family conferences. Competing time demands, lack of space, cultural differences, language barriers, and clinicians who are inadequately trained in communication skills are barriers to family conferences in the ICU setting.[45] Families are more satisfied with ICU communication when relational comments outweigh informational content (i.e., physiological data), when clinicians spend more time listening to and less time talking at the family members, when the family members feel their perspective is valued, and when their emotions are acknowledged and supported.[5] The APRN can use the *Care and Communication Bundle*[2] developed by the IPAL-ICU project. This bundle is a systematized set of activities that culminate in a structured family meeting. It entails several crucial steps, including time frames that are evidence-based. Strategies for improving communication in the ICU are shown in Box 9.2.

Finally, authentic teamwork that involves communication among all team members, regardless of rank or position,

is essential to improve palliative care integration in the ICU. Experts assert that interdisciplinary collaboration based on open communication and mutual respect is the single most important element for success.[2] The palliative APRN should drive such team collaboration based on an understanding of the ICU culture and the evidence behind proactive, structured communication between patients, families, and the ICU team.

RESUSCITATION OUTCOMES AND THE WITHHOLDING AND DISCONTINUING LIFE-SUSTAINING TREATMENTS

A strong working knowledge of resuscitation outcomes and guidelines for discontinuation of life-sustaining treatments is a required element of the palliative APRN's practice in the ICU. This knowledge is essential for optimal outcomes in patient/family meetings, for prognostication, and to achieve congruence between the patient's preferences for treatment and the ICU treatment goals.

Since cardiopulmonary resuscitation (CPR) was first reported in a 1960 study,[46] overall survival to hospital discharge has remained essentially unchanged for decades.[47] The American Heart Association issued 2013 consensus recommendations to improve survival after in-hospital cardiac arrest.[47] The current prevalence of in-hospital cardiac arrests outside the ICU setting is 3.66 in 1,000 adult admissions and 1.14 in pediatric admissions, with 45% of adult and 65% of pediatric arrests occurring in ICUs. Adult survival to discharge after an in-hospital cardiac arrest is 18%, with a 1-year survival of 6.6%. This survival rate was similar to the survival rate of 17% that Weil and Freis reported in 2005 in their analysis of more than 14,000 in-hospital cardiac arrests[48] and in an earlier study by Peberdy and colleagues of 14,720 cardiac arrests.[49] More recent studies of out-of-hospital cardiac arrests show similar outcomes. A study conducted in Sweden analyzed more than 30,000 out-of-hospital cardiac arrests to determine whether bystander CPR performed before the arrival of Emergency Medical Services (EMS) correlated with survival and found that 30-day survival was 10.5% versus 4.0% when no CPR was performed.[50] Yan and colleagues conducted a systematic review and meta-analysis of 141 studies and 1.5 million incidents of out-of-hospital cardiac arrest completed between 1975 and 2019.[51] They found that return of spontaneous circulation after CPR was 29.7%, survival to hospital admission 22%, survival to hospital discharge 8.8%, 1-month survival 10.7%, and 1-year survival 7.7%. Survival was more likely if the out-of-hospital cardiac arrest was witnessed, the victim received bystander CPR, and they were living in Europe or North America. The investigators concluded that global survival rates have increased over the past 40 years, but it should be noted that this survival-to-discharge rate of 8.8% in out-of-hospital cardiac arrests compares to the 17% survival rate of in-hospital cardiac arrest reported in earlier studies.

The American Heart Association has raised concerns that the current culture of hopelessness in outcomes after

---

Box 9.2 EVIDENCE-BASED COMMUNICATION STRATEGIES

1. Train clinicians in communication skills.

2. Conduct family meetings early in the ICU admission.

3. Increase proportion of time spent listening to family members.

4. Use VALUE mnemonic during family meetings:

   a. *Value* statements by family members

   b. *Acknowledge* emotions

   c. *Listen* to family members

   d. *Understand* who the patient is as a person

   e. *Elicit questions* from the family members

Adapted from Troug et al.[5]

in-hospital cardiac arrests may lead to the early discontinuation of life-sustaining treatment and has noted that CPR outcomes should be interpreted with caution due to the lack of consistency in reporting these events.[47] Also, the rising use of therapeutic hypothermia is changing resuscitation outcomes. Three studies, conducted between 2002 and 2011 with a total of 1,391 participants, show better outcomes in the setting of the shockable rhythms of ventricular tachycardia and ventricular fibrillation; survival in this population ranged from 55% to 66%. For patients presenting with asystole or pulseless electrical activity, 8% had a favorable outcome from therapeutic hypothermia.[52-54] Worse outcomes were associated with advanced age, low ejection fraction, seizures, and hemodynamic instability.[52-54]

The palliative APRN should keep abreast of resuscitation outcomes in the ICU and the difference in outcomes between in- and out-of-hospital cardiac arrests or whether therapeutic hypothermia was performed. The APRN should use this prognostic data in combination with the patient's preferences and advance directives as the basis for discussions about whether to withhold or discontinue life-sustaining treatment. Such decisions are commonly made in the ICU setting, and the palliative APRN may be consulted to drive such decisions. There is no ethical distinction between withholding or discontinuing life-sustaining treatment, and experts consider that it is morally and legally permissible for a patient or his or her surrogate to make such life-limiting choices.[55-57] Discontinuation of life-sustaining treatment has broad support in the United States and is based on three principles: discontinuing and withholding are equivalent, allowing death and killing are clearly distinct, and the doctrine of double effect.[5]

Even though there is no ethical distinction between withholding and discontinuing treatment, clinicians are generally more comfortable with the former. The decision to offer or discontinue an intervention should be based solely on a honest risk–benefit analysis in light of the patient's goals and preferences. High courts have upheld a person's right to refuse any unwanted medical treatment, even if life-sustaining.[5] Thus, discontinuing such treatment, even if death follows, is considered to be allowing the person to die from the underlying condition and not to be killing. Finally, the principle of double effect applies to discontinuing or withholding life-sustaining treatment. The philosophical doctrine of double effect draws a moral distinction between giving medications with the intent to allow a natural death free from suffering and giving medications with the direct intent to kill the patient.[5,56]

If the palliative APRN is coordinating discontinuation of life-sustaining treatment, several principles guide care. First, words matter. The APRN should be careful to use the words "discontinuation of technology," avoiding the phrase "discontinuation of care." Language is important, especially to family members who will live with the memory of their loved one's death. Second, there is no single, universally accepted protocol for discontinuation of treatment, so the APRN should be aware of unit or system policies and procedures. Acceptable strategies include nonescalation of current therapies and discontinuation of some or all current support.

The process of discontinuation may be gradual or immediate. Communication with the family and among the team should occur prior to removal of life-sustaining treatment. Third, the palliative APRN should anticipate symptom management needs, especially respiratory distress, if the patient is removed from mechanical ventilation and extubated. The possibility of stridor and airway compromise should be anticipated, and interventions, such as racemic epinephrine, should be readily available. Cook and Rocker[3] found that no or only a low risk of physical distress is associated with discontinuation of renal replacement therapy and inotropes or vasopressors, but a risk of dyspnea is associated with removal of the endotracheal tube and mechanical ventilation. Again, the APRN should be prepared for distressing symptoms in order to act quickly.

Finally, multidisciplinary team members, such as the chaplain or social worker, should be recruited to offer additional support for the family and the ICU team.[3] Cook and Rocker outline activities of dignity-conserving care in the setting of discontinuation of life-sustaining technology: awareness of one's attitudes and assumptions, dignity-enhancing behaviors such as sitting down and not rushing, using compassion to be sensitive to the suffering of others, and engaging in dialogue that acknowledges the personhood of the patient.[3] The palliative APRN can serve as a role model for these dignity-enhancing behaviors to the ICU team when such treatments are discontinued.

THE PALLIATIVE APRN'S ROLE IN QUALITY IMPROVEMENT IN THE ICU

Due to several national initiatives, the palliative APRN has multiple resources for QI in the ICU. In 2002, the Robert Wood Johnson Foundation established the Promoting Palliative Care Excellence in Intensive Care project. The aim was to balance medically aggressive or even futile care with goal-directed palliative care. Seven domains were identified for QI: patient- and family-centered decision-making, communication, continuity of care, emotional and practical support, symptom management, spiritual support, and emotional and organizational support for ICU clinicians. The IPAL-ICU project at the Center to Advance Palliative Care[55] provides a wealth of resources for the palliative APRN to use in QI initiatives. In the Improvement Tools section, there are templates for family meetings, pocket cards to use for family conferences, professional education materials, and other resources. Also, the palliative APRN could use the PADIS guidelines to monitor the quality of outcomes related to the management of pain, agitation, or delirium in the ICU population.

National educational programs are also available that could form the basis for QI. The End-of-Life Nursing Education Consortium (ELNEC) was established more than 10 years ago with the goal to educate nurses, thereby improving the care of patients at end of life. An ELNEC curriculum specific to critical care was developed in 2006. In a statewide effort to educate critical care nurses, ELNEC was shown to be an effective strategy to improve end-of-life care in the ICU.[58]

PALLIATIVE CARE AND CRITICAL CARE IN THE 2020 CORONAVIRUS PANDEMIC

The coronavirus global pandemic in 2020 presented unique challenges to the provision of palliative care in the ICU setting. In the early months, some ICUs and their teams, especially in the Northeast, were overwhelmed with critically ill patients suffering from COVID-19 infection. The consequences of this pandemic and the need to adjust care practices and family visitation policies had a direct effect on ICU and palliative care teams. These challenges included the evolving scientific understanding of the optimal way to treat patients with COVID-19, procedures to keep healthcare personnel safe with personal protective equipment (PPE), care practices that minimized exposure time, and mortality rates with the inherent proximity to the dying process that had a cumulative impact on the well-being of nurses and ICU teams.[59]

The morbidity and mortality rates associated with COVID-19 highlighted the need to integrate palliative care and critical care. Rosa, Ferrell, and Wiencek reported on the resources available to palliative care and critical care teams to optimally support patients and their families and, as importantly, their teams.[59] Many professional associations offered high-quality COVID-19 resources free of charge on their websites.[59] The palliative APRN is directed to those sites as the pandemic continues to be a challenge to holistic care and clinician well-being.

PALLIATIVE CARE IN THE EMERGENCY DEPARTMENT

Many of the conditions and challenges that the palliative APRN must manage in the ICU setting also apply to the emergency department (ED) setting. The challenges of balancing the goals of cure and aggressive interventions against the reality of life-limiting disease or injuries and providing holistic care that encompasses the physical, psychological, social, and spiritual dimensions of quality of life in a typically frenetic environment are the same. As discussed in this chapter, the palliative APRN should use evidence-based pain and symptom management, use skilled communication with patients and families and the ED team, be familiar with resuscitation outcomes, and be sensitive to the workflow of the ED setting. The APRN is directed to Chapter 10, The Palliative APRN in the Emergency Department and the rich resources provided by the Center to Advance Palliative Care's initiative to integrate palliative care practices in the emergency department.[55]

SUMMARY

Palliative care is now considered an essential component of high-quality critical care. ICU patients experience serious or life-threatening illnesses and the associated symptom burden. Distressing symptoms are common in the critically ill and are amenable to the intervention of palliative APRNs. Palliative APRNs, whether in a consultative or integrative role, can improve outcomes for the critically ill in the areas of pain and symptom management, communication enhancement and family meeting structures, withholding and discontinuation of life-sustaining treatments, and the planning and implementation of QI activities. The palliative APRN has the skills to help patients and families and the ICU team navigate the often-tumultuous transition from the ICU goals of rescue to the more palliative goals of comfort and quality of life. The time is now for the full integration of these two disciplines.

REFERENCES

1. Rothman DJ. Where we die. *N Engl J Med.* 2014;370(26):2457–2460. doi:10.1056/NEJMp140427
2. Nelson JE, Cortez TB, Curtis JR, et al. Integrating palliative care in the ICU: The nurse in a leading role. *J Hospice Palliat Nurs.* 2011;13(2):89–96. doi:10.1097/NJH.0b013e318203d9ff
3. Cook D, Rocker G. Dying with dignity in the intensive care unit. *N Engl J Med.* 2014;370(26):2506–2514. doi:10.1056/NEJMra1208795
4. American Association of Critical Care Nurses (AACN). Palliative care in the acute and critical care setting. 2021. https://www.aacn.org/clinical-resources/palliative-end-of-life
5. Troug RD, Campbell ML, Curtis JR, et al. Recommendations for end-of-life care in the intensive care unit: A consensus statement by the American College of Critical Care Medicine. *Crit Care Med.* 2008;36(3):953–963. doi:10.1097/CCM.0B013E3181659096
6. Lanken PN, Terry PB, Delisser HM, et al. An official American Thoracic Society clinical policy statement: Palliative care for patients with respiratory distress and critical illnesses. *Am J Respir Crit Care Med.* 2008;177(8):912–927. doi:10.1164/rccm.200605-587ST
7. Selecky PA, Eliasson CA, Hall RI, et al. Palliative and end-of-life care for patients with cardiopulmonary diseases: American College of Chest Physicians position statement. *Chest.* 2005;128(5):3599–3610. doi:10.1378/chest.128.5.3599
8. Nelson JE, Bassett R, Boss RD, et al. Models for structuring a clinical initiative to enhance palliative care in the intensive care unit: A report from the Improve Palliative Care in the ICU (IPAL-ICU) Project and the Center to Advance Palliative Care. *Crit Care Med.* 2010;38(9):1765–1772. doi:10.1097/ccm.0b013e3181e8ad23
9. National Consensus Project for Quality Palliative Care. *Clinical Practice Guidelines for Quality Palliative Care.* 4th ed. Richmond, VA: National Coalition for Hospice and Palliative Care; 2018. https:www.nationalcoalitionhpc.org/ncp
10. Institute of Medicine. *The Future of Nursing: Leading Change, Advancing Health.* Washington, DC: National Academies Press; 2011. https://www.nap.edu/catalog/12956/the-future-of-nursing-leading-change-advancing-health
11. Angus DC, Barnato AE, Linde-Zwirble WT, et al. Use of intensive care at the end of life in the United States. *Crit Care Med.* 2004;32(3):638–643. doi:10.1097/ccm0000114816.62331.08
12. SUPPORT Principal Investigators. A controlled trial to improve care for seriously ill hospitalized patients. The study to understand prognoses and preferences for outcomes and risks of treatments (SUPPORT). *JAMA.* 1995;274(20):1591–1598. PMID: 7474243
13. Field MJ, Cassell CK, eds. *Approaching Death: Improving Care at the End of Life.* Washington, DC: National Academies Press; 1997. https://www.nap.edu/catalog/5801/approaching-death-improving-care-at-the-end-of-life
14. White KR, Roczen ML, Coyne PJ, Wiencek C. Acute and critical care nurses' perceptions of palliative care competencies: A pilot study. *J Contin Educ Nursing.* 2014;45(6):265–277. doi:10.3928/00220124-20140528.01
15. Teno JM, Gozalo PL, Bynum JPW, et al. Change in end-of-life care for Medicare beneficiaries: Site of death, place of care, and health care transitions in 2000, 2005, and 2009. *JAMA.* 2013;309(5):470–477. doi:10.1001/jama.2012.207624

16. American Association of Critical Care Nurses. Family presence: Visitation in the Adult ICU. February 1, 2016. https://www.aacn.org/clinical-resources/practice-alerts/family-presence-visitation-in-the-adult-icu

17. Puntillo KA. Pain experiences of intensive care unit patients. *Heart Lung*. 1990;19(5):526–533. PMID: 2211161

18. Chanques G, Sebbane M, Barbotte E, et al. A prospective study of pain at rest: Incidence and characteristics of an unrecognized symptom in surgical and trauma versus medical intensive care unit patients. *Anesthesiology*. 2007;107(5):858–860. doi:10.1097/01.anes.0000287211.98642.51

19. Barr J, Fraser GL, Puntillo K, et al. Clinical practice guidelines for the management of pain, agitation, and delirium in adult patients in the Intensive Care Unit. *Crit Care Med*. 2013;41(1):263–306. doi:10.1097/ccm.0b013e3182783b72

20. Erstad BL, Puntillo K, Gilbert HC, et al. Pain management principles in the critically ill. *Chest*. 2009;135(4):1075–1086. doi:10.1378/chest.08-2264

21. Puntillo KA, White C, Morris AB, et al. Patients' perceptions and responses to procedural pain: Results from the Thunder Project II. *Am J Crit Care*. 2001(4);10:238–251. PMID: 11432212

22. Devlin J, Skrobik Y, Gelinas C, et al. Executive summary: Clinical practice guidelines for the prevention and management of pain, agitation/sedation, delirium, immobility, and sleep disruption in adult patients in the ICU. *Crit Care Med*. 2018;46(9):1532–1548. doi:10.1097/ccm.0000000000003259

23. Duran-Crane A, Laserna A, Lopez-Olivo M, et al. Clinical practice guidelines and consensus statements about pain management in critically ill end-of-life patients: A systematic review. *Crit Care Med*. 2019;47(11):1619–1626. doi:10.1097/ccm.0000000000003975

24. Chow K. Ethical dilemmas in the intensive care unit. *J Hosp Palliat Nurs*. 2014;16(5):256–260. doi:10.1097/NJH.0000000000000069

25. Herr K, Coyne P, Ely E, et al. ASPMN 2019 position statement: Pain assessment in the patient unable to self-report. *Pain Manage Nsg*. 2019;20(5):402–403. doi:10.1016/j.pmn2019.07.007

26. Chawla L, Bellomo R, Bihorac A, et al. Acute kidney disease and renal recovery: Consensus report of the Acute Disease Quality Initiative (ADQI) 16 Workgroup. *Nephrology* 2017;13(4):241–257. doi:10.1038/nrneph.2017.2

27. Arnold R, Verrico P, Kamell A. Fast facts #161. Opioid use in renal failure. Appleton, WI: Palliative Care Network of Wisconsin. 2020. https://www.mypcnow.org/fast-fact/opioid-use-in-renal-failure/

28. Chandok N, Watt KDS. Pain management in the cirrhotic patient: The clinical challenge. *Mayo Clin Proc*. 2010;85(5):451–458. doi:10.4065/mcp.2009.0534

29. Bernal W, Wendon J. Acute liver failure. *N Engl J Med*. 2013;369(26):2525–2534. doi:10.1056.NEJMra1208937

30. Oliverio C, Malone N, Rosielle D. Fast facts #260 Opioid use in liver failure. Appleton, WI: Palliative Care Network of Wisconsin. 2015 https://www.mypcnow.org/fast-fact/opioid-use-in-liver-failure/

31. Shehabi Y, Riker RR, Bokesch PM, et al. SEDCOM (Safety and Efficacy of Dexmedetomidine Compared with Midazolam) study group: Delirium duration and mortality in lightly sedated, mechanically ventilated intensive care patients. *Crit Care Med*. 2010;38(12):2311–2318. doi:10.1097/ccm.0b013e3181f85759

32. Girard TD, Jackson JC, Pandharipande PP, et al. Delirium as a predictor of long-term cognitive impairment in survivors of critical illness. *Crit Care Med*. 2010;38(7):1513–1520. doi:10.1097.CCM.0b013e3181e47be1

33. Puntillo K, Nelson JE, Weissman D, et al. Palliative care in the ICU: Relief of pain, dyspnea and thirst: A report from the IPAL-ICU Advisory Board. *Intensive Care Med*. 2014;40(2):235–248. doi:10.1007/s00134-013-3153-z

34. Lorenz KA, Lynn J, Dy SM, et al. Evidence for improving palliative care at the end-of-life: A systematic review. *Ann Intern Med*. 2008;148(2):147–159. doi:10.7326/0003-4819-148-2-200801150-00010

35. Leung JG, Nelson S, Leloux M. Pharmacotherapy during the end of life: Caring for the actively dying patient. *AACN Adv Crit Care*. 2014;25(2):79–88. doi:10.1097/NCI.0000000000000010

36. Mahler DA, Selecky PA, Harrod CG, et al. American College of Chest Physicians consensus statement on the management of dyspnea in patients with advanced lung or heart disease. *Chest*. 2010;137(3):674–691. doi:10.1378/chest.09-1543

37. Simon ST, Higginson IJ, Booth S, Harding R, Bausewein C. Benzodiazepines for the relief of breathlessness in advanced malignant and non-malignant diseases in adults. *Cochrane Database Syst Rev*. 2010;1:CD007354. doi:10.1002/14651858.CD007354.pub2

38. Munro CL, Savel RH. Communicating and connecting with patients and their families. *Am J Crit Care*. 2013;22(1):4–6. doi:10.4037/ajcc2013249

39. Fox MY. Improving communication with patients and families in the intensive care unit. *J Hosp Palliat Nurs*. 2014;16(2):93–98. doi:10.1097/NJH.0000000000000026

40. Daly BJ, Douglas SL, O'Toole E, et al. Effectiveness trial of an intensive communication structure for families of long-stay ICU patients. *Chest*. 2010;138(6):1340–1348. doi:10.1378/chest.10-0292

41. Lilly Cm, De Meo DL, Sonna LA, et al. An intensive communication intervention for the critically ill. *Am J Med*. 2000;109(6):469–475. doi:10.1016/s0002-9343(00)00524-6

42. Bosslet G, Pope T, Rubenfeld G, et al. An official ATS/AACN/ACCP/ESICM/SCCM policy statement: Responding to requests for potentially inappropriate treatments in Intensive Care Units. *Am J Respir Crit Care Med*. 2015;191(11):1318–1330. doi:10.1164/rccm.201505-0924st

43. Bibas L, Peretz-Larochelle M, Adhikari N, et al. Association of surrogate decision-making interventions for critically ill adults with patient, family, and resource use outcomes. A systematic review and meta analysis. *JAMA*. 2019;2(7):e197229. doi:10.1001/jamanetworkopen.2019.7229

44. Evans LR, Boyd EA, Malvar G, et al. Surrogate decision-makers' perceptions on discussing prognosis in the face of uncertainty. *Am J Respir Crit Care Med*. 2009;179(1):48–53. doi:10.1164/rccm.200806-969OC

45. Gay EB, Pronovost PJ, Bassett RD, Nelson JE. The intensive care unit family meeting: Making it happen. *J Crit Care*. 2009;24(4):629.e1–12. doi:10.1016/j.jrc.2008.10.003

46. Kouwenhoven WB, Jude JR, Knickerbocker GG. Closed-chest cardiac massage. *JAMA*. 1960;173:1064–1067. doi:10.1001/jama.1960.03020280004002

47. Morrison L, Neumar R, Zimmerman J, et al. Strategies for improving survival after in-hospital cardiac arrest in the United States: 2013 consensus recommendations: A consensus statement from the American Heart Association. *Circulation*. 2013;127(14):epub. doi: 10.1161/CIR.06013e31828b2770

48. Weil MH, Fries M. In-hospital cardiac arrest. *Crit Care Med*. 2005;33(12):2825–2830. doi:10.1097/01.ccm.0000191265.20007.9d

49. Peberdy MA, Kaye W, Ornato JP, et al. Cardiopulmonary resuscitation of adults in the hospital: A report of 14720 cardiac arrests from the National Registry of Cardiopulmonary Resuscitation. *Resuscitation*. 2003;58(3):297–308. doi:10.1016/s0300-9572(03)00215-6

50. Hasselqvist I, Riva G, Herlitz J, et al. Early cardiopulmonary resuscitation in out-of-hospital cardiac arrest. *N Eng J Med*. 2015;372:2307–2315. doi:10.1056/NEJMoa1405796

51. Yan S, Gan Y, Jiang N, et al. The global survival rate among adult out-of-hospital cardiac arrest patients who received CPR: A systematic review and meta analysis. *Critical Care*. 2020;24(1):61. doi:10.1186/s13054-020-2773-2

52. Laish-Farkash A, Matetzky S, Oieru D, et al. Usefulness of mild therapeutic hypothermia for hospitalized comatose patients having out-of-hospital cardiac arrest. *Am J Cardiol*. 2011;108(2):173–178. doi:10.1016/j.amjcard.2011.03.021

53. The Hypothermia After Cardiac Arrest Study Group. Mild therapeutic hypothermia to improve the neurologic outcome after cardiac arrest. *N Engl J Med*. 2002;346(8):549–556. doi:10.1056/NEJMoa012689

54. Dumas F, Grimaldi D, Zuber B, et al. Is hypothermia after cardiac arrest effective in both shockable and nonshockable patients? Insights from a large registry. *Circulation*. 2011;123:877–886. doi:10.1161/CIRCULATIONAHA.110.987347

55. Center to Advance Palliative Care. Integrating palliative care practices in the ICU. New York, NY: CAPC. Jun 22, 2020. https://www.capc.org/toolkits/integrating-palliative-care-practices-in-the-icu/

56. Berlinger N, Jennings B, Wolf S. *The Hastings Center Guidelines for Decisions on Life-Sustaining Treatment and Care Near the End-of-Life: Revised and Expanded second edition*. New York: Oxford University Press; 2013. https://www.thehastingscenter.org/publications-resources/books-by-hastings-scholars/the-hastings-center-guidelines-for-decisions-on-life-sustaining-treatment-and-care-near-the-end-of-life-revised-and-expanded-second-edition/

57. Wiegand DL, Grant MS. Bioethical issues related to limiting life-sustaining therapies in the Intensive Care Unit. *J Hospice Palliat Nurs*. 2014;16(2):60–64. doi:10.1097/NJH.0000000000000056

58. Grant M, Wiencek C, Virani R, et al. End-of-life care education in acute and critical care: The California ELNEC project. *AACN Adv Crit Care*. 2013;24(2):121–129. doi:10.1097/NCI.0b013e3182832a94

59. Rosa W, Ferrell B, Wiencek C. Increasing critical care nurse engagement of palliative care during the COVID-19 pandemic. *Crit Care Nurse*. 2020. Published online Jul 23, 2020. doi:https://doi.org/10.4037/ccn2020946

10.

THE PALLIATIVE APRN IN THE EMERGENCY DEPARTMENT

Sarah Loschiavo and Angela Starkweather

KEY POINTS

- The role of the palliative advanced practice registered nurse (APRN) in the emergency department (ED) incorporates expert provision of care that addresses the physical, psychological, emotional, and spiritual needs of patients with life-limiting illness and their family members.

- The ED often serves as a port of entry to palliative care services for patients with complex symptoms and/or care coordination, individuals with chronic or serious illness or injury, and individuals at the end of life.

- Models of palliative care in the ED may incorporate coordinated direct-admission services, palliative care team consultations, ED-based palliative APRN champions, and partnerships with external agencies that provide palliative care or hospice services.

- The palliative APRN can use systematic methods to identify patients with the greatest need for palliative care services or to initiate consultation/referral to palliative care in the ED setting.

- The palliative APRN has an important role in ED and telephonic communication because of the critical nature and timing of conversations that influence patient and family interactions with the healthcare team and ED palliative care outcomes.

CASE STUDY: EMERGENCY DEPARTMENT PALLIATIVE CARE

Mr. A was a 55-year-old man with a history of a glioblastoma multiforme who was found unconscious at home by his wife. En route to the hospital, the paramedics intubated him and provided basic life support. When he arrived in the ED, he immediately received a head computerized tomography (CT) scan and laboratory studies. The CT scan revealed a large tumor in the left temporal lobe, midline shift, and impending uncal herniation. Uncal herniation occurs secondary to large mass effect (glioblastoma) that will lead to increased intracranial pressure and herniation. Uncal herniation carries a lethal prognosis due to the direct compression of the vital midbrain centers. His wife was at the bedside, and, upon questioning, she stated that her husband complained of a headache over the past week but was otherwise

tolerating his cancer treatment. The attending neurosurgeon arrived at the bedside and recommended emergent neurosurgical decompression.

The palliative advanced practice registered nurse (APRN), Elizabeth, was called to provide support to Mr. A's wife and address the goals of care. On arrival at the bedside, Elizabeth realized she had cared for Mr. A during previous ED visits for complications related to his cancer and treatment. During his last ED visit, Elizabeth introduced palliative care and coordinated a referral to the outpatient palliative care clinic where he was being co-managed by medical oncology and palliative care in the setting of his aggressive cancer.

Without decision-making capacity, Mr. A's surrogate decision-maker was his wife. Elizabeth's initial priority was to ensure that Mrs. A understood her husband's condition, all treatment options available, and his prognosis. Elizabeth explained that while emergency medical treatments were keeping him alive, her husband was critically ill, and further interventions such as surgical decompression would only prolong his dying. Specifically, Elizabeth explained that there were three directions for his care: (1) surgical decompression for palliation (noncurative) with high risk of complications and immediate death, (2) sustaining life through artificial means as a short-term measure until brain death or cardiovascular arrest occurs, or (3) discontinuing life-prolonging therapies to allow a shift to comfort-focused care during the progression to natural death. Elizabeth asked Mrs. A the question "if your husband was here, what would he say?" Mrs. A responded "my husband's greatest fear was being in a coma and that he would not want to live in a way that he could not care for himself." His wife recalled a visit with his medical oncologist where they discussed cardiopulmonary resuscitation. When they arrived home that day, they had a discussion about what he would want done if there was clearly no chance of recovery from illness or injury. At the time, her husband stated that he hoped she would let him go, to allow natural death since he was certain he would be going to a better place rather than having to live out a life that was dependent on everyone else.

There were no advance directives present in the electronic medical record, and his wife stated they never completed the advance directive document. However, Mrs. A's statements regarding her husband's wishes and preferences provided adequate information to suggest that he would have made the decision to discontinue life-sustaining measures to allow natural death.

At this point, the wife asked if she should call their daughter to come to the hospital because she was a college freshman living in a different part of the state. Recognizing that Mr. A would likely face impending death upon discontinuation of life-sustaining medical treatment, the APRN directed the focus of care to the family. While immediate discontinuation of mechanical ventilation would avoid any further suffering and use of resources that would not contribute to the recovery of the patient, this approach did not provide time for the family to say their last goodbyes, deal with the psychological and emotional aspects of the unexpected death of their family member, or perform necessary spiritual or religious rituals.

Elizabeth discussed the benefits and burdens of having the patient's 18-year-old daughter see her father in this condition. Mrs. A and Elizabeth decided that allowing her daughter to see that all possible measures had been taken would provide emotional comfort and closure for her. Elizabeth offered to call Mrs. A's daughter, but she insisted that she wanted to communicate with her directly and make sure she could travel safely to the hospital. Elizabeth then offered information on the next steps. This included the dying process, either in the ED or after transfer to the ICU. After the discussion, a plan was created with his wife to continue mechanical ventilation until after the daughter arrived and had time with her father; however, if cardiac arrest occurred before she arrived, compressions would not be initiated.

In addition, Mrs. A was informed that since her husband had a catastrophic brain injury and remained on mechanical ventilation, the local organ procurement organization was contacted as part of hospital procedure. The ED staff left the discussion of organ donation to a trained designated requestor or the organ procurement organization representative (a process that depends on state policy and procedures).

Mrs. A was very decisive about her husband wanting to donate his organs, and his wishes were further indicated on his driver's license. The patient's daughter arrived and was greeted by the social worker who provides emotional support for anticipatory grief. The daughter agreed that her father would want to proceed with organ donation, as he had mentioned this on several occasions. The family members expressed their comfort in knowing that their loved one's last act was one of giving, something he would have wanted. Elizabeth used molding clay to create a handprint as a remembrance. She then contacted the hospital chaplain for prayer and to perform a religious ritual as requested by the patient's wife. The family members said their last goodbyes to their husband and father before he was transferred to the ICU for organ procurement. Elizabeth provided bereavement information, and the social worker and chaplain stayed with the family to provide support until they were ready to leave the ED.

In the scenario of an imminent fatal outcome, the ethical values of beneficence and nonmaleficence extend to the patient's family as well as to the patient. Confronted with an unexpected fatal event, it is often unreasonable to expect a grieving family to make immediate decisions. However, Elizabeth established the patient's and family's goals of care and created a treatment plan to align with their goals, which incorporated their religious rituals and allowed the patient's family time to be present with him during the dying process. This case demonstrates the vital role of the advanced practice registered nurse (APRN) in the ED to integrate palliative care for all patients who suffer from serious, chronic, and life-limiting illness. ED visits increase as serious illness progresses, regardless of the underlying disease, and as patients approach the end of life. The ED visit may present a unique opportunity for the APRN to connect patients in need with palliative care consultation and services. Early integration of palliative care concurrent with active treatment is optimal and recommended for all patients with advanced cancer.

This case also illustrates the decision-making process regarding palliative care and end-of-life care in a patient with an acute event. Advance directives were not available to help inform decisions, but the wife had previously discussed situations such as living in a coma and being incapacitated as well as whether her husband would want cardiopulmonary resuscitation when facing a terminal prognosis. The APRN utilized members of the interprofessional team to address the physical, emotional, psychological, and spiritual needs of the patient and family unit, thus providing holistic care.

Although not all scenarios are as clear-cut as this one, the APRN has a vital role in initiating such conversation in the ED, understanding disease trajectories of approaching death, establishing goals of care, and determining advance care planning. Often the patient's prognosis may not be clear until more invasive measures have taken place, which makes it challenging for the APRN to make the transition from the goals of cure to relieving suffering and providing comfort in death. In other situations, families may not agree with the goals of care, thus requiring lengthy discussions among the APRN, other consultants, and the family.

The scenario also demonstrates the process of shared decision-making between the provider and family. Once the prognosis is clear and the family understands the prognosis, this process can become much easier. However, establishing trust is imperative. Demonstrating that decisions will be made based on what the patient and family need, rather than the provider's goals, can take time. The APRN can serve as a consistent provider in these discussions (see Chapter 32, "Advance Care Planning" and Chapter 34, "Communication at End of Life" for further information).

INTRODUCTION

This chapter outlines the role of the palliative APRN in the emergency department (ED) and highlights strategies to identify patients at the greatest need for palliative care and the successful integration of palliative care in the ED setting, as well as common barriers to implementation. Various models that may be used are described, along with approaches to operationalize the provision of palliative care to patients in the ED. Methods to evaluate palliative care services in the emergency department are discussed, along with guidelines for delivering notification of death by telephone or use of other technologies.

Advances in disease-targeted therapies that have greatly enhanced survival and the world's aging demographics translate into a growing percentage of the overall population living with serious illnesses such that one in every three adults suffers from multiple chronic conditions.[1] A growing number of patients with serious illness(es) and complex needs present to the ED, with one of the most frequent users of ED services being individuals over the age of 65 years; more than 50% of older adults visit the ED in the last month of life, and many are subsequently admitted and die in the hospital.[2]

Emergency medicine has traditionally focused on preserving life by providing rapid, aggressive resuscitation and stabilization of acutely presenting health conditions or injuries while palliative care needs have been delegated to other professionals and excluded from standard ED services. However, many patients present to the ED with complex physical symptoms or nonphysical aspects of suffering, life-limiting disease, and/or injuries that necessitate an alignment of the clinician's prognostic evaluation, the patient's values, and realistic goals of care. In these cases, the limited focus on acute stabilization and determination of an appropriate disposition can generate additional confusion and frustration for patients and families whose needs remain unmet or who are provided with care that is incongruent with their values, goals, or preferences.

The interactions that occur in the ED present key decision points that can influence the patient's treatment trajectory and set them on a pathway that is not congruent with their goals of care. A key to resolving this dilemma is through integrating palliative care in the ED because palliative services can be incorporated into patient care at any time along the trajectory of any type of serious illness, concurrent with curative, restorative, and any life-prolonging therapies.[3] Because evidence has shown that early integration of palliative care into the care plan for seriously ill patients can improve quality of life and care coordination for the patient and family, there has been increased emphasis on identifying patients in the ED setting who would benefit from palliative care services.[4] In addition, because palliative care principles and practices can be delivered by all clinicians who provide care to seriously ill patients in any setting, there is an enormous need to ensure that ED providers and personnel are equipped with the knowledge, skills, attitudes, and collaborative infrastructure to coordinate palliative care at any stage of illness or injury.

Recognition of missed opportunities for initiating palliative care early in the patient's course of illness and the challenges in identifying patients and families with difficulty in managing symptoms or other nonphysical aspects of illness have spurred the need to integrate palliative care into the ED setting.[5,6] Management of physical suffering in the ED may entail symptomatic treatment of pain, dyspnea, loss of appetite, neurological deterioration, or general distress, which are typically part of a much longer trajectory of the patient's illness experience. In addition, assessment and management of nonphysical aspects of suffering are equally important and may involve cultural, psychological, social, spiritual, financial, ethical, and legal issues that influence the patient's care coordination.[3]

Palliative APRNs are leaders in clinical care, education, advocacy/policy, research, and administration/management, and this role can positively enhance holistic integration of palliative services in care provided within the ED.[7] Specific to the ED setting, the palliative APRN has an important clinical role in promoting care that is aligned with patient values and preferences. Major challenges to healthcare professionals in the ED include balancing the goal to cure against the context of life-limiting disease/injuries and incorporating physical, psychological, emotional, and spiritual needs in the provision of ED care. The palliative APRN can fill these gaps in care and address the multiple challenges to palliative care implementation that are frequently encountered in the ED setting as well as in other areas of healthcare.

Given the demands of making healthcare decisions in the ED, palliative APRNs can play an instrumental role in ensuring that patients and families are fully informed and understand the prognosis and its implications for management options; they can also foster a plan of care that is guided by the patient's values. With appropriate timing, education, palliative care models, and the increasing role of palliative APRNs in the ED, recent studies demonstrate the positive outcomes of palliative care initiation and coordination.[8] These include improved patient outcomes, family and patient communication and satisfaction, reduction in hospital costs and patient's length of stay, and increased appropriate direct hospice consults.[9–12]

PALLIATIVE CARE MANAGEMENT IN CRISES

In addition to serving the health needs of patients and families, the ED is a coordination hub for humanitarian crises and disaster management related to bioterrorism, geological and weather-related hazards (earthquakes, hurricanes, tornadoes, floods, and fires), mass casualty incidents, and public health emergencies such as COVID-19. Humanitarian crises that involve the sudden arrival of multiple critically ill patients require the implementation of multilevel triage, strategies to address surge capacity, and ability to manage resuscitation, stabilization, and palliation needs based on accessible resources, personnel, and infrastructure.[13] During the COVID-19 pandemic, palliative APRNs have been leading such coordination efforts, particularly in the integration of palliative care in the ED for patients with COVID-19, and implementing new models of triage, identification, and patient and family communication.[14]

Integrated ED palliative care during crises serves a vital role in establishing the patient's wishes for life-sustaining treatment such as intubation and resource-intensive cardiopulmonary resuscitation and ensure they are aligned with a patient's goals and values.[15] Having designated palliative care providers in the ED as well as providing palliative care education to all ED clinicians can help to avoid life-sustaining treatments in patients with a poor prognosis that are unlikely to be beneficial or that have a high risk of causing additional suffering.[16] The high volume and acuity of patients during a crisis makes it extremely challenging for ED clinicians to take adequate time to clarify goals of care. Palliative care providers have a critical role during crises in identifying patients at the point of triage or initial assessment who may benefit from having crucial conversations concerning goals of care, values, and preferences and in initiating communication with next of kin. Timely goals-of-care conversations by the palliative APRN can help avoid unwanted life-sustaining treatments for patients with a poor prognosis and provide comfort and support for families during their sudden and unanticipated loss.[17]

ADDRESSING RACISM AND HEALTH DISPARITIES IN THE ED

The ED serves as an entry point to the healthcare system, often due to lack of access to primary care, lack of insurance, and convenience of "on-demand" care.[18] Despite advances and the growth of palliative care programs, low-income and minority populations remain significantly underserved.[19] Research has documented racial differences in hospice use and end-of-life treatment intensity consistent with a broad range of disparities in healthcare use and health outcomes.[20] Reasons for these disparities include preferences for more aggressive care, mistrust of the healthcare system, lack of in-home resources, and miscommunication and misunderstanding of treatment options. There are several barriers to high-quality palliative and end-of-life care among racial/ethnic minority adults. Some of the barriers are due to institutional racism, including unfair profiling and denial of treatment or services, while other barriers are social or structural in nature, including economic insecurity, lack of adequate insurance, geographic location, cultural and spiritual values about health and medicine, underrepresentation of minorities in medicine, and the dismantling of affirmative action programs.[21] Additionally, provider-level barriers, including communication and perceptions of discrimination, exist.[22] Efforts to reduce disparities in the quality of palliative care must be prioritized. Targeted efforts to increase advance care planning, early palliative care integration, and hospice services among underrepresented populations should be expanded in order to improve health equity and ensure culturally sensitive care coordination.[23]

For millions of Americans living in vulnerable rural and urban communities, the ED is an important—and often their only—source of healthcare.[24] Transformation among hospitals and healthcare systems is needed to address communities at risk of losing access to the healthcare services and resources they need to improve and maintain their health.[24] A recent study by Hanchate et al.[25] measured the differences in ED destination by the race/ethnicity of patients transported by emergency medical services (EMS) from the same geographic area. The study found race/ethnicity variation in ED destination for patients using EMS transport, with Black and Hispanic patients more likely to be transported to a safety-net hospital ED compared with white patients living in the same ZIP Code. A study by Hanna et al. showed disparities in the utilization of advanced imaging during emergency room visits.[26] Institutional racism in funding community resources such as EMS, housing, schools, and transportation, along with an ongoing lack of education and financial opportunities, perpetuate the need for ED services in low income neighborhoods and individuals in minimum-wage positions who

often must hold down multiple jobs to make ends meet. The role of emergency medicine healthcare professionals is significant as racial and ethnic communities seek healthcare in the ED. An increase in the size of vulnerable populations served by EDs is an important contributor to increases in ED visits.[27] Language barriers and lack of interpreter services impede healthcare delivery in the ED setting.

According to the Centers for Disease Control and Prevention, despite years of attention to disparities, the racial gap in Americans' health continues to widen.[27] Evidence of disparities is most plentiful for African Americans. Of note, 80% of all heart failure hospitalizations originate in the ED. Racial disparities in hospitalization rates for ED patients with heart failure are well-documented.[28] African Americans are approximately 1.5 times more likely than white patients to be denied authorization for their ED visit.[27] Black individuals are significantly less likely to use hospice and more likely to have multiple ED visits and hospitalizations and undergo intensive treatment in the last 6 months of life compared with white individuals regardless of cause of death.[29] The top three causes of death in the United States are the same for Blacks and Whites, but the rates of death for Black people are strikingly higher: heart disease (30% higher), cancer (30% higher), and stroke (40% higher). African Americans prefer more "aggressive" care when seriously ill, which is influenced by cultural and religious values and perspectives.[30,31] Palliative care teams have a significant role in helping patients reframe the meaning of their spiritual beliefs in the context of their medical circumstances in ways that do not exclude care in hospice and palliative care settings. In 2010, the American Academy of Pediatrics released a report reviewing the extant literature on racial/ethnic health and healthcare disparities among US children, concluding that care disparities were "extensive, pervasive, and persistent." Black and Hispanic children faced disparities in emergency care across multiple dimensions when compared to non-Hispanic White children, while Asian children did not demonstrate such patterns.[32]

The COVID-19 pandemic and recent social justice movements in the United States have led to an important moment for the palliative care community to step back and consider opportunities for expansion and growth.[33] The COVID-19 pandemic has shown that communities of color are disproportionately affected, with a higher burden of morbidity and mortality seen among African Americans.[34] Death rates from COVID-19 are three times higher nationally in Black counties compared with White counties, with 70% of deaths occurring among Blacks in certain states. Cultural humility enables healthcare practitioners to remain present to the individual patient's reality and be able to assist them in making decisions that best align with their values regardless of prognosis or resource allocation limitations during a pandemic. In medical decision-making conversations, it is important to affirm a patient's life first and subsequently what is important to them. This builds a foundation of trust that bridges difference in culture, ethnicity, and religion.[35]

Due to long-standing systemic racism, the reasons for disparities in care and health outcomes are multifaceted, arising from individual and institutional sources that are conscious and unconscious.[35] The moral duty of all healthcare providers is to ensure equity across all realms of decision-making and within the healthcare system and to consistently demonstrate authentic trustworthiness to all people.[35] Only when the importance of palliative care in the ED is recognized by both those that work there and those in palliative care, and the necessary skills are acquired, can systems begin to change to enable an environment better suited to its delivery.[36] Additionally, targeted efforts to increase advance care planning among Black and other racial minority populations should be expanded.[29]

THE ROLE OF THE PALLIATIVE APRN IN THE ED

The role of the palliative APRN in the ED entails direct clinical care, education, and policy development and implementation, as well as research and administration.[7] The palliative APRN plays a major role in identifying patients with palliative care needs.[37] Unlike other settings in which the diagnosis is known and the plan of care is clear, patients arriving to the ED are often confronted with options of undergoing a range of diagnostic tests and procedures before the net benefit can be considered regarding patient/family goals of care, life expectancy, or improvement in quality of life.

The palliative APRN can play an instrumental role in eliciting information from the patient and family that can inform decisions regarding the workup and plan of care in the ED.[8] Palliative APRNs facilitate decisions that are aligned with the patient's values in the context of serious or life-limiting disease/injury as well as patient and family wishes and preferences when cure is no longer possible. The palliative APRN's assessment of the physical, psychological, emotional, and spiritual needs of the patient and family can have dramatic implications for the course of care provided. The role of the palliative APRN in the ED setting incorporates a process of negotiation among healthcare professionals, the patient, and family members to define realistic goals of care in the context of the patient's wishes and preferences.

A critically important role and prerequisite skill for aligning the goals of care with patient and family wishes and preferences is initiating difficult conversations. Palliative APRNs have exquisite skill in eliciting information from patients and family members as well as guiding crucial conversations that are culturally sensitivity and can inform the provision of patient-centered care in the ED.[37] The ED setting may be the first place in which the patient's prognosis is fully understood by the patient and family. Assisting the patient and family as they encounter limitations in life-preserving measures and the possibility or reality of death is a major role of the palliative APRN in the ED setting.

Coordination of care is another major role of the palliative APRN in the ED. This role incorporates navigating the healthcare system and accessing resources for the patient and family that support palliative care. Care transitions represent one of the most significant challenges to continuity of care and increase the risk of readmission.[38] Ensuring that all providers involved in the care of the patient are informed of the palliative care plan and making certain that adequate resources are provided to address the trajectory of declining health status, distressing symptoms, and caregiver needs are important aspects in the palliative APRN's coordination of care.

The unique perspective of the palliative APRN also provides a foundation for advancing palliative care in the ED setting. Although there is a movement toward incorporating palliative care principles and practices utilizing the End-of-Life Nursing Education Consortium (ELNEC) Critical Care Curriculum across healthcare disciplines,[39,40] the culture and infrastructure of the ED is currently based on rapid decision-making and determination of disposition to maximize revenue. The palliative APRN can be a resource and change agent by providing education to ED physicians, nurses, and staff regarding the identification of patients with palliative care needs, initiating conversations about palliative care with patients and families, and establishing palliative care services in the ED.

A change in the ED culture toward patient-centered care can result in an expansion of the palliative APRN's role in areas of policy development and implementation, research, and administration in order to integrate a care model that facilitates the goals of ED care while enhancing the ability to effectively provide palliative care services. Obtaining and analyzing data on patient palliative care needs in the ED as well as disposition and follow-up can initially inform the most relevant model of care to consider.[37] In addition, policies and procedures for identifying patients and families who would benefit from early palliative care services in the ED and quality improvement of the care coordination are other areas in which the palliative APRN can have great influence.

IDENTIFYING PATIENTS WHO NEED PALLIATIVE CARE IN THE ED

One of the major challenges to efficient implementation of palliative care services in the ED is identifying patients early in the patient encounter and trajectory of serious illness. Patients at high risk for needing palliative care can be identified through triggers or high-risk characteristics. Palliative APRNs may be responsible for selecting such triggers to embed in the electronic health record as well as educating triage nurses and EMS personnel on appropriate assignment to palliative care champions in the ED.

Triggers for palliative care consultation are listed in Table 10.1 and may include elderly patients with life-limiting conditions, such as advanced dementia, severe congestive heart failure, chronic obstructive pulmonary disease, advanced malignancy, and/or AIDS with at least moderate functional status limitations.[1] Additional criteria have been found to be applicable in identifying patients in need of palliative care, such as having recent losses in activities of daily living, high symptom distress, poor functional status, and high levels of caregiver burden.

Questions on these topics may be incorporated as part of the triage process to assist in identifying patients who need

Table 10.1 TRIGGERS TO IDENTIFY PATIENTS WHO NEED PALLIATIVE CARE

INDICATOR	CHARACTERISTICS
Serious illness, potentially life-limiting or life-threatening condition	Advanced cancer, dementia, severe congestive heart failure, chronic obstructive pulmonary disease, multi-organ disease, AIDS with at least moderate functional status limitations
Frequent admissions	More than one admission for same condition within several months or increasing frequency
Presentation due to difficult-to-manage physical or psychological symptoms	Moderate to severe symptom intensity/distress for more than 24–48 hours
Complex care requirements	Functional dependence, complex home support, high level of caregiver burden
Failure to thrive	Decline in function, feeding intolerance, or unintended decline in weight
Karnofsky Performance Scale	Performance status as predictor of survival
Palliative Performance Scale (PPS)	Predicts approximate 6-month survival
Palliative Prognostic Score (PaP)	Predicts 30-day mortality
Palliative Prognostic Index (PPI)	Predicts <3-week mortality

palliative care services and to inform assignment to the ED-based palliative APRN. Standardized screening tools have been shown to be feasible and increase the rates of palliative care referrals.[41] The Palliative Care and Rapid Emergency Screening (P-CaRES) Table 10.2 can be used for rapid screening in triage.[41] In addition, the 5-SPEED Box 10.1 screen was created for the purpose of identifying patients with the need for palliative care consultation.

However, because of the often urgent nature of care needs and brief encounter with triage nurses who have limited time to build rapport with patients and families, these questions are often difficult to administer. In addition, patients are often

too ill, too distressed, and unwilling to answer these screening questions in the ED setting.[40] Yet, when these factors are present on ED admission, a palliative care consultation may be beneficial. In addition, triggers may be embedded in the electronic health record to automatically ask the provider if a palliative care consultation is necessary.

One such approach is to use the surprise question as the threshold to initiate palliative care: "Would you be surprised if this patient died in the next 12 months?" When the provider answers "no" to this question (they would not be surprised), this can serve to alert the provider of the possible need for palliative care, and an automated notification to the palliative care team can be sent to initiate referral.[42] Other triggers or prognostic indicators may include

- The Karnofsky Performance Scale
- Palliative Performance Scale (PPS)
- Palliative Prognostic Score (PaP)
- Palliative Prognostic Index (PPI)[43]

These indicators can be used to consult palliative care services as well as initiate case management to assist in

Table 10.2 PALLIATIVE CARE AND RAPID EMERGENCY SCREENING (P-CARES) TOOL

STEP	QUESTION
Step 1	Does the patient have a life-limiting illness? *Select all that apply and proceed to Step 2 if one or more items are checked.* • Advanced dementia or central nervous system disease • Advanced cancer • Advanced heart failure • Advanced liver disease • Septic shock • Provider discretion: High chance of accelerated death
Step 2	Does the patient have two or more unmet palliative care needs? *Select all that apply. If two or more are checked, referral for palliative care is recommended.* • Frequent visits • Uncontrolled symptoms • Functional decline • Uncertainty about goals of care and/or caregiver distress Would you be surprised if the patient died in 12 months?[41]

Box 10.1 **5-SPEED SCREEN**

Questions to assess for unmet palliative care needs

- How much are you suffering from pain?
- How much difficulty do you have getting your care needs met at home?
- How much are you having difficulties with your medications?
- How much are you suffering with feeling overwhelmed?
- How much difficulty are you have getting medical care that fits with your goals of care?

coordination of care. Coordinating the ED system with triggers or indicators of the need for palliative care can be a major role of the palliative APRN and can help drive the delivery of palliative care in the ED setting.

DELIVERY OF PALLIATIVE CARE IN THE ED

Palliative APRNs play a vital role in the early recognition of critically ill patients requiring palliative care in the ED because the trajectory of resuscitation and stabilization using invasive diagnostic or treatment procedures as well as inpatient hospitalization is often set in the ED. Although 70% or more of older adults prefer quality of life over life extension, most individuals do not have advance directives on presentation to the ED.[2] Working from a framework of communication, the clinician in the ED can use a structured, stepwise approach to elicit information about patient and family goals of care by using open-ended questions such as, "Help me understand what you are hoping will happen?" Other tools, such as the REMAP framework (Reframe, Expect emotion, Map out the future, Align with values, Plan treatment that matches values),[44, 45] the Serious Illness Conversation Guide,[46] or the MVP (Medical situation, Values, Plan)[47] can also be useful for guiding conversations when there is limited time to build the patient–provider relationship and the plan of care needs to be quickly determined.[48]

In a patient with advanced illness who is unlikely to benefit from invasive interventions, the palliative APRN should address the goals of care before initiating aggressive therapies. Immediately upon the patient's presenting to the ED with a life-threatening emergency, full resuscitative efforts will occur unless the patient rejects treatment or an advance directive is in place. When resuscitative efforts cannot stabilize the patient's condition and offer virtually no chance of clinical benefit, prolonged survival, or quality-of-life improvement, the palliative APRN and patient or family/surrogate decision-maker should decide whether to make the transition from resuscitation to comfort measures.

APRNs play a vital role in facilitating communication regarding the patient's prognosis, patient and family wishes and preferences, and realistic goals of care in the ED. By following the steps in Box 10.2, they can promote communication and decision-making for patients with serious illness, acute devastating events, or individuals who are near the end of life. This process starts with determination of the patient's decision-making capacity, identification of surrogates, and interpretation of advance directives.[49] In addition, communication to empower the patient, family, or surrogate decision-maker at the end of life should include the following[50]:

1. Assess the patient's or family or surrogate decision-maker's understanding of what is happening.

2. Provide an honest view of the patient's condition and prognosis.

Box 10.2 **STEPS OF PALLIATIVE CARE COMMUNICATION**

Determine patient's diagnosis and prognosis, decision-making capacity, surrogate, and advance directives.

1. Determine patient's diagnosis and prognosis using assessment skills, documentation, or consultation with the patient's other healthcare providers.

2. Determine patient's decision-making capacity through documentation and/or verbal or written communication.

3. Identify the legal surrogate decision-maker.

4. Elicit patient values as expressed in completed advance directives or through verbal or written communication.

Discussion of integrating palliative care in the patient's care plan.

1. Determine patient's/surrogate's understanding of prognosis, limitations of curative treatment, and expected goals of care.

2. Explain palliative care as a means to address quality of life and congruence between palliative care and patient's goals of care.

3. Convey provider's understanding of patient's condition, prognosis, and treatment options with recommendation.

4. Share decisions regarding resuscitative efforts, invasive procedures designed to sustain life, and available resources to address patient/family physiological, psychological, social, and spiritual needs.

5. Consider options for organ donation.

6. Revise goals of treatment as necessary.

---

3. Elicit the patient's values or the family/surrogate decision-maker's best judgment of the patient's values regarding end-of-life decisions.

4. Communicate medical information using understandable language.

5. Build trust and make decisions with the family that incorporate the patient's values, beliefs, and preferences in determining the goals of care.

Continuity of care is cited as one of the most challenging aspects of palliative care from the perspective of patients and providers.[49,50] Regardless of how aggressive the goals of care are for the patient, addressing symptom management is paramount. APRNs play a vital role in this process. First, they can ensure that symptom management strategies are used and anticipatory guidance is provided regarding expected symptoms, stages of illness, and dying. These educational topics are critical for helping the patient and family to understand the patient's prognosis, how to obtain information and emotional support, and for reducing unnecessary ED visits. Education and planning should include the patient, family members, and other caregivers as well as the primary care and specialty providers involved in the patient's care. Clear instructions should be provided about accessing care when necessary. Communication should also take place between the palliative care team and the primary care provider and on-call provider regarding palliative care or end-of-life management and goals of care in case a subsequent ED visit is inevitable.

MODELS OF PALLIATIVE CARE DELIVERY IN THE ED

In response to the growing number of patients with advanced illness cared for in the ED, several health systems have initiated programs to deliver ED-based palliative care, consultation, and/or coordination. There are typically three types: embedded palliative care in the ED with palliative APRNs and physicians on staff, ED-based consultation programs initiated by the inpatient (hospital-based) palliative care team, and ED partnerships with palliative care or hospice providers.

A greater number of palliative APRNs are being hired for full-time clinical practice and in leadership roles in the ED in response to the recognized need. There has been a positive response to using this model reported by other clinicians in the ED setting.[51] An added benefit of having ED-based palliative APRNs is the ability to identify patients who may need palliative care as they arrive in the ED so that crucial conversations about the goals of care can take place early on. Education in palliative care practice is necessary so that uniform access to palliative care services can be provided in the ED. As more clinicians and healthcare systems are taking the opportunity to become adept at meeting the needs of palliative care patients in the ED, it is anticipated that there will be greater coordination of care. Palliative APRNs in the ED setting can play an instrumental role in advancing palliative care education and strengthening systems for the provision of palliative care in the ED, as well as in coordination of care and tracking palliative care outcomes.

Hospital-based palliative care teams routinely cover ED consultations, and the ED may provide a significant source of outpatient referrals or inpatient admissions to the palliative care team and/or unit. However, with increasing palliative care consultations throughout the hospital and time constraints in providing care on the inpatient side, ensuring timely consultation in the ED can be challenging. Regardless, patient management through palliative care services has been shown to decrease the number of ED visits. Billing and administrative data support the fact that ED-based palliative care consultation decreases hospital length of stay and costs for those who are admitted to and die in the hospital.[10,11]

ED partnerships with hospice providers can also provide a system for increasing access to palliative care services. When patients are identified in the ED as requiring palliative or end-of-life care, the palliative APRN can facilitate transfer to the in-patient palliative care or hospice unit or initiate referral and transfer to a hospice facility or hospice services. For patients who can be managed at home, palliative care outpatient services or palliative or hospice home services may be most useful. In addition, other services to enhance transitions in care, such as employing palliative APRNs and other providers after hours and on weekends, providing a palliative care hotline, or follow-up clinic/home services for patients recently seen in the ED, can be especially useful in improving care coordination.[28] Coordination of care can be easier to implement when partnerships are established between providers and institutions. An important competency of palliative APRNs is building systems and resources to ensure quality care during transitions and to support the patient and family while making these difficult decisions and through the process of bereavement.

EVALUATION OF PALLIATIVE CARE IN THE ED

The evaluation of palliative care services may involve operational, clinical, and patient/family satisfaction indicators (Table 10.3). *Operational indicators* are those that affect the operational aspects of providing palliative care in the ED.[52] These include the number of palliative care consultations and referrals, the response time of the palliative care team, and the number of clinicians who are certified in the specialty of palliative care.[53]

Clinical indicators represent actions carried out in the clinical setting that incorporate palliative measures. These include the number of patients screened for palliative care needs, documentation of advance directives, end-of-life decisions, and communication with patients and family concerning palliative and end-of-life care.

Patient and family satisfaction indicators are subjective assessments of how well the palliative care team addressed palliative care needs and the overall delivery of palliative care.[54] These indicators may include the level of care provided to address communication and decision-making, symptom management, and end-of-life support. Acquiring information from each of these realms is important to inform the quality of palliative care delivery from an organizational, a clinician, and an individual patient and family level.[55] The APRN may play a role in creating such assessments, initiating their use, following-up with patients and families, or evaluating and reporting the data.

NOTIFICATION OF DETERIORATION IN HEALTH STATUS OR DEATH

Communicating the deterioration and death of a family member is a difficult skill, particularly for providers with limited interactions with the patient or family. Although it is usually preferable to notify the family in person, APRNs must weigh the benefits of truthfulness against the risk of potential harm resulting from abrupt disclosure of the bad news. For instance, during the recent COVID-19 pandemic, these conversations were only allowed via phone using verbal or video communication due to restricted visitation.[53] Factors to consider in making this decision include whether the health

Table 10.3 METRICS INFORMING QUALITY OUTCOMES IN ED PALLIATIVE CARE

METRIC TYPE	PARAMETERS
Operational	Number of palliative care/hospice consultations/referrals
	Number of in-service education sessions provided, interprofessional participation, and ratings of the sessions, number of questions asked, and reports of application in practice
	Time from call for consultation to documented consultation
	Discharge status/disposition
	% palliative care patients returning to ED within 30 days
	% palliative care patients readmitted to hospital within 30 days
	Mean/median length of stay in ED
	% of patients admitted to palliative care services/unit
	Number of board-certified palliative care providers
	Hospital direct costs
Clinical	% of patients screened for need of palliative care services
	% of patients with advance directives in the EMR
	% of patients for whom the healthcare decision maker is documented in the EMR
	% of patients with documented pain assessment on presentation
	% of patients prescribed opioids with bowel regimen on discharge
	% of patient families with documented offer of spiritual support after ED death
	% of patient caregivers screened for caregiver strain
	% of patients with documented family meeting
	% of patients with documented family contact
Patient/family satisfaction	% of patients reporting excellent level of satisfaction with palliative care services/coordination
	% of patients reporting excellent pain/symptom management
	% of patients reporting excellent transition of care to palliative or hospice services
	% of patients discharged from ED who reported they were informed about their condition/prognosis/treatment options
	% of surrogates/families who reported excellent end-of-life care after ED death
	% of patient families who perceived that the management decisions were congruent with the patient's values

Adapted from Dundin A, Siegert C, Miller D, et al. A pivot to palliative: An interdisciplinary program development in preparation for a coronavirus patient surge in the emergency department. *Emerg Nurs.* 2020;doi:10.1016/p.jen.2020.08.003.

deterioration and death was expected or not, how well the provider knows the patient and the family, the relationship of the contact person to the patient, the anticipated emotional reaction of the contact person based on prior information, whether the contact person will be alone when receiving the information, the contact person's level of understanding, and the distance, availability of transport, time of day, and infection risk.[54] Communication between the palliative APRN and family takes place within the context of culture, language, and prior experiences and includes indirect cues (body language, facial expression, and gestures). When there is a need to update family members regarding the health status of the patient, particularly regarding deterioration in health or to inform them of the patient's death by telephone or other technology, the call should be made as soon as possible when changes occur or following the death.[55]

There are several key steps for the APRN to follow in notification of health deterioration or death. First, after positively identifying the patient, obtain relevant information about the patient (name, age, gender, patient identity numbers, and circumstances of deterioration in health or death).[56] Second, establish the relationship of the contact person to the patient;

Table 10.4 STEPS FOR TELEPHONIC COMMUNICATION WITH NEXT OF KIN WHEN PATIENT DETERIORATES OR DIES

Preparing for the call	Prepare for the call by gathering all information about the patient (name, gender, age, medical record number, circumstances of illness or death); verify information with colleagues who have cared for the individual to review events of the last few days.
	Review with a colleague what you will say, including the context of the call and history of care. Find a quiet place to call. Take a few minutes to prepare yourself using a mindfulness minute or deep breathing.
	Arrange for a medical interpreter, if needed.
	If using a personal phone, consider using technology to block the telephone number such as *67 or Doximity.
Determine next of kin as listed in the electronic health record or other source and ask an identifying question.	Identify yourself, your position, and ask to speak to the contact person indicated in the chart. If that person is not available, ask the identity of the person you are talking to, their relationship to the patient, and let them know you are urgently trying to reach the next of kin.
	Avoid responding to any direct questions until you have verified the identity of the person to whom you are speaking as the next of kin.
	Do not give health deterioration information or death notification to minor children.
	If you reach an answering machine or voice mail, only leave specific contact information for the family to call back (e.g., "This is Julie Smith, APRN at Shorline Hospital. Please call me back at the following number"). If you are unable to make contact within 1–2 hours, contact a hospital representative (e.g., social worker) to assist you in locating family or others.
Determine what the contact person knows about the patient's illness/injury.	Speak clearly and slowly, allowing time for questions.
	If you do not have a prior relationship with the person you are speaking with, ask what he or she knows about the patient's condition.
	"What has the healthcare team told you about [patient]'s condition?"
Provide a prelude to the conversation.	Provide a warning: "I'm afraid I have some bad news" or "I have some difficult news to share."
	Find out if the person is in a safe place, is driving, or has anyone with them. Allow them time to pull over on the road, get to a room with another person, or call another person. Once they are ready, prepare to proceed.
Use clear and direct language, avoiding medical jargon.	"[_____'s] condition has deteriorated and we believe that [_____] will not live much longer. Do you want to arrange to come in or we can hold the phone next to [_____]'s ear so that you can say your good-bye's?" If the family asks to see the patient via video, ensure that the platform is HIPAA compliant with the Health Insurance Portability and Accountability Act (HIPAA)and secure.
	"I'm sorry, [_____] has just died." Use the word "died" or "dead." Other terms, such as "expired," "passed away," or "didn't make it," can be misinterpreted.
Assess the person's emotional response.	Allow time and silence for the next of kin to take in the information. Be prepared for the expression of emotions.
	Offer simple details about the sudden deterioration of the patient, events leading to or reasons for the deterioration, and comfort provided. Allow the family to ask additional questions and express feelings.
	Provide therapeutic listening and support
Ask the family if they would like to come to the hospital to view the body (if possible).	If the family chooses to come to see the body, arrange to meet with them personally when they arrive. If you are unable, make arrangements for a colleague such as a social worker or chaplain to meet them.
	Provide contact information for the clinical team member who can meet with them and answer questions about the patient's death, funeral planning, and other administrative issues.
Closing the call.	Offer follow-up phone calls by the social worker or chaplaincy to help with support and funeral planning. Provide information about follow-up phone calls from the hospital, including the release of the body.
	Offer condolences and a statement for having to receive this information by phone. "Again, my condolences on the loss of your loved one. I wish I had been able to be with you in person during this time."
Communicate to the team.	Document the call in the chart.
	Notify the clinical team and bereavement liaison that the call has been completed.
	Take a moment to reflect and provide a positive affirmation for providing a difficulty call with empathy.[59]

obtain the full name, address, and telephone numbers of the person(s) who need to be informed from the chart and/or nursing staff. Third, find a quiet or private area with a phone and thoroughly review the information to be conveyed. When making the phone call, follow the steps listed in Table 10.4 to ensure best practices are utilized.[57–59] Telehealth technologies are being used more frequently to provide palliative care to patients and families, and, as they are being evaluated, it is anticipated that modifications to best practices will occur.[60]

SUMMARY

The ED is an important setting for the initiation of palliative care. The quickly changing status of ED patients makes access to palliative services an important element of care. Moreover, communication is different from that in other departments, as often patients present without family members. The palliative APRN has a significant role in identifying patients who need palliative care; assessing the patient's physical, psychological, emotional, and spiritual needs; initiating difficult conversations; and coordinating care that is culturally sensitive and congruent with the patient's values and goals.

Palliative APRNs are experts in designing and implementing system-based standardized methods for advancing palliative care services in settings such as the ED. Working with the interprofessional team, the palliative APRN may be the leader in developing triggers for recognizing palliative care needs in ED patients. This process can make the system of triage and referral more efficient so that crucial conversations can take place early in the ED visit. The palliative APRN can initiate difficult conversations and negotiate realistic goals of care among the patient, family, and other providers involved in the patient's care, a process that often takes time to build trust and constant presence as the patient and family work through difficult decisions.

Using a holistic assessment of the patient and family, the palliative APRN offers a unique perspective in the ED that is focused on patient-centered care and congruence between the goals of care and the patient's wishes and preferences. Coordination of palliative care is also a major role of the palliative APRN in the ED, which is critical for ensuring quality and safety throughout care transitions. The palliative APRN also has expertise in designing outcomes for system improvement using quality indicators to evaluate how palliative care is being used and implemented in the ED. This is a critically important process to achieve the best use of palliative care services and improve the ways it is implemented in the ED setting.

REFERENCES

1. Hajat C, Stein E. The global burden of multiple chronic conditions: A narrative review. *Prev Med Rep.* 2018;12(2):284–293. doi:10.1016/j.pmedr.2018.10.008

2. George N, Bowman J, Aaronson E, et al. The past, present, and future of palliative care in emergency medicine in the USA. *Acute Med Surg.* 2020;7(1):e497. doi:10.1002/ams2.497

3. National Coalition for Hospice and Palliative Care, National Consensus Project for Quality Palliative Care. *Clinical Practice Guidelines for Quality Palliative Care*, 4th ed. Richmond, VA: National Coalition for Hospice and Palliative Care; 2018. https://www.nationalcoalitionhpc.org/ncp/

4. Cooper E, Hutchinson A, Sheikh Z, et al. Palliative care in the emergency department: A systematic literature qualitative review and thematic synthesis. *Palliat Med.* 2018;32(9):1443–1454. doi:10.1177/0269216318783920

5. Mogul AS, Cline DM, Gabbard J, et al. Missed opportunities: Integrating palliative care into the emergency department for older adults presenting as level I triage priority from long term care facilities. *J Emerg Med.* 2019;56(2):145–152. doi:10.1016/j.jemermed.2018.10.020

6. Reuter Q, Marshall A, Zaidi H, et al. Emergency department-based palliative interventions: A novel approach to palliative care in the emergency department. *J Palliat Med.* 2019;22(6):649–655. doi:10.1089/jpm.2018.0341

7. Dahlin C, Coyne P. The palliative APRN leader. *Ann Palliative Med.* 2019;8(1):S30–S38. doi:10.21037/apm.2018.06.03

8. Collins CM, Small SP. The nurse practitioner role is ideally suited for palliative care practice: A qualitative descriptive study. *Can Oncol Nurs J.* 2019;29(1):4–9. doi:10.5737/2368807629149

9. Cassel JB, Garrido M, et al. Impact of specialist palliative care on re-admissions: A "competing risks" analysis to take mortality into account. TH341A. *J Pain Symptom Manage.* 2018;55(2):581. doi:10.1016/jpainsymman.2017.12.045

10. May P, Normand C, Cassel JB, et al. Economics of palliative care for hospitalized adults with serious illness: A meta-analysis. *JAMA Intern Med.* 2018;178(6):820–829. doi:10.1001/jamainternmed.2018.0750

11. Spettell CM, Rawlins WS, Krakauer R, et al. A comprehensive case management program to improve palliative care. *J Palliat Med.* 2019;12(9):827–832. doi:10.1089/jpm.2009.0089

12. Di Leo S, Alquati S, Autelitano C, et al. Palliative care in the emergency department as seen by providers and users: A qualitative study. *Scand J Trauma Resus Emerg Med.* 2019;27(1):88. doi:10.1186/s13049-019-0662-y

13. Stoltenberg M, Jacobsen J, Wilson E, et al. Emergency department-based palliative care during COVID. *J Palliative Med.* 2020;23(9):1151–1152. doi:10.1089/jpm.2020.0285

14. McNamara R. Emergency palliative care. *Emerg Med J.* 2020;37(1):260–261. doi:10.1136/emermed-2020-209464

15. Eygnor JK, Rosenau AM, Burmeister DB, et al. Palliative care in the emergency department during a COVID-19 pandemic. *Am J Emerg Med.* 2021;45:516–518. doi:10.1016/j.ajem.2020.07.004

16. Curtis JR, Kross EK, Stapleton RD. The importance of addressing advance care planning and decisions about do-not-resuscitate orders during novel Coronavirus 2019 (COVID-19). *JAMA.* March 27, 2020. doi:10.1001/jama.2020.4894

17. Lee J, Abrukin L, Flores S, et al. Early intervention of palliative care in the emergency department during the COVID-19 pandemic. *JAMA Intern Med.* 2020;180(9):1252–1254. doi:10.1001/jamainternmed.2020.2713

18. Rocovich C, Patel T. Emergency department visits: Why adults choose the emergency room over a primary care physician visit during regular office hours? *World J Emerg Med.* 2012;3(2):91–97. doi.org/10.5847/wjem.j.issn.1920-8642.2012.02.002

19. Gardner DS, Doherty M, Bates G, et al. Racial and ethnic disparities in palliative care: A systematic scoping review. *Families Soc.* 2018;99(4):301–316. doi.org/10.1177/1044389418809083

20. Ornstein KA, Roth DL, Huang J, et al. Evaluation of racial disparities in hospice use and end-of-life treatment intensity in the REGARDS cohort. *JAMA Netw Open.* 2020;3(8):e2014639. doi:10.1001/jamanetworkopen.2020.14639

21. Krakauer EL, Crenner C, Fox K. Barriers to optimum end-of-life care for minority patients. *J Am Geriatr Soc.* 2002;50(1):182–190. doi:10.1046/j.1532-5415.2002.50027.x

22. LoPresti MA, Dement F, Gold HT. End-of-life care for people with cancer from ethnic minority groups: A systematic review. *Am J Hosp Palliat Care.* 2016;33(3):291–305. doi:10.1177/1049909114565658

23. Pecanac KE, Repenshek MF, Tennenbaum D, et al. Respecting choices and advance directives in a diverse community. *J Palliat Med.* 2014;17(3):282–287. doi:10.1089/jpm.2013.0047

24. Bhatt J, Bathija P. Ensuring access to quality healthcare in vulnerable communities. *Acad Med.* 2018;93(9):1271–1275. doi:10.1097/ACM.0000000000002254

25. Hanchate AD, Paasche-Orlow MK, Baker WE, Lin MY, Banerjee S, Feldman J. (2019). Association of race/ethnicity with emergency department destination of emergency medical services transport. *JAMA Netw Open.* 2019;2(9):e1910816. doi:10.1001/jamanetworkopen.2019.10816

26. Hanna TN, Friedberg E, Dequesada IM, Chaves L, Pyatt R, Duszak R Jr, Hughes DR. (2021). Disparities in the use of emergency department advanced imaging in medicare beneficiaries. *AJR.* 2021;216(2):519–525. doi:10.2214/AJR.20.23161

27. Heron SL, Stettner E, Haley LL, Jr. Racial and ethnic disparities in the emergency department: A public health perspective. *Emer Med Clin North Amer.* 2006;24(4):905–923. doi:10.1016/j.emc.2006.06.009

28. Lo AX, Donnelly JP, Durant RW, Collins SP, Levitan EB, Storrow AB, Bittner V. A national study of U.S. emergency departments: Racial disparities in hospitalizations for heart failure. *Amer J Prev Med.* 2018;55(5 Suppl 1):S31–S39. doi:10.1016/j.amepre.2018.05.020

29. Ornstein KA, Roth DL, Huang J, et al. Evaluation of racial disparities in hospice use and end-of-life treatment intensity in the REGARDS cohort. *JAMA Netw Open.* 2020;3(8):e2014639. doi:10.1001/jamanetworkopen.2020.14639

30. Payne R. (2016). Racially associated disparities in hospice and palliative care access: Acknowledging the facts while addressing the opportunities to improve. *J Palliat Med.* 2016;19(2):131–133. doi:10.1089/jpm.2015.0475

31. Perry LM, Walsh LE, Horswell R, et al. Racial disparities in end-of-life care between black and white adults with metastatic cancer. *J Pain Symptom Manage.* 2021;61(2):342–349.e1. doi:10.1016/j.jpainsymman.2020.09.017

32. Zhang X, Carabello M, Hill T, He K, Friese CR, Mahajan P. Racial and ethnic disparities in emergency department care and health outcomes among children in the United States. *Front Pediatric.* 2019;7:525. doi:10.3389/fped.2019.00525

33. Nelson KE, Wright R, Fisher M, et al. A call to action to address disparities in palliative care access: A conceptual framework for individualizing care needs. *J Palliat Med.* 2021;24(2):177–180. doi:10.1089/jpm.2020.0435

34. Johnson KA, Quest T, Curseen K. Will you hear me? Have you heard me? Do you see me? Adding cultural humility to resource allocation and priority setting discussions in the care of African American patients with COVID-19. *J Pain Symptom Manage.* 2020;60(5):e11–e14. doi:10.1016/j.jpainsymman.2020.08.036

35. Krakauer EL, Crenner C, Fox K. Barriers to optimum end-of-life care for minority patients. *J Am Ger Soc.* 2002;50(1):182–190. doi:10.1046/j.1532-5415.2002.50027.x

36. Cooper E, Hutchinson A, Sheikh Z, Taylor P, Townend W, Johnson MJ. Palliative care in the emergency department: A systematic literature qualitative review and thematic synthesis. *Palliat Med.* 2018;32(9):1443–1454. doi:10.1177/0269216318783920

37. Nigolian L, Gantioque R, Dexheimer J. Palliative care in emergency medicine. What are we missing? *Open J Emerg Med.* 2019;7(1), 1–10. doi:10/4236/ojem.2019.71002

38. Reuter Q, Marshall A, Zaidi H, et al. Emergency department-based palliative interventions: A novel approach to palliative care in the emergency department. *J Palliat Med.* 2019;22(6):649–655. doi:10.1089/jpm.2018.0341

39. Northwestern University. *EPEC: Education in Palliative and End-of-life Care for Emergency Medicine (EPEC-EM) curriculum.* Chicago, IL: Northwestern University; 2019. https://www.bioethics.northwestern.edu/programs/epec/

40. Shoenberger, J, Lamba S, Goett R, et al. Development of hospice and palliative medicine knowledge and skills for emergency medicine residents: Using the accreditation council for graduate medical education milestone framework. *AEM Educ Train.* 2018:2(1):130–145. doi:10.1002/ae2.10088

41. George N, Phillips E, Zaurova M, et al. Palliative care screening and assessment in the emergency department: A systematic review. *J Pain Symptom Manage.* 2016;15(1):108–119. doi:10.1016.j.jpainsymman.2015.07.017

42. Zeng H, Eugene P, Supino M. Would you be surprised if this patient died in the next 12 months? Using the surprise question to increase palliative care consults from the emergency department. *J Palliat Care.* 2020;35(4):221–225. doi:10.1177/0825859719866698

43. Ouchi K, Strout T, Haydar S, et al. Association of emergency clinicians' assessment of mortality risk with actual 1-month mortality among older adults admitted to the hospital. *JAMA Netw Open.* 2019;2:e1911139. doi:10.1001/jamanetworkopen.2019.11139

44. Childers JW, Back AL, Tulsky JA, et al. REMAP: A framework for goals of care conversations. *J Oncol Pract.* 13(10):e844–e850. doi:10/1200/JOP.2016.018796

45. Vitaltalk. Addressing goals of care: Using the REMAP tool. *Seattle, WA: VitalTalk.* 2019. https://www.vitaltalk.org/guides/transitionsgoals-of-care/

46. Ariadne Labs. Serious illness conversation guide. Boston, MA: Ariadne Labs. 2017. https://www.ariadnelabs.org/wp-content/uploads/sites/2/2017/05/SI-CG-2017-04-21_FINAL.pdf

47. Horowitz RK, Hogan LA, Carroll T. MVP-medical situation, values and plan: A memorable and useful model for all serious illness conversations. *J Pain Symptom Manage.* 2020;doi:10.1016/j.jpainsymman.2020.07.022

48. Jain N. Bernacki RE. Goals of care conversations in serious illness: A practical guide. *Med Clin No Amer.* 2020;104(3):375–389. doi:10.1016/j.mcna.2019.12.001

49. Cote AJ, Payot A, Gaucher N. Palliative care in the pediatric emergency department: Findings from a qualitative study. *Ann Emerg Med.* 2019;74(4):481–490. doi:10/1016/j.annemergmed.2019.03.008

50. Verhoef MJ, de Nijs E, Horeweg N, et al. Palliative care needs of advanced cancer patients in the emergency department at the end of life: An observational cohort study. *Support Care Cancer.* 2020;28(3):1097–1107. doi:10.1007/s00520-019-04906-x

51. Loving Aaronson E, Petrillo L, Stoltenberg M, et al. The experience of emergency department providers with embedded palliative care during COVID. *J Pain Symptom Manage.* 2020;doi:10.1016/j.jpainsymman.2020.08.007

52. Koh MYH, Lee JF, Montalban S, et al. ED-PALS: A comprehensive palliative care service for oncology patients in the emergency department. *Am J Hosp Palliat Med.* 2019;36(7):571–576. doi:10.1177/1049909119825847

53. World Health Organization. Palliative care. Key Facts. August 5, 2020. Geneva, Switzerland. https://www.who.int/news-room/factsheets/detail/palliative-care

54. National Hospice and Palliative Care Organization. Home Page. Advancing healthcare with a model that works. 2021. https://www.nhpco.org/about-nhpco//

55. Center to Advance Palliative Care. The case for palliative care. New York, NY: CAPC. 2019. https://www.capc.org/the-case-for-palliative-care/

56. Pfeifer M, Head BA. Which critical communication skills are essential for interdisciplinary end-of-life discussions? *AMA J Ethics.* 2018;20(8):E724–731. doi:10.1001/amajethics.2018.724

57. Back AL. Patient-clinician communication issues in palliative care for patients with advanced cancer. *J Clin Oncol.* 2020;38(9):866–876. https://doi.org/10.1200/JCO.19.00128

58. Anderson RJ, Bloch S, Armstrong M, et al. Communication between healthcare professionals and relatives of patients approaching the

end-of-life: A systematic review of qualitative evidence. *Palliat Med.* 2019;33(8):926–941. doi:10.1177/0269216319852007

59. Dahlin C. ELNEC COVID-19 communication resource guide: An APRN telephone death notification to family tool. 2020. AACN ELNEC webpage. https://www.aacnnursing.org/Portals/42/ELNEC/PDF/APRN-Death-Notification-Resource-Guide.pdf

60. Grudzen CR, Shim DJ, Schmucker AM, et al. Emergency medicine palliative care access (EMPallA): Protocol for a multicenter randomized controlled trial comparing the effectiveness of specialty outpatient versus nurse-led telephonic palliative care of older adults with advanced illness. *BMJ Open.* 2019;9(1):e025692. doi:10.1136/bmjopen-2018-025692

11.

THE PALLIATIVE APRN IN THE PALLIATIVE CARE CLINIC

Brooke Smith and Lisa A. Stephens

KEY POINTS

- The palliative advanced practice registered nurse (APRN) in a palliative care clinic provides continuity of care and symptom management concurrent with disease-modifying treatment that enhances patient satisfaction and reduces healthcare utilization.

- The palliative APRN offers collaborative decision support at key points along the disease trajectory to offer patient-centered, preference-sensitive treatment options.

- The palliative APRN's longitudinal relationship with the patient and family, as well as with other members of the patient's healthcare team, enhances their coping and fosters resilience.

CASE STUDY: THE PALLIATIVE CARE CLINIC APRN

Eileen was a 35-year-old woman with a history of asthma and obesity, status post gastric bypass surgery. She was admitted to the hospital with progressive, severe shortness of breath. She was diagnosed with pulmonary hypertension due to dermatomyositis-associated interstitial lung disease. Six years prior to her diagnosis, Eileen left her position as a bank manager and moved closer to her aged, ailing parents, with her fiancé and his two sons. She was estranged from her two sisters, who both struggled with alcoholism. Over the next 2 years, her mother and father died. One year prior to her admission, her fiancé died suddenly after a viral illness, leaving behind his 14- and 11-year-old sons. In the aftermath of that loss, their mother continued the previous custody arrangement, allowing the boys to stay with Eileen every other weekend.

In the first year after her diagnosis, despite treatment for her dermatomyositis, Eileen's pulmonary hypertension progressed significantly, resulting in cor pulmonale and New York Heart Association (NYHA) functional Class III–IV disease. In the setting of chronic steroid use, she gained more than 100 pounds, reaching a body mass index (BMI) of 38. She was admitted for initiation of vasodilator therapy, epoprostenol, which resulted in significant headache and muscle and joint pain. During this admission, she learned that she had been denied transplant listing by two different regional heart/lung transplant centers due to her weight. Faced with the progression of her disease and lack

of apparent options to treat it, she presented as hopeless and distressed. Her pulmonologist requested a consultation from the inpatient palliative care team to establish a longitudinal relationship for ongoing goals-of-care discussions, pain management, and psychosocial support. For continuity, she was seen by the outpatient palliative advanced practice register nurse (APRN) during that admission and then followed closely in the outpatient clinic.

Over the second year, Eileen was seen monthly by the palliative APRN. Eileen's severe dyspnea made it difficult to navigate the healthcare campus, so the APRN saw her during monthly infusion therapy for dermatomyositis. It was hoped this would stabilize enough to again pursue heart/lung transplantation. A co-management model allowed the palliative APRN to assess and manage Eileen's pain and symptoms and provide appropriate prescriptions and nonpharmacologic interventions. Eileen suffered from headache, jaw pain, and shoulder aches secondary to epoprostenol but feared opioid addiction given her family history. The palliative APRN provided education regarding opioid misconceptions and counseling regarding coping strategies. Eileen was also followed closely by the outpatient palliative social worker. Knowledge of community resources on the part of the APRN and the social worker enhanced Eileen's access to services and allowed her to stay home longer. Emotionally, Eileen struggled to maintain hope without a certain plan for heart/lung transplant. She told the social worker, "I feel as if I have no past (referencing the death of her fiancé and parents), no future (referencing survival without a transplant), and the present sucks." Both the palliative APRN and social worker simultaneously enhanced Eileen's resilience in the face of physical debility and medical uncertainty and supported her coping with her changing physical abilities as a stepmother.

As she began the third year of her illness, now 37 years old, Eileen suffered increasingly with dyspnea and pain and worsening functional ability. Eileen's pulmonary, cardiology, and rheumatology teams shared with her that her disease was not responding as they had hoped. A transplant was no longer a possibility. She began to ask theoretical questions about stopping treatment of her pulmonary hypertension, stating, "I don't think I can do this anymore," but she was not ready to stop life-sustaining treatments out of concern that her stepsons would think she was a "quitter."

In response to Eileen's distress, the palliative APRN organized and led a multidisciplinary outpatient team meeting to discuss Eileen's goals of care. Eileen and her close friend, along with her primary pulmonologist, cardiologist, and rheumatologist, were in attendance. Eileen described the misery of her home situation and made the request that someone "give me an achievable goal or let me go." Her subspecialists responded that ongoing therapy of her pulmonary hypertension would only slow the rate of her inevitable decline and death. She asked what would happen if her epoprostenol was discontinued. The reply was she might die quickly and might suffer significantly worsened dyspnea or chest pain after withdrawal. She was offered the option of admission to the medical center's cardiology floor for discontinuation of the drug in a monitored setting, with the expectation that she would die, which she accepted. She requested the admission be arranged after one last Christmas with her stepsons, at a time when all of her medical subspecialists, including the palliative APRN, could be present.

When Eileen was ultimately admitted, as requested, all her known providers were available including the palliative APRN and her primary cardiologist, pulmonologist, and rheumatologist. Before the epoprostenol was discontinued, she spent a wonderful day and a half with her close family and dear friend at her side. Each family member had an opportunity to say goodbye to her. The palliative social worker assessed the coping of each family member and ensured they had adequate supports going forward. The palliative APRN was the primary clinician responsible for Eileen's comfort medications during the discontinuation process and provided intensive emotional support to the nursing staff. Eileen died peacefully several hours after her epoprostenol was discontinued, with her stepsons, aunt and uncle, and best friend at her side.

CONCURRENT CARE
FROM DIAGNOSIS ONWARD

The prevalence of inpatient palliative care programs continues to rise in the United States. From 2000 to 2016, among hospitals with more than 50 beds, the number of palliative care teams increased by 178%.[1] While hospital-based palliative care has grown substantially over the years, continuity across all settings has been slower to grow. Outpatient palliative care often extends the impact of an inpatient program "upstream" by providing concurrent care from the time of diagnosis across the illness to end of life. The most common model of outpatient clinics has been the academic medical center model of outpatient palliative care clinics as a growth of inpatient palliative care services. Newer clinic models have emerged from a more community-based perspective. In these settings, palliative care clinics are developing from a breadth of community partnerships, such as hospice, home health agencies, independent practices, and community service agencies.

All along a patient's disease trajectory, a palliative care clinic can enhance continuity of care, improve symptom management, increase patient satisfaction, and reduce healthcare utilization, particularly at the end of life.[2–10] As the case study demonstrates, the initial palliative care consultation was requested during an inpatient admission,

but the referring team recognized that this patient needed longitudinal care. The patient, Eileen, had a high symptom burden and poor social support. Her goals were to continue pursuing disease-modifying treatment with the hope of prolonging her life. Her prognosis was poor, and she was overwhelmed. Outpatient palliative care clinics are often started as an extension of the inpatient palliative care team to enhance the quality and continuity of care throughout the disease trajectory.[7]

Palliative advanced practice registered nurse (APRN) play a pivotal role in the delivery of high-quality palliative care concurrent with disease-modifying treatments. A key component of quality is continuity of care, which is enhanced by a continuous patient–APRN relationship. This promotes the APRN's ability to provide ongoing assessment and management of pain and symptoms, counseling regarding adjustment to illness, advance care planning (ACP), and education regarding the side effects of treatments and medications. Moreover, the palliative APRN is poised, through education and experience, to assess the patient's emotional history and coping and to provide supportive counseling and screening for spiritual concerns.[8,11–15] A pilot study, looking at the effects of integrating a palliative APRN into a community oncology center, found that, when compared to usual care, patients were six times less likely to be hospitalized and possibly even lived longer.[8] In this study, the palliative APRN was integrated into the care of patients with advanced cancer at the time of diagnosis and followed the patient and family throughout the disease trajectory. This study, as well as other research, demonstrates the value of a continuous relationship with a palliative APRN who has specialized knowledge and experience.[6,8,13]

The trust that is built by the palliative APRN over time also acts as a foundation for the difficult conversations that will come later in the disease trajectory. A preexisting relationship brings comfort to the patient, family, and caregivers when these conversations are revisited in times of crisis. Since most patients are ambulatory at the time of diagnosis and continue treatments on an outpatient basis, an outpatient palliative care clinic is the ideal place for the APRN to develop such relationships. In addition to improving patient satisfaction and quality of life and decreasing hospital admissions, concurrent palliative care has been proved, in a population of lung cancer patients, to increase survival.[16–18] Box 11.1 lists the benefits of a clinic or outpatient palliative care services.

CORE SERVICES AND
PRACTICE CONSIDERATIONS

The first step in building a palliative care clinic is to determine the primary population of patients to be served and the core services to be provided. This is best achieved by a needs assessment done with stakeholder. Most palliative care clinics serve patients with serious or life-limiting illness who have one or more of the following needs: complex pain and symptom management, complex medical decision support, assistance with goals of care clarification, assistance with ACP, and/or

Box 11.1 BENEFITS OF A PALLIATIVE CLINIC OR OUTPATIENT SERVICES

- Allows for earlier involvement of palliative care at the time of diagnosis

- Builds relationship with patient and family before a crisis

- Improves symptom burden and quality of life for the patient

- Increases earlier advance care planning

- Allows for continuity of care over time

- Increases patient, family, and caregiver satisfaction and reduces caregiver burden

- Increases psychosocial support

- Often increases skills of other caregivers and providers

- Provides decision support at key points along the disease trajectory

- Improves transitions of care

- Often reduces unwanted healthcare utilization, such as hospital admissions and emergency room visits

- Reduces healthcare costs

- Increases hospice utilization and earlier hospice involvement

From Rabow et al.[2,4,17]; Cunningham et al.[3,19]; Kluger et al.[5]; Fulton et al.[6]; Smith et al.[7]; Prince-Paul et al.[8]; Hui and Bruera[9]; National Consensus Project[15]; Bakitas et al.[16]; and Temel et al.[18]

complex social and family dynamics, including substance use disorder and mental health needs (see Chapter 46, "Serious Mental Illness," and Chapter 47, "Patients with Substance Use Disorder and Dual Diagnoses"). It is important to determine whether outpatient palliative care services will be provided to a certain disease-specific population based on a needs assessment that reveals challenges with patient populations or based on pain and symptoms.[10]

The most common reasons for referrals are management of pain and non-pain symptoms, prognosis and determining goals of care, end-of-life planning, and support for psychological issues.[7,20] Often patients may be referred for one reason and additional needs may be discovered and addressed during the course of their visit.[7] Defining the delivery model and core services is imperative to help guide referral sources and define the mission of the clinic. However, addressing unmet needs is often welcomed by the referring providers and patients and families. Prior to initiating an outpatient clinic, there must be well-defined descriptions of appropriate palliative patients, triggers that may warrant referral, and clear expectations of the services to be provided.

Palliative APRNs' scope of practice may determine their role in a palliative care clinic. Specifically, individual state nurse practice acts and statutes, as well as institutional bylaws, need to be considered when designing the palliative care clinic. Furthermore, there may be differences between the role of a clinical nurse specialist (CNS) and a nurse practitioner (NP) in state nurse practice acts. Some states may allow autonomy through full independent practice without physician oversight; other states may have more restrictive practice acts requiring physician supervision. Another important

aspect of a palliative care clinic is prescription medications. There is state variation on prescriptive authority, with some states more progressive than others.[21] The APRN in a more restrictive state will need to develop a plan for prescription writing. Due to COVID-19, some states have temporarily suspended or waived practice agreements and implemented temporary changes to prescriptive authority.[22] It will be necessary to stay abreast of whether these changes become permanent.

Despite these state differences, the palliative APRN can function at the highest scope of practice and provide advanced knowledge of the physical, emotional, social, and spiritual needs of seriously ill patients. Moreover, palliative APRNs institute comprehensive care and provide communication to healthcare providers. In states where APRNs have full independent practice, collaborative practice with physician colleagues is still an important consideration for palliative care. Indeed, for optimizing the management of patients who need highly complex symptom management, a physician colleague can co-manage patients to assist with problem-solving and decision-making.

The ongoing shortage of board-certified hospice and palliative medicine physicians should not be a barrier to finding the right fit with a collaborating physician. If the palliative APRN is providing palliative care services to primarily heart failure or oncology patients, they may choose to collaborate with a cardiologist or an oncologist. A non-hospice and palliative medicine collaborating physician provides expertise in complex diagnostic and specific disease management issues that may arise, while the palliative APRN provides expertise on the assessment and treatment of symptoms and offers psychosocial and spiritual counseling as well as coordination of care.

MODELS OF OUTPATIENT PALLIATIVE CARE CLINICS

Across the United States, a wide variety of models are used to deliver outpatient palliative care services, ranging from outpatient clinics to home and nursing home visits. Once the scope of services is determined, the setting for the care can easily be identified. New models are emerging in the growth of community-based outpatient palliative care clinics. See Table 11.1 for a summary of three current palliative care clinic models: embedded, stand-alone, and co-located.

The *embedded model* is often used to start a palliative care clinic. Several successful and innovative embedded models have been described that use a palliative APRN as the core team member.[8,11,13,24,25] Embedding a palliative APRN in an outpatient clinic has been associated with measurable benefits such as improved symptom management, decreased emergency department visits and hospital admissions, and possibly a decrease in mortality rate.[8,11]

In the embedded model, palliative care is available as standard treatment for any clinic patient with a life-limiting illness. This patient-centered approach allows the palliative APRN to get a "foot in the door" with reluctant referrers and patients, decreasing the perception that palliative care is only for the imminently dying. Fairly quickly, referrers note the benefits of being supported in the arenas of complex symptom management, coordination of care, and complex goals-of-care discussions. Often, in the embedded clinic model, the palliative APRN becomes an informal teacher for other healthcare providers by modeling complex conversations or coaching other providers through these conversations, thus enhancing the care delivered. The embedded clinic model not only enhances the satisfaction of the referrers but may also provide support to the palliative APRN who, by practicing in collaboration with others, develops specialty-level knowledge of the disease state.

There are several disadvantages to an embedded clinic model and these are centered on lack of control for patient flow issues. The palliative APRN's schedule depends on another clinician's timeliness, and there is a higher likelihood of unscheduled add-on appointments and a higher number of cancellations. Despite these inefficiencies, embedding an APRN in a clinic is often a cost-effective way to establish credibility and build relationships while slowly increasing referrals, possibly with a goal of developing a sustainable stand-alone clinic.

A recent review of the literature of models of outpatient palliative care in oncology concluded that the *stand-alone interdisciplinary palliative care clinic* has improved patient outcomes.[26,27] Patients with cancer or non-cancer diagnoses can be easily cared for in a stand-alone clinic. In addition to the APRN, other team members, such as a chaplain or social worker, are highly valuable members of the palliative care team and should be available to see patients and family members on a part- or full-time basis. Palliative physicians may also see patients in tandem with the palliative APRN or may just consult on occasion.

Some strengths of the stand-alone model include its strong evidence of impact on patient outcomes; in addition, this model allows for more continuity and resource utilization, consistent referral criteria, and it is a visible space for the palliative care outpatient service. In a stand-alone clinic, the palliative APRN becomes an important consultant. Patients and families will see the added value of the palliative APRN separate from their other specialty or primary care providers.

Some palliative care clinics are *co-located* in a cancer clinic or an HIV or congestive heart failure clinic. The advantage to the host clinic is quick and easy access to the palliative APRN and other palliative care team members. This model may save costs for the palliative care service in terms of overhead and allow more incremental growth.[23]

Outpatient palliative care services can also be provided as a combination of embedded and stand-alone clinics. In institutions where specialty outpatient clinics are in close proximity, palliative APRNs can float to multiple different clinics in the same day. An example might include seeing his or her own panel of patients in a stand-alone clinic, traveling to see others in the oncology infusion suite, and then joining a heart failure clinician for a joint visit. Advantages include in-time coordination and collaboration of care, allowing those

Table 11.1 MODELS OF PALLIATIVE CARE CLINICS

DESCRIPTION	FINANCING
Independent clinic. These are independently functioning, specialty clinics where patients receive specialty palliative care services. Referrals are received from physicians, APRNs, and PAs per CMS guidelines.	Palliative care clinic responsible for all costs.
Co-located. These palliative care clinics operate in a shared space with other medical services. Referrals to palliative care services may come from physicians, APRNs, and PAs within the specialty clinic in other specialties, or from other practices entirely.	Costs may be shared between the palliative care clinic and the host clinic.
Embedded. These palliative care services share similar characteristics with outpatient co-located clinics. Palliative care providers share space and work closely with other providers. There may be protocols that define how palliative care functions in tandem with other medical services.	The host clinic is typically responsible for all costs.

Adapted from: Cunningham et al.[19] and Barbour et al.[23]

patients who have long days with infusions or have a harder time getting from place to place to have palliative care services come to them.

This approach has the value of being extremely patient-centered by going to where the patient is, but it can be inefficient, as the palliative APRN loses valuable documentation time while in transit between clinics. The palliative APRN is again at the discretion of another clinic's schedule changes or appointment delays. For certain populations, however, having the palliative APRN travel to the patient is indispensable. Some instances include the reluctant or fearful patient who might not be willing to come to a stand-alone clinic visit or a patient with complex chronic illness who does not yet understand the role that palliative care can play in his or her care.

No matter what type of palliative care clinic, there may come a time when it is difficult for a patient to travel to a clinic. In these situations, the APRN must have knowledge about community resources to ease the transition of care to the home. Home palliative care services may include hospice when appropriate or desired, home health when the homebound criteria are met and/or the patient declines hospice, and home palliative care from either hospice or independent providers (see Chapter 14, "The Palliative APRN in the Community Setting," and Chapter 15, "The Palliative and Hospice APRN in Hospice and Home Health Programs").

ROLE OF OTHER TEAM MEMBERS

Other team members may be embedded in the palliative care clinic or may require referral, notably social work and chaplaincy. However, dedicated team members such as a social worker or chaplain can enhance whole-person care, a tenet of providing palliative care.[28] In addition to providing in-depth counseling and support, social workers can help patients to complete advance directive forms and assist with finding resources for those with financial, insurance, or transportation needs. If a social worker and chaplain are not fully dedicated to a palliative care clinic, a plan must be in place for timely referrals. Early joint visits with the chaplain or social worker can facilitate rapport, allowing for subsequent visits to be completed separately from the palliative APRN.

Other team members who can be invaluable to the clinic include nurses and pharmacists. Pharmacists can provide valuable support with comprehensive assessments of medications, assistance with dose conversions, and assessment for any possible medication-related adverse events.[29,30] Registered nurses can serve many roles in a palliative care clinic including education and support for staff, patients, families, and caregivers; help with ACP; and scheduling.[31] Ideally, the palliative APRN will have institutional or local access to nutrition services; rehabilitative therapies, such as physical therapy, occupational therapy, and speech and language pathology; chronic pain management (if not covered by the palliative APRN); child life specialists; grief counseling for their patients; psychologists; psychiatrists; and addiction specialists.

FINANCES

A variety of funding sources are generally necessary to run a palliative care clinic. APRN billing and reimbursement will vary depending on whether a clinic is an independent practice, a hospital-owned clinic, or part of another entity. See the Appendix I for details on billing and coding issues. Typically, given low rates of reimbursement and relatively low clinic appointment volumes, billing revenues do not cover the full cost of an outpatient clinic practice and at least one other source of funding will be needed. In a survey of 20 outpatient palliative care practices, funding sources varied among the programs, but the most common was a combination of institutional support and billing revenues.[7] Commonly, justification for a palliative APRN may include cost avoidance through decreased hospital admissions, decreased emergency department visits, decreased lengths of stay, and early admission to hospice. This cost avoidance may translate into financial support from the institution at large. Embedding an APRN in an oncology or primary care clinic has shown such cost avoidance through decreased healthcare utilization.[8,11] Philanthropy, research, and private foundation support are also common funding sources. Funding will be required for staff (medical and nonmedical), overhead (space and supplies), billing, budgeting and information systems, and tracking of outcomes.[19]

LAUNCHING THE PALLIATIVE CARE CLINIC

ESTABLISHING VISIT TIMES

Once a model is chosen for the palliative care clinic, funding has been located, and a staffing plan has been identified, decisions should be made about clinic flow and practice, in particular establishing visit times. Visit times may need to be longer to accommodate travel time, lack of support staff, and documentation time. A survey of 20 outpatient palliative care programs showed that new consultation times were 40–120 minutes, with an average of 65 minutes, and follow-up visit times were 20–90 minutes, with an average of 37 minutes.[11] In another oncology-embedded APRN-run palliative care clinic visits were on average 56 minutes in length.[13] In general, a good rule is to begin with 90 minutes for a new patient or new consultation and 45 minutes for a follow-up visit, unless more time is needed to travel from clinic to clinic. These appointment times provide a cushion for those days when a follow-up patient may have complex issues and extensive care coordination is needed. Clinic times may be adjusted on a case-by-case basis or shortened if needed to accommodate same-day appointments. Due to the COVID-19 pandemic, video visits have become frequently utilized as another way to offer palliative care to patients, families, and caregivers while maintaining social distance. These visits are often scheduled for the same time duration as usual in-person clinic visits (see Chapter 17, "The Palliative APRN in Telehealth").

REFERRALS AND SCHEDULING

Referrals can come from many sources, such as registered nurses, physician's assistants, physicians, social workers, rehabilitation therapists (physical therapy or occupational therapy), chaplains, other APRNs, or patient and family self-referral. Scheduling guidelines developed by the palliative care team members should be established prior to the startup of the palliative care clinic. Screening for inappropriate referrals should be outlined within these guidelines. In some practices, screening questions can be used by the scheduling secretary: the reason for the consult and the urgency.[23] These questions, as well as self-referrals, may trigger the palliative APRN to interview the patient or referring provider about the appropriateness of the consultation. Some self-referred patients may not have a serious, life-limiting illness but are looking for a new opioid prescriber or may be asking for patient care coordination that would be better provided by their primary care provider's team.

As a way of building clinic volumes or to reach a specific high-needs population, outpatient palliative care clinics can be part of disease-specific or algorithm-driven triggered consultations. Scheduling pathways can then be developed for automatic referrals in these groups. As an example, an automatic palliative care consultation could be scheduled for patients with newly diagnosed Stage IIIB or stage IV lung cancers, pancreatic cancer, New York Heart Association (NYHA) Stage III or IV heart failure, advanced chronic obstructive pulmonary disease, or amyotrophic lateral sclerosis. Automatic referrals require close collaboration with the specialty group. These automatic referrals not only make palliative care consultation part of the routine care provided by the specialty group but also decrease the perception that palliative care is only for patients at the very end of life. Hui et al.[32] performed a Delphi study to develop international consensus on a list of referral criteria to outpatient palliative care for cancer patients. Box 11.2 lists these criteria that may assist in the development of automatic referral criteria.

PATIENT CARE RESPONSIBILITIES

The palliative APRN should explicitly communicate with referring clinicians about role expectations. The role may vary on a case-by-case basis, ranging from consultation only to co-management and even sometimes assuming primary responsibility for the patient.

Co-management is an ideal model for providing specialty palliative care for patients with serious illness. These patients have intense needs, and a co-management approach allows team members to lean on each other along the disease trajectory to off-load work and support each other emotionally, thus decreasing the risk of burnout. This collaboration also avoids a "handoff" when the patient's care needs tip toward a more palliative focus, away from disease-modifying therapies. This integrated, co-management model prevents the patient from feeling abandoned and enhances the concept that palliative care is an "extra layer of support" that is offered to many patients at the time of diagnosis.[33] Other providers

---

Box 11.2 REFERRAL CRITERIA FOR OUTPATIENT SPECIALTY PALLIATIVE CANCER CARE

- Severe physical symptoms (pain, nausea and vomiting, fatigue, dyspnea, etc)
- Severe emotional symptoms (depression, anxiety)
- Delirium
- Requests for assisted death
- Spiritual or existential crisis
- Assistance with decision-making or care planning
- Patient request for referral
- Oncology issues
  o Spinal cord compression
  o Brain or leptomeningeal disease
- Within 3 months of advanced diagnosis in patient with median survival of 1 year or less

From Hui et al.[32]

---

may request consultation for a specific issue only (such as pain management) or for the palliative APRN to take over full care of the patient.

Consultation-only requests that require the referring provider to implement recommendations may not improve symptom control outcomes.[17] The embedded model is the ideal setting for a consultation-only role as the APRN can work closely with the referring provider to guide the implementation of the recommendations. Assuming sole care for a patient can be time-intensive for the palliative APRN. However, it may be appropriate for a patient who has no primary care provider and is no longer receiving disease-modifying treatment or is referred to hospice care without a primary care provider.[23] Defining these roles up front, at the time of consultation, not only helps the patient clarify whom to call with specific issues but also improves collaboration between team members, ultimately benefiting the patient and increasing satisfaction among all team members.

THE INITIAL OUTPATIENT CONSULTATION

Prior to the visit, the palliative APRN should gain a comprehensive understanding of the patient's medical history, likely prognosis, and disease trajectory through chart review and discussion with primary specialists and/or the primary care provider. The underlying goal of the initial visit is to introduce the patient and family to the role of palliative care to establish rapport and to screen for and address the most pressing needs, whether those are physical symptoms, emotional distress, or decision-making support. During the initial visit, the palliative APRN performs a comprehensive assessment of symptoms. Tools such as the Edmonton Symptom Assessment Scale,[34] the Memorial Symptom Assessment Scale,[35] and the Patient Health Questionnaire (PHQ-9)[36] can help can help identify patient-reported symptoms and assist with a comprehensive evaluation of physical and psychological symptoms.

The APRN should also assess, to the extent possible, the patient's and family's understanding of the illness and prognostic awareness, mentally bookmarking areas of significant disconnect between what the patient believes and what chart review has revealed. Communication about serious illness care goals should happen early in the course of a serious illness and be revisited at various times along the illness trajectory. The American College of Physicians High Value Task Force recommends having these conversations in the outpatient setting before a crisis and using a check list or conversation guide.[37] Ariadne Labs offers resources and tools to develop a Serious Illness Care Program and offers a tool, the *Serious Illness Conversation Guide*, that can be used to support best practices in having these conversations.[38] The guide helps to identify understanding of illness, information preferences, prognostic awareness, goals in the face of worsening health, fears and worries, critical functions, tradeoffs, and family awareness of priorities and wishes (see Chapter 32, "Advance Care Planning") and can assist the APRN in counseling regarding end-of-life preferences. The palliative APRN should perform a social assessment to determine the patient's and family's coping strengths and deficiencies.

After the initial consultation, the palliative APRN can identify longitudinal goals for addressing the identified areas of coping and symptom management needs and can suggest a frequency of follow-up visits. For example, if a patient is emotionally resilient, fully understands his or her disease trajectory and prognosis, and has no symptom issues, the palliative APRN might offer to see the patient every 1 to 2 months, in conjunction with surveillance, restaging diagnostics, or visits with the primary specialist. If, however, the palliative APRN identifies a number of coping needs, or there is a high likelihood that symptom burden may change rapidly due to beginning new disease-directed therapies (chemotherapy or radiation), the patient might need to be seen as soon as a few days or a week following the consult.

Above all, the palliative APRN should set realistic personal expectations himself in an initial consultation to avoid forcing an agenda on the patient and family members, potentially alienating them. The philosophy of promoting quality of life, maximizing functional status, optimizing psychosocial coping, and assisting with care management can guide care and help the patient and family understand the support of palliative care. If the patient/family is willing to return, the palliative APRN has succeeded and the work can continue. Box 11.3 lists unique components of the initial consultation note.

OPIOID AND CONTROLLED SUBSTANCES MANAGEMENT

It is imperative that the palliative APRN provide skillful pain and symptom management that mitigates risks when prescribing opioids or other controlled substances.[39] (See Chapter 43 on pain and Chapter 47 on substance use disorder for a more detailed approach to prescribing opioids and other controlled substances and mitigating risks.) The use of universal precautions is recommended for all patients, even in the palliative care clinic, and can mitigate risks and help develop an individualized ongoing assessment and monitoring plan.[40] Universal precautions include the use of an opioid risk screening tool, opioid agreement, calculating the morphine equivalent daily dose (MEDD), performing urine drug screening (UDS), and reviewing prescription drug monitoring programs (PDMP).[40] See Table 11.2 for an example of types of screening actions, risk stratification, and monitoring plans based on initial and ongoing assessments. In Table 11.2, the Opioid Risk Tool (ORT)[39,41] is used.

SUBSEQUENT OUTPATIENT VISITS

Depending on the disease type and trajectory, the middle phase of outpatient palliative care work can last weeks, months, or even years. During this time, in addition to ongoing symptom management as indicated, the palliative APRN should work on fostering resilience and developing prognostic awareness in the patient and their caregivers.[42,43] This work increases the patient's tolerance for difficult discussions and

---

***Box 11.3* UNIQUE OUTPATIENT PALLIATIVE CARE DOCUMENTATION CHARACTERISTICS**

Understanding of Illness or Illness Understanding

Goals of care: Hopes, worries, and priorities
Preferences: Communication, decision making, and advance directives
Social context: Social determinants of health, place of residence, important family members, occupation, and hobbies, employment status, insurance status
Emotional history: Existing coping strategies and their effectiveness; sources of strength, pride, meaning, and connection; fears; areas of significant personal distress (e.g., financial concerns, worries about family members' coping)
Spiritual history: Include a screening tool for spirituality
Cultural history: Meaning of current illness, cultural aspects of health, illness, and death within context of care

Table 11.2 DARTMOUTH-HITCHCOCK PALLIATIVE CARE OPIOID UNIVERSAL PRECAUTIONS: QUICK REFERENCE GUIDELINES

INITIAL ACTION (WITHIN 1ST–2ND VISIT)	PDMP REVIEW ORT CALCULATE & DOCUMENT MEDD TREATMENT AGREEMENT SIGNED AND SCANNED (ORIGINAL TO PATIENT) UDS		
ACTIONS EVERY VISIT	PDMP REVIEW/DOCUMENT AND CALCULATE & DOCUMENT MEDD		
RISK STRATIFICATION CRITERIA	LOW ("STANDARD")	MODERATE	HIGH
Follow-up visits (minimum frequency)	Monthly; if stable alternate APRN visit	Monthly; APRN visit clinician discretion	Every 2 weeks until stable; APRN visit clinician discretion
Palliative social worker participation in care	Clinician discretion	Clinician discretion	Engage for evaluation
Random UDS (minimum)	Yearly	Every 6 months	Every 3 months
Pill count	Clinician discretion	Random	Every visit
Naloxone	Consider offering prescription (based on comorbidities)	Prescribe	Prescribe

From Wilson MM. Dartmouth-Hitchcock Medical Center, Section of Palliative Medicine, Palliative Care Opioid Universal Precautions: Quick Reference Guidelines, October 12, 2020. Used with permission.

lays a foundation of trust in the relationship for the later, challenging work of end-of-life decision-making. The APRN should partner with the patient in celebrating the happy moments and solving problems through the tough times, effectively banking a store of goodwill in the relationship that increases the patient's willingness to engage in less comfortable conversations when they are needed.

Once patients and families can rely on adequate coping skills and have appropriate prognostic awareness, they have the emotional energy to participate in legacy work: preparing for leave-taking. For those patients with adequate coping and strong familial and financial supports at diagnosis, this work may be engaged in much earlier, but for some particularly challenged patients or family members, the capacity may never evolve.[44]

FOSTERING RESILIENCE

Addressing coping throughout the disease trajectory has been associated with improved patient-reported outcomes of improved quality of life and decreased depressive symptoms.[45] Early in the course of the relationship, the palliative APRN should inquire about, explicitly name, and validate the patient's existing and past coping strategies and assess how well they worked in the past and are working now. If past strategies are no longer effective, offer alternatives and offer to brainstorm how new behaviors might work for the patient.[42] Table 11.3 lists different coping strategies patients might employ. The palliative APRN relies on his or her ability to synthesize the coping history, prognosis, and emotional response to the illness in order to reflect core strengths

back to the patient. This approach will not only foster resiliency in the patient but also strengthen the patient–APRN relationship.

In addition to identifying existing coping styles and developing new ones, the palliative APRN should foster the experience of positive emotion. Facilitating discussions about things that bring joy and meaning to the patient provides important coping support.[42] When patients report happy events, the APRN should celebrate those moments with them and, at other times, help them to recognize and enjoy those things they are grateful for.

Finally, the palliative APRN should strategically interpose challenging conversations or difficult encounters with more lighthearted interludes or matter-of-fact visits. This careful titration of discomfort is critical to avoid overwhelming the patient's and family's ability to cope, and it fosters the resilience needed to engage in the next difficult conversation to come.

IDENTIFICATION OF HIGH EMOTIONAL DISTRESS

One challenge is handling patients who struggle to adapt to these circumstances and who require more in-depth services. The palliative APRN should identify the patient with high emotional distress when they are first screened in palliative care and enlist the help of a skilled social worker or other counselor to engage more intensively in counseling around coping strategies. Box 11.4 lists a number of "red flag" characteristics that should prompt referral to a social worker or other

Table 11.3 SAMPLE COPING BEHAVIORS AND EXAMPLES[42]

BEHAVIOR	DEFINITION	ACTIVITY
Distraction	Diverting attention from a stressor	Reading poetry, books or religious books. Listening to music, singing and poetry. Dancing and exercising.
Optimism	Focusing on the positive in life	Looking for the good or positive in situations, such as a serious illness, in terms of what it has meant or brought. Planning for the future and the good things it will bring.
Gratitude	Being thankful for the benefits in life	Communicating appreciation and thankfulness to loved ones, family circle of friends, and health care providers through expressions of verbal or written expressions of gratitude.
Joy	Enjoying the elements of life	Engaging in activities that bring happiness - time in nature, time with loved ones, time with art (painting, singing, dancing, building) or time with sports.
Meditation	Engaging the mind in a focused quietness	Reading, practicing yoga. Listening to guided meditation. Walking a labyrinth. Reading or attending religious rituals.
Humor	Finding amusement in a situation	Finding humor in current situation. Appreciating the absurd, irony, or silly side of life. Making jokes.
Problem-solving	Creating solutions to problems	Planning for the future with financial and legal planning. Embarking on closure.

Adapted from Jacobsen J et al.[42]

clinician skilled in problem-solving therapies or cognitive-behavioral therapy.[46]

COPING AND DENIAL

A common reason for referral is concern that the patient is in "denial." In the face of life-threatening illness, patients cope by avoiding their painful new reality as a way of preserving psychological equanimity. Denial is adaptive until it is proved otherwise, and the palliative APRN should not seek to correct the denial by forcing the patient to discuss topics that are clearly causing discomfort. In patients with incurable lung cancer or non-colorectal cancer, Nipp et al. found that patient denial and self-blame correlated with worse quality of life and mood.[46] The palliative APRN in the clinic is afforded multiple visits over time to support a patient's transition from denial to adaptive acceptance.

DEEPENING PROGNOSTIC AWARENESS

Most patients experience an acute stress response driven by a nervous system sympathetic discharge when they are first told they have a life-limiting illness. For many patients, this sympathetic response overloads their cognitive capacities and much of what they are subsequently told may be heard but not comprehended. Over time, the majority of patients pass through this sympathetically charged, fear-driven stage and into a cognitively intact phase in which they have achieved an accurate understanding of their prognosis. Having this awareness facilitates goal-directed medical decision-making, as when discontinuing chemotherapy prior to enrolling in hospice or when electing not to pursue an implanted defibrillator in NYHA Class IV heart failure.[47]

The minority of patients who struggle with this comprehension phase should be referred to a palliative care clinic to assist with improving prognostic awareness and establishing a relationship for future decision support. With the combination of education and experience in compassionate nursing care and expertise in symptom management, the APRN is well prepared to address "a patient's capacity to understand his or her prognosis and the likely illness trajectory" (prognostic awareness).[43] When palliative care has been involved early in the course of the disease, or when the patient has a slowly progressive disease, the palliative APRN has time to work on fostering resilience, as described earlier. The APRN can intermittently test the patient's tolerance for discussions of prognosis by asking him or her to imagine worse health states, making use of a "hope for the best, prepare for the worst" framework: "I'm really hopeful that this new chemotherapy regimen will do the trick, and I also wonder, though, if we should plan for what you might do if it doesn't."

When the patient's disease progresses rapidly, or when he or she is referred late to palliative care, the patient may be faced with decisions that depend on adequate prognostic understanding even if he or she is not there yet. The palliative APRN should consider "naming the dilemma" as a way of aligning with the patient but ensuring the conversation is opened. "I can tell that talking about a time when your cancer is worse is really hard to do and I wish we didn't have to, but I worry that if we don't we won't be able to make good decisions together. Can you help me think about a way to discuss this that would feel OK to you?"43

SUPPORTING THE RESILIENCE OF REFERRING CLINICIANS

Palliative APRNs are well-positioned to support their referring colleagues and reduce the risk of compassion fatigue and burnout. The palliative APRN can lighten the referring APRN's or physician's workload and time pressures by handling intensive symptom management or by exploring goals and preferences. As a co-manager of complex cases, the palliative APRN serves as a mentor for difficult communication, and the palliative care team-at-large acts as a supportive community for other APRNs and physicians. The palliative APRN can also support the resiliency of other referring APRNs through relationship building that fosters informal discussions of complex cases, which may lead to requests for formal case reviews. Providing shadowing experiences for new APRNs during orientation can also bolster APRN colleagues' confidence in discussing palliative care services with patients and their families.

COMPREHENSIVE, COORDINATED, CONTINUOUS CARE

An important aspect of quality palliative care is to provide a coordinated assessment and continuity of care along the disease trajectory. The National Consensus Project for Quality Palliative Care *Clinical Practice Guidelines* discuss domains of quality that form the basis of practice. Under Domain 1, Structure and Processes of Care, there is an emphasis on coordinated assessment and continuity of care across all healthcare settings.15 Moreover, a recent review of the literature supporting the integration of palliative care into oncology care for patients with advanced cancer found that specialty palliative care that was team-based, initiated early in the disease trajectory, and targeted to those patients who may benefit (use of triggers for automatic referrals) improves patient outcomes.26 Patients may have complex pain or symptoms requiring frequent medication adjustments and education; they may have multiple specialists involved in their care and experience increased vulnerability during transitions of care. The palliative APRN is well-suited to address this challenge and provide continuity of care.

A skilled coordinating RN is a critical support to the APRN. This RN is primarily responsible for phone triage in ensuring that patients' symptoms are managed and psychosocial needs are met in a timely manner in between visits. The nurse also communicates with patients' other providers and helps to coordinate hospital admissions. The RN acts to "extend" the reach of the APRN, handling basic symptom assessment and management (such as bowel medication titration), using appropriate guidelines to allow one to practice within one's professional nursing scope of practice. When patients are undergoing dose titration of pain medications or require close monitoring for other reasons, the coordinating nurse can make routine phone calls to check in with the patient, ensuring that the correct protocol is followed and optimal results are achieved. Because this RN acts as the "right hand" of the APRN, they are best located in the clinic to ensure optimal communication and collaboration with the APRN and the team. Depending on workload, the nurse may also assist with checking patients in before visits, reconciling medications, assessing and evaluating the effectiveness of interventions, monitoring for adverse effects of medications, and screening for new symptoms or problems.

Another important aspect of providing coordinated care and continuity of care is through the interdisciplinary meeting. The expectation for an inpatient palliative care staff is similar to that for outpatient palliative care staff: the need to meet at least weekly to discuss patients and review new consults and particularly challenging situations. This ensures that the palliative care roles are defined, that handoffs through transition of care are thorough, and that care goals are in alignment. This meeting also provides support to clinicians in the ongoing clinical care.

When providing quality palliative care in the outpatient setting, access to a specialty palliative care provider should be available 24 hours a day, 7 days a week. This service is helpful not only for patients who have active symptoms but also for referring providers who may need phone consultation about a complex symptom management situation. This is especially important when the palliative APRN dispenses prescriptions to enable follow-up care.

APPROACHING END OF LIFE: LATE WORK

As a patient's life approaches its close, the palliative APRN partners with other clinicians and discusses the perceived benefits and burdens of further disease-directed therapy. This discussion may trigger awareness that the patient's goals need further clarification. Chapter 33, "Family Meetings," offers a thorough review of conducting these discussions. In general, a goals-of-care discussion must be informed by the patient's values and goals and the medically available and/or appropriate treatment options that will meet those goals.

Most patients choose to continue disease-directed therapy as long as they perceive the treatment as beneficial (i.e., it is helping them to meet their goals) and not significantly limiting their quality of life. When a patient's scales tip such that the benefit is outweighed by the burdens, it is often the palliative APRN who learns, through the longitudinal relationship developed in the clinic, that a transition to purely palliative therapies is needed. Some patients may be perceived by their primary specialists as desiring inappropriately aggressive care. Palliative APRNs can elucidate the reasons for these choices: in one typical scenario, a patient is willing to temporarily accept an otherwise unacceptably low quality of life in order to meet certain goals, such as living long enough to be present for a major life event, like the birth of a grandchild. By sharing these motivations with the treatment team(s), the palliative APRN can ease some of the moral distress experienced by clinicians who worry the patient "just doesn't get it."

Increasingly, palliative APRNs are incorporated into the care team of patients with multiple chronic illnesses and multiple specialty providers. The palliative APRN is well-positioned to arrange and facilitate multidisciplinary meetings in the outpatient setting. The palliative APRN serves to translate medical information to the patient and family and helps to elicit the patient's goals, which are reflected back to the medical team. The benefits to patients are clear, given the often fragmented care and communication they experience because they have multiple specialists.

In addition to supporting patients through the transition to end-of-life care, the palliative APRN is in an optimal position to support the patient's primary provider, who may be struggling with anticipatory grief at the thought of losing a patient or guilt that he or she could not cure or forestall the disease's progression. The palliative APRN helps team members to cope through debriefing conversations that allow for expression of emotions and for thorough discussion of the patient's goals and preferences. Knowledge and acceptance of the patient's goals facilitate adaptive coping in the provider.

REFERRALS TO HOSPICE

The rapport and trust developed over time in the longitudinal relationship described in this chapter become the foundation for emotionally charged discussions closer to the end of life. Helping a patient and family make the transition to hospice is one of those complex conversations. In addition to skill in communicating empathically, the palliative APRN should have a thorough understanding of hospice eligibility criteria for the patient's diagnosis and the services provided in the patient's community. Assuming hospice eligibility criteria are met, a patient should be referred to hospice once they are no longer receiving disease-modifying therapy or when coming back and forth to the clinic has become burdensome. At the time of the hospice referral, the palliative APRN should review the patient's medication list to identify medications that might not be on the hospice formulary and suggest alternatives and should prepare for crisis events in the home by prescribing medications for crescendo pain, dyspnea, seizures, or agitation.

Prior to making a hospice referral, the palliative APRN should identify which provider will oversee the patient's care once on hospice. To promote quality care within the transition, the palliative APRN should be explicit that he or she remains available as a consultant to the hospice medical director and should state whether they will serve as the Provider Attending of Record for hospice care. This ongoing consultative relationship helps patients and families feel that they are not being abandoned once a referral to hospice is made and provides expert-level guidance to the clinician managing the patient's care going forward. It is important that the Attending of Record feels comfortable with the current plan of care and feels prepared to manage any foreseeable complex pain or symptom issues. Carefully communicated handoffs at the time of hospice referral are imperative to ensure a smooth transition.

SUMMARY

Embedded in the culture of nursing and APRN education are the skills of communication, assessment and management of symptoms, psychosocial and spiritual support, and coordination of care. The palliative APRN in the clinic draws on these skills, improving patient satisfaction and decreasing healthcare utilization. The longitudinal APRN–patient relationship enhances communication with patients and families, thereby improving the ability to offer patient-centered, preference-sensitive treatment options. Palliative APRNs deliver coordinated, comprehensive care that can lessen the burden of illness on patients and families and may improve the resilience of the clinicians who co-manage these patients with the palliative APRN.

REFERENCES

1. Center to Advance Palliative Care. Palliative care continues its annual growth trend, according to latest center to advance palliative

care analysis. Press Release. February 28. 2018. https://www.capc.org/about/press-media/press-releases/2018-2-28/palliative-care-continues-its-annual-growth-trend-according-latest-center-advance-palliative-care-analysis/

2. Rabow M, Kvale E, Barbour L, et al. Moving upstream: A review of the evidence of the impact of outpatient palliative care. *J Palliat Med.* 2013;16(12):1540–1549. doi:10.1089/jpm.2013.0153

3. Cunningham C, Ollendorf D, Travers K. The effectiveness and value of palliative care in the outpatient setting. *JAMA Intern Med.* 2017;177(2):264–265. doi:10.1001/jamainternmed.2016.8177

4. Rabow MW, Dahlin C, Calton B, Bischoff K, Ritchie C. New frontiers in outpatient palliative care for patients with cancer. *Cancer Control.* 2015;22(4):465–474. doi:10.1177/107327481502200412

5. Kluger BM, Miyasaki J, Katz M, et al. Comparison of integrated outpatient palliative care with standard care in patients with parkinson disease and related disorders: A randomized clinical trial. *JAMA Neurol.* 2020;77(5):551–560. doi:10.1001/jamaneurol.2019.4992

6. Fulton JJ, LeBlanc TW, Cutson TM, et al. Integrated outpatient palliative care for patients with advanced cancer: A systematic review and meta-analysis. *Palliat Med.* 2019;33(2):123–134. doi:10.1177/0269216318812633

7. Smith AK, Thai JN, Bakitas MA, et al. The diverse landscape of palliative care clinics. *J Palliat Med.* 2013;16(6):661–668. doi:10.1089/jpm.2012.0469

8. Prince-Paul M, Burant CJ, Saltzman JN, Teston LJ, Matthews CR. The effects of integrating an advanced practice palliative care nurse in a community oncology center: A pilot study. *J Support Oncol.* 2010;8(1):21–27. PMID: 20235420

9. Hui D, Bruera E. Models of palliative care delivery for patients with cancer. *J Clin Oncol.* 2020;38(9):852–865. doi:10.1200/JCO.18.02123

10. Finlay E, Rabow MW, Buss MK. Filling the gap: Creating an outpatient palliative care program in your institution *Am Soc Clin Oncol Educ Book.* 2018;38:111–121. doi:10.1200/EDBK_200775

11. Owens D, Eby K, Burson S, Green M, McGoodwin W, Isaac M. Primary palliative care clinic pilot project demonstrates benefits of a nurse practitioner-directed clinic providing primary and palliative care. *J Am Acad Nurse Pract.* 2012;24:52–58. doi:10.1111/j.1745-7599.2011.00664.x

12. Heinle R, McNulty J, Hebert RS. Nurse practitioners and the growth of palliative medicine. *Am J Hosp Palliat Care.* 2013;31(3):287–291. doi:10.1177/1049909113489163

13. Walling AM, D'Ambruoso SF, Malin JL, et al. Effect and efficiency of an embedded palliative care nurse practitioner in an oncology clinic. *J Oncol Pract.* 2017;13(9):e792–e799. https://ascopubs.org/doi/pdfdirect/10.1200%2FJOP.2017.020990.

14. Sherman DW, Free DC. Nursing and palliative care. In: Cherney NI, Fallon MT, Kaasa S, Portenoy RK, Currow DC, eds. *Oxford Textbook of Palliative Medicine.* 5th ed. New York: Oxford University Press; 2015: 160–161.

15. National Consensus Project for Quality Palliative Care. *Clinical Practice Guidelines for Quality Palliative Care.* 4th ed. Richmond, VA: National Coalition for Hospice and Palliative Care; 2018. https://www.nationalcoalitionhpc.org/ncp.

16. Bakitas M, Lyons KD, Hegel MT, et al. The project ENABLE II randomized controlled trial to improve palliative care for rural patients with advanced cancer: Baseline findings, methodological challenges, and solutions. *Palliat Support Care.* 2009;7(1):75–86. doi:10.1017/S1478951509000108

17. Rabow M, Dibble SL, Pantilat SZ, McPhee SJ. The comprehensive care team: A controlled trial for outpatient palliative medicine consultation. *Arch Intern Med.* 2004;164:83–91. doi:10.1001/archinte.164.1.83

18. Temel JS, Greer JA, Muzikansky A, et al. Early palliative care for patients with metastatic non-small-cell lung cancer. *N Engl J Med.* 2010;363(8):733–742. doi:10.1056/NEJMoa1000678

19. Cunningham C, Travers K, Chapman R, et al. Palliative care in the outpatient setting: A comparative effectiveness report. Final report. Institute for Clinical and Economic Review; April 27 2016.

20. Hui D, Meng Y, Bruera S, et al. Referral criteria for outpatient palliative cancer care: A systematic review. *Oncologist.* 2016;21(7):895–901. doi:10.1634/theoncologist.2016-0006

21. American Association of Nurse Practitioners. State practice environment. 2019. Updated January 1. 2021. https://www.aanp.org/advocacy/state/state-practice-environment

22. American Association of Nurse Practitioners. COVID-19 state emergency response: Temporarily suspended and waived practice agreement requirements. 2020. Updated December 7, 2020. https://www.aanp.org/advocacy/state/covid-19-state-emergency-response-temporarily-suspended-and-waived-practice-agreement-requirements

23. Barbour L, Cohen SE, Jackson V, et al. *Getting Started: The Outpatient Palliative Care Clinic: A Technical Assistance Monograph from the IPAL-OP Project.* New York: Center to Advance Palliative Care; 2012. https://www.yumpu.com/en/document/view/30287447/the-outpatient-palliative-care-clinic-the-ipal-project-center-to-

24. Meier DE, Beresford L. Outpatient clinics are a new frontier for palliative care. *J Palliat Med.* 2008;11(6):823–828. doi:10.1089/jpm.2008.9886

25. Bakitas MA, Bishop MF, Caron P, Stephens L. Developing successful models of cancer palliative care services. *Semin Oncol Nurs.* 2010;26(4):266–284. doi:10.1016/j.soncn.2010.08.006

26. Hui D, Hannon BL, Zimmermann C, Bruera E. Improving patient and caregiver outcomes in oncology: Team-based, timely, and targeted palliative care. *CA Cancer J Clin.* 2018;68(5):356–376. doi:10.3322/caac.21490

27. Hui D. Palliative cancer care in the outpatient setting: Which model works best? *Curr Treat Options Oncol.* 2019;20(17):1–13. doi:10.1007/s11864-019-0615-8

28. Benton K, Zerbo KR, Decker M, Buck B. Development and evaluation of an outpatient palliative care clinic. *J Hosp Palliat Nurs.* 2019;21(2):160–166. doi:10.1097/NJH.0000000000000544

29. McPherson ML, Walker K. How to include a pharmacist in the palliative care mix. Center to Advance Palliative Care Blog. September 25, 2019. Available at https://www.capc.org/blog/how-include-pharmacist-palliative-care-mix/

30. Lehn JM, Gerkin RD, Pinderhughes S, Kisiel SC. Center to Advance Palliative Care, National Seminar Poster session 2017. Pharmacists providing palliative care: Showing positive ROI. 2017. https://www.capc.org/seminar/poster-sessions/pharmacists-providing-pall-care-showing-positive-roi/

31. Price C. The role of a nurse on an outpatient palliative care team to increase provider productivity and improve communication. Center to Advance Palliative Care National Seminar Poster Session 2018. https://www.capc.org/seminar/poster-sessions/the-role-of-a-nurse-on-an-outpatient-palliative-care-team-to-increase-provider-productivity-and-improve-communication/

32. Hui D, Mori M, Watanabe SM, et al. Referral criteria for outpatient specialty palliative cancer care: An international consensus. *Lancet Oncol.* 2016;17(12):e552–e559. doi:10.1016/S1470-2045(16)30577-0

33. Vergo MT, Cullinan AM. Joining together to improve outcomes: Integrating specialty palliative care into the care of cancer patients. *J Natl Compr Canc Netw.* 2013;11(Suppl 4):S1–S9. doi:10.6004/jnccn.2013.0220

34. Hui D, Bruera E. The Edmonton Symptom Assessment System 25 years later: Past, present and future developments. *J Pain Symptom Manage.* 2017;53(3):630–643. doi:10.1016/j.jpainsymman.2016.10.370

35. Portenoy RK, Thaler HT, Kornblith AB, et al. The Memorial Symptom Assessment Scale: An instrument for the evaluation of symptom prevalence, characteristics and distress. *Eur J Cancer.* 1994;30A(9):1326–1336. doi:10.1016/0959-8049(94)90182-1

36. Kroenke K, Spitzer RL, Williams JB. The PHQ-9: Validity of a brief depression severity measure. *J Gen Intern Med.* 2001;16(9):606–613. doi:10.1046/j.1525-1497.2001.016009606.x

37. Bernacki RE, Block SD, American College of Physicians High Value Care Task Force. Communication about serious illness care

goals: A review and synthesis of best practices. *JAMA Intern Med.* 2014;174(12):1994–2003. doi:10.1001/jamainternmed.2014.5271

38. Ariadne Labs. Serious illness care conversation guide. Boston, MA. 2017. https://www.ariadnelabs.org/serious-illness-care/for-clinicians/

39. Tuelings L, Broglio K. Opioid misuse risk: Implementing screening protocols in an ambulatory oncology clinic. *Clin J Oncol Nurs.* 2020;24(1):11–14. doi:10.1188/20.CJON.11-14

40. Paice JA. Risk assessment and monitoring of patients with cancer receiving opioid therapy. *Oncologist.* 2019;24(10):1294–1298. doi:10.1634/theoncologist.2019-0301

41. Ma JD, Horton JM, Hwang M, Atayee RS, Roeland EJ. A Single-center, retrospective analysis evaluating the utilization of the opioid risk tool in opioid-treated cancer patients. *J Pain Palliat Care Pharmacother.* 2014;28(1):4–9. doi:10.3109/15360288.2013.869647

42. Jacobsen J, Kvale E, Rabow M, et al. Helping patients with serious illness live well through the promotion of adaptive coping: A report from the Improving Outpatient Palliative Care (IPAL-OP) initiative. *J Palliat Med.* 2014;17(4):463–468. doi:10.1089/jpm.2013.0254

43. Jackson VA, Jacobsen J, Greer JA, Pirl WF, Temel JS, Black AL. The cultivation of prognostic awareness through the provision of early palliative care in the ambulatory setting: A communication guide. *J Palliat Med.* 2013;16(8):894–900. doi:10.1089/jpm.2012.0547

44. Block SD. Psychological considerations, growth, and transcendence at the end of life: The art of the possible. *JAMA.* 2001;285(22):2898–2905. doi:10.1001/jama.285.22.2898

45. Hoerger M, Greer JA, Jackson V, et al. Defining the elements of early palliative care that are associated with patient-reported outcomes and delivery of end-of-life care. *J Clin Oncol.* 2018;36(11):1096–1102. doi:10.1200/JCO.2017.75.6676

46. Nipp RD, El-Jawahri A, Fishbein JN, et al. The relationship between coping strategies, quality of life, and mood in patients with incurable cancer. *Cancer.* 2016;122(13):2110–2116. doi:10.1002/cncr.30025

47. Knight SJ, Emanuel L. Processes of adjustment to end-of-life losses: A reintegration model. *J Palliat Med.* 2007;10(5):1190–1198. doi:10.1089/jpm.2006.0068

12.

THE PALLIATIVE APRN IN PRIMARY CARE

Rosemary Gorman, Dorothy Wholihan, and Sarah Bender

KEY POINTS

- The advanced practice registered nurse (APRN) in primary care requires a generalist (primary) palliative care skill set and an understanding of referral criteria to hospice and specialist palliative care.

- Primary palliative care skills include knowledge of disease trajectories and the management of multidimensional symptoms, as well as communication skills needed for determination of goals of care and advance care planning.

- Given their long-standing relationships with patients, primary care providers are well-suited to facilitate values-based conversations concerning goals of care.

CASE STUDY: TRANSITIONAL CARE MANAGEMENT

Mary was an 88-year-old woman with history of congestive heart failure (CHF), atrial fibrillation, hypertension, and chronic kidney disease (CKD) Stage 3, who was recently discharged from the hospital after a 7-day admission for lower extremity edema and acute kidney injury. Mary was taking double her Lasix dosing for her lower extremity edema and therefore became volume-depleted. She was treated with gentle oral and IV hydration until her creatinine was back to her baseline. Her furosemide and blood pressure medications were held at discharge. The primary care APRN was notified of her hospitalization and made an appointment within 7 days for high-complexity transitional care management (discussed in the billing and coding section).

During the transitional care management visit, Mary and the APRN discussed her hospitalization and treatment for her chronic conditions. Using palliative care communication skills, the advanced practice registered nurse (APRN) discussed prognostication with the patient, given her most recent symptoms. The APRN proposed a plan going forward for managing the patient's multiple comorbidities and addressed goals of care in this plan. Mary expressed that she values spending time with her family and being at home. She wished to be pain free and comfortable and not be readmitted to the hospital. A medical order for life-sustaining treatments (MOLST) form was filled out by the APRN, who spent an additional 30 minutes discussing advance care planning. The APRN bills for high-complexity transitional care management (99496) with an additional 30 minutes spend discussing advance care planning (99498).

Mary's condition continued to decline at home in the next few weeks, and the APRN referred her to hospice after having a discussion with Mary and her family. Mary had her symptoms closely managed and spent her final months surrounded by her family and friends.

INTRODUCTION

The Healthy People 2020 Report, published by The Office of Disease Prevention and Health Promotion, uses the The National Academies of Sciences, Engineering, and Medicine (NASEM) (formerly known as the Institute of Medicine) definition of primary care which is "the provision of integrated, accessible healthcare services by clinicians who are accountable for addressing a large majority of personal healthcare needs, developing a sustained partnership with patients, and practicing in the context of family and community."[1] Clinicians who provide such care are called primary care providers (PCPs). PCPs offer routine physicals, preventive care, chronic disease management, and referrals for specialty care. APRNs frequently serve as the PCP for patients throughout the life span, often being the first point of contact for a patient's medical care needs. The advanced practice registered nurse (APRN) PCP is therefore in a prime position to identify patients who could benefit from palliative care services. The APRN has the added benefit of working with patients and families over long periods of time with frequent interactions, therefore having well-established relationships.[2] This gives the APRN the opportunity to deliver primary palliative care by recognizing those patients who could benefit from symptom management of chronic diseases, prognostication, advance care planning (ACP), and timely hospice referrals.[3]

The implementation of the *Affordable Care Act (ACA)* in 2010 supported legislation to give nurse practitioners full practice authority in many states. The ACA highlighted the need for increased access to primary care as more people in the United States gained health insurance. At the same time, the United States is experiencing an increasing number of people over the age of 65 years who have increased health needs.[4] Due to advances in medical therapies and technology, our population is living with chronic illnesses for longer. As of 2014,

60% of Americans has at least one chronic condition, and 42% had more than one chronic condition.[5] This highlights the potential for primary palliative care to improve quality of life as the population ages.

According to *Palliative Nursing: Scope and Standards*,[6] as nurses, all APRNs practice primary palliative care. Basic palliative care is inherent in the definition of nursing: alleviation of suffering through the diagnosis and treatment of human response and advocacy for patients and their families. Furthermore, all nurses provide psychosocial and spiritual support and assist with ACP within the context of a patient's cultural background.[6] The National Consensus Project for Quality Palliative Care identifies four major domains for primary palliative care: assessment/treatment of physical symptoms; psychological, social, cultural, and spiritual aspects of care; serious illness communication issues; and care coordination.[6] This includes basic management of physical symptoms, exploring religious beliefs and psychological suffering, ACP conversations, coordination with specialists, and appropriate and timely referrals. There has been a long-documented gap of palliative care demand compared to the availability of palliative care specialty providers.[2] APRN PCPs are uniquely suited to help fill the gap of palliative care needs within the primary care environment. This chapter discusses how to integrate palliative care skills into the primary care setting, including identifying patients who need palliative care, palliative care for common chronic illnesses, ACP in primary care, billing/coding, prognostication in primary care, and the emerging telehealth trend.

WHO NEEDS PALLIATIVE CARE?

The National Consensus Project for Quality Palliative Care *Clinical Practice Guidelines* defines palliative care as follows: "Beneficial at any stage of a serious illness, palliative care is an interdisciplinary care delivery system designed to anticipate, prevent, and manage physical, psychological, social, and spiritual suffering to optimize quality of life for patients, their families and caregivers."[7 (p. 8)] APRN PCPs must be cognizant that palliative care is not the same as hospice care. Moreover, in primary care, both are important and will support the care offered by the PCP.

Palliative care can be applicable early in the course of illness and is also appropriate in conjunction with treatment intended to prolong life. Palliative care focuses on the management of both physical and emotional symptoms experienced by those with serious illness. Palliative care helps to match treatment with a patient's self-identified goals. Since primary care is comprehensive care, basic palliative care must be incorporated as an integral part of primary care. When it is time for hospice, the APRN PCP will need to work with hospice nurses to develop a plan of care and will often continue to order medications and supervise the plan of care. There are numerous resources available to help PCPs determine when hospice referral is indicated.[3,8]

Today's APRN PCPs must understand primary palliative care principles. Vigilant symptom management for patients with multiple comorbid diseases can optimize quality of life and minimize unnecessary admissions. Communication skills essential to the determination of individual and family goals can ensure person-centered care. The awareness of and ability to connect with community resources assists patients to access appropriate services, which can help them remain at home. The primary care APRN PCP can provide background and guidance in the ongoing management of long-term patients referred to ambulatory or home-based palliative care or hospice.

The specialist palliative APRN has an important role in collaborating with PCPs in the community. When a patient is hospitalized, inpatient palliative care specialist consultants can assist with appropriate discharge and follow-up planning, providing essential but often-neglected care coordination by maintaining clear, open communication with community providers. Outpatient palliative care specialty clinics and office practices are expanding, and palliative APRNs in these settings need to increase awareness among PCPs about their contributions and how they can develop partnerships for patient care. Palliative care can be translated to the community settings through a variety of models. Outpatient palliative care improves access to early care by providing consultative services to primary care practices, home care agencies, and community residential agencies like assisted living. Early evidence reveals encouraging outcomes, such as increased caregiver support, decreased hospitalization rates, and improved symptom management and quality of life.[9]

Palliative APRNs also need to develop their teaching skills. Providing interprofessional educational opportunities for care partners can facilitate the development of working relationships, increase professional awareness of the benefits of palliative care, and improve the general levels of palliative care knowledge among PCPs. In addition, both primary care nurse practitioners and palliative APRN clinical nurse specialists are well-suited to provide public education in order to increase public awareness of the benefits and availability of palliative care in the community.

The aging of America's "baby boomers" will have a significant impact on healthcare. The number of Americans ages 65 and older is projected to nearly double from 52 million in 2018 to 95 million by 2060, and the 65-and-older age group's share of the total population will rise from 16% to 23%.[10] Technological advances in both the pharmaceutical and medical device industries have improved medical care and resulted in the increased survival of individuals with chronic conditions. An estimated 50% of people older than 60 have more than one chronic condition.[11] Diseases previously considered terminal, such as HIV, end-stage renal disease, liver failure, heart failure, chronic obstructive pulmonary disease (COPD), and cancer, are now chronic long-term health problems, with basic healthcare managed by APRN PCPs in specialty consultation as needed.

Progressive chronic disease can have an uncertain illness trajectory, one characterized by intermittent disease exacerbations and progressive decline in functional status, together with an associated high symptom burden. This care requires palliative interventions to maintain quality of life. There is a dearth of evidence for the management of patients with multiple coexisting chronic conditions, which adds to the complexity of treatment and difficulty with prognostication. The principles of palliative care can guide the APRN PCP in basic symptom management and the establishment of treatment plans based on realistic goals.

INTEGRATING PALLIATIVE CARE INTO THE PRIMARY CARE OF COMMON CHRONIC ILLNESS

HEART DISEASE IN PRIMARY CARE

The Centers for Disease Control and Prevention (CDC) identifies heart disease as the number one cause of death in the United States, with 6.2 million adults identified as having heart failure.[12] With evolving pharmacologic and technologic therapies, these patients are living longer The symptom burden identified by those with heart failure has been reported to include general discomfort and fatigue, anorexia, dyspnea, depression, and anxiety. In addition, patients with advanced congestive heart failure routinely have multiple comorbidities and multiple symptoms. Primary palliative care can facilitate coping with complex symptoms, decrease frequency of exacerbation and hospitalization, and help with ongoing determination of care goals in the context of evolving specialized therapies[13] (see Chapter 13, "The Palliative APRN in Specialty Cardiology" and Chapter 54, "Discontinuation of Cardiac Therapies" for more details on heart disease management).

CHRONIC OBSTRUCTIVE PULMONARY DISEASE IN PRIMARY CARE

COPD refers to a group of diseases that cause obstruction of the airways with resulting breathing problems; COPD includes emphysema and chronic bronchitis. The CDC cites COPD as the third leading cause of death in the United States, affecting more than 16 million Americans.[14] COPD is a crippling disease and significantly affects quality of life. Breathlessness is the primary symptom of advanced COPD and can be accompanied by pain, fatigue, and insomnia. Anxiety, depression, and social isolation contribute to psychological suffering and the high symptom burden. Primary palliative care skills are integral to successful symptom management, but also help the PCP with the difficult issue of prognostication in this disease.[15] Further discussion of palliative care issues in advanced respiratory disease can be found in Chapters 44 and 55.

CANCER AND SURVIVORSHIP IN PRIMARY CARE

The American Cancer Society reports that cancer survival rates have improved within almost all of the most common cancers. The 5-year relative survival rate for all cancers diagnosed from 2009 to 2015 was 67% overall, 68% in Whites, and 62% in Blacks.[16] As these numbers grow, health professionals are learning that there are a wide array of clinical issues which may arise, both physical and psychological. Some survivors will have little sequelae, while others may experience a higher probability of cancer recurrence, long-lasting emotional difficulties, or symptoms related to treatment side effects. These side effects may not occur until years after treatment is completed. Cardiac problems, neuropathy, osteoporosis, and liver or lung problems can arise, as well as an increased risk of other cancers. Anxiety and depression can also have a significant impact on quality of life. PCPs should determine who is at high risk for recurrence or late symptoms to provide appropriate surveillance and support.[17] *Cancer survivorship care plans* are individualized treatment and follow-up plans which are now recommended by the major cancer care organizations and can be helpful for patients and PCPs who may not be not familiar with chemotherapeutic agents and the possible long-term effects of cancer and cancer treatment.[18]

The American Society of Clinical Oncology (ASCO) and the National Comprehensive Cancer Network (NCCN) have issued evidence-based clinical practice guidelines for common symptom issues facing cancer survivors, including fatigue, anxiety, depression, chemotherapy-induced peripheral neuropathy, sexual dysfunction, and menopausal symptoms.[17] In addition, the American Academy of Family Physicians has published a helpful series on the primary care of patients surviving specific types of cancer, detailing surveillance and symptom issues for those surviving cancers of the breast, prostate, and colorectal.[19-22] While reimbursement is currently not available for the completion of the Survivorship Care Plan—composed of the treatment summary and long-term care plan—ASCO and others are actively working on legislation to enable providers to bill for this service, and the organization does provide some guidance on billing for survivor-related symptoms.[23] The APRN PCP should maintain awareness of ongoing survivorship issues and coordinate care with oncology services as needed (see Chapter 24 for more detail on specific care issues).

FRAILTY

The aging population and better long-term management of chronic conditions create a focus on frailty in the elderly. Although there is no consensus on definition, frailty is understood to be a state of increased vulnerability to adverse health outcomes in a defined age group.[24] Two primary tools used to evaluate for frailty are the Frailty Index, which is a ratio of deficits in a particular age group, and the Frailty Phenotype, which consists of three or more of the following traits: unintentional weight loss, fatigue, weakness, low walking speed, and low physical activity.[25] Similarities between frailty measurements and the Palliative Performance Scale (see section on Prognostication) shows the relevance of primary palliative care for frail patients.

Frail patients are at a higher risk of adverse health outcomes, including falls, hospitalizations, and even death.[25] Furthermore, frail patients have a higher symptom burden than their non-frail counterparts, which can decrease quality of life. Weight loss, weakness/slowness, fatigue, depression, falls, and pain are the most common symptoms among frail patients.[25] Knowing that frailty contributes to worse health outcomes, it is less likely that aggressive medical interventions will be of value. Although frailty cannot be used as a primary hospice diagnosis, it often coincides with other chronic illnesses that can qualify a patient for hospice.

Recognition of frailty, optimization of community resources, and early ACP are essential. A scoping review of communication about frailty in the primary care setting found that older adults wish to discuss ways to prevent or improve their condition, potential complications, and prognosis.[26] APRN PCPs should recognize and address frailty as a syndrome and understand its effect on functionality and prognosis because it may have clear implications in terms of treatment decisions and goals of care. APRNs have the opportunity to improve the patient's quality of life by addressing symptoms of frailty and leading goals-of-care discussions accordingly in the primary care setting.

DEMENTIA

According to the Alzheimer's Association, Alzheimer's disease accounts for 60–80% of the cases of dementia and is now the sixth leading cause of death in the United States.[27] There are more than 5.8 million people age 65 or older living with Alzheimer's disease in 2020, with 13.8 million people expected to be living with the disease by 2050.[27] PCPs are on the frontlines of providing dementia care. Early recognition is key, and dementia should be addressed as a terminal disease. Patients with Alzheimer's disease and other dementias and their caregivers require complex symptom management and support.

Dementia is an incurable and life-limiting illness; it is characterized by a slow progressive decline of cognitive abilities and functional decline that ultimately limits participation in activities of daily living. This neurodegenerative disorder leads to severe cognitive deficits, gradual functional decline, and death. Currently, there is no cure or therapy to halt or reverse this devastating disease. Delirium and behavioral problems associated with dementia can be challenging to attribute to the disease itself versus other common etiologies, such as adverse drug effects, infection, dehydration, hyponatremia, and a wide variety of other chronic conditions.[28] Caregivers who report these symptoms often have their own degree of distress, reflecting the importance of managing the dyad of needs of both caregiver and patient.

Primary palliative care for people with advanced dementia can reduce symptom burden, prevent unnecessary interventions, improve caregiver burden, and increase quality of life.[29] Challenging prognostication issues and strict requirements for hospice admission leave dementia patients and their caregivers with few resources. The length of time from diagnosis to advance-staged illness means that APRN PCPs provide care for longer periods, with different types of interventions and support needed. The APRN PCP should guide care in line with palliative care principles that focus on proactive management of symptoms, caregiver support, and ACP.

Emphasis is placed on early recognition and management of behaviors and caregiver assistance in medical decision-making. Coordination of care among providers can also ensure that benefit versus burden is fully understood when treatment goals are determined (see Chapter 45, "Cognitive Impairment").

RENAL DISEASE

CKD affects approximately 15%—or 37 million—of US adults.[30,31] Most patient with CKD will remain in Stages I–V, however some progress to end-stage renal disease (ESRD), as defined as a glomerular filtration rate (GFR) of less than 15 mL/min. ESRD is seen in approximately 650,000 patients per years in the United States, with the number increasing by 5% annually.[32] Many of these patient are on hemodialysis for survival, which has a high symptom burden and is costly for the healthcare system. APRN PCPs have the obligation to discuss all treatment options for CKD and ESRD with their patients and develop a plan aligning with goals of care.

Shared decision-making is beneficial in the primary care setting when patients are healthy enough to participate and can discuss the benefits and burdens of treatment options.[33] APRN PCPs will often see renal disease patients throughout their illness trajectory and have the opportunity to have continuing goals-of-care discussions with their patients in which they outline symptoms burden and quality of life. These conversations often happen in collaboration with a nephrologist, family members, social workers, and anyone else familiar with the patient's CKD course. Information should include an estimated prognosis and a clear description of dialysis and conservative treatment options, including risks and benefits as well as side effects of all options.[34] Patients should be assured that ongoing symptom management and care will continue regardless of treatment course.

High symptoms burden in CKD appears to be as common in conservatively managed patients as in those managed with dialysis.[34] The myriad of symptoms may include pain, fatigue, pruritus, dyspnea, edema, dry mouth, muscle cramps, restless leg syndrome, sleep disturbance, and constipation.[31] PCPs or a palliative care specialist, depending on the complexity, can manage these symptoms. Patients with ESRD are good candidates for palliative care referral given their large symptom burden, poor quality of life, and need for ACP. The trusted APRN PCP may be most suitable to suggest referral to palliative care specialists (see Chapter 8 to learn more about renal care).

PROGNOSTICATION

"How long do I have?" This is the question most frequently asked by patients facing a terminal illness or debilitating condition. *Prognosis* is a prediction of the outcome of a disease based on medical knowledge and experience.[35] Prognosis can affect treatment decisions as well as eligibility for hospice care. Diseases that result in chronic organ failure can have multiple exacerbations, any one of which could result in death, thus making prognostication extremely difficult even for skilled palliative care specialists. The rate of decline in functional status can be a key indicator in determining prognosis. These tools can help palliative care specialists with prognostication:

- *The Palliative Performance Scale* (PPS) is a reliable and valid tool for the measurement of performance status in palliative care. It uses the patient's functional status to predict survival. The PPS evaluates ambulatory status, activity level, evidence of disease, level of consciousness, and the ability to perform self-care. Periodic measurements document the evolving physical deterioration of an individual. The rapidity of the functional decline likely corresponds with rapid deterioration and ultimately a shorter survival.[36]

- *The "surprise question"*: "Would I be surprised if this patient died in the next year?" This simple question has been recognized as a tool to improve end-of-life care in both primary care and dialysis populations. A "no" answer to this question can serve to identify patients with a poor prognosis who would be appropriate for palliative care. Although research shows that the accuracy of the surprise question varies, it is a tool recommended and widely used.[35]

- Mobile applications and online resources containing prognostic information and tools exist for a multitude of individual medical conditions. Box 12.1 lists useful resources to assist in prognostication in primary care.

A patient's relationship with a PCP develops over time. Due to advances in medical technology and pharmacotherapy, patients with chronic illness and multimorbidities can experience a long trajectory, with multiple exacerbations of each chronic disease. Given their long-standing relationships with patients, PCPs are well-suited to facilitate values-based communication concerning goals of care. ACP is a process that is ideally developed over multiple interactions, not during a period of crisis. Changes in a patient's condition warrant evolving discussions of treatment, including the specific impact of the treatment on the patient's quality of life and ongoing reassessment of ACP. An informed PCP can consider the synergistic symptom burden, along with the patient's specific goals and values, and counsel the patient accordingly. Racial and ethnic differences must also be considered; knowledge of a patient's cultural beliefs and practices may influence their care choices and define their decision-makers.[37,38]

Patient-centered care requires that patients are well-informed about their condition. The success rate of proposed treatment, the overall prognosis with and without treatment, and the expected impact on quality of life are all important aspects for an individual to consider in making a decision regarding treatment and goals of care. Such information may help patients establish their priorities, make informed decisions regarding treatment, and ultimately formulate an advance directive. ACP is best done in the primary care setting because the established ongoing patient–practitioner relationship in the primary care setting gives the practitioner

Box 12.1 TOOLS TO ASSIST IN PROGNOSTICATION OF SERIOUS ILLNESS IN PRIMARY CARE PRACTICE

Palliative Care Network of Wisconsin; Palliative Care Fast Facts and Concepts[37]

- Fast Fact #213: Prognosis in HIV and AIDS
- Fast Fact #191: Prognostication in Patients Receiving Dialysis
- Fast Fact #189: Prognosis in Decompensated Chronic Liver Failure
- Fast Fact #150: Prognostication in Dementia
- Fast Fact #143: Prognostication in Heart Failure
- Fast Fact #141: Prognosis in End-Stage COPD
- Fast Fact #099: Chemotherapy: Response and Survival
- Fast Fact #013: Determining Prognosis in Advanced Cancer

Mobile Apps

I. MPI (Multidimensional Prognostic Index), a prognostic tool based on a standard geriatric assessment, predicts short- and long-term mortality in the elderly.

II. Qx Calculate, an app focused on highlighting tools used in clinical practice that affect diagnosis, treatment, and prognosis. It includes prognostic indicators for heart failure, lymphoma, myeloma, hemodialysis, COPD, transient ischemic attacks, pancreatitis, and many others.

insight into the patient's support system and values. This familiarity opens the door for an honest, nonintimidating discussion about values, ultimately leading to an advance care plan. Because goals and preference change over time, this is best done as an ongoing conversation between patients and providers.[39]

The Conversation Project National Survey 2018 reports that 92% of Americans say that it is important to discuss wishes for end-of-life care, but only 32% have had this conversation. Ninety-five percent stated they would be willing to have this conversation, and 53% stated they would be relieved to discuss their end-of-life wishes.[40] ACP often involved completion of an advance directive (AD), which is a written document, varying by state, of a patient's assigned health care proxy (HCP) and their goals, values, and wishes for future healthcare, sometimes referred to as a Living Will.[39] Advance directives are typically followed if a patient loses decision-making capacity. Because goals and circumstances can change, it is important that the AD is an ongoing conversation with the patient. It is equally as important to assign an HCP who understands the patient's goals and values. The National Hospice and Palliative Care Organization website, CaringInfo,[41] has a list of advance directives and instructions for each state. It is important that the PCP keeps an easily accessible and updated record of this document for all of their patients.

The ACA expanded access to high-quality end-of-life care for Americans with serious illness.[42] Reimbursement for end-of-life discussions was one of the provisions of the ACA. Repeal or replacement of the ACA is a possibility, and this may shift the risk and responsibility for healthcare payments to individual states, healthcare organizations, commercial payers, and possibly even patients and families. State policy may be expected to play an increased role in determining who gets care and how it is paid for within the standards of quality and safety. Individually, some states have policies that require information on palliative care be made available to patients with serious illness, and other states are requiring hospitals, skilled nursing facilities, and long-term care facilities to identify those patients who could benefit from palliative care and distribute information regarding its availability. Many states are using their authority over professional licensure to increase access to palliative care by mandating that clinicians pursue continuing education in pain management, palliative care, and addiction.[43] Individual states vary in their acceptable ACP documents and the practitioners who can sign them to make them valid. Nurse practitioners can check the American Association of Nurse Practitioners website (www.aanp.org) to view the Nurse Practice Act for their individual state's restrictions.

The goal of ACP is to help ensure that people receive medical care that is consistent with their values, goals, and preferences during serious and chronic illness.[44] ACP has been proved to decrease healthcare costs, hospitalizations and prolonged intensive care unit admissions, do-not-resuscitate orders, and cardiopulmonary resuscitations, mechanical ventilation, and use of feeding tubes.[45] Families also report higher satisfaction when ACP has taken place. Given that PCPs can now bill for having these discussions, and ACP is considered a low-risk high-value intervention,[46] it is essential that the APRN PCP initiate these important conversations (for more information on the process, see Chapter 32).

ACP requires substantial communication skills and can be challenging. Healthcare professionals who have established long-term relationships with their patients may face the difficulty of "letting go." Furthermore, end-of-life preferences can be complicated and influenced by religion, race, and culture, requiring providers to be culturally sensitive to the population they serve. When discussions about Ads become a routine part of a primary care visit, the interactions can be calm and nonthreatening.[47] APRNs can improve their comfort and competence in addressing goals of care through formal academic or continuing education programs that emphasize communication skills. The use of simulation has become increasingly popular in teaching communication strategies (see Chapter 2 for discussion of strategies to improve palliative APRN education). Strategies to improve completion rates of ADs in primary care include improved reimbursement, increased patient awareness, and educational efforts geared to improving communication skills among providers.[48] Chapter 33 discusses advance directives. Box 12.2 lists educational resources for professionals to facilitate ACP discussions in primary care settings. Box 12.3 presents resources for patients and families.

Box 12.2 EDUCATIONAL RESOURCES FOR ADVANCE CARE PLANNING DISCUSSIONS IN PRIMARY CARE

1. End-of-Life Nursing Education Consortium (ELNEC): ELNEC is a national education initiative to improve palliative care. ELNEC offers a 2-day course to prepare APRNs to deliver appropriate palliative and end-of-life care, including symptom management and communication. An additional intensive course on communication has also been developed. Free COVID-related materials available.[49]

2. Palliative Care Network of Wisconsin Palliative Care Fast Facts and Concepts[37]

   - Fast Fact #06 and #011: Delivering Bad News, Parts 1 and 2
   - Fast Fact #017: Patient-Centered Interviewing
   - Fast Fact #021: Hope and Truth Telling
   - Fast Fact #023 and #024: Discussing DNR Orders, Parts 1 and 2
   - Fast Fact #065: Establishing End-of-Life Goals: The Living Will Interview
   - Fast Fact #162: Advance Care Planning in Chronic Illness

3. Vital Talk: Addressing Goals of Care[50] Communication tools, with extensive video examples and "Quick Guide" resources. More extensive training available for a fee.

BILLING AND CODING FOR PALLIATIVE CARE WITHIN THE PRIMARY CARE VISIT

There are a number of opportunities for APRNs to bill for time spent performing palliative care skills during a visit, including ACP, transitional care management, and prolonged services. Providing palliative care in the primary care setting often requires an extended amount of time beyond the allotted visit time, and it is important for the APRN to learn how to be reimbursed for these services. To bill for these discussions, documentation must meet specific criteria under Medicare regulations. Private insurers may have specific codes, thus making these discussions reimbursable with specific criteria. Evaluation/management and diagnosis codes are based on location, complexity, and effort. When counseling/information-giving represents more than 50% of the patient visit, it may be most appropriate to bill by time, and the provider should select an evaluation and management code that corresponds to the total time of the face-to-face visit.[51]

BILLING FOR ADVANCE CARE PLANNING

ACP is defined as "the process that supports adults at any age or stage of health in understanding and sharing their personal

The *Five Wishes* tool is available in 28 languages and Braille; it is written in simple language and is legal in 42 states. Available through Aging with Dignity, which provides tools and guides for discussions with individuals, families, children, adolescents, and young adults (http://agingwithdignity.org).

PREPARE is a patient-friendly online resource to assist individuals in making complex medical decisions by using video. Videos are used to help identify values and how to communicate them with family and physician. The content is developed at a fifth-grade reading level and is easy to use (http://prepareforyourcare.org).

Mydirectives.com is a free online advance care planning service. My Directives is a global advance care planning digital platform and repository that allows patients and practices to develop their own documents or upload existing ones (https://mydirectives.com/en/).

Caring Conversations provides a workbook in Spanish and English to guide patients through the advance care planning process. Individual guidance is also available if needed (https://practicalbioethics.org/programs/advance-care-planning.html).

The Conversation Project is an initiative of the Institute of Healthcare Improvement (IHI), which emphasizes public engagement in values-based care planning and provides practical resources for public use, including a *What Matters to Me* workbook (https://the conversationproject.org/).

values, life goals, and preferences regarding future medical care. The goal of ACP is to help ensure that people receive medical care that is consistent with their values, goals and preferences during serious and chronic illness."[52] There are two current procedural terminology (CPT) codes that can be used for ACP, either in addition to or independently from an E/M code. The code 99497 is "Advance care planning including the explanation and discussion of advance directives such as standard forms (with completion of such forms, when performed), by the physician or other qualified health care professional; first 30 minutes, face-to-face with the patient, family member(s), and/or surrogate."[53] Code 99498 may be added to 99497 for each additional 30 minutes of time spent.

There is no limit to the number of times the code can be billed for a patient, as long as the documentation supports a change in health status or directives. ACP can include discussed goals/preferences of care, making complex decisions about life-limiting illness, and introducing and/or completing forms such as a health care proxy, durable power of attorney, living will, and medical orders for life sustaining treatment (MOLST).[51] It is important for the APRN to document a brief summary of the conversation, who was present, total time in minutes (including start and end times), and if any forms were introduced or completed. More information about ACP can be found in Chapter 33 and billing and coding in Appendix I.

BILLING FOR TRANSITIONAL CARE MANAGEMENT

Transitional care management (TCM) was designed to allow health professions to provide postdischarge care for patients who were hospitalized for moderate to high-complexity medical conditions. Patient are especially vulnerable during the transition, especially elderly patients with chronic health conditions.[54] TCM was adopted by Medicare in 2013 to improve patient outcomes after being discharged to the community from a medical facility. This involves follow-up on patients discharged from an inpatient facility and their transition to home, as well as a face-to-face visit within a required time-frame. This face-to-face visit allows the practitioner to discuss the condition or exacerbation of the condition precipitating the admission, the treatment that was rendered, and its impact on the patient's quality of life and/or functional status. The potential for repeat exacerbations and the implications for further care can also be discussed. For example, an end-stage COPD patient who was recently hospitalized with an exacerbation requiring intubation may verbalize a request to never endure intubation again, leading to a pertinent goals' discussion and the implementation of an AD document.

Clinicians can receive an enhanced reimbursement for office visits following an eligible discharge. There is a specific 30-day period for TCM which begins on the date the patient is discharged from a medical facility. Patients with high-complexity needs must be seen within 7 days of discharge and within 14 days for moderate-complexity needs.[55] Three components must be met: (1) interactive contact within 2 business days of discharge, (2) non–face-to-face services throughout the 30-day period, and (3) required face-to-face visit within 7 or 14 days of discharge. To complete non–face-to-face services throughout the 30-day period, the APRN may obtain and review discharge information, coordinate care with all clinicians treating the patient, educate patients and their families, establish referrals within the community, and assist with follow-up care.[56]

There are two CPT codes that can be used for TCM: 99495 is used for services with moderate medical decision complexity within 14 days of discharge, and 99496 may be used for high medical decision complexity within 7 days of discharge. This visit may be done via telehealth, in accordance with existing Medicare regulations for telehealth services. Medicare beneficiaries who receive TCM services have been shown to have lower Medicare costs and decreased mortality in the subsequent month as compared to patients who do not receive these services.[54] APRNs can utilize TCM billing codes not only for higher reimbursement rates, but also to improve their patients' coordination of care and outcomes.

BILLING FOR PROLONGED SERVICES

Providing palliative care services often requires APRNs to spend more face-to-face time than captured by E/M codes. *Prolonged services codes* are used to capture this time spent.

Examples of this include a family meeting to discuss treatment options or explaining complex treatments or additional factors (need for interpreters, visual aids, etc.). Prolonged service codes are *add-on* codes that can be used in conjunction with an E/M code. These codes are only billed when the time involved exceeds the typical time of E/M service by more than 30 minutes. The highest level of E/M code must be billed prior to billing for prolonged services.[57] For example, if the APRN saw a patient with moderate-complexity medical decision-making for approximately 25 minutes and 99214 was billed as the E/M code, the APRN would have to spend an additional 30 minutes (for a total 55 minutes) to bill for prolonged services. The CPT code used for prolonged services of 31- to 75-minute visits is 99354. Visits that last 76–105 minutes can use the codes 99354 and 99355. The APRN must be with the patient during all of the time being billed for prolonged services. The start and stop times must be documented, as well as the content of the prolonged services. The APRN who spends prolonged time providing palliative care skills to the patient should utilize these codes to get reimbursement for time spent.

Table 12.1 summarizes the CPT codes that can be used to bill for palliative care provided in the primary care setting. Further details of reimbursement for APRN palliative care are detailed in Appendix 1, Palliative APRN Billing and Coding.

TELEHEALTH

Telehealth is a new and emerging trend in primary care, one accelerated during the COVID-19 pandemic. Telehealth, sometimes referred to as *telemedicine*, consists of using telecommunications and digital communication technologies to deliver and facilitate health and health-related services.[58] Video platforms, including Apple Face Time, Google Hangouts, Zoom, Skype, Doximity, and EMR platforms, are commonly used to provide telehealth services. The use of these different video platforms was liberalized during the COVID-19 pandemic by the US Department of Health and Human Services.[59] Furthermore, Medicare and Medicaid expanded insurance coverage to allow providers to bill for telehealth visits for the same reimbursement as face-to-face visits during the COVID-19 pandemic under the 1135 Waiver.[59] This transition toward telehealth in primary care is pivotal for providing access to care for vulnerable populations that often have difficulty accessing traditional medical services.[60]

Table 12.1 COMMON CODES FOR PALLIATIVE CARE INTERVENTIONS

CPT CODE	DESCRIPTION	REQUIRED ELEMENTS	TIME-BASED CODING THRESHOLD	TIPS-NOTES
99497	Advance Care Planning (ACP) – first 30 minutes	Explanation and discussion of advance directives such as standard forms (including the completion of such forms) by the APRN; first 30 minutes, face-to-face with the patient, family members and/or surrogate.	First 30 minutes (16–45 min)	Forms do not have to be completed to bill this code.
99498	ACP – additional 30 minutes	ACP each additional 30 minutes	Each additional 30 minutes (>45 minutes)	Billed with 99497.
99495	Transitional Care Management Services – Moderate Level Decision Making	Three components – 1. Call required as initial interaction within 2 days of discharge; 2. F2F visit within 14 days; 3. Non F2F interaction throughout 30 days after discharge.	Face-to-face visit within 14 days of discharge	F2F must be completed within 14 days of discharge to bill for service.
99496	Transitional Care Management Services – High Level Decision Making	Three components – 1. Required initial interaction within 2 day - phone, telehealth, IT; 2. Non F2F interaction; 3. F2F visit within 7 days.	Face-to-face visit within 7 days of discharge	For more complex patients, who must be seen within 7 days of discharge.
99354	Office/Outpatient prolonged discussion with direct patient contact – first 30 minutes	Prolonged evaluation and management service before and/or after direct patient care; first 60 minutes	30 minutes beyond the usual service	Counseling, education or exploration of goals of care >50% of the encounter; the visit maybe billed based on time.
99355	Office/Outpatient prolonged discussion with direct patient contact – additional 30 minutes	Prolonged evaluation and management service each additional 30 minutes	Each additional 30 minutes	Billed with 99354.

Adapted from CAPC[51,55–57]

Telehealth visits provide a unique opportunity to have a face-to-face interaction with patients in their own environment, much like home-based care. Palliative care patients are often seriously ill and benefit from the ease and convenience of having a video visit in their home. The APRN has the chance to observe the patient's daily life, social supports, and functionality at home. For example, the APRN may observe the elderly patient ambulating down a hall or up the steps to assess their gait stability and use of assistive devices at home versus outside the home. The APRN might also ask to review the patient's medications by showing them how they store and take their medications for an accurate medication reconciliation. If family members can participate in the visit, the APRN might use the occasion to discuss ACP. These types of opportunities provide similar benefits to home care without the logistical challenges of a home visit. Furthermore, studies show that patients are highly satisfied with the quality of care they receive using telehealth platforms.[58] See Chapter 17 on the APRN in Telehealth for more information.

SUMMARY

Growing evidence demonstrates the benefits of early palliative care for patients with serious illness, and palliative care shares many common goals with primary care. Primary and palliative care address the patient with serious illness within the context of their diagnosis and their community, emphasizing symptom support and communication, with a focus on care over time[7-8, 32]

APRN PCPs are well-suited to incorporate palliative care into their practices. Their unique blend of medical knowledge with an educational background based on a holistic nursing model makes the APRN a prime candidate to assume the role of PCP, able to deliver high-quality, patient-centered healthcare. Practicing within a primary care framework allows the APRN to establish an ongoing relationship with the patient and family, which facilitates an honest, trusting bond and positions the APRN to monitor the patient's progress over time. This ongoing relationship can allow the primary care APRN to discuss goals of care with an educated patient/family in a nonemergent environment, revising the advance care plan as needed. APRNs who integrate palliative care into their primary care practices should understand the range of disease trajectories and multidimensional symptoms, as well as the communication skills needed for ACP and end-of-life decision making. Once adept at these skills of symptom management and care planning, primary care APRNs can play an integral role in incorporating primary palliative care into their practice and serving as a role model to others.

REFERENCES

1. Office of Disease Prevention and Health Promotion. Access to Primary Care. Healthy People. Updated August 27, 2021. Washington, DC: U.S. Department of Health and Human Services. https://www.healthypeople.gov/2020/topics-objectives/topic/social-determinants-health/interventions-resources/access-to-primary#1

2. Ghosh A, Dzeng E, Cheng MJ. Interaction of palliative care and primary care. Clin Geriatr Med. 2015;31(2):207–218. doi:10.1016/j.cger.2015.01.001

3. Buss MK, Rock LK, McCarthy EP. Understanding palliative care and hospice: A review for primary care providers [published correction appears in Mayo Clin Proc. 2017 May;92(5):853]. Mayo Clin Proc. 2017;92(2):280–286. doi:10.1016/j.mayocp.2016.11.007

4. Brom HM, Salsberry PJ, Graham MC. Leveraging health care reform to accelerate nurse practitioner full practice authority [published correction appears in J Am Assoc Nurse Pract. 2018 Nov;30(11):662]. J Am Assoc Nurse Pract. 2018;30(3):120–130. doi:10.1097/JXX.0000000000000023

5. Buttorff C, Ruder T, Bauman M. Multiple Chronic Conditions in the United States. Santa Monica, CA: RAND; 2017. https://www.rand.org/content/dam/rand/pubs/tools/TL200/TL221/RAND_TL221.pdf

6. Dahlin C. Palliative Nursing: Scope and Standards of Practice. 6th ed. Pittsburgh, PA: Hospice and Palliative Nurses Association; 2021.

7. National Consensus Project for Quality Palliative Care. Clinical Practice Guidelines for Quality Palliative Care. 4th ed. Richmond, VA: National Coalition of Hospice and Palliative Care; 2018. https://www.nationalcoalitionhpc.org/ncp/.

8. Greenstein JE, Policzer JS, Shaban ES. Hospice for the primary care physician. Prim Care Clin Office Prac. 2019;46(3):303–317. doi:10.1016/j.cger.2015.01.009.

9. Robinson N, Sutton B. Palliative care in the community. In Ferrell BR, Paice JA, eds. Oxford Textbook of Palliative Nursing. 5th ed. New York: Oxford University Press; 2019: 615–623.

10. Mather M, Scommegna P, Kilduff L. Fact Sheet: Aging in the United States. Population Reference Bureau. July 15, 2019. https://www.prb.org/aging-unitedstates-fact-sheet/

11. Long CO. The older adult in the community. In Ferrell BR, Paice JA, eds. Oxford Textbook of Palliative Nursing. 5th ed. New York: Oxford University Press; 2019: 483–489.

12. Centers for Disease Control and Prevention. Heart Failure Fact Sheet. Updated September 8, 2020. https://www.cdc.gov/heartdisease/heart_failure.htm

13. Dionne-Odom JN, Wells R, Swetz KM. Palliative care in heart failure. In Ferrell BR, Paice JA, eds. Oxford Textbook of Palliative Nursing. 5th ed. New York: Oxford University Press; 2019: 555–570.

14. Centers for Disease Control and Prevention. Chronic Obstructive Pulmonary Disease. February 22, 2021. https://www.cdc.gov/copd/index.html

15. Ansari AA, Pomerantz DH, Jayes RL, Aguirre EA, Havyer RD. Promoting primary palliative care in severe chronic obstructive pulmonary disease: Symptom management and preparedness planning. J Palliat Care. 2019;34(2):85–91. doi:10.1177/0825859718819437

16. Siegel RL, Miller KD, Jemal A. Cancer statistics, 2020. CA Cancer J Clin. 2020;70(1):7–30. doi:10.3322/caac.21590

17. Reb A, Economou D. Cancer survivorship. In Ferrell BR, Paice JA, eds. Oxford Textbook of Palliative Nursing. 5th ed. New York: Oxford University Press; 2019: 530–538.

18. American Society of Clinical Oncology. Cancer Treatment and Survivorship Care Plans. 2021. https://www.cancer.net/survivorship/follow-care-after-cancer-treatment/asco-cancer-treatment-and-survivorship-care-plans

19. Wilbur J. Surveillance of the adult cancer survivor. Am Fam Physician. 2015;91:29–36.

20. Zoberi K, Tucker J. Primary care of breast cancer survivors. Am Fam Physician. 2019;99(6):370–375.

21. Noonan EM, Farrell TW. Primary care of the prostate cancer survivor. Am Fam Physician. 2016;93(9):764–770.

22. Burgers K, Moore C, Bednash L. Care of the colorectal cancer survivor. Am Fam Physician. 2018;97(5):331–336.

23. American Society of Clinical Oncology. Coverage & Reimbursement for Survivorship Care Services. 2016. https://www.asco.org/node/6526

24. Rockwood K, Howlett SE. Fifteen years of progress in understanding frailty and health in aging. BMC Med. 2018;16(1):220. doi:10.1186/s12916-018-1223-3

25. Crooms RC, Gelfman LP. Palliative care and end-of-life considerations for the frail patient. *Anesth Analg*. 2020;130(6):1504–1515. doi:10.1213/ANE.0000000000004763

26. Lawless MT, Archibald MM, Ambagtsheer RC, Kitson AL. Factors influencing communication about frailty in primary care: A scoping review. *Patient Educ Couns*. 2020;103(3):436–450. doi:10.1016/j.pec.2019.09.014

27. Alzheimer's Association. 2021 Alzheimer's Disease Facts and Figures. *Alzheimers Dement*. 2021. 17(3).

28. Stewart JT, Schultz SK. Palliative care for dementia. *Psychiatr Clin North Am*. 2018;41(1):141–151. doi:10.1016/j.psc.2017.10.011

29. Eisenmann Y, Golla H, Schmidt H, Voltz R, Perrar KM. Palliative care in advanced dementia. *Front Psychiatry*. 2020;11:699. doi:10.3389/fpsyt.2020.00699

30. Center for Disease Control and Prevention. Chronic Kidney Disease Initiative. Chronic kidney disease in the United States, 2021. https://www.cdc.gov/kidneydisease/pdf/Chronic-Kidney-Disease-in-the-US-2021-h.pdf

31. Mechler K, Liantonio J. Palliative care approach to chronic diseases: End stages of heart failure, chronic obstructive pulmonary disease, liver failure, and renal failure. *Prim Care*. 2019;46(3):415–432. doi:10.1016/j.pop.2019.05.008

32. University of San Francisco. The Kidney Project: Statistics. 2019. https://pharm.ucsf.edu/kidney/need/statistics

33. Rosansky SJ, Schell J, Shega J, et al. Treatment decisions for older adults with advanced chronic kidney disease. *BMC Nephrol*. 2017;18(1):200. doi:10.1186/s12882-017-0617-3

34. Raghavan D, Holley JL. Conservative care of the elderly CKD patient: A practical guide. *Adv Chronic Kidney Dis*. 2016;23(1):51–56. doi:10.1053/j.ackd.2015.08.003

35. Chu C, White N, Stone P. Prognostication in palliative care. *Clin Med (Lond)*. 2019;19(4):306–310. doi:10.7861/clinmedicine.19-4-306

36. Baik D, Russell D, Jordan L, Dooley F, Bowles KH, Masterson Creber RM. Using the Palliative Performance Scale to estimate survival for patients at the end of life: A systematic review of the literature. *J Palliat Med*. 2018;21(11):1651–1661. doi:10.1089/jpm.2018.0141

37. Palliative Care Network of Wisconsin. *Palliative Care Fast Facts and Concepts*. Appleton, WI: Palliative Care Network of Wisconsin. 2021. https://www.mypcnow.org/fast-facts/

38. Cain CL, Surbone A, Elk R, Kagawa-Singer M. Culture and palliative care: Preferences, communication, meaning, and mutual decision making. *J Pain Symptom Manage*. 2018;55(5):1408–1419. doi:10.1016/j.jpainsymman.2018.01.007

39. Thompson K, Shi S, Kiraly C. Primary care for the older adult patient: Common geriatric issues and syndromes. *Obstet Gynecol Clin North Am*. 2016;43(2):367–379. doi:10.1016/j.ogc.2016.01.010

40. The Conversation Project. Institute of Health Improvement. Boston, MA. www.theconversationproject.org. Accessed September 12, 2021.

41. Caring Information. Advanced Directives. National Hospice and Palliative Care Organization. Alexandria, Va. https://www.nhpco.org/advancedirective/

42. Parikh RB, Wright AA. The Affordable Care Act and end-of-life care for patients with cancer. *Cancer J*. 2017;23(3):190–193. doi:10.1097/PPO.0000000000000264

43. Sinclair S, Meier D. How states can expand access to palliative care. Health Affairs Blog. 2017. Available at https://www.healthaffairs.org/do/10.1377/hblog20170130.058531/full/ doi:10.1377/hblog20170130.058531

44. Sudore RL, Lum HD, You JJ, et al. Defining advance care planning for adults: A consensus definition from a multidisciplinary delphi panel. *J Pain Symptom Manage*. 2017;53(5):821–832.e1. doi:10.1016/j.jpainsymman.2016.12.331.

45. Barkley A, Liquori M, Cunningham A, Liantonio J, Worster B, Parks S. Advance care planning in a geriatric primary care clinic: A retrospective chart review. *Am J Hosp Palliat Care*. 2019;36(1):24–27. doi:10.1177/1049909118791126.

46. Lakin JR, Block SD, Billings JA, et al. Improving communication about serious illness in primary care: A review. *JAMA Intern Med*. 2016;176(9):1380–1387. doi:10.1001/jamainternmed.2016.3212

47. Solis GR, Mancera BM, Shen MJ. Strategies used to facilitate the discussion of advance care planning with older adults in primary care settings: A literature review. *J Am Assoc Nurse Pract*. 2018;30(5):270–279. doi:10.1097/JXX.0000000000000025

48. Rose BL, Leung S, Gustin J, Childers J. Initiating advance care planning in primary care: A model for success. *J Palliat Med*. 2019;22(4):427–431. doi:10.1089/jpm.2018.0380

49. American Association of Colleges of Nursing. End-of-Life Nursing Education Consortium (ELNEC). 2021. https://www.aacnnursing.org/ELNEC/About/ELNEC-Curricula

50. Childers JW, Back AL, Tulsky JA, Arnold RM. REMAP: A Framework for Goals of Care Conversations. *J Oncol Pract*. 2017;13(10):e844–e850. doi:10.1200/JOP.2016.018796

51. Center to Advance Palliative Care. Optimizing Billing and Coding. Billing and coding for advance care planning (ACP) services. June 20, 2020. https://www.capc.org/toolkits/optimizing-billing-practices/

52. Sudore RL, Lum HD, You JJ, et al. Defining advance care planning for adults: A consensus definition from a multidisciplinary delphi panel. *J Pain Symptom Manage*. 2017;53(5):821–832.e1. doi:10.1016/j.jpainsymman.2016.12.331

53. Center to Advance Palliative Care. Advance Care Planning (The ABCs of Getting Paid. February 3, 2019. https://www.capc.org/documents/354/

54. Bindman AB, Cox DF. Changes in health care costs and mortality associated with transitional care management services after a discharge among Medicare beneficiaries. *JAMA Intern Med*. 2018;178(9):1165–1171. doi:10.1001/jamainternmed.2018.2572

55. Center to Advance Palliative Care. Optimizing Billing and Coding. Billing and coding for transitional care management (TCM). June 22, 2020. https://www.capc.org/toolkits/optimizing-billing-practices/

56. Center to Advance Palliative Care. Optimizing Billing and Coding. Prolonged Services. June 22, 2020. https://www.capc.org/toolkits/optimizing-billing-practices/

57. Center to Advance Palliative Care. Optimizing Billing and Coding. Evaluation and Management for Clinic Visits. June 22, 2020. https://www.capc.org/toolkits/optimizing-billing-practices/

58. NEJM Catalyst. What is telehealth? NEJM Catalyst. February 1, 2018. Available at https://catalyst.nejm.org/doi/full/10.1056/CAT.18.0268

59. Calton B, Abedini N, Fratkin M. Telemedicine in the time of coronavirus. *J Pain Symptom Manage*. 2020;60(1):e12–e14. doi:10.1016/j.jpainsymman.2020.03.019

60. Lau J, Knudsen J, Jackson H, et al. Staying connected in the COVID-19 pandemic: Telehealth at the largest safety-net system in the United States. *Health Affairs (Millwood)*. 2020;39(8):1437–1442. doi:10.1377/hlthaff.2020.00903

13.

THE PALLIATIVE APRN IN SPECIALTY CARDIOLOGY

Beth Fahlberg, Ann Laramee, and Erin Donaho

KEY POINTS

- Patients with cardiac conditions have unique needs, experiences, pathophysiologies, and devices that necessitate a specialized approach to palliative care.

- The palliative advanced practice registered nurse (APRN) facilitates individualized discussions about goals of care and treatment considerations with patients and families.

- Effective teamwork is enhanced by the palliative APRN's understanding of common cardiac diagnoses, tests, treatments, and medications, as well as the patient with serious cardiac disease and the cardiology mindset.

CASE STUDY: IMPLANTABLE CARDIOVERTER DEFIBRILLATOR

RB was a 72-year-old retired bank executive with advanced heart failure whose history included myocardial infarction (MI) with cardiogenic shock and coronary artery bypass graft 15 years ago. He was admitted with a new MI, with an ejection fraction of 20% after experiencing several months of fatigue. He was not a candidate for bypass surgery or stent, so his medications were adjusted to make him more comfortable. Two months later, an implantable cardioverter defibrillator (ICD) was placed to prevent sudden death.

After ICD placement, RB was hospitalized for heart failure (HF) three times and his ICD shocked him on five separate occasions for ventricular fibrillation. To prevent additional shocks, his cardiologist prescribed the antiarrhythmic drug amiodarone. However, 1 month after starting this medication, RB developed worsening shortness of breath caused by amiodarone pulmonary toxicity. The amiodarone was discontinued, and his treatment was changed to oral prednisone and continuous home oxygen to treat his pulmonary symptoms. The prednisone caused fluid retention, exacerbating RB's HF. As the amiodarone wore off, RB's heart went into frequent arrhythmias.

One day, his ICD shocked him every 2 minutes five times in a row. He was alert through the incident, crying out in distress. When the paramedics arrived, they deactivated the ICD by placing a magnet on it and transported him to the hospital with continuous cardiac monitoring, advanced cardiac life support (ACLS) drugs, and external defibrillator ready for immediate use. Upon arrival to the emergency department an electrophysiologist and device nurse interrogated his ICD. He had received two appropriate shocks for slow ventricular tachycardia while three were unexplained, likely due to a faulty lead. His daughter, who witnessed the episode at home, was traumatized, saying she would never forget that horrible experience.

RB's cardiologist placed a palliative care consult to clarify his goals of care and treatment options. Two treatment options were presented to RB and his family. The first was to replace his malfunctioning ICD with cardiac resynchronization therapy (CRT), with goal of improving his functional status and prolonging his life. The cardiologist explained that CRT had a 60% chance of improving his quality of life and functional status. However, the procedure imposed several important risks, including kidney injury and potential dialysis, infection, or HF exacerbation. It was also likely that RB would still receive shocks from a new ICD since he continued to have ventricular arrhythmias without the benefit of additional antiarrhythmic medications.

The second option would be to discontinue the ICD to prevent further shocks. This could result in sudden death at any time, but he would avoid further surgery, potential complications, and complex medical interventions as well as increased medical and insurance costs. The goal would be comfort with enrollment in hospice.

When the palliative advanced practice registered nurse (APRN) met RB, she assessed that he demonstrated signs of severe anxiety any time the ICD was mentioned. Knowing patients could develop posttraumatic stress disorder after repeated ICD shocks, she explored his feelings about the ICD. RB cried, "I just want this thing out of my body!" When asked about his goals of care, he exclaimed "I'm so tired of this! I just want to go home and be left in peace! My dad died in his sleep. That's the way to go. The life I've got now is hell on earth!"

Based on RB's goals, and with the agreement of the cardiac team, the palliative APRN facilitated a discharge plan with hospice focused on comfort. His ICD was deactivated. Five weeks later, RB died suddenly while watching a football game with his family.

INTRODUCTION

Heart disease is the leading cause of mortality in the United States for both men and women, accounting for approximately 655,000 deaths per year. As of 2016, approximately 6.2 million Americans had heart failure and sudden cardiac death appears on 13.5% of death certificates.[1] Cardiovascular disease continues to grow in prevalence and cost. By 2035, it is estimated that 45% of the US population will have some form of cardiovascular disease, with total costs reaching $1.1 trillion, rising from $351.3 billion in 2015.[1] Even so, only 10–16% of inpatient patients with cardiac conditions receive a palliative care consult,[2] and patients with heart problems represent only 17.6% of Medicare patients who receive the support of hospice.[3]

The purpose of this chapter is to describe the role of the palliative advanced practice registered nurse (APRN) in an acute cardiac unit. The palliative APRN working with patients with cardiac disease must understand the cardiology mindset, the trajectory of cardiac disease, common symptoms, shared decision-making specific to cardiac tests and treatments, and the barriers to the use of palliative care.

The palliative APRN has a unique set of skills and perspectives that are beneficial within cardiology. Thus far, most efforts to integrate palliative care in cardiology have focused on patients with heart failure (HF) and advanced HF treatments. However, palliative care is also needed in acute care cardiac specialty units, as well as cardiology and cardiac surgery clinics. Many patients and their families are faced with decisions about potential interventions that pose significant risk, particularly in patients with significant comorbidities

or frailty or of advanced age. It is essential to have a foundational understanding of common cardiac medications, tests, and treatments, and the risks and benefits of each. The APRN should be familiar with tools for risk stratification and shared decision-making associated with common and challenging decisions about cardiac medications, procedures, and devices.

PALLIATIVE CARE FOR PATIENTS WITH ADVANCED CARDIAC DISEASE

Over the past 15 years, palliative care for patients with advanced cardiac disease has become widely accepted and increasingly evidence- and guideline-based due to the unflagging and coordinated efforts of both cardiology and palliative care clinicians, providers, and researchers.[4] Despite these advancements, barriers exist to palliative care for patients with cardiac conditions. Due to the uncertainty of the cardiac illness trajectory, referrals to hospice care are often too late to benefit the patient and family.

Palliative care for advanced cardiac disease should be a seamless collaborative process with referrals to palliative specialists at key points in the disease trajectory, as illustrated by the stars in Figure 13.1. Early in the trajectory, the cardiac

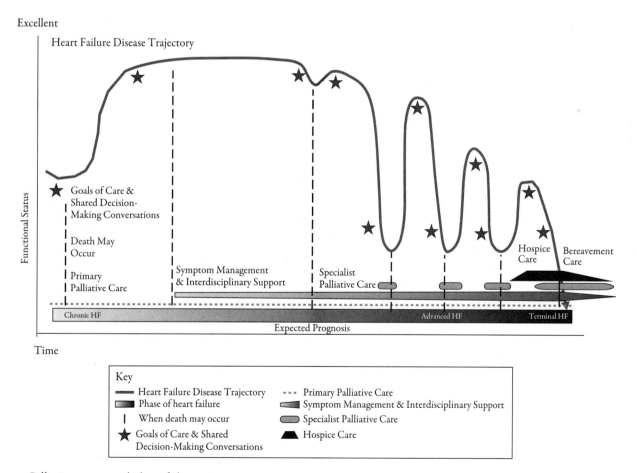

Figure 13.1 Palliative care across the heart failure trajectory.

specialty team is responsible for providing primary palliative care, referring to palliative specialists as needed. When the cardiac disease progresses to advanced HF, which has a poor prognosis, the patient should be referred to palliative specialists because symptoms and shared decision-making become more complex.[5,6]

Despite widespread recognition of palliative care as important, integration of palliative care in routine cardiology decision-making and practices can be challenging. Many barriers to specialist palliative care referral for patients with cardiac conditions have been described.[7,8] These barriers include cardiology providers' lack of understanding of palliative care and its benefits, their discomfort communicating about palliative care issues, and reimbursement limitations. At any given time, the high volume of patients with cardiac issues in any healthcare organization may be an issue for a palliative care program. Smaller palliative care teams may become overwhelmed by referrals for patients with advanced heart disease and the complex situations they encounter. Evidence shows that HF outcomes can be improved using both primary and specialty palliative care.[4] As a result, most palliative care within a cardiology population is often implemented using a primary or integrated palliative care model by cardiac nurses and primary care providers. Table 13.1 provides detailed information about cardiac medications.

The responsibility for the care of patients with HF falls within the circle of health providers that includes primary care, cardiology, and mental health as well as community supports. They will provide primary palliative care. This includes the assessment and treatment of physical, psychological, spiritual, emotional, and cultural aspects of care.[4] This should begin at the diagnosis of the cardiac condition and be integrated throughout the continuum of cardiac disease and HF. The collaboration of a cardiology and HF team and palliative care facilitates better understanding of the illness and a more informed understanding of treatment options, with the goal of informed decision-making.[9]

Over the past several years, evidence has accumulated supporting the integration of palliative care into the management of patients with cardiac disease.[4] Expert consensus guidelines in cardiology recommend the integration of palliative care throughout the patient's trajectory of illness, particularly when decisions are being made for advanced therapies such as mechanical circulatory devices or transplantation.[9] However, the care of patients with advanced cardiac disease may be fraught with moral distress. While there have been improvements in care as a result of advancements and technology in cardiology, there is the potential for moral distress for clinicians surrounding care decisions. Therefore, it is important to learn from the experiences of patients and their families as well as clinicians to inform the translation of evidence into practice. Within palliative care, the goal is to optimize function and promote quality of life while the patient lives with advanced heart disease. At the end of life, the focus changes to dying well through the promotion of comfort and dignity at the end of life.

THE UNPREDICTABLE CARDIAC DISEASE TRAJECTORY

Heart disease may affect someone for 30 days or 30 years, and, in the midst of an acute cardiac event, it can be difficult to predict which outcome is more likely. This uncertainty can have a marked impact on patients and their families, who may not know what their future holds, how to plan, or which testing and treatment options will be best for them.[7]

A key barrier to the use of both palliative care and hospice for patients with HF is the unpredictability of the cardiac trajectory and experience (see Figure 13.1).[10,11] The last several years of life for a person with HF have been described as "ambiguous dying."[12] Providers are often uncertain about whether the patient is dying and when death is likely to occur.[12] The patient with HF often has fluctuating symptoms and functional status and has experienced numerous life-threatening events, such as myocardial infarction, acute exacerbation, or sudden cardiac arrest. The decline of patients with heart disease is often subtle, occurring over years rather than months. Death may seem sudden, occurring within a few days of stability. This uncertainty extends to their providers, who may feel they have few objective predictors to determine prognosis other than the gradual development of frailty in their patients.[13] One challenge is that most respected tools used to predict mortality in patients with cardiac disease are inaccurate.[14]

The second case study illustrates the fact that while patients are sick, their providers often overestimate survival. Therefore, they are unlikely to describe them as "dying" or to talk with them about planning for the possibility of a sudden death.[15] This ambiguity about when or whether someone is dying also makes it difficult for providers to discuss prognosis or when to apply hospice admission criteria compared to diagnoses with more predictable trajectories leading to death. To complicate manners, patients also experience ambiguity and are overly optimistic about their life expectancy,[16] and this can have serious consequences.

In addition, families live in confusion for years about their loved one's future and their own prospects and plans, not knowing how long their situation will last, what to expect, or how to prepare for what is to come. Even if the patient and family understand the future, their distress may be compounded when healthcare providers are not straightforward with them about the prognosis. This can be particularly distressing when the patient dies, yet the provider has communicated only messages of hope for a transplant, ventricular assist device (VAD), or other "fix" without providing anticipatory guidance about the very real and simultaneous risk of sudden death. Rather than relying on timing for palliative care involvement, one approach emphasized in the literature is using specific clinical markers such as hospitalization or not tolerating guideline-directed medical therapy (GDMT) and "need-based" referrals utilizing triggers such as refractory symptoms or family distress.[17]

Open, honest, and regular communication acknowledging the uncertainties,[18] with a "hope for the best, plan for the worst" approach facilitates legacy-building and end-of-life

Table 13.1 GUIDELINE-BASED CARDIAC MEDICATIONS: PALLIATIVE CONSIDERATIONS

DIURETICS, LOOP: *FUROSEMIDE, TORSEMIDE, BUMETANIDE*

DOSING	BENEFITS	DECISIONS	RISKS	MONITORING	SELF-CARE
Furosemide 20–40 mg 1–2 ×/day Up to 600 mg/day Torsemide 10–20 mg 1–2 ×/day Up to 200 mg/day Bumetanide 0.5–1 mg 1–2 ×/day Up to 10 mg/day Need both maintenance and PRN orders	Fluid status control: (maintenance dose) Diuresis: Increase dose or add metolazone Alternatives to furosemide can be more effective in diuretic resistance	↓ sx vs ↓ renal function and diuretic resistance Diuretic resistance: ↑ oral dose, change diuretic, add oral metolazone, IV bolus or IV infusion	↓ renal function ↓BP, over-diuresis and falls in patients with poor intake, anorexia, nausea, or vomiting. May need to pause diuretics or dose diuretics only for ↑ wt until intake improves	Weights HF sx For ↑ wt/sx add prn dose until return to dry wt goal. ↑ or ↓ K Dosage of K replacement or aldosterone antagonist ↑ Creatinine	Daily wt ↓ Na diet Dose adjusted often: prescribed dose on container may not reflect the current dosing Diuretics may work best when supine: try dosing in early a.m. before getting up and early afternoon before nap to ↑ effect and ↓ nocturia

DIURETICS, THIAZIDE-LIKE: *METOLAZONE*

DOSING	BENEFITS	DECISIONS	RISKS	MONITORING	SELF-CARE
Dosed PRN for fluid overload. Administer 30 minutes before furosemide. Start at 2.5 mg	Potent diuretic to treat fluid overload	Requires daily communication with patient, especially when initiating Tx	Marked diuresis, K loss, symptomatic hypotension	Relief of dyspnea and orthopnea Wt, K, signs of dehydration	Daily wt ↓ Na diet

ANGIOTENSIN CONVERTING ENZYME (ACEI): *ENALAPRIL, LISINOPRIL*

DOSING	BENEFITS	DECISIONS	RISKS	MONITORING	SELF-CARE
For HFrEF: Titrate up to highest tolerable dose Enalapril 20 mg BID, start at 2.5 mg BID Lisinopril 40 mg daily, start at 2.5 mg daily	Prevent HF sx and ↑ survival in all patients with ↓EF	Advanced HF: May need to stop ACE for symptomatic hypotension, yet ACEs are key for sx mgt	↓ renal function ↑ K with ↓ renal function or aldosterone antagonists Cough: 5–20% try ARB if bothersome	K, Cr. ↑ dose may ↑ creatinine: If Cr ↑ >30% consider d/c ACEI or ↓dose	Stopping may cause rapid ↓ of heart function and sx

ANGIOTENSIN-RECEPTOR BLOCKERS (ARBS): *LOSARTAN, VALSARTAN, CANDESARTAN*

DOSING	BENEFITS	DECISIONS	RISK	MONITORING	SELF-CARE
For HFrEF titrate up to highest tolerable target dose Losartan 50 mg daily Valsartan 160 mg BID Candesartan 32 mg daily	Prevent HF sx and ↑ survival in patient with ↓EF ↓ cough than ACEI	Advanced HF: May need to d/c ARB for symptomatic ↓ BP, yet ARBs are key for sx mgt	↓ BP ↓ renal function Risk of ↑ K with ↓ renal function/K-sparing diuretics	K, Cr. ↑ dose may ↑ creatinine If Cr ↑ >30% consider d/c or reducing dose	Stopping may cause rapid ↓ of heart function, ↑ Sx

BETA-BLOCKERS: *METOPROLOL SUCCINATE, CARVEDILOL, BISOPROLOL*

DOSING	BENEFITS	DECISIONS	RISKS	MONITORING	SELF-CARE
For HFrEF: titrate up to highest tolerated dose Metoprolol succinate 200 mg daily, start at 25 mg Carvedilol 25 mg BID, start at 3.125 mg BID Bisoprolol 10 mg daily, start at 1.25 mg	↓ EF in HFrEF: ↓ HF sx risk ↑survival in CAD Controls ischemic sx by ↓cardiac work. Arrhythmia Tx and HR control in AF, HTN	Consider ↓ dose or d/c if symptomatic ↓ HR (<55) ↓ BP (SBP <80) Should not d/c suddenly: reflex tachycardia	↓ HR, ↓ BP fatigue ↓lung function in asthma/chronic obstructive pulmonary disease Blunted hypoglycemia sx in diabetes	Monitor HR, BP at each visit and sx of light-headedness, fatigue	Patient should know how to check pulse and check it periodically or if symptomatic

(continued)

Table 13.1 CONTINUED

VASODILATORS/NITRATES: *ISOSORBIDE DINITRATE AND HYDRALAZINE*

DOSING	BENEFITS	DECISIONS	RISKS	MONITORING	SELF-CARE
For HFrEF: Isosorbide dinitrate 20–40 mg TID Hydralazine 25–100 mg TID; dose based on BP tolerance	↑ survival ↑ QOL ↓ admissions	Use in HFrEF patients: -Who self-identify as Black -Who cannot take ACEI, ARB, or ARNI (i.e., angioedema) with NYHA class III or IV sx despite GDMTs	Common AEs: ↓ BP, headache and chest pain Hydralazine: drug-induced lupus Contraindicated with phosphodiesterase 5 inhibitors (i.e., sildenafil)	BP Antinuclear antibody before starting	Avoid dehydration TID dosing: Adherence is important but difficult

DIRECT ORAL ANTICOAGULANTS/FACTOR XA INHIBITORS: *APIXABAN, RIVAROXABAN*

DOSING	BENEFITS	DECISIONS	RISKS	MONITORING	SELF-CARE
Based on age, weight, and renal function Apixaban 2.5–5 mg BID Rivaroxaban 20 mg once daily	Prevent and treat venous thrombotic emboli and stroke in atrial fibrillation	Severe renal dysfunction: renal dosing or consider warfarin Severe liver disease: contraindicated	↑ bleeding Antidote to reverse Factor Xa inhibitors is exanet alfa	No blood monitoring required so adherence is critical, renal function	Prevent falls and injuries

CARDIAC GLYCOSIDE: *DIGOXIN*

DOSING	BENEFITS	DECISIONS	RISKS	MONITORING	SELF-CARE
Low dose recommended: high risk of toxicity (i.e., elderly, renal failure) May need to ↓ dose for progressive wt loss and cachexia at EOL	Atrial fibrillation: HR control adjunct to beta-blocker or calcium channel blocker. HFrEF: May ↑ functional status, ↑ quality of life and ↓ admissions in patient with HF sx with GDMTs	Risk vs. benefit: May help HF sx but toxicity risk, particularly with ↓ K, ↓ Mg, ↓ body mass, ↓ renal function, ↑ age	Many drug interactions Toxicity: Slow arrhythmias Heart block GI and neuro sx. Contraindicated in heart block without pacemaker.	HR should be ≥60 (lower may indicate toxicity) Digoxin levels Goal digoxin level: 0.5–0.9 ng/mL K, Mg, renal function	Accurate dosing essential to avoid toxicity

ANTICOAGULANTS: *WARFARIN (COUMADIN)*

DOSING	BENEFITS	DECISIONS	RISKS	MONITORING	SELF-CARE
Complex dosing guided by algorithms and INR results, often managed by AC service Typical INR goals: Atrial fibrillation: INR 2–3 Thrombosis Tx and prevention: INR 2–3 Mechanical heart valve 2.5–3.5	↓ risk embolic stroke in atrial fibrillation and prosthetic valve Thrombus Tx	Individualized using shared decision-making High risk: previous CVA, TIA. Risk calculator for nonvalvular Afib: CHA_2DS_2-VASc Anticoagulation bleeding risk: HAS-BLED ATRIA	Many drug interactions ↓ INR: stroke ↑ INR: bleeding Heparin bridge for invasive tests and txs. Risk of bleeding/ hemorrhagic stroke in patient at risk for falls. Aspirin/antiplatelet may be used when AC risk > benefit	INR fluctuates with changing health status, diet, medication changes. Many drug interactions.	INR blood test ≥1 ×/week when starting, monthly when stable. Vitamin K-balanced diet

Table 13.1 CONTINUED

SODIUM-GLUCOSE COTRANSPORTER 2 (SGLT2) INHIBITORS: *EMPAGLIFLOZIN, DAPAGLIFLOZIN*

DOSING	BENEFITS	DECISIONS	RISKS	MONITORING	SELF-CARE
Empagliflozin 25 mg daily, starting dose 10 mg Dapagliflozin 10 mg daily, starting dose 5 mg	Diuresis and Tx of fluid overload ↓mortality ↓ admissions ↓serious renal issues and progression of renal disease in HFrEF patients with or without diabetes.	Evidence only for HFrEF but with or without diabetes; coordinate care with endocrine Avoid if GFR 30–44 Contraindicated if GFR<30, dialysis or type 1 diabetes	Overdiuresis ↓ renal function UTI genital mycotic infections	Baseline renal function fluid status, watch for overdiuresis	Daily wt Watch for fluid overload/ dehydration, Hold 3 days before surgery

ALDOSTERONE RECEPTOR ANTAGONIST: *SPIRONOLACTONE, EPLERENONE*

DOSING	BENEFITS	DECISIONS	RISKS	MONITORING	SELF-CARE
For HFrEF: Titrate up to highest tolerated dose Spironolactone: 12.5 mg 25 mg 50 mg	↑ survival ↓ admissions in HFrEF ↓ BP ↓ K with loop diuretics	Spironolactone is less expensive	↑ K ↓ renal function For gynecomastia change to eplerenone	K BP renal function Fluid balance	Daily wt ↓Na diet Avoid ↑ K rich foods

ANGIOTENSIN RECEPTOR BLOCKER-NEPRILYSIN INHIBITOR (ARNI): *SACUBITRIL/VALSARTAN*

DOSING	BENEFITS	DECISIONS	RISKS	MONITORING	SELF-CARE
For HFrEF: Titrate up to highest tolerated dose Start at: 24 mg/26 mg, Target dose: 97 mg/103 mg	↑ survival with patients with HFrEF; ↓ admissions and sx	May start while in hospital; Assure ACEI or ARB are stopped at least 36 hours prior to starting. May cause hypotension	Same as ACEI. Angioedema possible at any time but especially with first dose 2% risk in black patients	Same as ACEI	Same as ACEI, orthostatic hypotension common

LIPID-LOWERING AGENTS: *ATORVASTATIN, LOVASTATIN, SIMVASTATIN, ETC.*

DOSING	BENEFIT	DECISIONS	RISK	MONITORING	SELF-CARE
Titrated to lipid goals varying by patient's cardiac risk profile In CAD, LDL should be ↓ >50% with the highest tolerated dose of high- intensity statin	↓ CV events	cvriskcalculator.com Safe to d/c at EOL[60]	Myositis: muscle aches. Hold drug and check for ↑ creatinine kinase	Lipid levels	Diet Exercise Wt loss

↑: increase(d); ↓: decrease(d). ACEI, angiotensin-converting enzyme inhibitor; AC: anticoagulation; AE: adverse effects; BP, blood pressure; CAD: coronary artery disease; Cr: creatinine; CV, cardiovascular; EF, ejection fraction; EOL: end of life; GDMT, guideline-directed medical therapy; HF, heart failure; HFrEF: heart failure with reduced EF; HR, heart rate; ICD: Implantable cardioverter-defibrillator; INR, International Normalized Ratio; K: potassium; Mg: magnesium; Mgt: management; Na: sodium; Sx: symptoms; Tx: treatment; Wt: weight.

From Fahlberg B, Laramee A, Donaho E. 2021. Used with permission.

"closure" all along the trajectory. Discussing future "what-ifs" can start an ongoing dialogue to help assure that the patient's business is complete and opportunities to say goodbye are not missed[4] (see Chapter 32, "Advance Care Planning" and Chapter 33, "Family Meetings").

REFERRING PATIENTS WITH ADVANCED CARDIAC DISEASE TO PALLIATIVE CARE

While palliative care is now recognized as a guideline-based intervention in advanced HF, the number of patients being referred to specialist palliative care remains low. Moreover, the percentage of patients with HF referred to hospice remains low.[3] Factors limiting cardiology referrals to specialty palliative care and the incorporation of palliative care interventions include:

1. Ongoing confusion between palliative care and hospice and when to refer patients for each[7]

2. The perception that cardiac symptom control requires specialty cardiac training and experience[18]

3. The sudden onset of new life-threatening cardiac and noncardiac events that require rapid decision-making based on guideline-focused algorithms[18]

4. The misperception that specialty palliative providers mainly guide patients into hospice, leading to specialist palliative care referrals being delayed until the end of life[18]

5. Lack of cardiology knowledge and experience for palliative care and hospice specialists, particularly for patients who require advanced therapies such as inotrope infusion or VAD.[4]

THE PALLIATIVE APRN IN CARE OF PATIENTS WITH CARDIOLOGY AT END OF LIFE

The palliative APRN working in a cardiac specialty unit is in an ideal position to bridge the gap between cardiac and palliative care. Shared viewpoints, knowledge, and experiences between cardiac and palliative care providers will promote effective implementation of team-based palliative care in cardiac settings. The role of the palliative APRN within the cardiac care team is still developing, yet there is great opportunity for palliative APRNs to bridge the divide between cardiology and specialty palliative care to improve the experience of patients with cardiac disease and their families during this challenging and unpredictable journey.

Palliative APRNs can play a key role in promoting quality of life and facilitating "a good death" for patients with cardiac disease. They can encourage the development of positive memories and prevent traumatic end-of-life experiences and complicated grief for family members by:[4]

- Engaging in open, honest communication about what to expect using a "hope for the best, prepare for the worst" approach

- Assuring current, specific documentation of patient preferences for emergency care and resuscitation that can be easily retrieved by any provider in any setting, including the community

- Having early conversations about end-of-life choices, such as specialist palliative care referral, hospice, and resuscitation options, including specific preferences about devices

- Facilitating patient and family decision-making meetings when patients are faced with high-risk options or advanced treatments, such as VADs, transplant, and risky treatment choices

- Supporting family members and patients with complicated advanced heart problems (such as VAD) and/or while waiting transplant

- Facilitating hospice referral when the patient with advanced HF has chosen to forgo further procedural and device "fixes"

- Learning cardiac-specific, guideline-based policies and procedures and training for specialty palliative care and hospice providers

- Assuring goal-concordant care, whether that is access to outpatient palliative care for patients who choose that their cardiac devices, such as implantable cardioverter defibrillator (ICD) or VAD, remain active or, if not, that they are referred to hospice.

CASE STUDY 2: OVERESTIMATED PROGNOSIS

JD was a 34-year-old survivor of Hodgkin's lymphoma. Ten years after his remission, he was diagnosed with doxorubicin-induced cardiomyopathy, with an ejection fraction of 15%. Once guideline-directed medical therapy was implemented, JD continued to have New York Heart Association (NYHA) Class III–IV symptoms, and he was placed on the cardiac transplant list with a plan for a ventricular assist device (VAD) as a bridge to transplant. JD was clinically stable and was scheduled for a biventricular pacer/implantable cardioverter defibrillator (ICD) placement in 2 weeks. However, because he was unable to work, his wife worked overtime hours at her job in addition to caring for their two young children and trying to do all the household chores that JD did in the past.

One night when cooking dinner with his family, JD collapsed on the kitchen floor. His wife called 911 and started cardiopulmonary resuscitation (CPR), yelling at him and crying the whole time, while his kids watched, not knowing what was going on. When the paramedics arrived, JD was in a fine ventricular fibrillation. Despite multiple shocks and advanced cardiac life support (ACLS) drugs, he could not be resuscitated.

After his death, JD's wife tried to keep the family going, but she struggled with what she thought should be simple tasks, such as paying the bills and accessing their online bank accounts. JD had never compiled their account information in one place, and the passwords were all in his head. She was still trying to piece together their financial records and was frequently surprised by unpaid bills and calls from collection agencies. She was angry with JD for not planning ahead so they would stable financially without him. She also worried about her children. Her younger child had night terrors, reliving the memory of seeing her father die. Her older child had become detached and acted indifferently, indicating he had some deep emotional wounds.

The cardiac disease trajectory may be described as "stuttering," with symptom exacerbations and remissions punctuated by significant events. These might include a new myocardial infarction (MI), an arrhythmia, or a serious infection, any of which could lead to death, particularly when the body's taxed compensatory mechanisms fail. When the patient with advanced cardiac disease is stable, the body's physiologic systems and compensatory mechanisms are in a delicately balanced homeostasis. A minor health issue, such as getting the flu, may trigger a rapid decline, leading to hospitalization, intensive care, or even death. In some cases, patients with advanced cardiac disease die within a few days of being stable.

Therefore, prior advance care planning and regular communication, including shared-decision-making, is essential to promote care that is realistic and based on the patient's current condition and consistent with their wishes. Hospitalizations and health status changes should be used to trigger discussions about goals of care where shared decision-making is applied and, in some instances, conversations about hospice referral.[4]

UNDERSTANDING THE CARDIOLOGY MINDSET

HEALTHCARE PROFESSIONALS IN CARDIOLOGY

Healthcare professionals working in cardiology respond rapidly to emergent changes in their patients' condition, employing algorithms, medications, devices, and procedures to save their patients' lives. A "good" outcome is life and a "bad" outcome is death. The word "death" or "dying" is not used; instead, the words used are "code," "cardiac arrest," ventricular fibrillation," or "asystole." Those professionals working in cardiac specialty units are trained in cardiac monitoring, are certified in advanced cardiac life support (ACLS), and regularly demonstrate their competency in providing appropriate care in a cardiac emergency. Therefore, they are constantly on the alert and prepared to rapidly intervene when the patient is "crashing" so they won't die. Many healthcare professionals may have difficulty identifying the patient who is "actively dying" because the processes that cause this, usually arrhythmias and cardiogenic shock, happen quickly and prompt immediate action. Understandably, and similar to a health professional working in critical care, not intervening is difficult because it goes against the training and mindset of "doing something." As a result, it can be difficult for cardiac providers to accept, understand, or implement the idea of letting "nature take its course." When confronted with a patient who has an acute cardiac event but who has a do-not-resuscitate (DNR) order or a comfort-directed plan of care, it can be difficult to switch from a lifesaving to a palliative mindset.

PATIENTS AND THEIR FAMILIES

A challenge in providing palliative care for patients with cardiac disease is that advance care planning may not be straightforward. One example of this is the conversation regarding resuscitation. Resuscitation options in patients with cardiac conditions may be more complex that in other patient populations. The patient may have survived cardiac arrest because someone did CPR and shocked him with an automated external defibrillator (AED). After the initial hospitalization and recovery, the patient may report a happy, healthy life for years afterward, with an ICD providing a safety net in case cardiac arrest happens again. Patients often express their gratitude to the person who did CPR and state that the additional years were a gift they do not take for granted. With this experience in mind, the cardiac survivor with advanced HF may not be interested in a DNR order. He or she is likely to remember the positive outcome and assume that the next time CPR is needed, the outcome will be the same, although not considering more recent changes in the patient's health.

PREVENTING RECURRENT ADMISSIONS

Preventing the readmission of HF patients is one of the top organizational priorities at hospitals across the United States. The *Affordable Care Act* (ACA) imposes Medicare reimbursement penalties for hospitals with HF 30-day readmission rates above the national benchmark.[5] However, predicting the future can be a significant challenge because advanced HF is characterized by recurrent exacerbations despite meticulous HF care. In addition, social and behavioral factors are often predictive of recurrent HF hospitalization, yet these can be difficult or impossible to change. When a patient with advanced heart disease is hospitalized, a global comprehensive transition to plan of care at home offers opportunities to prevent future readmissions. One strategy is using "trajectory checks" at key periods to identify when palliative care should be consulted.[4,5] Palliative specialty care and early hospice referral have been shown to reduce readmission rates over a period of 9 months.[19]

PALLIATIVE MANAGEMENT OF CARDIAC SYMPTOMS

As illustrated in the first case study, pain may not be the most common cause of physical distress among patients in the later stages of heart disease, in contrast to traditional palliative care priorities for other conditions. Fatigue, functional limitations, difficulty breathing, and ischemia-related chest discomfort are common and often distressing physical symptoms of advanced heart disease.[4] These symptoms may have an insidious onset, slowly worsening over time. Patients may report "a lack of energy," "slowing down," "having to pace myself," or difficulty sleeping, and it can be difficult for both patients and providers to distinguish whether these symptoms are due to heart problems or another cause. Therefore, palliative APRNs must understand the common symptoms of HF and other cardiac conditions, as well as the medications and other interventions appropriate to the underlying cause of these symptoms. Box 13.1 provides a comprehensive list of symptoms to guide assessment.

DYSPNEA AND DIFFICULTY SLEEPING

Dyspnea is a common and distressing symptom in patients with cardiac disease and can be exacerbated by exertion or lying supine, or it may occur when sleeping. People with dyspnea on exertion often reduce their activity to avoid this symptom; therefore, an accurate assessment of the patient's actual recent physical activity is a key element of the history that can help identify problems and treat symptoms. *Orthopnea, paroxysmal nocturnal dyspnea*, and *bendopnea* (a novel symptom that occurs when patients bend forward) are hallmark signs of

Box 13.1 CLINICAL SIGNS OF HEART FAILURE

- Weight gain

- Elevated jugular vein pressure

- Hepatic congestion or enlargement

- Ascites with evidence of fluid wave

- Hepatojugular reflux

- Peripheral or dependent edema

- Crackles with lung auscultation

- Decreased breath sounds related to pleural effusions

- Signs of low cardiac output such as fatigue, dizziness, hypotension, tachycardia

- Elevated B-type natriuretic peptide (BNP)/N-terminal prohormone of brain natriuretic peptide (NT proBNP)

fluid overload in the patient with cardiac disease, warranting careful assessment and the possible need for diuresis (see Box 13.2 for further details). The absence of edema and crackles should not be used as sole indicators of fluid status as they may be absent in the patient with chronic HF who has fluid overload.

Fluid overload-related dyspnea requires diuresis for symptom management. This is usually accomplished with loop diuretics (see Table 13.1). Morphine and lorazepam can be used to alleviate feelings of air hunger and anxiety while diuresis is being accomplished. Yet, these drugs should not be used as the sole treatments for fluid-related dyspnea as they will only mask the cause of the symptoms rather than treating it, producing ongoing symptom distress.

Another source of dyspnea that should not be ignored is the possibility of a new cardiac event, such as a MI and/or acute pulmonary edema. The sudden onset of new symptoms should prompt rapid assessment and treatment as well as

Box 13.2 TYPES OF DYSPNEA CHARACTERISTIC OF HEART FAILURE

- *Dyspnea on exertion*: Feeling of shortness of breath while doing a mild or moderate activity

- *Orthopnea*: Shortness of breath that is exacerbated when lying flat; feeling of suffocation, or drowning prompts patients to sit up so they can breathe and prop themselves up in bed with pillows or sleep in a recliner

- *Paroxysmal nocturnal dyspnea (PND)*: Occurs while sleeping; the patient wakes up at night unable to breathe or feeling claustrophobic, alleviated by sitting upright or getting up

- *Bendopnea*: Sensation of feeling short of breath while leaning forward, associated with elevated ventricular filling pressures

communication with the family so that treatments are consistent with the patient's goals and plan of care.

An exception to the use of diuretics in treating fluid-related dyspnea may be the person who is actively dying as the result of a new cardiac event and whose expected prognosis is hours to a day. Diuretics are unlikely to provide symptomatic benefit if this person is in cardiogenic shock as the weakened heart will not adequately perfuse the body, severely limiting the absorption, distribution, and metabolism of drugs like diuretics and preventing excretion of excess fluid. In this end-of-life situation, the opioid-naïve patient with end-stage cardiac disease may benefit from small doses of opioids (and benzodiazepines if the opioids fail) to provide comfort while the patient and family say goodbye.

CARDIAC PAIN

In the patient with cardiac disease who reports pain, it is important to distinguish between "cardiac" and "noncardiac" pain, as the causes, treatments, and short-term implications are quite different. Assessment should not be limited to using the word "pain" as this may not prompt the patient to report his or her cardiac symptoms. Patients may perceive their cardiac ischemic symptoms in different ways and may describe their symptoms with terms like "discomfort," "pressure," or "heaviness."

Cardiac "pain" or "discomfort," also called *angina*, is a sign of poor perfusion to the heart muscle (ischemia or infarction). It is commonly aggravated by exertion and alleviated with rest (or stopping the activity), nitroglycerin, oxygen, and opioids. Cardiac symptoms may indicate serious problems, such as a new MI; therefore, in the absence of a treatment plan for symptomatic relief, the patient should be promptly evaluated for the cause and treated until the symptoms are completely relieved. Prompt treatment of cardiac symptoms with a goal of complete relief and ongoing prevention with medications that promote coronary perfusion will promote positive patient outcomes, including better quality of life and functional status.

Stable cardiac symptoms often present in the same way from one episode to the next; however, symptoms may differ markedly between patients. Higher risks for atypical symptoms or silent ischemia include being female, a diagnosis of diabetes, and being older than 65 years. In the absence of chest discomfort, patients with silent ischemia may have other symptoms, such as shortness of breath, lightheadedness, gastrointestinal upset, falls, or sudden decline in functional status. Dramatic changes in health status with these types of symptoms should raise a high index of suspicion for a new cardiac event, prompting rapid evaluation and treatment or implementation of the agreed-upon plan.

NONCARDIAC PAIN

Noncardiac pain is common in people with heart disease, usually associated with coexisting conditions such as arthritis, diabetic neuropathy, and back problems. However, nonsteroidal antiinflammatory drugs (NSAIDs) should be avoided in heart disease patients if possible because they carry a higher risk of serious cardiovascular events, such as MI, stroke, and death.[20] NSAIDs block renal prostaglandin synthesis, which can compromise renal function and contribute to fluid retention in patients with HF and older adults. Many patients with cardiac disease take anticoagulants and antiplatelet medications, which are also contraindications to NSAIDs because of the additive risk of bleeding. Being aware of other medications to avoid in HF is also key to preventing exacerbation or causing new symptoms.[21]

SHARED DECISION-MAKING IN CARDIAC SPECIALTY CARE

When patients with cardiac disease and their families are faced with decisions related to cardiac medications, procedures, and devices, a shared decision-making approach should be used, one informed by a palliative perspective that prioritizes patient's goals, preferences, and resources with a realistic evaluation of potential benefits and risks.[22] This is particularly important in patients with significant comorbid conditions, frailty, dementia, and advanced age.[23]

Many life-saving treatments, and devices, such as cardiac interventions, surgery, VAD, and transplant, can alleviate symptoms and prolong life in even the sickest patients with cardiac disease, and these should be acknowledged as an important part of cardiac decision-making. With so many effective disease-directed therapies and devices available, providers must take care to avoid offering a laundry list of treatment options to patients and first determine a person's overall goals of care to assure that treatments are goal-concordant.

Common cardiac diagnoses for patients admitted to the hospital include MI, atrial fibrillation, and acute exacerbations of chronic HF. Many of these patients are elderly, with multiple comorbid conditions such as chronic kidney disease, dementia, and lung disease. Palliative consults often focus on shared decision-making around specific medications, diagnostic tests, procedures, or surgeries. Some tests and treatments have the potential to cause more burden than benefit. For example, with ischemic heart disease, a heart catheterization may be indicated, but for those with severe kidney disease contrast dye nephrotoxicity could lead to dialysis. Patients with atrial fibrillation may require anticoagulation or antiarrhythmic medications or a cardioversion, all with potential for serious adverse effects. Those who are frail and elderly could have significant consequences with certain medications, procedures, or advanced therapies, requiring thoughtful discussion of the options, risks, and benefits. Palliative specialists are also increasingly called upon to assist with shared decision-making around advanced therapies such as heart transplant, VADs, and heart valve procedures such as transaortic valve replacement (TAVR).

Evidence-based patient decision aids can assist patients and families faced with difficult decisions about medical treatments. Numerous decision aids are available for cardiac treatments, tests, and devices (e.g., medications for hypertension,

atrial fibrillation, high cholesterol, coronary angiogram, ablation, pacemaker, ICD, TAVR, and VAD) as well as for hospice.[24,25]

Advance care planning prior to hospitalization is critical because patients and their families are faced with complex decisions. Discussion with the patient and family before an emergent event and documentation of patient preferences can facilitate the decision-making process in a critical situation. Cardiac technologies and treatment developments have outpaced communication, documentation, and policies for patients with cardiac disease, particularly those with devices like ICDs and VADs. Therefore, the one-size-fits-most approach to advance care planning that is reflected in most legal documents does not apply to the patient with cardiac disease and their family. They may want more options, all while considering previous experiences, as well as the risks and benefits of each.[4]

Unfortunately, most advance care planning documents and DNR orders do not easily accommodate "special requests." Considering this, early advance care planning with patients with advanced cardiac conditions is important to address potential treatment decisions in the patient's future. Cardiac care options may include:

- CPR

- Emergency drugs

- ICD shock and pacing

- Defibrillation

- External pacing

- Mechanical ventilation

- Temporary suspension of DNR/do-not-intubate (DNI) for procedures or surgery

- Mechanical circulatory support

- Inotropes

- Coronary angioplasty and stent

- Dialysis

- Other invasive tests or treatments such as coronary angiogram, TAVR, or pacemaker

- Repeat hospitalizations

- Intensive care.

The palliative APRN working with patients with advanced cardiac conditions should be prepared to discuss the risks, burdens, and benefits of each option with the individual and legally document and effectively communicate the patient's specific goals of care and preferences.

CARDIAC HOSPITALIZATION

If a new cardiac hospitalization occurs, the patient's proxy, goals of care, and advance care plan documents should be immediately available to direct treatment decisions. Because patients can die within a short time of being stable, a rapid change in the patient's condition should prompt quick intervention, consistent with the patient's wishes. If the patient has chosen a comfort approach, the team's interventions should be directed toward promoting open, honest, empathetic communication and comfort for the patient and support for the family. Most important is realizing that the period when the patient is "actively dying" may be short and the end may come suddenly.

If an advance care plan has not been identified or if the patient has elected to have some or all resuscitative or life support measures employed, the palliative care team should facilitate ongoing communication about the patient's and family's decisions. Topics include the need for monitoring and intensive care, as well as anticipated tests and treatments. As the patient's condition declines, the palliative APRN can assist in clarifying the code status and begin preparing for resuscitation or activating a rapid response. The palliative APRN can ensure that the patient and family have adequate information, support, and resources to assist in shared decision-making and can promote their psychological, spiritual, and physical well-being throughout this challenging period.

CARDIAC PROCEDURES: ANGIOGRAM AND STENT

When a patient has a heart attack or worsening symptoms of coronary ischemia, testing often includes coronary angiogram, also called a "cardiac cath." Coronary angiogram involves inserting a catheter in a blood vessel in the groin, neck, or arm and threading it to the heart, where the coronary arteries are injected with dye to identify narrowed or blocked blood vessels. In many cases, another catheter with a balloon and metal coil called a "stent" can then be used to open the blocked artery, thus restoring blood flow to the affected area of the heart.[26,27] This is the least invasive approach to treating coronary artery disease. Cardiac catheterization can also be used for other diagnostic tests and interventions including measuring pressures and oxygen levels inside the heart, determining pumping function (EF), cardiac tissue sampling (biopsy), and treating heart valve conditions.[26]

CORONARY ARTERY BYPASS GRAFT SURGERY

Coronary artery bypass grafting (CABG), a surgical procedure to improve poor blood flow to the heart, is performed when the arteries supplying blood to heart tissue are narrowed or blocked, causing symptoms of cardiac ischemia or heart attack. CABG may prevent serious complications such as heart attack, stroke, and death in people with severe coronary artery disease. It may also be used emergently in a severe heart attack to save the person's life. The surgery involves using blood vessels from another part of the body, usually from the arm or chest or veins from the legs, to connect blood vessels above and below the blocked artery, bypassing the blockage and restoring adequate blood flow to the heart. Bypass is usually performed when multiple blockages are present, making stent treatment less realistic. CABG is a treatment, but not a cure, for ischemic heart disease. Postoperative recommendations include taking prescribed cardiac medications, making heart-healthy lifestyle changes, and clinical follow-up to control symptoms, treat disease, and prevent complications.[28]

HEART VALVE REPAIR AND REPLACEMENT

Heart valve repair or replacement is used to treat symptoms and preserve cardiac function in the person with symptomatic heart valve disease. There are two primary types of heart valve defects: stenosis and regurgitation. Stenosis is a narrowed valve, as seen in aortic stenosis, that prevents blood from being pushed out to the body. Regurgitation is a leaky valve (such as mitral regurgitation) that causes blood to back up in the heart and lungs. Both problems cause symptoms of HF such as fatigue, weakness, pulmonary congestion, and edema. Heart valve procedures are used to repair or replace the affected heart valves.

Surgical options to valve repair or replacement include open-heart surgery and minimally invasive heart surgery, as well as cardiac catheter-based procedures. Valve surgery may also be performed in conjunction with CABG in patients with both arterial and valvular disease. Palliative procedures such as TAVR or a "mitral clip" may be options if the patient is not a surgical candidate, with the goal of improving their functional status and quality of life. The palliative procedures can also carry significant risks for complications as patients often have a long history of symptomatic HF and multiple comorbidities. Procedural risks should be weighed against potential benefits using shared decision-making. This is when a palliative care consultation may be requested, weighing the procedure against a palliative medical/hospice care option.

The three common types of valve procedures are repair using annuloplasty or valvuloplasty and valve replacement. Annuloplasty is used to repair a regurgitant valve by reducing the diameter of the valve's fibrous ring. Valvuloplasty, the other repair option, is used to open a stiff, stenotic valve by using a heart catheter to place a balloon into the valve opening, where it is inflated to push open the stiff valve leaflets. Once the valve has been opened, the balloon is deflated and the catheter removed.[29]

Valve replacement involves replacing the entire heart valve with either a mechanical or bioprosthetic valve. Decision-making about the type of valve usually focuses on two issues: anticoagulant requirements and the expected life of the implanted valve. While short-term anticoagulation with warfarin or a similar drug is needed with the bioprosthetic valve to prevent stroke or other embolic events, the mechanical valve requires long-term anticoagulation. If the patient with a bioprosthetic valve has or develops atrial fibrillation, a common postsurgical complication, anticoagulation will be needed while the arrhythmia persists. The expected life of the two types of valves differs: while a mechanical valve may last for decades, a bioprosthetic valve usually has a shorter life expectancy. Therefore, mechanical valves are preferred for patients who are younger—with the tradeoff anticoagulant requirements—so they can avoid repeated valve replacement surgeries in the future, each with increasing risks of complications. Decision-making about valve repair or replacement should consider factors including the patient's age, life expectancy, comorbidities, indications, or contraindications for anticoagulant therapy and, perhaps most important, the patient's preference for the valve procedure.[30]

Transcatheter Aortic Valve Replacement

Severe aortic stenosis typically occurs in older individuals. Once patients become symptomatic, those treated with medications alone have mortality rates of approximately 25% in 1 year and 50% in 2 years, with sudden death in 50%.[31] While traditional surgical aortic replacement may be offered, the growing and evolving catheter-based TAVR procedure may be an option for many patients with severe aortic stenosis. However, patients with a life expectancy of 12 months or less or poor quality of life due to noncardiac comorbid conditions are unlikely to improve with a TAVR and may instead benefit more from a medical palliative approach.[32] For patients who are high and intermediate surgical risk, TAVR may be the appropriate option if it is consistent with their goals of care. In patients with low surgical risk, the choice of surgical aortic replacement versus TAVR is not clear at this time as the evidence continues to evolve. Outcomes for patients who received a TAVR compared to medical management have demonstrated improved survival and increased functional status but with increased risk of stroke in the procedural phase. Compared to surgical aortic valve replacement, patients who have had a TAVR also had improved survival, especially women, and had decreased risk of kidney injury, new atrial fibrillation, or major bleeding. However, major vascular complications, need for a permanent pacemaker, and paravalvular regurgitation were less frequent with surgery.[32] A critical part of the pre-TAVR checklist is assessment of the patients' preferences, values, goals, expectations, and advance care planning, ensuring that documents are in place before the procedure.[30]

Mitral Clip

Patients with symptomatic mitral regurgitation typically have comorbidities that put them at high surgical risk, and they have typically been treated with medical therapy alone. However, the transcatheter mitral clip provides a palliative option to improve the patient's symptoms and quality of life while reducing the risk of hospitalization for patients who are poor surgical candidates.[33] As with TAVR, which is also used in a very sick patient population, the mitral clip has been associated with high rates of adverse events in the first 30 days after the procedure.[34] Surgical or transcatheter treatment for mitral regurgitation secondary to other heart problems is recommended only after other medical and device therapies have been instituted and optimized.[35]

CARDIAC IMPLANTED ELECTRONIC DEVICES

Cardiac implantable electrical devices (CIEDs) include pacemakers, ICDs, and cardiac resynchronization therapy + defibrillator devices (CRTDs). These devices are widely used to treat cardiac electrical problems such as bradycardias, symptomatic and life-threatening arrhythmias, and cardiac dyssynchrony. All these devices can monitor, record, and treat the heart's electrical activity. When a patient has symptoms suggestive of device malfunction, the device can be interrogated by a specially trained cardiac professional or company representative, and the recorded heart activity and device interventions are reviewed to determine whether there are problems with the device or its programmed functions. Toward the end of life, patients with ICD often choose to have the shocking capabilities discontinued to prevent distressing shocks as they are dying. Palliative APRNs can play a key role in deactivation discussions.[15]

ICD shocks in a terminally ill patient are painful and distressing, serve no medical purpose, and should be avoided.[4] Discussions regarding prognosis, end-of-life symptom management, and ICD deactivation may take place in the acute care setting, cardiology, or primary care office, and information about the option of deactivation should be included in pre-implantation teaching.[15] In patients with a DNR order in place, deactivation of an ICD's shocking function should be discussed. Deactivating the pacemaker function of an ICD or a pacemaker itself should be avoided, as it can result in symptoms like dizziness and even syncopal episodes (passing out) due to inadequate cardiac output.[15]

Deactivation or reprogramming of a CEID requires a medical order, and proper etiquette is to notify the cardiologist managing the device. Deactivation may be done by a cardiac device specialist or a representative from the company that made the device. In an emergent situation, such when an ICD is shocking a patient who is DNR and who is dying, ICD deactivation may be accomplished by taping a medical-grade magnet over the device, but this is not the case for all devices. Palliative APRNs should be aware of any CIEDs in their patients because patients with cardiac disease are at risk for rapid changes in their health, during which the CIED may need to be addressed.

IMPLANTABLE HEMODYNAMIC MONITOR

Implantable pulmonary artery (PA) pressure ambulatory monitoring devices can help healthcare providers proactively determine changes indicating worsening HF. The implantable hemodynamic monitor (IHM) device is used to remotely monitor PA pressures and is placed in the PA using a percutaneous procedure. Adjustments of guideline-based HF medications based on PA pressures can promote better quality of life and fewer hospitalizations for patients with HF compared to medication titration alone.[36] The ideal patient for PA pressure monitoring is someone who has ongoing symptoms of HF despite optimized GDMT.[37] Patients who may not be good candidates for PA pressure monitoring are those with end-stage HF or heading to advanced therapies or palliative care, Stage IV–V chronic kidney disease who are not responding well to diuretics, a body mass index (BMI) greater than 35, and/or history of pulmonary emboli or deep vein thromboses (DVTs) making implantation difficult.[37]

INOTROPE INFUSION

Inotropes are medications that help the heart beat more strongly by increasing contractility. They are used for temporary symptom palliation in select patients with advanced HF.[23,38] Despite many attempts to develop oral inotropes that are safe and effective, inotropes are still only available as intravenous infusions. Inotropes are used in conjunction with guideline-based medications and cardiac device-based treatments in advanced HF to improve symptoms of poor cardiac output such as fatigue and breathlessness as well as the patient's functional status. Inotropes may be used in patients awaiting transplant or VAD implantation, giving them time to address key decisions while providing relief from distressing symptoms.[39] However, despite this symptom benefit, inotropes do not extend life,[40] and they may increase the risk of dangerous cardiac events such as arrhythmias, MI, and hypotension by forcing an already weakened heart to pump more vigorously.[41]

Advanced HF specialists may offer inotropes as a palliative treatment, explaining that their goal is to "improve symptoms but not survival."[40] Palliative care issues to address with patients being considered for or receiving inotropes for symptom relief may include shared decision-making regarding ongoing use of these agents, the potential for inotrope discontinuation with disease progression, and the discussion of potential adverse events such as arrhythmias that may be life-threatening or that could cause ICD shocks. For patients who are not eligible for inotropes or do not wish to elect other advanced heart therapies, the involvement of palliative care is critically important to assist with decisions about home healthcare or hospice. All providers should emphasize at the beginning of inotrope therapy the different scenarios that may lead to the need to discontinue the medication. These include deteriorating health status as evidenced by decreased quality of life, functional status, increased symptoms, and arrhythmias.

An ongoing challenge with inotropes is access to hospice for these patients. Hospices that can provide inotropes for a period of time in addition to oral GDMT medications for symptom relief must have providers and nurses skilled in HF management. Hospice management of inotrope infusions requires coordination of care between the hospice and the infusion company, with periodic clinical reevaluation of the infusion's clinical efficacy. Weekly goals-of-care conversations are important, with assessment of the patient's functional and quality of life status. The clinical exam may consist of monitoring serial pulse pressures and proportional pulse pressure readings as a clinical parameter to determine the inotropes' ongoing efficacy.[4,42]

VENTRICULAR ASSIST DEVICE

VADs are increasingly used in advanced HF to alleviate symptoms and improve functional status in patients with advanced HF whose heart function continues to deteriorate on GDMT and other treatments. While VAD has the potential to significantly benefit patients, there are also many risks and obligations associated with VAD therapy. The risk of serious complications or death may be underrecognized by patients who may see this as a "miracle" being offered when they have become very symptomatic and disabled.

In 2013, the Centers for Medicare and Medicaid Services mandated palliative specialist involvement in the care of patients being considered for VADs used as a bridge to transplant and destination therapy, working with patients before and after placement of a VAD in collaboration with the multidisciplinary HF team.[43] Palliative care is key to improving preparation of the patient and their family/caregivers for this device and the outcomes they may experience.

Patients who are offered VAD often have multiple comorbidities with a significant symptom burden that needs to be addressed throughout the trajectory. Palliative interventions for VAD patients include treating physical and psychological symptoms, providing emotional and practical support for caregivers, and alleviating suffering.[4,44] Palliative APRNs who work with a VAD program should learn about common VAD complications such as driveline infections, stroke, bleeding, and symptoms of persistent HF such as nausea and edema. APRNs should also gain experience in promoting support and alleviating distress during VAD deactivation, as well as managing advanced HF symptoms, especially treating dyspnea with diuretics and opiates.

Palliative APRNs are often consulted by potential VAD recipients to discuss quality of life, and this discussion does not routinely move to end-of-life discussions. Instead, palliative discussions center on "what matters most" to the patient regarding hopes for life and their goals of care with the device.[45] Palliative care discussions pre- and post-implant should be nuanced, evolving as the patient and family journey through the VAD process. The pre-implantation palliative care consult focuses on preparing patients to better understand VAD therapy and its tradeoffs. Issues that should be discussed may include expected outcomes and risks, advance care planning, postoperative symptom management, and caregiver support. An evidence-based VAD decision aid, available at patient decisionaid.org/VAD,[45] is recommended by the Patient-Centered Outcomes Research Institute as an essential tool for palliative practice with this population. Research with this tool found that patients in the intervention group had better decision quality, with closer alignment of the VAD medical decision and the patients' care preferences. Interestingly fewer patients in the intervention arm went on to have VAD implantation (54% vs. 80%, p < 0.01). Post-implant palliative discussions may focus more on code status, VAD-specific symptoms, end-of-life symptom management, and comfort-focused care such as hospice.[46]

A challenging part of VAD care is the issue of deactivation. Patients with VAD are dependent on the device for survival. Both intentional deactivation as well as accidental discontinuation of the VAD's external energy source can cause rapid decompensation and death. For this reason, a VAD device has a loud alarm that sounds if the energy supply is cut off;

patients and their caregivers must practice responding to the alarms troubleshooting issues, knowing that the patient's life is hanging in the balance. Deactivation of a VAD device may be either medically indicated, such as when a patient has a catastrophic event following implantation, or deactivation may be requested by the patient (e.g., if their quality of life is poor).[47] Ethically, it is important to recognize that the cause of death following VAD deactivation is the underlying advanced HF syndrome and not the act of deactivating the device[48] (see Chapter 53, "Navigating Ethical Dilemmas").

Palliative APRNs working with VAD patients should collaborate with HF clinicians to gain experience in deactivating commonly implanted VADs when the need arises. It is important to anticipate and treat the common symptoms that patients experience after VAD withdrawal.[4] Deactivation decisions may be complicated when the VAD patient is not necessarily terminally ill, but they have chosen deactivation due to a poor quality of life, psychological distress, or existential suffering. It is important to work toward shared goals between the patient and family, ensuring adequate symptom management and support at the time of deactivation.[4,45]

HEART TRANSPLANT

Heart transplant is a treatment of choice for some patients with advanced HF who remain symptomatic despite GDMT optimization. As of 2017, median survival after heart transplant was 11.8 years. In 2019, there were more than 55,000 heart transplants worldwide, but the number is limited by the availability of donor hearts. Absolute contraindications for heart transplant are systemic illness with life expectancy of less than 2 years, irreversible pulmonary hypertension, severe cerebrovascular disease, active substance abuse, and multisystem disease with severe organ dysfunction. Relative contraindications include advanced age (70 or older), BMI greater than 35, diabetes with poor control or end organ damage, neoplasm, infection, pulmonary embolism within 6–8 weeks, irreversible renal dysfunction, tobacco or substance abuse within 6 months, and inadequate support system to comply with treatment plan.[49] Palliative care consultation is recommended by clinical practice guidelines pre- and post-heart transplant, especially for progression of cardiac disease.[50]

HOSPICE IN ADVANCED HEART DISEASE

One of the greatest challenges in working with patients with advanced cardiac disease can be determining when they are at the end of the testing and treatment process and ready to consider hospice. While a 6-month prognosis can be challenging to accurately determine, a pattern of worsening functional status with little improvement despite GDMT titration is a key indicator of limited life expectancy that has consistently emerged in the research. Other hospice eligibility criteria for the patient with advanced HF include:

- Symptoms of recurrent HF or angina at rest, discomfort with any activity despite optimal treatment with guideline-directed medications such as diuretics, beta-blockers, and angiotensin-converting-enzyme inhibitors a (ACEIs)

- Ejection of less than 20%

- Symptomatic arrhythmias

- History of cardiac arrest and CPR

- Unexplained syncope.

The use of hospice in patients with advanced HF, as well as in patients who are not interested in pursuing advanced treatment options, may prevent unwanted hospital admissions and nonbeneficial tests and treatments while reducing healthcare costs.[18] A decision aid to assist patients and their family considering hospice care is available at patientdecisionaid.org/hospice.[24]

Hospice can be a fearful prospect for the HF patient and family if the medications they are used to taking to manage their symptoms are stopped. Many cardiology providers incorrectly believe that GDMTs, including medications and some devices, must be stopped upon hospice admission, which may prevent them from entertaining the idea of hospice for their patients.[4] The American College of Cardiology Foundation/American Heart Association and the Heart Failure Society of America (HFSA) have guidelines for end-of-life care in the HF patient.[23,38] In addition, in 2014, the HFSA published *Consensus Statement: End-of-Life Care in Patients with Heart Failure*,[51] while the American Heart Association issued a policy statement in 2016 providing guidance for the development and growth of palliative care in cardiovascular disease and stroke.[43] While guidelines specific to hospice and palliative care for patients with advanced heart disease have yet to be clearly articulated, these statements and guidelines are essential foundations for palliative care practice.

For the hospice-appropriate patient with advanced HF, the guidelines recommend care that includes[23,38]

1. Clinical assessment of hemodynamic status, blood pressure, and weight with adjustment of GDMT

2. Continue guideline-based cardiac medications including ACEIs, angiotensin receptor blockers (ARBs), angiotensin receptor neprilysin inhibitors (ARNIs), beta-blockers, calcium channel blockers, nitrates, oral and intravenous diuretics, antiarrhythmics, and anticoagulants (see Table 13.1)

3. Intravenous inotrope infusion (milrinone, dobutamine, dopamine) for symptom palliation in select patients (see Table 13.1)

4. Intravenous administration of diuretics (furosemide or bumetanide) to relieve pulmonary congestion; thiazide/loop combination may also be helpful for symptom relief

5. Device deactivation including ICDs at the end of life

6. Ongoing advance care planning and discussions about goals of care

There are many challenges and opportunities as the HF and the hospice care communities interface to provide the best evidenced-based care throughout the entire trajectory of HF, from diagnosis to death. Intravenous inotropes, including dobutamine, milrinone, or, in rare cases, dopamine, are sometimes offered to patients with HF with reduce ejection fraction as an advanced palliative therapy. Palliative inotropes can be cost-prohibitive for some hospices, and many hospice agencies hesitate to accept patients on inotropes due to the capitated per diem model of hospice reimbursement.[52]

It is important that HF teams develop partnerships with hospices that can provide palliative inotrope infusions for select patients while on hospice care. Patients likely to benefit from inotropes while in hospice are those who have demonstrated favorable hemodynamic or symptomatic benefit from inotropes, who have not tolerated an attempt at weaning, and whose goals are aligned with hospice care.[52]

CARE OF THE PATIENT WHO IS IMMINENTLY DYING

The final phase of a person's life is an especially important time. Palliative APRNs have an opportunity and an obligation to help patients have a good death. There are three main commitments at the end of life

- expert symptom management

- supporting and preparing the patient and family

- intensive comfort-focused care

It is essential to recognize when someone is within hours to days of dying. The mode of death for cardiac disease can be very sudden with arrhythmias; however, patients are more likely to die from progressive symptoms related to cardiovascular or noncardiovascular causes, though these can cause death within a few days of being stable. A new cardiac event in the patient with comfort-focused care may cause a rapid change in the patient's condition. They may exhibit signs of progressive cardiogenic shock as the compensatory mechanisms fail, and death may happen within 24 hours of symptom onset. While the patient in this scenario is actively dying, ICD shock may occur if they have an active ICD. Deactivation of the ICD's shocking function should be a priority to prevent patient, family, and caregiver distress. However, if the patient has a pacemaker, this device will not prevent the person from dying a natural death and it will not cause distressing symptoms. In fact, deactivation of a pacemaker in someone pacer-dependent can *worsen* distressing symptoms, so pacemaker deactivation is not indicated. (Funeral homes should be notified about implanted pacemakers or ICDs because devices must be removed before cremation.)

Three symptoms that may abruptly worsen as the patient is dying are secretions, delirium, and shortness of breath. Symptom distress should be treated as an emergency, requiring thoughtful escalation of medications and close bedside monitoring. At such a time in someone's life, it is more about them, less about the disease, and the priority is intensive, comfort-focused care.[53]

Sensitive expert communication skills should be used to prepare and support the patient and their family. There are several principles in working with families.

1. Do not assume the family knows that the person is dying.

2. Assess what is important to the family, such as seeing a chaplain or wishes for family presence during resuscitation.

3. Explain what they can expect with the person's condition and management.

4. If the patient has transitioned to a comfort-directed plan of care, provide a specific description about what this means.

5. Using a shared decision-making approach, talk about the care that will and will not be provided.

6. Assess for factors that may contribute to complicated grief such as surrogate-made treatment decisions, discontinuation of life-sustaining treatments, or unresolved family issues.

THE PALLIATIVE APRN-AN INTEGRAL MEMBER OF THE CARDIAC TEAM

SUPPORT, COMMUNICATION, AND SYMPTOM MANAGEMENT

The palliative APRN in the cardiac setting should provide ongoing support for the patient and family while facilitating important discussions and advocating for the patient's goals and preferences in treatment decisions. At the same time, they may also be an important source of support for the members of the cardiac care team, especially those experiencing moral distress or grief resulting from complex and heartbreaking situations. The palliative APRN should also be a role model and teacher of palliative care communication, shared decision-making, and symptom management strategies, disseminating primary palliative care knowledge, skills, and attitudes throughout the cardiac care environment.

FAMILY LIAISON IN EMERGENT EVENTS

The palliative APRN with an understanding of ACLS and emergent cardiac care can play an important role in supporting the family and providing information during a code, rapid response, or other emergent event, while the cardiac team is busy caring for the patient. The family that is present should be offered the option of watching resuscitation efforts, though always accompanied by a clinician who can explain what is happening. They can provide anticipatory guidance based on what is happening with the patient's response to medical efforts and facilitate decision-making, such as whether resuscitation efforts should be stopped when futile. The palliative APRN can also assist with contacting support systems and spiritual care.[54]

Anticipatory guidance may be used early in the code to prepare the family for the possibility that the patient may die and about the option to stop resuscitation efforts at some point. As the code progresses, the palliative APRN can explain to the family what is happening and what they are seeing and hearing, according to their needs and answering their questions. The family may experience comfort in knowing that the team did all they could to save their loved one. This type of support during a family-witnessed resuscitation can prevent complicated grief and posttraumatic stress disorder in bereaved family members.[55] The palliative APRN can fill this important yet underimplemented role of family liaison for the code and rapid response teams.

EMERGING OPPORTUNITIES

In this chapter we envisioned the role of palliative APRNs on the cardiac specialty unit, yet this vision has been limited to patients with advanced HF. As this role becomes established, there is ample opportunity for expansion of the role to include decisional support and holistic symptom management care for many more types of cardiac issues.[56] The role of the palliative APRN in the care of patients being worked up for VAD is currently being identified. Another emerging APRN role in cardiac palliative care is decisional support for any high-risk patients who are considering their testing and treatment options. These roles will require greater understanding of cardiology as well as the risks, benefits, and nuances of different options. As evidence grows and more clinicians experience the complexities and rewards of this exciting area of clinical practice, the palliative APRN role on the cardiac specialty unit will continue to evolve.

SUMMARY

This chapter has delineated the many ways in which the patient with cardiac disease in the acute care setting can benefit from specialist palliative care. The palliative APRN plays an important role in the care of patients on the acute cardiac specialty unit by promoting a focus on comfort, quality of life, communication, shared decision-making, advance care planning, and family support. Patients with advanced cardiac disease and their families are challenged by needs, experiences, and pathophysiologic changes that are unique to this population, affecting their quality of life, decisions, and the advance care plans that are appropriate for them. An understanding of the cardiac provider's mindset and common cardiac diagnoses, tests, treatments, and decisions will enable the palliative APRN to become a trusted, effective member of the interdisciplinary cardiac team

so that, one day, specialty palliative care will be available to all patients with cardiac conditions, from diagnosis to death.

REFERENCES

1. Virani SS, Alonso A, Benjamin EJ, et al. Heart disease and stroke statistics: 2020 update: A report from the American Heart Association. *Circulation*. 2020;141(9):E139–E596. doi:10.1161/CIR.0000000000000757
2. Warraich HJ, Wolf SP, Mentz RJ, Rogers JG, Samsa G, Kamal AH. Characteristics and trends among patients with cardiovascular disease referred to palliative care. *JAMA Network Open*. 2019;2(5):e192375. doi:10.1001/jamanetworkopen.2019.2375
3. National Hospice and Palliative Care Organization. *Facts and Figures: Hospice are in America, 2020 edition. Alexandria*: National Hospice and Palliative Care Organization. August 2020. https://www.nhpco.org/factsfigures/
4. Fahlberg B, Panke J, Donaho E. Advanced heart failure. In: Whitehead P, Dahlin C, eds. *Compendium of Nursing Care for Common Serious Illnesses*. 3rd ed, Pittsburgh: Hospice and Palliative Nurses Association; 2019: 120–192.
5. Hollenberg SM, Warner Stevenson L, Ahmad T, et al. 2019 ACC expert consensus decision pathway on risk assessment, management, and clinical trajectory of patients hospitalized with heart failure: A report of the American College of Cardiology Solution Set Oversight Committee. *J Am Coll Cardiol*. 2019;74(15):1966–2011. doi:10.1016/j.jacc.2019.08.001
6. Singh GK, Davidson PM, Macdonald PS, Newton PJ. The perspectives of health care professionals on providing end of life care and palliative care for patients with chronic heart failure: An integrative review. *Heart Lung Circ*. 2019;28(4):539–552. doi:10.1016/j.hlc.2018.10.009
7. Lindvall C, Hultman TD, Jackson VA. Overcoming the barriers to palliative care referral for patients with advanced heart failure. *J Am Heart Assoc*. 2014;3(1):e000742. doi:10.1161/JAHA.113.000742
8. van den Heuvel LA, Hoving C, Schols JM, Spruit MA, Wouters EF, Janssen DJ. Barriers and facilitators to end-of-life communication in advanced chronic organ failure. *Int J Palliat Nurs*. 2016;22(5):222–229. doi:10.12968/ijpn.2016.22.5.222
9. Kavalieratos D, Gelfman LP, Tycon LE, et al. Palliative care in heart failure: Rationale, evidence, and future priorities. *J Am Coll Cardiol*. 2017;70(15):1919–1930. doi:10.1016/j.jacc.2017.08.036
10. Lunney JR, Lynn J, Foley DJ, Lipson S, Guralnik JM. Patterns of functional decline at the end of life. *JAMA*. 2003;289(18):2387–2392. doi:10.1001/jama.289.18.2387
11. Im J, Mak S, Upshur R, Steinberg L, Kuluski K. "The future is probably now": Understanding of illness, uncertainty and end-of-life discussions in older adults with heart failure and family caregivers. *Health Expect*. 2019;22(6):1331–1340. doi:10.1111/hex.12980
12. Bern-Klug M. The ambiguous dying syndrome. *Health Social Work*. 2004;29(1):55–65. doi: 10.1093/hsw/29.1.55
13. Jha SR, Hannu MK, Chang S, et al. The prevalence and prognostic significance of frailty in patients with advanced heart failure referred for heart transplantation. *Transplantation*. 2016;100(2):429–436. doi:10.1097/TP.0000000000000991
14. Allen LA, Matlock DD, Shetterly SM, et al. Use of risk models to predict death in the next year among individual ambulatory patients with heart failure. *JAMA Cardiol*. 2017;2(4):435–441. doi:10.1001/jamacardio.2016.5036
15. Benjamin MM, Sorkness CA. Practical and ethical considerations in the management of pacemaker and implantable cardiac defibrillator devices in terminally ill patients. Proc (*Bayl Univ Med Cent*). 2017;30(2):157–160. doi:10.1080/08998280.2017.11929566
16. Carlsson J, Paul NW, Dann M, Neuzner J, Pfeiffer D. The deactivation of implantable cardioverter-defibrillators. *Dtsch Arztebl Int*. 2012;109(33–34):535–541. doi:10.3238/arztebl.2012.0535

17. Chang YK, Kaplan H, Geng Y, et al. Referral criteria to palliative care for patients with heart failure: A systematic review. *Circ Heart Fail*. 2020;13(9):382–392. doi:10.1161/CIRCHEARTFAILURE.120.006881

18. Gelfman LP, Kalman J, Goldstein NE. Engaging heart failure clinicians to increase palliative care referrals: Overcoming barriers, improving techniques. *J Palliat Med*. 2014;17(7):753–760. doi:10.1089/jpm.2013.0675

19. Wiskar K, Celi LA, Walley KR, Fruhstorfer C, Rush B. Inpatient palliative care referral and 9-month hospital readmission in patients with congestive heart failure: A linked nationwide analysis. *J Intern Med*. 2017;282(5):445–451. doi:10.1111/joim.12657

20. Solomon DH. In Furst D, Cannon C, eds. Nonselective NSAIDs: Adverse cardiovascular effects. UpToDate. Waltham, MA: UpToDate. Updated September 13, 2021. http://www.uptodate.com/contents/nonselective-nsaids-adverse-cardiovascular-effects

21. Page K, Marwick TH, Lee R, et al. A systematic approach to chronic heart failure care: A consensus statement. *Med J Aust*. 2014;201(3):146–150. doi: 10.5694/mja14.00032.

22. Allen LA, Stevenson LW, Grady KL, et al. Decision making in advanced heart failure: A scientific statement from the American Heart Association. *Circulation*. 2012;125(15):1928–1952. doi:10.1161/CIR.0b013e31824f2173

23. WRITING COMMITTEE MEMBERS, Yancy CW, Jessup M, et al. 2013 ACCF/AHA guideline for the management of heart failure: a report of the American College of Cardiology Foundation/American Heart Association Task Force on practice guidelines. *Circulation*. 2013;128(16):e240–e327. doi:10.1161/CIR.0b013e31829e8776

24. Colorado Program for Patient Centered Decisions. Decision aids. Aurora, CO. 2021. Available at https://patientdecisionaid.org/decision-aids/

25. Ottawa Hospital Research Institute. Patient Decision Aids. A to Z inventory. Modified June 26, 2019. Available at https://decisionaid.ohri.ca/AZinvent.php

26. Mayo Clinic Staff. Patient Care and Information. Tests and Procedures. Cardiac catheterization website. June 4, 2019. Available at https://www.mayoclinic.org/tests-procedures/cardiac-catheterization/about/pac-20384695

27. Pietrangelo A. Cardiac stent: Benefits and how it works. Healthline. Updated March 22, 2019. Available at https://www.healthline.com/health/heart-disease/stent#benefits

28. Mayo Clinic Staff. Patient Care and Information. Tests and Procedures. Heart valve surgery. Website. August 7, 2020. Available at https://www.mayoclinic.org/tests-procedures/heart-valve-surgery/about/pac-20384901

29. Johns Hopkins Medicine. Health. Treatments, Tests, and Therapies. Website. Valvuloplasty. Available at https://www.hopkinsmedicine.org/health/treatment-tests-and-therapies/valvuloplasty

30. Nishimura RA, Otto CM, Bonow RO, et al. 2017 AHA/ACC focused update of the 2014 AHA/ACC guideline for the management of patients with valvular heart disease: A report of the American College of Cardiology/American Heart Association Task Force on Clinical Practice Guidelines. *Circulation*. 2017;135(25):e1159–e1195. doi:10.1161/CIR.0000000000000503

31. Turina J, Hess, O, Sepulcri F, Krayenbuehl HP. Spontaneous course of aortic valve disease. *Eur Heart J*. 1987;8(5):471–483. doi:10.1093/oxfordjournals.eurheartj.a062307

32. Otto CM, Kumbhani DJ, Alexander KP, et al. 2017 ACC expert consensus decision pathway for transcatheter aortic valve replacement in the management of adults with aortic stenosis: A report of the American College of Cardiology Task Force on Clinical Expert Consensus Documents. *J Am Coll Cardiol*. 2017;69(10):1313–1346. doi:10.1016/j.jacc.2016.12.006

33. Berardini A, Biagini E, Saia F, et al. Percutaneous mitral valve repair: The last chance for symptoms improvement in advanced refractory chronic heart failure? *Int J Cardiol*. 2017;228:191–197. doi:10.1016/j.ijcard.2016.11.241

34. Philip F, Athappan G, Tuzcu EM, Svensson LG, Kapadia SR. MitraClip for severe symptomatic mitral regurgitation in patients at high surgical risk. *Catheter Cardiovasc Interv*. 2014;84(4):581–590. doi:10.1002/ccd.25564

35. Bonow RO, O'Gara PT, Adams DH, et al. 2020 Focused update of the 2017 ACC expert consensus decision pathway on the management of mitral regurgitation: A report of the American College of Cardiology Solution Set Oversight Committee. *J Am Coll Cardiol*. 2020;75(17):2236–2270. doi:10.1016/j.jacc.2020.02.005

36. Abraham WT, Perl L. Implantable hemodynamic monitoring for heart failure patients. *J Am Coll Cardiol*. 2017;70(3):389–398. doi:10.1016/j.jacc.2017.05.052

37. Leung CC. Current role of the CardioMEMS device for management of patients with heart failure. *Curr Cardiol Rep*. 2019;21(9):98. doi:10.1007/s11886-019-1194-9

38. Lindenfeld J, Albert NM, Boehmer JP, et al. HFSA 2010 comprehensive heart failure practice guideline. *J Card Fail*. 2010;16(6):e1–e194. doi:10.1016/j.cardfail.2010.04.004

39. Francis GS, Bartos JA, Adatya S. Inotropes. *J Am Coll Cardiol*. 2014;63(20):2069–2078. doi:10.1016/j.jacc.2014.01.016

40. Nizamic T, Murad MH, Allen LA, et al. Ambulatory inotrope infusions in advanced heart failure: A systematic review and meta-analysis. *JACC Heart Fail*. 2018;6(9):757–767. doi:10.1016/j.jchf.2018.03.019

41. Amin A, Maleki M. Positive inotropes in heart failure: A review article. *Heart Asia*. 2012;4(1):16–22. doi:10.1136/heartasia-2011-010068

42. Yildiran T, Koc M, Bozkurt A, Sahin DY, Unal I, Acarturk E. Low pulse pressure as a predictor of death in patients with mild to advanced heart failure. *Texas Heart Inst J*. 2010;37(3):284–290.

43. Braun LT, Grady KL, Kutner JS, et al. Palliative care and cardiovascular disease and stroke: A policy statement from the American Heart Association/American Stroke Association. *Circulation*. 2016;134(11):e198–e225. doi:10.1161/CIR.0000000000000438

44. Allen LA, McIlvennan CK, Thompson JS, et al. Effectiveness of an intervention supporting shared decision making for destination therapy left ventricular assist device the DECIDE-LVAD randomized clinical trial. *JAMA Int Med*. 2018;178(4):520–529. doi:10.1001/jamainternmed.2017.8713

45. Thompson JS, Matlock DD, McIlvennan CK, Jenkins AR, Allen LA. Development of a decision aid for patients with advanced heart failure considering a destination therapy left ventricular assist device. *JACC Heart Fail*. 2015;3(12):965–976. doi:10.1016/j.jchf.2015.09.007

46. Warraich HJ, Maurer MS, Patel CB, Mentz RJ, Swetz KM. Top ten tips palliative care clinicians should know about caring for patients with left ventricular assist devices. *J Palliat Med*. 2019;22(4):437–441. doi:10.1089/jpm.2019.0044

47. Panke JT, Ruiz G, Elliott T, et al. Discontinuation of a left ventricular assist device in the home hospice setting. *J Pain Symptom Manage*. 2016;52(2):313–317. doi:10.1016/j.jpainsymman.2016.02.010

48. Mueller PS, Swetz KM, Freeman MR, et al. Ethical analysis of withdrawing ventricular assist device support. *Mayo Clin Proc*. 2010;85:791–797. doi:10.4065/mcp.2010.0113

49. Mehra MR, Canter CE, Hannan MM, et al. The 2016 International Society for Heart Lung Transplantation listing criteria for heart transplantation: A 10-year update. *J Heart Lung Transplant*. 2016;35(1):1–23. doi:10.1016/j.healun.2015.10.023

50. Owen MI, Braun LT, Hamilton RJ, Grady KL, Gary RA, Quest TE. Palliative care in heart transplantation. *Prog Transplant*. 2020;30(2):144–146. doi:10.1177/1526924820913521

51. Whellan DJ, Goodlin SJ, Dickinson MG, et al. End-of-life care in patients with heart failure. *J Card Fail*. 2014;20(2):121–134. doi:10.1016/j.cardfail.2013.12.003

52. Warraich HJ, Rogers JG, Dunlay SM, Hummel E, Mentz RJ. Top ten tips for palliative care clinicians caring for heart failure patients. *J Palliat Med*. 2018;21(11):1646–1650. doi:10.1089/jpm.2018.0453

53. Blinderman CD, Billings JA. Comfort care for patients dying in the hospital. Longo DL, ed. *N Engl J Med.* 2015;373(26):2549–2561. doi:10.1056/NEJMra1411746

54. Porter J, Cooper SJ, Sellick K. Attitudes, implementation and practice of family presence during resuscitation (FPDR): A quantitative literature review. *Int Emerg Nurs.* 2013;21(1):26–34. doi:10.1016/j.ienj.2012.04.002

55. Kentish-Barnes N, Davidson JE, Cox CE. Family presence during cardiopulmonary resuscitation: An opportunity for meaning-making in bereavement. *Intensive Care Med.* 2014;40(12):1954–1956. doi:10.1007/s00134-014-3396-3

56. Yancy CW, Januzzi JL Jr, Allen LA, et al. 2017 ACC expert consensus decision pathway for optimization of heart failure treatment: Answers to 10 pivotal issues about heart failure with reduced ejection fraction: A report of the American College of Cardiology Task Force on Clinical Expert Consensus Decision Pathways. *J Am Coll Cardiol.* 2018;71(2):201–230. doi:10.1016/j.jacc.2017.11.025

14.

THE PALLIATIVE APRN IN THE COMMUNITY SETTING

Nicole DePace

KEY POINTS

- The palliative advanced practice registered nurse (APRN) possesses unique skills and abilities to meet the complex needs of seriously ill patients and their caregivers in the community setting.

- The palliative APRN practices in a variety of roles in the community setting and must advocate to practice at the highest level of their ability and scope of practice.

- Models of community-based palliative care are changing and evolving quickly, and APRNs continue to struggle with scalable and sustainable reimbursement structures.

CASE STUDY 1: MULTISITE PALLIATIVE CARE

Theo is a palliative advanced practice registered nurse (APRN) working for a multisite hospice organization providing palliative consultation services to patients with advanced serious illness living in senior housing communities, assisted living facilities, and private residences in a large suburban county. On Tuesday, Theo consulted on the following patients.

- An initial or new consultation at a residence for complex pain management in a 56-year-old man with esophageal cancer who was treated with chemotherapy and radiation. The man lived at home with his partner. Theo completed a comprehensive history and physical, a holistic and comprehensive pain assessment, an opioid risk assessment and initiated opioid therapy, and a bowel regimen. He communicated the plan to the primary oncology team, provided patient and caregiver education about safe medication administration and storage, counseled about potential side effects, coordinated the opioid prescription with the community pharmacy, and communicated a plan for follow-up with the patient and his caregiver.

- A subsequent or follow-up visit in senior housing where he addressed the needs for psychosocial support and clarified the wishes for a feeding tube in a 72-year-old veteran with amyotrophic lateral sclerosis (ALS) who lived alone. Theo spent an hour in ongoing discussion and counseling with this patient about his expected disease trajectory, the benefits and risks of a feeding tube, the caregiving considerations to manage a feeding tube at home as his illness progresses, and he provided psychosocial support. Theo contacted the ALS clinic and the VA social worker at the close of the visit to coordinate a home

health referral for an in-home speech and swallow evaluation, updated the team about this patient's decisions, and advocated for increased home-based services to support his independent living in his apartment.

- Two subsequent or follow-up visits within a memory care unit of an assisted living facility (ALF) to complete discussions regarding prognosis and hospice transition in a patient with end-stage vascular dementia, and he completed advance directives with the healthcare agent of a patient with advanced Parkinson's dementia. Theo conducted two family meetings, collaborated with the nursing staff in the wellness office at the ALF community, coordinated a hospice referral with the hospice organization, completed advance directives, updated each patient's primary care provider about the outcomes of each visit, and ensured that each patient's family understood who to call for further questions.

Theo typically spends 75–120 minutes with his new patients and 45–90 minutes in each follow-up visit. Most days he sees 3–4 patients, depending on their location and the balance of new consults to follow-up visits on his schedule. He typically sees his patients for 2–3 visits before (1) they are referred to hospice or home health services, (2) symptoms are stabilized and management is taken over by the primary care team, (3) adequate counseling and education is provided to the patient, family, and care team about expected disease trajectory and prognosis, and/or (4) an advance directive is completed. Theo manages all aspects of patient care at each visit including empathetic communication and comprehensive documentation within the electronic health record (EHR). He attempted to make phone calls for coordination of care during his patient encounters or immediately after. He communicated with his program manager on a regular basis to review his schedule to cluster patients geographically and minimize his daily drive time between visits to reduce the documentation burden at the end of each day.

INTRODUCTION

Community-based palliative care (CBPC) is the integration of palliative and serious illness care outside of the acute care setting which continues to develop in terms of program design, resources, reimbursement, and emerging models. Individuals living with serious illness require holistic support focused on meeting their complex needs where they live. These patients and families need access to palliative care services that can follow them for longer periods of time and with flexible levels of intensity based on their often changing condition and needs. Failing to meet these long-term needs places patients and families at risk of unnecessary suffering, burdensome emergency room visits, and hospitalizations. Advanced practice registered nurses (APRNs) possess the necessary knowledge, skills, and abilities to provide palliative care in the community setting and are uniquely and rightly positioned to improve access to palliative care services for patients and families living with serious illness. This chapter focuses on CBPC provision in a home environment (e.g., residence, assisted living, nursing home, group home etc.) while recognizing that community-based care can and should entail any palliative care required outside of the hospital setting.

DEVELOPMENT OF PALLIATIVE CARE IN THE COMMUNITY

Every person living with serious illness deserves access to palliative care, regardless of the setting.[1] Because most patients want to receive care in their home and community, currently, CBPC serves to fill the gaps in care for seriously ill patients.[2] As CBPC matures, it may serve as the primary area of palliative care, although as CBPC programs evolve, they are designed to meet the unique characteristics of the communities they serve. Development is guided by a needs assessment of the specific community, as well as the organizational objectives and resources available to support the program's existence and growth. This flexibility has led to individual programs and services development unique to various markets. Moreover, there have been significant opportunities for the palliative APRN to serve as a direct care provider and clinical leader in this arena.

The lack of federal regulation or conditions of participation for palliative care in the community has the potential to contribute to market variability, if not confusion. Confusion may arise due to variability in program design and objectives. A majority of CBPC programs are administered by hospice and home health organizations. This can lead to misunderstanding or avoidance of using these services due to fears surrounding hospice and end-of-life care,[3] worries about services meeting homebound criteria, or having limitations in the types of treatments that would remain available to patients. It is necessary for CBPC programs to fully differentiate themselves from hospice services and home health services and not base program eligibility on prognosis or homebound criteria.[4] There is also a need to continue to educate the general public about palliative care because significant knowledge gaps exist about what palliative care is, how it is paid for, and how to access services.[3,5] The patient, family, and community education is a role that the APRN must address both informally and formally. Once patients and caregivers are educated, they may be interested in palliative care with the reassurance that decisions will be based on their needs and not their prognosis.[5]

In 2018, the National Hospice and Palliative Care Organization (NHPCO) surveyed its members and found that at least half of its organizations were providing CBPC services and another third were considering or in the process of developing services.[6] The majority of accountable care organizations (ACOs) have implemented efforts to identify their seriously ill patient populations, but only 8% were offering CBPC.[7] In 2019, the Center to Advance Palliative Care (CAPC) released *Mapping Community Palliative Care,* with 890 CBPC programs identifying themselves across the United States, and with 65% percent of these programs providing home visits.[8] This proliferation still only leaves 39% of the counties in the United States with home-visiting palliative care services.[2]

The National Consensus Project for Quality Palliative Care (NCP) *Clinical Practice Guidelines* provide best practices for palliative program structure and processes.[9] These guidelines, initially developed in 2004, are a consensus process that includes major hospice and palliative care organization, home health organizations, professional clinical organizations, and consumer organizations, and are endorsed by 100 organizations. These guidelines are widely recognized in inpatient settings, however, to date, these guidelines are less recognized in the CBPC setting. For both acute care and CBPC, there are barriers to adherence to the guidelines, especially those aimed at programs delivering fully staffed interdisciplinary teams and 24/7 availability.[10] Yet, these are the distinct characteristics of effective specialty palliative care. This is due to market variability and the inability of the fee-for-service (FFS) model to cover the cost of interdisciplinary team members. However, in the community, the nonbillable team members—nursing aides, social workers, and counselors—may be most needed.[2] It is imperative that policymakers, payers, organizations, and clinicians work to reduce the burdens of people living with serious illness. APRNs must advocate for strategies and take actions that make it easier for patients, caregivers, and healthcare providers to work together, address social service needs, and make care accessible and affordable.[11]

DISPARITY IN PALLIATIVE CARE

Further gaps in CBPC exist in meeting the needs of diverse patient populations. In 2020, the COVID-19 pandemic and social justice movements highlighted the undeniable racial and socioeconomic inequality in healthcare. This is an important moment to consider the past, present, and future of palliative care, which focuses on equitable growth and development of our services.[12] There is evidence that demonstrates lower quality palliative care for minority populations in various domains, yet there is not robust research data to describe racial disparities in nonhospice palliative care.[13] Two facts are known: (1) 82% of hospice patients identify as White[14] and (2) there are numerous structural barriers that prevent end-of-life care from being accessible and acceptable to all patients, especially racial minority and vulnerable patient populations. Moreover, LGBTQ + individuals, persons who experience homelessness, persons who are incarcerated, and individuals with comorbid substance use disorders or serious psychiatric illness are at greater risk for lower quality palliative care (see

Chapter 20, "Health Disparities," Chapter 22, "LGBTQ+ Inclusive Palliative Care," Chapter 46, "Serious Mental Illness," and Chapter 47, "Patients with Substance Use Disorder and Dual Diagnoses.") These patient populations also lack access to providers who possess the skills and knowledge to adequately address their needs and provide care that is concordant with their wishes and respects their inherent dignity.

While the individual palliative APRN may not have the immediate ability to adequately address the disparity in care to minority and vulnerable populations, they can immediately begin to identify and partner with community providers and agencies who are doing the work of caring for diverse patient populations. Palliative APRNs can forge relationships and offer consultation and education to their clinician peers to improve the primary palliative care skills of their colleagues practicing in diverse clinical settings. Palliative APRNs must be willing to learn about the structural barriers that prevent adequate palliative care services from being provided to minority and vulnerable patient populations (Box 14.1). Once informed, the palliative APRN must commit to act to remove structural barriers to access to quality palliative care for all patients. Palliative APRNs and CBPC organizations should (1) participate in diverse community activities, (2) engage in dialogue with community organizations including faith leaders and clergy, and (3) demonstrate a culture of humility, caring, and service with diverse groups.[15] Being a visible and supportive presence in the community is an essential component of CBPC and is necessary to become a trustworthy community resource for palliative care.

MODELS OF PALLIATIVE CARE IN THE COMMUNITY

CBPC fills the gap in care for patients living with serious illness and for those who have high disease burden, high healthcare utilization, and who are neither hospice eligible, hospice accepting, nor require or desire hospitalization. CBPC may focus on meeting the needs of these patients over years or the last months of their lives, depending on program structure and objectives. The reality is that, too often, patients with serious illness are not extended palliative care support until they experience a crisis and are in the hospital. This inconsistency in palliative care access leaves patients and families with little or no support to remain in their community and home setting. There has been a proliferation of community programs to meet the needs of these patients and their families. Yet not all patients with serious illness have access to reliable CBPC.

The majority of CBPC is administered by hospice and home health organizations and provided to patients in their homes, which includes assisted living communities.[6,8] Progress has been made in program development in recent years. Many CBPC teams are interdisciplinary, including some combination of APRNs, physicians, registered nurses (RNs), and social workers. Many programs report having three or more clinicians included in their CBPC teams.[6] Palliative APRNs

are most often the dedicated full-time employees for these programs.[8,16]

There are clearly identified needs for new payment models, beyond FFS payment. Most programs rely on FFS reimbursement as a single-payer source.[6] An FFS payment structure alone does not cover program expenses or take into account reimbursement for interdisciplinary care or the time-intensive and repetitive nature of the discussions required by this patient population.[2] In the FFS model, there is no reimbursement structure for spiritual care, and reimbursement is limited for social work outside of the certified home health benefit.

An increasing numbers of programs have diversified their payment structures and are pursuing contracts with payers and other risk-sharing models, such as ACOs.[17] Transitioning to other payment structures, such as case rate payment for service or per member per month models, has been suggested. Assistance with negotiation, strategic guidance, and national comparison of such payment structures and model design is necessary for programs to succeed.[2,18,21] Despite these financial challenges, when executed well, CBPC improves symptom management, improves coordination of care, and reduces unnecessary ED visits and hospitalizations in the months before death.[19,20,22] Sustainability of high-quality CBPC programs requires alignment of fiscal and quality incentives, and there is a continued need to see creative partnerships with health systems, service providers, and payers (Table 14.1).[18]

KEY ELEMENTS OF THE APRN ROLE IN THE COMMUNITY

Patients living with serious illness experience high disease-related burdens: complex and significant symptom burden, poor care coordination, poor understanding of their illness trajectory and options for care, and unmet psychosocial needs.[21,22] Frequently, CBPC programs are asked to assist with goals-of-care discussions, patient and family education, symptom management, comprehensive assessments, advance care planning, and care coordination.[6] Unfortunately, there is often poor awareness and understanding of CBPC services by non-palliative care clinicians and laypeople,[22,23] which can delay access to care. The APRN responds to the needs of this patient population with expertise in comprehensive assessment, care management and coordination, clinical management, psychosocial support of patient and family, communication about goals of care, and advance care planning and education (Table 14.2).[20,24–28]

MODELS OF COMMUNITY PALLIATIVE CARE USING APRNS

VNA CARE OF NEW ENGLAND

The VNA Care of New England (nonprofit home health and hospice agency) established a CBPC program in response to the needs of their health system. This Rhode Island health

Box 14.1 HEALTHCARE DISPARITIES IN COMMUNITY-BASED PALLIATIVE CARE

What is known:

- There is mistrust of the healthcare system and medical providers by minority and vulnerable populations that is rooted in historical mistreatment of these populations by the healthcare system and providers.[12,29,30]

- Differences in healthcare outcomes, quality of care, and access to care exist across racial and ethnic groups and other vulnerable populations.[13,29,31]

- There is documentation of lower quality palliative care for minorities across the domains of satisfaction, communication, and pain management.[13,31]

- Studies demonstrated lower rates of hospice utilization among non-White adults.[13,15]

- Research and data are minimal on disparities in the use of non-hospice palliative care in minority populations[13,31] and in other vulnerable populations.[29]

- Minority patient populations do not have equal access to pain care in the United States.[13,31]

- There are opportunities for community-based palliative care programs to improve access, reduce barriers, and reduce inequities in palliative care.[12]

What can be done to reduce and eliminate disparities in community based-palliative care:

- Provide resources and support to palliative care clinicians who care for minority and vulnerable patient populations in primary palliative care skills and on end-of-life care issues.[29]

- Promote community-based partnerships with stakeholders and leaders in minority communities, including clergy, and with community agencies without expecting a payback.[13,15,29]

- Address language barriers for specific groups of patients through the use of interpretive services in the community.[13,15]

- Evaluate and measure the racial/ethnic composition of palliative care staff, goals, and culture pertinent to diversity and inclusion.[13,15]

- Facilitate research and interventions that aim to understand and address health literacy, communication skills, and culturally specific models of care to meet the needs of diverse patient populations.[13]

What the community-based palliative APRN can do to reduce disparities:

- Provide affirmative nonjudgmental care, and approach cultural differences with humility and sensitivity.[30]

- Create a trusting relationship and safe environment for all patients and families.

- Commit to learning the historical events and context that affect current interactions of minority and vulnerable populations with healthcare providers and systems.

- Learn principles of trauma-informed care as part of professional development.

- Provide peer support to clinician colleagues who are working with minority and vulnerable populations to increase their primary palliative care skills.[16,31]

- Engage in community outreach and education to increase awareness and understanding of palliative care, advance care planning, and community bereavement resources.[13,16,17]

- Address and reduce barriers to completion of advance directives in vulnerable populations.[13,30,32]

Recommended resources to inform and improve palliative care in diverse and vulnerable communities:

- The Nurse's Pledge to Champion Diversity, Equity, and Inclusivity (https://www.aonl.org/news/nurses-diversity-equity-and-inclusivity-pledge)

- NHPCO Inclusion and Access Toolkit: Professional Development and Resources Series (https://www.nhpco.org/wp-content/uploads/Inclusion_Access_Toolkit.pdf)

- National LGBT Cancer Network (https://cancer-network.org/)

- The Conversation Project, The Other Conversation (https://theconversationproject.org/tcp-blog/the-other-conversation/)

- Us Against Alzheimer's (https://www.usagainstalzheimers.org/center-brain-health-equity)

- Humane Prison Hospice Project (https://humaneprisonhospiceproject.org/)

Table 14.1 PAYMENT MODELS FOR COMMUNITY-BASED PALLIATIVE CARE (CBPC)

	KEY FEATURES	OPPORTUNITIES	RISKS
Fee for service (FFS)	Payment based on volume of services/number of visits. Paid for by Medicare Part B and other insurers.	Accounts for the majority of CBPC Medicare payments. Well-established and understood payment structure. Any provider eligible to bill Medicare Part B can provide palliative care services in this model.	Limits billing to services provided by physicians or advance practice providers. Variations by state regarding which clinicians can be reimbursed.
FFS linked to value-based payment supplements	A portion of payment is based on the quality or efficiency of service delivery.	Providers are rewarded or penalized based on performance. Providers can self-select the quality measures they choose to report on.	There are no palliative care specialty specific measures sets. Increases the complexity and expertise needed for billing and CMS data submission. Requires Medicare certified EHR.
Alternative payment models (APMs)	Payment is based on quality and cost, structure built on FFS model.	Shared risk and payment savings shared between Medicare and accountable care organizations. Organizations can include palliative care in bundled payment. Payment corresponds to a specific condition or episode of care. Allows for interdisciplinary structure.	Program assumes financial risk for the specific condition. Most bundled payments are in early phases and therefore not as well understood by CBPC programs.
Population-based payment	Payment is determined for an episode of care for each patient assigned to a care provider.	Supports service delivery for prolonged periods of time. Allows for interdisciplinary structure.	Payment is fixed. The service provider owns financial risk for providing all palliative services with allotted payment.

Adapted from CAPC.[33]

system is comprised of hospitals, outpatient services, accountable care organization, and a community substance abuse treatment program. A catalyst for the development of the CBPC program was a taxed and overwhelmed inpatient palliative care consultation program.[24] The program relies on both the APRN and RN being allowed to operate to the full extent of their license and experience, with adequate support.

The CBPC program was designed and led by Therese Rochon, a palliative APRN responsible for program development, direct patient care, mentoring, and palliative care education for home healthcare nursing staff. The APRN used population health principles to identify patients at highest risk for hospitalization and poor prognosis. This was accomplished using data analytics software and Outcome and Assessment Information Set (OASIS) data.[24] The APRN led case conferences, provided real-time education to the nursing staff regarding disease trajectory, guided symptom management, and coached nurses about how to begin to address goals-of-care conversations with these medically frail patients. The APRN completed in-person home consultations with patients with the most complex needs and billed for services using the FFS model.

The palliative care referral stream, as built into this model, has a flow of patients across the system's continuum of care. Referrals to the palliative care program came from the inpatient team, RNs in the home health program, and primary and specialty medical providers, and from self-directed referrals from patients and families. Over the course of 5 years, the palliative care program has demonstrated a striking increase in the number of referrals to the hospice program and, more importantly, a meaningful increase in the average hospice length of stay.[24] VNA Care New England has been able to create a robust referral stream to CBPC from their community partners in care (home health nurses and physicians), meaning it is not solely dependent on the inpatient team to direct palliative care referrals.

One marker of program success is that completion of advance care planning conversations and documents increased from 8% to 78% over the course of 5 years.[24] This program has proved its ability to improve the quality of care of medically frail patients within the health system and grow the hospice program with appropriate and timely referrals. Engagement and collaboration with stakeholders across the health system have secured adequate infrastructure and support to sustain

Table 14.2 KEY ELEMENTS OF THE PALLIATIVE APRN ROLE IN THE COMMUNITY

Comprehensive assessment	Complete a comprehensive history and physical exam, a psychosocial assessment including risk for isolation, home safety evaluation, caregiver burden assessment, opioid risk assessment when appropriate.
Patient and family education	Conduct the necessary counseling to help patients and families understand the illness and its expected trajectory, prognosis, treatment options, community resources including hospice, home safety, and advance care planning. The palliative APRN has acquired advanced communication skills to ensure effective and empathetic communication with the seriously ill patient population.
Symptom management	Direct the plan of care to ensure adequate pharmacologic and nonpharmacologic management of distressing symptoms that is line with the patient's goals of care and treatment options. Ensure the patient has access to medications and treatments. Ensure an adequate plan for follow-up is established and communicated. Ensure the plan of care is patient-centered and family-focused.
Advance care planning	Conduct conversations with patients and families to determine wishes and preferences for future healthcare. Provide counseling about risks and benefits of life-prolonging medical treatment options. Document patient wishes in the medical record. Complete advance care planning documents including: a) surrogate decision maker forms- healthcare proxy forms, durable power of attorney forms, b) advance directives or living wills c) out of hospital orders for living sustaining treatments -POLST/MOLST forms, do-not-resuscitate orders. Repeat conversations and update documentations as frequently as necessary based on the patient's changing condition and priorities.
Care coordination	Facilitate communication between primary and specialty providers, direct referrals to home health and hospice, direct referrals to community service providers. Refer to and collaborate with interdisciplinary team (IDT) members, meet with IDT on a scheduled basis to review and update the plan of care to meet the patient's changing needs.
Community outreach	Informally or formally engage in community education about palliative care and advance care planning. Provide peer support to non-palliative care clinicians in primary palliative care skills. Form relationships with community service providers.

MOLST, medical orders for life-sustaining treatment; POLST, physician orders for life-sustaining treatment.

Adapted from Melhado[34]; Rotundo[35]; Frier[36]; and Dahlin.[37]

the program. The palliative APRN was successful in this program because institutional barriers to practice to the full extent of licensure and education (within the context of state and federal regulations) were removed.

PALLIATIVE CARE HOMEBOUND PROGRAM

The Mayo Clinic Palliative Care Homebound Program (PCHP) in Rochester, Minnesota, is an ACO-funded program focusing on the palliative care needs of a high-risk, frail, homebound population. Patients served in this program had higher rates of moderate to advanced dementia.[38] The interdisciplinary team consisted of nurse practitioners (NPs), RNs, and physicians. One RN was assigned to two NPs, and the team met with the physician weekly. The program also had access to the system's geriatricians, social services department, case managers, and pharmacists.

Each full-time NP was responsible for 20–35 high-acuity patients. This program aimed to provide early palliative care and has the capacity to care for this patient population in the months to years leading up to the terminal phase of their illness, when hospice would become appropriate. The NPs provided scheduled and acute in-home visits. Physicians were available for consultation and more limited home visitation. The program was committed to providing NP visits for acute symptom management needs within 24 hours. Additional

responsibilities included chronic disease management, home safety assessments, care coordination, goals of care, and advance care planning conversations.

PCHP reduced annual Medicare expenditures by $18,251 per program participant compared with matched control patients.[39] Patients enrolled in this program had high rates of advance directive completion, documentation of frequent discussions regarding goals of care, decreased hospitalization rates, and fewer overall days spent in the hospital setting. Additionally, the team provided patient and family education and support.[38] This model demonstrated significant financial value, and the quality outcomes for patients were striking and contributed to more time at home with a higher quality of life. This model of a CBPC allowed NPs to function as primary palliative care providers in the home and delivered interdisciplinary high-value care to high-risk older adults (Table 14.3).

APRN ROLES IN COMMUNITY-BASED PALLIATIVE CARE

APRNs may practice in CBPC settings that do not support their practice within the full scope of their role as either an NP or a clinical nurse specialist (CNS) (see Chapters 2 and 3). They may function as a program coordinator, liaison between providers, educator, in telephonic management, and/or as support to patients and families. Successful CBPC programs rely

Table 14.3 COMPARING AND CONTRASTING TWO CBPC MODELS USING APRNS

	VNA CARE NEW ENGLAND	MAYO CLINIC HOMEBOUND PROGRAM
Organizational structure	Nonprofit home-health and hospice agency within a regional health system	Accountable care organization (ACO)
Role of APRN	Program design and leadership Leads case conference and interdisciplinary team (IDT) meetings Staff education and development Consultant for symptom management, advance care planning (ACP), and goals of care	Primary care provider for frail, homebound patients Chronic disease management Acute and chronic symptom management ACP, goals of care, care coordination
Payment/Funding source	Medicare Part B fee-for-service (FFS) billing Indirect revenue related to hospice transitions	ACO funding
Key outcomes	High completion rate of ACP conversations and documents Referrals from across the health system to the palliative care program Increase in referrals to hospice Increase of hospice length of stay	High completion rates of ACP conversation and documents Significant reduction in Medicare spending Frequent goals of care conversations Decreased hospitalizations and fewer days in hospital
Benefits	Access to IDT Sustainability through indirect financial benefit to hospice Leadership opportunity for APRN	Nurse practitioner (NP) and registered nurse (RN) partnership Access to physician, geriatrician pharmacist, social service consultants Early palliative care involvement allowed NP to care for patients for months to years
Challenges	Model is not sustainable without indirect hospice revenue Adequate support for Medicare Part B billing and support Differentiation of CBPC from hospice	Model is not sustainable without ACO funding Financial risk for program if outcomes are not favorable

Adapted from Rochon, Emard[24]; Chen et al.[38,39]

on the APRN's full scope of practice and expertise[17,19,20,25,38] and benefit from the APRN's comprehensive clinical assessment and consideration of all aspects of the patient's illness, including psychosocial distress and functional capabilities.[26,27] Patients with serious illness often experience fluctuating and protracted disease trajectories with needs that can change frequently over time. APRNs in CBPC provide insight into home environments, barriers to successful self-management, and caregiver function, and create patient and family-centered plans of care. These complex patients require a team of providers to address their diverse needs, and the APRN is central to care coordination, collaboration, and providing specialty-level palliative care in the home setting.

CARE MANAGEMENT AND COORDINATION

CASE STUDY 2: COMPREHENSIVE ASSESSMENT

Ben was an 84-year-old man with end-stage renal disease on hemodialysis, congestive heart failure (CHF), chronic obstructive pulmonary disease, diabetes, and transient ischemic attacks. Ben initiated dialysis in the setting of increasingly difficult to manage fluid volume status and diuretic resistance. Initially, dialysis helped to reduce the number of hospitalizations for his CHF, and he felt dialysis was beneficial. He continued to make urine and his course was complicated by urinary retention and frequent complex urinary tract infections. His daughter, who was his primary healthcare agent, expressed distress around medical decision-making and balancing caring for her parents and her school-age children. Ben was hospitalized three times in 6 months for several healthcare issues and expressed increasing distress about being separated from his family. Following the third hospitalizations, Ben was referred by his primary care physician to the palliative APRN for consultation to assist with clarifying the goals of medical care and coordination of care. The APRN was able to provide a comprehensive assessment of Ben's physical, social, and psychological needs and explore the caregiver's source and level of distress. Through a series of conversations, the APRN was able to elicit Ben's goals to live for as long as he could if he was able to spend more days at home and if he could ensure adequate help at home without feeling that he was burdening his children. He was also able to identify that he would not want to live for as long as he could if he lost his ability to eat his favorite foods or walk to the bathroom. Through coordination of care with his multiple medical providers, home health clinicians, and his dialysis center, the APRN was able to guide Ben's decision-making around outpatient tests and treatment that were tolerable and in line with his goals. A referral was placed to social work to assist with resource connection and additional family counseling and support.

Ben was able to remain at home for the next 18 months, with only one hospitalization and continuation of his dialysis treatment. His daughter expressed feeling relieved and better prepared to meet the needs of his changing functional status and increased personal caregiving needs. Unfortunately, Ben suffered from a stroke during dialysis treatment and was hospitalized. Once the effects of the stroke were understood by Ben's children, they were able to decide for Ben to return home with hospice services and focus his care on comfort. Ben died peacefully at home with his children and wife at his bedside.

A critical role of the palliative APRN is aligning the patient's treatment options with their goals of care and helping patients and families prepare for eventual decline or complications from their illness. The APRN must recognize that patients with organ failure experience disease-related burdens similar to patients with metastatic cancer yet often do not have access to early palliative care services.[28] These patients are less likely to have adequate information about their disease and do not always fully understand their prognosis and treatment options.[21,28] This patient population is at greater risk for acute high-burden symptoms and caregiver burden.[21] The CBPC palliative APRN can spend time with these patients and families and address goals of care and crisis planning, place timely referrals, and support proxy decision-makers.

COMMUNICATION AND EDUCATION

CASE STUDY 3: ADVANCE CARE PLANNING

Jennie was a 93-year-old woman with advanced vascular dementia who had been hospitalized four times in the past 5 months for complications related to her frail status and advancing dementia. The palliative APRN was asked to see Jennie by her home care RN to help Jennie's daughter with advance care planning and education regarding the dementia disease process. The home care RN expressed feeling frustrated that despite frequent education, she could not seem to get through to Jennie's daughter about the progression of Jennie's dementia.

The palliative APRN planned a co-visit with the home care RN. The APRN found that Jennie has been bed-bound for 2 years since a stroke left her unable to walk. She was incontinent, had chronic lower extremity contractures, and was lovingly hand-fed by her daughter for each meal. Through a process of obtaining a history from Jennie's daughter and discussion about what the daughter understands about Jennie's dementia, it became clear that Jennie's daughter did not understand her mother's illness. She revealed that Jennies' husband (her father) died of Lewy body dementia, and that was a very different experience. She also revealed that her dad died very quickly in the hospital of pneumonia after aspirating

at home, and she continues to worry that she missed something or waited too long to seek help for her dad.

Over a series of three home visits, the palliative APRN provided counseling and education to Jennie's daughter about vascular dementia, its expected trajectory and complications, options for managing complications in the home setting, expert consensus statements on the use of feeding tubes in a person with advanced dementia, and hospice services. The palliative APRN coached the home care RN about indicators for hospice eligibility and communication strategies to provide follow-up education and support to Jennie's daughter. The palliative APRN managed Jennie's symptoms, supported the home care RN, and completed advance directives. At the third and final visit with the APRN, the daughter expressed readiness for hospice transition and relief from her worry about not providing adequate care to her mom. Jennie remained at home, comfortable and lovingly cared for her by her dedicated daughter for the remaining months of her life.

One of the most important functions of an APRN is the ability to understand complex pathophysiology, prognostic indicators, and treatment options and to integrate this information into the context of the unique patient and family system. The palliative APRN has a specialized ability to see the "big picture" and to communicate this information in a way that can be understood by the patient, family, and other clinicians. The palliative APRN can model empathetic and honest communication strategies and coach other clinicians in providing manageable "chunks" of information to assist patients and families in their understanding of and coping with the progression of a serious illness. The palliative APRN is versatile in their ability to respond to emotional cues and continue to engage in conversations that are difficult but necessary to provide patient-centered care and honor patient's wishes. In the third case study, Jennie exhibited signs of disease progression and complications associated with nearing the end of life. The palliative APRN provided a comprehensive assessment of the physical, social, and emotional needs of Jennie, her daughter, and the RN. This led to the development of a plan of care that was patient-centered, honored Jennie's wishes, addressed the caregiver's needs, and allowed Jennie to remain in her home through the end of her life.

Many community RNs express a lack of confidence or uncertainty in communicating with patients and families regarding disease trajectory or about initiating conversations about advance care planning.[24,40] Having the ability to request the consultation of a palliative APRN to assist in the care of these patients at home is invaluable to patients and families and to the nursing staff who have the most frequent contact and are responsible for direct care provision.

Patients with dementia are less likely to receive specialist-level palliative care despite disease and symptom burdens that are similar to or greater than that of patients with cancer, especially as they near end of life.[41,42] There is often a lack of understanding of the progressive and ultimately terminal nature of the disease and higher levels of functional impairment and caregiver distress, and end-of-life decision-making is likely to be made by a proxy decision-maker.[26] Emergency department use at end of life is associated with poor quality of care and with reduced quality of life for people living with dementia.[41] Acute care encounters are associated with negative consequences for the patient population in advanced disease. Unfortunately, as many as 70% of people with dementia will visit an ED in the last year of life, and the risk increases as they get closer to death.[43] Involvement of CBPC in the care of people with dementia allows for timely access to counseling and education about the disease process and expected complications of the illness, establishing and continuous evaluation of the goals of care, treatment of recurring symptoms in the home setting, and care coordination.[44] Providing access to CBPC in this patient population has been shown to prevent avoidable ED encounters and hospital admissions, especially as people living with dementia approach end of life,[43,44] and better-coordinated care.[40]

SYMPTOM MANAGEMENT AND ADVANCE CARE PLANNING

CASE STUDY 4: COMPLEX SYMPTOM MANAGEMENT

Michelle was a 50-year-old woman with metastatic breast cancer. She had been living with her cancer illness for 12 years and had undergone numerous treatment lines and clinical trials. She was married and had a 10-year-old daughter. Her Jewish faith was important to her, and she expressed her belief that all life is sacred. She wanted to pursue all treatment options available to preserve her life and to be present for her daughter for as long as possible. She had new brain metastases that caused her to experience seizures and headaches and new bony metastases in her right ribs and thoracic spine, necessitating a course of palliative radiation.

The palliative APRN was asked to see her by the primary oncology team to assist with complex symptom management and coordination of care. The APRN met Michelle at home, during the context of the COVID-19 pandemic. Michelle had not seen her primary oncologist in person for 2 months, and the majority of her care had been coordinated by telehealth encounters. In preparation for the initial home visit, the palliative APRN spoke with the oncologist who shared that there were no additional cancer-directed treatments available to Michelle and felt the best plan for Michelle would be a transition to hospice care at home. The oncologist had difficulty initiating this conversation with Michelle and her husband and worried about the effects of doing so during a telehealth consultation. The palliative APRN provided hands-on assessment of Michelle's symptoms and assessed the family dynamics and the ability to manage symptoms in the home setting. Michelle's husband was a paramedic and expressed comfort with performing personal care and medication management. His biggest worry was managing further seizure activity.

A trusting relationship was built with the APRN over a course of weeks, symptom management was optimized, and an emergency plan was developed for both a pain crisis and breakthrough seizure activity. Michelle and her husband agreed to let the palliative APRN coordinate a co-visit with the oncologist via a telehealth consult. Michelle expressed that she would not want to die at home and wanted to focus on living for as long as possible, even if life-support were required. The palliative APRN and the oncologist were able to discuss options for hospital admission if there was uncontrollable seizure activity or symptoms become too much to manage at home. They discussed a plan to include the inpatient palliative care team if Michelle was admitted to the hospital. Michelle and her husband agreed with the APRN's recommendation to seek counsel from their Rabbi regarding Jewish teaching and end-of-life decision-making.

The goal of CBPC is to address the needs of patients and families living with serious illness and provide patient-driven family-centered care. The art of this practice is to meet patients where they are, to make good use of the resources at hand, and to build trust and help patients and families fully understand their options. Patients with advanced and terminal cancer may have significant fear and difficulty accepting their prognosis or approaching death.[45] APRNs can be effective in assessing and understanding the patient's complex psychological and spiritual experiences. Community clergy often minister to patients and families suffering during a terminal illness,[46] and the APRN must be aware of this. An opportunity exists for APRNs in CBPC to engage with community clergy to build informal networks and explore their educational needs around palliative and end-of-life care. An expressed desire by community clergy for end-of-life care provides palliative APRNs an opportunity to apply the NCP *Clinical Practice Guidelines* for interdisciplinary care and create informal networks of spiritual care services for their patients.[9,46]

PRACTICING AT FULL SCOPE AND ABILITY

CASE STUDY 5: PROGRAM DEVELOPMENT

Lucia was an APRN employed by a system-based hospice and palliative care organization. Her organization had been awarded a 3-year grant to implement a population health model of CBPC care delivery. The focus of this project was to meet the palliative care needs of a high-morbidity patient population. Lucia took on the role of palliative care coordinator for a team of two RNs, one social worker, and a very part-time physician. She was responsible for care delivery and oversight of the team's ability to provide patient and caregiver outreach, consults for prognostication and hospice eligibility, complex symptom management, and running the weekly interdisciplinary team meeting. In her first year in the role, she was able to implement team-based training and establish program metrics. The program demonstrated a reduction in hospital admissions, but not ED encounters. The program also showed an increase in referrals to the hospice program. Lucia identified confusion among non–palliative care clinicians (physicians and nurses) regarding the differences between hospice and palliative care, which led to a reluctance to refer patients to the palliative care program. The benefits of the program to the system

Table 14.4 OPERATIONAL CONSIDERATIONS OF CBPC

	FOCUS	DESCRIBE	ROLE OF THE APRN
Clinical care model and patient population	Determine consultation only, co-management, primary care, or some combination of these models. Define referral criteria and patient population.	Define whether consultations will result in recommendations only, prescriptive authority, or taking on primary care responsibility for the patient. Medicare Part B billing criteria requires that a written request for consultation is provided by the referring provider. The program may receive referrals from a variety of sources including community primary care providers (PCPs), specialty providers, hospital discharge planning staff, complex care and transition management coordinators, and home care services, as well as patients and caregivers themselves.	Adheres to state practice requirements. Establishes collaborative relationships with referral sources and community organizations. Communicates with the PCP if the referral was not initiated by the PCP.
Patient eligibility	May differ between programs.	Criteria often include adults with serious illness and need for: Complex pain and symptom management Advance care planning Establishing or clarifying goals of care Risk for burnout of caregiver of frail elder.	Provides in-person evaluation of patient's clinical presentation, healthcare utilization, and psychosocial needs to best determine their level of acuity and complexity.
Patient encounters	Ensure continuity and individualized care.	Time and frequency will be determined by program design and patient needs.	Explains palliative care and the role of the APRN. Determines and communicates a plan for subsequent, follow-up care.
Catchment area	A determining factor in caseload and visits per day	Travel time may restrict productivity, should be regionalized whenever possible.	Communicates needs to program manager or coordinator to balance productivity, quality, and safety.
Visit preparation	Ensuring access to adequate clinical information.	Depending on practice structure, the APRN may review records from a variety of sources (e.g., electronic health record, fax or scanned documents, phone or email communication, etc.).	Ensures an adequate understanding of the patient's history, current situation and expectations of the referring provider to ensure safe and satisfying care.
Communication	Provide safe, comprehensive, and well-understood care.	Comprehensive assessments are documented in the electronic health record. Patients, families, and clinicians will have access to contact information for the CBPC program and know how and when to contact the APRN.	Provides verbal and written communication to referring provider/agency. Clinical notes are finished in a timely manner. Coordinates and communicates with IDT and community organizations. Documents advance directives in the patient record and shared with referring providers/agencies.

Adapted from Meier et al.[33]; Melhado[34]; Dahlin.[37]

were demonstrable, and Lucia advocated for the addition of another APRN to the team. This allowed for more focus on complex pain and symptom management and more timely consultation for prognostication and hospice transition planning. With this additional resource, the program was better able to meet the needs of the patient population and plan for targeted education to clinicians in the system to help increase the understanding of the palliative care program and increase referrals. In preparation for the second year of the program, the APRN made plans to meet with the organization's data analytics, business development leaders, and clinical operations stakeholders to evaluate the program's current progress and reach consensus on additional metrics that can be measured to demonstrate the sustainability of the program.

To ensure the future of APRNs' contributions to healthcare, the workforce must be able to protect and advance the APRN role. Palliative APRNs in all settings, including those outside of academic settings, must be allowed to overcome the threats to their scope of practice, reimbursement, and full practice authority.[47] The work of CBPC palliative APRNs needs to be visible, and their accomplishments need to be publicized (Table 14.4).[47]

OPERATIONAL CONSIDERATIONS OF PALLIATIVE CARE IN THE COMMUNITY

INITIATING CARE

CBPC programs must be clear about the services they are offering to referring providers: consultation only, co-management, primary care, or some combination of these options. It is important to establish the prescribing capabilities and responsibilities of the program. Referrals to palliative care programs can be received from a variety of sources, including community primary care providers, specialty providers, hospital discharge planning staff, complex care and transition management coordinators, and home care services, as well as patients and caregivers themselves. Medicare Part B and most managed care payer source referrals require a form request/order from the requesting provider to receive payment for services rendered. Proper consultation etiquette suggests that the primary care provider be alerted if he or she has not initiated the referral. This establishes collaboration, which is an important aspect of any home palliative care program. Referrals should be managed by a clinically trained professional to assess eligibility and triage symptom management concerns and psychosocial needs.

The criteria for patient eligibility for palliative care differ between programs and are influenced by the needs of the local community. Criteria often include adults with serious illness including metastatic and progressing cancer, organ failure, and dementia. Eligibility for palliative care should take into consideration the patient's clinical presentation, healthcare utilization, and psychosocial needs to best determine his or her level of acuity and complexity.

PATIENT ENCOUNTERS

The patient's length of stay in a palliative care program depends on symptom burden, disease progression, and the psychosocial needs of the patient and family. Program design will also determine the length of stay on the CBPC program. Some initial consults may only require one visit due to an immediate transition to hospice. Visit frequency for each patient varies and should be determined at each appointment depending on the patient's current clinical and psychosocial needs as well as the staffing and resources of each practice. Visits can be scheduled between appointments with the patient's primary care provider or specialist to maintain continuity of care.

The amount of time spent completing initial palliative care consults and subsequent visits depends on the complexity and acuteness of the patient's needs. On meeting the patient and family for the first time, the palliative APRN explains the palliative care home-based service and clarifies the APRN's role. A working relationship with the patient and family is subsequently established, with the focus of care being patient-centered and patient-driven. With this approach, patients often prioritize their greatest health concerns early in the visit. Time is allowed for patients to describe their experience of living with chronic illness, their coping mechanisms, and their life's journey.

EFFECTS OF CATCHMENT AREA

Geography is an important consideration for both the size of caseload and the number of visits per day. In addition to the length of time spent with each patient, the travel time between patients restricts the number of patient visits each day. Travel time is affected by whether the catchment area is urban, suburban, or rural. Practices with multiple providers should consider regionalizing providers to improve efficiency and in consideration of quality-of-life factors for staff.

PREPARATION AND COMMUNICATION

To make safe and beneficial clinical decisions, the palliative APRN practicing in the home setting must have access to adequate clinical information. Practicing in the home environment presents unique challenges in that it is not a controlled environment and can be unpredictable. Preparation is key for efficient and safe encounters. Preparation involves reviewing the patient's medical record and communicating with providers to clearly understand the patient's overall situation and the expectations of the consultation by the referring provider. The palliative APRN should have access to pertinent primary and medical specialty notes, recent hospital or ED discharge summaries, lab results and diagnostic reports, and medication lists before making in-home visits. A copy of the palliative APRN's consultation note should be sent to the referring provider after each encounter. This is a core component of consultation etiquette and is required to meet conditions for FFS billing.

Specialty-level palliative care consultation notes should be comprehensive and illustrate the holistic and comprehensive assessments and unique characteristics of palliative assessments. In the community setting, it is especially important to ensure that notes include detailed information about symptom status, cognitive status, functional and nutritional status, home safety and fall history, caregiver status and community supports, goals of care, and advance care planning discussions and documents.

Per the NCP *Clinical Practice Guidelines*, the palliative care team should meet regularly to discuss and collaborate on difficult cases.[9] Team meetings provide an opportunity for interdisciplinary teams to discuss and address complex issues, identify referral resources for care coordination, and establish plans to address caregiver distress. Team meetings also offer opportunities to address conflicts in care and maintain team and professional caregiver wellness (Box 14.2).

SUMMARY

Palliative APRNs are instrumental in providing comprehensive care for patients with serious illness. Their advanced education and nursing experience allow them to bring a unique patient-centered approach to care into the home environment.

Box 14.2 APRN CONSIDERATIONS FOR CBPC HOME VISITING PROGRAM DESIGN

Patient Population

- Needs assessment of the community and organization/health system
- Community assessment of demographics and resources
- Analysis of potential patient populations (e.g., by risk, diagnosis, prognosis)
- Geographic catchment area

Palliative Care Service Delivery

- Model of clinical responsibility of the palliative care service: Consultative, co-management, primary provider, or mix of all three
- Coverage and Accessibility for After hours – evenings, weekends and holidays coverage of patients (by palliative care team or covering team)
- Scheduling: Frequency and duration of patient encounters
- Staffing of team members: Clinical staff, interdisciplinary team, and administrative support staff
- Design a comprehensive palliative care clinical note

Types of Services

- Management of physical needs - Pain and symptom management
- Management of psychological, spiritual, emotional needs of the patient and caregiver
- Skilled communication and support for complex medical decision making
- Advance care planning and goals of care conversations and advocacy for care delivery congruent with these conversations
- Conversations in context of culture, ethnicity and religion to reduce disparities of care
- Care coordination and management of quality transitions of care
- Medication management, reconciliation, and monitoring
- Planning for end-of-life care, with appropriate and timely referral to hospice when requested by the patient and family
- 24/7 accessibility to palliative care expertise and staff

Community Collaboration

- Establishment of relationships with primary care and specialty health providers
- Establishment of relationships with community services: Elder service programs, community alternative programs, community clergy, parish nurses, behavioral health service providers, legal services, interpreter services, transportation services, respite services, home health agencies, hospices
- Education to community partners: Address fears about hospice directly
- Education to lay community: Address fears related to prognosis and treatment directly

Administrative

- Electronic health record implementation and integration
- Reimbursement process
- Development of data and metrics by which to measure success and support financial viability
- Staff continuing education, certification, and retention

Adapted from Fitzgerald et al.[48]

The palliative APRN provides individualized care through undivided attention and understanding of the complexity of serious illness, support systems, and home environment. Providing care to someone in their home is intimate, and the palliative APRN is successful in the environment by offering continuity of care, support, and trust. This unique relationship and setting allow for meaningful conversations regarding a patient's values and wishes. Palliative APRNs improve the quality of life of patients with serious illness by managing complex symptoms, addressing psychosocial needs, providing counseling and education, discussing goals care over time as needs change, and reducing the frequency of burdensome and unnecessary transitions. Functioning to the full extent of education, licensure, and skill is integral to the ability of the APRN in CBPC to expand the opportunities to meet the needs of patients and families living with serious illness at home.

REFERENCES

1. Meghani S, Hinds P. Policy brief: The institute of medicine report dying in America: Improving quality and honoring individual preferences near the end of life. *Nurs Outlook*. 2015;63(1):51–59. doi:10.1016/j.outlook.2014.11.007
2. Bowman B, Twohig J, Meier D. Overcoming barriers to growth in home-based palliative care. *J Palliat Med*. 2019;22(4):408–412. doi:10.1089/jpm.2018.0478
3. Boucher N, Bull J, Cross S, Kirby C, Davis J, Taylor D. Patient, caregiver, and taxpayer knowledge of palliative care and views on a model of community-based palliative care. *J Pain Symptom Manage*. 2018;56(6):951–956. doi:10.1016/j.jpainsymman.2018.08.007
4. Rahman A. Let's not muddle the message about home-and community-based palliative care. *Health Aff*. 2019. doi:10.1377/hblog20190206.338341
5. Center to Advance Palliative Care. Public Opinion Research Key Findings. New York, NY: CAPC. Updated April 15, 2021. https://www.capc.org/documents/651/
6. National Hospice and Palliative Care Organization. Palliative care needs survey results. Alexandria, VA: National Hospice and Palliative Care Organization. 2018. https://www.nhpco.org/wp-content/uploads/2019/04/Palliative_Care_Needs_Report_NHPCO.pdf
7. Bleser W, Saunders R, Winfield L et al. ACO serious illness care: Survey and case studies depict current challenges and future opportunities. *Health Aff*. 2019;38(6):1011–1020. doi:10.1377/hlthaff.2019.00013
8. Center to Advance Palliative Care. Mapping community palliative care -A Sanpshot. New York, NY: Center to Advance Palliative Care. 2019. https://www.capc.org/mapping-community-palliative-care/
9. National Consensus Project for Quality Palliative Care. *Clinical Practice Guidelines for Quality Palliative Care*. 4th ed. Richmond, VA: National Coalition for Hospice and Palliative Care; 2018. https://www.nationalcoalitionhpc.org/ncp
10. Rogers M, Meier D, Heitner R et al. The national palliative care registry: A decade of supporting growth and sustainability of palliative care programs. *J Palliat Med*. 2019;22(9):1026–1031. doi:10.1089/jpm.2019.0262
11. Schneider E, Abrams M, Shah A, Lewis C, Shah T. Healthcare in America: The experience of people with serious illness. New York, NY: Commonwealth Fund. 2018. https://www.commonwealthfund.org/sites/default/files/2018-10/Schneider_HealthCareinAmerica.pdf
12. Nelson K, Wright R, Fisher M et al. A call to action to address disparities in palliative care access: A conceptual framework for individualizing care needs. *J Palliat Med*. 2020. doi:10.1089/jpm.2020.0435
13. Johnson K. Racial and ethnic disparities in palliative care. *J Palliat Med*. 2013;16(11):1329–1334. doi:10.1089/jpm.2013.9468
14. National Hospice and Palliative Care Organization. NHPCO facts and figures 2020 ed. Alexandria, VA: National Hospice and Palliative Care Organization. August 20. 2020. https://www.nhpco.org/wp-content/uploads/NHPCO-Facts-Figures-2020-edition.pdf
15. National Hospice and Palliative Care Organization. Inclusion and access tool kit. Professional development and resource series. Alexandria, VA: National Hospice and Palliative Care Organization. October 2020. https://www.nhpco.org/wp-content/uploads/Inclusion_Access_Toolkit.pdf
16. Ernecoff N, Hanson L, Fox A, Daaleman T, Kistler C. Palliative care in a community-based serious-illness care program. *J Palliat Med*. 2020;23(5):692–697. doi:10.1089/jpm.2019.0174
17. Yosick L, Crook R, Gatto M et al. Effects of a population health community-based palliative care program on cost and utilization. *J Palliat Med*. 2019;22(9):1075–1081. doi:10.1089/jpm.2018.0489
18. Cassel J, Kerr K, Kalman N, Smith T. The business case for palliative care: Translating research into program development in the U.S. *J Pain Symptom Manage*. 2015;50(6):741–749. doi:10.1016/j.jpainsymman.2015.06.013
19. Ruiz S, Snyder L, Rotondo C, Cross-Barnet C, Colligan E, Giuriceo K. Innovative home visit models associated with reductions in costs, hospitalizations, and emergency department use. *Health Aff*. 2017;36(3):425–432. doi:10.1377/hlthaff.2016.1305
20. Coppa D, Winchester S, Roberts M. Home-based nurse practitioners demonstrate reductions in rehospitalizations and emergency department visits in a clinically complex patient population through an academic–clinical partnership. *J Am Assoc Nurse Pract*. 2018;30(6):335–343. doi:10.1097/jxx.0000000000000060
21. Kavalieratos D, Kamal A, Abernethy A et al. Comparing unmet needs between community-based palliative care patients with heart failure and patients with cancer. *J Palliat Med*. 2014;17(4):475–481. doi:10.1089/jpm.2013.0526
22. Siler S, Mamier I, Winslow B. The perceived facilitators and challenges of translating a lung cancer palliative care intervention into community-based settings. *J Hospice Palliat Nurs*. 2018, 20(4):407–415. doi:10.1097/njh.0000000000000470. PMID: 30063635; PMCID: PMC6070356.
23. Singh G, Ramjan L, Ferguson C, Davidson P, Newton P. Access and referral to palliative care for patients with chronic heart failure: A qualitative study of healthcare professionals. *J Clin Nurs*. 2020;29(9–10):1576–1589. doi:10.1111/jocn.15222
24. Rochon T, Emard E. End-of-life care: Redesigning access through leveraging the institute of medicine future of nursing recommendations. *Home Healthc Now*. 2019;37(4):208–212.
25. Constantine L, Dichiacchio T, Falkenstine E, Moss A. Nurse practitioners' completion of physician orders for scope of treatment forms in West Virginia. *J Am Assoc Nurse Pract*. 2018;30(1):10–16. doi:10.1097/jxx.0000000000000012
26. Collins C, Small S. The nurse practitioner role is ideally suited for palliative care practice: A qualitative descriptive study. *Can Oncol Nurs J*. 2019;29(1):4–9. doi:10.5737/2368807629149
27. Howell D, Hardy B, Boyd C, Ward C, Roman E, Johnson M. Community palliative care clinical nurse specialists: A descriptive study of nurse–patient interactions. *Int J Palliat Nurs*. 2014;20(5):246–253. doi:10.12968/ijpn.2014.20.5.246
28. Watson S, Yeboah W. The role of the renal palliative care clinical nurse specialist. *J Renal Nurs*. 2013;5(5):258–261.
29. Huynh L, Henry B, Dosani N. Minding the gap: Access to palliative care and the homeless. *BMC Palliat Care*. 2015;14(1):62. Published 2015 Nov 18. doi:10.1186/s12904-015-0059-2
30. Haviland K, Burrows Walters C, Newman S. Barriers to palliative care in sexual and gender minority patients with cancer: A scoping review of the literature. *Health Soc Care Community*. 2020. doi:10.1111/hsc.13126

31. Smith C, Brawley O. Health equity disparities in access to palliative care. *Health Affairs Blog.* 2014. doi:10.1377/hblog20140730.040327

32. Rosa W, Shook A, Acquaviva K. LGBTQ + inclusive palliative care in the context of covid-19: Pragmatic recommendations for clinicians. *J Pain Symptom Manage.* 2020;60(2):e44–e47. doi:10.1016/j.jpainsymman.2020.04.155

33. Meier D, Bowman B, Collins K, Dahlin C, Sheils Twohig J. *Palliative Care in the Home: A Guide to Program Design.* New York: Center to Advance Palliative Care; 2016. https://www.capc.org/shop/palliative-care-in-the-home-a-guide-to-program-design_3/

34. Melhado L. The nursing process in palliative care. In: Dahlin C, Tycon Moreines L, Root M, eds. *Core Curriculum for the Hospice and Palliative APRN.* 3rd ed. Pittsburgh, PA: Hospice and Palliative Nurses Association; 2020: 3–13.

35. Rotundo E. Communication in advanced palliative nursing practice. In: Dahlin C, Tycone Moreines L, Root M, eds. *Core Curriculum for the Hospice and Palliative APRN.* 3rd ed. Pittsburgh, PA: Hospice and Palliative Nurses Association; 2020: 691–702.

36. Frier K. Advance Care Planning. In: Dahlin C, Tycone Moreines L, Root M, eds. *Core Curriculum for the Hospice And Palliative APRN.* 3rd ed. Pittsburgh, PA: Hospice and Palliative Nurses Association; 2020: 705–714.

37. Dahlin C. National Guidelines and APRN Practice. In: Dahlin C, Tycone Moreines L, Root M, eds. *Core Curriculum for the Hospice and Palliative APRN.* 3rd ed. Pittsburgh, PA: Hospice and Palliative Nurses Association; 2020: 773–779.

38. Chen C, Thorsteinsdottir B, Cha S et al. Health care outcomes and advance care planning in older adults who receive home-based palliative care: A pilot cohort study. *J Palliat Med.* 2015;18(1):38–44. doi:10.1089/jpm.2014.0150

39. Chen C, Naessens J, Takahashi P et al. Improving value of care for older adults with advanced medical illness and functional decline: Cost analyses of a home-based palliative care program. *J Pain Symptom Manage.* 2018;56(6):928–935. doi:10.1016/j.jpainsymman.2018.08.015

40. Smith C, Newbury G. Palliative care for community patients diagnosed with dementia: A systematic review. *Br J Community Nurs.* 2019;24(12):570–575. doi:10.12968/bjcn.2019.24.12.570

41. Rosenwax L, Spilsbury K, Arendts G, McNamara B, Semmens J. Community-based palliative care is associated with reduced emergency department use by people with dementia in their last year of life: A retrospective cohort study. *Palliat Med.* 2015;29(8):727–736. doi:10.1177/0269216315576309

42. Martinsson L, Lundström S, Sundelöf J. Quality of end-of-life care in patients with dementia compared to patients with cancer: A population-based register study. *PLoS One.* 2018;13(7):e0201051. doi:10.1371/journal.pone.0201051

43. Harrison K, Bull J, Garrett S et al. Community-based palliative care consultations: Comparing dementia to nondementia serious illnesses. *J Palliat Med.* 2020;23(8):1021–1029. doi:10.1089/jpm.2019.0250

44. Spilsbury K, Rosenwax L. Community-based specialist palliative care is associated with reduced hospital costs for people with non-cancer conditions during the last year of life. *BMC Palliat Care.* 2017;16(1):1–12. doi:10.1186/s12904-017-0256-2

45. Kyota A, Kanda K. How to come to terms with facing death: A qualitative study examining the experiences of patients with terminal cancer. *BMC Palliat Care.* 2019;18(1):33. doi:10.1186/s12904-019-0417-6. PMID: 30947725; PMCID: PMC6449951.

46. LeBaron V, Smith P, Quiñones R et al. How community clergy provide spiritual care: Toward a conceptual framework for clergy end-of-life education. *J Pain Symptom Manage.* 2016;51(4):673–681. doi:10.1016/j.jpainsymman.2015.11.016

47. Berg J, Ruppert S. Fostering promotion and protection of the professional nurse practitioner role. *J Am Assoc Nurse Pract.* 2019;31(1):3–5. doi:10.1097/jxx.0000000000000180

48. Fitzgerald G, Naugle M, Wolf J. The Palliative Advanced Practice Registered Nurse in the Home Setting. In: Dahlin C, Coyne P, Ferrell B, eds. *Advanced Practice Palliative Nursing.* 1st ed. New York: Oxford University Press; 2016: 180–187.

15.

THE PALLIATIVE AND HOSPICE APRN IN HOSPICE AND HOME HEALTH PROGRAMS

Rikki N. Hooper, Chari Price, and Jamie Lee Rouse

KEY POINTS

- Palliative advanced practice registered nurses (APRNs) in hospice and home health organizations are in an ideal position to extend palliative care in the community, achieving improved symptom management, effective communication, successful collaboration, decreased use of hospital services at the end of life, and earlier hospice transitions.

- An APRN is a leader and advocate for hospice care of patients with life-limiting illnesses, working within an interdisciplinary, holistic, and compassionate model of care focused on promoting quality of life. This model of care demands that APRNs function at the highest level of their education and training.

- Palliative and hospice APRN encounters are reimbursable services across settings and services through Medicare, private insurance, and Medicaid programs.

CASE STUDY 1: TRANSITION FROM PALLIATIVE CARE TO HOSPICE

Mr. A was a 46-year-old Native American man referred to palliative care services for symptom management and goals of care. Mr. A's medical history included end-stage renal disease (ESRD), new to hemodialysis, with congestive heart failure (CHF), hepatitis C, and a history of substance misuse. Mr. A had a history of multiple lengthy hospitalizations in the prior year and was recently discharged home from a skilled nursing facility after completing rehabilitation services. He had intermittently missed dialysis treatments because of nausea and anxiety.

He was not partnered and had three children. Mr. A lived with his aunt on disability insurance, retiring from the Forestry Service due to ESRD. His substance misuse consisted of cannabis and methamphetamine. Mr. A had completed advance care planning (ACP) and named his aunt as his surrogate decision-maker. His code status was do not intubate (DNI), and he wanted to continue dialysis in spite of his frequent missed appointments. His symptoms included bilateral pedal neuropathy and a triad of symptoms related to his dialysis, including nausea, fatigue, and anxiety. His Palliative Performance Scale was 60%. He received care at the Tribal Hospital.

Mr. A was followed by the palliative nurse practitioner (NP) over 5 months to control his nausea, anxiety, and fatigue with medication adjustments. He subsequently moved in with his brother and began using cannabis because he felt it helped his symptoms. Over the next 3 months, Mr. A had several emergency department (ED) visits and hospitalizations secondary to cannabis hyperemesis syndrome. Mr. A continued to decline over the course of the following 2 months with significant worsening of his nausea, anxiety, and neuropathy resulting in missed dialysis treatments. Discussions regarding dialysis continuation versus discontinuation occurred at each palliative care visit during this time period because medication no longer managed his symptoms. Mr. A had weekly ED evaluations for significant symptom burden. Although dialysis discontinuation was strongly encouraged, he struggled with the decision until after the third visit.

Mr. A then shifted his focus to comfort measures only and was admitted to the Tribal Hospital for general inpatient hospice care. He chose the palliative NP to serve as his hospice attending of record as he appreciated her consistent support to him and his family. The palliative NP—in serving in the hospice role—provided recommendations to the hospitalists regarding symptom management medications. Several members of the hospital team struggled with Mr. A's decision to discontinue dialysis at his age. The staff was provided with hospice support and education by the NP and the hospice team to navigate their feelings about the death of this younger patient in his pursuit of comfort measures. Mr. A spent 18 days under hospice care, which managed his progressive pain, nausea, and agitation through medication adjustments until he died peacefully, surrounded by his family.

INTRODUCTION

Advanced practice registered nurses (APRNs) have a unique skill set ideally suited to working with people who are chronically seriously ill or at the end of life, being cared for either through a hospice or home health program, by providing a well-organized, consistent approach that is both comprehensive and proactive in providing symptom management. A position statement from nurse leaders described the APRN in both moving the field forward and preparing for the graying of America.[1] Usually the APRN, in either home health or hospice organizations, is a nurse practitioner (NP) or clinical nurse specialist (CNS). APRNs working within hospice or home health organizations have the opportunity to work to the full extent of their potential while providing compassionate care to seriously chronically or terminally ill individuals and their families.

Using the nursing process, APRNs address the complex issues of seriously ill people by synthesizing complex data to develop and implement advanced person-centered care plans.[2,3] APRNs combine palliative nursing's focus on the whole person[4] and their advanced education to perform comprehensive physical evaluations and order and interpret diagnostic tests, in addition to prescribing medications (depending on state-specific APRN practice regulations).[5,6] The palliative APRN acts as a case manager, involves other members of the interdisciplinary team when appropriate, and educates the patient and family, empowering them to fully participate in the plan of care and encouraging self-management whenever possible. Part of this assessment includes exploring the patient's value system and their culture, as well as leading discussions regarding goals of medical treatment and explaining different options for care or intervention which are set in context of the individual's advanced illness and preferences for care. These discussions often include choices regarding end-of-life care or resuscitation. By virtue of the nursing code of ethics and both scope and standards for nursing and palliative nursing, the APRN is accountable for advocating for the person's preferences.

HISTORY OF APRN ROLE IN SERIOUS ILLNESS CARE

This model of using advanced practice nurses in serious illness or end-of-life care is not new: the British Macmillan Nurse Model has existed for many years. In this model, advanced practice and specialty training offers registered general nurses (RGNs) an in-depth knowledge of advanced disease pathophysiology, as well as the psychological, social, and spiritual needs of patients with a life-threatening disease.[7] Originally developed for nurses caring for cancer patients, the Macmillan Model has nurses follow people through their disease, from diagnosis onward, whether the treatment course is thought to be curative or palliative in nature. This model provides continuity for patients and families; it involves home visits and the nurse's presence at physician specialist appointments when an advocate might be beneficial. Macmillan nurses identified the following components as part of their role[7]: expert practitioner, consultant, educator, researcher, and leader. These components are also identified in the 2021 third edition of *Competencies for Palliative and Hospice APRN*, published by the Hospice and Palliative Nurses Association (HPNA), with the addition of case manager, advocate, program developer, and policymaker.[8,9]

APRNs have consistently demonstrated commitment to providing excellent care to vulnerable populations in the United States: frail, poor, rural, and culturally diverse.[7] They have performed this care with a high degree of autonomy, collaborating with physician colleagues when appropriate but exercising their excellent skills in critical thinking and implementing strategies to provide improved care.[9] APRNs apply an evidence-based approach to care delivery, incorporating physical, emotional, psychosocial, spiritual, and existential

aspects.[10] Using this multifaceted assessment, the APRN can apply a holistic approach to advance care planning with patients and families.

The role of palliative APRNs in these principally community-based organizations can be primarily clinical, but there are also roles in leadership such as clinical team leader, clinical director, chief clinical officer, and even chief executive officer. Clearly, palliative APRNs have roles not only in clinical work but also in leadership areas, and they have a role in influencing change in nursing practice and within organizations as a whole.[3]

THE HOSPICE MODEL OF CARE

Palliation of distressing symptoms at the end of life through hospice care has been available to people with terminal illnesses in the United States since the early 1970s, after interest was sparked during a 1963 visit by Dame Cicely Saunders from England. She has been referred to as the matriarch of the modern hospice model of care and Dr. Florence Wald is the mother of hospice in the United States. Hospice services were not reimbursable under the insurance system in the United States until 1982, so early hospice services were provided by volunteers, mostly nurses. The number of people accessing services has increased through the years, with most recent data reporting an increase in the number of Medicare beneficiaries receiving hospice care from 1.32 million to 1.55 million between 2014 and 2018.[11] This represented an average increase of 4% each year.[11] In 2011, the number of Medicare decedents enrolled in hospice care was 44.6%; by 2014, this was up to 47.8% and, in 2018, reached greater than half at 50.8%.[11] Additionally, people who enrolled in Medicare Advantage the same year they accessed hospice plans accounted for 36.9% of recipients, an increase of 6.5% between 2014 and 2018.[11] Although the total number of people receiving hospice services has increased, they are still only receiving services for around half of the benefit time, with average length of stay being 89.6 days in 2018, but median length of stay being 18 days, a decrease since 2011, when it was 18.7 days.[11]

Hospice is a model of healthcare delivery that provides palliative care, defined by the National Consensus Project for Quality Palliative Care (NCP) as "patient and family-centered care that optimizes quality of life by anticipating, preventing, and treating suffering. Palliative care throughout the continuum of illness involves addressing the physical, intellectual, emotional, social and spiritual needs and to facilitate patient autonomy, access to information, and choice."[12] Since its inception, hospice care has matured into both an advanced model of care for terminally ill patients and a philosophy of care. The hospice model of care focuses on all dimensions of quality of life for both the patient and family; this model started in England in the 1960s, migrating to the United States in the 1970s. The first American hospice was opened in 1974, heavily influenced by the vision of an APRN, Dr. Florence Wald, Dean of the Yale School of Nursing. As a distinguished APRN, she collaborated with two pediatricians and a chaplain to start the first home hospice program in New Haven, Connecticut.[13]

Today in the United States, hospice services are a guaranteed benefit for individuals over the age of 65, with a prognosis of 6 months or less to live if their terminal disease takes its natural course and they choose to focus on comfort only rather than curative interventions. The Centers for Medicare and Medicaid Services (CMS) oversees the provision of hospice services. Medicaid and many commercial and private insurance companies mirror the *Medicare Hospice Benefit* (MHB) for individuals younger than 65. In October 2020, changes to the hospice benefit began with the addition of the *Addendum to the Hospice Beneficiary Election Statement*, which allows for beneficiaries or their proxies to request an explanation of medications or services not covered by the hospice organization. This is described in the FY2020 Hospice Final Rule 84 FR 38508.[14,15]

In 2021, changes to the Medicare Advantage (MA) coverage of hospice services occurred, using data from a demonstration project testing the inclusion of hospice benefits in the value-based insurance design model (VBID). This is often referred to as the *Medicare Advantage hospice carve-in* and is a 4-year project sponsored by the Center for Medicare and Medicaid Innovation (CMMI).[16,17] The intent of this project is to increase access to hospice services and improve coordination between hospice providers and other clinicians caring for patients, with the goal of identifying and reducing gaps in hospice care. With more Americans choosing to enroll in MA plans rather than traditional Medicare, this proposal respects beneficiary choice and seeks to bridge needs and resources to ensure more seamless transitions of care and supportive services. The focus will continue to be on the provision of high-quality, person-centered care that has a higher level of integration. An underlying goal is to bring a broader range of palliative and supportive services upstream for individuals with serious life-limiting illness, with possible options for concurrent care.[18]

The demonstration project includes nine Medicare Advantage Organizations (MAOs) that applied to participate, covering care provided in 13 states and Puerto Rico during the first year with additional opportunities to apply for the 2022 enrollment.[19] With the evolution of hospice care in the United States from a volunteer-based to small local organizations to even multistate organizations, payment structures have advanced as well and may be influenced by the outcomes of the VBID demonstration project. An overview of the different types of hospice providers can be seen in Table 15.1.

These agencies vary considerably in their organizational structure (not-for-profit vs. for profit), the communities they serve (rural vs. urban), size (from large to small), and setting (stand-alone and independent vs. beds within a nursing home).[11,13] Hospice services are provided in any setting, anywhere along the age continuum, to individuals with a variety of diseases. In 2017, 94.9% of recipients were over the age of 65, demonstrating that most recipients are indeed eligible for Medicare benefits. However, as illustrated in Table 15.2, 81.2% of individuals received care at their place of residence, and approximately 82.3% had a non-cancer diagnosis spanning all organ systems.[11]

Reimbursement for services varies across the country and whether it is provided in rural or urban settings. Routine-level care is reimbursed at much lower rates than inpatient-level care, reflecting the lower amount of resources needed for care provision. For example, in Western North Carolina, a predominantly rural area with a town, the routine level of care is reimbursed at $178.20 per day ($174.64 after sequestration) while inpatient-level care is reimbursed at $941.50 ($922.67 after sequestration). *Respite care*, which can be provided for 5 days per benefit period, is reimbursed at a rate of $420.38 per day ($411.97 after sequestration). It should be noted that the decreases for sequestration have been suspended during the 2020 COVID-19 pandemic.[20] Table 15.3 shows the difference in qualifications for each of these levels of care.

Hospice eligibility is based on benefit periods, with the first two periods of 90 days each, with subsequent periods of 60 days in length. Each of these subsequent benefit periods requires that a provider, either a physician or NP, has a face-to-face encounter with the patient to attest that there is continued eligibility for service. These requirements were initiated as part of the *Affordable Care Act* (ACA) in 2011.[21,22] This documentation is key to continued payment for services provided and must paint the picture of continued eligibility in as objective a way possible. Descriptive expansion on elements such as appetite, functional status, and body habitus can be very helpful. For example, rather than describing the patient as "thin," the NP could expand by describing the patient has having sunken orbits, temporal wasting, and generalized

Table 15.1 HOSPICE PROVIDERS BY TYPE

Provider by tax status type	% in 2012	% in 2018
For-profit providers	63.	69.95
Not-for-profit providers	31.9	26.94
Government providers	4.9	3.41

Adapted from NHPCO Facts and Figures 2020.[11]

Table 15.2 2018 SPENDING AND DAYS OF HOSPICE CARE PERCENTAGES BY PRINCIPAL DIAGNOSIS

DIAGNOSIS GROUP	% OF MEDICARE SPENDING BY PRINCIPAL DIAGNOSIS	DAYS OF HOSPICE CARE BY PRINCIPAL DIAGNOSIS
Dementia	25.3	105.2
Circulatory/Heart	20.2	80.2
Cancer	17.7	45.6
Other	13.3	64.3
Respiratory	10.9	71.8
Stroke	11.5	82.8
Chronic kidney disease	1.1	38.1

Adapted from NHPCO Facts and Figures 2020.[11]

Table 15.3 LEVELS OF HOSPICE CARE

LEVELS OF HOSPICE CARE	DESCRIPTION	SETTINGS
Routine	Visits by nursing, social work, and spiritual care as per care plan. Comprehensive nursing assessment visits at least every 15 days.	Home, ALF, SNF
Continuous care	Hospice provider crisis intervention, must include at least 8 hours continuous nursing care. May also receive hospice aide care as part of plan.	Home
Inpatient respite care	Short-term, up to 5 days in a contracted facility to give caregivers a break. Routine-level hospice care is provided during this time.	SNF, ALF, hospice in-patient unit
General inpatient care	Short-term care to manage uncontrolled symptoms that cannot be managed in another location. Generally requires frequent changes in symptom management plan of care. 24-hour nursing services are provided.	Hospice in-patient unit, hospital or SNF (if 24-hr registered nurse on site)

ALF, assisted living facility; SNF, skilled nursing facility.

Adapted from Medicare Regulations for Hospice Care.[23]

muscle wasting and wearing ill-fitting clothes. Instead of saying that the patient is eating 25% of meals, a more accurate way of demonstrating this could be that the patient requires the assistance of a caregiver to eat, with multiple cues being given and much encouragement. Despite this and supplements being offered, the patient is still only ingesting 25% of recommended caloric intake.[22]

Death is a natural part of life and can occur at any point in life, but in the United States it is predominantly associated with aging, and the aging population is growing. In 2014, 46 million adults in the United States were over age 65, but it is estimated that, by 2030, this will increase to 74 million individuals, almost 21% of the population.[24] In the United States, prior to death, most terminally ill individuals find themselves caught in a fragmented healthcare system, relying on complex medical interventions and burdened by rising costs. In contrast, when given a choice about end-of-life care, many Americans would prefer medical care that is coordinated and comprehensive; they want their care to reflect their wishes for comfort and quality of life, and they want information about what lies ahead for them and their family.[25] Hospice is the healthcare delivery model that provides this type of care. The demand for hospice services will likely increase, resulting in an increased demand for a skilled workforce. However, the shortage of hospice and palliative medicine physicians has led to an increased demand for palliative APRNs and will continue to do so.[26,27]

THE USE OF APRNS IN HOSPICE CARE

The clinical APRN is an evolving role in hospice care, with most APRNs providing clinical care in hospices either as NPs or CNSs. APRNs are able to work in influential positions in hospice programs throughout the United States. In addition to clinical care, other roles includes chief clinical officer, chief executive officer, chief operating officer, clinical director, administrator, quality and performance improvement officer, and clinical manager, to name a few. APRNs in these

roles combine a tradition of advocacy and teaching, a broad clinical knowledge base, and their critical thinking skills to make complex decisions related to the structure and processes of patient care in the hospice setting.[28] This includes issues related to organizational and workforce excellence, as well as compliance with laws and regulations. Stewardship, accountability, and quality and performance improvement are all important elements of these roles.[29] As leaders at all organizational levels in hospice, APRNs understand the importance of patient-centered, whole-person, interdisciplinary care delivered within a framework of high-quality, evidence-based practice[30] along with expert communication skills that enable them to collaborate not only with clinical teams but also with administrative leaders of their own and other organizations. Specific tasks that rely on these skills are gathering and relaying information, negotiating, teaching, and resolving conflicts. APRNs in leadership roles must bring the unique care needs of hospice patients to the attention of the larger healthcare community through advocacy and education. Discussing end-of-life care even at an institutional level can be fraught with pitfalls, so the APRN must have expert guidance and coaching skills and a solid knowledge of the ethical issues associated with end-of-life care in the hospice setting.

In hospice, APRNs combine common theoretical concepts of both nursing practice and the hospice philosophy, including whole-person care and the impact of health on quality of life, with the skills needed to provide expert care at the end of life. The HPNA published the *Palliative Nursing: Scope and Standards of Practice*, which establish the competencies necessary to meet these standards. These standards are divided into Standards of Practice for Palliative Nursing, which incorporates the nursing process, and Standards of Professional Performance. The competencies are advanced clinical judgment, use of evidence and research, expert communication skills, collaboration, knowledge of ethical principles and professional standards, respect for cultural and spiritual diversity, advocacy, systems thinking, and an understanding of the importance of ongoing education in creating a professional practice that delivers expert end-of-life care.[8] To demonstrate their specialty practice, it is recommended that APRNs obtain certification as an advanced certified hospice and palliative nurse (ACHPN).

These standards and associated competencies are closely aligned with both the eight domains of quality palliative care as outlined in the NCP *Clinical Practice Guidelines for Quality Palliative Care*[12] and the National Hospice and Palliative Care Organization's (NHPCO) *Standards of Practice for Hospice Programs*, which stipulate that for hospice providers to provide high-quality patient- and family-centered palliative care, they must incorporate either the NCP *Clinical Practice Guidelines* or the NHPCO *Standards of Practice for Hospice Programs* into the delivery of hospice services.[29] This comparison can be seen in Table 15.4.

In addition, familiarity with the hospice local coverage determinations (LCDs), which are published by the local geographic area's Medicare administration contractor, and the hospice conditions of participation (COPs) criteria set forth by the CMS is essential. The LCDs are guidelines for determining eligibility and prognosis.[23] The COPs delineate the services that a certified hospice provider must provide to a patient as it relates to his or her terminal diagnosis and related conditions and set the standards for the delivery of hospice services, such as clinical record-keeping and staff credentials. To receive reimbursement from the CMS, a hospice provider must comply with these standards and requirements.[23] Private insurers usually follow the CMS hospice guidelines for eligibility, the type of services provided, and reimbursement. The NHPCO works closely with these agencies to create these guidelines and requirements.

An extensive clinical knowledge base is essential for practice in a hospice setting. APRNs are expected to provide care for diverse patients of all ages in a variety of settings, with any and all terminal illnesses and within a finite reimbursement system. Such a broad sphere of practice demands creativity, flexibility, and a high level of critical thinking skills to produce good outcomes in such a multitude of situations. Some hospices provide services not required under the regulations set forth by CMS (e.g., specialized wound care or disease-specific care programs for individuals with cardiac or pulmonary conditions or dementia), which in turn requires a broader APRN expertise. Moreover, essential components of professional practice are the foundation of a comprehensive knowledge base for advanced practice nursing in hospice care. These guidelines, standards, and competencies guide the hospice APRN to care for the patient and family as the unit of care. Figure 15.1 illustrates these components, clearly showing the multifaceted dimensions of professional practice that contribute to the provision of expert end-of-life care by APRNs within the hospice model of care.

Table 15.4 HOSPICE APRN PRACTICE, AND COMPETENCIES AND HOSPICE STANDARDS AND GUIDELINES

PALLIATIVE NURSING: SCOPE AND STANDARDS OF PRACTICE[2]			HPNA COMPETENCIES FOR THE PALLIATIVE AND HOSPICE APRN[8]	NHPCO STANDARDS OF PRACTICE FOR HOSPICE PROGRAMS[29]	NCP CLINICAL PRACTICE GUIDELINES[12]
Communication	Education[a]	Standards of practice Evidence-based practice and research Collaboration Leadership Environmental health	Clinical judgment Evidence-based practice and research	Clinical excellence and safety	Physical care Care of the patient at the end of life
		Ethics	Advocacy and ethics	Ethical behavior and consumer rights	Ethical and legal
		Quality of practice Evidence-based practice and research Resource utilization Professional practice evaluation Collaboration Leadership	Professionalism Systems thinking Collaboration Evidence-based practice and research Systems	Organizational excellence Workforce excellence Standards Compliance with laws and regulations Stewardship and accountability Performance measurement	Structure and processes of care
		Collaboration Standards of practice	Cultural and spiritual Evidence-based practice and research	Patient- and Family-centered care Standards Inclusion and access	Cultural Psychological and psychiatric Social spiritual, religious, and existential

[a]Facilitator of learning.

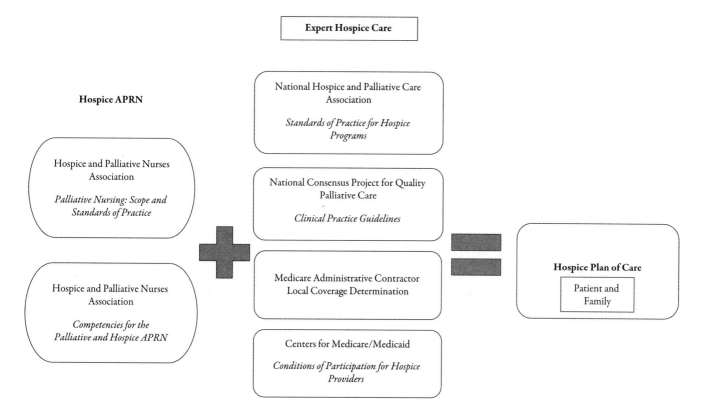

Figure 15.1 Overview of the requirements for expert professional practice for the hospice APRN.

Although hospice services are predominantly used by individuals over the age of 65, services are available to neonates, young children, adolescents, young adults, and middle-aged individuals.[11] Understanding each age group's developmental stage and cognitive capacity as well as physical and intellectual abilities is critical. Caring for individuals across the age continuum necessitates that palliative APRNs manage a multitude of disease states. This demands a comprehensive knowledge of many illnesses and conditions as well as their pathophysiology, manifestations, progression, and associated pharmacology.

The hospice APRN will also encounter a wide diversity of patients, such as military veterans; individuals with developmental or cognitive disabilities; individuals experiencing serious mental illness; individuals who are incarcerated; lesbian, gay, bisexual, transgender, and intersex individuals; individuals with substance use disorders; individuals experiencing homeless; and individuals of low socioeconomic status. Cultural humility and sensitivity specific to these populations are essential. The COVID-19 pandemic has highlighted social injustices and systematic racism in healthcare as well as the clear differences in the way that individuals with different social and ethnic backgrounds have been affected by the Coronavirus[31] (see Chapter 20, "Social Determinants of Health").

The setting in which hospice services are provided plays an important role in the delivery of hospice care. In 2018, 51.5% of people received care in their homes, whereas 12.3% were in an assisted living facility and 17.4% in a skilled facility.[11]

These patients received care at the routine level, whereas the majority of the 12.8% of patients in a hospice inpatient facility or unit would have received the higher level of care provided under the general inpatient level, which is reimbursed at a much higher rate (almost five times that of routine-level care).

Caring for an individual in his or her home presents different challenges than in another type of conjugate care setting, such as an acute or skilled care facility. Stepping into a person's home is a privilege, as the APRN is a visitor. In the private home, family members are usually the primary caregivers. Their caregiver burden is significant due to little knowledge, training, or support to assess symptoms and then apply interventions. Paid caregivers, often with limited scope of practice and frequently minimal training, may also be providing the care in private homes. Hospice houses, or hospice inpatient units, depending on the population they serve, may have only paid unlicensed caregivers or highly skilled licensed and unlicensed personnel, or a mixture of both. All these scenarios present advantages and disadvantages in terms of symptom assessment and management, medication administration, and delivery of personal care. The hospice APRN must consider these when developing a plan of care unique to the patient and caregiver.

The hospice APRN must determine the knowledge and expertise of the caregivers in settings other than the private home. Moreover, each physical location outside of the home has regulatory oversight by state and federal licensing agencies based on their designation. The hospice APRN must understand how these regulations affect the treatment and management of the patient's symptoms. For example, nursing homes often have strict regulations regarding the use of certain antipsychotics, thus influencing the APRN's choice of medications and how they might be prescribed in these facilities. In another example, many residential care facilities do not have the licensed staff to dispense medications like opiates. Therefore, these medications cannot be prescribed for use on an as-needed basis. In both cases, the hospice APRN must balance regulatory restrictions with recommended standards of care to develop an appropriate care plan.

In addition to physical location, the four CMS-mandated hospice levels of care that a hospice provider must offer strongly influence the delivery of hospice care. These four levels of care are routine home care; continuous home care for patients in crisis; inpatient respite care, usually provided in a contracted facility, for patients whose families need respite from caregiving; and general inpatient care for patients in crisis who cannot be managed at home.[32]

In July 2015, Congress approved significant changes to hospice reimbursement, the first since the Medicare Hospice benefit went into effect in 1983. The changes went into effect January 1, 2016, and included a two-tiered routine home care rate and a service intensity add-on payment, as can be seen in Table 15.5. The two-tiered payment model for routine home care translates into a higher hospice reimbursement rate for the first 60 days of hospice care and a lower rate for any additional days of hospice care. Using the prior geographical example, the rates for the first 60 days are highlighted at $178.20, but the rates decrease to $140.83 on day 61 and thereafter for routine care.[20]

The service intensity add-on payment reflects the higher acuity and needs of dying patients and their families in the last 7 days of life. It is calculated retrospectively based on nursing and social work visits and is equal to the continuous home care hourly rate up to 4 hours per day. For the region in the example, this is an hourly rate of $53.27 prior to sequestration.[20] These reimbursement changes reflect the reality of short lengths of stay and a higher intensity of care in the last week of life that many hospices encounter.[33] Clearly, the hospice APRN must be able to assess the patient's and family's needs and the skill of the caregivers, then incorporate this information into a care plan that meets regulatory oversight, all within finite monetary compensation to the hospice provider.

There is also the additional limitation of a capitated reimbursement for hospice services, which also affects the treatment plan. Appropriate resource utilization while achieving good outcomes is a standard of professional practice. The hospice organization is responsible for the cost of all the care of an individual as it relates to his or her terminal diagnosis. The latest rule from CMS reflects the right of an individual and their family to request a written rationale of non-coverage of medications, items, and services, otherwise known as the *addendum*, which became effective October 1, 2020. This additionally adds a time limit for when this care must be provided to patients: 5 days when requested upon admission or election of the benefit or 3 days when requested at a later time. This list of services or medications must be provided upon request to the patient or family and any other non-hospice medical providers if requested.[14] Therefore, an extensive knowledge of pain and symptom management options is necessary to enable the creation of a care plan that provides comfort in any setting to any individual in a fiscally responsible manner. De-prescribing of medications is part of this plan, with the knowledge that individuals taking more than five medications are at higher risk for drug interactions.

Hospice APRNs must be aware of some of the barriers to accessing hospice services, including lack of healthcare provider and community knowledge, the predominant culture's death-denying beliefs, the influence of an individual's culture, and insurance issues, among others.[7] The delivery of end-of-life care in a hospice setting is governed by financial restraints and regulatory issues, as discussed previously. Hospice APRNs must integrate these factors into their clinical decision-making when creating, maintaining, or changing hospice programs. Providing compassionate, evidence-based, patient- and family-centered care within these confines can be challenging.

The NHPCO has an extensive compilation of resources designed to help hospice providers and clinicians achieve good clinical outcomes within these regulatory and financial constraints; these can be accessed at NHPCO.org. Interpretation of the eligibility criteria has also been noted to be a barrier to service because many clinicians have trouble interpreting the LCDs or prognosticating accurately.[34] Tools often utilized by hospice providers to document this are not widely available to the general medical population; one such tool is the *International Classification of Functioning, Disability and Health* (ICF),[35] which goes beyond an individual's terminal diagnosis and encompasses other determinants of health such as living situation and emotional well-being. This tool is used more widely in Europe than the United States but has some useful elements to examine when determining eligibility for hospice.[35]

Table 15.5 HOSPICE LEVELS OF CARE AND REIMBURSEMENT

LEVEL OF CARE	REIMBURSEMENT RULES	REIMBURSEMENT AMOUNTS
Routine	Days 1-60	$199.25
	Days 61+	$157.49
	Last 7 days of life	Additional payment RN and SW
Continuous care	Full rate (24 hrs of care)	$1,432.41
	Hourly rate	$59.68
Respite	Per day	$461.09
General inpatient	Per day	$1,045.66

Adapted from CMS.gov.[23]

CASE STUDY 2: HOME HEALTH

Mr. S was a 65-year-old man referred to palliative care/home health by his oncologist to assist with medical decision-making and symptom management in the setting of metastatic prostate cancer detected 3 years prior. Mr. S received 45 treatments of radiation therapy and achieved remission. Two years later, he developed left hip pain. Imaging revealed metastasis to the lung, hips, skull, and bladder. He was then hospitalized, during which an indwelling catheter was placed in the right lung to manage malignant effusions. Home health services were ordered for education and management of the catheter and pain control.

Mr. S was married to Amy, his second wife. He was retired, although his wife continued to work part-time. They both had children from previous marriages who lived out of state. He had completed paperwork designating his wife as his surrogate decision-maker. He wanted no extraordinary measures and an out of hospital DNR form was signed. The palliative APRN initiated discussion about a provider out-of-hospital order for life-sustaining treatment (POLST) form.

Mr. S's symptoms included pain, dyspnea, debility, insomnia, and anorexia. His Palliative Performance Scale (PPS) is 70%. His pain was in his right hip, and he was on morphine extended-release (ER) tablets 30 mg every 8 hours and oxycodone immediate-release (IR) tablets 10 mg every 4 hours with usual use 2–3 times daily. His oncologist asked for the palliative APRN to partner with him and take over prescribing Mr. S's pain medications. To assure safe prescribing, he was assessed for opioid narcotic abuse risk using an Opioid Risk Tool (ORT). He scored 0, indicating a low risk of abuse. He signed an agreement to have the palliative APRN as his sole prescriber of opioids. His dyspnea was related to his malignant pleural effusion, which was managed with use of the indwelling catheter that kept excess pleural fluid drained. Because he was weak, he received home health physical therapy. His insomnia was related to anxiety and dyspnea. Although he had zolpidem 5 mg prescribed by the oncologist, it had been unnecessary with the placement of the catheter. For his anorexia, he was prescribed prednisone 5 mg twice daily, which helped his appetite as well as his energy, his mood, and his pain.

Mr. S continued palliative chemotherapy with full understanding that his cancer was metastatic and had a poor prognosis. He had conveyed this to his family. He has begun financial planning for his wife and family. He had also informed his family that he wanted to focus on quality of life and remain at home, but wanted to continue life-sustaining therapies at the current time. The palliative APRN continued to check in and monitor his symptoms and support the family.

Over the following 18 months, Mr. S's functional status continued to decline as his PSA level increased despite treatment. Amy retired to be home with him full-time. She provided all the meals, housekeeping, and assisted with Mr. S's personal care. They had their bathroom adapted to allow Mr. S to use it more easily. The palliative APRN adjusted his pain medications to morphine sulfate ER 45 mg every 8 hours and morphine sulfate IR 15 mg 1–2 tabs every 4 hours as needed for pain.

One day, Mr. S had a fall and Amy could not get him up. She summoned the fire department and they came to the home and helped him up. Later, as he walked to the bathroom, he fell again, and emergency medical services (EMS) arrived and took him to the hospital. Work-up revealed a meningioma, and he underwent surgery for removal. After hospitalization, he was discharged to home with his wife to restart home health services to facilitate ambulation, strengthening, and balance.

Mr. S had mentioned wanting to stop cancer-directed treatments and "let nature take its course." However, his oncologist urged him to continue treatments. The palliative APRN initiated conversations about goals and the transition to hospice. His wife left the decisions up to Mr. S, but tearfully stated she would support his decisions. He planned the transition from his current level of supportive service at that time. His goal was to make it to Thanksgiving, when he could see his children and grandchildren again.

The *Medicare Hospice Benefit* structure is limiting for patients desiring treatments or interventions deemed to be aggressive or "curative" in nature by a particular hospice, even when they are clearly used to palliate symptoms (e.g., palliative chemotherapy, inotropes for heart failure, or medications for amyotrophic lateral sclerosis are just a few examples). These limitations led to the development of the palliative care movement in the 1990s, when it became clear that technology had outgrown the underpinnings of the hospice benefit which was grounded in incurable cancers. Hospice principles moved into the acute care and community settings to become palliative care programs. In the community, palliative care is often provided within a home health organizational framework, where other therapies are also provided to support a patient's desire for independence at home. Home health services are provided by members of a multidisciplinary team in order to meet the patient's needs; however, unlike hospice, there is not the mandate for interdisciplinary care. Therefore, palliative APRNs may provide supportive care often without the benefit of a team designed around this purpose. In general, the goal of home healthcare is to provide treatment for an illness or injury. Where possible, home healthcare helps a person get better, regain their independence, and become as self-sufficient as possible. However, home healthcare may help a patient maintain a current condition or level of function or slow decline.

The *Home Health Care Benefit* is available to individuals with Medicare who meet certain criteria. This includes being under the care of a medical provider (until recently this had to be a physician) and have a need for some type of care, such as skilled nursing care, speech therapy, or physical or occupational therapy. These services must be deemed medically necessary as part of the plan of care, and the patient must be certified as being "homebound," as defined in the Medicare Home Health information booklet.[36]

- A person has difficulty leaving their home without help (like using a cane, wheelchair, walker, or crutches; special transportation; or help from another person) because of an illness or injury, or leaving the home isn't recommended because of their condition.

- A person is normally unable to leave their home, but if they do it requires a major effort.

- A person may leave home for medical treatment or short, infrequent absences for no-medical reasons, like an occasional trip to the barber, a walk around the block or a drive, or attendance at a family reunion, funeral, graduation, or other infrequent or unique event. The person can still get home healthcare if they attend adult day care or religious services.

Services are often time-limited, lasting only a few weeks following an acute event or hospitalization. Additionally, home healthcare must be ordered by a physician who has had a face-to-face visit with the patient within the past 30 days.[37] Often when a patient is discharged following a hospitalization, home healthcare is ordered, but the physician ordering this is not usually the one who must complete the paperwork associated with the ongoing plan of care. This medically necessary visit was determined to be necessary as part of the ACA due to occurrences of fraudulent billing for services.[38] By virtue of being homebound, in that leaving requires considerable and taxing effort (see CMS definition), many individuals have difficulty accessing a physician at their office. Even though APRNs provide high-quality care to individuals in communities across the country, especially in rural or underserved areas, they have not in the past been permitted to sign certifications for home health services.[39]

The COVID-19 pandemic in 2020 led to a relaxation of this rule, and NPs were granted the ability to order and certify home healthcare services through the passing of H.R.2150/S.296 *Home Health Care Planning Improvement Act*, as part of the *Coronavirus Aid, Relief, and Economic Security* (CARE) Act in May of 2020, though this is still state-dependent.[40] Though a relatively new development, it has become evident that billing for APRNs performing the care plan oversight has been successfully accomplished. Some home health organizations had difficulty grasping this concept, and some continue to refuse to accept orders and certifications from non-physician providers (NPPs), despite the provider being the individual who has provided all that patient's primary care services. Another area where APRNs have been able to successfully provide care for is in wound care, particularly in rural areas. These patients often have limited access to wound care experts and have difficulty getting to a wound center. APRNs can assist with this management and further utilize telehealth platforms to access consultations with wound specialists.[41]

It has become abundantly clear that, with advances in healthcare and technology, Americans are living longer. However, as the average life span has increased, so has the number of people living with chronic progressive disease. These individuals have multiple chronic medical conditions requiring longer and more sustained care and have psychosocial situations requiring additional support and assistance. Heart failure, for example, has become a leading factor in chronic complex illness, with technological and pharmaceutical advances delaying the progression of the disease and leading to longer lives, but often with significant symptom burden and associated medical costs. The American Heart Association projects that direct costs for heart failure may be more than $75 billion by 2030. Approximately 50% of people die within 5 years of being diagnosed with heart failure.[42] Within a home health organization, the palliative APRN can facilitate services to maximize functional abilities and foster independence while addressing any palliative symptom needs. They can also provide case management services and coordinate the team. Within a home healthcare organization, the team should be most familiar with treatments for heart failure and the associated 30-day readmission rates.[42] The palliative APRN is able to address not only the medical treatment needs of the individual and coordinate the interdisciplinary team but also address the goals of medical care and complete appropriate documentation as indicated in the individual state. The palliative APRN is uniquely qualified to provide education and support to individuals as they determine their goals of care and whether a transition to hospice care is appropriate. These decisions are often among the most difficult decisions they will make regarding their healthcare, and it is imperative that they are provided as much support as possible as they work through these decisions.[43]

This role could be filled by either an NP or a CNS, although NPs could bill for some services, such as medical visits, advance care planning discussions, and, now, care plan oversight, a once-monthly service. This would elevate the quality of care for homebound patients, which is often uncoordinated, inaccessible, and ineffective.[41] It has been shown that palliative care provided in the home setting is associated not only with a reduction in symptom burden, but also with increases patient and family satisfaction. Furthermore, studies in the United States and other countries have shown decreased utilization of healthcare resources and associated costs. Some organizations have developed disease-specific programs for individuals with heart failure, chronic obstructive pulmonary disease, and HIV/AIDS, as well as for those living with advanced cancer.[44] Individuals in these programs may not yet meet eligibility criteria for hospice care, want expensive life-sustaining therapies that may diminish quality of life, or want to pursue a curative plan of care. Thus, their palliative APRN facilitates the establishment of goals of care and advance care planning documents and completes orders for life-sustaining treatments as consistent and available within their state scope of practice.[45] These forms may be termed provider/physician orders for life-sustaining treatment (POLSTs), portable orders for life-sustaining treatment, medical orders for life-sustaining treatment (MOLSTs), or medical orders for scope of treatment (MOSTs) depending on the state. Many states have legislation allowing the completion of these documents by APRNs. Specific up-to-date information can be found at Post.org.

The inclusion of palliative APRNs as part of the team promotes nursing and guides the plan of care to truly enable the right care to be provided at the right time using a person-centered approach.[46] Goals-of-care discussions allow patients and their families to make the decision about when to make a change to their plan of care. This may include a transition to hospice care services, and studies have shown that patients access these services for a longer period and have decreased hospitalizations during the last weeks and months of their life when a palliative care approach is incorporated into the home health model.[47] Individuals receiving palliative care as part of their home healthcare plan are also more likely to die at home.[44]

SUMMARY

The demand for home health and hospice services will grow, and the roles available to APRNs in these organizations are rich and varied. These types of care are not limited by age, disease, or population, and hospice is not limited by setting. Even though the work is challenging, demanding that palliative APRNs work to their fullest professional capacity, caring for individuals living with and dying from serious illness and their families is a great privilege that offers many rewards. Palliative APRNs represent an invaluable resource for the healthcare field, particularly in these fields, and it is clear that it is time for core palliative care competencies to be incorporated into all APRN education programs.[48] Even though there has recently been an increased focus on education through fellowships with the passing of the *Palliative Care and Hospice Education Act* (PCHETA), it is unclear how much this would provide for APRN education in addition to that for physicians.[48] As far back as 2011, the Institute of Medicine highlighted the need for more APRNs and recommended maximizing their use to improve quality, cost-effective care through advanced care management programs.[49,50] Both hospice and home health organizations provide opportunities for palliative APRNs to achieve these goals, and educational programs need to plan accordingly. Staffing will continue to be a major challenge for healthcare organizations, particularly following the pandemic in 2020, as will opportunities to leverage technology to expand options to increase patient access, not only in hospice care, but also in home healthcare. Utilizing telehealth platforms can be a more efficient way of reaching patients, especially in rural areas.[51]

REFERENCES

1. Promoting Excellence in End-of-Life Care. Advanced practice nurses role in palliative care: A position statement from American nursing leaders. 2002. https://repository.library.georgetown.edu/handle/10822/941899
2. Dahlin C. *Palliative Nursing Scope and Standards of Practice.* 6th ed. Pittsburgh, PA: Hospice and Palliative Nurses Association; 2021.
3. Dahlin C, Coyne P. The palliative APRN leader. *Ann Palliat Med.* 2019;8(Suppl 1):S30–S38.doi:10.21037/apm.2018.06.03
4. Meier D, Beresford L. Advanced practice nurses in palliative care; a pivotal role and perspective. *J Palliat Med.* 2003;9(3):624–627. doi:10.1089/jpm.2006.9.624.
5. National Council of State Boards of Nursing. Consensus Model for APRN Regulation: Licensure, accreditation, certification and education. Chicago, IL: NCSBN. 2008. https://www.ncsbn.org/aprn-consensus.htm
6. American Nurses Association (ANA). ANA position statement: Nursing care and do-not-resuscitate (DNR) decisions. Silver Spring, MD; ANA. 2020. https://www.nursingworld.org/certification/aprn-consensus-model/
7. Kuebler K. The palliative care advanced practice nurse. *J Palliat Med.* 2003;6(5):707–712. doi:013/10.1089.109662103322515211
8. Dahlin C. *Competencies for Palliative and Hospice APRN (3rd ed.).* Pittsburgh, PA: Hospice and Palliative Nurses Association; 2021.
9. Coyne P. The evolution of the advanced practice nurse within palliative care. *J Palliat Med.* 2003;6(5):769–770. doi:10.1089/109662103322515275
10. Dahlin C, Moreines LT, Root M. Evolution of the advanced practice nurse in palliative care. In: Dahlin C, ed. Core Curriculum for the Advanced Practice Hospice and Palliative Registered Nurse. 3rd ed. Pittsburgh, PA: Hospice and Palliative Nurses Association; 2020: xv–xvii.
11. National Hospice and Palliative Care Organization (NHPCO). *NHPCO facts and figures on hospice care in America.* 2020 ed. National Hospice and Palliative Care Organization. August 20, 2020. https://www.nhpco.org/factsfigures/
12. National Consensus Project for Quality Palliative Care. *Clinical Practice Guidelines,* 4th ed. Richmond, VA: National Coalition for Hospice and Palliative Care. 2018. https://www.nationalcoalitionhpc.org/ncp/
13. National Hospice and Palliative Care Organization. History of hospice. 2021. https://www.nhpco.org/hospice-care-overview/history-of-hospice/
14. Centers for Medicare and Medicaid Services. CMS.gov. FY21 hospice wage index final rule. July 30. 2020. https://www.govinfo.gov/content/pkg/FR-2020-08-04/pdf/2020-16991.pdf
15. Centers for Medicare and Medicaid Services. CMS.gov. Model Example of Hospice Election Statement 2020. https://www.cms.gov/files/document/model-hospice-election-statement-modified-july-2020.pdf
16. Fields T, Silvers A. Explaining the newly-released medicare advantage "carve-in" model. *CAPC Blog.* March 5, 2020. https://www.capc.org/blog/explaining-hospice-benefit-medicare-advantage-carve-in-model/
17. Parker J. Medicare advantage hospice carve-in starting small in 2021. *Hospice News.* September 28, 2020. https://hospicenews.com/2020/09/28/medicare-advantage-hospice-carve-in-starting-small-in-2021-%EF%BB%BF/
18. Bacher G, Atalla M, Ozcelik S, Driessen J. Introduction to the CY2021 hospice component. *VBID Model Information Session. Centers for Medicare & Medicaid Services Innovation Center.* 2020. https://innovation.cms.gov/iniyiatives/vbid/
19. Rosenthal S. CMMI releases hospice carve-in participating plans. *Blog to Transform Advanced Care.* C-TAC News. September 20, 2020. https://www.thectac.org/2020/09/cmmi-releases-hospice-carve-in-participating-plans/
20. Palmetto GBA. 2021. https://www.palmettogba.com/palmetto/calculators/hospicerateday.nsf/Calculator_N/OpenForm
21. English T C, Mazaner P. Hospice face-to-face recertification. *J Hosp Palliat Nurs.* 2016;18(4):317–323. doi:10.1097/NJH.0000000000000249.
22. Quinlin L. Face-to-face documentation using the face-2-face method. *J Hosp Palliat Nurs.* 2019;21(4):305–311. doi:10.1097/NJH.0000000000000572.
23. Horton J, Indelicato R. The advanced practice nurse. In Ferrell B, Coyle N eds. *Oxford Textbook of Palliative Nursing.* 3rd ed. Oxford, New York: Oxford University Press; 2010:1121–1129.
24. National Prevention Council Healthy aging in action. *Healthy Aging in Action.* Washington, DC: U.S. Department of Health and Human Services, Office of the Surgeon General, 2016. cdc.gov/aging/pdf/healthy-aging-in-action508.pdf
25. Dahlin C. National Consensus Project: Assuring quality palliative care through clinical practice guidelines. In: Ferrell B, Paice J, eds.

Oxford Textbook of Palliative Nursing. 5th ed. New York: Oxford University Press; 2019: 5–12.

26. Lupu D, Quigley L, Mehfoud N, Salsberg E. The growing demand for hospice and palliative medicine physicians: Will the supply keep up? *J Pain Symptom Manage.* 2018;55(4):1216–1223. jpsmjournal.com/article/S0885-3924(18)30031-9/pdf

27. Lupu D. Estimate of current hospice and palliative medicine physician workforce shortage. *J Pain Symptom Manage.* 2010;40(6):899–911. doi:10.1016/j.jpainsymman.2010.07.004.

28. Horton J, Indelicato R. The advanced practice nurse. In Ferrell B, Coyle N eds. *Oxford Textbook of Palliative Nursing.*3rd ed. Oxford, New York: Oxford University Press; 2010:1121–1129.

29. National Hospice and Palliative Care Organization (NHPCO). Standards of practice for hospice programs nhpco 2018. https://www.nhpco.org/wp-content/uploads/2019/04/Standards_Hospice_2018.pdf

30. Tracy M, Hanson C. Leadership. In: Hamric A, Hanson C, Tracy M, O'Grady E, eds. *Advanced Practice Nursing. An Integrated Approach.* 6th ed. St. Louis, MO: Elsevier. 2019:256–285.

31. Stokes E, Zambrano L, Anderson K, et al. Coronavirus disease 2019 case surveillance: United States, January 22–May 30, 2020. *MMWR Morb Mortal Wkly* 2020;69(24):759–765. Published 2020 Jun 19. doi:10.15585/mmwr.mm6924e2

32. Lysaght S, Ersak M. Settings of care within hospice, new options and questions about dying "at home." *J Hosp Palliat Nurs.* 2013;15(3):171–176. doi:10.1097/NJH.06013e3182765a17.

33. Federal Register. Medicare Program; FY 2016 Hospice Wage Index and Payment Rate Update and Hospice Quality Reporting Requirements; Correcting Amendment. August 31, 2020. https://www.federalregister.gov/documents/2015/08/06/2015-19033-medicare-program-fy-2016-hospice-wage-index-and-payment-rate-update-and-hospice-quality-reporting

34. Fine Perry G. MD. Hospice underutilization in the U.S.: The misalignment of regulatory policy and clinical reality.*J Pain Symptom Manage.* 2018;56(5):808–815. doi:10.1016/j.jpainsymman. 2108.08.005.

35. Nation L. Using the international classification of functioning, disability and health to document hospice eligibility. *J Hosp Palliat Nurs.* 2019;21(3):237–244. doi:10.1097/NJH.0000000000000516.

36. Centers for Medicare & Medicaid Services. Medicare and home health. *CMS Product No. 10969 Revised September 2020.* https://www.medicare.gov/Pubs/pdf/10969-medicare-and-home-health-care.pdf

37. Leff B, Carlson C, Saliba D, Ritchie C. The invisible homebound: Setting quality-of-care standards for home-based primary and palliative care. *Health Aff.* 2015;34(1):21–29. doi:https://doi.org/10.1377/hlthaff.2014.1008

38. Jaffe S. Home health care providers struggle with state laws and medicare rules as demand rises. *Health Aff.* 2019;38(6):981–986. doi:https://doi.org/10.377/hlthaff.2019.00529

39. Brassard A. *Removing barriers to advanced practice registered nurse care: Home health and hospice services.* AARP Policy Institute. 2012. https://www.aarp.org/content/dam/aarp/research/public_policy_institute/health/removing-barriers-advanced-practice-registered-nurse-home-health-hospice-insight-july-2012-AARP-ppi-health.pdf

40. Madeline Morr. PAS and NPS celebrate home health care planning improvement act in covid-19 legislation. Clin Advis. April 1, 2020. https://www.clinicaladvisor.com/home/topics/practice-management-information-center/pas-and-nps-celebrates-home-health-care-planning-improvement-act-in-covid-19-legislation/

41. Roche RL. *Store and forward wound teleconsultation in rural home health: A practice improvement project.* 2019. https://scholarworks.montana.edu/xmlui/handle/1/15589?show=full

42. Gasper AM, Magdic K, Ren D, Fennimore L. Development of a home health-based palliative care program for patients with heart failure. *Home Healthcare Now.* 2018;36(2):84–92. doi:10.1097/NHH.0000000000000634

43. Finnigan-Fox G, Matlock D, Tate C, Knoepke C, Allen L. Hospice, she yelped: Examining the quantity and quality of decision support available to patent and families considering hospice. *J Pain Symptom Manage.* 2017;54(6):916–921. doi:10.1016/j.jpainsymman.2017.08.002.

44. Twaddle, M. McCormick, E. In: Ritchie, Silveira M. UpToDate. *Palliative care delivery in the home.* February 22, 2021. https://www.uptodate.com/contents/palliative-care-delivery-in-the-home

45. Hayes S, Zive D, Ferrell B, Tolle S. The role of advance practice registered nurses in the completion of physician orders for life-sustaining treatment. *J Palliat Med.* 2017;20(4):415–419. doi:10.1089/jpm.2016.0228

46. Young H, Siegel E. The right person at the right time: Ensuring person-centered care. *Generations.* 2016;40(1):47–55.

47. Jackson M, Mecklenburg J, Feshzion A. Palliative care at the doorstep: A community based model. *J Hosp Palliat Nurs.* 2017;19(3):282–286. doi:10.1097/NJH.0000000000000344.

48. Parker J. *House approves Hospice Education Act.* Hospice News. October 28, 2019. https://hospicenews.com/2019/10/28/house-to-vote-on-hospice-education-act/

49. Safriet B. Federal options for maximizing the value of advanced practice nurses in providing quality, cost effective health care. In: Institute of Medicine. *The Future of Nursing: Leading Change, Advancing Health*; Washington, DC: The National Academies Press. 2011: 443–475. doi:10.17226/12956

50. Scholaski J, Weiner J. Health care system reform and the nursing workforce: Matching nursing practice and skills to future needs, not past demands. In: Institute of Medicine. *The Future of Nursing: Leading Change, Advancing Health*; Washington, DC: The National Academies Press. 2011: 375–400. doi:https://doi.org/10.17226/12956

51. Parker J. *New hospice news report details industry outlook for 2021. Hospice News.* February 4 2021. https://www.prweb.com/releases/new_hospice_news_report_deatils_industry_outlook_for_2021/prweb17704420.htm

16.

THE PALLIATIVE APRN IN REHABILITATION

Lorie Resendes Trainor

KEY POINTS

- Rehabilitation and palliative care share similar values in providing patient-centered care with a focus on improving quality of life.

- Rehabilitation can be beneficial at all stages of palliative care involvement—including hospice.

- The palliative advanced practice registered nurse (APRN) is an important partner in the rehabilitation team, providing expert symptom management and education to staff and ensuring the patient's goals remain relevant throughout their rehabilitation journey.

CASE STUDY 1: HIP FRACTURE RECOVERY

Mark was an 80-year-old man with hypertension but otherwise healthy. He was hospitalized for a fall at home resulting in a hip fracture and was found to have newly diagnosed metastatic lung cancer. Mark lives with his elderly wife in a split-level home. They have limited support, and Mark is the primary caretaker in the home. Mark's recovery from his surgery was unremarkable, and he was sent to short-term rehabilitation due to his inability to navigate the stairs at his home.

The rehabilitation team and the palliative advanced practice registered nurse (APRN) met with Mark and his wife frequently throughout his rehabilitation stay. The team reviewed patient and family goals, which included safely returning home. The physical therapist provided a tailored exercise program for Mark and provided recommendations regarding assistive devices and fall prevention. Recommendations were made by the palliative APRN for a short-acting opioid to be given prior to therapy and as needed. The occupational therapist made recommendations to make bathing and dressing easier while expending less energy. The palliative APRN provided education regarding his new underlying disease and explored what matters most to him and his wife. Documents including a health care proxy and orders for life-sustaining treatment were completed. The palliative APRN placed these in the medical record and sent them home with Mark to ensure that his wishes were honored. The social worker facilitated discharge planning to a palliative care program within a VNA program and assisted with ensuring the proper equipment was at home, including bathroom handrails. The social worker also provided a referral to community-based resources with the local Council on Aging to support both Mark and his wife, given their limited support.

Mark was able to increase his strength and was able to safely ambulate around his home. He and his wife felt adequately prepared at discharge to manage his care. Documentation of his rehabilitation stay and advance directives were sent to his new oncology team, thus ensuring continuity of care.

INTRODUCTION

Physical rehabilitation aims to maximize and restore function for those with disabilities.[1] It utilizes an interdisciplinary approach to optimize functional ability and improve quality of life.[2] There has been a steady increase in the utilization of rehabilitation services in the United States. In 2017, Medicare spent $58.9 billion in payments to post-acute care facilities, including skilled nursing facilities (SNFs), home health agencies, inpatient rehabilitation facilities, and long-term care hospitals.[3] Patients who utilize rehabilitation services represent a diverse group and include those with acute illness, traumatic injuries, and progressive chronic illnesses such as cardiopulmonary disease and cancer.[1] The Medicare rehabilitation benefit is widely used; almost 2.4 million beneficiaries accessed the benefit in 2017, representing 4.2% of all Medicare users.[3] The majority of this rehabilitation will take place in an SNF.[3] Beneficiaries increase rehabilitation utilization as they become more ill; one in three Medicare users access their SNF benefit in the last 6 months of life.[4] Overall, patients entering these SNFs represent a more frail and medically complex population.[5,6]

Palliative care and physical rehabilitation share similar goals (Table 16.1). Both are interdisciplinary and focused on improving a patient's quality of life.[7] The palliative care population experiences a significant level of functional loss with disease progression, and this disability may lead to difficulty coping and increased healthcare utilization and caregiver stress.[8] Similar to the palliative care population, rehabilitation patients also have diagnoses associated with high symptom burden.[1] Rehabilitation in the palliative care setting is focused on patients reaching their maximum physical and psychosocial potential within the constraints of their disease.[8] Palliative care and rehabilitation also have a shared value of supporting caregivers through education;

Table 16.1 COMPARISON OF REHABILITATION AND PALLIATIVE CARE

REHABILITATION CARE	PALLIATIVE CARE
A set of interventions designed to optimize functioning and reduce disability in individuals with health conditions in interaction with their environment.[9]	Palliative care is an approach that improves the quality of life of patients (adults and children) and their families who are facing problems associated with life-threatening illness. It prevents and relieves suffering through the early identification, correct assessment and treatment of pain and other problems, whether physical, psychosocial or spiritual.[10]

professional rehabilitation staff are skilled in teaching care-givers proper body mechanics, use of adaptive equipment, and fall prevention.[8–10]

Despite all their shared principles, palliative care is underutilized in rehabilitation. Conversely, rehabilitation care may be overlooked by palliative care providers as a tool which improves patient and family quality of life. Greater understanding of rehabilitation can broaden the palliative advanced practice registered nurse's (APRN) perspective of the many benefits that rehabilitation has to offer those with serious illness.

Even in the setting of advanced illness, patients have expressed a desire to remain physically active and wish to maintain independence for as long as possible.[7,8] Rehabilitation provided to patients with advanced illness has demonstrated benefit. Studies have shown improved quality of life along with better control of pain, dyspnea, and mood.[8] Rehabilitation and palliative goals of care can include both comfort and maximizing independence.[1] The collaboration between rehabilitation and palliative care offers patients a greater potential to reach their goals while also reducing caregiver burden.[1,2]

FOCUS OF REHABILITATION

There are distinctions on the focus of rehabilitation based on a patient's clinical status and functional prognosis: preventative, restorative, supportive, and palliative (Table 16.2).[8,11]

Providing education to the staff, patient, and family regarding the focus of rehabilitation will help to clarify expectations.

LOCATIONS FOR REHABILITATION

Patients can receive rehabilitation services in a variety of settings based on specific admission criteria according to their needs and goals. Long-term acute care hospitals (LTACHs) maintain a complex level of medical care while offering more therapy than the inpatient setting.[1] In 2018, the most common diagnoses for patients admitted to an LTACH were pulmonary edema and respiratory diagnoses requiring mechanical ventilation.[3] LTACHs represent the smallest population of post-acute care facilities; they care for those who are critically ill, caring for 102,288 Medicare patients in 2018.[3]

Inpatient rehabilitation facilities (IRFs) require patients be able to participate in greater than 15 hours per week of physical and occupational therapy.[1] These patients are expected to make significant functional improvement.[8] Because of this requirement, few Medicare beneficiaries are able to tolerate the intensity of an IRF.[1] The most common diagnoses for IRFs are stroke and other neurological disorders.[3] Patients in IRFs are less medically complex and are able to participate more intensely with therapy than those in an LTACH. In 2018, more than 408,000 Medicare patients were cared for in an IRF.

The most utilized post-acute care location by far is the SNF.[3] The SNF offers interdisciplinary collaboration for

Table 16.2 TYPES OF REHABILITATION AND THEIR FOCUS

TYPE	FOCUS	EXAMPLE
Preventative	To prevent or lessen the morbidity caused by treatment.	Patient with lung cancer attends rehabilitation prior to chemotherapy and surgery to optimize functional outcomes.
Restorative	To return a patient to their previous level of function when long-term impairment is not anticipated.	Patient with osteoarthritis undergoes hip replacement to improve their ability to walk without pain.
Supportive	To maximize function after permanent impairment.	Patient status post a stroke with hemiparesis adapting to new ways to ambulate and care for self.
Palliative	To reduce dependence in activity in self-care in setting of progressive disease.	Patient with metastatic cancer who wishes to be able to sit at dining room table with her family but is limited due to pain and low energy.

Table 16.3 LOCATIONS FOR REHABILITATION SERVICES

LOCATION	REQUIREMENTS	EXAMPLE
LTACH	Hospital level of care	Patient discharged from a prolonged hospitalization with a tracheostomy with goal of weaning from mechanical ventilation. He will participate with therapy as tolerated.
IRF	3 hours of PT/OT 5 days per week or 15 hours PT/OT per week	Patient with stroke resulting in severe functional deficits. She is physically able to participate in daily, intensive therapy to reach goal of returning home.
SNF	One hour of PT, OT +/− SLP per day	Elderly female with hip fracture. Goal is to return to her assisted living facility; she is not physically capable of intensive therapy.

SNF, Skilled Nursing Facility; IRF, inpatient rehabilitation facility; LTACH, long-term acute care hospital.

those with less intense rehabilitation needs, with requirements of 1 hour per day of therapy.[8] In 2018, 4% of Medicare beneficiaries—more than 2.3 million patients—utilized their SNF benefit, with an average length of stay of 25 days (Table 16.3).[3]

THE APRN IN THE REHABILITATION SETTING

The role of the rehabilitation APRN in all post-acute care settings is supported by the Association of Rehabilitation Nurses.[12] The rehabilitation APRN serves to manage patients with complex rehabilitation needs, collaborate with the interdisciplinary team, and provide education for staff.[13,14] The value of the APRN can be seen in improved cost-effectiveness of care, reduced frequency of complications for the rehabilitation patient, and increased quality of nursing care.[13]

The rehabilitation APRN also provides comprehensive medication management. This is of importance given the high risk of polypharmacy since patients are medically complex.[1] There is evidence of decreased antipsychotic use and indwelling catheter use in facilities with a dedicated APRN.[15] The facility APRN is better able to understand the processes of the facility and develop closer working relationships with the staff to improve patient experiences and outcomes.[15] When an APRN is embedded in a SNF, hospital transfers can be reduced because the clinician is more easily accessible and can provide complex care in the facility.[13,14]

The palliative APRN has been shown to provide quality, comprehensive palliative care.[16] While the rehabilitation APRN role encompasses many of the tenets of primary palliative care, such as basic symptom management and goals of care, the palliative specialist is more strongly associated with decreased symptom burden.[17] The palliative APRN has the ability to help patients and families navigate goals of care in the setting of serious illness and coordinate care.[7] Patients in the rehabilitation setting often experience significant symptom burden, which the palliative APRN is equipped to address.[2] Working together, the rehabilitation and palliative APRNs can optimize quality of care for patients.

THE REHABILITATION TEAM

THE PHYSIATRIST

Physical medicine and rehabilitation (PM&R) physicians are also known as *physiatrists*. This specialty aims to optimize, restore, and maintain functional ability for those with physical impairments and disabilities.[1] The skill set of the PM&R physician includes pain and symptom management along with helping patients to set functional goals. The goals are individualized and based on the patient's prognosis and ability to regain function.[8] PM&R physicians are able to provide bedside pain management interventions and provide prognosis regarding functional outcomes.[1] The palliative APRN has an opportunity for collaboration with the PM&R physician in improving patient symptom control and setting realistic expectations, particularly for patients with complicated medical problems.[1]

THE PHYSICAL THERAPIST

The intent of physical therapy is to optimize physical functioning.[18] Physical therapists (PTs) are trained to improve functional quality of life through interventions that reduce discomfort, improve functional ability, and promote independence.[19] They are trained to manage functional issues including muscle weakness, deconditioning, and motor deficits.[8] Interventions include providing adaptive and assistive equipment and environmental modification.[8] PTs also play a key role in providing symptom management in nonpharmacological ways (see Box 16.1). This is important because patients often report a preference for nonpharmacological management for certain symptoms such as fatigue.[1] Interventions includes education on energy conservation and exercise, which is utilized in the maintenance of muscle strength, range of motion, and balance.[8]

Another important role for the PT is assisting the patient and family with setting functional goals.[19] The goals of the patient may shift in the setting of progressive debility; the PT is trained to modify their plan given the patient's limitations and focus on the priorities of the patient.[19]

Box 16.1 PHYSICAL THERAPY INTERVENTIONS
FOR PAIN MANAGEMENT

- Massage
- Heat
- Cold
- Ultrasound
- Transcutaneous electronic nerve stimulation
- Diathermy
- Splinting and braces
- Positioning and exercise

In palliative care, physical therapy is often underutilized.[18] Even in the setting of progressive and serious illness, PTs can contribute to improving quality of life through significant reductions in pain, improved performance of activities of daily living (ADLs), and improvement in mood and fatigue.[18] However, the payment structure for physical therapy requires sustainable improvements in function.[18] This may not be feasible in the setting of serious illness and terminal disease. Patients with gradually declining diseases may benefit from intermittent physical therapy for reevaluation and intervention as their care needs evolve.[18]

The American Physical Therapy Association recognizes the importance of PTs partnering with palliative care,[20] and there is awareness of the need to expose physical therapy students to palliative care early in their training.[21] However, there is currently limited education of palliative care among physical therapists.[18] Given that there is not a palliative care specialization for rehabilitation, the palliative APRN is critical in providing ongoing staff education and collaboration to improve palliative care awareness and enhance quality of care. The palliative APRN can collaborate with the PT to ensure symptoms are managed using a multimodal approach, allowing the patient to comfortably participate in therapy.

THE OCCUPATIONAL THERAPIST

The occupational therapist (OT) provides assessment and management to improve fine motor skills performance with ADLs, work tasks, and recreation.[8] Occupational therapy contributes to quality of life by enabling patients to lead fulfilling lives within the limitations of their disease.[22] It decreases isolation, enabling patients to redefine their social roles and how they participate in activities.[23] This contributes to enhanced social relationships and personal dignity.[22] OTs accomplish this through instructing patients on the use of aids and adaptive equipment in addition to developing strategies to accommodate their limitations and conserve energy.[23] Examples include built-up handles on toothbrushes and utensils, sock donners, grab bars, and raised toilet seats.[1] The OT works with patients and caregivers in setting activity-related

goals surrounding self-care, transfers, and home management.[8] The OT works within the interdisciplinary team to inform others of the level of help the patient requires to make activity possible.[23]

The role of the OT in enhancing quality of life is complementary to palliative care involvement. This is recognized by the American Occupational Therapy Association: "Occupational therapy services . . . integrate the physical, cognitive, emotional, and spiritual aspects of clients' experiences so they may participate in their life roles regardless of the stage of their disease process."[24] The palliative APRN works jointly with the OT to facilitate discussions of meaningful functional goals for the patient.

THE SPEECH LANGUAGE PATHOLOGIST

The speech language pathologist (SLP) provides rehabilitation services to patients with conditions impacting their communication, cognition, or swallowing.[25] While SLPs have not traditionally been associated with palliative care, they have an important role in maintaining quality of life for patients with serious illness and those who are terminally ill.[25] Patients may have impaired abilities to communicate as a result of their disease process. Impaired communication can affect the patient's ability to make their preferences known and influence their emotional status and even their symptom management.[25,26] The SLP provides a comprehensive assessment and strategies to enhance communication.[25] Strategies include providing appropriate alternative communication tools (see Table 16.2).[25,27] These interventions allow patients to continue to direct their own care and socially interact (Table 16.4).[1]

Dysphagia management is another way that the SLP can facilitate quality of life in those with a serious illness. As patients enter the later stages of disease, decisions may need to be made regarding optimal routes of nutrition, which can lead to conflict within families and teams.[25] The SLP provides direction to the patient and team regarding modifying diets for safety and teaching safer and more comfortable swallowing techniques, allowing the patient to enjoy eating for as long as possible.[25] Decisions regarding risks and benefits of enteral nutrition and tracheostomy should be considered in conjunction with the entire interdisciplinary team, including the SLP, with respect to the patient's prognosis and goals of care[25] (see Chapter 56, "Discontinuation of Other Life-Sustaining Therapies"). As with other therapy disciplines, the palliative APRN plays a key role in educating the SLP regarding palliative care and participating in discussions regarding patient-centered goals of care.

Table 16.4 AUGMENTATIVE AND ALTERNATIVE COMMUNICATION (AAC)[27]

Unaided systems	Aided systems
• Gestures	• Pen and paper
• Body language	• Picture/alphabet boards
• Facial expressions	• Computer generating speech devices

Adapted from American Speech-Language-Hearing Association.[27]

THE DIETICIAN

Registered dieticians are specialized professionals trained to evaluate a patient's nutritional needs, prevent malnutrition, and improve nutritional status.[28] There can be confusion between the titles *dieticians* and *nutritionists*; registered dieticians must have at minimum a bachelor's degree and must pass a national certifying exam after completing specific academic and clinical requirements.[29] The more generic title "nutritionist" is not regulated in some states, and those with simply an interest in nutrition can use this label; in acute and long-term care settings, the dietician is the designated professional to oversee food and nutrition services.[29]

In rehabilitation care, the caloric needs of patients vary greatly, and malnutrition can lead to functional decline. For example, in patients with a hip fracture, malnutrition can lead to postoperative complications, poor functional improvement, and higher rates of rehospitalization.[30] For patients with dementia, nutritional issues will arise over the course of the disease including difficulty swallowing and taste changes.[15] Given that one in four elderly patients admitted to rehabilitation with a hip fracture have insufficient caloric intake, problems with nutrition in this setting are significant.[30] Studies have shown increased dietary intake is associated with improved ADLs after hip fracture surgery.[30] The dietician often works with the SLP to tailor a plan for the patient to optimize nutrition, including flexibility for patient preferences and caloric needs.[31]

THE SOCIAL WORKER

The needs of the rehabilitation patient are multidimensional and include psychosocial support.[32] The role of the social worker (SW) in the rehabilitation setting is to empower residents and enhance their coping ability.[32] Particularly in the SNF setting, the SW is a key part of the interdisciplinary team supporting the patient, family, and staff both formally and informally.[32] SWs have comprehensive assessment skills and are able to engage the patient and family in eliciting what matters most to them.[33] These needs, including adequate treatment of depression and anxiety, can influence physical symptoms.[34] SWs support a patient's autonomy, emotional well-being, and quality of life.[31] In palliative care, social workers are valued professionals who establish trust with patients and families to explore goals of care and validate concerns in the setting of serious illness.[34,35] In the rehabilitation setting, SWs provide this support in addition to facilitating a safe discharge plan with the patient and family.[32]

REHABILITATION DISEASE-SPECIFIC GROUPS

THE CANCER POPULATION

Patients with cancer may be admitted to rehabilitation facilities related to disability from the cancer itself, treatment-related debility, or complications such as pathologic fracture.[36]

They may also be admitted to rehabilitation with the goal of "getting stronger" to pursue cancer-directed treatment.[37] Exercise during and after cancer treatment has been shown to be safe and is effective in decreasing fatigue, improving sleep quality, reducing long-term side effects, and even decreasing risk of recurrence.[38] The positive effects of rehabilitation can be seen across all stages of cancer, including survivorship.[39] Even in advanced cancer, rehabilitation techniques used for palliation can prevent decline and even improve ADLs.[40,41] Such gains in function can be maintained several weeks after rehabilitation discharge.[41] Maximizing independence, while important to patients, also plays a role in reducing caregiver burden.[36]

In the setting of advanced cancer, the palliative APRN assists the rehabilitation team in setting realistic goals. For instance "getting stronger" for treatment may unfairly burden patients who are in the later stages of their disease and unable to stop their increasing frailty.[36] Among patients at one hospital who were discharged to rehabilitation with the goal of getting stronger for immunotherapy, only one-third received additional treatment.[37] Average survival of those who did not receive additional treatment was only 51 days, and 30-day readmission rates were high at 28%.[37] The palliative APRN can help the patient and rehabilitation team set expectations of possible improvement in symptoms such as fatigue while simultaneously having ongoing goals-of-care discussions.[36] The social worker also works with the patient in acknowledging the patient's desire to maintain a sense of self while coping with their changing body and roles.[42] The palliative APRN can also optimize symptom management in this population, including management of fatigue, pain, and nausea that may interfere with a patient's ability to participate in rehabilitation. The palliative APRN also provides support with advance care planning and discussion of priorities in the setting of advanced disease.[36,39] Coordination of symptom management should ideally occur among the oncology, rehabilitation, and palliative care teams.[40]

THE PULMONARY POPULATION

Patients who have pulmonary disease may avoid activity due to dyspnea and can consequently become deconditioned.[43] Pulmonary rehabilitation serves to rebuild the functional capacity of patients who experience dyspnea and deconditioning.[43] Tools used to achieve this include addressing the underlying pulmonary disease and breathing retraining to improve gas exchange, along with airway clearance techniques.[43] Rather than being solely an exercise program, it is a comprehensive way of managing the disabling aspects of respiratory disease and has been shown to improve quality of life and symptom control.[43] Benefits include less dyspnea and fatigue, improved endurance, and better ability to perform ADLs. These benefits extend to those with limited life expectancy due to chronic obstructive pulmonary disease (COPD) and lung cancer.[43] The pulmonary patient receiving rehabilitation provides an opportunity to discuss advanced directives; this discussion can also alleviate anxiety regarding end of life and increase goals-of-care discussions.[44]

THE CARDIAC POPULATION

Evidence shows that palliative care for patients with heart failure improves quality of life, patient satisfaction, and documentation of preferences and decreases rehospitalization.[45] The American College of Cardiology has recognized the importance of integrating palliative care throughout the course of management in patients with heart failure[46] and recommends considering referral to specialty palliative care when patients develop New York Heart Association (NYHA) Class III–IV symptoms.[45]

Cardiac rehabilitation is a specialized program which combines exercise with addressing modifiable risk factors such as smoking, nutrition, and management of comorbid conditions such as hypertension and diabetes.[46] For patients with heart failure and NYHA Class II–III symptoms, exercise training improves exercise tolerance and health-related quality of life.[47] It has also been shown to decrease hospitalizations for those with reduced ejection fraction.[47] Cardiac rehabilitation is underutilized in the Medicare population, with only 1 in 4 eligible beneficiaries participating.[48]

THE NEUROLOGY POPULATION

The course of neurological disease can be challenging for patients, families, and clinicians. The involvement of palliative care often depends on a patient's prognosis and the natural history of the illness.[49] Patients in the rehabilitation setting may have experienced a sudden event, such as a stroke, while others are grappling with the complications of their underlying progressive disease. In the setting of a sudden event such as stroke, prognosis can be uncertain and variable, leading to difficulty in decision-making among patients and families.[50] Patients can be faced with focusing on rehabilitation while preparing for a life that may include severe disability.[50] Surrogates may find themselves in a role of decision-making that they were not prepared for and may be hearing conflicting information regarding prognosis, thus contributing to their distress.[50,51] A model of "preparing for survival, decline or death and hoping for the best" may be helpful, allowing patients and families to work through these life-altering events.[50]

Patients with progressive neurological disorders such as Parkinson's disease can experience high symptom burden related to their motor dysfunction along with social and emotional distress.[52] Neuropsychiatric symptoms such as dementia, depression, and apathy can also impair communication and social interactions.[52] Proactive intervention is recommended to reduce symptom intensity, symptom frequency, and the need for crisis-level intervention.[52] Therapies may be focused on treating underlying issues such as SLP for speech-amplifying devices in the setting of hypophonia, social worker support for anxiety, and PT and OT for activity modification. As with other diseases, physical activity remains important for those with neurological disorders—even if a person is wheelchair-bound.[52] Rehabilitation interventions have been shown to maintain residual ability and prevent complications such as pressure ulcers, contractures, and pneumonia.[52] Symptom management may include optimizing dopaminergic medications in collaboration with the neurologist and monitoring for medication-induced side effects, such as sedation and orthostatic hypotension.[52] Ensuring that inappropriate medications are not prescribed also supports quality symptom management. This includes avoiding certain neuroleptics and antiemetics that are dopamine receptor blocking agents that can worsen motor dysfunction.[52]

THE DEMENTIA POPULATION

The treatment of patients with dementia requires comprehensive medical and social support.[53] Patients with dementia may be unable to express their preferences for care or verbalize their symptom needs.[54] Despite these limitations, patients with dementia can benefit from rehabilitation services.[55] The rehabilitation is focused on achieving goals important to the patient within the limitations of their disease.[55] All members of the rehabilitation team have the ability to improve the quality of life for the patient with dementia. Given that dysphagia develops in a majority of patients with dementia, the SLP is able to offer strategies to optimize swallowing and make it more comfortable.[31] The dietician and SLP can work together to identify food and drink preferences to maximize nutrition while providing flexibility in the setting of decreased oral intake.[31] The OT can provide equipment to make getting food to the mouth easier by offering modified cutlery and plates,[31] in addition to strategies to minimize social isolation.[23] Hand feeding can be provided by staff and family once the SLP has identified the safest way for the patient to eat. The PT can provide an exercise program and interventions for fall reduction.[2] The focus of rehabilitation may be to maintain function and independence for as long as possible rather than making significant functional gains.[19]

SETTING GOALS OF CARE IN THE REHABILITATION SETTING

There can be misguided expectations from patients and family when a patient enters rehabilitation care. Patients may not have a clear understanding of the progressive nature of their illness because they are in rehabilitation care with the goal of improvement[18] and may expect to leave rehabilitation "stronger and better."[7] Despite the many benefits of rehabilitation, many older patients who are discharged from the hospital to a facility have serious illnesses associated with poor prognoses.[56] The goal of regaining function and returning to independence may only be met in a minority of patients who have received palliative care in the hospital,[57] and overall survival is poor.[58] Transitions of care can be high in this population; studies show high rates of 30-day readmissions for patients who received a palliative care consultation in the hospital and are discharged to a SNF.[58] For Medicare patients in 2015, more than 43% had a nursing home stay in the last 90 days of life—almost 24 million people.[59] Such transitions can be burdensome to patients, leading to inadequate symptom management, pressure ulcers, and poorer end-of-life outcomes.[56,57]

These transitions can also be difficult for family members and can exclude them from the end-of-life process.[60]

Reasons for increased transitions for seriously ill patients in the SNF setting are varied. Patients with chronic diseases such as heart, lung, and kidney issues are at elevated risk for transitions due to poor coordination of care.[61] Up to 49% of patients who receive a palliative care consultation in the hospital are discharged to an SNF[58]; SNF staff may not have adequate symptom management training and often lack access to a palliative care clinican.[57] Lack of continuity of palliative care support can lead to poor communication and disruption of ongoing goals-of-care discussions.[57] Palliative care involvement in the SNF setting has been shown to lower rates of potentially burdensome care transitions.[62]

Patients and families benefit from ongoing disease and prognostic information to make appropriate healthcare decisions.[56] The goal of the palliative APRN is to ensure patient-centered goals are consistently addressed and there is communication with the patient and family in setting realistic expectations.[7] In the rehabilitation setting, this involves ensuring documentation of goals and values and ensuring these are conveyed across settings to avoid unwanted care.[63] Coordination with the rehabilitation staff to recognize decline and lack of progression is vital in these goals-of-care discussions.[7] In situations of prognostic uncertainty, a *time-limited trial* may be helpful. A time-limited trial allows the patients, families, and staff to establish mutual expectations regarding how a patient is progressing based on an intervention and an established time frame for assessing outcomes.[64] Collaboration with rehabilitation staff and reassessment of goals is important throughout the patient's rehabilitation care.

CASE STUDY 2: DEMENTIA

Mary was a 90-year-old nursing home resident with advanced Alzheimer's dementia. She was sent to the hospital after falling while attempting to get up from her chair. She was noted to have a right hip fracture on imaging. Orthopedic surgery was consulted, and she underwent hip repair due to severe pain. She was sent back to her nursing home under the Medicare rehabilitation benefit.

At baseline, Mary is a one-person assist with transfers from bed to chair. She speaks a few words and eats a pureed diet with thickened liquids. She will occasionally have sundowning behaviors in which she becomes more confused and occasionally refuses care. Her healthcare proxy is her daughter Jennifer, and this proxy is activated.

The rehabilitation team and palliative APRN met with Jennifer to review the plan and elicit goals of care. Jennifer expressed her wish that her mother return to her baseline prior to the hip fracture, and she was worried that her mother had become increasingly anxious and uncomfortable since the hospital. PT began working toward Mary returning to her previous status of being able to transfer with assistance. Over time, it became clear that Mary was not making any progress, and goals were shifted to provide comfortable transfer with a mechanical lift. Her pain was managed by the palliative APRN with scheduled acetaminophen and oxycodone as needed. Mary was experiencing delirium from the hospital, and the palliative APRN ensured her pain was managed and that she was not experiencing reversible sources of delirium such as opioid-induced constipation.

The palliative APRN communicated frequently with the rehabilitation staff as Mary continued to functionally decline. Since Mary's hospitalization, the dietician noted a 10% weight loss and continued poor oral intake despite supplementation. Mary also seemed to be sleeping more and was no longer speaking.

The team met with Jennifer to readdress goals of care. Jennifer did not want her mother to undergo any further hospitalizations and did not want any invasive measures such as a feeding tube. Goals were shifted solely to comfort care. The SLP worked with Mary to liberalize her food and drink consistency to allow comfort feeding. The staff nurses were educated on the importance of assessing and managing nonverbal signs of pain. The palliative APRN ensured wishes for no further hospitalizations were documented in the medical record, nonessential medications were stopped, and comfort medications were in place. Mary passed away comfortably while under her rehabilitation benefit with the support of the entire team.

END OF LIFE IN THE SKILLED NURSING FACILITY SETTING

The payment structure of rehabilitation favors functional progression rather than a focus on comfort.[57] Despite the functional improvement goal of rehabilitation, more than 9% of Medicare beneficiaries will die while utilizing their SNF rehabilitation benefit.[57] Financially, nursing homes are reimbursed at a higher rate for rehabilitation than for long-term care.[57] This may lead to interventions that support the goals of rehabilitation but not the patient's changing needs at end of life.[4] For families, rehabilitation facilities may be the only financial option to cover the needed 24-hour care of their loved one after a hospitalization.[4] Patients who are utilizing their rehabilitation benefit are not able to access their hospice benefit, leaving those who are at end of life without all the support hospice offers.[57] In the rehabilitation setting, APRNs are able to provide palliative care consultations through Medicare Part B billing[62] without impacting the revenue of the rehabilitation facility, thus filling an important gap in end-of-life care in this setting.

The palliative APRN can address changes in a patient's condition that may not be recognized as end-of-life deterioration by rehabilitation staff.[65] This recognition is essential in providing the appropriate level of support for the patient and families[49] in addition to the symptom management that may be lacking from the rehabilitation staff.[58] The APRN can provide support to families who may be unprepared for their loved one's end of life due to the expectation of recovery with rehabilitation care. The APRN can also work with the rehabilitation staff to ensure that interventions are aligned with the patient's and family's goals of care at end of life and decrease the risk of hospitalization.[66]

SUMMARY

Patients entering rehabilitation care often have complex medical and psychosocial needs. They may be facing debility due to a sudden event such as a stroke or experiencing ongoing debility from chronic illness. Rehabilitation care provides a comprehensive interdisciplinary team approach which includes physiatrists, PTs, OTs, SLPs, dieticians, and medical social workers. The benefits of rehabilitation can be seen at all stages of disease and has been shown to improve a patient's quality of life. The palliative APRN is a key member of the team and facilitates symptom management and ongoing goals-of-care discussions in collaboration with the rehabilitation staff. They are critical in eliciting patient-centered goals of care and helping patients and staff establish realistic expectations for rehabilitation. The palliative APRN assists the patient and family in navigating the complexities of both sudden and progressive diseases and provides ongoing support during uncertainty and shifting goals. They also provide expert end-of-life care for patients who die during rehabilitation and are unable to access their hospice benefit. Palliative care in the rehabilitation setting is underutilized and represents an opportunity to improve quality of life and coordination of care.

REFERENCES

1. Brassil M, Cheville A, Zheng J, et al. Top ten tips palliative care clinicians should know about physical medicine and rehabilitation. *J Palliat Med*. 2020;23(1):129–135. doi:10.1089/jpm.2019.0440

2. Wittry S, Lam N, McNalley T. The value of rehabilitation medicine for patients receiving palliative care. *Am J Hosp Palliat Care*. 2017;35(6):889–896. doi:10.1177/1049909117742896

3. Medicare Payment Advisory Commission. A Data Book. Healthcare Spending and the Medicare Program. 2020 Meid. http://medpac.gov/docs/default-source/data-book/july2020_databook_entireport_sec.pdf?sfvrsn=0

4. Carpenter J. Forced to choose: When medicare policy disrupts end-of-life care. [published online ahead of print, 2020 Mar 29]. *J Aging Soc Policy*. 2020:1–8. doi:10.1080/08959420.2020.1745737. Epub ahead of print. PMID: 32223534; PMCID: PMC7679051.

5. Gonella S, Basso I, De Marinis M, Campagna S, Di Giulio P. Good end-of-life care in nursing home according to the family carers' perspective: A systematic review of qualitative findings. *Palliat Med*. 2019;33(6):589–606. doi:10.1177/0269216319840275

6. Wallace C, Adorno G, Stewart D. End-of-life care in nursing homes: A qualitative interpretive meta-synthesis. *J Palliat Med*. 2018;21(4):503–512. doi:10.1089/jpm.2017.0211

7. Runacres F, Gregory H, Ugalde A. "The horse has bolted I suspect": A qualitative study of clinicians' attitudes and perceptions regarding palliative rehabilitation. *Palliat Med*. 2016;31(7):642–650. doi:10.1177/0269216316670288

8. Javier N, Montagnini M. The role of palliative rehabilitation in serious illness #364. *J Palliat Med*. 2018;21(12):1808–1809. doi:10.1089/jpm.2018.0541

9. World Health Organization. Rehabilitation Fact Sheet. Updated July 16, 2021. https://www.who.int/news-room/fact-sheets/detail/rehabilitation

10. World Health Organization Palliative Care Fact Sheet. Updated August 5, 2020. https://www.who.int/news-room/fact-sheets/detail/palliative-care

11. Montagnini M, Javier NM. The role of rehabilitation in patients receiving hospice and palliative care. *Rehab Oncology*. 2020;(38):9–21.

12. Association of Rehabilitation Nurses. Position statement: Advanced practice in rehab nursing. Chicago, IL: ARN. Updated 2020. https://rehabnurse.org/about/position-statements/advanced-practice-in-rehab-nursing

13. Association of Rehabilitation Nurses. Position statement: Advanced practice rehabilitation nurse. Chicago, IL: ARN. Updated 2020. https://rehabnurse.org/about/roles/advanced-practice-rehab-nurse

14. Robatin K, Robatin M, Robatin K, Reed S. Role of the advanced practitioner in the delivery of quality care in the post-acute care setting. *J Am Med Dir Assoc*. 2019;20(3):B11–B12. doi:10.1016/j.jamda.2019.01.062

15. Ryskina K, Lam C, Jung H. Association between clinician specialization in nursing home care and nursing home clinical quality scores. *J Am Med Dir Assoc*. 2019;20(8):1007–1012.e2. doi:10.1016/j.jamda.2018.12.017

16. Opitz S, Hebert R. Nurse practitioners as disruptive innovators in palliative medicine. *J Palliat Care*. 2018;33(4):191–193. doi:10.1177/0825859718785227

17. Ernecoff N, Check D, Bannon M, et al. Comparing specialty and primary palliative care interventions: Analysis of a systematic review. *J Palliat Med*. 2020;23(3):389–396.

18. Wilson C, Mueller K, Briggs R. Physical therapists' contribution to the hospice and palliative care interdisciplinary team. *J Hosp Palliat Nurs*. 2017;19(6):588–596. doi:10.1097/njh.0000000000000394

19. Wilson C, Stiller C, Doherty D, Thompson K, Smith A, Turczynski K. Physical therapists in integrated palliative care: A qualitative study. *BMJ Support Palliat Care*. Published Online First: 20 February 2020. doi:10.1136/bmjspcare-2019-002161

20. American Physical Therapy Association. The role of physical therapy in palliative care and hospice. Alexandria, VA: APTA. Updated September 20, 2019. https://www.apta.org/apta-and-you/leadership-and-governance/policies/role-of-physical-therapy-in-palliative-care-and-hospice

21. Chiarelli P, Johnston C, Osmotherly P. Introducing palliative care into entry-level physical therapy education. *J Palliat Med*. 2014;17(2):152–158.

22. Eva G, Morgan D. Mapping the scope of occupational therapy practice in palliative care: A European association for palliative care cross-sectional survey. *Palliat Med*. 2018;32(5):960–968. doi:10.1177/0269216318758928

23. Tavemark S, Hermansson L, Blomberg K. Enabling activity in palliative care: Focus groups among occupational therapists. *BMC Palliat Care*. 2019;18(1). doi:10.1186/s12904-019-0394-9

24. The American Occupational Therapy Association. The role of occupational therapy in palliative and hospice care. Bethesda, MD: AOTA. 2015. https://www.aota.org/~/media/Corporate/Files/AboutOT/Professionals/WhatIsOT/PA/Facts/FactSheet_PalliativeCare.pdf

25. Chahda L, Mathisen B, Carey L. The role of speech-language pathologists in adult palliative care. *Int J Speech Lang Pathol*. 2016;19(1):58–68. doi:10.1080/17549507.2016.1241301

26. American Speech-Language-Hearing Association. End-of-life issues in speech language pathology. 2004. https://www.asha.org/slp/clinical/endoflife/

27. American Speech-Language-Hearing Association. Augmentative and alternative communication (AAC). 2019. https://www.asha.org/public/speech/disorders/aac/

28. Holmes R. Role of dietitians in reducing malnutrition in hospital. *Can Med Assoc J*. 2019;191(5):E139–E139. doi:10.1503/cmaj.71130

29. Institute of Medicine (US) Committee on Nutrition Services for Medicare Beneficiaries. The role of nutrition in maintaining health in the nation's elderly: Evaluating coverage of nutrition services for the medicare population. Washington, DC: National Academies Press. 2000. https://www.ncbi.nlm.nih.gov/books/NBK225286/

30. Umezawa H, Kokura Y, Abe S, et al. Relationship between performance improvement in activities of daily living and energy intake in older patients with hip fracture undergoing rehabilitation. *Ann Rehabil Med*. 2019;43(5):562–569. doi:10.5535/arm.2019.43.5.562

31. Murphy J, Holmes J, Brooks C. Nutrition and dementia care: Developing an evidence-based model for nutritional care in nursing homes. *BMC Geriatr.* 2017;17(1):55. doi:10.1186/s12877-017-0443-2. PMID: 28196475; PMCID: PMC5309970.

32. Lev S, Ayalon L. Coping with the obligation dilemma: Prototypes of social workers in the nursing home. *Br J Soc Work.* 2015;46(5):1318–1335. doi:10.1093/bjsw/bcv038

33. Giuffrida J. Palliative care in your nursing home: Program development and innovation in transitional care. *J Soc Work End Life Palliat Care.* 2015;11(2):167–177. doi:10.1080/15524256.2015.1074143

34. Almada A, Casquinha P, Cotovio V, Heitor dos Santos M, Caixeiro A. The potential role of psychosocial rehabilitation in palliative care. *J Royal Coll Phys Edin.* 2018;48(4):311–317. doi:10.4997/jrcpe.2018.405

35. Social Work Hospice and Palliative Care Network 2021. https://www.swhpn.org/

36. Padgett L, Asher A, Cheville A. The intersection of rehabilitation and palliative care. *Rehabil Nurs.* 2018;43(4):219–228. doi:10.1097/rnj.0000000000000171

37. Yeh J, Knight L, Kane J, Doberman D, Gupta A, Smith T. Has there been a shift in use of subacute rehabilitation instead of hospice referral since immunotherapy has become available? *J Oncol Pract.* 2019;15(10):e849–e855. doi:10.1200/jop.19.00044

38. Lopez G, Eddy C, Liu W, et al. Physical therapist–led exercise assessment and counseling in integrative cancer care: Effects on patient self-reported symptoms and quality of life. *Integr Cancer Ther.* 2019;18:1–7. doi:10.1177/1534735419832360

39. Silver J, Stout N, Fu J, Pratt-Chapman M, Haylock P, Sharma R. The state of cancer rehabilitation in the United States. *J Cancer Rehabil.* 2018;1(1):1–8.

40. Zhu Y. Value-based practice: Integration of cancer rehabilitation and palliative care in oncology services. *Chin Med Sci J.* 2018;33(4):204–209. doi:10.24920/003523

41. Guo Y, Fu J, Guo H, et al. Postacute care in cancer rehabilitation. *Phys Med Rehabil Clin N Am.* 2017;28(1):19–34. doi:10.1016/j.pmr.2016.09.004

42. Morgan D, Currow D, Denehy L, Aranda S. Living actively in the face of impending death: Constantly adjusting to bodily decline at the end-of-life. *BMJ Support Palliat Care.* 2015;7(2):179–188. doi:10.1136/bmjspcare-2014-000744

43. Tiep B, Sun V, Koczywas M, et al. Pulmonary rehabilitation and palliative care for the lung cancer patient. *J Hosp Palliat Nurs.* 2015;17(5):462–468. doi:10.1097/njh.0000000000000187

44. Grossman D, Katz A, Lock K, Caraiscos V. A retrospective study reviewing interprofessional advance care planning group discussions in pulmonary rehabilitation: A proof-of-concept and feasibility study. *J Palliat Care.* 2019. doi:10.1177/0825859719896421

45. Diop M, Rudolph J, Zimmerman K, Richter M, Skarf M. Palliative care interventions for patients with heart failure: A systematic review and meta-analysis. *J Palliat Med.* Jan 2017;20(1):84–92. doi:org/10.1089/jpm.2016.0330

46. Goodlin S. Palliative care in congestive heart failure. *J Am Coll Cardiol.* July 2009;54(5):386–396.

47. Pina I. In: Gottlieb, S. Ed. Cardiac rehabilitation in patients with heart failure. In: Gottlieb S, Yeon S, eds. *UpToDate.* Waltham, MA:UpToDate.Updated June 21, 2020. From https://www.uptodate.com/contents/cardiac-rehabilitation-in-patients-with-heart-failure

48. Braun L. Wegner, N, Rosenson R. In: Gersh, R. Cardiac rehabilitation programs. In: Gersh B, Saperia G, eds. *UpToDate.* Waltham, MA: UpToDate. Updated July 13, 2021. https://www.uptodate.com/contents/cardiac-rehabilitation-programs/print

49. Oliver D, Borasio G, Caraceni A, et al. A consensus review on the development of palliative care for patients with chronic and progressive neurological disease. *Eur J Neurol.* 2015;23(1):30–38. doi:10.1111/ene.12889

50. Kendall M, Cowey E, Mead G, et al. Outcomes, experiences and palliative care in major stroke: A multicentre, mixed-method, longitudinal study. *Can Med Assoc J.* 2018;190(9):E238–E246. doi:10.1503/cmaj.170604

51. Zahuranec D, Anspach R, Roney M, et al. Surrogate decision makers' perspectives on family members' prognosis after intracerebral hemorrhage. *J Palliat Med.* 2018;21(7):956–962. doi:10.1089/jpm.2017.0604

52. Katz M, Goto Y, Kluger B, et al. Top ten tips palliative care clinicians should know about Parkinson's disease and related disorders. *J Palliat Med.* 2018;21(10):1507–1517. doi:10.1089/jpm.2018.0390

53. Jennings L, Laffan A, Schlissel A, et al. Health care utilization and cost outcomes of a comprehensive dementia care program for medicare beneficiaries. *JAMA Intern Med.* 2019;179(2):161. doi:10.1001/jamainternmed.2018.5579

54. Fox S, FitzGerald C, Harrison Dening K, et al. Better palliative care for people with a dementia: Summary of interdisciplinary workshop highlighting current gaps and recommendations for future research. *BMC Palliat Care.* 2017;17(1). doi:10.1186/s12904-017-0221-0

55. Clare L. Rehabilitation for people living with dementia: A practical framework of positive support. *PLoS Med.* 2017;14(3):e1002245. doi:10.1371/journal.pmed.1002245

56. Carpenter J, Berry P, Ersek M. Care in nursing facilities after palliative consult. *J Hosp Palliat Nurs.* 2018;20(2):153–159. doi:10.1097/njh.0000000000000420

57. Carpenter J, Berry P, Ersek M. Nursing home care trajectories for older adults following in-hospital palliative care consultation. *Geriatr Nurs.* 2017;38(6):531–536. doi:10.1016/j.gerinurse.2017.03.016

58. Carpenter J. Hospital palliative care teams and post-acute care in nursing facilities: An integrative review. *Res Gerontol Nurs.* 2017;10(1):25–34. doi:10.3928/19404921-20161209-02

59. Teno J, Gozalo P, Trivedi A, et al. Site of death, place of care, and health care transitions among us medicare beneficiaries, 2000-2015. *JAMA.* 2018;320(3):264. doi:10.1001/jama.2018.8981

60. Fleming J, Calloway R, Perrels A, Farquhar M, Barclay S, Brayne C. Dying comfortably in very old age with or without dementia in different care settings: A representative "older old" population study. *BMC Geriatr.* 2017;17(1). doi:10.1186/s12877-017-0605-2

61. Wang S, Aldridge M, Gross C, Canavan M, Cherlin E, Bradley E. End-of-life care transition patterns of medicare beneficiaries. *J Am Geriatr Soc.* 2017;65(7):1406–1413. doi:10.1111/jgs.14891

62. Miller S, Lima J, Intrator O, Martin E, Bull J, Hanson L. Palliative care consultations in nursing homes and reductions in acute care use and potentially burdensome end-of-life transitions. *J Am Geriatr Soc.* 2016;64(11):2280–2287. doi:10.1111/jgs.14469

63. Meisenberg B, Zaidi S, Franks L, Moller D, Mooradian D. Discrepant advanced directives and code status orders: A preventable medical error. *J Hosp Med.* 2019;14(11):716–718. doi:10.12788/jhm.3244

64. Quill T, Holloway R. Time-limited trials near the end of life. *JAMA.* 2011;306(13):1483. doi:10.1001/jama.2011.1413

65. Bloomer M, Botti M, Runacres F, Poon P, Barnfield J, Hutchinson A. Communicating end-of-life care goals and decision-making among a multidisciplinary geriatric inpatient rehabilitation team: A qualitative descriptive study. *Palliat Med.* 2018;32(10):1615–1623. doi:10.1177/0269216318790353

66. Ouslander J, Berenson R. Reducing unnecessary hospitalizations of nursing home residents. *N Engl J Med.* 2011;365(13):1165–1167. doi:10.1056/nejmp1105449

17.

THE PALLIATIVE APRN IN TELEHEALTH

Katherine Kyle and Constance Dahlin

KEY POINTS

- Telehealth palliative care extends the boundaries of palliative care by promoting access to individuals previously limited by geography and providers while simultaneously complementing in-person provider visits.

- Telehealth has experienced recent rapid proliferation, offering opportunities of palliative care growth and expansion to marginalized populations.

- Palliative advanced practice registered nurses (APRNs) may provide telehealth delivery because it is within their scope of practice and reimbursement eligibility.

- Providing telehealth requires education, planning, and the use of skillful communication.

CASE STUDY: TELEHEALTH CONSULTATION

Mrs. K was a 68-year-old woman with metastatic pancreatic cancer referred to palliative care for symptom management for cancer-/treatment-related symptoms. At the time of visit, she was on her second-line chemotherapy with a high performance status. Her symptoms included abdominal pain, for which she was prescribed oxycodone 5 mg every 4 hours. She also had intermittent nausea and vomiting in the hours and days immediately following chemotherapy. For this, she was prescribed aprepitant on the day of infusions as well as Ondansetron ODT 8 mg as needed. The patient shared concern over her weight loss related to decreased appetite and intermittent bouts of nausea and vomiting in the days following chemotherapy infusions. Her decline and symptoms were causing her some symptoms of depression included sadness, anhedonia, and hopelessness, which was different for her.

The palliative advanced practice registered nurse (APRN) recommended adjusting her medications to long-acting oxycodone 30 mg scheduled twice daily with a breakthrough dose of oxycodone to 10 mg every 4 hours. The APRN prescribed mirtazapine 7.5 mg at bedside for appetite stimulation as well as to assist with depression management. A referral was also made by the palliative APRN to an interventional pain clinic for celiac plexus nerve block. These interventions provided relief.

In-person follow-up was disrupted by the COVID-19 outbreak, so the palliative APRN conducted video visits. Since the nerve block, Mrs. K reported only needing breakthrough medication once a day. The palliative APRN monitored her symptoms and adjusted medications. In addition, the palliative APRN initiated advance care planning. Family members were able to attend the meeting. Mrs. K was able to share her goal of continuing treatments as long as they were helpful. When they were not longer helpful, she wanted to focus on staying at home and focusing on comfort.

The palliative APRN continued to monitor Mrs. K, who was still receiving chemotherapy infusions. She developed further nausea and vomiting and was admitted. Work-up revealed liver metastases. The palliative APRN followed her care in the hospital and provided inpatient telehealth visits so family members could be present in the care.

INTRODUCTION

DEFINITION OF TELEHEALTH

Telehealth is broadly defined as the delivery of health and health-related services using digital information and telecommunication technologies.[1–4] The Health Resource Services Administration (HRSA) defines *telehealth* as "the use of electronic information and telecommunications technologies to support and promote long-distance clinical healthcare, patient and professional health-related education, public health and health administration. Technologies include videoconferencing, the internet, store-and-forward imaging, streaming media, and terrestrial and wireless communications."[5]

The terms *telehealth* and *telemedicine* are often used interchangeably but there are some key distinctions. Healthcare institutions and professional organizations also vary in their definitions but this adds emphasis to the fact that telehealth is a constant and rapidly evolving specialty that adapts to contemporary innovations in technology and to the healthcare needs of populations and societal conditions.[6,7]

Telehealth is considered to be a more encompassing and holistic term, referring to a broad range of health services delivered remotely or from a distance through the use of electronic information and telecommunication technologies.[1–4,7] *Telemedicine* means "healing at a distance" and refers to actual patient care through telehealth or the provision of clinical services using telecommunication technologies.[6] The American Telemedicine Association (ATA) describes telemedicine as the exchange of medical information from one site to another or between providers using electronic communication with the intention of improving a patient's clinical health status.[8]

There are six modalities of telecommunication technology used in telehealth as outlined here (Table 17.1).

Synchronous telecommunication refers to live or two-way interactions between a person (patient, caregiver, or provider) and a provider through audio-visual technologies that allows the exchange of health information in real time.[1,7–10] Through the advancement of peripheral technology devices, such as electronic stethoscopes and otoscopes, these visits provide a comparable alternative to in-person visits. Synchronous telehealth can also include educational programs between providers or from provider to patient.

Store-and-forward or *asynchronous telecommunication* involves the exchange of prerecorded health information or data through secure electronic communications between two or more individuals at different times.[7,8]

A provider may use this technology for consultation. A patient's diagnostic imaging or case description may be sent through secure email to a specialist or expert to review and recommend treatment options.

Table 17.1 TELEHEALTH MODALITIES

MODALITY	DEFINITION	EXAMPLE
Synchronous	Live or two-way interactions between a person (patient, caregiver, or provider) and a provider through audio-visual technologies that allow the exchange of health information in real time	A referring provider places an order for a telepalliative care consult for patient hospitalized at satellite campus with COVID-19. Telepalliative care provider connects with patient using real-time videoconferencing to discuss goals of care.
Asynchronous	Exchange of prerecorded health information or data through secure electronic communications between two or more individuals at different times	A referring provider sends diagnostic imaging or case description of a patient through secure email to a specialist or expert who later reviews information and replies back with a probable diagnosis and options for treatment.[2,7–10] Another common use of asynchronous care involves virtual visits that use a standard set of clinically based questions to obtain specific information about present illness or health complaint in order to identify to probable diagnosis, provide recommendations for treatment, and, if appropriate, prescribe medications.[8,11]
Remote patient monitoring (RPM)	Technology to gather patient medical and other forms of data and electronically send that information to providers for assessment in order to create, track, and make changes to a patient's treatment and plan of care	A patient with congestive heart failure wears a remote monitor to track their activity level and changes in functional status, pulse oximetry, and dyspnea.
mHealth	Asynchronous and synchronous through mobile technology; mHealth is medical and public health practices supported by mobile devices or other wireless technologies including health apps for smartphones or tablets and devices used at home or wearable to monitor the patient	Mobile applications are used to assist with the assessment and monitoring of patient symptoms to improve management and communication between patient and provider.[12]
eConsult	Secure electronic communication and consultations between providers and specialists	Providers connect with each other for asynchronous or store-and-forward consultations; this allows the primary team providers to connect with specialist to obtain expertise in managing complex patients. Primary care provider is electronically consulted by a palliative care specialist to discuss intractable abdominal pain in a patient with Stage IV pancreatic adenocarcinoma. The palliative care specialist reviews patient chart, medication history, imaging, and recommends provider and refers the patient to an interventional pain specialist for adjustment in opioids and celiac plexus nerve block.
Project ECHO (Extension for Community Health Outcomes)	Clinician links with expert issues in "virtual grand rounds"	A provider seeking continuing education uses the Project ECHO technology and platform to address global health disparities.

Remote patient monitoring (RPM) uses technology to gather patient medical information and other forms of data and electronically send that information to providers for assessment to create, track, and make changes to a patients' treatment and plan of care.[7,8] Remote patient monitoring is commonly used to follow patients at home for chronic disease management and following hospitalizations to reduce escalation of care (hospital admissions and readmissions) with timely interventions in response to changes in patient information.[7,8] There are a number of RPM monitoring devices and technologies that can be either synchronous or asynchronous. Targets of RPM include monitoring of a specific vital sign (blood pressure), pulse oximetry, electrocardiogram, and blood glucose levels.[8,10] Very commonly, but not always, RPM is prescribed by a provider for both short- and long-term periods for data collection.[8]

mHealth, also referred to as *mobile health*, has become an increasingly utilized form of telehealth. This subset refers to both asynchronous and synchronous communication through mobile technology. mHealth comprises medical and public health practices supported by mobile devices or other wireless technologies including health apps for smartphones or tablets and monitoring devices used at home or worn by the patient.[6-8] Applications can also be helpful in promote the adoption and maintenance of healthy lifestyle behaviors and safety with alerts, updates, and reminders.[7]

eConsult or electronic consults are secure electronic communication and consultations between providers and between providers and patients.[8] Frequently, eConsults are used to connect primary care providers to specialists in order to receive expert assessment and recommendations for patients.[7,13] eConsults can be cost-effective, eliminating unnecessary in-person subspecialty clinic visits that can be expensive for patients and health organizations.[7,13] eConsults are delivered through synchronous communication technology with real-time video or through asynchronous communications through store-and-forward technology.[7] Electronic consults in the outpatient setting are common practice, but inpatient e-consults are a relatively new practice. Academic medical centers have increased their use of e-consults where the availability of specialists cannot be maintained across growing health systems stretched across multiple sites.[13,14] The options for specialist involvement in the inpatient setting traditionally have been a time-consuming in-person consult or the informal "curbside consult" that may have limited documentation in the patient's electronic health record.[13,14]

Project ECHO (Extension for Community Health Outcomes) is a provider-focused education program that occurs within a free platform developed at the University of New Mexico. The focus is on shared knowledge to improve patient outcomes. It utilizes technology to share and promote health education, particularly in rural and underserved areas. It also allows for case-based learning and telementoring. It can be focused on a particular topic area, such as hospice and palliative medicine, or between organizations.

In 2016, telehealth visits accounted for 0.5% of Medicare billing. In 2017, the America Hospital Association (AHA) reported that approximately 76% of hospitals had partially or fully instituted a telehealth program, a substantial increase from the reported 35% in 2010.[15] However, telehealth only accounted for a small fraction of billable visits.[16,17] Evidence demonstrates that telehealth increases access to care, improves patient satisfaction, increases the quality of care, and reduces overall healthcare costs.[1,15,16]

TELEHEALTH IN THE UNITED STATES

Telehealth has a history dating back to the use of the telegraph during the Civil War.[8] Throughout its evolution, the focus has been on connectivity between those in need of care and those who are able to attend to them,[11] as in an underserved community or rural area, or to reach individuals who have a hard time traveling to healthcare appointments. Over the past 50 years, telehealth has evolved from the transmission of health data between healthcare organizations to the creation of a network of health organizations in which telehealth interventions offer healthcare to individuals in the military, prison systems, and rural areas.[1,8,18]

The federal government placed more emphasis on telehealth beginning with the *Balanced Budget Act of 1997*, which introduced Medicare reimbursement for telehealth and telehealth projects.[8] However, reimbursement was limited to members who lived in medically underserved rural areas and to specific providers using billing codes established by the Centers for Medicare and Medicaid Services (CMS).[8] This led to the establishment of the American Telemedicine Association (ATA), which assists with collaborations, development of standards, and working on legislation.[8]

When healthcare as an institution began to shift away from volume of care to value in terms of quality, efficiency, and cost, new modes of care delivery were required. With this change, telehealth has been embraced by the AHA. While there had been a slow increase in the development of telehealth within healthcare organizations, the COVID-19 pandemic accelerated telehealth with unprecedented expediency. Telehealth became essential to reduce rates of transmission, decrease contact in vulnerable patient populations, and preserve personal protective equipment.[19]

CURRENT STATE OF TELEHEALTH IN PALLIATIVE CARE

Regardless of setting, every individual with a serious illness has the right to palliative care.[20] The World Health Organization (WHO) estimates that, worldwide, only 14% of those individuals needing palliative care actually receive it.[21] Despite the extensive need for palliative care, seriously ill patients continue experience difficulty with accessing hospice and palliative care services. The number of patients in need of palliative care services greatly exceeds the workforce of palliative care specialists.[22,23] With a greater number of people living into advanced age and a palliative care workforce shortage, telehealth is one solution.

Telepalliative care refers to the use of telehealth to deliver palliative care services.[24-26] This includes telephone-based programs, video conferencing, and remote patient monitoring. The use of telemedicine in palliative care has been found to improve access to care and symptom management and increase patient and family satisfaction with care. However, the amount of evidence available is limited and fails to define how best to provide telepalliative services and other limitations.[25,27]

Early applications of telehealth in the field of palliative care focused on using remote communication technology to provide hospice care and services to patients at a distance, also referred to as *telehospice*.[28] In the late 1990s, the University of Kansas Center for Telemedicine and Telehealth (KUCTT) established one of the first telehospice programs.[29]

Palliative telehealth been used in the inpatient setting,[24,26,30] and a home-based palliative care (HPBC) program implemented in a New York metropolitan area provides telehealth service that includes 24/7 access to providers by phone or videoconference.[27,31] Compared to patients who received usual care, patients in the telepalliative program had a 34% lower rate of hospital admissions in last month of life, a 35% increase in hospice enrollments, and a significant increase in the median hospice length of stay.[27,31]

Prior to the COVID-19 pandemic, telepalliative services were concentrated in the outpatient setting, often within specific patient populations including oncology, heart failure, and advanced lung disease, and for those in rural or geographically isolated environments. Palliative care in the outpatient setting is crucial in assessing and managing physical and psychosocial symptoms, establishing goals of care, assisting with medical decision-making regarding treatments, and coordinating care on the basis of the individual needs of the patient and their families.[32] Telehealth be used to promote early transitions to hospice and to assist patients in completing advance care planning and clarifying preferences for hospitalization.[23]

Telehealth has also been useful in providing online palliative care education through videoconferencing, training, and peer mentoring.[33,34] Although there is lack of consensus on the ideal use and limitations of telepalliative care, evidence suggests that telepalliative care improves primary care access, reduces patient and family caregiver illness-related burden, offers remote monitoring and better management of symptoms, identifies anticipated or unexpected health decline, reduces escalations of care, and reduces unnecessary utilization of healthcare resource.[27,30,31,33,35–38] In recent years, palliative telehealth has focused on rural areas.

IMPLEMENTATION OF PALLIATIVE TELEHEALTH

For any telehealth program, a well-planned implementation is essential. There must be collaboration from palliative care clinicians, administrative leadership, and informational technology experts. It will be important to validate professional licensing, prescribing limitations, healthcare malpractice, and privacy and security requirements.[39] Overall, planning must be done to consider reimbursement by patient insurers, the telehealth modality, and the roles and responsibilities of participants. The program must be designed to provide a good clinical experience and proper documentation and coding, and be able to measure quality and satisfaction.

Scheduling of a telehealth visit can occur through several methods. These include creating 4-hour blocks of time similar to clinic schedules; devoting a full day to telehealth visits as needed, as for in-hospital visits based on the needs of patients, visitor restrictions, or distance of facility from patient family; on-call scheduling during evenings or weekends; or a mixed model of in-person and telehealth visits. Clinicians must remember to allow time to take breaks between virtual calls because the work is as demanding as in-person visits due to the co-management of technology, "reading" the patient, and leading the call.

It is important to assess the effectiveness of palliative telehealth visits. For a healthcare organization, this may include looking at overall telehealth metrics such as palliative care virtual visit volume and number of palliative providers trained and using virtual services. For population-specific metrics, it may include which types of patients do best in accessing palliative care (e.g., oncology, heart failure, pulmonary failure, neurocognitive disorders, etc.). Palliative care–specific metrics include reduction of no-show palliative care appointments, number of additional appointments available as a result of virtual visits, and number of advance care planning conversations as well as the documents completed. For patients and families, metrics also includes patient satisfaction in terms of access and wait time for a scheduled appointment.

OPPORTUNITIES AND CHALLENGES OF TELEHEALTH

There are a number of opportunities for palliative telehealth to enhance patient and clinician access; patient, family, and clinician travel times; and quality of care. With a focus on assuring palliative care across communities and rural areas, patients can experience an increased number of visits rather than clinic visits or home visits. Moreover, telehealth offers more care to individuals in long-term care settings, on reservations, or in prisons. It increases access for patients for whom travel is too expensive or difficult. Telehealth allows palliative care to decrease health inequities by offering care to marginalized patient populations as well.[40] Quality has been improved by more frequent follow-up and by using professionals to their full scope of practices. For instance, a registered nurse can do a telehealth visit for medication reconciliation and need for prescriptions. Advanced practice providers and physicians can do clinical visits.

Challenges exist as well. The move from in-person to virtual encounters with patients requires new skill development. The transition for palliative care providers who cherish in-person visits to establish an effective and therapeutic provider–patient relationship through "reading" nonverbal body language and real-time verbal expression has taken time. Inherent in web communications are connection delays and forced pauses. Moreover, the organization for a telehealth visit requires different planning. Specifically, there are requirements for platforms and devices that are compliant with the *Health Insurance Portability and Accountability Act* (HIPAA). These requirements translate to start-up costs for implementing an organization-wide platform, buying smart devices, and educating providers on how to use them, as well as costs for robust internet and broadband connections to support the visits. For patients, education is required on how to use the technology and the visit platform, to obtain access to devices, and to access the internet and broadband networks. Older patients may have difficulty with technology and need coaching prior to visits (Table 17.2). Within the COVID-19 pandemic, some community palliative care agencies have redeployed staff to bring devices to patient's homes and teach them how to use them. Other patients have been forced driven to known businesses (libraries or town offices) with guest access to internet.

TELEHEALTH ADVANCED PRACTICE NURSING

Telehealth provides opportunities to expand the reach of the omnipresent workforce of nurses. Project Enable (Educate, Nurture, Advise Before Life Ends) is one the earliest telehealth approaches in providing early palliative care intervention to rural patients with serious illness and their family caregivers.[41-44] Palliative advanced practice registered nurses (APRNs) were central to the study, which focused on symptom management for patients in the community and laid groundwork for telehealth advanced practice nursing.

Telehealth provides APRNs with the opportunity to improve access to care for patients, but it also increases options for clinical practice.[45] The American Association of Nurse Practitioners (AANP) position statement on telehealth acknowledges the support of providing healthcare services through telehealth but does not considers that services provided through telehealth are a separate specialty or are confined to the practice of one profession.[46] The shortage of palliative care specialist providers makes telehealth an attractive option for hospice and palliative care organizations, and the recent COVID-19 pandemic made the intervention integral. Integration of telehealth curricula has been developing rapidly in both generalist and specialist palliative APRN education.

Within a telehealth practice, palliative APRNs can provide the same services they would in-person: advance care planning, pain and symptom management, medication management, goals-of-care discussions, counseling, discharge planning, and planning for end of life.

PROVIDING A PALLIATIVE TELEHEALTH VISIT

The palliative APRN needs to plan for a telehealth visit.[47-51] Ideally, this includes prior education about an organization's capacities for telehealth, including the platform, device, and documentation.[39,50] It may also include the downloading of any applications or creating an account for a platform.

STEPS TO A TELEHEALTH ENCOUNTER

Preparation

1. Prepare for the appointment ahead of time by connecting with the platform. The platform must be HIPAA compliant.

2. Choose the device you plan to use. It can be a computer, laptop, smartphone, or tablet. It is important to discern whether the device is Apple-, Google-, Windows-, or Android-based. Make sure it is compliant with the platform.

3. Use a high definition web camera and microphone.

4. Ensure a reliable internet connection.

5. Find a private area for the visit.

6. Consider your environment.
   a. Consider lighting: Keep it neutral and well-lit.
   b. Ensure a private space for the appointment to occur, to meet HIPAA regulations.
   c. Make sure the space is quiet, and turn off cellphones and beepers.

7. Remember to dress appropriately for the clinical visit.

8. Set up the computer at eye level and check sound.

9. Review the patient's chart ahead of time, including history, medications, and advance care plans.

Table 17.1 PALLIATIVE TELEHEALTH OPPORTUNITIES AND CHALLENGES

OPPORTUNITIES	CHALLENGES
Access	Provider education on conducting effective visit
Time: Decreased travel and transportation time for patients and families and provider	Legal variability by state
Quality: Patient satisfaction, increased interactions	Redesign of work flow; changing clinical encounter
More frequent interactions	Cost of equipment
Use of palliative care team members to the fullest scope of practice	Internet and broadband access for patients, providers, and, potentially, healthcare facilities
	Lack of equipment for patient, family, or providers (smart devices, computers)

Initiation of Visit

1. Remember to allow for transmission delay.

2. Provide introductions for everyone on the visit. Ask who else is in the room.

3. Confirm if translation services are needed.

4. Start the appointment with the patient. Ask the patient if they are new to virtual visits.

5. Ensure they have strong broadband and internet capacity. Speak loud and clear.

6. Ask them to gather anything they might need (e.g., their medication bottles and supplements).

7. Ask for permission to take notes or type while the patient is talking.

8. Let the patient know how long the visit will be. Establish the agenda (e.g., "We have 20 minutes for today's visit"; "My schedule states this is an appointment for X"; "What brings you to today's visit?").

9. Ask the patient what topic is most important to discuss. Add what is important for you to discuss (e.g., "What are your most important concerns?").

10. Perform the visit. This includes the palliative care questions about how they are doing, and their level of function. Make sure to review the plan at the end. Remember to pause due to internet connectivity lapses.

11. Perform an exam by helping them to move the device. Review vital signs.

12. Let the patient talk about their concerns.

13. Demonstrate empathy. Validate the patient's concerns ("I wish I could be there in person"). Use the SAVE Model[50]:
    Support the patient: " I'm here for you." "I'm here to help you or guide you."
    Acknowledge the situation: "This has been really hard." "I wish there were better alternatives." "I can hear your worry."
    Validate the emotions and experience: "Given your situation, I think many people would feel that way."
    Emotion: "I can imagine how difficult this has been." "You sound frustrated/scared/anxious, etc."

14. Tell the patient when you need to access computer files. Or share information on the screen as appropriate.

15. Review medications.

16. Give a warning shot when visit will close to ask if there are other issues to cover.

17. Make sure there is a follow-up plan.

18. Thank the patient and family for the encounter.

After the Visit

1. Provide a post visit summary and plan

2. Document the encounter.

3. Submit a charge for the encounter

DOCUMENTATION AND BILLING

The reimbursement for telehealth has been in flux over the years.[50,51] CMS and private insurance organizations have covered telehealth in rural areas. During the COVID-19 pandemic, CMS offered waivers for telehealth and allowed for increased eligibility and scope beyond rural practice. Private payers also have adopted some coverage of telehealth services.[14,50,51] It is unclear how telehealth reimbursement will level out. Even if they are not submitted, providing charges to your organization assists in the collection of information about the use of palliative telehealth.

In terms of actual charges, CMS allows APRNs to be reimbursed for telecommunication hospital, office, and home visits that generally occur in person. The APRN must use an interactive audio and video telecommunication platform. Telehealth cannot occur by email or telephone.

CMS allows billing for telehealth in a fee-for-service model. Commercial providers may allow telehealth under alternative payment models for enhanced case management and improved efficiency. Best practice suggests that palliative APRNs document and bill similarly to face-to-face visits (Box 17.1).

Box 17.1 DOCUMENTATION ELEMENTS OF PALLIATIVE TELEHEALTH PATIENT ENCOUNTERS

1. Patient consent: Need to document the patient's consent of the visit (e.g., "Patient provided with patient risks and benefits of telehealth, verbal consent given for the telehealth visit").

2. Participants in the visit: This should include who was present, what was discussed, and the start and stop times of the visit.

3. Essential components of a note: Document the history, physical examination, and medical decision-making. Patient presents with X problem. Nurse reports physical findings (e.g., "Patient is calm, color is good, lips are pale. Breathing unlabored and even or using accessory muscles. Abdomen is distended when patient reveals stomach").

4. Document counseling and topics: If more than 50% of time was spent on counseling and care coordination, this should be documented.

5. Include impression and recommendations or plan.

6. Document visit start times and stop times.

Adapted from Cleveland Clinic[50]; and Lampert.[51]

Table 17.3 PALLIATIVE TELEHEALTH CODING

Video visits	New patients 99201–99205
	New patients 99201–99205
Telephone visits	May be a temporary basis
	G20212
Online eVisit	99241–99423
Interprofessional eConsult	Palliative Consulting Provider codes 99446–99451
Telehealth evaluation and management codes	99441–99443

Adapted from American Academy of Family Physicians[39]; and Lampert.[51]

There are consistent telehealth codes that the palliative APRN may use in the appropriate situations; see Table 17.3.

SUMMARY

Telehealth has been an emerging form of palliative care brought to the forefront by the COVID-19 pandemic. From a patient perspective, it offers an opportunity to facilitate early access to quality palliative care. Moreover, it allows delivery to individuals with serious illness for whom social determinants of care make in-person visits difficult. From a team perspective, telehealth allows the full participation of the palliative interdisciplinary team, which is the basis of holistic care. It also connects specialists, thus using people to maximum of their expertise and combining the expertise from different professions. From a policy perspective, telehealth is a cost-effective method of patient care delivery for appropriate patients.

Previously, there has been a lack of focus on telehealth in palliative care education. Palliative APRNs will need to ensure that their knowledge and skills are adequate to provide effective telehealthcare. They will need to monitor legislation about its application, guidelines, and reimbursement.

REFERENCES

1. Dorsey ER, Topol EJ. State of telehealth. *N Engl J Med.* 2016;375(2):154–161. doi:10.1056/nejmra1601705
2. Gogia S. *Fundamentals of Telemedicine and Telehealth.* San Diego: Elsevier Science and Technology; 2019.
3. Henderson K, Carlisle Davis T, Smith M, King M. Nurse practitioners in telehealth: Bridging the gaps in healthcare delivery. *J Nurse Practit.* 2014;10(10):845–850. doi:10.1016/j.nurpra.2014.09.003
4. Rutledge CM, Kott K, Schweickert PA, Poston R, Fowler C, Haney TS. Telehealth and ehealth in nurse practitioner training: Current perspectives. *Adv Med Educ Pract.* 2017;8:399–409. doi:10.2147/AMEP.S116071
5. Office of the National Coordinator for Health Information Technology (ONC) U.S. department of health and human services. What is telehealth? How is telehealth different from telemedicine? Updated October 17, 2019. https://www.healthit.gov/faq/what-telehealth-how-telehealth-different-telemedicine
6. World Health Organization. Telemedicine: Opportunities and developments in member states. https://www.who.int/goe/publications/goe_telemedicine_2010.pdf
7. Schweickert PA, Rutledge CM. *Telehealth Essentials for Advanced Practice Nurses.* 1st ed. West Deptford, NJ: Slack Incorporated; 2020.
8. Rheuban KS, Rheuban KS, Krupinsk EA. *Understanding Telehealth.* 3rd ed. New York: McGraw-Hill Education; 2018.
9. National Consortium of Telehealth Resource Centers. Telehealth Basics. Frameing telehealth? June 28, 2021. https://telehealthresourcecenter.org/resources/fact-sheets/framing-telehealth/
10. Telligen, Great Plains Resource and Assistance Center. Telehealth: Start-up and resource guide. Version 1.1, October 2014. https://www.healthit.gov/sites/default/files/playbook/pdf/telehealth-startup-and-resource-guide.pdf
11. Ryu S. History of telemedicine: Evolution, context, and transformation. *Healthc Inform Res.* 2010;16(1):65–66. doi:10.4258/hir.2010.16.1.65
12. Bienfait F, Petit M, Pardenaud R, Guineberteau C, Pignon A. Applying m-health to palliative care: A systematic review on the use of m-health in monitoring patients with chronic diseases and its transposition in palliative care. *Am J Hosp Palliat Care.* 2020;37(7):549–564. doi:10.1177/1049909119885655
13. Najafi N, Harrison JD, Duong J, Greenberg A, Cheng HQ. It all just clicks: Development of an inpatient e-consult program. *J Hosp Med.* 2017;12(5):332–334. doi:10.12788/jhm.2740
14. Vimalananda VG, Gupte G, Seraj SM, et al. Electronic consultations (e-consults) to improve access to specialty care: A systematic review and narrative synthesis. *J Telemed Telecare.* 2015;21(6):323–330. doi:10.1177/1357633X15582108
15. American Hospital Association. Factsheet: Telehealth. February 2019. https://www.aha.org/system/files/2019-02/fact-sheet-telehealth-2-4-19.pdf
16. Kane CK, Gillis K. The use of telemedicine by physicians: Still the exception rather than the rule. *Health Aff (Millwood).* 2018;37(12):1923–1930. doi:10.1377/hlthaff.2018.05077
17. Mehrotra A, Jena AB, Busch AB, Souza J, Uscher-Pines L, Landon BE. Utilization of telemedicine among rural medicare beneficiaries. *JAMA.* 2016;315(18):2015–2016. doi:10.1001/jama.2016.2186
18. Weinstein RS, Lopez, Ana Maria, Joseph BA, et al. Telemedicine, telehealth, and mobile health applications that work: Opportunities and barriers. *Am J Med.* 2014;127(3):183–187. doi:10.1016/j.amjmed.2013.09.032
19. Jaffe DH, Lee L, Huynh S, Haskell TP. Health inequalities in the use of telehealth in the United States in the lens of covid-19. *Popul Health Manag.* 2020;23(5):368–377. doi:10.1089/pop.2020.0186
20. Dahlin C, Coyne PJ, Ferrell BR. *Advanced Practice Palliative Nursing.* Kindle ed. New York: Oxford University Press; 2016.
21. World Health Organization. Palliative care. Key facts. Updated August 5, 2020. https://www.who.int/news-room/fact-sheets/detail/palliative-care
22. Worster B, Swartz K. Telemedicine and palliative care: An increasing role in supportive oncology. *Curr Oncol Rep.* 2017;19(6):1. doi:10.1007/s11912-017-0600-y
23. Silva MD, Schack EE. Outpatient palliative care practice for cancer patients during covid-19 pandemic: Benefits and barriers of using telemedicine. *Am J Hosp Palliat Care.* 2021:1049909121997358. doi:10.1177/1049909121997358
24. Calton B, Abedini N, Fratkin M. Telemedicine in the time of coronavirus. *J Pain Symptom Manage.* 2020;60(1):e12–e14. doi:10.1016/j.jpainsymman.2020.03.019
25. Calton BA, Rabow MW, Branagan L, et al. Top ten tips palliative care clinicians should know about telepalliative care. *J Palliat Med.* 2019;22(8):981–985. doi:10.1089/jpm.2019.0278
26. Humphreys J, Schoenherr L, Elia G, et al. Rapid implementation of inpatient telepalliative medicine consultations during covid-19 pandemic. *J Pain Symptom Manage.* 2020;60(1):e54–e59. doi:10.1016/j.jpainsymman.2020.04.001
27. Bonsignore L, Bloom N, Steinhauser K, et al. Evaluating the feasibility and acceptability of a telehealth program in a rural palliative care

population: Tapcloud for palliative care. *J Pain Symptom Manage.* 2018;56(1):7–14. doi:10.1016/j.jpainsymman.2018.03.013

28. Gurp JLP, Selm M, Leeuwen E, Vissers K, Hasselaar GJ. Teleconsultation for integrated palliative care at home: A qualitative study. *Palliat Med.* 2016;30(3):257–269. doi:10.1177/0269216315598068

29. Doolittle GC, Nelson E, Spaulding AO, et al. Telehospice: A community-engaged model for utilizing mobile tablets to enhance rural hospice care. *Am J Hosp Palliat Care.* 2019;36(9):795–800. doi:10.1177/1049909119829458

30. Jess M, Timm H, Dieperink KB. Video consultations in palliative care: A systematic integrative review. *Palliat Med.* 2019;33(8):942–958. doi:10.1177/0269216319854938

31. Lustbader D, Mudra M, Romano C, et al. The impact of a home-based palliative care program in an accountable care organization. *J Palliat Med.* 2017;20(1):23–28. doi:10.1089/jpm.2016.0265

32. Jacobsen J, Kvale E, Rabow M, et al. Helping patients with serious illness live well through the promotion of adaptive coping: A report from the improving outpatient palliative care (IPAL-OP) initiative. *J Palliat Med.* 2014;17(4):463–468. doi:10.1089/jpm.2013.0254

33. Gordon B, Mason B, Smith SLH. Leveraging telehealth for delivery of palliative care to remote communities: A rapid review. *J Palliat Care.* 2021:82585972110011. doi:10.1177/08258597211001184

34. Kidd L, Cayless S, Johnston B, Wengstrom Y. Telehealth in palliative care in the UK: A review of the evidence. *J Telemed Telecare.* 2010;16(7):394–402. doi:10.1258/jtt.2010.091108

35. Head BA, Schapmire TJ, Zheng Y. Telehealth in palliative care: A systematic review of patient-reported outcomes. *J Hospice Palliat Nurs.* 2017;19(2):130–139. doi:10.1097/NJH.0000000000000319

36. Rabow MW, Dahlin C, Calton B, Bischoff K, Ritchie C. New frontiers in outpatient palliative care for patients with cancer. *Cancer Control.* 2015;22(4):465–474. doi:10.1177/107327481502200412

37. Calton B, Shibley WP, Cohen E, et al. Patient and caregiver experience with outpatient palliative care telemedicine visits. *Palliat Med Rep.* 2020;1(1). https://doi.org/10.1089/pmr.2020.0075

38. Rogante M, Giacomozzi C, Grigioni M, Kairy D. Telemedicine in palliative care: A review of systematic reviews. *Ann Ist Super Sanita*;52(3):434–442. doi:10.4415/ANN_16_03_16

39. American Academy of Family Physicians. A toolkit for building and growing a sustainable telehealth program in your practice. September 2020. https://www.aafp.org/dam/AAFP/documents/practice_management/telehealth/2020-AAFP-Telehealth-Toolkit.pdf

40. Shigekawa E, Fix M, Corbett G, Roby DH, Coffman J. The current state of telehealth evidence: A rapid review. *Health Aff (Millwood).* 2018;37(12):1975–1982. doi:10.1377/hlthaff.2018.05132

41. Bakitas MA, Dionne-Odom J, Ejem DB, et al. Effect of an early palliative care telehealth intervention vs usual care on patients with heart failure: The enable CHF-PC randomized clinical trial. *JAMA Intern Med.* 2020;180(9):1203–1213. doi:10.1001/jamainternmed.2020.2861

42. Watts KA, Malone E, Dionne-Oden N, et al. Can you hear me now?: Improving palliative care access through telehealth. *Res Nurs Health.* 2021;44(1). doi:10.1002/nur.22105

43. Elk R, Emanuel L, Hauser J, Bakitas M, Levkoff S. Developing and testing the feasibility of a culturally based tele-palliative care consult based on the cultural values and preferences of southern, rural African American and white community members: A program by and for the community. *Health Equity.* 2020;4(1):52–83. doi:10.1089/heq.2019.0120

44. Dionne-Odom J, Ejem DB, Wells R, et al. Effects of a telehealth early palliative care intervention for family caregivers of persons with advanced heart failure: The enable chf-pc randomized clinical trial. *JAMA Netw Open.* 2020;3(4):e202583. doi:10.1001/jamanetworkopen.2020.2583

45. NCSBN's environmental scan: A portrait of nursing and healthcare in 2020 and beyond. *J Nurs Regul.* 2020 10(4):S1–S35. doi:10.1016/S2155-8256(20)30022-3.

46. American Association for Nurse Practitioners. Position statement: Telehealth. Austin, TX; AANP 2019. https://storage.aanp.org/www/documents/advocacy/position-papers/Telehealth.pdf

47. eVisit. Technical tips for a successful telemedicine visit. 2021. https://evisit.com/resources/technical-tips-for-a-successful-telemedicine-visit/

48. Cooley L. Fostering human connection in the covid-19 virtual healthcare realm. *NEJM Catalyst.* May 20, 2020. https://catalyst.nejm.org/doi/pdf/10.1056/CAT.20.0166

49. Centers for Medicare and Medicaid Services. Newsroom. Medicare telemedicine health care provider fact sheet. March 17, 2020. CMS.gov. https://www.cms.gov/newsroom/fact-sheets/medicare-telemedicine-health-care-provider-fact-sheet

50. Cleveland Clinic. Centers for excellence in healthcare communication. Communication. Top 10 Tips for Virtual Clinician Communications. May 20, 2020. https://consultqd.cleveland-clinic.org/communicating-with-patients-in-a-new-world-of-virtual-visits/

51. Lampert H. Telemedicine documentation guidance during the covid-19 pandemic. May 7, 2020. TEAMHealth. https://www.teamhealth.com/wp-content/uploads/2020/07/TeamHealth_Telehealth-documentation-during-the-COVID-19-pandemic.pdf

18.

THE PALLIATIVE APRN IN THE RURAL COMMUNITY

Traci Sickich

KEY POINTS

- Individuals with serious illness who live in rural areas face unique challenges.

- The palliative advanced practice registered nurse (APRN) has the potential to improve the care of these individuals and become a vital resource for patients, families, and the medical community.

- Palliative care can be woven into the social fabric of the rural community and provide a bridge to rural hospice services.

CASE STUDY: RURAL PALLIATIVE CARE

Tom is a 60-year-old man who was evaluated by his primary care provider for persistent abdominal pain, weight loss over 3 months, and frequent episodes of diarrhea with incontinence. Tom lives in a remote town, with the nearest clinic 80 miles away, and he is only able to see a rotating primary care provider when they make scheduled monthly visits. Tom was given a referral for further evaluation at a large medical center 200 miles away, which required travel by air. There, he was found to have metastatic gastric cancer after imaging, labs, and biopsy were completed. Tom proceeded with cancer-directed treatment, including chemotherapy, radiation, and surgical resection of abdominal masses. These treatments required frequent travel out of his rural town to the larger medical community, and, after 2 years, Tom was referred to the palliative care team, who assisted with telehealth visits when Tom was home.

The palliative advanced practice registered nurse (APRN) assisted Tom with navigating local resources in his small community, as well as with coordinating clinic visits when Tom traveled to the city for oncology appointments. In addition, the APRN facilitated navigating goals-of-care discussions, provided support with completion of advance directives, and managed Tom's symptom burden. Balancing in-person clinic visits with rural telehealth visits provided a continuity of care for Tom, who was not only navigating advanced serious illness but also the challenges of rural living. After a number of months, Tom started reporting feeling burdened by having to travel such a long distance for care, stating he was not sure "how much more of this I can take."

Tom's cancer progressed while on chemotherapy, and he chose to pursue immunotherapy that was offered. Unfortunately, immunotherapy was poorly tolerated. At this point, Tom was cachectic, taking hours to eat small meals and balancing nausea

and pain with his oral intake. Tom stated he was spending all day trying to find the energy to eat. As the palliative APRN had a long-standing relationship with Tom, she provided guidance regarding his current functional status. Reminding him that in previous goals-of-care discussions Tom had stated that if he could no longer travel to the large city for care then he would want to spend his final days in his remote town. Tom chose to no longer pursue cancer treatment and decided to focus on comfort, spending all of his time with his family. Tom stated he felt validated and supported in his medical decisions, and he valued the medical input and recommendations shared by the palliative APRN. At his final clinic visit, Tom was suffering from large malignant pleural effusions. The palliative APRN was able to coordinate with the oncology team to have a Pleurx drain inserted for comfort before Tom traveled back home one last time.

Tom's remote town did not have a Medicare-certified hospice but did have a network of volunteers who helped those who wanted to stay in their rural town at end of life. The palliative APRN served a vital role in facilitating the delivery of necessary durable medical equipment and comfort medications and continued to provide virtual visits to Tom's family to assist with end-of-life symptom management. Because Tom was able to stay in his rural town for his final 3 months of life, he was able to participate in meaningful activities, such as being carried by his family to see his daughter graduate high school. He died peacefully 2 days later. The family shared with the palliative care team how important it was for Tom to be home and how thankful they were for the resources and support provided by the palliative care team despite their remote location.

INTRODUCTION

Rural communities across the United States face their own unique challenges that extend beyond the isolated setting. In the context of healthcare, rural populations experience a variety of factors affecting access to care, challenges with models of delivery, and resource limitations, which can lead to disproportionately high levels of healthcare burden and even mortality. There are approximately 60 million Americans who live in a rural setting.[1] Rural America is facing growing health disparities, with an increase in incidence of heart disease, cancer, respiratory disease, and stroke.[2] These poorer outcomes have been linked to numerous challenges facing rural communities, including an aging population, increasing rates of poverty, and poor access to healthcare, including fewer available healthcare providers as well as closure of rural hospitals.[2] In addition to a lack of primary medical facilities, there is a shortage in specialty services, including palliative care. In fact, 90% of hospitals that offer palliative care services are located in urban areas.[3]

Palliative care is a basic human right, fundamental to health and human dignity for all individuals regardless of geographic location, socioeconomic status, or racial or cultural background.[4] Access to healthcare, and specifically palliative and hospice care in rural communities, is challenged by geography, provider availability, and rural culture. The rural palliative APRN is identified as meeting a unique need for those facing serious illness compounded by the challenging factors of rural life.

In a healthcare context, populations at risk, such as those in rural areas, have an increased risk of or susceptibility to adverse health outcomes, as evidenced by higher morbidity, premature mortality, and diminished quality of life. Low socioeconomic level and lack of external and environmental resources may contribute to disease susceptibility and are therefore indicators of vulnerability.[5] The purpose of this chapter is to describe barriers to access and delivery of palliative and hospice care in rural and remote areas, discuss the unique characteristics of rural culture, offer suggestions for developing a rural community palliative care program, provide an update on the current status of rural delivery of palliative and hospice care, and discuss future implications.

The National Consensus Project for Quality Palliative Care (NCP) *Clinical Practice Guidelines* establish a foundation on which quality palliative care is delivered. In relation to rural healthcare delivery, the social determinants of health can have an overwhelming influence on patients who are living with serious illness.[6] The palliative APRN needs to be cognizant of the impacts of financial constraints, including lack of insurance, and skilled in identifying and addressing the social implications of a serious illness. This assessment is amplified in a rural setting, where it may require more time and increased communication to understand the community resources available or lack thereof. Additionally, the palliative advanced practice registered nurse (APRN) needs to be aware of the influence of culture on how patients and families navigate serious illness and medical decision-making, as evidenced by the NCP domain on culture.[6] It is imperative for the palliative care team to understand the needs of the community and provide culturally appropriate care by performing a thorough needs assessment of patients who are part of an underserved population.

Significant barriers exist in the United States, as well as in other countries, that limit access to healthcare and palliative care for rural dwellers. For decades there has been a known shortage of healthcare providers in rural areas.[7] In response, health centers were built, and rural healthcare became a specialty for physicians and APRNs. Federal legislation was created to address the issue of rural healthcare access, which led to the development of Area Health Education Centers (AHECs), National Health Service Corps (NHSC), and Federally Qualified Heath Centers (FQHCs), as well as the creation of critical access hospitals (CAHs).[7,8] Despite all of these measures, there continues to be a physician shortage in rural settings, with an estimated 80% of rural counties reporting a lack of primary care doctors and concern that this number will rise given the number of those physicians who are age 60 or older.[9]

With the declining number of family practice physicians, changes in reimbursement, and a limited number of professionals who desire to work in rural areas, APRNs have assumed the role of primary care provider for many of these rural patients.[10] According to the American Nurses Association, the *Affordable Care Act* (ACA) fosters the growth of independent practices for the APRN because their skills will be in demand to meet the healthcare needs of those in rural regions and other areas of health disparity.[11] Recent research has shown that APRNs working within a full-practice state have a greater impact on access to healthcare, especially in rural communities, which can decrease healthcare disparities in these settings.[12]

However, rural care delivery is different from urban care delivery. Barriers to healthcare access in the rural setting exist at the system, provider, and individual levels and are reflected in the lack of availability of palliative care in these areas.[13] According to the Center to Advance Palliative Care (CAPC), linear growth is reported for the prevalence of palliative care across the country, now with 72% of US hospitals with more than 50 beds having a palliative care team—an increase from the 7% reported in 2001.[3] Research from rural hospitals has shown clinical and financial findings that support the need for and potential benefit of rural palliative care programs.[14,15] Unfortunately, complicating access to care even further is the recent development of a high concentration of rural hospital closures due to shrinking inpatient volume and more documented revenue occurring from outpatient care.[16] Even though hospital-based palliative care programs are increasing, rural dwellers experience significant barriers to accessing palliative care and hospice services.[13]

Literature review of the role of palliative care in the rural community is limited, with most studies focusing on countries outside of the United States. Systematic reviews have identified barriers that include the geographical dispersion of residents, inadequate financial resources, limited support systems, and lack of qualified medical, psychosocial, and spiritual support to meet the needs of the patient, caregiver, and family.[17,18] These research findings are consistent with the limited number of studies conducted in the United States and document the same barriers to access and delivery of palliative care.

THE RURAL COMMUNITY

There are three governing bodies that have established the definition of "rural." The US Census Bureau uses "rural" to encompass all population, housing, and territory not included within an urbanized area (UA) of 50,000 or more people or an urban cluster (UC) of 2,500 to 50,000 people.[19] The Office of Management and Budget uses metropolitan statistical areas (MSAs) to define urban and rural areas. An MSA is a city with 50,000 or more residents and a surrounding metropolitan area of at least 100,000 people. All non-MSA areas are considered rural. The US Department of Agriculture Economic Research Service collaborated with the Federal Office of Rural Health Policy to develop the Rural Urban Commuting Area (RUCA) System.[20] This method utilizes the Census UAs and UCs together with information on commuting to further delineate metropolitan, micropolitan, small town, and rural areas.[20] According to the US Census Bureau, in the 2010 Census, 19.3% of the population was classified as rural (59,492,276), while greater than 95% of the land area was classified as rural; by contrast, 80.7% of the population was classified as urban (249,253,271), while 5% of the land was classified as urban.[20] In addition to a rural designation, areas may be known as *frontier*. According to the National Rural Health Association, "frontier" is defined as an area with fewer than six people per square mile.[20] No matter the definition one chooses, a rural area involves a small population spread over a large distance. The distance and the terrain present unique barriers to healthcare service delivery, including palliative care.

In addition to unique geographical considerations, rural life is a culture within itself, and this cultural lens has its own application to healthcare specifically. The culture of rural living is not bound to a specific geographic location or population but based on "social, structural, and behavioral norms that represent a continuum based on the degrees to which individuals internalize rural culture."[21 (p. 6)] How a rural dweller defines health affects how they will seek out healthcare as well as influencing how they prefer to live.[22] Rural life constructs are centered within rural nursing theory, first developed by Long and Weinert in 1989, who assert that rural-dwelling people define health "as the ability to be productive, to do, not necessarily as the absence of disease."[23 (p. 120)] There is a resiliency in rural people, a desire to be in control of their own decisions, to do and care for themselves.[24] Additional distinctive attributes found in studies of rural population include a strong sense of independence, a connection to the land, the influence of faith, and the use of informal networks.[21]

In rural communities, the healthcare provider may encounter clients with low health literacy, especially among individuals who have previously chosen to not seek out providers to address their healthcare needs. Health literacy plays a key role in a patient's ability to discuss end-of-life care and must be considered and assessed by the palliative APRN. For example, in a family meeting with the goal to create a care plan, the patient or family members may have trouble understanding details the provider is sharing but may be too proud to ask for clarification. Members of the palliative care team can bridge the gap between the patient/caregiver and healthcare providers, eliminating confusion and frustration. They can provide essential support to patients who have never received healthcare but who have been diagnosed with a life-threatening illness and do not know what to do or how to cope with the diagnosis. In these situations, it often takes time to develop trust among the clinician, patient, and medical community, and the palliative care team may serve as a vital intermediary.[25] It is important to approach the rural patient

and family with a willingness to listen, rather than judge, in order to keep the path to trust open. Purposeful listening and being fully present are vital to the spiritual and emotional care of the rural palliative care patient.

ACCESS AND COORDINATION OF CARE

Chronic disease is among the most prevalent and costly health condition in the United States, killing an estimated 1.7 million Americans per year and accounting for nearly 75% of aggregate healthcare spending.[26] It is estimated that 81% of adults age 65 and older have two or more chronic disease conditions.[27] Based on the latest report of *The Older Population in Rural America*: 2012–2016, of the 46.2 million older adults in the United States, 10.6 million of them reside in rural areas, which is an increase from the last report in 2007.[28] In addition, the Medicare Payment Advisory Commission (MedPAC) report to Congress illustrates that 20% of Medicare beneficiaries live in a rural setting.[29] In a juxtaposition to who in the rural setting is receiving hospice care, the National Hospice and Palliative Care Organization illustrates how the percentage of Medicare beneficiaries enrolled varies from 60% in Utah to 22% in Alaska.[30]

As the population ages, the number of adults who experience multiple chronic illnesses, cognitive impairment, and related disability and increasing dependency will increase. Many of these older adults in the rural community will be cared for in their home by family members with the support of both formal and informal care systems. There are both benefits and challenges to providing home palliative care in a rural setting. The rural APRN is in the unique position of having amplified social connections and may be called on to care for a close friend. These fluid professional and personal boundaries in the rural palliative care setting create a dual relationship in rural practice of provider and friend, which can create conflicting demands between work and personal requirements.[32]

According to Hanson and colleagues, the benefits of palliative care in the rural setting include a familiarity between patient, primary family caregivers, and the formal care provider; flexibility in organizational support; and a vast informal support network of family, church members, neighbors, and friends.[32] Challenges to end-of-life care relate to limited resources and caregiver stressors, including service boundaries leading to limited hours or availability of formal services and a lack of qualified caregivers, which increases primary family caregiver stress.[32]

Accessing and coordinating palliative care services can be difficult in rural areas. Persistent barriers to accessing palliative care in the rural setting include fragmented services, unclear referral pathway, and lack of available providers.[33] The goal is for palliative care to be patient-centered and family-focused within the context of the patient's home, thereby addressing the needs of the patient and caregivers. In the rural community, these needs are met through both formal and informal care providers.

Formal care refers to healthcare services commonly provided in the rural areas by a generalist practitioner, a nurse practitioner (NP), clinical nurse specialist (CNS), or a physician assistant (PA). From 2008 to 2016, there has been an increase of 43% of rural nurse practitioners providing care.[34] All rural healthcare providers are engaged in "expert generalist" care with their patients, providing a range of healthcare in a limited resource setting.[31] Rural patients are faced with limited access to formal care and sometimes need to make decisions on how far to travel to access care based on road or driving conditions.[35]

Informal care refers to services that are provided by unpaid family members, friends, volunteers, or organizations. Informal care and networks may be a necessity rather than a choice. They reflect some of the strengths of rural relationships, such as social solidarity, close-knit relationships, and community commitments, and they may result in high-quality, integrated palliative and end-of-life services despite scarce resources (Table 18.1).[36]

RURAL PALLIATIVE CARE PROGRAMS: CONSIDERATIONS

A rural palliative care program must be based on a thorough understanding of the rural community, including its beliefs and customs, prevalent medical diagnoses, and available community resources, including financial and human capital. Rural dwellers tend to have lower financial stability. They experience a consistently higher rate of poverty compared to urban counterparts, earning about 4% less than the median income for urban households.[37] Rural Americans are more likely to live below the poverty level and to rely heavily on the Federal Food Stamp Program at a rate of 16% per household compared to 13% in urban areas.[38] Disparity in incomes is even greater for minorities living in rural areas. Compared

Table 18.1 BARRIERS TO RURAL PALLIATIVE CARE

BARRIER	INDICATOR
Provider shortages	Difficulty with retention Low provider comfort with palliative care Limited APRN scope of practice
Education	Lack of formal palliative care education Lack of understanding referral criteria
Financial/Policy constraints	Reimbursement regulations Decrease reimbursement rate for rural setting Medicare constraints on definition of hospice care
Geography	Decreased socioeconomic status Lack of resources/accessibility Isolated providers
Patient	Misunderstanding of services Fear of unknown Rural culture

Data adapted from Tedder et al.[17]

to the urban population, rural dwellers are less likely to have employer-provided healthcare coverage or prescription drug coverage or to be covered by Medicare benefits, which in turn limits medical service availability.[39]

There are 4,485 health professional shortage areas in rural and frontier areas, compared to 2,323 in urban areas.[40] Although nearly one-fourth of the population lives in these areas, only about 10% of physicians practice in rural America.[41] A 2013 survey of family medicine physicians found that, of the 3,000 surveyed, only 33% stated they provided some palliative care. Additionally, the workforce distribution report of hospice and palliative boarded physicians found large disparities in the availability of those working in rural settings, noting a maldistribution problem because many tend to work near large university centers.[39] A perspective analysis of rural hospice medical directors illustrated common themes of heavy workloads, limited options for training, physical and emotional stress, and safety concerns related to travel when caring for rural patients at end of life.[42] It can be extrapolated that APRNs who practice in rural areas mirror these statistics and share these concerns.

DESIGNING A RURAL PALLIATIVE CARE PROGRAM

An important first step in designing a successful palliative care program in a rural community is performing a needs assessment for the program within the community. This focuses on the current state of caring for patients with serious illness, local assets, resources, and stakeholders who recognize the need for palliative and hospice services. High-quality community-based palliative care requires clinical expertise in the field, knowledge around community care delivery, understanding of caregiver assessment, and support, as well as a thorough assessment of the home environment.[43] Community engagement is crucial to the success of a rural palliative care program, ensuring community buy-in of palliative care and an understanding of what these services can offer to the community.[44] Focusing on identifying community values using a respectful lens allows for a collaborative relationship between relevant stakeholders, community members, and palliative care providers.

Understanding the nature of family and community support is crucial to the success of the program. Studies have found that rural dwellers are accepting of barriers to healthcare due to their rurality and therefore are reticent about seeking care. Rural residents tend to *make do* with available resources, *solve their problems* independently, and be *self-reliant*. The sense of *community belonging* in rural culture means that "neighbors know and look out for each other," and individuals in *close-knit communities* fear sharing their health-related issues and seek care due to privacy issues. These attributes are a source of strength and personal control for rural dwellers but may also be a barrier to seeking out palliative care at end of life.[45] However, acceptance and knowledge of the unique beliefs, customs, and rituals of rural culture will promote acceptance of the APRN and the palliative care program (Table 18.2).

Table 18.2 RURAL CULTURE INFLUENCE

POSITIVE INFLUENCE	NEGATIVE INFLUENCE
Resiliency	Increase in caregiver burden
Self-reliance	Lack of local support services
Community support networks Friends involved at end of life	Low expectations; "make do"
Attitude of acceptance of death with desire for less interventions	Reluctance to seek care

Data adapted from Kirby et al.[45]

For a palliative care program to succeed in a rural community, healthcare providers must possess cultural competency and communication skills and be able to deliver effective care for patients with diverse values, beliefs, and behaviors. Mass media can be used as a health promotion tool to build community trust. The goal of public education and social marketing is to help people change their health behaviors by acquiring information and education they lack or through verbal and visual messaging that can shift the individual's thinking, attitudes, and values. Effective use of the media requires positioning oneself as an expert in palliative care and being available *formally* and *informally* to explain, promote, and be a resource for information, referrals, and services.[46]

Not all healthcare can be provided in the rural community itself, and travel may present unique barriers and challenges for the patient and family. As the expert in palliative care, the APRN must understand who to contact for services; how and where to obtain medications, equipment, and supplies; and ways to offer appropriate care that is within the financial means of the rural population. The APRN must also appreciate the benefits and burden of care, recognize when care needs exceed the rural area's capacity, and when referral to a larger town or city is appropriate and necessary (Table 18.3).

Table 18.3 CORE COMPONENTS OF A RURAL PALLIATIVE CARE PROGRAM

COMPONENT	DESCRIPTION
Training and education	Offers local rural opportunities for providers and staff
Telehealth utilization	Increases patient access in rural setting
Clinical pathways	Creates accessible bridges between hospital, clinic, and home care
Concise payment/ Reimbursement structure	Leverages state and federal guidelines
Inclusion of community stakeholders	Creates a model based on each community, tailored to specific resources and needs

Data adapted from Hawkins-Taylor et al.[48]; and Crooks et al.[68]

TRAVEL FOR SPECIALTY HEALTHCARE SERVICES

Distance, roadways, and weather conditions are significant factors when patients consider the commute for specialized healthcare services not available in the rural community. In a mountainous area, a 50-mile commute may take 3 hours. Early in the disease process, this may be acceptable to the patient, but as the disease progresses and treatments continue, the patient may decide the time burden is too much and may decide not to leave the community for care or may relocate to the urban area to be closer to specialized services. The costs for transportation, food, and lodging, as well as the time commitment are important considerations.[17]

Transportation is a common barrier for the rural dweller because public transportation may not exist or may exist for local areas only. Moreover, such transportation may be costly and time-consuming. The patient may already be experiencing financial hardships due to treatment and must then rely on family and friends for support and transportation. Family and friends must take time from work to drive the patient to the city and stay with the patient either for the day or several days, depending on the treatments required. Financial support is generally shared by family and friends. Many treatment facilities have agreements with agencies that provide lodging and meals for patients and caregivers at a reduced rate.

In addition to the considerations of time and cost, commuting may be anxiety-provoking for the patient who feels he or she is a burden to the family and community. Travel can also create significant anxiety for the caregiver. Strategies for coping with commuting include careful preparation for the trip, maximizing a routine, managing time, and maintaining significant relationships. Additionally, it may require care coordination to consolidate multiple provider appointments in the same day to ease the burden of travel. Anticipation of weather and traffic delays, planning for food and rest stops, scheduling pain medications and other pharmacologic agents to maintain analgesic coverage during the commute, and sharing quality time together may decrease the patient's anxiety.[47] Worries about the feasibility of continuing the care plan once the patient returns home may also cause anxiety, and these concerns should be specifically addressed by the palliative APRN. The patient may not spontaneously provide information about relevant stressors, so the APRN will need to elicit this insight with sensitive and careful questioning.

Conversely, from the provider perspective, it is not the mileage alone but the road conditions (e.g., curves, elevation) and weather conditions (e.g., flooding, mud, snow and ice) that make it daunting for a provider to make a house call or for the patient to make a clinic visit. Considerations must be given to distance, travel time, and visit time. A community APRNs in rural areas may be only able to do 1-2 visits as day.

SITUATIONS OF LOST TO FOLLOW-UP CARE AND ABANDONMENT

Being "lost to follow- up" in their own community is another concern for patients who choose to travel out of the rural area for care. Such patients may lose contact with their local provider. The APRN can bridge this gap by assuming "ownership" of the patient's case (acting as case manager) when the patient is referred, while the patient is under the care of providers in distant cities, and when the patient returns to the community. Frequently, the APRN serves as the communication link by providing continuity of care for the patient and family, including providing the referring provider with updates on the patient's status and plan of care. Communication, either in person or by telephone, is paramount with this patient population to prevent the patient from being "lost to follow-up care."[48]

Another way in which patients may be "lost to follow-up care" may occur when there are limited or no palliative care providers in their rural area. If there are no defined palliative care services, their primary healthcare professional is expected to provide these services and coordinate their care. If their healthcare professional lacks primary palliative care education and training, the treatment plan that was established when the patient was discharged may not be continued. The patient may experience untreated, undertreated, or overtreated pain and symptoms, both physical and psychological.

The patient who does not have a primary care provider and who was not referred to a primary care provider by the discharging facility is at a great disadvantage. If the lack of a primary care provider is not recognized by the family and friends, the patient will truly be "lost to follow-up care." To avoid these situations, a *rural–urban referral system* needs to be established. The APRN formulates and maintains a list of contacts in other facilities, communicates with the facility when a patient is referred, maintains verbal and written contact during the admission, monitors for the expected time of discharge, and anticipates the patient's needs prior to their return to the rural community.

Second, the unfamiliar language of palliative care may be a barrier to rural patients, family members, and healthcare professionals who equate palliative care to hospice care. Hawkins-Taylor found that, in rural South Dakota, 73% of rural residents were unable to define the concept of palliative care.[48] Lack of understanding around the definition of palliative care can lead to rural patients experiencing disproportionate access to palliative care services. The existence of documented low health literacy among rural patients, combined with a rural culture of resiliency, individualism, and reticence in seeking care, may negatively affect the ways in which rural patients perceive specialized palliative care and discourage them from accessing these services.

Third, navigating the bureaucratic healthcare system may be a challenge for members of rural populations. It can be difficult to know what agencies to contact for help with securing medical services, obtaining financial resources to pay for medications and living expenses, and coordinating home health services and equipment. Challenges related to navigating the complex and often fractured healthcare system can cause emotional and psychological stress for the patient and family members who have always been self-sufficient and "do whatever it takes" to make things work. To address this concern, a community resource information flyer or magnet can

be developed, including the name of the facility or organization with relevant contact addresses and telephone numbers. If there are no hospice services in the patient's rural area, the APRN should coordinate alternate providers for services, such as grief support to be provided by the funeral home or local clergy; pain and symptom management to be provided by emergency medical personnel or community members with appropriate medical skills; and support services, such as meals, respite care, transportation, and performing necessary errands to be coordinated through local churches and service organizations. Importantly, the ongoing development of coordinated palliative services and the provision of fundamental palliative education for healthcare professionals and the community will help to alleviate this stress and ultimately change the cultural attitude toward palliative care.

SITES OF CARE AND WORKFORCE

Many rural dwellers prefer to die at home, in their community or village, with family and friends present at the time of death because there is a strong connection between place and self in the rural setting.[49] The ethnography work of Rainsford found that rural patients equate a "good death" with that of a "safe death," meaning that one's identity was preserved, autonomy respected, and control maintained over decisions around end-of-life care.[49] The perception of a "safe death" is also rooted in creating a safe physical place, whether that be the rural homestead where one has a connection to self and memories or the rural hospital where a patient may still receive personal attention from well-known caregivers. The limited number of healthcare professionals trained in primary or specialty palliative care, homecare and volunteer services, nursing home beds, and/ or alternate sites of care may create barriers to rural palliative care. If the family cannot care for the patient, it may be difficult to locate a skilled nursing facility close to the patient's home. This scenario is common in rural areas in Alaskan villages as well as in Appalachia and other mountainous regions.

As noted earlier, the shortage of healthcare professionals and facilities in rural communities continues to be an issue for the APRN to address in order to provide continuity of care. MacDowell and colleagues conducted a nationwide survey of 1,031 rural hospital CEOs to determine if they perceived a shortage of healthcare professionals in their area.[50] Seventy-five percent of the responders reported shortages of all healthcare professionals (the survey did not address palliative care specialists.)[50] To address the shortage of rural physicians in the United States, the "Conrad State 30" program was developed to recruit foreign-trained physicians to work in rural areas in exchange for permanent residence. A similar program exists for APRNs and nursing faculty to serve in critical shortage facilities and accredited schools of nursing. The program pays 60% of their unpaid nursing student loans for 2 years of service and an additional 25% of the original balance for an optional third year.[51] Continuing to pave the way for advancement in education, work in Congress continues to push for the *Palliative Care and Hospice Education and Training Act* (PCHETA). This act, if passed, allows for an increase in the number of permanent faculty in palliative care at accredited programs, awards grants or contracts to academic programs (medical schools and nursing schools) and teaching hospitals, provides career incentive awards, and creates special preferences in existing nurse education to promote retention projects and workforce development.[52]

Given the economic burden that serious illness places on rural dwellers, it is important to note the potential cost savings that a palliative care program can have at multiple system levels. Palliative care programs save hospitals money through cost avoidance (decreased daily costs, decreased length of stay, increased hospice referrals), as well as by supporting a home healthcare model to reduce emergency room visits and hospitalizations in general. One study found that a hospital with more than 50 beds that has a palliative care service can see a savings per patient per admission of $2,659, which translates to an estimated $1.2 billion in savings per year nationally.[53] In the rural setting, this economic savings would be seen at the hospital level due to decreased need to seek tertiary care if health needs are addressed in the community setting. Significant cost savings can occur for the patient as well, who will not have to travel as far for supportive health care.

FAMILY AND COMMUNITY SUPPORT

The challenge for the palliative APRN and the interdisciplinary team in the rural community is to coordinate formal and informal services to meet the needs of patients and caregivers. As noted earlier, rural dwellers tend to be reticent to seek care, possibly in part due to their inability to access and understand healthcare information (low health literacy), which impedes their acceptance of healthcare interventions.

Communication is a critical component of this coordination and is paramount to the peace of mind of the patient and caregiver. Additionally, communication around end-of-life concerns, critical medical decision-making, and the many stressors related to the experience of serious illness requires an additional skill set for the healthcare provider. Patient- and family-centered communication requires that the APRN is comfortable and competent in meeting the complex needs of patients with a life-limiting illness.[54]

Frequently, the APRN is the leader of the palliative care team (officially or unofficially) and is responsible for care coordination from the patient and family perspective. By holding a family meeting to explore goals of care, the APRN can ensure that the patient's and family's perceived needs are met, including medical, financial, physical, and spiritual needs, as well as other requirements specific to the patient/family culture and belief systems. As part of the family meeting, the palliative APRN should discuss each member's perception of the shared information, should help determine what services are needed, should make necessary referrals, and, within 24 hours, should provide the patient and family with a written plan of care.

Providing information about the patient's illness, including how the condition will progress, the patient's life expectancy, and specific treatment options is an important aspect of care. As health literacy levels are reported to be low in many rural populations, patients and families may be confused about the disease process and treatment options, and their understanding and perceptions are often overshadowed by cultural beliefs and rituals. Assessing understanding and filling in knowledge gaps is a critical function of the APRN and is even more pronounced in the fractured rural healthcare system.

Teamwork is essential to the delivery of rural palliative care. The independence, cooperation, and collaboration evident in rural communities are the strengths that allow the APRN and healthcare professionals, family, and community to meet the needs of the patient, even though resources may be lacking.

COMPETENCIES FOR THE RURAL APRN

Whether palliative services are delivered using a specialist or generalist model, the APRN's educational needs are essentially the same. The American Nurses Association and the Hospice and Palliative Nurses Association jointly state that nursing education is rooted in primary palliative nursing skills, including advance care planning, basic pain and symptom management, and assessment of patient and family needs.[55] However, in the community, competence is necessary in pain and symptom management, addressing spiritual needs, assisting with the creation of advance directives, identifying psychosocial concerns, and providing family support. Barriers to professional development for rural practitioners include geographic and professional isolation, time constraints, workload, and lack of professional coverage during absences. Various modalities exist to acquire training and maintain skills; unfortunately, one-on-one and classroom presentations appear to be both the most rewarding for rural healthcare practitioners and the least accessible.

In the generalist model, there has been consistent evidence citing a lack of providers trained in primary palliative care. Core competencies of primary palliative care include physical, psychological, social, and spiritual assessment, as well as communication.[56] Even specialist palliative APRNs described a lack of palliative care education in their graduate curriculum.[57] Identified barriers for providers training in primary palliative care include lack of knowledge of the field of palliative care, absence of an interdisciplinary team, professional time constraints, lack of funding for educational opportunities, and lack of access to a palliative specialist.[44]

The American Association of Colleges of Nursing has addressed this by developing competencies for all APRNs who pursue graduate education. These competencies include the assessments previously listed, as well as interprofessional collaboration to provide patient-centered and family-focused care, application of evidence-based care, legal and ethical issues in prescribing and de-prescribing medications, communication expertise in primary palliative care skills, and complex symptom management related to serious illness.[58]

The role of the palliative care specialist is further complicated by the tendency of some rural populations to have more trust in their "local expert" and therefore be less likely to seek care from specialists not known to their community.[59] Studies on APRN autonomy and satisfaction have found that while rural APRNs work more hours, this is balanced with greater practice autonomy, and APRNs report being highly satisfied with their work in rural communities, which improves retention.[60] The culture of a rural APRN has its own challenges and benefits, just as the rural culture does itself.

Given the importance of communication and collaboration in palliative care, as well as the geographic challenges just identified, generalist and specialist palliative APRNs should be able to incorporate telemedicine into their practice. *Telemedicine*, also known as *telehealth* or *health information technology*, is a rapidly developing application of clinical medicine using telephone, computers, the internet, and other networks to advance the delivery of rural and remote healthcare. Telehealth facilitates the exchange of information and knowledge regardless of geographic or environmental barriers while reducing access time and costs. Holland and colleagues demonstrated positive results using health information technology for rural palliative care and hospice patients and families, such as improved quality of life and satisfaction with care, reduced hospital readmissions, and reduced healthcare costs.[61] The use of telehealth has increased despite ongoing rural barriers such as the availability of internet or broadband connectivity in remote locations and variable reimbursement from Centers for Medicare and Medicaid Services (CMS) for telemedicine services. CMS announced in 2020 an initiative to improve rural and telehealth access, the *Community Health Access and Rural Transformation (CHART)* model.[62] This model aims to modify reimbursement to help ensure financial stability for rural providers and provide waivers that increase operational and regulatory flexibility, thereby enhancing beneficiaries' access to services by increasing the ability for rural providers to stay in practice.[62] Additionally, during the COVID-19 pandemic, CMS adapted telehealth policies to allow for increased reimbursement while limiting restrictions on telehealth related to its use by rural providers.[63] It is hoped that these regulations will continue after the pandemic (see Chapter 17 on the "Palliative APRN in Telehealth").

RURAL HOSPICE

In the United States, the number of hospice agencies has decreased in the past 10 years. Currently, there are 878 rural hospices per the *2019 MedPAC Report to Congress*.[64] While there was a 2.6% decrease from 2016 to 2017 alone, there was a simultaneous increase in the percentage of rural Medicare beneficiaries who utilize hospice services.[64] Hospice care in the rural community has unique elements, including staffing by local citizens or volunteers, limited resources, and large geographic areas. Rural hospices are often a real part of the social fabric of their communities.

Changes from CMS as mentioned earlier have provided an updated wage index model and payment allocation for the different types of hospice care. Historically, hospices were reimbursed at a daily rate at $17 less per day than their urban counterparts.[42] The new proposed payment model is forecasted to provide a 3% increase in revenue for nonprofit and a 0.8% increase in for-profit hospice agencies.[65]

Historically the role of the APRN has been limited in hospice as the eligibility form known as Certificate of Terminal Illness requires a physician signature. The rural community may benefit from a wider scope of practice for APRNs to provide continuity of care from the palliative care setting by creating a bridge to the hospice setting, particularly as an estimated 16% of Medicare beneficiaries report seeing an APRN or PA for their primary care services, which is a higher percentage than for urban beneficiaries.[66]

Difficulties with maintaining financial stability may be accelerating the recent decline in the number of rural hospice agencies. Other healthcare delivery factors that affect rural hospice care include demographic changes in the rural community (i.e., availability of volunteers or an aging workforce), rural economics, and travel time for the hospice staff. Frequently, "windshield time" or lengthy drive times in rural locations can have a negative impact on care and present a reimbursement challenge. Time lost to driving may increase a nurse's workload and result in lost productivity as well as in the ability of a provider to respond to a hospice emergency.[42] With the aforementioned reimbursement changes, these historic difficulties may be changing the future landscape of rural hospice programs.

THE REALITY OF RURAL LIFE

Imagine a patient in a rural area with no access to healthcare. The patient receives a terminal diagnosis after visiting a city following a bad fall. The patient views the healthcare providers as haughty and only wanting money. A specialist offers aggressive treatment that may cure the patient's disease. After several meetings and treatments, the patient gradually lets down his defenses and finds he not only trusts this clinician, but has also developed a sense of dependency on her because she offers a possible cure. However, the treatments stop working or do not achieve cure and actually make the patient sicker. At some point, the patient is told there is nothing more to be done, and he should go home and die. Imagine the level of distrust with the larger medical community that could result, as well as potential feelings of abandonment and thoughts around missed time with loved ones. Quality of life needs to be addressed early, especially in rural patients whose persistent barriers to healthcare can lead to poor outcomes.

The remedy is to begin palliative care early, soon after the diagnosis, and to collaborate with rural care providers. A shift toward seeing palliative care as part and parcel of care, rather than a last resort, is very welcome. In this way, palliative care becomes concurrent care, a bridge to support the patient and family throughout the journey of serious illness, whatever its length. Palliative care should be woven seamlessly into treatment to reduce families' stress levels and improve patients' quality of life throughout their illness and in their final days.[67]

SUMMARY

Palliative care is both a specialty and a philosophy of care that has evolved over many decades. Central to its practice is the development of an informed and compassionate approach to care for the chronically ill patient and family. Palliative care views the patient and family as a unit. Its goal is to improve the quality of life for both by treating pain and other symptoms; providing time-intensive communication; supporting complex medical decision-making; ensuring practical, spiritual, and psychological support; and coordinating care across all settings.

The palliative APRN serves a vital role in addressing whole-person care for those with serious illness, and this role is amplified in the rural community. The rural palliative APRN is woven into the social fabric of the rural community, addressing physical, spiritual, and at times complex social needs, thereby requiring an expert generalist model in order to provide competent care. In larger communities where resources are "just around the corner," this is more easily accomplished. However, in rural communities, where 80% of palliative care is provided by non-physician providers, the challenge for the APRN and members of the healthcare team is to design a community-based palliative care program that allows a seamless transition from curative care to comfort care while meeting the needs, wishes, and expectations of the patient and family.

REFERENCES

1. Garcia MC, Rossen LM, Bastian B, et al. Potentially excess deaths from the five leading causes of death in metropolitan and non-metropolitan counties: United States, 2010–2017. *MMWR Surveill Summ*. 2019;68: (SS-10):1–11. doi: http://dx. doi.org/10.15585/mmwr.ss6810a1
2. Capriotti T, Pearson T, Dufour L. Health disparities in rural America: Current challenges and future solutions. Clinical Advisor. February 3, 2020. https://www.clinicaladvisor.com/home/topics/practice-management-information-center/health-disparities-in-rural-america-current-challenges-and-future-solutions/
3. Center to Advance Palliative Care, National Palliative Care Research Center. America's care of serious illness: A state by state report card on access to palliative care in our nation's hospitals. New York, NY: Center to Advance Palliative Care and National Palliative Care Research Center. 2019. https://reportcard.capc.org/wp-content/uploads/2020/05/CAPC_State-by-State-Report-Card_051120.pdf
4. Open Society Foundations. Public health fact sheet. Palliative care as a human right: A fact sheet. Updated February 2016. https://www.opensocietyfoundations.org/publications/palliative-care-human-right-fact-sheet#publications_download
5. Brundisini F, Giacomini M, DeJean D, Vanstone M, Winsor SSA. Chronic disease patients' experiences with accessing health care in rural and remote areas: A systematic review and qualitative meta-synthesis. *Ont Health Technol Assess Ser*. 2013;13(15):1–33.
6. National Consensus Project for Quality Palliative Care. *Clinical Practice Guidelines for Quality Palliative Care*. 4th ed. Richmond, VA: National Coalition for Hospice and Palliative Care. 2018; https://www.nationalcoalitionhpc.org/wp-content/uploads/2020/07/NCHPC-NCPGuidelines_4thED_web_FINAL.pdf
7. Deligiannidis K. Primary care issues in rural populations. *Prim Care Clin Office Pract*. 2017;44(1):11–19. doi:10.1016/j.pop.2016.09.003
8. Bolin J, Bellamy G, Ferdinand A, Vuong A, Kash B, Schulze A, Helduser J. Rural health people 2020. New decade, same challenges. *J Rural Health*. 2015;31(3):326–333. doi:10.1111/jrh.12116
9. Ollove M. Rural America's health crisis seizes attention. Stateline; Pew Trusts. January 31,2020. https://www.pewtrusts.org/en/research-and-analysis/blogs/stateline/2020/01/31/rural-americas-health-crisis-seizes-states-attention
10. Emnett J, Byock I, Twohig JS. Advanced practice nursing: Pioneering practices in palliative care. Promoting excellence in end-of-life care, a national program. Robert Wood Johnson Foundation. 2002; 1–13. https://www.yumpu.com/en/document/view/37527925/advanced-practice-nursing-pioneering-practices-in-dying-well
11. Cleveland KA, Motter T, Smith Y. Affordable care: Harnessing the power of nurses. *Online J Issues Nurs*. 2019;24(2):manuscript 2. doi:10.3912/OJIN.Vol24No02Man02
12. Ortiz J, Hofler R, Bushy A, Lin Y, Khanijahani A, Bitney A. Impact of nurse practitioner practice regulations on rural population health outcomes. *Healthcare (Basel)*. 2018;6(2):65. doi:10.3390/healthcare6020065
13. Loftus J, Allen E, Call K, Everson-Rose S. Rural-urban differences in access to preventative healthcare among publicly insured Minnesotans. *J Rural Health*. 2018;Feb 34(suppl 1):S48–s55. doi:10.1111/jrh.12235
14. Armstrong B, Jenigiri B, Hutson SP, Wachs PM, Lambe CE. The impact of a palliative care program in a rural Appalachian community hospital: A quality improvement process. *Am J Hosp Palliat Med*. 2013;30(4):380–387. doi:10.1177/1049909112458720
15. Mcgrath LS, Gar D, Frith KH, Hall WM. Cost effectiveness of a palliative care program in a rural community hospital. *Nurs Econ*. 2013;31(4):176–183. PMID: 24069717
16. Rosenberg J. Understanding the health challenges facing rural communities. AJMC. February 9, 2019. https://www.ajmc.com/view/understanding-the-health-challenges-facing-rural-communities
17. Tedder T, Elliott L, Lewis K. Analysis of common barriers to rural patients utilizing hospice and palliative care services: An integrated literature review. *J Am Assoc Nurse Practit*. 2017;29(6):356–362. doi:10.1002/2327-6924.12475
18. Bakitas M, Elk R, Astin M, et al. Systematic review of palliative care in rural setting. *Cancer Control*. 2015;22(4):450–464. doi:10.1177/107327481502200411
19. The United States Census Bureau. Urban and rural. 2020. https://www.census.gov/programs-surveys/geography/guidance/geo-areas/urban-rural.html
20. Rural Health Information Hub. What is rural? 2019; last reviewed April 8, 2019. https://www.ruralhealthinfo.org/topics/what-is-rural#ruca
21. Holms C, Levy M. Rural culture competency in health care white paper. Lawrence, KS: University of Kansas School of Social Welfare. 2015; https://reachhealth.org/wp-content/uploads/2016/12/REACH-RCC-White-Paper-Final.pdf
22. Tasseff T, Tavernier S, Watkins P, Neill K. Exploring perceptions of palliative care among rural dwelling providers, nurses, and adults using a convergent parallel design. *Online J Rural Nurs Health Care*. 2018;18(2):152–188. doi:Http://dx. doi.org/10.14574/ojrnhc.v18i2.527
23. Long KA, Weinert C. Rural nursing: developing the theory base. *Sch Inq Nurs Pract*. 1989;3(2):113–127.
24. Christensen K, Winters C, Colclough Y, Oley E, Luparell S. Advance care planning in rural montana. *J Hosp Palliat Nurs*. 2019;21(4):264–271. doi:10.1097/NJH.0000000000000556
25. Parker J. Improving health literacy could boost access to hospice, palliative care. Hospice News. January 2, 2020. https://hospicenews.

com/2020/01/02/improving-health-literacy-could-boost-access-to-hospice-palliative-care/

26. Raghupathi W, Raghupathi V. An empirical study of chronic diseases in the United States: A visual analytics approach to public health. *Int J Environ Res Public Health*. 2018;15(3):431. doi:10.3390/ijerph15030431

27. Buttorff C, Ruder T, Bauman M. Multiple chronic conditions in the United States. Santa Monica, CA: Rand Corporation. 2017. https://www.rand.org/content/dam/rand/pubs/tools/TL200/TL221/RAND_TL221.pdf

28. Symens Smith A, Trevelyan, E. The older population in rural America: 2012-2016, report number acs-41. 2019; The United States Census Bureau. September 23, 2019. https://www.census.gov/library/publications/2019/acs/acs-41.html.

29. Medicare Payment Advisory Commission. Chapter 2-medicare beneficiary demographics. A data book: Health care spending and the Medicare Program. July 2020. http://www.medpac.gov/docs/default-source/data-book/july2020_databook_sec2_sec.pdf?sfvrsn=0

30. National Hospice and Palliative Care Organization. NHPCO facts and figures 2020 ed. Alexandria, VA: NHPC). August 20, 2020. https://www.nhpco.org/wp-content/uploads/NHPCO-Facts-Figures-2020-edition.pdf

31. Schlairet M. Complexity compression in rural nursing. *Online J Rural Nurs Health Care*. 2017;17(2): 2–33. doi:Http://dx. doi:org/10.14574/ojrnhc.v17i2.445

32. Hansen L, Cartwright JC, Craig CE. End-of-life care for rural-dwelling older adults and their primary family caregivers. *Res Gerontol Nurs*. 2012;5(1):6–15. doi:10.3928/19404921-20111213-01

33. Bakitas M, Watts K, Malone E, Dionne-Odom J, McCammon S, Taylor R, Tucker R, Elk R. Forging a new frontier: Providing palliative care to people with cancer in rural and remote areas. *J Clin Oncol*. 2020;38(9):963–973. doi:Https://doi.org/10.1200/JCO.18.02432

34. Barnes H, Richards M, McHugh M, Martsolf G. Rural and nonrural primary care physician practices increasingly rely on nurse practitioners. *Health Aff (Millwood)*. 2018;37(6):908–914. doi:10.1377/hlthaff.2017.1158

35. Lee H, Winters C. Testing rural nursing theory: Perceptions and needs of service providers *Online J Rural Nurs Health Care*. 2004;4(1):51–63. doi:Https://doi.org/10.14574/ojrnhc.v4i1.212

36. Spelten E, Timmis J, Heald S, Duigts S. Rural palliative care to support dying at home can be realized; experiences of family members and nurses with a new model of care. *Aust J Rural Health*. 2019;27:336–343. doi:10.1111/ajr.12518

37. Bishaw A, Posey K. A comparison of rural and urban America: Household income and poverty. Census Blogs. The US Census Bureau. December 8, 2016. Available at https://www.census.gov/newsroom/blogs/random-samplings/2016/12/a_comparison_of_rura.html

38. Food Research and Action Center. Rural hunger in America: Supplemental nutrition assistance program. 2018. https://frac.org/wp-content/uploads/rural-hunger-in-america-snap-get-the-facts.pdf

39. Rural Health Information Hub. Healthcare access in rural communities. Last reviewed August 18, 2021. https://www.ruralhealthinfo.org/topics/healthcare-access

40. U.S. Department Health and Human Services. Health and Human Resources Administration. data.HRSA.gov Designated health professional shortage areas statistics. First quarter of Fiscal year 2021; Designated HPSA Quarterly Summary December 31, 2020. https://data.hrsa.gov/topics/health-workforce/shortage-areas

41. Brundisini F, Giacomini M, DeJean D, Vanstone M, Winsor S, Smith A. Chronic disease patients' experiences with accessing health care in rural and remote areas: A systematic review and qualitative meta-synthesis. *Ont Health Technol Assess Ser*. 2013;13(15):1–33. Published 2013 Sept 24228078; PMID PMC3817950.

42. Gibbens B, Schroeder S, Knudson A, Hart G. Perspectives of rural hospice directors. Rural Health Research Gateway. Policy Brief,

March 2015. https://www.ruralhealthresearch.org/publications/962

43. Meier D, Bowman B, Collins K, Dahlin C, Twohig J. *Palliative Care in the Home: A Guide to Program Design*. New York: Center to Advance Palliative Care; 2016. https://www.capc.org/shop/palliative-care-in-the-home-a-guide-to-program-design_3/

44. Parrish M, Kerr K. Country road; bringing palliative care to rural California. Sacramento, CA: California Health Care Foundation. July 18, 2016. https://www.chcf.org/wp-content/uploads/2017/12/PDF-CountryRoadPalliativeCare.pdf

45. Kirby S, Barlow V, Saurman E, Lyle D, Passey M, Currow D. Systematic review: Are rural and remote patients, families and caregivers needs in life-limiting illness different from those of urban dwellers? A narrative synthesis of the evidence. *Aust J Rural Health*. 2016;24:289–299. doi:10.1111/ajr.12312

46. Mason DJ, Gardner D, Outlaw F, O'Grady E. *Policy and Politics in Nursing and Health Care*. 7th ed. St. Louis, MO: Elsevier; 2015. http://evolve.elsevier.com

47. Pesut B, Robinson CA, Bottorff JL, Fyles G, Broughton S. On the road again: Patient perspectives on commuting for palliative care. *Palliat Support Care*. 2010;8(2):187–195. doi:10.1017/S1478951509990940

48. Hawkins-Taylor C, Mollmon S, Walstrom B, Kerkvliet J, Minton M, Anderson D, Berke C. Perceptions of palliative care: Voices from rural South Dakota. *Am J Hospice Palliat Care*. 2020:1–9. doi:10.1177/1049909120953808

49. Rainsford S, Phillips C, Glasgow N, MacLeod R, Wiles R. The "safe death": An ethnography study exploring perspectives of rural palliative care patients and family caregivers. *J Palliat Med*. 2018;32(10):1575–1583. doi:10.1177/0269216318800613

50. MacDowell M. Glasser M, Fitts M, Neilsen K, Hunsaker M. A national view of rural health workforce issues in the USA. *Rural Remote Heal*. 2013;10(3):1–16. PMID: 2065889

51. Health Resources and Service Administration. HRSA Health Workforce. Nurse corps loan repayment program. https://bhw.hrsa.gov/loans-scholarships/nurse-corps/loan-repayment-program/determine-eligibility-and-apply

52. American Academy of Hospice and Palliative Medicine. Palliative care and hospice training act. 2019. Available at: http://aahpm.org/uploads/advocacy/PCHETA_Summary.pdf

53. Mckinley D, Shearer J, Weng K. Palliative care in rural minnesota: Findings from stratis health's minnesota rural palliative care initiative. *Clin Health Aff*. 2016:39–41. PMID: 26897897

54. Isaacson M, Minton M, DaRosa P, Harming S. Nurse comfort with palliative and end-of-life communication; a rural and urban comparison. *J Hosp Palliat Nurs*. 2019;21(1):38–45. doi:10.1188/11.ONF.E229–E239

55. American Nurses Association, Hospice and Palliative Nurses Association. A call for action-nurses lead and transform palliative care. Silver Spring, MD: American Nurses Association. 2017. http://www.nursingworld.org/~497158/globalassets/practiceandpolicy/health-policy/palliativecareprofessionalissuespanelcallforaction.pdf

56. Parrish M, Kinderman A, Rabow M. Weaving palliative care into primary care: A guide for community health centers. Sacramento, CA: California Health Care Foundation. 2015. https://www.chcf.org/wp-content/uploads/2017/12/PDF-WeavingPalliativeCarePrimaryCare.pdf

57. Pawlow P, Dahlin C, Doherty CL, Ersek M. The hospice and palliative care advanced practice registered nurse workforce: Results of a national survey. *J Hosp Palliat Nurs*. 2018;20(4):349–357. doi:10.1097/NJH.0000000000000449.

58. American Association of Colleges of Nursing, Primary palliative care competencies for masters and DNP nursing students: (G- CARES). Graduate competencies and recommendations for educating nursing students. American Association of Colleges of Nursing. 2019. https://www.aacnnursing.org/Portals/42/ELNEC/PEF/Graduate-CARES.pdf

59. Robinson C, Pesut B, Bottorff J. Issues in rural palliative care: Views from the countryside. *J Rural Health*. 2010;36:78–84. doi:10.1111/j.1748-0361.2009.00268.x

60. Spetz J, Skillman S, Andrilla C. Nurse practitioner autonomy and satisfaction in rural settings. *Med Care Res Rev*. 2017;74(2):227–235. doi:10.1177/10775558716629584

61. Holland DE, Vanderboom CE, Ingram CJ, et al. The feasibility of using technology to enhance the transition of palliative care for rural patients. *Comput Inform Nurs*. 2014;32(6):257–266. doi:10.1097/CIN.0000000000000066

62. Centers for Medicare and Medicaid Services. Innovation models: Chart model. CMS.gov. Updated September 10, 2021. https://innovation.cms.gov/innovation-models/chart-model.

63. Centers for Medicare and Medicaid Services. Trump administration finalizes permanent expansion of medicare telehealth services and improved payment for time doctors spend with patients. Last edited December 1, 2020. CMS.gov. https://www.cms.gov/newsroom/press-releases/trump-administration-finalizes-permanent-expansion-medicare-telehealth-services-and-improved-payment

64. Medicare Payment Advisory Commission. Chapter 12. Hospice services. Report to the Congress: Medicare Payment Policy. March 2019. http://www.medpac.gov/docs/default-source/reports/mar19_medpac_ch12_sec.pdf.

65. Healthcare Financial Management Association. Medicare Program: FY 2020 Hospice Wage index and Payment Rate update and Hospice Quality Reporting Requirements. [CMS-1714-f]. https://www.hfma.org/content/dam/hfma/Documents/industry-initiatives/fact-sheets/fs-fy2020-hospice-final-rule-summary.pdf

66. Medicare Payment Advisory Commission. Chapter 4. Physician and other health professional services: Report to the congress: Medicare payment policy. March 2017. http://www.medpac.gov/docs/default-source/reports/mar17_medpac_ch4.pdf

67. Ledwick M. Palliative care isn't "giving up": It improves quality of life and dignity, and maybe even survival. Cancer Research UK. Blog. August 23, 2010. Available at https://news.cancerresearchuk.org/2010/08/23/palliative-care-isnt-giving-up-it-improves-quality-of-life-and-dignity-and-maybe-even-survival/

68. Crooks VA, Giesbrecht M, Castleden H, Schuurman N, Skinner M, Williams A. Community readiness and momentum: Identifying and including community driven variables in a mixed-method rural palliative care service siting model. *BMC Palliat Care*. 2018;17:59. doi:10.1186/s12904-018-0313-5

19.

THE PALLIATIVE APRN IN RESIDENTIAL FACILITIES

Melissa McClean and Victoria Nalls

KEY POINTS

- There is growing evidence that advanced practice registered nurses (APRNs) in residential facility settings such as assisted living facilities and nursing homes improve clinical outcomes for residents with advanced illness.

- APRNs with specialized training in palliative care are uniquely suited to elevate the quality of care for facility-dwelling individuals by assisting in the continuum of care: facilitating advance care planning, providing expert symptom management, and coordinating care during transitions.

- Implementing and sustaining APRN-led care models in these settings can be challenging due to regulatory restrictions on APRNs that impact scope of practice, variability in care delivery models, and a shortage of professionals educated and trained to support residents requiring palliative and end-of-life care.

- APRNs have the potential to lead facilities in education and training, process improvements, and culture change initiatives.

CASE STUDY: GOALS OF CARE

Ralph was an 87-year-old African American man who lived in a nursing home. Ralph's past medical history included hypertension, history of myocardial infarction, diabetes, peripheral vascular disease, chronic obstructive pulmonary disease (COPD), chronic kidney disease (CKD) Stage II, osteoarthritis, peripheral neuropathy, and mild dementia. Prior to residing in a nursing home, Ralph lived at home but had trouble managing his complicated medication regimen. Due to misunderstanding his medications, Ralph endured several hospitalizations. His daughter, Ralph's surrogate decision-maker, decided it was unsafe for him to live alone and moved him into the nursing home. Upon admission to the nursing home, the facility medical director completed Ralph's admission assessment. The facility-employed advanced practice registered nurse (APRN) continued to see Ralph for ongoing care. He initially received skilled therapy services for debility after the hospital. However, a short time later, he declined to participate because he resented being placed in a nursing home.

Three months into his stay, his nurse reported to the APRN that she has noticed Ralph huffing and puffing on occasion. Ralph reported he found it hard to breath in the afternoon if he wheeled

himself around the facility "too much." He felt much better after pausing, taking some deep breaths, and resting. He denied any pain or difficulty getting air. Ralph still actively smoked and told the APRN, "Don't even tell me about stopping . . . going outside and smoking is the only thing that makes me happy in this awful place." His vital signs were stable at rest, but became elevated after activity. His mini-mental status examination (MMSE) was 24/30. His exam revealed displaced point of maximal impulse (PMI) with regular heart sounds, noted rales in the lung bases, normal bowel sounds, and +1 bilateral pedal edema.

To determine the plan of care, the APRN asked him what was most important to him, to which he replied, "I just want to go home." The APRN explored this sentiment a little further and learned that Ralph valued independence and disliked that staff dictated his day. Since he could not return home, he wanted to make sure that he could continue to go outside and smoke. When asked what he understood about his current medical situation, he stated, "I am old, and I haven't always taken good care of my body. If it's my time, then I want to go." The APRN attempted to explore this further, but Ralph was reluctant to talk about end-of-life wishes. When asked about his time in the hospital, Ralph shared that he disliked the hospital even more than the nursing home. The APRN shared with Ralph that she thought he may have heart failure, but they could manage his symptoms in the nursing home. Ralph was skeptical about the diagnosis of heart failure and asked for further evidence. The APRN provided two options that aligned with Ralph's preferences: facility work-up or cardiology consult. Ralph declined the cardiology consult, stating "I don't need any more doctors in my life." The APRN ordered an echocardiogram, chest x-ray, and lab work to be done in the facility. She also started Ralph on a diuretic.

The chest x-ray showed cardiomegaly with no active disease. Ralph's ejection fraction was 30%, and his blood work showed mild hyponatremia, CKD Stage III, and mild anemia. The APRN asked Ralph if she could include his daughter in a conversation for next steps. He confirmed his daughter as his medical power of attorney. A family meeting was held to plan the most appropriate treatment course.

At the end of a long conversation, the APRN summarized what she heard to be most important to Ralph. His daughter acknowledged his requests, and they completed an advance directive and a provider/physician order for life-sustaining treatment (POLST) form. The APRN also reviewed Ralph's medications and discontinued some medications that were no longer congruent with his goals of care. The most difficult topic was Ralph's smoking, which he was adamant he would not stop. The APRN helped the daughter understand that, although it is not the healthiest choice, it made Ralph happy. The final plan included a do-not-resuscitate/do-not-intubate (DNR/DNI) order, transfer to a hospital for acute injury only, and managing Ralph's symptoms based on maintaining his ability to get outside and smoke. The APRN documented the conversation and billed for an advance care planning visit of longer than 30 minutes. She also communicated the changes to the physician, nurse, nursing assistant, and social worker of the facility.

A few months later, the APRN walked into the facility and found the nurses on Ralph's unit slightly panicked and reaching to call 911. Ralph had been found in his room lethargic, febrile, and with difficulty breathing. There was a concern he may have had COVID-19. The APRN reminded the staff of Ralph's preferred wishes and insisted on reviewing his POLST form and calling the daughter before calling emergency medical services (EMS). After a brief report from the APRN, the daughter agreed that Ralph would not be transferred to the hospital and comfort measures would be instituted in the nursing home. The APRN followed facility protocol regarding possible SARS-CoV-2 and adjusted Ralph's medications to include only those needed for symptom management. She donned her appropriate personal protective equipment (PPE) and assisted staff in making Ralph comfortable. She connected Ralph with his daughter through video chat. Ralph's daughter saw her father and asked if he was dying, to which the APRN replied, "Yes, I think he is dying." The daughter said good-bye to her father and thanked the APRN for engaging them in that important conversation months ago. Although Ralph's daughter was sad to lose her father, she stated that she felt some peace knowing she was able to follow her father's instructions. Ralph died within 2 days, in the comfort of familiar faces, voices, and surroundings.

INTRODUCTION

Currently, in the United States, people are living longer despite the occurrence and progression of chronic diseases. The fastest growing age group in the Unites States are those 65 and older, with one in five people expected to be 65 or older by the year 2030.[1] Currently, 49 million Americans are 65 and older. These older adults are disproportionately affected by chronic disease that impacts their ability to remain independent.[2] The leading causes of death among older adults—cardiovascular disease, diabetes, lower respiratory diseases, and dementia—can limit older adults' ability to perform daily activities and result in the need for long-term services such as institutional or residential care.[3] This chapter focuses on the care provided by advanced practice registered nurses (APRNs), specifically nurse practitioners (NPs) and clinical nurse specialists (CNSs), in two long-term care settings: assisted living facilities and nursing homes (see Table 19.1). NPs and CNSs have been practicing in various facility settings for more than three decades and demonstrate the ability to successfully manage the complex conditions of residents in long-term care settings.

DESCRIPTION OF FACILITY SETTINGS

ASSISTED LIVING

Assisted living (AL) facilities provide a variety of services for individuals who can no longer live independently but do not require continuous skilled nursing. AL facilities may be associated with skilled nursing homes or be a component of continuing care retirement communities and/or independent communities. Often the living arrangements resemble an apartment or private room, and typically AL facilities are private pay. Currently, there are approximately 28,900 AL communities with nearly 1 million licensed beds in the United States. The median stay of an individual in AL is about 22 months, and about 60% of AL residents will transition from an AL environment to a nursing home.[4]

NURSING HOMES

Like AL facilities, nursing homes (NH) provide a wide range of services, but additionally they offer continuous nursing care and rehabilitation services. NH residents typically have more complex health conditions and reside in a bedroom

Table 19.1 RESIDENTIAL FACILITY DEFINITIONS

Long-term care	A broad term that describes any facility where residents receive assistance with their medical needs and/or daily activities over a long period of time. Types of facilities include board and care homes, assisted living facilities, nursing homes, and continuing care retirement communities (CCRCs).
Assisted living	A facility that offers residents assistance with daily activities and some medical care but does not provide 24-hour nursing care. These facilities are usually regulated by the state and typically private pay, although some states may provide coverage via Medicaid waivers. Residents often live in apartments or private rooms with shared common areas.
Nursing home	A facility that offers residents assistance with daily activities, continuous nursing care, and supervision. These facilities are mostly both state and federally regulated and typically funded by Medicaid or private pay. Residents can live in private or shared rooms with shared common areas.
Skilled nursing facility	A nursing home that provides short-term post-acute skilled rehabilitation and/or daily skilled nursing service under the Medicare Part A benefit. Often the goal for residents on the skilled unit is to return home. Most nursing homes function and provide services as both nursing facility and skilled nursing facility.

within the facility rather than in an independent apartment. These residents require 24-hour skilled nursing care and supervision. NHs are mostly funded by Medicare and/or Medicaid programs depending on the services offered by the nursing facility. There are approximately 15,600 NHs with 1.7 million licensed beds in the United States. Approximately 1.4 million individuals live in NHs, with 84% of these residents over the age of 66, predominantly female, and non-Hispanic White.[5]

THE APRN IN FACILITY SETTINGS

APRNs including NPs and CNSs have been directing and delivering care in NHs since the 1970s. Those with enhanced training in the medical complexity of long-term care residents have positively impacted resident and facility outcomes.[6] Prepared with a foundation in baccalaureate nursing, APRNs achieve an advanced level of knowledge through either graduate- or doctoral-level education. Upon successful completion of their program, APRNs also obtain national certification in advanced nursing practice and, often, specialty practice.

NURSE PRACTITIONERS

NPs participate in both direct and indirect care roles in facility settings. The number of these providers working in NHs has steadily increased over the past few decades.[7] According to the American Academy of Nurse Practitioners (AANP), approximately 11.7% of the 290,000 NPs licensed in the United States hold privileges in long-term care.[8] Of the NPs designated by certification, approximately 1.5% hold a specialty certification in hospice and palliative care. It should be noted that specialty certification is not mandatory, and therefore NPs who practice primary palliative care as part of general primary care or geriatrics are not recognized by this statistic. As direct care providers, NPs have expertise in assessing, diagnosing, and managing patients with complex health conditions, with a focus on interdisciplinary coordination of care.

CLINICAL NURSE SPECIALISTS

CNSs have expertise in affecting systems of care, including planning for, implementing, and evaluating improvements in quality and safety. Based on a recent systematic review, Salamanca-Balen et al. conclude that the role of the CNS in palliative care, and specifically in long-term care settings, is poorly recognized and not clearly defined.[9] Furthermore, the National Association of Clinical Nurse Specialists (NACNS) does not differentiate the number of licensed CNS providers working in long-term care settings, nor does it differentiate the CNS providers holding certification in hospice and palliative care.[10] Though these statistics are unclear, the education and certification required of a CNS complements the quality of care provided to residents in facility settings.

THE INFLUENCE OF STATE AND FEDERAL REGULATIONS

State and federal regulations significantly impact the management and day-to-day operations of long-term care facilities. It is important that an APRN practicing in either an AL or NH has a working knowledge of these regulations to ensure compliance and successful functioning within the facilities.

ASSISTED LIVING

The licensing and certification requirements for AL, along with the requirements for AL administrators, are dictated and enforced predominately at the state level. There are a few federal laws that apply to AL facilities, but mostly each state specifies which facilities qualify as AL communities. Between 2018 and 2019, many states updated plans to prevent or address potential abuse or neglect, requirements for staff training, emergency preparedness, and life safety plans.[11] APRNs practicing within an AL settings should become familiar with their state-specific regulations.

NURSING HOMES

NHs are governed by both state and federal regulations. The Foundation for Nursing Home Regulations was established in 1987 by the *Omnibus Budget Reconciliation Act*, also known as the Nursing Home Reform Act. For an NH to participate in Medicare and Medicaid, it must comply with requirements from the Centers for Medicare and Medicaid (CMS) for long-term care facilities. Some example requirements include having sufficient nursing staff, developing a comprehensive plan for each resident, maintaining the dignity and respect of each resident, providing activities of daily living assistance as appropriate, and promoting each resident's qualify of life.[12]

REGULATIONS AND STANDARDS

As a federal entity, CMS is responsible for monitoring the quality of care and enforcing care standards at a national level. State surveyors employed by CMS conduct an on-site evaluation of the facility at least annually and investigate complaints from the public, residents, or facility employees should they occur. On-site evaluations are unannounced and involve a team of healthcare professionals. The focus of the evaluation includes assessment of patients' conditions, rights, and needs; assessment of facility's policies and procedures; assessment of medication management and skin care; and assessment of the facility environment, including food and service. Information is gathered from the medical record, interviews with patients (or patients' legal representative), and discussions with facility staff and medical providers caring for patients. If an evaluation reveals a failure to meet a standard(s), the facility may be issued a deficiency citation that requires action; this is called a *plan of correction* (POC). The POC must include corrective actions for (1) those patients affected by the deficiency, (2) identifying other patients who are also potentially affected by the deficiency, and (3) ensuring that the deficiency will not recur. The POC must also include use of the facility's quality assurance program to monitor the systems, policies, and procedures for ongoing compliance.

Deficiencies are classified on the seriousness of the offense, from being isolated and less serious to being widespread and very serious. Deficiencies are also judged according to severity, ranging from "no actual harm with potential for minimal harm" to the patient to "immediate jeopardy to resident health or safety." Remedies are imposed based on the scope and severity of detected deficiencies and include required in-service training for the staff, fines to the facility or denial of payments for services provided, replacement of the facility administrator with temporary management, or installation of a state monitor in the facility. Ultimately, the failure of the facility to comply with standards can result in CMS revoking the facility's certification.

CARE OF RESIDENTS

Long-term care facilities are compromised largely of frail older adults with several comorbid conditions. As such, these facilities are a challenging setting for clinical practice. CMS began the National Nursing Home Quality Initiative (NHQI) in 2002. From this initiative, NHs created Quality Measures based on the resident's assessment data to include the resident's physical and clinical conditions, their preferences, and life care wishes. In 2003, the Quality Measures were added to the Nursing Home Compare website, which is a site that allows the public to review and compare Medicare- and Medicaid-certified nursing homes' inspection results across the country.[13] In 2008, CMS implemented the Five Star Nursing Home Quality Rating System to facilitate easier interpretation of Quality Measures. The rating system is a 1- to 5-star scale, with NHs receiving 1 star considered to have below average quality care and NHs with 5 stars considered to have above average quality care. NHs receive a star rating for three types of performance measures domains, as well as an overall star rating. The three performance measures include Health Inspections, Staffing, and Quality Measures.[14]

Under regulation *483.25 Quality of Care in the State Operations Manual*, CMS provides guidance on the assessment, management, and care planning for an NH resident approaching end of life.[12] Additionally, use of the ABCDE mnemonic is suggested as an approach to manage symptoms of residents with serious illness (see Table 19.2). The following must be accomplished and documented for NH residents approaching end of life: (1) identify the resident's prognosis on the basis of a comprehensive assessment, (2) advise and educate the resident and family about palliative care and hospice, (3) discuss advance care planning (ACP) and document those parties involved (resident, family, interdisciplinary team), and (4) delineate the resident's preferences regarding care. The developed plan of care must be reviewed and revised on a consistent basis to ensure services provided to the resident align with the wishes of the resident and family. Should an NH resident or designated healthcare surrogate elect hospice, documentation should reflect coordination of care between the facility and hospice.[15]

Table 19.2 **ABCDE MNEMONIC**

A	Ask the resident or legal representative about pain and other symptoms related to end of life on admission and periodically thereafter. Assess regularly and systematically for symptoms and their impact on the resident.
B	Believe the resident's report of pain or other symptoms, then inquire what causes it and what makes it better or worse.
C	Choose symptom control options that are person-centered.
D	Deliver timely, coordinated interventions.
E	Empower the resident to participate in advance care planning to the extent possible. Evaluate the effectiveness of implemented interventions.

Adapted from CMS: State Operations Manual Appendix PP – Guidance to Surveyors for Long-Term Care Facilities.[12]

In 2016, CMS's *Requirements for Participation for NHs* were revised to reflect the advances of medicine, service delivery, and safety. The changes included reducing the number of avoidable hospitalizations and healthcare-associated infections, enhancing person-centered care and behavioral/mental health management, providing culturally competent trauma-informed care, and utilizing technology and electronic health information exchange.[16] Care provided by APRNs in long-term care has been shown to positively impact quality measures.[17] For example, APRNs have successfully reduced avoidable hospitalizations.[18] They have also led quality improvement projects addressing antibiotic stewardship and de-prescribing that positively impact the above-mentioned quality measures.[17] Other possible roles for APRNs in long-term care include pressure ulcer prevention, overseeing wound rounds, providing staff education, and strategies to minimize psychotropics for behavioral and psychological symptoms of dementia.

REGULATORY RESTRICTIONS ON APRNS

Leveraging APRNs to care for residents in long-term care has been met with regulatory and cultural barriers. The scope of practice for APRNS varies by state, and some states limit the autonomy and prescribing practices of APRNs. Additionally, CMS has specific limitations for APRNs working in NHs. For example, APRNs are not allowed to conduct and bill for the initial skilled nursing facility admission visit nor write the admission orders. This limitation could impact the quality of care for the short-stay resident who is at risk of hospital readmission within the first 30 days of skilled nursing facility care. APRNs performing initial assessments could help mitigate this risk by identifying a resident's decline sooner. APRNs also cannot sign a *Certification of Terminal Illness* required by the *Medicare Hospice Benefit* that allows a patient to transition to hospice care. These assessments are deemed complete only when performed by a physician. Other limitations to the APRN practice in NHs are outlined in Table 19.3.

Table 19.3 APRN APPROVED VISITS AND ACTIVITIES IN SKILLED NURSING FACILITIES

	INITIAL COMPREHENSIVE VISIT AND ADMISSION ORDERS	REQUIRED VISITS AS OUTLINED IN 483.30(C)(1)	MEDICALLY NECESSARY VISITS	CERTIFICATION AND RECERTIFICATION FOR MEDICARE A
Skilled nursing facility (Medicare A stay)				
APRN employed by the facility	May NOT perform or sign	May perform alternating visits	May perform and sign	May NOT sign
APRN NOT employed by facility	May NOT perform and sign	May perform alternating visits	May perform and sign	May sign subject to State regulation
Direct admission to nursing facility/LTC (NOT Medicare A stay)				
APRN employed by the facility	May NOT perform or sign	May NOT perform	May perform and sign	NA
APRN NOT employed by facility	May perform and sign if a physician approved in writing a recommendation for admission to the facility prior to admission	May perform	May perform and sign	NA

Adapted from CMS: State Operations Manual Appendix PP–Guidance to Surveyors for Long Term Care Facilities.[12]

Culturally, the acceptance of APRNs as providers within the long-term care settings is still evolving. Some residents, families, and staff struggle to understand the difference between a registered nurse (RN) and an APRN. There is also confusion given that the APRN can function similarly to the physician for medical management of the resident. The role and function of the APRN varies greatly among facilities and states. Some facilities utilize the APRN for more administrative roles, others for more clinical roles. Despite the ambiguity, more facilities are hiring APRNs in long-term care given their value in delivering quality resident- and family-centered care.

MODELS OF CARE DELIVERY IN FACILITY SETTINGS

As an interdisciplinary model of advanced illness care, palliative care entrusts various disciplines to holistically address the medical, psychosocial, and spiritual needs of individuals. With robust global efforts to incorporate aspects of palliative care into the standard of care in facility settings, a wide variety of practice models exist.[19,20] These models can be aptly categorized by examining the discipline of the provider rendering care, the entity with fiscal responsibility of the provider, and determining whether palliative care is delivered to individuals with terminal illness through a federally regulated hospice program.

NON-APRN MODELS

A diverse array of healthcare professionals has demonstrated the capacity to lead palliative care efforts in facility settings, including physicians, nurses, social workers, and chaplains. For example, Morris and Galicia-Castillo presented a consultant model of palliative care, also known as the CARES Program, intended to serve 170 nursing home residents in Virginia using two physicians and a chaplain.[21] Additionally, Giuffrida presented an example of a palliative care program at a 364-bed skilled nursing and rehabilitation facility in New York where social workers were integral leaders in the program's success.[22] As part of a federal effort to affect hospitalizations rates of facility residents, CMS supported two RN-led programs in their Initiative to Reduce Avoidable Hospitalizations among Nursing Facility Residents.[23] Since palliative care is inherently interdisciplinary, various healthcare professionals within the team are capable of operationalizing various modalities, and examples of these models exist in the literature.

MODEL OF EMBEDDED APRN

By virtue of their education and training, APRNs also lead and manage either primary or specialty-level palliative care delivery programs.[24] APRNs employed in facility settings take an active part in direct patient care including disease-specific treatment, medication reconciliation, wound management, and care coordination. Additionally, facility-employed APRNs can provide ongoing staff education and lead quality improvement efforts.[20] Perhaps most importantly, APRNs embedded in the facility can rapidly respond to acute changes in a patient's condition consistent with the resident and family's expressed preferences for care.[19] APRNs working full-time in the facility build ongoing relationships with residents and their families, which improves communication, education, and establishing goals of care.[17] In these cases, the facility assumes full financial responsibility for the APRN employee but gains a valued and reliable team member.

MODEL OF CONTRACTED APRN

Facilities can also incorporate APRN-led care by contracting with physician groups, hospital systems, managed care organizations, or consultant services, often as part of a hospice organization. In 2016, the Center to Advance Palliative Care (CAPC) began conducting a 3-year project to assess community-based palliative care programs across the United States.[25] In the final report *Mapping Community Palliative Care*, Heitner et al. concluded that 28% of survey respondents serve long-term care settings. The following statement provides further detail:

> Of the programs delivering palliative care in long-term care settings, 38% are operated by long-term care facilities, 32% are operated by hospices, 21% are operated by hospitals, 5% are operated by office practices or clinics, and 4% are operated by home health agencies.[25 (p. 4)]

In these models, facilities assume minimal to no financial responsibility for the APRN employee. APRNs utilize fee-for-service billing reimbursable under Medicare Part B, Medicaid, and most commercial insurers. Consultant or contract models have been shown to influence facilities' processes in palliative care referral, document the presence of pain and other symptoms, and increase hospice utilization.[26] However, gaps in quality care coordination can exist when APRNs work in multiple settings or facilities to maintain or increase revenue. Furthermore, sustainability of these models depends on the facility's ability to embrace cultural shifts in care leaders and the funder's ability to ensure longevity of the program.[20,27]

HOSPICE MODEL

Hospice is the most common model of palliative care delivery in facility settings.[28,29] Hospice services are provided in 80.7% of NHs and 67.7% of residential care communities, including AL facilities.[5] Despite the prevalence, not all residents have access to standardized end-of-life care. According to a report from the National Hospice and Palliative Care Organization (NHPCO), approximately 19.7% of recipients of hospice care resided in AL facilities and 17.3% resided in NHs, including skilled nursing facilities.[30] Lack of access to hospice services can impact symptom management and limit much-needed psychosocial support.[28]

For NH residents who elect the hospice benefit, the facility and the hospice agency are jointly responsible for developing, implementing, and evaluating a coordinated plan of care. The facility maintains the responsibility for the overall care of the patient and must notify hospice if the patient experiences an acute change in condition. Value-added services demonstrated by hospice, beyond standard palliative care approaches

in the plan of care, include volunteer, pastoral care, bereavement services, and interdisciplinary staff who have specialized training and skills in providing end-of-life care. Research investigations have demonstrated fewer hospital admissions, fewer unmet needs, and improved pain and other symptom assessment and management when patients are admitted to hospice in the NH. As previously mentioned, APRNs cannot certify residents with a terminal illness to initiate hospice services. They also cannot provide reimbursable care to hospice-enrolled residents unless they are designated as the attending of record.

APRN CLINICAL PRACTICE IN FACILITY SETTINGS

Approximately 25% of US residents will die in a facility setting, despite residents' overwhelming preference to live their last moments at home.[28] A facility environment, either AL or NH, is perhaps a close second choice for residents who would prefer not to die in the hospital. Since the NH will inevitably be the final place of residence for many frail and elderly individuals with terminal illness who require continuous nursing care, integration of high-quality palliative care seems crucial. Many of CMS's regulations and standards of care for NHs align with the philosophy of palliative care and support that palliative care may be appropriate rather than seeking a cure for residents who have chronic, progressive illnesses.[31] Additionally, high-quality palliative care initiatives can be developed by interpreting and adapting the National Consensus Project for Quality Palliative *Clinical Practice Guidelines*.[32] The following sections highlight clinical practice considerations for the APRN delivering palliative care in ALs and NHs.

CONTINUUM OF ILLNESS

Given the stringent regulations around preventing decline, meticulous documentation by the APRN is crucial when providing palliative and end-of-life care to residents in the NH. Decline due to a natural disease trajectory must be reflected in the provider's note through the patient's history, the physical exam, and any pertinent diagnostic testing. For example, CMS revised its regulatory guidance around pressure injuries and acknowledged that pressure injuries may be unavoidable at end of life. However, a provider's documentation must still reflect standard of care for pressure injury prevention and interventions to prevent further decline. Additionally, the APRN must note that the patient has nonmodifiable physiology contributing to the formation of pressure injuries and note appropriate efforts to stabilize the resident's condition. Finally, the patient's plan of care must be resident-centered and aligned with the advance directives of the resident.[12] When defined and expected findings of disease progression are considered, the APRN should incorporate palliative management strategies into the plan of care.

ADVANCE CARE PLANNING

While true across all care settings, close attention to ACP is especially important in ALs and NHs. Patient preferences must be ascertained, documented, and followed by all care providers in a facility setting. It is important to initiate and continue discussions with facility-dwelling residents who, because of advanced frailty and multiple life-limiting illnesses, are expected to have a decreased life expectancy. With astute attention to disease trajectory and prognostication, APRNs can assist residents in identifying a power of attorney for healthcare or surrogate decision-maker before the resident becomes acutely ill or loses decision-making capacity. In this setting, preferences such as a do-not-resuscitate (DNR), do-not-intubate (DNI), or do-not-transfer (DNT) order are especially important to discuss and document according to the resident's stated goals of care. However, a DNR/DNI/DNT order does not preclude the need for discussions with the resident and family regarding other medical treatments. In these instances, it may be appropriate for the APRN to discuss whether the resident would elect other potentially life-saving medical treatments such as medically administered nutrition; intravenous antibiotics, fluids, or blood products; or dialysis. After the discussion, the APRN can note the resident's preferences into a portable medical order, national provider/physician order for life-sustaining treatment (POLST) form or similar form in the resident's state.[33]

A recent systematic review conducted by Martin et al. explains that the type of ACP document utilized may vary from facility to facility but that the incidence of unwanted interventions reduces with use of the POLST form.[34] ACP also may lead to earlier and more frequent palliative care and hospice referrals.[34] The APRN can be instrumental in creating policies that make ACP part of the standard practice with every resident admitted to and residing in the facility. Such interventions work to identify and uphold residents' expressed wishes and can encourage more dignified end-of-life care with hospice.

SYMPTOM MANAGEMENT

Many residents experience undesirable symptoms as a result of chronic and advanced illnesses. In these instances, ongoing assessment of symptoms, management of symptoms according to evidence-based practices, and evaluation of selected interventions are necessary. APRNs working in ALs and NHs are in an ideal position to manage the complex symptoms associated with progressive illnesses because they are regularly on site and available for immediate attention, if necessary. Additionally, they can educate staff at the bedside, as well as have conversations with families regarding goals of care. The assessment and management of pain is of utmost importance when approximately 40–83% of residents' experience pain due to musculoskeletal conditions (e.g., osteoarthritis, post-stroke disabilities), cancer, and neuropathy.[35] Many barriers to pain assessment and management in the facility setting exist, especially in the care of residents with cognitive impairment whose self-reports of pain are more difficulty to ascertain.[36]

The current opioid epidemic also poses challenges to transparent reporting of pain.[37] APRNs possess the skills and knowledge to both adequately assess and treat pain symptoms. In an example of an APRN-led pain management intervention in a long-term care setting, Kasssalainen et al. found that NPs are effective in reducing residents' pain and subsequently improving residents' function.[35] The study also reported that the facility relied on the NP's ability to educate staff on pain management assessment and intervention. Expert symptom management is one of the trademark skills of specialty palliative APRNs, and they can therefore target barriers to adequate pain management and advocate for the highest quality of care for residents.

TRANSITIONAL CARE AND CARE COORDINATION

APRNs have demonstrated the capacity to assist residents who transition from one care setting to another (e.g., from hospital to skilled nursing facility or from NH to the emergency room) in the event of a change in condition. APRNs, as care coordinators, influence greater communication between care providers and care settings to avoid unnecessary errors through medication reconciliation processes. Also, APRNs can provide the resident or family with anticipatory guidance to impact a resident's experience of care in a more favorable way. There are also times when transfer to an acute level of care is not congruent with the resident's expressed goals of care. In these instances, APRNs have been instrumental in reducing unavoidable hospitalizations by as much as 17%.[18] These positive outcomes occur when the embedded APRN participates in daily rounding and can respond to acute changes in a timely manner or when an APRN consultant introduces specialty-level palliative care to address symptom management and initiates earlier conversations on the resident's goals of care.[38] By leveraging the APRN's role in care coordination and other palliative care interventions, the resident and family are likely to report more positive experiences with care and ultimately decrease healthcare spending.[20,39]

CURRENT IMPLICATIONS AND FUTURE OPPORTUNITIES FOR APRNS

In 2017, the American Nurses Association (ANA) and the Hospice and Palliative Nurses Association (HPNA) partnered to issue a publication titled *Call for Action: Nurses Lead and Transform Palliative Care*. This document urges nurses, including all APRNs, to consider the role of palliative care in practice, education, administration, research, and policy in order to improve care to individuals with serious illness. APRNs are encouraged to assist in increasing access to specialist palliative care in all practice settings, including long-term care.[40] APRNs are also charged with elevating their practice in other areas, as described next. The following sections review two current implications in facility settings and explore ways in which APRNs can contribute to future efforts.

REFORMING CARE DELIVERY

Variability in care delivery models occurs when institutions are required to adapt to the characteristics of their setting. Aspects such as the geographic location of the facility, the health condition of residents, the vitality of the workforce, and the institutional culture created by administrators, medical directors, and payers all influence care in various ways, particularly in the operationalization of care models. For example, there existed a misalignment between the realities of institutionalized care and reimbursement for quality measures in the post-acute care setting. As such, legislation including the *Improving Medicare Post-Acute Transformation Act (IMPACT Act) of 2014* and *Protecting Access to Medicare Act (PAMA)* have influenced care standards, quality measures, and reimbursement for a wide array medical services including diagnostic imaging.[41-43] Additionally, recent advances in technology have also contributed to a shift in care delivery. The wide acceptance of telehealth, as a response to the COVID-19 pandemic, prompted CMS to adopt temporary regulatory waivers and enact policy changes to increase access to and reimbursement for telehealth services. In rural setting, the use of telehealth allowed residents access to services not otherwise available.[43-45] APRNs in facility settings will be challenged to adapt the ways in which they deliver care in these complex settings as policymakers cycle through the processes, innovation, legislation, and reformation efforts. As APRNs practice in concert with ongoing developments in healthcare, they can not only influence the quality of care delivered to residents, but they can also contribute to policy and research at local and national levels.

WORKFORCE CONSIDERATIONS

A stable and educated workforce is vital to caring for an aging population. However, building a strong force means overcoming existing obstacles such as staff turnover. Turnover in facility settings occurs widely, and the negative impact is multifaceted and well-documented.[29] Consistent turnover of nursing staff, administrators, and medical directors leads to knowledge deficits and increased training needs. For example, the indirect cost of training and education can negatively impact a palliative program's sustainability and cause financial hardship. Transitioning staff take with them institutional knowledge that would help inform coordinators or directors of effective strategies for sustainability and critical feedback to improve initiatives. Turnover also impacts efforts to understand the outcomes of palliative initiatives.[46] The validity and quality of clinical trials investigating the effects of symptom management, ACP, care coordination, and the resident's or family's experience can be weakened by staff turnover.[29,46] Having knowledge of care that is safe, efficient, and quality-driven improves healthcare expenditures. A systematic review by Carpenter et al. found minimal high-quality evidence from 13 clinical trials investigating the effects of palliative care interventions in NHs, and staff turnover is cited as one of the many contributing factors.[26] In the end, the economic impact of this issue cannot be ignored. APRNs, as clinical leaders in facility settings, can work to mitigate staff turnover by encouraging collaborative and interdisciplinary team-based interventions, educating staff on compassion fatigue and burnout, and promoting a culture of transparency and resilience. Future opportunities for practice and research include piloting and investigating APRNs as clinical leaders, such as medical directors in facility settings, to relieve today's facility administrators of the unrelenting challenges. There has never been a more appropriate time to reimagine the care delivered to a most precious generation.

SUMMARY

APRNs are ideally positioned to advance the delivery of evidence-based palliative care to residents in facility settings. Their education of advanced chronic disease management and their communication skills promote collaboration with resident's, families, and other members of the healthcare team. In their care of residents in facility settings, APRNs lead and participate in the continuum of care by facilitating ACP, providing expert symptom management, and coordinating care during transitions. While challenges to practicing in this setting exist, ample evidence confirms numerous positive outcomes when APRNs are involved in the care of facility-dwelling residents. There are tremendous opportunities for APRNs to affect the quality of living and dying for residents in these settings.

REFERENCES

1. The United States Census Bureau. Newsroom. 65 and older population grows rapidly as baby boomers age. The United States Census Bureau. June 25, 2020. https://www.census.gov/newsroom/press-releases/2020/65-older-population-grows.html
2. U.S. Department of Health and Human Services. Administration of Community Living. Administration on Aging. Profile of older Americans: 2017. April 2018. https://acl.gov/sites/default/files/Aging%20and%20Disability%20in%20America/2017OlderAmericansProfile.pdf
3. Kochanek KD, Murphy SL, Xu J, Arias E. Mortality in the United States, 2016. *NCHS Data Brief.* 2017;(293):1–8.
4. American Health Care Association. National Center for Assisted Living. Facts and figures. 2020. https://www.ahcancal.org/Assisted-Living/Facts-and-Figures/Pages/default.aspx
5. Harris-Kojetin L, Sengupta M, Lendon JP, Rome V, Valverde R, Caffrey C. Long-term care providers and services users in the United States, 2015–2016. *National Center for Health Statistics. Vital Health Stat.* 2019;3(43). https://www.cdc.gov/nchs/data/series/sr_03/sr03_43-508.pdf
6. Barker RO, Craig D, Spiers G, Kunonga P, Hanratty B. Who should deliver primary care in long-term care facilities to optimize resident outcomes? A systematic review. *J Am Med Dir Assoc.* 2018;19(12):1069–1079. doi:10.1016/j.jamda.2018.07.006
7. Intrator O, Miller EA, Gadbois E, Acquah JK, Makineni R, Tyler D. Trends in nurse practitioner and physician assistant practice in nursing homes, 2000–2010. *Health Serv Res.* 2015;50(6):1772–1786. doi:10.1111/1475-6773.12410
8. American Association of Nurse Practitioners. NP fact sheet. Austin, TX: AANP. Updated May 2021. https://www.aanp.org/about/all-about-nps/np-fact-sheet

9. Salamanca-Balen N, Seymour J, Caswell G, Whynes D, Tod A. The costs, resource use and cost-effectiveness of clinical nurse specialist–led interventions for patients with palliative care needs: A systematic review of international evidence. *Palliat Med.* 2018;32(2):447–465. doi:10.1177/0269216317711570

10. National Association of Clinical Nurse Specialists What is a CNS? 2021. https://nacns.org/about-us/what-is-a-cns/

11. National Center for Assisted Living. 2019 Assisted living state regulatory review. Washington, DC: NCAL. https://www.ahcancal.org/Assisted-Living/Policy/Documents/2019_reg_review.pdf

12. U. S. Department of Health and Human Services. Centers for Medicare and Medicaid Services. State operations manual: Appendix PP: Guidance to surveyors for long term care facilities. Rev. 173, 11-22-2017. https://www.cms.gov/Regulations-and-Guidance/Guidance/Manuals/downloads/som107ap_pp_guidelines_ltcf.pdf

13. U.S. Centers for Medicare and Medicaid Services. Medicare.gov. Find and compare nursing homes, hospitals and other providers near you. 2021. https://www.medicare.gov/nursinghomecompare/search.html

14. U.S. Centers for Medicare and Medicaid Services. CMS.gov. Five-Star Quality Rating System. October 7, 2019. https://www.cms.gov/medicare/provider-enrollment-and-certification/certificationandcomplianc/fsqrs

15. U.S. Centers for Medicare and Medicaid Services. State operations manual: Appendix M: Guidance to surveyors for hospice. Rev.200, 2-21-20. https://www.cms.gov/Regulations-and-Guidance/Guidance/Manuals/downloads/som107ap_m_hospice.pdf

16. Department of Health and Medicare Services. Centers for Medicaid and Medicare Services. Medicare and Medicaid programs: Reform of regulations for long-term care facilities. *Federal Register.* 81(192). October 4, 2016. https://www.govinfo.gov/content/pkg/FR-2016-10-04/pdf/2016-23503.pdf

17. Rantz MJ, Popejoy L, Vogelsmeier A, et al. Impact of advanced practice registered nurses on quality measures: The Missouri quality initiative experience. *J Am Med Dir Assoc.* 2018;19(6):541–550. doi:10.1016/j.jamda.2017.10.014

18. Mileski M, Pannu U, Payne B, Sterling E, McClay R. The impact of nurse practitioners on hospitalizations and discharges from long-term nursing facilities: A systematic review. *Healthcare.* 2020;8(2):114. doi:10.3390/healthcare8020114

19. Kaasalainen S, Sussman T, McCleary L, et al. Palliative care models in long-term care: A scoping review. *Nurs Leadersh.* 2019;32(3):8–26.

20. Rantz MJ, Birtley NM, Flesner M, Crecelius C, Murray C. Call to action: APRNs in U.S. Nursing homes to improve care and reduce costs. *Nurs Outlook.* 2017;65(6):689–696. doi:10.1016/j.outlook.2017.08.011

21. Morris DA, Galicia-Castillo M. Caring about residents' experiences and symptoms (cares) program: A model of palliative care consultation in the nursing home. *Am J Hosp Palliat Med.* 2017;34(5):466–469. doi:10.1177/1049909116641606

22. Giuffrida J. Palliative care in your nursing home: Program development and innovation in transitional care. *J Soc Work End-Life Palliat Care.* 2015;11(2):167–177. doi:10.1080/15524256.2015.1074143

23. U. S. Centers for Medicare and Medicaid Services. CMS.gov. Initiative to reduce avoidable hospitalizations among nursing facility residents. Last updated May 4, 2021. https://innovation.cms.gov/innovation-models/rahnfr

24. Dahlin C, Coyne P. The palliative APRN leader. *Ann Palliat Med.* 2019;8(S1):S30–S38. doi:10.21037/apm.2018.06.03

25. Heitner R, Rogers M, Meier DE. *Mapping Community Palliative Care: A Snapshot.* New York: Center to Advance Palliative Care; 2019. https://www.capc.org/mapping-community-palliative-care/

26. Carpenter JG, Lam K, Ritter AZ, Ersek M. A systematic review of nursing home palliative care interventions: Characteristics and outcomes. *J Am Med Dir Assoc.* 2020;21(5):583–596.e2. doi:10.1016/j.jamda.2019.11.015

27. Carlson MDA, Lim B, Meier DE. Strategies and innovative models for delivering palliative care in nursing homes. *J Am Med Dir Assoc.* 2011;12(2):91–98. doi:10.1016/j.jamda.2010.07.016

28. Hunt LJ, Stephens CE, Smith AK. Palliative care in the nursing home: Shifting paradigms. *JAMA Intern Med.* 2020;180(2):243. doi:10.1001/jamainternmed.2019.5359

29. Norton SA, Ladwig S, Caprio TV, Quill TE, Temkin-Greener H. Staff experiences forming and sustaining palliative care teams in nursing homes. *Gerontologist.* 2018;58(4):e218–e225. doi:10.1093/geront/gnx201

30. National Hospice and Palliative Care Organization. NHPCO facts and figures. 2020 edition. Alexandria, VA: National Hospice and Palliative Care Organization. August 20, 2020. https://www.nhpco.org/wp-content/uploads/NHPCO-Facts-Figures-2020-edition.pdf

31. Department of Health and Human Services. Centers for Medicare and Medicaid services. Center for Clinical Standards and Quality/Survey and Certification Group. Quality of Care. Pub 10-07 State Operations Provider Certification. Revisions to Appendix PP – "Interpretive Guidelines for Long-Term Care Facilities F tag 309 Quality of Care" September 27, 2012. https://www.cms.gov/Medicare/Provider-Enrollment-and-Certification/SurveyCertificationGenInfo/Downloads/Survey-and-Cert-Letter-12-48.pdf

32. National Consensus Project for Quality Palliative Care. *Clinical Practice Guidelines for Quality Palliative Care.* 4th ed. Richmond, VA: National Coalition for Hospice and Palliative Care; 2018. https://www.nationalcoalitionhpc.org/wp-content/uploads/2018/10/NCHPC-NCPGuidelines_4thED_web_FINAL.pdf

33. National POLST. National POLST form: Portable medical order. 2021. https://polst.org/national-form/

34. Martin RS, Hayes B, Gregorevic K, Lim WK. The effects of advance care planning interventions on nursing home residents: A systematic review. *J Am Med Dir Assoc.* 2016;17(4):284–293. doi:10.1016/j.jamda.2015.12.017

35. Kaasalainen S, Wickson-Griffiths A, Akhtar-Danesh N, et al. The effectiveness of a nurse practitioner-led pain management team in long-term care: A mixed methods study. *Int J Nurs Stud.* 2016;62:156–167. doi:10.1016/j.ijnurstu.2016.07.022

36. Kaasalainen S, Ploeg J, Donald F, et al. Positioning clinical nurse specialists and nurse practitioners as change champions to implement a pain protocol in long-term care. *Pain Manag Nurs.* 2015;16(2):78–88. doi:10.1016/j.pmn.2014.04.002

37. U.S. Centers for Medicare and Medicaid Services. Quality Measures. CMS.gov. October 19, 2020. https://www.cms.gov/Medicare/Quality-Initiatives-Patient-Assessment-Instruments/NursingHomeQualityInits/NHQIQualityMeasures

38. Miller SC, Lima JC, Intrator O, Martin E, Bull J, Hanson LC. Palliative care consultations in nursing homes and reductions in acute care use and potentially burdensome end-of-life transitions. *J Am Geriatr Soc.* 2016;64(11):2280–2287. doi:10.1111/jgs.14469

39. Wichmann AB, Adang EMM, Vissers KCP, et al. Decreased costs and retained qol due to the "pace steps to success" intervention in ltcfs: Cost-effectiveness analysis of a randomized controlled trial. *BMC Med.* 2020;18(1):258. doi:10.1186/s12916-020-01720-9

40. American Nurses Association and Hospice and Palliative Nurses Association. *Call for Action: Nurses Lead and Transform Palliative Care.* Silver Spring, MD: American Nurses Association; 2017. https://www.nursingworld.org/~497158/globalassets/practiceandpolicy/health-policy/palliativecareprofessionalissuespanelcallforaction.pdf

41. American Hospital Association. Fact sheet: Reset IMPACT Act to account for Covid-19 lessons on post-acute care. Updated April 28, 2021. https://www.aha.org/fact-sheets/2020-06-24-fact-sheet-reset-impact-act-account-covid-19-lessons-post-acute-care

42. Care Select. The protecting access to Medicare Act: Appropriate use criteria consultation mandate for advanced diagnostic imaging. National Decision Support Company. 2019. https://nationaldecisionsupport.com/blog/wp-content/uploads/2019/09/PAMA-Flyer-August-2019-1.pdf

43. Jones CD, Nearing KA, Burke RE, et al. "What would it take to transform post-acute care?" 2019 conference proceedings on re-envisioning post-acute care. *J Am Med Dir Assoc.* 2020;21(8):1012–1014. doi:10.1016/j.jamda.2020.02.004

44. U.S. Centers for Medicare and Medicaid Services. CMS.gov. Long-term care nursing homes telehealth and telemedicine tool kit. March 27, 2020. https://www.cms.gov/files/document/covid-19-nursing-home-telehealth-toolkit.pdf

45. U.S. Centers for Medicare and Medicaid. Rural health clinics (RHCS) and federally qualified health centers (FQHCS): CMS flexibilities to fight covid-19. Baltimore, MD: CMS. May 21, 2021. https://www.cms.gov/files/document/omh-rural-crosswalk-5-21-21.pdf

46. Van den Block L, Honinx E, Pivodic L, et al. Evaluation of a palliative care program for nursing homes in 7 countries: The pace cluster-randomized clinical trial. *JAMA Intern Med*. 2020;180(2):233. doi:10.1001/jamainternmed.2019.5349

SECTION IV

POPULATIONS AT RISK

20.

HEALTH DISPARITIES IN PALLIATIVE CARE AND SOCIAL DETERMINANTS OF HEALTH

Alma Y. Dixon and Cecilia R. Motschenbacher

KEY POINTS

- Awareness of structural vulnerability allows clinicians to view the social conditions that undermine the capacity of patients to access healthcare, adhere to treatment, and successfully modify lifestyles.

- In assessing the structurally vulnerable patient, clinicians need to be mindful and question if the patient elicits a potential stigma or stereotypical bias or if the patient's appearance, ethnicity, accent, addiction status, or behaviors cause the clinician to think this person does not deserve, want, nor be willing to participate in a treatment regime.

- The palliative advanced practice registered nurse (APRN) is a patient and family advocate who assesses the patient for structural vulnerability.

- The interdisciplinary team plays a key role in securing needed resources for the structurally vulnerable patient and for self-monitoring to determine if implicit biases exist.

CASE STUDY: SOCIAL DETERMINANTS OF HEALTH

Mr. J was a 62-year-old African American man recently diagnosed with recurrent metastatic head and neck cancer. He was referred to the supportive and palliative care (SPC) clinic by his oncologist for pain and symptom management. Upon initial assessment, it was noted that he was unable to read instructions provided to him and could not operate his smartphone, rendering him functionally illiterate. These challenges made it difficult for him to adhere to his complicated medication regimen. He had not completed high school, and his employment history included various jobs within the construction industry. He had married and had two estranged adult children. A brother lived nearby, but was not overly involved. Mr. J had a history of substance use disorder and had experienced homelessness. However, he had secured low-income housing. It was relatively close to his medical care, but he was without reliable transportation. As a result, he spent much of his time walking to the local food bank and to his necessary appointments.

Mr. J admitted that although his appetite was good, he could not afford enough food to keep him satiated. At times, he had to decide between paying for his prescribed medications or paying for food. Mr. J endorsed right-sided cervical pain, which correlated with an enlarged malignant mass. The pain was relatively controlled with opioids and adjuvant therapy. He also had opioid-induced constipation. The palliative advanced practice registered nurse (APRN) referred Mr. J to the SPC social worker (LCSW), who performed a thorough psychosocial and needs assessment. She provided him with nutritional shakes from oncology and bus tokens for the local transportation system. She also requested support from the team registered nurse (RN) to reconcile his medication list, provide further education about medication administration, and create a system for him to label his bottles so he knew which medications were for which symptoms.

For many months, the palliative APRN ensured adequate symptom relief for Mr. J while the LCSW partnered with him for emotional, nutritional, and transportation support. Then suddenly, there was a 3-month gap of care during which Mr. J disappeared. He did not attend any of his medical appointments and his phone number was disconnected. Concerned, the APRN contacted Mr. J's brother to ensure his safety and encourage continued follow-up with his medical team. When Mr. J attended his next visit, the cervical mass had grown considerably and was now impeding his ability to swallow and receive adequate nutrition. Attempts to reconnect him to oncology services proved difficult because of he did not keep appointments with his specialists and primary care provider.

One afternoon, the SPC team was contacted regarding a patient whose family was at the front desk demanding he be seen urgently. Mr. J, cachectic and weak, had been transported to the clinic in a wheelchair by his brother who was afraid his brother was dying. He did not know what to do nor did he have the capacity to care for Mr. J. The palliative APRN arranged to have Mr. J admitted to the palliative care unit although this was complicated when a urine drug screen was positive for cocaine. The attending physician was conflicted about continued opioid utilization considering concurrent substance misuse and subsequently discontinued opioids during his inpatient stay. The APRN held a meeting between the inpatient and outpatient teams to advocate for the patient and determine a path forward. They determined that since he was dying and would be under the service of hospice, pain medications could be controlled. The pain regimen was reinitiated with opioid therapy, and Mr. J's pain was well-controlled. Coordination was made to transfer him to a skilled nursing facility with hospice services, and he was ultimately reconnected with his estranged daughter.

This chapter discusses how social determinants of health undermine many patients' capacity to access healthcare, adhere to treatment, and modify lifestyles successfully. The foundation of understanding social determinants of health is that healthcare providers often have preconceived notions about a patient which limits their ability to develop an effective plan of care.[1] In the case study presented, Mr. J's homelessness, illiteracy, poverty, and social isolation need to be viewed as the social constructs that impeded his ability to actively engage in a plan of care. Because of these social determinants, he was placed at a lower rung of political and social hierarchies and, in fact, faced unique barriers in accessing and actively participating in his care. In addition, his race, social condition, and diagnosis may have resulted in negative preconceptions by healthcare providers. These preconceptions can result in clinicians prejudging patients like Mr. J's willingness to modify behavior. The collaboration of the palliative interdisciplinary team (IDT) is essential to ensure that patients like Mr. J are viewed as individuals with significant challenges rather than as individuals who are noncompliant and willfully choose not to adhere to their treatment regime.

Structural vulnerability refers to an individual or group being at risk for adverse health outcomes due to their position within interconnecting socioeconomic, political, and cultural hierarchies that constrain the ability to pursue healthy lifestyles.[1] It occurs due to a combination of socioeconomic and demographic characteristics such as gender, gender expression, sexual orientation, socioeconomic status, race, ethnicity, sexuality, citizenship status, and physical location. Structural vulnerabilities vary depending on context but can include poverty, homelessness, social isolation, HIV status, ongoing trauma and violence, mental health and addictions, and experience with the criminal justice system.

Social determinants of health (SDOH) are conditions that determine individual and population health, as depicted in Figure 20.1. Individuals with structurally vulnerability may experience lack of income, inability to pay medical bills, substandard housing, homelessness, limited or no access to healthcare, lack of social support, illiteracy, and hunger.[2]

Health disparities represent the impact of race, socioeconomic status, gender, gender expression, sexual orientation, age, diagnosis, and mental ability on an individual's or group's ability to achieve positive health outcomes. They are

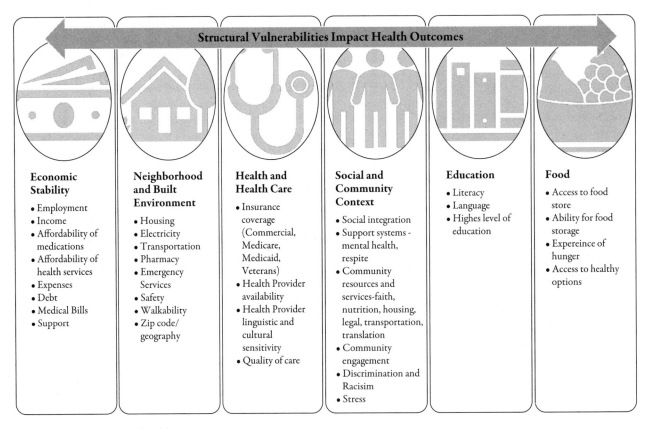

Figure 20.1 Social determinants of health.
Infographic adapted from Artiga S, Hinton E. Beyond health care: The role of social determinants in promoting health and health equity. May, 10, 2018. Kaiser Family Foundation.[3]

a direct result of political and economic structures that create inequality.[1]

Implicit bias refers to the negative preconceptions that an individual has based on a patient's gender, ethnicity, sexual orientation, socioeconomic status, or diagnosis. Implicit negative biases are reflected in verbal judgments and nonverbal behavior. Patients who can be classified as structurally vulnerable often fall prey to healthcare providers' implicit bias. Implicit biases contribute to health disparities by adversely affecting patient assessment, treatment decisions, and healthcare follow-up.[4]

PALLIATIVE CARE AND THE TEAM

Individuals seeking palliative care tend to share similar socioeconomic and demographic profiles. For example, they reside in homes or assisted living facilities and have diagnoses with predictable outcomes, such as cancer, heart failure, or pulmonary disease. However, individuals who are structurally vulnerable do not fit this picture, especially people who are experiencing homelessness, poverty, serious mental illness, substance abuse, or stigmatized illnesses such as HIV and AIDS. These individuals tend to be unnoticed, and their needs go unmet.[5]

The palliative care team focuses on symptom management, care coordination, and advance care planning. This can be especially challenging when working with patients disproportionately affected by poverty, housing instability, food insecurity, behavioral health conditions, and substance use disorder. The team may adhere to the belief that, at the end of life, patients may wish to die at home, without pain, with family surrounding them. However, patients like Mr. J require that this mindset be examined. The notion of "at home" must be expanded to include homelessness, the idea of "without pain" needs to include pain management within a history of substance abuse, and "family" requires identification of supportive persons rather than biological ties.[6] Patients like Mr. J rely on the collaboration of palliative team members to work as a cohesive whole to address their complex problems. Within the palliative care team, members can name and challenge implicit biases by asking tough questions.

- Does this patient elicit a sense of distrust because of behavior or lack of adherence to a plan of care?

- Does this patient's behavior indicate a lack of desire to participate in a plan of care?

- Does this patient's ethnicity, gender, gender expression, sexual orientation, or past behavior produce negative expectations of ability to engage in a plan of care?

By asking these questions, the team is empowered to acknowledge the impact of structural vulnerability on the outcomes of care.[1] Through the work of the IDT, the perception of Mr. J moved from an unreliable drug-seeking patient to a man with complex medical and social needs.

IMPLICATIONS FOR PALLIATIVE CARE

An exhaustive array of research has qualified the platitude that structurally vulnerable individuals receive a different standard of care and therefore achieve poorer health outcomes (see Chapter 18, "Palliative and Hospice Care in Rural Areas"; Chapter 47, "Patients with Substance Use Disorder and Dual Diagnoses"; Chapter 21, "Economically Disadvantaged Urban Dwellers"; and Chapter 23, Care of Veterans with Palliative Care Needs").[1,2,4–12] Awareness of such health disparities and inequities within the palliative care domain is essential to impart radical change that expands across care systems. A microcosm of the healthcare system at large reveals that hospice and palliative services are often not accessible to the most structurally vulnerable patients, specifically, those individuals who are lacking vital resources and supports as defined by their SDOH. The intersection between health outcomes and SDOH requires clinicians who are both adept at identifying a patient's and family's psychosocial needs and have a foundational understanding of the resources available to support their journey.[7] The 2018 National Consensus Project for Quality Palliative Care (NCP), *Clinical Practice Guidelines,* Domain 4: Social Aspects acknowledges the importance of SDOH as an essential element to individualized care. It states that "social determinants of health, hereafter encompassed in the term 'social factors,' have a strong and sometimes overriding influence on patients with a serious illness. Palliative care addresses environmental and social factors that affect patient and family functioning and quality of life."[10 (p. 26)]

Patient advocacy is a core tenet of palliative advanced practice nursing. Palliative APRNs must be prepared to promote patient engagement, protect individual autonomy, and champion social justice.[8] This can be performed at the individual, organizational, community, and national levels. Although the systematic challenges may seem insurmountable, the palliative APRN can impart practical interventions that can have a dramatic impact on patient access and well-being. It is vital to utilize and lean on the strengths of the IDT and local organizations to facilitate the identification of care gaps and the resources that may be utilized to address them.[9] Within the public health arena, palliative APRNs have opportunities to participate within their organizations as well as within local and national legislative bodies to promote awareness and social equity.

ASSESSMENT

Traditional clinical assessments do not accurately identify patients with complex social and structural needs. As a palliative APRN, it is important to delve deeper into a patient's history to determine barriers and opportunities to improve healthcare access. This includes assessing environmental aspects of care, financial aspects of care, and community aspects of care (see Table 20.1). The National Hospice and

Table 20.1 SOCIAL DETERMINANT OF HEALTH ASSESSMENT

SOCIAL DETERMINANT DOMAIN	ASSESSMENT QUESTION

Economic stability	• How much of financial hardship is your illness for you or your family?[13]
	• Are you able to pay for your medical care and medicine?
	• Are you receiving any government or financial assistance?
	• What is your current work situation?
	• Do you have money to pay your rent or get food?
	• Do you run out of money by the end of the month?
	• Have you or any of your family members been unable to get any of the following when it was needed in the past year?
	  • Food
	  • Clothing
	  • Utilities
	  • Childcare
	  • Medications or any healthcare services
	  • Phone

Education	• What is the best way to share health information with you? • How far did you go in school? Did you graduate? • Is English your first language? In what language would you prefer to receive your medical information?
Social and community context	• Do you have friends or family who can help you if you need it? • Do you have people with whom you can talk and feel supported? • Do you feel safe in your current living situation? • Have you ever felt discrimination has impacted your care? • Have you ever been arrested or incarcerated? • Are you exposed to illegal drug use or violence? • Are you a veteran?
Health and healthcare	• How much trouble do you have getting the medical care you need? • Where do you go for your medical care? • Do you have a primary care provider, and how often do you see them? • Do you have adequate medical insurance? • How do you get to your medical appointments? How reliable is your transportation? • Are there any situations that make it difficult to access healthcare?
Neighborhood and built environment	• Where do you live and with whom? • Is it a safe place to sleep and store your possessions? • Are you worried about losing your housing? • Do you have a safe place to spend your time? • Do you have access to transportation? • Do you have access to telephone services? • Do you have access to emergency services?
Food insecurity	• Do you have access to food storage? • Do you have access to cold food and safe food storage? • Do you have access to food banks? • Over the past 12 months, how often were you worried whether the food would run out before you had money to buy more? Or how often did the food not last and you didn't have money to get more?[14–15]

From Centers for Disease Control and Prevention [2]; Artiga S and Hinton E [3]; and Grindrod.[5]

Palliative Care Organization challenges clinicians to maintain awareness surrounding social constraints and the degree to which a patient's circumstances directly impact their health outcomes.[10] Deficits in any of these areas may contribute to the concept of total pain and suffering, whereby lack of recognition about the significance of these attributes can directly impact the patient's well-being. If a patient cannot satisfy the prerequisites for care, medical access and adherence will decline accordingly.[11–12]

Although there has been a considerable focus on SDOH at the national and global scales, there is limited research surrounding hospice and palliative care implications. There are several resources that define the importance of identifying patient SDOH and structural vulnerability to promote health outcomes, but valid and reliable clinical tools are lacking. Table 20.1 depicts a consolidation of assessment questions the APRN can utilize to facilitate identification of essential structural variables such as poverty, food insecurity, literacy, safety, and legal status. Universal screening is not recommended because it may activate an inappropriate social prescribing pathway and negatively impact the patient–provider relationship. The general guidance is to seek clarity if a patient is exhibiting clinical concerns indicative of social constraint and inquire based on the individual context.[13] Some questions may elicit responses from several of the overarching domains.

The palliative APRN needs to approach these sensitive topics in a caring, tactful, and culturally acceptable way to promote candid conversations and build rapport with the patient. The development of a trusting therapeutic alliance is essential to this practice because historically marginalized populations may be skeptical of the medical system at large. The APRN must also acknowledge, manage, and mitigate their inherent beliefs, which may contribute to the broader context of implicit bias and structural vulnerabilities. Once this information is obtained, it should be well-documented within the patient record to facilitate communication across care teams and facilitate comprehensive care planning in which social constructs are fully considered.[16]

PALLIATIVE CARE INTERVENTIONS

When a social need has been identified, connection to appropriate referral sources is paramount. If working within a robust organizational setting, leveraging the strengths and resources of the IDT is crucial. The NCP *Clinical Practice Guidelines* state that the palliative care IDT partners with the patient and family to identify and support their strengths and address areas of need (Box 20.1). Social workers are well-poised to assess complex psychosocial needs, provide emotional support, and connect patients to institutional and community resources. Institutions that recognize the importance of social equality have successfully implemented the role of community resource specialists who are knowledgeable about local and national assistance programs for financial, transportation, caregiver, food, housing, and legal needs. Community health workers function similarly, with the added benefit of case management to assist patients in navigating the health system.[11] Staff registered nurses (RNs) are invaluable for patient education, care coordination, and more frequent nurse–patient encounters to monitor the patient's health status. Chaplains can assist the APRN in assessing the spiritual, cultural, and religious SDOH and in connecting patients and families with their faith community.

PALLIATIVE INTERVENTIONS

It can be challenging for clinicians to broach structural vulnerabilities and, this is understandable given the issue's complexity and depth. The hospice and palliative APRN's skill set, rooted in high-quality communication, allows for adaptability and interpretation of complex medical terminology in an understandable way. Patients with low health literacy or language barriers are well-served when information-sharing is adapted to suit their needs. Patient handouts should be simple, clear, concise, and in the patient's preferred language.

Consideration should be given to using words or pictures depending on the patient's literacy. Utilization of interpreter services ensures that medical terminology is conveyed and provides patients the opportunity to share their health concerns with the APRN. Visual aids, easy-to-understand instructions, and verbal teachback methods are helpful. They foster education and afford the clinician an opportunity to clarify information as necessary. Navigating patients through the healthcare system through simplification of treatment regimens and alignment of medical appointments across specialties are additional ways in which an APRN can bridge the gap of social inequity (see Box 20.2).

There are several considerations for patients with financial and transportation concerns. Cost of medications and medical supplies, copays, and transportation arrangements must be considered when developing a patient-centered plan of care. Coordination with the patient's specialty and primary care provider to align visits can reduce the logistical burden and cost associated with frequent medical appointments. If appropriate and accessible by the patient, transition to intermittent telemedicine communication may also offset some stressors and allow for continued safety through remote monitoring. If financial concerns are a barrier to medication adherence, it is equally important to account for this when deciding on a treatment plan and avoid cost-prohibitive therapies.[11]

PALLIATIVE CARE TEAM INTERVENTIONS

Palliative APRNs can work with their teams to promote more education on social determinants of care. This will necessitate some difficult conversations about health inequities. One important step is for the team to do some reflection on individual and team implicit biases and consider more culturally sensitive treatment planning. Then they can perform outreach within the community.[17] This includes more education about the communities that the team is serving. The team also needs to be mindful of communities not being served (e.g., individuals with dual diagnoses such as serious illness and substance use disorders or serious mental illness). An assessment of these communities will need to consider the resources and collaborations necessary to include those populations.

SUMMARY

It is imperative that palliative APRNs understand the impact of structural vulnerabilities on their patients' well-being and global health outcomes. Awareness of health inequities should allow the provider to identify social needs and connect patients to appropriate resources within the team, organization, and community. Although rectifying the social determinants for a patient may seem insurmountable, palliative APRNs are empowered to provide tailored interventions to mitigate healthcare barriers within their own practice. They can work with their teams to ensure access to quality palliative care and reduce health disparities caused by social determinants of care.

Box 20.1 NATIONAL CONSENSUS PROJECT DOMAIN 4 SOCIAL ASPECTS OF CARE

Domain 4: Social Aspects of Care

Social determinants of health, hereafter encompassed in the term "social factors," have a strong and sometimes overriding influence on patients with a serious illness. Palliative care addresses environmental and social factors that affect patient and family functioning and quality of life. The palliative care interdisciplinary team (IDT) partners with the patient and family to identify and support their strengths and to address areas of need. The IDT includes a social worker to maximize patient functional capacity and achieve patient and family goals.

GUIDELINE 4.1 GLOBAL

The palliative care IDT has the skills and resources to identify and address, either directly or in collaboration with other service providers, the social factors that affect patient and family quality of life and well-being.

CRITERIA

4.1.1 The palliative care IDT includes a social worker with expertise and experience in:

  a. Assessing and supporting emotional aspects of care and improving quality of life (see Domain 3: Psychological and Psychiatric Aspects of Care)

  b. Identifying and addressing social consequences of a serious illness

  c. Collaborating with community-based services and supports and the organizations providing them

  d. Applying care management and care coordination techniques and evidence-based models of care transitions

  e. Working as part of an interdisciplinary team

  f. Utilizing patient- and family-centered and developmentally appropriate approaches to assessment, care planning, care management, and care delivery

4.1.2 All members of the IDT understand the impact of social factors on seriously ill patients and family members. The IDT:

  a. Is aware of the implications on care when patients are uninsured, under-insured, undocumented, homeless, or under the custody of the county or state

  b. Is cognizant of the financial impact of serious illness, including the cost of medications and other treatment, as well as the costs to the family

  c. Provides, directly or through referral, access to follow-up appointments, treatments, medications, nutrition, and other resources, as indicated in the plan of care

GUIDELINE 4.2 SCREENING AND ASSESSMENT

The IDT screens for and assesses patient and family social supports, social relationships, resources, and care environment based on the best available evidence to maximize coping and quality of life.

CRITERIA

4.2.1 Before involving family or caregivers, the patient or legal decision-maker identifies who can participate in the assessment and care planning process, as well as their level of involvement.

4.2.2 The IDT performs developmentally and culturally sensitive screening and assessment in the setting in which the patient receives care.

4.2.3 The social assessment includes:

  a. Family structure and function, including roles, quality of relationships, communication, and decision-making preferences and patterns, as well as an assessment of those involved if the patient is in the custody of the county or state

  b. Patient and family strengths, resiliency, social and cultural support, and spirituality

c. The availability and ability of a support system to provide respite, assist with errands and chores, and guard against social vulnerability

d. The effect of illness or injury on intimacy and sexual expression, prior experiences with illness, disability and loss, risk of abuse, neglect or exploitation, incarceration, or risk of social isolation

e. Functional limitations that impact activities of daily living (ADLs), instrumental activities of daily living (IADLs), and cognition

f. Changes in patient or family members' school enrollment, employment or vocational roles, recreational activities, and economic security

g. Identification and documentation if the adult patient or a family member served in the military, and whether the patient or family member may be eligible for VA benefits

h. Living arrangements and perceived impact of the living environment on patient and family quality of life, including safety issues

i. Patient and family perceptions about caregiving needs, including caregiver availability and capacity

j. The need for adaptive equipment, home modifications, or transportation.

k. Financial vulnerability (e.g., ability to pay rent or mortgage and other bills).

l. Ability to access prescription and over-the-counter medications for any reason, including functional or financial issues

m. Nutritional needs and food insecurity

n. Advance care planning and legal concerns (see Domain 8: Ethical and Legal Aspects of Care)

o. Patient and caregiver ability to read and understand information from health and social service providers, insurance companies, and the IDT, as well as the ability of the patient and family to ask questions and advocate for their needs

p. The ability of the patient and/or family to adhere to medication or treatment regimens

q. Patient and family willingness and ability to engage or accept resources and referrals.

4.2.4 A separate assessment of the family's needs, resources, resiliency, and capacity to provide care is also conducted.

GUIDELINE 4.3 TREATMENT

In partnership with the patient, family, and other providers, the IDT develops a care plan for social services and supports in alignment with the patient's condition, goals, social environment, culture, and setting to maximize patient and family coping and quality of life across all care settings.

CRITERIA

4.3.1 The IDT engages the patient and family in developing a care plan that addresses the social needs and is in alignment with their goals. The care plan:

a. Reflects patient and family culture, values, strengths, goals, and preferences, which may change over time

b. Assesses factors that prevent the patient from remaining independent and connected with family and friends

c. Specifies the role and contributions of family members and the types and sources of support that will be provided to the family

d. Identifies community service providers and the type and amount of care they will provide

e. Includes developmentally appropriate support for the patient and family, including children and adolescents

f. Identifies outcomes specific to each goal

4.3.2 The IDT coordinates care with care manager(s) and care team(s) to address patient- and family-identified social needs, providing referrals to resources and services as needed.

From National Consensus Project for Quality Palliative Care.[10]

Box 20.2 SOCIAL DETERMINANTS OF HEALTH RESOURCES

Agency for Healthcare Research and Quality: Compilation of research and practice improvement projects as well as links to governmental programs that address SDOH.[18]
https://www.ahrq.gov/sdoh/resources.html

CLEAR toolkit: Clinical decision aid developed to help physicians, nurses, and other health workers assess different aspects of patient vulnerability in a contextually appropriate and caring way and easily identify key referral resources in their local area. Available in multiple languages.[19]
https://Mcgill.ca/clear/

The EveryONE Project: Social determinants of health guide to social needs screening.[20]
https://www.aafp.org/family-physician/patient-care/the-everyone-project.html

Provider Training: Addressing Social Determinants of Health: Beyond the Clinic Walls. Sponsored by the American Medical Association.[21]
https://edhub.ama-assn.org/steps-forward/module/2702762?token=a8ab0a54-c1af-4797-af22-8ae2d9111849

Find Help: Search tool connection patients with a social care network of nonprofit organizations and verified social care providers in their area.[22]
https://findhelp.org

REFERENCES

1. Bourgois P, Holmes SM, Sue K, Quesada J. Structural vulnerability: Operationalizing the concept to address health disparities in clinical care. *Acad Med.* 2017;92(3):299–307. doi:10.1097/ACM.0000000000001294

2. Centers for Disease Control and Prevention. Social determinants of health: Know what affects health. About Social Determinants of Health. March 10, 2021. https://www.cdc.gov/socialdeterminants/about.html

3. Artiga S, Hinton E. Beyond health care: The role of social determinants in promoting health and health equity. Issue Brief. Kaiser Family Foundation May, 10, 2018. https://www.kff.org/racial-equity-and-health-policy/issue-brief/beyond-health-care-the-role-of-social-determinants-in-promoting-health-and-health-equity/

4. FitzGerald C, Hurst S. Implicit bias in healthcare professionals: A systematic review. *BMC Med Ethics.* 2017;18(1):19. doi:10.1186/s12910-017-0179-8

5. Grindrod A. Choice depends on options: A public health framework incorporating the social determinants of dying to create options at end of life. *Prog Palliat Care.* 2020;28(2):94–100. doi:10.1080/09699260.2019.1705539

6. Stajduhar KI, Mollison A, Giesbrecht M, et al. "Just too busy living in the moment and surviving": Barriers to accessing health care for structurally vulnerable populations at end-of-life. *BMC Palliat Care.* 2019;18(1):11. doi:10.1186/s12904-019-0396-7

7. Asare M, Flannery M, Kamen C. Social determinants of health: A framework for studying cancer health disparities and minority participation in research. *Oncol Nurs Forum.* 2017;44(1):20–23. doi:10.1188/17.ONF.20-23

8. De Chesnay M, Anderson BA, eds. *Caring for the Vulnerable: Perspectives in Nursing Theory, Practice, and Research.* 4th ed. Burlington, MA: Jones and Bartlett Learning; 2016.

9. McHugh M, Arnold J, Buschman P. Nurses leading the response to the crisis of palliative care for vulnerable populations. *Nurs Econ.* 2012;30(3):140–147.

10. National Consensus Project for Quality Palliative Care. *Clinical Practice Guidelines for Quality Palliative Care.* 4th ed. Richmond, VA: National Coalition for Hospice and Palliative Care; 2018. https://www.nationalcoalitionhpc.org/ncp/

11. Frier A, Devine S, Barnett F, Dunning T. Utilising clinical settings to identify and respond to the social determinants of health of individuals with type 2 diabetes: A review of the literature. *Health Soc Care Community.* 2020;28(4):1119–1133. doi:10.1111/hsc.12932

12. Ruiz-Pérez I, Rodríguez-Gómez M, Pastor-Moreno G, Escribá-Agüir V, Petrova D. Effectiveness of interventions to improve cancer treatment and follow-up care in socially disadvantaged groups. *Psychooncology.* 2019;28(4):665–674. doi:10.1002/pon.5011

13. Andermann A. Taking action on the social determinants of health in clinical practice: A framework for health professionals. *CMAJ.* 2016;188(17–18):E474–E483. doi:10.1503/cmaj.160177

14. Scandrett KG, Reitschuler-Cross EB, Nelson L, et al. Feasibility and effectiveness of the nest13 + as a screening tool for advanced illness care needs. *J Palliat Med.* 2009;13(2):161–169. doi:10.1089/jpm.2009.0170

15. Pooler JA, Hartline-Grafton H, DeBor M, Sudore RL, Seligman HK. Food insecurity: A key social determinant of health for older adults. *J Am Geriatr Soc.* 2019;67(3):421–424. doi:10.1111/jgs.15736

16. Berkowitz SA, Hulberg AC, Placzek H, et al. Mechanisms associated with clinical improvement in interventions that address health-related social needs: A mixed-methods analysis. *Popul Health Manag.* 2019;22(5):399–405. doi:10.1089/pop.2018.0162

17. Sinclair S, Chambers B. Using palliative care to support equitable care in the midst of covid-19. Center to Advance Palliative Care Blog. Updated June 15, 2020. https://www.capc.org/blog/using-palliative-care-support-equitable-care-midst-covid-19/

18. U.S. Department of Health and Human Services. Agency for Healthcare and Research Quality. SDOH resources. Page last reviewed January 2021. Available at https://www.ahrq.gov/sdoh/resources.html

19. McGill University. Department of Family Medicine. Clear collaboration project. 2021. Health workers address the social causes of poor health. Available at https://Mcgill.ca/clear/

20. American Academy of Family Physicians. The Everyone Project™. 2020. https://www.aafp.org/family-physician/patient-care/the-everyone-project.html

21. American Medical Association. Steps forward. Addressing social determinants of health (SDOH): Beyond the clinic walls. August 30, 2018. https://edhub.ama-assn.org/steps-forward/module/2702762?token=a8ab0a54-c1af-4797-af22-8ae2d9111849

22. Findhelp.org. Powered by Aunt Bertha. 2021. https://www.findhelp.org/?ref=ab_redirect

21.

ECONOMICALLY DISADVANTAGED URBAN DWELLERS

Natasha Curry

KEY POINTS

- Economically disadvantaged persons living with serious illness are ethnically, culturally, and linguistically diverse, with differing resources and unique challenges.

- By practicing cultural humility, the advanced practice registered nurse (APRN) is better able to understand the impact of serious illness on those who are economically disadvantaged and gain an appreciation of their worldviews.

- Collaboration with community health, social services, housing, substance use treatment services, mental health services, and, at times, the legal system, is vital if APRNs are to truly meet the palliative care needs of the economically disadvantaged population.

CASE STUDY: CARE FOR INDIVIDUALS EXPERIENCING HOMELESSNESS

Danny was born in 1967 to an African American single mother in Oakland, California. His mother, Grace, had seven other children when Danny was born, all under the age of 10 with four different fathers, two of whom were incarcerated at the time and two of whom had "disappeared." Grace received no form of child support for any of her children.

She loved her children, but caring for eight children in the increasingly expensive Bay Area was very difficult for Grace. She often turned to alcohol to help numb the pain and help her relax. Although they were all crammed into a two-bedroom apartment, Grace felt so fortunate that she had this stable, rent-controlled housing. Then, when Danny was 11 their elderly landlord died and his son decided to sell the property; the family became homeless. Danny and three of his siblings entered the foster care system, and Grace moved away. Danny never saw or heard from her again. Danny lived in more than seven different foster homes. Some families he liked, some he thought were only in it for the money and treated him like an annoyance.

As the years passed, Danny dropped out of school, left the foster care system to fend for himself, and fathered his first child when he was 17. He did not establish a relationship with the mother and would go on to have four other children with different women. Danny spent some years in and out of prison, held a number of minimum wage jobs in Oakland, and reunited with his father in his mid-30s. He would say, he was mostly "running the streets with the others."

In his mid-40s Danny met Marcia, 15 years his junior, and for the first time he felt this was a woman he could trust. They had three children together, close in age. Danny took a job unloading fruits and vegetables for an organic delivery service while Marcia stayed in their small studio apartment in San Francisco's Tenderloin district with the children. Danny said it felt as though his life was stabilizing. He was dreaming of returning to night school to get his GED; he wanted to teach, a dream he had held onto for many years. Save for an assault in 2017, which resulted in a fractured arm and leg, both of which required surgery, Danny had no health issues.

At the end of 2018, Danny found himself incarcerated again for a minor drug charge. Marcia and the three young boys lost their housing because there was no income coming in. They moved in with friends in the North Bay area, occasionally sleeping in their car or on friends' couches. At the beginning of 2019, while still in prison, Danny noticed he was losing weight. He felt as though something was stuck in his throat, struggling to swallow, and he thought his voice was starting to sound odd, as if he "was a frog." He went to the medical service, where he was given a rapid strep test and was told there was nothing wrong.

When he was released in March 2019, he started working under the table, the only job available to a felon, to send money to his kids. He moved in with his dad in San Francisco, sleeping on the couch. He still couldn't swallow well and was mostly just drinking Mountain Dew to give him the energy to get through the day. Danny was losing weight rapidly. He knew it was time to see a medical provider again. His job obviously offered no benefits, so he had no commercial health insurance. However, he was able to make an appointment with a primary care nurse practitioner (NP) at an urban health clinic in San Francisco. It took 6 weeks until he could be seen, so he waited, increasingly unable to eat or drink much without pain or vomiting.

His primary care nurse practitioner (NP) was appropriately concerned and sent Danny to the otolaryngology team at the local safety net hospital for expedited evaluation and workup. The clinic squeezed him in in 10 weeks, the earliest available appointment. A computed tomography (CT) scan and fine needle aspiration (FNA) showed what his providers had feared: supraglottic squamous cell carcinoma, at least a Stage III. With only local advancement, oncology was going for a cure with total laryngectomy, likely to be followed by concurrent radiation and chemotherapy. To get him nutrition, an order was placed for a feeding tube, and Danny was scheduled for a full mouth dental extraction to get ready for radiation. Danny had gold grills—a type of dental jewelry worn over the teeth—and he loved his grills. To Danny, his grills symbolized his enduring love for hip hop music, and, because they had cost him over a thousand dollars, they were also a symbol of the wealth he hoped to achieve for himself and his sons. He fought long and hard with his doctors to keep his teeth; he lost, and his teeth were removed.

Danny had been staying with his father to satisfy his parole expectations and taking public transport to spend time with his kids. There was no room for the entire family to stay with Danny's father. Marcia and the boys were now sleeping in the car every night. The kids were not enrolled in school because they kept getting moved on by the police, which meant Marcia had no way of knowing where they would spend the night.

Danny hated being in the hospital, not knowing where his kids were. He would spend hours on the hospital telephone trying to track his family down. He threatened on more than one occasion to go AMA because he couldn't locate them. At the end of May 2019, Danny had his surgery. He woke up in the ICU with a trach, no vocal cords, and a feeding tube. What's more, pathology showed positive margins; Danny was going to need radiation and chemotherapy.

With a long history of methamphetamine and alcohol use, most providers in the hospital were leery of giving him opioids. The palliative advanced practice registered nurse (APRN) was consulted, and the terror in Danny's eyes filled the room. This was someone who needed more opioids because of his substance use history, not fewer. At the APRN's suggestion, Danny was started on patient-controlled analgesia (PCA) and finally got some relief.

Two weeks later, Danny came to the palliative APRN's outpatient clinic. He still had the laryngeal tube and the percutaneous endoscopic gastrostomy (PEG), and in his hand he had a burger, fries, and milkshake. Danny pulled up the trash can, chewed then spat his burger and milkshake into it. Danny found himself back in the OR for an esophageal dilation. This was getting too much for him. Danny missed all of his follow-up appointments with oncology and was never started on treatment for the residual cancer. Calls to his phone either went straight to voice mail if he had been able to pay for his phone that month or went nowhere.

In February 2020, Danny passed out in the bathroom of a local grocery store. There was blood on the floor, and he showed signs of an infected groin abscess where he had been injecting methamphetamine. His PEG tube was also infected, and his trach ties were filthy. He was brought back into the hospital.

Danny's cancer had progressed and was now incurable. Radiation and chemotherapy could offer some relief and extra time, but he had missed the window for complete remission. The palliative APRN sat with Danny. His only way of communication was writing, and this took time. He became frustrated whenever anyone tried to hurry him along, and especially when people tried to finish his sentences for him. He told her how tired he was, how he just wanted to "end it all," but felt he needed to stay strong for his kids. He expressed his frustration at having lost his voice, and his sadness at being told he had less than a year to live. But he was going to make it to all his treatments this time; he had to, for his kids.

Then, in March 2020, everything was put on hold when the coronavirus hit his city. In-person clinic appointments were cancelled—all visits were now to be either telephone or video visits, challenging for someone with no vocal cords. Danny's kids were to be schooled from home, Marcia lost her job, and the bus service was slashed, making it almost impossible for Danny to get to his daily radiation and weekly chemo treatments. Danny began missing treatments. The palliative APRN tried obtaining taxi vouchers, but these were now in short supply. One day in April, at 4 AM, Marcia left a message for the APRN: "I think Danny just died."

INTRODUCTION

In 2018, the official poverty rate in the United States stood at 11.8%, or 38.1 million people.[1] For a family of four in 2020, poverty is determined to be an income of less than $26,200, and less than $12,760 for an individual.[2] While these data showed the fourth consecutive annual decline, it was an unevenly shared experience. Some groups continue to face much higher levels of economic hardship, particularly Black and Hispanic populations, those with the lowest levels of education, and among individuals and families living in neighborhoods of concentrated poverty. The poverty rate for non-Hispanic Whites was 8.1% in 2018, with 15.7 million individuals in poverty; for Blacks in the same year, it was 20.8%, representing 8.9 million people; for the Latinx community it was 17.6%, representing 10.5 million. In addition, while the median income in 2018 for White households was at $66,943, it was just $43,161 for Black households.

Of the 31.1 million people living in poverty, more than 50%, or 15.3 million live in cities.[3] There are many studies that show how poverty can lead to adverse health outcomes, both by increasing illness burden (morbidity) and leading to premature death.[4,5] A seminal public health paper published in 2011 found that deaths attributable to social factors such as lack of education, racial segregation, limited social support, individual-level poverty, and area-level poverty were comparable to the number attributed to pathophysiological and behavioral causes.[6] Basically, the economically disadvantaged are more likely to get sick, become seriously sick, and die younger. Clearly the urban poor are a population in need of the interdisciplinary approach offered by palliative care; however, low-income communities have traditionally underutilized palliative care services.[7]

Figure 21.1 shows just some of the factors associated with decreased survival in poor and medically underserved communities. Recent social and environmental factors that support health and longevity have been shown to have biological correlates that may ultimately provide a mechanistic understanding of the ways in which psychological stress associated with poverty, racial discrimination, and other social ills influence excessive mortality.

Barriers to palliative care for the urban poor are multifactorial: lack of health insurance, mistrust of the healthcare system, comorbid mental illness, drug and/or alcohol dependence, lack of transportation, competing demands of finding

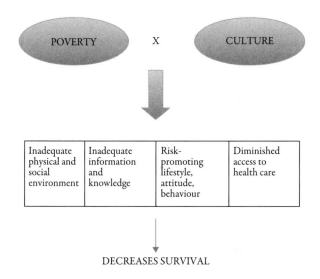

Figure 21.1 Medical neglect syndrome.
Reprinted with permission from David Wendell Moller, *Dying at the Margins*. New York: Oxford University Press; 2018: 65.[8]

food and shelter, and insufficient social support.[8,9] Other issues include availability, accessibility, and affordability.

1. *Availability*: One-third of US hospitals with 50 or more beds have no palliative care services, and, in the states reporting the greatest poverty (Alabama, Mississippi, New Mexico), fewer than 40% of the hospitals have palliative care teams. Nationwide, only 60% of public hospitals, often the only option for the urban poor, have palliative care programs, a number that has remained unchanged for the past 4 years.[10]

2. *Accessibility*: Most outpatient palliative care is provided at home, not in a clinic. Although many patients at comprehensive cancer centers have access to outpatient palliative care, access outside of these academic centers is very limited.[11] For the urban poor, "home" may be on the streets, may vary from week to week, or may be so run down and shabby that they do not want professionals visiting. And, if they are lucky enough to find a palliative care provider to order something to help with the metastatic cancer, it is a strong possibility that the pharmacy in the low-income neighborhood has chosen not to stock opioids out of concern that this will make them targets for theft.[8]

3. *Acceptability*: Is it any surprise that people who have endured deprivation all their lives would be suspicious of a medical team that does not revolve around life-saving and life-prolonging treatments?[8] As stated by David Wendell Moller in *Dying at the Margins*, "Victimized by structural racism, poverty and discrimination, they are wary of mainstream institutions and how they represent the interests of a status quo that has been unhelpful to them throughout life."[8 (p. 39)]

4. *Affordability*: The current fragmentation of health care can result in multiple outpatient visits, each of which often requires money for transportation. Just getting to the clinic or hospital for care is an especially difficult

challenge for the urban poor. For individuals with serious illness or who are dying, the obstacles are even more formidable.

As a result of these barriers, providing palliative care to the economically disenfranchised requires the palliative advanced practice registered nurse (APRN) to wear many hats: clinician, advocate, educator, therapist, care coordinator, social worker, and researcher.

The stereotype of the urban poor is a mentally ill, substance-using person, often male, who is living on the streets or in a single-room occupancy hotel. However, as with many stereotypes, this is not an accurate picture. They may have housing, although not in a place that many would think of as a "home." Cowboy, the charming character featured Moller's seminal work *Dancing with Broken Bones*, has lived under a bridge in a Midwestern city for decades and adamantly denies being homeless.[12] Some are working poor who may be undocumented or otherwise living on the margins of society. An increasing number of urban poor are single mothers.[2]

Danny's story introduces several issues that are common in the care of urban poor: the role of safety net hospitals and community health systems in care delivery, the frequency with which patients are often "lost to follow-up," the skills needed to manage pain in those with a substance use disorder, and the need to be an advocate for the patient living within the chaos, stress, and indignity of inner-city poverty.

A growing body of literature identifies the challenges of providing palliative care to the urban poor, such as illness-related issues, resource limitations, healthcare system interactions, and end-of-life preferences (see Table 21.1).

PRIMARY CARE FOR THE ECONOMICALLY DISADVANTAGED

Community health centers play a critical role in providing comprehensive primary healthcare services, chronic illness management, cancer screening, and other healthcare maintenance for underserved and vulnerable populations. But if the location of the clinic is inconvenient and its hours are not conducive to work schedules, the urban poor may have difficulty even getting there. Taking time off from work to obtain medical care is a problem for someone who does not have a car, does not have sick leave, is paid on an hourly basis, has more than one job, and does not have coworkers to cover their workload. It is especially difficult if the person's income supports many other individuals. Lacking a medical home, many of the urban poor rely on the emergency department (ED), with its open-door access to medical care 24 hours a day, 365 days a year. A 2016 study of homeless patients who presented to the ED of a Bay Area hospital found that only 7.3% of visits resulted in hospitalization and that close to 50% of participants had made another ED visit in the past 6 months, significantly higher than the US age-matched population.[13]

Given these challenges, it is no surprise that Danny had no long-term relationship with a primary care provider. Sadly, with his initial presentation of oral symptoms while

Table 21.1 CHALLENGES OF PROVIDING PALLIATIVE CARE TO THE ECONOMICALLY DISADVANTAGED

Illness-related	Prevalence of concurrent mental illness and substance use disorder Lack of decision-making capacity Presentation with advanced disease Multiple comorbidities End-organ diseases altering pharmacodynamics
Resource challenges	Health literacy Language discordance with health care providers Family or friend caregiver availability Need for designated surrogate decision-maker in the event of loss of decision making Chaotic lives with little room for day-to-day illness demands Adverse childhood or adulthood events (trauma histories) Limited ongoing therapeutic relationships with health or social service providers Survival or addiction that overshadows illness management Competing role responsibilities Functional impairments, geographic distances, & transportation
Relationships with healthcare system or providers	Cultural history of racism, discrimination, or rejection in health care system As a result of disrespectful, rude, or dismissive interactions in past, patients may present as angry, avoidant, suspicious, or nonadherent with care recommendations Healthcare providers often have different cultural & ethnic backgrounds/worldviews
End-of-life preferences	Reluctance to relinquish aggressive medical management Different assumptions about optimal end-of-life care, particularly in communities of color Lack of advance care planning as life is survived moment to moment Tendency to equate goals of care modification with abandonment or continued poor care Spirituality may be a hidden resource for comfort and in guiding decision-making

Adapted from Dahlin et al.[14]

incarcerated, he was merely given a test for rapid strep then dismissed with no follow-up. More importantly, he had never participated in an advance care planning conversation with a trusted provider, nor had he been given the chance to nominate Marcia as his surrogate decision-maker.

Given that Danny presented with clinical "red flags" (weight loss and severe dysphagia), the clinic APRN in the neighborhood health center appropriately referred Danny to otolaryngology, where her suspicion of a malignancy was confirmed. Due to lack of resources in both community health and the safety net hospital, for an oncology treatment plan to be developed; a picture common across the United States. A 2018 report showed that the shortage of specialists working within the safety net can mean wait times of up to 8 months.[15]

By the time Danny met the palliative APRN, he had literally lost the ability to speak for himself. How does a palliative APRN meeting a patient for the first time provide information, support, and anticipatory guidance in this situation, particularly for a patient like Danny who lives on the margins of the dominant society? Very fortunately for Danny, this APRN was able to assess and understand his needs and advocate for him. She was able to get him pain medication when he needed it, after his surgical team had deemed him to be just another drug seeker. The APRN was able to get him the esophageal dilation when she discovered a postop stricture. The APRN was able to hold the space for him to explore, through writing, his fears, anxieties, and frustrations, and learn of his overarching love for his children above all. All this took time, and a clinician focused on hurrying through

the appointment to empty out the waiting room would have missed much of it.

The palliative APRN must complete a comprehensive social and cultural assessment while simultaneously being truly "present" for patients, listening to their story, attending to their immediate self-identified needs, and creating a therapeutic environment in which they feel valued, safe, and cared for as human beings. This is a population too often ignored by the biomedical healthcare model, a model that tends to miss the whole person while focusing on lab values and checklists.[8]

The National Consensus Project for Quality Palliative Care (NCP) *Clinical Practice Guidelines* outlines social and cultural assessment components relevant to the care of patients (Table 21.2).

ROLE OF SAFETY NET HOSPITALS AND PUBLIC HEALTH CARE SYSTEMS

In 2000, the Institute of Medicine defined *safety-net hospitals* (SNHs) as hospitals that, by mission or mandate, provide care to a substantial share of vulnerable patients regardless of their ability to pay.[16] In short, these hospitals care for patients and communities who would otherwise "fall through the cracks." Safety net providers serve vulnerable populations at risk for health disparities, such as communities of color, immigrants, and the uninsured or underinsured, and they play a critical role as training sites for physician trainees, undergraduate and graduate nursing students, and other allied health students. APRNs may be particularly drawn to practice in safety net

Table 21.2 SELECTED APRN ROLES AND BEHAVIORS IN CARING FOR THE URBAN POOR

ROLE	ADVANCED CORE BEHAVIORS
Advocacy and moral agency	Assesses the individual with serious illness with attention to populations at risk (e.g., older adults; children and youths; persons experiencing homelessness; persons of color; LGBTQ+ persons; persons experiencing substance abuse disorders; persons with serious mental illness; individuals without legal validation; individuals incarcerated in jails, prisons, and detention centers; persons with cognitive impairment, as well as developmental, intellectual, and physical disabilities) in an age-, cognitive-, and developmentally appropriate manner.
	Collaborates with the palliative interdisciplinary team, other health team professionals, and the public to protect human rights, promote health diplomacy, enhance cultural sensitivity and congruence, and reduce health disparities.
	Collaborates with other health professionals to ensure ethically sound organizational systems for access to and fair distribution of healthcare resources across all populations.
	Uses a systematic approach to ethical and legal review of clinical and palliative-related healthcare issues in collaboration with an ethics committee and legal counsel, particularly in the development of palliative-related policies and procedures, incorporating ethical principles (i.e., beneficence, autonomy, justice, nonmaleficence, veracity), and consulting ethics resources/services as appropriate.
Collaboration	Builds trusting and collaborative relationships with interdisciplinary team members, health colleagues of all disciplines, healthcare staff, and the community.
	Collaborates with community agencies to facilitate care in the setting preferred by the individual and family, when feasible, including both hospice and home care services provided in a variety of settings.
Systems thinking	Analyzes systems-level policies considering issues of access, quality and cost, and health disparities through the development and implementation of policies.
	Develops strategies of palliative care programs and systems to meet the needs of its communities, patient populations, and care locations, with particular attention to health, racial, and social disparities.
	Articulates the importance of population health principles and apply them to palliative care.
	Utilizes systematic methods to assess the palliative care needs of healthcare systems, healthcare organizations, individuals, and families.
Response to diversity	Practices with cultural awareness, sensitivity, and humility by performing self-examination of cultural beliefs and values and how they relate to healthcare and the environment in which one works.
	Identifies and responds to health disparities, social injustices and racism within palliative care and leads initiatives to mitigate them.
	Demonstrates ability to collect relevant cultural data related to the individual and family presenting health condition and unmet needs; accurately performs culturally specific assessment to deliver culturally competent interdisciplinary palliative care.
	Assesses, identifies, and addresses cultural, spiritual, and existential beliefs, behaviors, practices, needs, and concerns of individuals with serious illness and family members according to established protocols and documents in the interdisciplinary care plan.
	Accesses appropriate cultural, spiritual, and religious resources to deliver palliative care to individuals and families.
	Addresses conflicts that may arise between individuals, families, and healthcare providers resulting from differences in cultural and spiritual perspectives related to palliative care, and plans for effective strategies to allow for and accommodate those differences.
	Recognizes and educates others about diverse systems of belief and the role of diversity in the application of professional health provider obligations, including information on diagnosis; disclosure; decisional authority; care; and acceptance of decisions to continue, discontinue, or forgo treatments.

From Dahlin.[14,17]

---

systems, given their social justice mission of improving the health and well-being of marginalized or underserved communities. In fact, a commitment to social justice is written into the American Nurses Association *Code of Ethics for Nurses*: "All nurses, through organizations and accrediting bodies involved in nurse formation, education, and development, must firmly anchor students in nursing's professional responsibility to address unjust systems and structures, modeling the profession's commitment to social justice and health through content, clinical and field experiences, and critical thought."[18 (p. 36)]

In fiscal year 2018, safety net hospitals reported that more than half (54%) of their discharges were from racial/ethnic minorities and three-quarters of patients were uninsured or covered by Medicaid or Medicare. Safety net hospitals provided nonemergent outpatient care to 80 million patients in 2018, and treated more than 14 million in EDs. Inpatient admissions averaged 18,000 per hospital, nearly three times more than the inpatient volume of other hospitals.[19]

The enactment of the *Affordable Care Act* (ACA) in 2010 and implemented in 2014 led to historic gains in health insurance coverage by extending Medicaid coverage to many low-income individuals. The number of uninsured nonelderly Americans decreased from more than 46.5 million in 2010 to just below 27 million in 2016, a historic low.[20] However, since 2016, the number of uninsured has increased by half a million every year, and undocumented immigrants still remain ineligible for coverage. People of color are at higher risk of being uninsured than Whites; while they make up 43% of the nonelderly US population, they account for more than a half of uninsured population.[21]

While this expansion of newly covered Medicaid patients may appear on the surface to be a boon for safety net hospitals, early data have actually shown that non–safety net hospitals are now also attracting Medicaid patients. Although reimbursement rates are typically lower than treatment costs, because the majority of hospital costs are fixed and tend not to vary by patient volume, Medicaid admissions can contribute to overall hospital profitability.[20] The uninsured, however, will likely continue to receive the vast majority of their care from safety net hospitals.[19]

Safety net hospitals have generally been slower to initiate a palliative care service. The Center to Advance Palliative Care has found that far fewer public hospitals report palliative care services, compared to similarly sized not-for-profit hospitals.[10] However, nurses in safety net hospitals are increasingly receiving training from the End-of-Life Nursing Education Consortium for Public Hospitals (ELNEC-PH), launched in 2012.[22] Geography also plays a major role in the availability of palliative care for the poor. People living with a serious illness who reside in the northeastern United States have access to significantly more hospital palliative care programs than those living in other regions. However, these numbers continue to increase as safety net hospitals recognize the benefits of palliative care.

OVERCOMING LANGUAGE BARRIERS

The United States is linguistically and culturally diverse. The US Census Bureau's *American Community Survey of 2018* revealed that one in five of the population speaks a language other than English at home, and 8.3% of the US population speaks English "less than well," with numbers significantly higher in patients older than 65.[23] Certain states have disproportionately large numbers of persons with limited English proficiency, from 9% of total households in California to 0.9% in Maine.[23]

These numbers are expected to increase in the 2020 US Census Bureau survey, suggesting that healthcare professionals will care for an increasing number of patients with limited English proficiency. The overlap between English proficiency and poverty is striking. Of the 38 million living below the poverty level in 2018, close to 30% speak a language other than English at home.[23]

Discussing end-of-life wishes, goals of care, giving bad news, prognostication—these conversations, frequent in the palliative care setting, require clear, straight forward communication skills and can be challenging for all practitioners. Language barriers are known to contribute to worse healthcare quality and outcomes, with non–English speaking patients reporting lower satisfaction with care, often being vulnerable to inadequate pain assessment and management

and overall suffering from unnecessary physical emotional and spiritual suffering, particularly at the end of life.[24] The *1964 Civil Rights Act* required all hospitals to provide language services to patients with limited English proficiency.[25] This was reinforced in 2020, by Section 1557 of the ACA, which requires healthcare providers to provide patients with access to qualified interpreters. If a qualified interpreter is not provided, patients have the right to sue the provider for language access violations.[26] Given the complexity and emotional weight of the information being communicated in many palliative care encounters, modifications in meaning can still occur even when professional interpreters are used.

CASE STUDY: LANGUAGE BARRIERS

Mr. X and his family were meeting with his palliative APRN to review his latest imaging and lab results. He had been losing weight for some months, and he had some new back pain that just wouldn't go away, even if he took his pain medications. Recognizing that the patient and his family did not speak English well enough to properly understand his diagnosis, the APRN called the language line and put the Cantonese interpreter on speakerphone. She carefully explained that Mr. X has multiple myeloma and that he would be started on treatment by the oncology team. She waited while the interpreter explained, then sat silently to allow the family time to process what had just been said. The family looked confused. The teenage son spoke up, in English: "Does my dad have two cancers now? Did it spread to his skin?" After exploring with the son what had been said, it became evident that the interpreter had told the X family that he had a diagnosis of melanoma, not myeloma, two very different diagnoses and prognoses.

Indeed, the very term "palliative" does not translate smoothly into many other languages. Dr. Pan, writing on the Geriatrics and Palliative Care blog *Geripal* tells us that

> The Google translation of Palliative Care is "姑息治疗." Back translated, the meaning is essentially "*Do Nothing Care.*" Similarly, the Google translation of Hospice is "临终关怀," literally meaning "*Last Minute Care.*" Is it any wonder that patients whose goals are comfort oriented end up declining hospice and palliative care once they hear the translated words?[27]

Translations are not much better in Spanish. The Spanish-language page of the National Institute of Health translates hospice as *hospicio*, a term also used by many medical interpreters.[28] While the Spanish and English words have the same Latin root, *hospes*, in Spanish the word came to mean a place for the destitute.[29] As we discussed earlier, the Latinx community has lower use of hospice and palliative care services: Is it any a surprise, given the translation?[10] The Spanish phrase "cuidados paliativos" has no negative connotations, but it remains an unfamiliar term for many. A 2019 survey by the Center to Advance Palliative Care (CAPC) found that almost half of all adults in America have never heard of palliative care.[30]

Surveys of professional interpreters with extensive experience in end-of-life discussions have identified specific techniques to optimize providers' patient encounters.[31] Guidelines for optimizing communication with healthcare interpreters are summarized in Box 21.1. The California Health Care Foundation also offers comprehensive recommendations for working with interpreters, specifically in a palliative care setting.[32] These best practices emphasize direct communication with the interpreter and outline basic principles of interacting with interpreters, including structural and practical aspects of communication.

NEGOTIATING HOSPITALIZATION AND TREATMENT

Given the limited access to and availability of outpatient and community-based palliative care for the urban poor,[10] it is most likely that patients will encounter palliative APRNs in the acute care setting. The patient in the case study, Danny, might receive education from an oncology APRN about his cancer diagnosis, treatment side effects, and recovery trajectory; a palliative APRN might assist with symptom management

---

Box 21.1 GENERAL GUIDELINES FOR WORKING WITH HEALTHCARE INTERPRETERS

- Use a professional interpreter (in person or via technology), unless an emergency or not available due to rare language dialect.

- Always brief the interpreter beforehand about the goal of the meeting and the issues to be discussed to make sure they are culturally appropriate.

- Introduce the interpreter to the family, set expectations, and address confidentiality concerns.

- Make eye contact at and speak directly to the patient, not the interpreter.

- Use short sentences or phrases and let the interpreter translate those into smaller sentences. Break up lengthy explanations or responses into multiple shorter responses.

- Avoid using euphemisms, proverbs, or cultural references, as they can lead to confusion or may not carry similar meaning when interpreted.

- Check for patient/family understanding frequently, either directly (e.g., teachback technique) or indirectly (checking with interpreter if he or she perceives that patient is or is not understanding).

- When trying to get the attention of the interpreter, start your comment with "Interpreter" to make it easier for the interpreter to distinguish the person you are addressing.

From Schenker et al.[33]; and Association of American Medical Colleges.[34]

---

and clarification of goals of care; a wound care APRN might be consulted regarding ostomy teaching or complex surgical wound management; and a psychiatric mental health APRN might help Danny identify coping resources for managing his new diagnosis and to acknowledge the impact of past traumas in his life. Regardless of the particular APRN role, an understanding of the hospitalization experience for Danny and others who are economically disadvantaged will be necessary to appreciate their understanding of the illness and its treatment demands.

Like many economically disadvantaged persons with serious illness, Danny had a difficult life story. Born in poverty, he was then passed from foster home to foster home, eventually ending up on the streets. He was incarcerated countless times, usually for minor drug charges. It's worth noting that while African Americans and Whites use drugs at similar rates, the imprisonment rate of African Americans for drug charges is almost six times that of Whites. For many, release from prison compounds preexisting disadvantage because people have difficulty finding stable accommodation and employment, accessing health services, and reconnecting with families, social groups, and communities.

Furthermore, the risk of premature mortality for adults released from incarceration is substantially higher than in the general population.[35] A 2017 study on the impact of socioeconomic status (SES) on esophageal cancer—Danny's diagnosis—found that the 5-year survival of patients with low SES is significantly lower than in patients with high SES.[36] The same pattern is seen in patients with other malignancies.[37,38]

Moller describes how the illness narrative of so many urban poor is one of "disempowerment, neglect and fear."[8(p. 61)] This mirrors Danny's situation:

a) disempowered—Danny did not fully understand his prognosis or even treatment regimen; b) neglect—Danny had no transportation, his housing was unstable with his kids living in car; c) fear—fear of abandoning his kids, concerned that Marcia would leave him, fear of death.

Many patients cared for by safety net systems have been exposed to unimaginable life events prior to the diagnosis of a life-threatening illness, such as child abuse, intimate partner violence, homelessness, incarceration, sexual assault, wartime exposure, homicides and suicides of family and friends, and substance abuse. Epidemiological surveys show that more than 70% of men and 80% of women (aged 15–54 years) in the general population have experienced at least one psychological trauma in their lifetime.[39] While there are no official data specific to the urban poor, it is not difficult to imagine significantly higher numbers; their lives are often trauma-filled.[40] Add to this the inherent trauma to all palliative care patients—the threat to life itself—and it becomes clear that this is an area that needs to be addressed in all safety net palliative care patients.

There is a growing awareness of the physical, psychological, emotional, and existential toll trauma exposure has on individuals, communities, and even healthcare professionals themselves. A healthcare setting poses unique risk for distress given the complex, invasive, and repetitive nature of traumatic exposure in this environment: persistent questioning by unfamiliar faces, unexpected tests in the dark hours of the night, the need to wear a dehumanizing hospital gown, endless blood draws—and during the COVID-19 pandemic, no visitors. What's more, patient care may be compromised because patients struggling with trauma histories are more likely to be anxious, depressed, distrustful, and angry, as well as avoidant of trauma reminders, which may include medical settings and medical personnel.[41] What might this look like in clinical practice? For example, a patient with a history of rape may become combative and anxious, as well as depressed if they are not adequately prepared for a switch from oral medication to suppository-based medication.[41]

Recognizing this risk, mental health experts and organizations such as the Substance Abuse and Mental Health Services Association (SAMHSA) have developed a framework of *trauma-informed care* (TIC) to prevent and treat trauma responses. TIC recognizes and responds in meaningful ways to individuals who have experienced trauma and is based on the principles of safety, trustworthiness, collaboration, empowerment, and choice.[42] While this remains a relatively new model of care, it undoubtedly will shape palliative care and other services for the economically disadvantaged and other vulnerable populations at high risk for posttraumatic stress disorder, as well as the healthcare and social service professionals working with them.

Perhaps because of their difficult biographies, many persons with limited resources have a remarkable resiliency.[43] When one lives at the financial edge, where daily life is shaped by constant struggle, a cancer diagnosis is often just one more bad thing to happen this week. According to Moller: "Poor patients can often show remarkable equanimity when told they are dying, in large part because their life-long experiences have taught them to expect bad news."[8 (p. 6)]

Some of this resilience may be understood by spiritual and religious beliefs and practices that connect patients' experiences to something greater than their everyday existence. When looking at the populations most represented in the urban poor, 96% of African Americans say they believe in God and 75% say that God is "very important" in their life; in the Latinx community these numbers are 91% and 59%, respectively. Compare this with the White communities: 86% and 49%.[44]

Let's review Danny and his family: as an African American, previously incarcerated male with little formal education, he was able to raise his children in one of the most expensive rental areas in the United States. His children were always well-dressed when they accompanied him to his appointments and polite to a T. Despite having no transportation, Danny made it on time to almost all of his appointments; he always had scraps of paper in his pocket to write on after his laryngectomy, and he joked with his palliative APRN that he would "buy us both steaks when I'm better." The palliative APRN is pivotal in helping to draw on this resiliency within patients to help them face serious illness and navigate complex healthcare systems.

Beyond linguistic and cultural barriers, the urban poor face many difficulties in the healthcare system, including logistical and bureaucratic difficulties accessing care, insensitive or dismissive interactions with healthcare professionals and support staff, and delays in nursing and medical care that result in patients being made to feel less than human.[45] It is also well-documented that minority patients are more likely to receive inadequate pain treatment compared with White patients.[46] During the COVID-19 pandemic, many healthcare providers switched to telemedicine, a delivery method that has been gaining in popularity over the past decade. This in itself assumes technological literacy, equipment availability, income, a stable housing situation, and it means that many underserved populations are being excluded from this shift in healthcare delivery.[47]

APRN COMPETENCIES IN CARING FOR ECONOMICALLY DISADVANTAGED PERSONS

For palliative APRNs caring for those who are economically disadvantaged, the knowledge and skills (competencies) are in many ways similar to the competencies required when caring for other palliative care populations, but there are some important differences to keep in mind. The Hospice and Palliative Nurses Association's *Competencies for the Palliative and Hospice APRN* with particular relevance to the urban poor are noted in Box 21.2.

ADVOCACY AND ETHICS

Moller states, "To be poor does not mean that one needs to die poorly."[8] One of the most important tenets of all health and social service professionals is advocacy for patients, families, and communities. This holds particular salience for palliative APRNs working with vulnerable or marginalized populations. Good palliative care embraces cultural, ethnic, and faith differences and preferences while interweaving the principles of ethics, humanities, and human values into every patient- and family-care experience.[48] This is reflective of the American Nursing Association *Standards of Professional Performance* that name advocacy as the "pillar of nursing" and requires *culturally congruent practice*: "The registered nurse practices in a manner that is congruent with cultural diversity and inclusion principles."[49 (pp. 69–70)]

In March 2017, the American Nurses Association and Hospice and Palliative Nurses Association (HPNA) published *A Call to Action: Nurses Lead and Transform Palliative Care*. This seminal document called for the funding, development, and evaluation of innovative palliative care models to address "the needs of communities of color, underserved populations, and other vulnerable groups, such as Native Americans, persons with intellectual and developmental disabilities, and others in rural and urban areas."[50 (p. 4)] The palliative APRN is encouraged to lead and transform palliative care in practice, education, research, administration, and policy.

Box 21.2 NATIONAL CONSENSUS PROJECT: SOCIAL AND CULTURAL DOMAINS

Domain 4: Social Aspects of Care

GUIDELINE 4.2

Social determinants of health have a strong and sometimes overriding influence on patients with a serious illness. Palliative care addresses environmental and social factors that affect patient and family functioning and quality of life. The palliative care interdisciplinary team (IDT) partners with the patient and family to identify and support their strengths and to address areas of need.

CRITERIA [SELECTED]

- The interdisciplinary team (IDT) performs developmentally and culturally sensitive screening and assessment in the setting in which the patient receives care. This includes:

- Family structure and function, including roles, quality of relationships, communication, and decision-making preferences and patterns, as well as an assessment of those involved if the patient is in the custody of the county or state

- Patient and family strengths, resiliency, social and cultural support, and spirituality

- The availability and ability of a support system to provide respite, assist with errands and chores, and guard against social vulnerability

- The effect of illness or injury on intimacy and sexual expression, prior experiences with illness, disability and loss, risk of abuse, neglect or exploitation, incarceration, or risk of social isolation

- Functional limitations that impact activities of daily living (ADLs), instrumental activities of daily living (IADLs), and cognition

- Changes in patient or family members' school enrollment, employment or vocational roles, recreational activities, and economic security

- Living arrangements and perceived impact of the living environment on patient and family quality of life, including safety issues

- Patient and family perceptions about caregiving needs, including caregiver availability and capacity

- Financial vulnerability (e.g., ability to pay rent or mortgage and other bills)

- Ability to access prescription and over-the-counter medications for any reason, including functional or financial issues

- Nutritional needs and food insecurity

- Advance care planning and legal concerns

- Patient and caregiver ability to read and understand information from health and social service providers, insurance companies, and the IDT, as well as the ability of the patient and family to ask questions and advocate for their needs

- The ability of the patient and/or family to adhere to medication or treatment regimens

- Patient and family willingness and ability to engage or accept resources and referrals

Domain 6: Cultural Aspects of Care

GUIDELINE 6.1

The palliative care program serves each patient, family and community in a culturally and linguistically appropriate manner.

CRITERIA [SELECTED]

- The IDT delivers care that respects patient and family cultural beliefs, values, traditional practices, language, and communication preferences and builds upon the unique strengths of the patient and family. Members of the IDT works to increase awareness of their own biases and seeks opportunities to learn about the provision of culturally sensitive care. The care team ensures that its environment, policies, procedures, and practices are culturally respectful.

- IDT members recognize that the provision of quality palliative care requires an understanding of the patient's and family's culture and how it relates to their decision-making process, and their approach to illness, pain, psychological, social, and spiritual factors, grief, dying, death, and bereavement.

- The IDT understands that each person's self-identified culture includes the intersections of race, ethnicity, gender identity and expression, sexual orientation, immigration and refugee status, social class, religion, spirituality, physical appearance, and abilities.

- The IDT recognizes that patients and families may have experienced barriers to receiving culturally respectful health care, and that these prior experiences may result in mistrust of the healthcare system.

- The IDT commits to continuously practice cultural humility and celebrate diversity.

From National Consensus Project for Quality Palliative Care.[17]

And while one may be unable to fix the problems of poverty, it is incumbent on all palliative APRNs to improve the care of individual patients. Working with the urban poor requires creative, in-the-moment problem-solving to honor patients' preferences and goals. To effectively care for vulnerable populations, palliative APRNs must develop collaborative relationships with a wide range of social services and other safety net providers, and they need to have a good working knowledge of Medicaid, to avoid presenting plans that are not possible to achieve logistically.

Palliative APRNs must relearn how the art of caring can intersect with the science of treatment. One can see how poverty is a major risk for morbidity and mortality. However, the healthcare system too often looks past our more vulnerable patients, focusing on lab results and imaging rather than seeing them as a whole person. One needs to see beyond the biomedical model and take the time to really get to know our patients, listen to their stories, and provide culturally, socially, and linguistically appropriate treatment for the whole person.

SUMMARY

Caring for persons who are economically disadvantaged and in need of palliative care demands not only expert clinical acumen but also—and equally important—an appreciation of their community and their everyday lives. This chapter examines (1) palliative care across settings, (2) the role of safety net providers, (3) the challenges of communicating through an interpreter, and (4) the competencies needed by hospice and palliative APRNs who care for this special population.

REFERENCES

1. United States Census Bureau. Tables. Poverty status in the past 12 months. Last update for 2019. https://data.census.gov/cedsci/table?q=S17&d=ACS%201-Year%20Estimates%20Subject%20Tables&tid=ACSST1Y2018.S1701
2. Chaudry A, Wimer C, Macartney S, et al. Poverty in the United States: 50-Year trends and safety net impacts. 2016: 47. Washington, DC: Office of Human Services Policy Office of the Assistant Secretary for Planning and Evaluation US Department of Health and Human Services. https://aspe.hhs.gov/system/files/pdf/154286/50YearTrends.pdf
3. Semega J, Kollar M, Creamer J, Mohanty A. U.S. Census Bureau, Current Population Reports, P60-266(RV), Income and Poverty in the United States: 2018, Washington, DC: U.S. Government Printing Office, 2020. https://www.census.gov/library/visualizations/2019/demo/p60-266.html
4. Hughes A, McMunn A, Bartley M, Kumari M. Elevated inflammatory biomarkers during unemployment: Modification by age and country in the UK. *J Epidemiol Community Health*. 2015;69(7):673–679. doi:10.1136/jech-2014-204404
5. Fleisch Marcus A, Illescas AH, Hohl BC, Llanos AAM. Relationships between social isolation, neighborhood poverty, and cancer mortality in a population-based study of US adults. Buchowski M, ed. Plos One. 2017;12(3):e0173370. doi:10.1371/journal.pone.0173370
6. Galea S, Tracy M, Hoggatt KJ, DiMaggio C, Karpati A. Estimated deaths attributable to social factors in the United States. *Am J Public Health*. 2011;101(8):1456–1465. doi:10.2105/AJPH.2010.300086
7. Reimer-Kirkham S, Stajduhar K, Pauly B, et al. Death is a social justice issue: Perspectives on equity-informed palliative care. *Adv Nurs Sci*. 2016;39(4):293–307. doi:10.1097/ANS.0000000000000146
8. Wendell Moller D. *Dying at the Margins*. New York: Oxford University Press; 2018.
9. Klop HT, de Veer AJE, van Dongen SI, Francke AL, Rietjens JAC, Onwuteaka-Philipsen BD. Palliative care for homeless people: A systematic review of the concerns, care needs and preferences, and the barriers and facilitators for providing palliative care. *BMC Palliat Care*. 2018;17(1):67. doi:10.1186/s12904-018-0320-6
10. Morrison S, Meier D, Rogers M, Heitner R. Center to Advance Palliative Care and the National Palliative Care Research Center. America's care of serious illness: A state-by-state report card on access to palliative care in our nation's hospitals. New York: NY: CAPC. 2019. https://capc.org/report-card
11. Finlay E, Rabow MW, Buss MK. Filling the gap: Creating an outpatient palliative care program in your institution. *Am Soc Clin Oncol Educ Book*. 2018;(38):111–121. doi:10.1200/EDBK_200775
12. Wendell Moller D. *Dancing with Broken Bones: Portraits of Death and Dying Among Inner-City Poor*. New York: Oxford University Press; 2004.
13. Raven MC, Tieu L, Lee CT, Ponath C, Guzman D, Kushel M. Emergency department use in a cohort of older homeless adults: Results from the HOPE HOME Study. Kuehl D, ed. *Acad Emerg Med*. 2017;24(1):63–74. doi:10.1111/acem.13070
14. Dahlin C, ed. *Competencies for the Palliative and Hospice APRN, 3rd ed*. Pittsburgh, PA: Hospice and Palliative Nurses Association; 2021.
15. Ezeonwu MC. Specialty-care access for community health clinic patients: Processes and barriers. *J Multidiscip Healthc*. 2018;11:109–119. doi:10.2147/JMDH.S152594
16. Popescu I, Fingar KR, Cutler E, Guo J, Jiang HJ. Comparison of 3 safety-net hospital definitions and association with hospital characteristics. *JAMA Netw Open*. 2019;2(8):e198577. doi:10.1001/jamanetworkopen.2019.8577
17. National Consensus Project for Quality Palliative Care. *Clinical Practice Guidelines for Quality Palliative Care*. 4th ed. 2018. Richmond, VA: National Coalition for Hospice and Palliative Care. https://www.nationalcoalitionhpc.org/ncp/
18. American Nurses Association. *Code of Ethics for Nurses*. 2nd ed. Silver Spring, MD: Nursebooks.org; 2015.
19. America's Essential Hospitals. Essential data: Our hospitals, our patients. Results of America's Essential Hospitals 2018 annual member characteristics survey. Washington, DC: America's Essential Hospitals. May 2020. https://essentialhospitals.org/wp-content/uploads/2020/05/Essential-Data-2020_spreads.pdf
20. Wu VY, Fingar KR, Jiang HJ, et al. Early impact of the Affordable Care Act coverage expansion on safety-net hospital inpatient payer mix and market shares. *Health Serv Res*. 2018;53(5):3617–3639. doi:10.1111/1475-6773.12812
21. Tolbert J, Orgera K, Singer N, Damico A. Key facts about the uninsured population. Issue Brief. Appendix. Kaiser Family Foundation. November 6, 2020. https://www.kff.org/report-section/key-facts-about-the-uninsured-population-appendix/
22. Virani R, Malloy P, Dahlin C, Coyne P. Creating a fabric for palliative care in safety net hospitals: End-of-Life Nursing Education Consortium for public hospitals. *J Hosp Palliat Nurs*. 2014;16(5):312–319. doi:10.1097/NJH.0000000000000074
23. United States Census Bureau. Language spoken at home. Last updated for 2019. https://data.census.gov/cedsci/table?q=language&tid=ACSST1Y2018.S1601&hidePreview=false
24. Silva MD, Genoff M BS, Zaballa A BS, et al. Interpreting at the end of life: A systematic review of the impact of interpreters on the delivery of palliative care services to cancer patients with limited English proficiency. *J Pain Symptom Manage*. 2015;51(3):569–580. doi:10.1016/j.jpainsymman.2015.10.011
25. US Congress. *US Civil Rights Act in 88-352*. 1964. Washington, CD: Government Printing Office. https://www.govinfo.gov/content/pkg/STATUTE-78/pdf/STATUTE-78-Pg241.pdf#page=1

26. US Department of Health and Human Services. Fact sheet: HHS finalizes ACA Section 1557 Rule. HHS.gov. June 12, 2020. https://www.hhs.gov/sites/default/files/1557-final-rule-factsheet.pdf

27. Pan, C. Lost in translation: Google's translation of palliative care to "do-nothing care." *GeriPal Blog*. May 20, 2019. https://www.geripal.org/2019/05/lost-in-translation-googles-translation-of-palliative-care.html

28. U.S. Department of Health and Huma Services. National Institute of Health. ¿Qué son los cuidados paliativos y los cuidados de hospicio? Revised May 19, 2017. https://www.nia.nih.gov/espanol/son-cuidados-paliativos-cuidados-hospicio

29. Gerson, D. What happens when the doctor says "hospice" and you understand "poorhouse"? The World. Heath and Medicine. May 29, 2014. https://www.pri.org/stories/2014-05-29/what-happens-when-doctor-says-hospice-and-you-understand-poorhouse

30. Ladwig S, Quill T, Horowitz R, Weibel A, Bell Dickson R. Public opinions about palliative care in 2019: The needle hasn't moved. Poster Session for CAPC National Seminar. 2019. https://www.capc.org/seminar/poster-sessions/public-opinions-about-palliative-care-in-2019-the-needle-hasnt-moved/

31. Wu MS, Rawal S. "It's the difference between life and death": The views of professional medical interpreters on their role in the delivery of safe care to patients with limited English proficiency. *PloS One*. 2017;12(10):e0185659. doi:10.1371/journal.pone.0185659

32. Roat C, Kinderman A, Fernandez A. Interpreting in palliative care: Continuing education workshop for interpreters in health care. *Sacramento, CA*: California HealthCare Foundation. Version 3-19-12. 2011. https://www.chcf.org/wp-content/uploads/2017/12/PDF-InterpretingPalliativeCareLessons.pdf

33. Schenker Y, Smith AK, Arnold RM, Fernandez A. "Her husband doesn't speak much English": Conducting a family meeting with an interpreter. *J Palliat Med*. 2012;15(4):494–498. doi:10.1089/jpm.2011.0169

34. Association of American Medical Colleges. Guidelines for use of medical interpreter services. Available at https://www.aamc.org/system/files/c/2/70338-interpreter-guidelines.pdf

35. Borschmann R, Tibble H, Spittal MJ, et al. The Mortality After Release from Incarceration Consortium (MARIC): Protocol for a multi-national, individual participant data meta-analysis. *Int J Popul Data Sci*. 2020;5(1):1145. Published 2020 Jan 25. doi:10.23889/ijpds.v5i1.1145

36. Lineback CM, Mervak CM, Revels SL, Kemp MT, Reddy RM. Barriers to accessing optimal esophageal cancer care for socioeconomically disadvantaged patients. *Ann Thorac Surg*. 2017;103(2):416–421. doi:10.1016/j.athoracsur.2016.08.085

37. Dhahri A, Kaplan JL, Ntiri S, et al. The impact of census-tract socioeconomic status on survival in stage III colon cancer. *J Clin Oncol*. 2020;38(15 Suppl):7032–7032. doi:10.1200/JCO.2020.38.15_suppl.7032

38. Wiese D, Stroup AM, Maiti A, et al. Socioeconomic disparities in colon cancer survival: Revisiting neighborhood poverty using residential histories. *Epidemiology*. 2020;31(5):728–735. doi:10.1097/EDE.0000000000001216

39. Frissa S, Hatch SL, Fear NT, Dorrington S, Goodwin L, Hotopf M. Challenges in the retrospective assessment of trauma: Comparing a checklist approach to a single item trauma experience screening question. *BMC Psychiatry*. 2016;16:20. Published 2016 Feb 1. doi:10.1186/s12888-016-0720-1

40. Hudson N. The trauma of poverty as social identity. *J Loss Trauma*. 2016;21(2):111–123. doi:10.1080/15325024.2014.965979

41. Ganzel BL. Trauma-informed hospice and palliative care. *Gerontologist*. 2018;58(3):409–419. doi:10.1093/geront/gnw146

42. Levy-Carrick NC, Lewis-O'Connor A, Rittenberg E, Manosalvas K, Stoklosa HM, Silbersweig DA. Promoting health equity through trauma-informed care: Critical role for physicians in policy and program development. *Fam Community Health*. 2019;42(2):104–108. doi:10.1097/FCH.0000000000000214

43. Kok AAL, van Nes F, Deeg DJH, Widdershoven G, Huisman M. "Tough times have become good times": Resilience in older adults with a low socioeconomic position. *Gerontologist*. 2018;58(5):843–852. doi:10.1093/geront/gny007

44. Pew Research Center. America's Changing Religious Landscape study. May 12, 2015. https://www.pewforum.org/2015/05/12/americas-changing-religious-landscape/

45. Hagiwara N, Elston Lafata J, Mezuk B, Vrana SR, Fetters MD. Detecting implicit racial bias in provider communication behaviors to reduce disparities in healthcare: Challenges, solutions, and future directions for provider communication training. *Patient Educ Couns*. 2019;102(9):1738–1743. doi:10.1016/j.pec.2019.04.023

46. Anderson SR, Gianola M, Perry JM, Losin EAR. Clinician-patient racial/ethnic concordance influences racial/ethnic minority pain: Evidence from simulated clinical interactions. *Pain Med*. 2020;21(11):3109–3125. doi:10.1093/pm/pnaa258

47. Latulippe K, Hamel C, Giroux D. Social health inequalities and eHealth: A literature review with qualitative synthesis of theoretical and empirical studies. *J Med Internet Res*. 2017;19(4):e136. doi:10.2196/jmir.6731

48. Matzo M, Witt Sherman D. *Palliative Care Nursing: Quality Care to the End of Life*. 5th ed. New York: Springer; 2019. http://search.ebscohost.com/login.aspx?direct=true&db=nlebk&AN=1834353&site=ehost-live

49. American Nurses Association. *Nursing Scope and Standards of Practice*. 4th ed. 2021. Silver Spring, MD: Nursebooks.org.

50. American Nurses Association, Hospice and Palliative Nurses Association. *Call for action: Nurses lead and transform palliative care*. Silver Spring, MD: ANA. 2017. http://www.nursingworld.org/~497158/globalassets/practiceandpolicy/health-policy/palliativecareprofessionalissuespanelcallforaction.pdf

22.

LGBTQ+ INCLUSIVE PALLIATIVE CARE

Jessica Nymeyer

KEY POINTS

- The palliative advanced practice registered nurse (APRN) is conscious of the importance of tailoring the care plan for each patient based on the patient's and their family's goals and values.

- An individual's sexual and gender identity are essential components of their lived experience and should not be overlooked while they are receiving care for a serious illness.

- The palliative APRN must understand the context of the LGBTQ community and the challenges for an individual with serious illness.

CASE STUDY 1: INCLUSIVE CARE

Mr. G, a 68-year-old man, was admitted to the hospital with respiratory distress and is suspected of having COVID-19. He was a new patient to the health system so there was no information in the electronic medical record. For the safety of staff and other patients, he was placed in an isolation room with the door closed and not allowed to have any visitors. He reported his health history of type-2 diabetes, hypertension, and high cholesterol; however his ability to participate in prolonged discussion was limited by shortness of breath. The advanced practice registered nurse (APRN) overheard staff discussing that his SARS-CoV-2 PCR came back positive and that he was having progressive hypoxia requiring increasing oxygen. The primary medical team was overwhelmed and asked for assistance from the palliative APRN because they were worried Mr. G's condition could rapidly decline. How should the APRN approach him?

In any situation where there is a possibility for rapid decline, there is limited opportunity to develop a relationship and establish goals of care with a patient. Best practices guide clinicians to use LGBTQ-inclusive language for every patient encounter to avoid marginalizing a patient.[1]

Recommended initial interview questions include:

1. What would you like me to call you?

2. What gender pronoun do you go by (he/him, she/her, them/their, etc.)?

3. Who do you consider to be your family?

4. Who is available to help you when you are sick?

It is important to establish an appropriate surrogate decision-maker for patients with serious medical conditions as soon as possible. Inclusive language may include:

1. If there comes a time when you are too sick to make your own decisions about your care, whom do you want to make decisions on your behalf? Have you already put that in writing? If not, can we do that today?

2. Do you have any concerns about a different person trying to step in to make decisions for you?

3. Have you spoken to them about your concerns? Does your chosen healthcare decision-maker know your concerns?

4. Privacy rules under the Health Insurance Portability and Accountability Act (HIPAA) guide that we can share information with your family and friends only with your permission. What information would you like us to share about your illness and medical condition and with whom?

INTRODUCTION

Delivering inclusive care to patients who identify as LGBTQ+ (lesbian, gay, bisexual, transgender, queer/questioning with+ representing other sexual or gender identities that are not named in the acronym) is not a political or religious statement; it has been clearly defined as a marker of best practices in delivering high-quality healthcare. The Joint Commission has issued guidance directing all healthcare facilities to consider the needs of the LGBTQ population in their policies and procedures with the goal to "advance effective communication, cultural competence, and patient-and family-centered care for all patients."[2]

As an advanced practice registered nurse (APRN), practice is guided by the American Nurses Association, which explicated the necessity for all nurses to provide inclusive care to sexual and gender minority (SGM) individuals in a 2018 position statement which states, "nurses must deliver culturally congruent care and advocate for lesbian, gay, bisexual, transgender, queer, or questioning (LGBTQ+) populations. . . . ANA is committed to the elimination of health disparities and discrimination based on sexual orientation, gender identity, and/or expression within health care."[3]

The goal of this chapter on LGBTQ+ inclusive palliative care is not to suggest a prescriptive approach to caring for any specific SGM but to ensure that all care delivered by the palliative APRN is inclusive. Every clinician should presume that they care for patients who identify as LGBTQ+ and not assume that these individuals can be identified by external characteristics or life experiences, such as having children.[4] This chapter describes physical and mental health issues that disproportionately impact the LGBTQ+ community, unique challenges SGM face while living with serious illness, raise the APRN's consciousness of the pervasive nature of heteronormative language and assumptions, and highlight techniques that individuals and institutions should use with all patients to provide inclusive care. Moreover, there may be some legal and financial issues for the palliative APRN to attend to when caring for patients that identify as SGM. Through the process of developing a knowledge base about the LGBTQ+ community and making an effort to thoughtfully reflect on their own behaviors and potential biases, the palliative APRN will be prepared to be a leader within their institutions in the care of SGM patients with serious illness.

DEFINITIONS AND LANGUAGE

Being familiar with the language associated with sexual and gender minorities has been shown to lead to more positive attitudes among healthcare providers when caring for LGBTQ+ individuals.[5] However, an emphasis on learning facts about any population of people assumes that individuals within the population are homogenous and that language is static. It is understandable that the palliative APRN may not have a detailed understanding of all of the words individuals use to describe their sexuality and gender identity. The emphasis should not be on memorizing terms or assuming how a person would prefer to be described but instead on approaching each individual with an open heart and willingness to learn from them about their experiences.

The palliative APRN should strive for an attitude of *cultural humility* which directs focus on self-reflection and actively listening to individuals to more clearly understand their unique perspective.[6] Key terms related to sexual and gender minorities, as defined by the Human Rights Campaign, are listed in Table 22.1. Terms, like the word "queer," which many believe has been "reclaimed" from being a slur to becoming an inclusive term of SGM identity, have changed in meaning over time and are likely to continue to evolve.[7] While some may perceive that patients would respond negatively, most patients are comfortable being asked questions about their sexual orientation and gender identity and understand what the questions mean.[8] The palliative APRN should be empowered to recognize that emphasizing equality by ignoring sexual and gender identity represents a failure to provide person-centered care.[9]

The terms "men who have sex with men" (MSM) and "women who have sex with women" (WSW) have been used in public health literature; however, this only serves to describe a behavior and does not address sexual identity or gender. Up to 50% of individuals who have reported sexual encounters with someone of the same sex identify themselves as heterosexual.[10]

Younger people who identify as sexual or gender minorities may be more open than older individuals to disclose their identity given increased acceptance of LGBTQ+ in recent years. They may still likely face significant challenges in their families and communities due to ongoing stigma and have higher rates of homelessness, suicidal ideation, and sexual abuse than heterosexual peers.[11] A telephone survey of a nationally representative sample of US residents conducted in 2017 found that slurs, *microaggressions* (often unintentional actions or comments based on stereotypes), sexual harassment, and violence were experienced by more than 50% of LGBTQ survey participants.[12]

HISTORY OF CHALLENGES FOR LGBTQ INDIVIDUALS WITH SERIOUS ILLNESS

In 2011, the National Institutes of Health (NIH) published the Institute of Medicine (IOM – now known as the National Academy of Medicine) a report on the *Health of Lesbian, Gay, Bisexual and Transgender (LGBT) People*, which cited lack of social support and legal protections as barriers to access and quality of palliative care among sexual and gender minorities.[13] The report recognized that improving the health of the LGBT community requires appreciation of their lived experience. While acknowledging the diversity of LGBT individuals, the report found that long-term discrimination, inadequate training of healthcare workers, and stigma associated with the HIV/AIDS epidemic have caused significant negative impact on the health of the population overall. The IOM described the ongoing HIV/AIDS epidemic as illustrative of the overall status of the LGBT population: unified and resilient in the face of stigma but with disparities exacerbated by race and ethnicity and limited understanding complicated by inadequate research funding.

Although legal protections have evolved since the IOM report, including the Supreme Court ruling in 2015 legalizing same-sex marriage[14] and the June 2020 ruling that Title VII of the constitution includes protection for sexual and gender minorities against employment discrimination,[15] the consequences of historical barriers remain, including state surrogacy laws that often prioritize biologic family over chosen family with lack of recognition of non-married partners. Box 22.1 describes some of the legal issues that disproportionately impact SGM that the palliative APRN should be aware of when providing care to LGBTQ+ individuals and their families. Lack of understanding of legal issues that disproportionately impact advance care planning for SGM can be a form of institutional discrimination inadvertently propagated by the palliative APRN.[16]

In addition to evidence of legal and social inequity, a record of discrimination against LGBTQ+ individuals exists within the healthcare system in the United States. Historically, identifying as a sexual or gender minority led to a psychiatric diagnosis. The American Psychiatric Association's *Diagnostic and Statistical Manual of Mental Disorders* (DSM) identified homosexuality as a "sociopathic personality disturbance" until 1973, and it wasn't until 1987 that diagnoses related to same-sex attraction were removed from the DSM.[17]

Table 22.1 GLOSSARY OF TERMS BASED ON HUMAN RIGHTS CAMPAIGN DEFINITIONS

TERM	DEFINITION
Androgynous	Identifying and/or presenting as neither distinguishably masculine nor feminine.
Asexual	The lack of a sexual attraction or desire for other people.
Bisexual	A person emotionally, romantically, or sexually attracted to more than one sex, gender, or gender identity though not necessarily simultaneously, in the same way or to the same degree.
Cis-gender	A term used to describe a person whose gender identity aligns with those typically associated with the sex assigned to them at birth.
Closeted	Describes an LGBTQ person who has not disclosed their sexual orientation or gender identity.
Coming out	The process in which a person first acknowledges, accepts, and appreciates his or her sexual orientation or gender identity and begins to share that with others.
Gay	A person who is emotionally, romantically, or sexually attracted to members of the same gender.
Gender dysphoria	Clinically significant distress caused when a person's assigned birth gender is not the same as the one with which they identify. According to the American Psychiatric Association's *Diagnostic and Statistical Manual of Mental Disorders* (DSM-5), the term—which replaces Gender Identity Disorder—"is intended to better characterize the experiences of affected children, adolescents, and adults."
Gender expression	External appearance of one's gender identity, usually expressed through behavior, clothing, haircut, or voice, and which may or may not conform to socially defined behaviors and characteristics typically associated with being either masculine or feminine.
Gender-fluid	According to the *Oxford English Dictionary*, a person who does not identify with a single fixed gender; of or relating to a person having or expressing a fluid or unfixed gender identity.
Gender identity	One's innermost concept of self as male, female, a blend of both or neither—how individuals perceive themselves and what they call themselves. One's gender identity can be the same or different from their sex assigned at birth.
Gender non-conforming	A broad term referring to people who do not behave in a way that conforms to the traditional expectations of their gender or whose gender expression does not fit neatly into a category.
Homophobia	The fear and hatred of or discomfort with people who are attracted to members of the same sex.
Lesbian	A woman who is emotionally, romantically, or sexually attracted to other women.
LGBTQ	An acronym for "lesbian, gay, bisexual, transgender and queer."
Living openly	A state in which LGBTQ people are comfortably out about their sexual orientation or gender identity— where and when it feels appropriate to them.
Outing	Exposing someone's lesbian, gay, bisexual, or transgender identity to others without their permission. Outing someone can have serious repercussions on employment, economic stability, personal safety, or religious or family situations.
Queer	A term people often use to express fluid identities and orientations. Often used interchangeably with "LGBTQ."
Questioning	A term used to describe people who are in the process of exploring their sexual orientation or gender identity.
Sexual orientation	An inherent or immutable enduring emotional, romantic, or sexual attraction to other people.
Transgender	An umbrella term for people whose gender identity and/or expression is different from cultural expectations based on the sex they were assigned at birth. Being transgender does not imply any specific sexual orientation. Therefore, transgender people may identify as straight, gay, lesbian, bisexual, etc.
Transphobia	The fear and hatred of, or discomfort with, transgender people.

From Human Rights Campaign.[52]

In 2014, the Department of Health and Human Services Departmental Appeals Board overruled a National Coverage Determination made in 1981 that designated "transsexual surgery" as "experimental," allowing costs associated with transition to now be covered by the Centers for Medicare and Medicaid Services (CMS).[18] In the most recent edition of the DSM (DSM-5; 2015), diagnoses associated with being transgender were specifically worded to ensure individuals could maintain access to care (which requires a medical diagnosis) while attempting to reduce the stigma associated with having a psychiatric diagnosis by creating a new term, *gender dysphoria*.[17] This terminology clarifies that it is not a mental illness that causes the person to desire a different identity but nonpathologic distress in the context of the physical body not aligning with the individual's self-perception.[5]

Heteronormative views presume that heterosexual orientation is the normal or preferred sexual orientation. The nurse practitioners in one study emphasized sexual behaviors and risk of sexually transmitted infections as the primary healthcare issue differentiating care of sexual minorities from heterosexual patients and described their belief in the importance of treating all sexual minorities "the same" as heterosexual patients.[19] This perspective demonstrates a knowledge gap of the unique psychosocial stressors and medical issues faced by SGM and highlights the prevalence of heteronormative assumptions. Box 22.2 highlights research findings about discrimination against SGM in the healthcare setting. An encouraging factor is that most healthcare staff want to provide high-quality care to all patients they work with and are open to receiving more information about issues impacting the LGBTQ community.[20] The opening case study reviews how the APRN may approach a patient with complex palliative care needs utilizing language that avoids heteronormative assumptions and moves to establish a trusting relationship in a short period of time.

COMING OUT, DISCLOSURE, OR FORTHCOMING LGBTQ+ IDENTITY

Given the complex history of discrimination some SGM have encountered in the healthcare system, individuals may not reveal their LGBTQ+ identity even if they are "out" in other areas of their life. Some individuals will feel comfortable revealing their sexual and gender identity or naming their same-sex partner before being specifically asked by the palliative APRN; however, others may be hesitant to reveal due to concerns about stigma or episodes of past rejection related to their identity.[21] An individual should not be forced to out themselves if they choose not to disclose their sexual or gender minority status.

Qualitative research has revealed a range of reasons a patient may choose not to be forthcoming to their medical team, many of which are described in Table 22.2.[22] Disclosing sexual or gender identity may be perceived as unnecessary by some individuals who prefer to maintain privacy and instead focus on the pathology of their disease as the nature of the healthcare transaction. Others may disclose on their own terms for ease of interaction, including maintaining control of the timing of information sharing and allowing for discussion about other aspects of their life without feeling the stress of withholding sexual or gender identity or not being able to receive appropriate psychosocial support consistent with their lived experience. Partnered LGBTQ+ individuals may disclose to ensure their significant other is able to be involved as a support person; if the partner is not included by healthcare staff there may be significant distress. The presence of visible symbols of acceptance, including public display of nondiscrimination policies or rainbow pins or insignia, helps some individuals feel more comfortable forthcoming. Microaggressions including overheard comments or heteronormative assumptions made by staff or other patients may make the environment feel unsafe for disclosure.

Table 22.2 CONTRIBUTING FACTORS OF INDIVIUDALS WITH SERIOUS ILLNESS TO DISCLOSE SEXUAL AND GENGER MINORITY STATUS TO THE PALLIATIVE APRN

PROMOTING	DISCOURAGING
Welcoming physical space with markers of inclusion (i.e., rainbow flag, inclusive pictures and information in waiting and exam rooms)	Patient's previous experience of discrimination in healthcare environment
Intake process with inclusive documents	Lack of markers of inclusion for LGBTQ population
Inclusive language used by all staff	Gender-specific or noninclusive intake documents
APRN asks about sexual and gender identity	APRN doesn't ask about sexual or gender identity
APRN includes support person/partner during encounter, asking their role, and encourages participation in goals-of-care discussions as appropriate	APRN uses heteronormative language
	Overheard homophobic comments
Strong self-identity by patient and sense that disclosure is important or "easier"	APRN assumes role of support person (i.e., a sibling or friend instead of partner)
Patient perception that disclosure will result in better care	Hierarchical power differential between patient and clinician, especially when patient is seriously ill and vulnerable
	Patient perception that sexuality and gender identity are not relevant to treatment

From Fish et al.[22]

HEALTH DISPARITIES

There is evidence that the LGBTQ+ population has higher rates of physical illnesses and mental health issues including anxiety, depression, and suicide attempts than do individuals who identify as heterosexual and *cis-gendered* (i.e., having a gender identity aligning with the one assigned at birth). In multiple studies researchers have identified that SGM have higher rates of cardiovascular disease, particularly among people of color.[23] The cause of these disparities is not completely understood, but it is recognized that they contribute to the complexity of serious illness among SGM individuals. One theoretical model to explain this phenomenon is *minority stress theory*, which describes an exacerbation of stress and mental health challenges among a minority population due to chronic discrimination, stigma, and prejudice. Conversely, for some individuals, identifying as a member of a minority group may build resilience and provide a positive protective factor.[24]

Another theory, *intersectionality*, describes that each individual has multiple social identities including sexual and gender identity, age, race/ethnicity, education level, and physical ability, among others, that may be outwardly visible or hidden.[25] Intersectionality related to membership in multiple minority groups is one way to frame the additive challenges some SGM individuals may face and can help explain the health disparities that they experience.

Researchers have also found evidence that experiencing multiple psychological health risks can lead to additive negative health effects among LGBTQ+ individuals. In one study, participants who experienced three or more psychosocial risks including sexual assault, intimate partner violence, posttraumatic stress disorder (PTSD), substance use, or depression, all of which disproportionately impact the SGM community, had exponential risk of physical health conditions.[26]

It is known that individuals in the United States who identify as SGM are more likely than cis-gendered heterosexual individuals to use tobacco, alcohol, and drugs, with some evidence that the highest risk is among those who identify as bisexual.[27] Using data from the 2015–2018 National Survey on Drug Use and Health, researchers noted significant disparities in cigarette smoking, heavy episodic drinking (four or more drinks per day for women or five or more drinks per day for men), and marijuana use between lesbian and bisexual women when compared to heterosexual women.[28] These effects were significantly more pronounced between lesbian and bisexual women who identified as Black or Hispanic than those who identified as White. In contrast, both sexual minority status and identifying as a racial or ethnic minority had a smaller effect on the rates of smoking, drug, and alcohol use on male participants. Study authors highlight the importance of recognizing the heterogeneity of the LGBTQ+ population and suggest that intersectionality theory may serve as a partial explanation for these differences. Increased rates of substance use may contribute to stereotyping and discrimination of the LGBTQ+ community.

There are a variety of social factors that also contribute to health inequalities. In the past it was very difficult for LGBTQ+ individuals to obtain health insurance. Rates of health insurance coverage have significantly improved since the implementation of the *Affordable Care Act* (ACA) and the legalization of marriage for same-sex couples, which allows families to access insurance through an employer; however, LGBTQ families continue to have lower rates of insurance and report avoiding care due to cost.[29] Employment discrimination due to sexual and gender identity was ruled to be illegal by the Supreme Court in 2020, but a prolonged history of legal discrimination and stigma has resulted in unequal pay and increased rates of poverty among SGM. Older LGBTQ+ women have identified poverty and social isolation as some of their top concerns when living with serious illness.[30] These complex social factors and high rates of poverty have contributed to the fact that 20–40% of the homeless population identifies as LGBTQ+.[31]

Although it is now known that SGM face increased risk of many mental and physical health conditions, research about health issues facing LGBTQ+ individuals historically focused only on sexually transmitted infections, most notably

HIV/AIDS. Unfortunately, HIV continues to have a disproportionate impact on the health of SGM. MSM, including all sexual and gender identities, make up the highest number of new HIV diagnosis in the United States. The Centers for Disease Control and Prevention (CDC) reports that, in 2018, 69% of new HIV diagnoses were between MSM. Most new infections occurred in men aged 25–34 and disproportionately impacted Black and Hispanic/Latino individuals.[32] Access to improved treatment regimens with antiviral medications has changed HIV from a near certain cause of death to a chronic condition that individuals may live with for decades; however, it continues to be an illness that carries significant stigma and can be a contributing factor to many health complications. In an analysis of insurance claims data from 2007 to 2016, researchers found significantly higher rates of diabetes, hypertension, stroke, cancer, and lung and cardiovascular diseases as well as cognitive impairment among individuals living with HIV when controlled for demographics, behavioral risk factors, and other comorbidities.[33]

SPECIAL ISSUES IN CANCER CARE

There is clear evidence that sexual and gender minorities have higher rates of cancer than their heterosexual peers, although, due to a history of poor data collection, true rates of cancer incidence, survivorship, and mortality among SGM are not known. Stress-related factors, higher rates of chronic illness, and substance use likely contribute, but there appear to be additional, unexplained factors that contribute to cancer risk.[34]

One factor is decreased cancer screening rates resulting in advanced stages of cancer at time of diagnosis. Major barriers to cancer screening by SGM include knowledge deficits of screening guidelines by both LGBTQ+ individuals and healthcare providers. Improved rates of cancer screening have been associated with well-informed clinicians who establish welcoming clinical environments and include the patient's preferred caregivers.[35]

Another likely cause of higher rates of cancer for SGM is decreased access to quality healthcare due to stigma and barriers. While LGBTQ+ patients may have the opportunity and time to search for a primary care provider they feel will be accepting of their sexual and gender identity, referrals to specialty care for a serious medical condition, like cancer care or palliative care, may limit choice. This places the individual in a position of needing to balance the risks and benefits of disclosing their SGM status and risk of discrimination.[22]

Heteronormative language and behaviors can be especially challenging in gender-specific cancers. For example, SGM with prostate cancer are less likely to self-disclose their sexual orientation and therefore may experience negative consequences ranging from embarrassment to inadequate side-effect management related to incontinence or erectile dysfunction, miss opportunities to receive meaningful psychosocial interventions from the care team, or have their preferred support person participate in difficult decision-making.[36] Research on oncology clinicians reveals a discomfort and lack of training about asking their seriously ill patients about sexual issues related to their illness or treatment course, citing limited time during encounters, fear of offending their patient, and uncertainty about how to respond to disclosure of minority sexual or gender status as barriers.[37] This provides an opportunity for the palliative APRN to offer support and education to both patients and clinicians. Having an oncologist who lacks LGBT competence has been associated with unmet psychosocial needs and even posttraumatic stress among SGM cancer survivors.[38]

CONSIDERATIONS IN THE CARE OF TRANSGENDERED INDIVIDUALS WITH SERIOUS ILLNESS

Gender identity exists on a continuum and choice of outward expression of gender identity may change over time for all individuals.[5,39] It is important to note that having a gender identity that does not match the gender assigned at birth is a deeply held part of an individual's sense of self and is not the same as a "drag queen" or "drag king" who is a performer who entertains by presenting in exaggeratedly feminine or masculine ways.[40] An individual who does not identify as their assigned gender at birth may or may not be interested in hormone therapy or surgical intervention, also known as *gender affirmation therapies*, with the goal of aligning the physical body with the individual's self-identity.

In the event an individual does desire to pursue gender affirmation interventions, they are dependent on healthcare providers to deliver transition-related care, including prescription refills for hormone therapy, which creates a profound power imbalance with the medical system directly related to that person's sexual and gender identity. Long-term health implications of estrogen, antiandrogen, or testosterone therapy among transgender people who chose to use them are not clearly understood.

The ability to continue gender affirmation therapies while receiving care for a serious illness or at the end of life may be limited for a variety of reasons, including inability to tolerate medications, contraindication in the setting of hormone-sensitive cancers, or challenges associated with the cost or logistics of obtaining treatment while physically debilitated as a result of illness. An individual who is unable to complete or continue the process of gender affirmation therapy due to their illness may face significant grief due to an inability to maintain an outward appearance that is consistent with their self-identity. A transgendered individual may also choose to revert to their birth gender around biologic family members to maintain a challenged relationship.[21] An individual nearing the end of life may also be concerned that their surrogate will honor their wish to be buried as their chosen gender.[30]

As discussed in the opening case study, palliative APRN should ask each person in their care their preferred name, *preferred pronouns* (e.g., she/her, he/his, they/their, ze/zir, among others), and what language the individual prefers to use for their body anatomy if an exam of sexual organs is required. Care for diseases of sexual organs exacerbates the vulnerability of transgendered individuals and requires additional sensitivity. Inclusion of a support person may be very helpful during exams. Language used to describe body organs should be as gender-neutral as possible. Comments about how masculine or feminine an individual or parts of their body appear are not helpful and contribute to objectifying their body. Screening exams should focus on the organ being evaluated and not the gender of the individual; a trans woman may benefit from both prostate cancer and breast cancer screening.

Transgender men have rates of cancer more closely related to cis-gender women, which is significantly higher than that of cis-gender men.[41] Inadequate knowledge of screening recommendations for trans-masculine individuals who are at risk of HPV and cervical cancer may lead healthcare providers to wrongly assume that their risks are lower than cis-gendered women and not recommend regular screening. Personal and physical vulnerability may limit the trans individual's desire to seek screening tests like Pap smears.[39] An individual who feels confident or self-affirmed in their gender identity may be comfortable asking a healthcare provider to change their behavior or language; however, a patient who has experienced a history of trauma or oppression related to other aspects of their identity, such as race/ethnicity, poverty, or level of education, may further shift power balance to healthcare staff.

CASE STUDY 2: CARING FOR A TRANSGENDER PATIENT

A palliative care consult was placed for assistance with symptom management for a patient named Joanne, with newly diagnosed cervical cancer. The patient was admitted to the hospital from the chemotherapy suite with severe nausea, vomiting, and abdominal pain. The palliative APRN worked frequently with the GYN-oncology team and always enjoyed going to the newly remodeled Women's Health wing in the hospital to assist with the care of their patients. The APRN was surprised to see an ill-appearing man lying in the hospital bed when they passed the room and walked to the nurses station to double-check the room number for the consult. Staff confirmed the room number and explained that the patient is transmasculine. Joanne's assigned gender at birth was female; however, he identifies as a male and prefers to be called Joel with the pronouns "he" or "him."

Given that the patient is transmasculine, what can you safely assume about their identity?

a. The gender of their sexual partners

b. They have had surgical alteration of their sexual organs, called *gender correction* or *gender affirming surgery*

c. They take hormone therapy with testosterone

d. They are unlikely to be religious or spiritual

e. You cannot assume anything and should address them as a unique individual

Making assumptions about any person limits the ability of the palliative APRN to provide person-centered care. The correct answer is "e." In order to learn more about Joel's sexual partners, surgical history, current medications and sources of support, including spiritual beliefs, a thoughtful interview is necessary.

When the palliative APRN entered his room they introduced themselves and asked if he is Joel Johnson—he indicated that he was and asked to be called Joel. Since the nurses confirmed that his preferred gender pronoun was he or him, the APRN did not need to ask him again but ensured they addressed him as he requests. Joel described his symptoms of chemotherapy associated nausea and abdominal pain. He described the experience of receiving chemotherapy as very upsetting and distressing. With further sensitive questioning, he explained that the chemotherapy suite in the women's cancer center was decorated with traditionally feminine designs, and he felt very uncomfortable as the only man in the room. He reported that he has noticed the staff and other patients staring at him and even the women's magazines and fliers in the lobby for wigs and special makeup events for cancer patients seemed to point out his gender. He felt like his cancer was a painful reminder of the emotional distress he suffered when he was living as a woman and he wondered if god is punishing him. When he thought about, it made his pain and nausea worsen. The palliative APRN recognized that Joel was suffering from emotional and spiritual distress as well as physical symptoms and would benefit from a team approach.

The interdisciplinary palliative care team worked closely with the GYN-onc team to support Joel during his hospitalization. The social worker and chaplain met with Joel regularly to provide emotional and spiritual support. He identified his partner and sister as his primary support people, and they were encouraged to visit regularly so that he would not feel so isolated. Fliers for the Women's Cancer Support Group were removed from the bulletin board in Joel's room and standard neutral-colored hospital gowns were obtained for him to wear instead of the mauve gowns designed especially for the women's health hospital wing. In coordination with the oncology department, plans were made for Joel to receive the remainder of his chemotherapy course in the general infusion center instead of the GYN-onc chemotherapy suite. Joel was referred to the palliative care outpatient clinic for ongoing symptom management and emotional support throughout his treatment course.

UNIQUE NEEDS OF OLDER LGBTQ+ INDIVIDUALS

Older SGM will experience similar challenges of aging as cis-gendered heterosexual adults, but they are less likely to be partnered or have children and are more likely to have *families of choice* as their primary supports, potentially raising the uncertainty of who may be available to act as a caregiver, if needed. Partners are the most common caregivers for older LGBTQ individuals, but about a quarter of caregivers for SGM are friends, a much higher rate than among heterosexual older adults.[42] Friends who serve as caregivers are less likely to receive formal support or have legal rights to make decisions on behalf of the patient without proper documentation. Unfortunately, some LGBTQ individuals may be estranged from their families, and this may be a source of distress at the end of life.

In the United States, surrogacy laws vary from state to state, and unless an individual has clearly identified and documented a surrogate decision-maker, important advance care planning decisions may defer to biologic relatives and not the desired chosen family member. However, this should not lead the palliative APRN to assume that an older LGBTQ+ individual does not have a positive relationship with their biologic family or does not have children. SGM may be legally married or partnered with biologic or adopted children, and some may have previously been in heterosexual marriages and remain close to their biologic children and extended family.

Older LGBTQ+ individuals with serious illness who are facing transition into an assisted living or skilled nursing facility may have concerns about the safety of revealing their SGM identity. Many have spent much of their lives facing stigma and discrimination, criminalization, and pathologization of their sexual or gender identity and have reasonable concerns about trusting the healthcare system to provide compassionate end-of-life care when they are most vulnerable, especially in institutions with conservative or religious emphasis.[9] This can be especially challenging for couples who would like to move to a facility together. This has been referred to as the "Gen Silent" phenomenon after a documentary film of the same name, released in 2010, highlighted the trend of elderly LGBTQ+ individuals hiding their identity to avoid discrimination when receiving long-term care.[43]

Palliative APRNs should assess for elder abuse in all patients and recognize that seriously ill SGM may be at increased risk due to vulnerabilities throughout their life span.[44] Disconnection from biologic family resulting in reduced access to caregivers and housing, history of abuse, income discrimination, and lack of spousal benefits leading to limited financial resources and health insurance are all factors that contribute to risk. A history of discriminating heteronormative experiences with law enforcement or the healthcare system may lead the individual to feel unsafe reporting their experiences of abuse and result in a lack of traditional support services or assistance with establishing long-term care resources.

END OF LIFE AND BEREAVEMENT

Receiving care for a serious illness involves encounters with a range of healthcare staff in multiple settings and may require making difficult decisions about end-of-life care. For LGBTQ+ individuals, the challenge of considering the safety of expressing one's sexual and gender minority status with each new clinical team can add distress during an already challenging time. When patients feel safe to reveal their identity, they report experiencing a higher quality of care.[45] Transitions in care location and goals require trusting relationships and clear communication between the healthcare team, the patient, and their identified supports; poorly coordinated transitions can be a point of great stress for SGM.[45]

The process of eliciting the patient's goals and values at the end of life is intensely personal. Honest and open communication is needed for the palliative APRN to successfully elicit the seriously ill individual's values and tailor a care plan to their needs. Identifying caregivers who are able to help a debilitated patient with activities of daily living may cause significant discomfort if, for example, a partner doesn't feel safe to explain that they share a bed with the patient and are willing to help them with personal care. Some individuals may not feel comfortable having hospice staff come into the safety of their home if they perceive the visit would reveal more than they are comfortable sharing about their sexual or gender identity.[45]

Spirituality is an important aspect of the human experience and may take increased prominence when individuals are facing the end of life. Conflict between religious beliefs and sexual or gender identity may result in psychological and spiritual distress. Some SGM have had negative experiences with organized religion and may be less engaged in religious communities than cis-gendered heterosexual individuals, but this is not a universal occurrence. A religious community that is affirming of LGBTQ+ members provides a positive source of support.[46]

Partners of SGM individuals who die are faced with the same bereavement challenges as heterosexual partners as well as specific experiences related to their sexual and gender identity. Additional stressors include experience of homophobia, exclusion from important decision-making, limited acknowledgment of the value of the relationship, ability to be present at the end of life, and financial and legal pressures.[47] These factors raise the risk of *disenfranchised grief*, or the inability of the bereaved to openly express their grief due to social stigma.[16] Transgender individuals who have their transition process interrupted or are not able to continue taking hormone therapy due to the severity of illness may experience their own forms of disenfranchised grief.

Many states stop recognizing a healthcare agent after death and custody of the body defaults to next of kin. The palliative APRN must be knowledgeable about the laws in the state where they practice and should ask all patients if they are comfortable with their next of kin having authority over their body after death. If a patient would prefer to name an alternative person, their wish must be documented appropriately to ensure it is honored after death.

IMPROVING CARE DELIVERY

Having an understanding of the origin of LGBTQ+ health disparities helps the palliative APRN appreciate the context within which the SGM individual with serious illness seeks care and highlights the value of creating safe spaces to provide inclusive, nonjudgmental care that affirms individuals as they define themselves.[48] In addition to being thoughtful and open about the needs of each patient in their care, a key component of cultural humility requires the palliative APRN to take time to reflect on their own response to caring for LGBTQ+ individuals and other minorities.

One tool for self-reflection during each clinical encounter is the mnemonic CAMPERS, outlined in Table 22.3.[49] The palliative APRN should enter the encounter with a

Table 22.3 CAMPERS TOOL FOR SELF-AWARENESS

STEP	DEFINITION
1. Know your **C**lear purpose	Understand the purpose of the interaction. Be conscious that this will likely evolve during the encounter based on patient needs
2. Know your **A**ttitudes and beliefs	Be aware of any assumptions you bring into the encounter; recognize that prejudgments are a natural human response but are often inaccurate. Be especially conscious if you feel more compassion for certain groups of people or specific illnesses
3. Know your **M**itigation plan	Identify the actions you will take to prevent the attitudes and beliefs you named from impacting your patient interaction, including a plan to minimize the power imbalance between you and the patient
4. Know the **P**atient	Learn about the patient as a person, including their gender and sexual identity—not only the patients you think are transgender
5. Know your **E**motions	Recognize your own feelings to prevent them from interfering with the quality of care you are providing
6. Know your **R**eactions	Be conscious of the way you express your emotions including body language, facial expressions, and tone
7. Know your **S**trategy	Pause to review each encounter and devise a plan for improving future interactions

From Acquaviva.[49]

Table 22.4 EVOLUTION OF NURSING ATTITUDES TOWARD SEXUAL AND GENDER MINORITY WITH SERIOUS ILLNESS

DECADE	PERCEPTION
1980s	Fear associated with high rates of death from HIV exacerbated homophobia and heteronormative perceptions with strong desire by many nurses to avoid caring for gay men with serious illness
1990s/2000s	Evidence of increased intellectual belief in equal rights for homosexual individuals at all stages of life; however, continued negative emotional reactions toward caring for SGM patients is associated with decreased quality of care
2010s	Increasing emphasis on treating all patients equally by focusing on physiologic illness and "ignoring" sexuality results in unintentional reinforcement of heteronormative assumptions and failure to provide individualized care in advanced disease

From Dorsen, Devanter.[19]

clear goal as well as the flexibility to understand that the goal will evolve based on the patient's needs. Awareness of the assumptions that naturally develop about others based on biases, social norms, and in response to certain disease states is critically important. However, equally valuable is taking time to develop plans to mitigate those assumptions and acknowledge the power the clinician inherently holds in the clinical interaction to ensure the encounter remains focused on the patient's needs and goals. The palliative APRN must make an effort to know each patient as an individual by asking questions, including clarifying the name they prefer, their sex assigned at birth and current gender identity with the pronouns they prefer, who they consider to be their family and supports, their current care needs, knowledge about their illness, and health-related goals. Being aware of the emotions that the encounter elicits as well as being conscious of the verbal and body language responses the emotion triggers are necessary to ensure the palliative APRN can remain focused on patient needs and does not allow personal responses to interfere with patient care. After each encounter, it is helpful to review the interaction to evaluate opportunities and challenges and consider what could be done differently to improve future encounters.

Table 22.4 describes ways the history of nurse's attitudes toward caring for sexual and gender minorities have evolved alongside the social norms and policies in the United States.[19] Research in the late 1980s found that significant negative attitudes toward LGBT persons were connected with the desire to avoid caring for patients with a diagnosis of AIDS. In the 1990s and 2000s, more nurse research participants identified the value of equal rights for all individuals but continued to report strongly negative emotional reactions to sexual minorities. More recent research has exposed a desire by nurses not to stereotype SGM; however, this has resulted in inadvertently furthering heternormative assumptions.

The palliative APRN has an obligation to ensure that the entire care team is providing inclusive care to all patients, including SGM. In addition to clinical teams, patients and their support persons interact with multiple staff members during each clinical encounter, including security guards, front desk staff, billing professionals, housekeepers, and more. Both clinical and nonclinical staff require education and reinforcement of the necessity to create an environment that is safe and welcoming.[50] One study found that members of the interdisciplinary hospice team had largely positive perceptions of SGM patients and their caregivers, with most positive attitudes associated with higher education and longer work experience and more negative perceptions associated with reported strong religious affiliation.[51] Encouraging individual and team reflection on biases and potential misunderstandings about caring for LGBTQ+ patients with serious illness and focusing on the importance of patient-centered care for all individuals are important steps in creating a welcoming space for SGM.

Including LGBTQ+ community members in the development of educational resources for healthcare staff and program development within the healthcare setting is an excellent way to improve care delivery and mitigate the risk of inadvertent exclusion of SGM.[9] Box 22.3 includes important insights elicited through a qualitative study describing what seriously ill LGBTQ patients felt their caregivers should understand in order to meet their needs. Teams should consider how marketing materials portray the services that are provided and whom they are provided to; including patients of racial and ethnic minority groups and sexual and gender minorities will demonstrate a welcoming attitude to future patients (Box 22.3).[4] For additional resources on caring for LGBTQ+ individuals with serious illness, see Table 22.5.

SUMMARY

Individuals who identify as sexual or gender minorities cannot be distinguished by exterior characteristics or health history. A history of discrimination in society and within the healthcare system may lead some SGM to avoid care or feel the need to withhold their identity from their clinicians. To provide holistic, inclusive, and supportive care to all patients they encounter, the palliative APRN must presume that each individual may be LGBTQ+ and approach with sensitivity and cultural humility. Recognizing that SGM are not a homogenous population is key to individualizing care; however, having an understanding of issues that disproportionately impact SGM with serious illnesses is necessary to provide quality care. Creating welcoming and inclusive settings for care delivery, avoiding heteronormative assumptions and language, and including the individual's partner or chosen family in their healthcare are important ways to establish a trusting relationship and develop a care plan that is consistent with the patient's goals and values. An understanding of legal issues, including the need for clearly documented healthcare agents if surrogates designated by state law are not consistent with the patient's preferences as well as documentation of wishes for care of their remains after death, allows the palliative APRN to fully support the patient's advance care planning needs. Keys to providing consistently high-quality care with all patients include acknowledging the emotions that arise when caring for SGM, being conscious of the verbal and body language reactions the APRN has during the encounter, and routinely reflecting on opportunities to improve care delivery.

Table 22.5 RESOURCES FOR THE PALLIATIVE APRN CARING FOR LGBTQ+ INDIVIDUALS

ORGANIZATION	RESOURCES	WEBSITE
Lambda Legal[53]	Nonprofit focusing on civil rights of LGBT individuals and those living with HIV through education and public policy	lambdalegal.org
LGBT HealthLink: Best and Most Promising Practices Throughout the Cancer Continuum[54]	Detailed and easy to use review of best practices throughout cancer care from surveillance to end of life care for sexual and gender minorities	Lgbthealthlink.org/ Cancer-Best-Practices
National LGBT Cancer Network[55]	Resources for LGBT individuals with cancer including provider referrals and resources for clinicians	cancer-network.org
National LGBTQIA+ Health Education Center[56]	Organization focused on advancing health equity for SGM thorough educational programs and resources for clinicians and health care organizations	lgbthealtheducation.org
Services and Advocacy for Gay, Lesbian, Bisexual & Transgender Elders (SAGE)[57]	National organization focused on supporting the needs of LGBT elders, including training on LGBT cultural competencies	sageusa.org
SAMHSA: Lesbian, Gay, Bisexual and Transgender[58]	Substance Abuse and Mental Health Services Administration (SAMHSA) resources focused on behavioral health equity	samhsa.gov/behavioral-health-equity/lgbt
UCSF Prevention Science: Center of Excellence For Transgender Health[59]	Excellent resource including training modules and detailed guidelines for clinicians caring for trans and gender non-binary individuals	prevention.ucsf.edu/ transhealth

REFERENCES

1. Rosa WE, Shook A, Acquaviva KD. LGBTQ+ Inclusive palliative care in the context of COVID-19: Pragmatic recommendations for clinicians. *J Pain Symptom Manage.* 2020;60(2):e44–e47. doi:10.1016/j.jpainsymman.2020.04.155

2. The Joint Commission. *Advancing Effective Communication, Cultural Competence, and Patient and Family Centered Care for the Lesbian, Gay, Bisexual, and Transgender (LGBT) Community: A Field Guide.* Oak Brook, IL: The Joint Commission, Oct. 2011. https://www.jointcommission.org/-/media/tjc/documents/resources/patient-safety-topics/health-equity/lgbtfieldguide_web_linked_verpdf.pdf?db=web&hash=FD725DC02CFE6E4F21A35EBD839BBE97&hash=FD725DC02CFE6E4F21A35EBD839BBE97

3. American Nurses Association. *Position Statement: Nursing Advocacy for the LGBTQ+ Population.* Silver Spring, MD: ANA; 2018. https://www.nursingworld.org/practice-policy/nursing-excellence/official-position-statements/id/nursing-advocacy-for-lgbtq-populations/

4. National Resource Center on LGBT Aging. Inclusive services for LGBT older adults: A practical guide to creating welcoming agencies. New York, NY: National Resource Center on LGBT Aging. May 20, 2020. https://www.lgbtagingcenter.org/resources/resource.cfm?r=487

5. Joseph A, Cliffe C, Hillyard M, Majeed A. Gender identity and the management of the transgender patient: A guide for non-specialists. *J R Soc Med.* 2017;110(4):144–152. doi:10.1177/0141076817696054

6. Sprik P, Gentile D. Cultural humility: A way to reduce LGBTQ health disparities at the end of life. *Am J Hosp Palliat Care.* 2020;37(6):404–408. doi:10.1177/1049909119880548

7. Collins C. Is queer OK to say? Here's why we use it. Teaching Tolerance. Learning for Justice Magazine. February 10, 2019. https://www.tolerance.org/magazine/is-queer-ok-to-say-heres-why-we-use-it

8. Alexander K, Walters CB, Banerjee SC. Oncology patients' preferences regarding sexual orientation and gender identity (SOGI) disclosure and room sharing. *Patient Educ Couns.* 2020;103(5):1041–1048. doi:10.1016/j.pec.2019.12.006

9. Higgins A, Downes C, Sheaf G, et al. Pedagogical principles and methods underpinning education of health and social care practitioners on experiences and needs of older LGBT+ people: Findings from a systematic review. *Nurse Educ Prac.* 2019;40:102625. doi:10.1016/j.nepr.2019.102625

10. Everett BG. Sexual orientation disparities in sexually transmitted infections: Examining the intersection between sexual identity and sexual behavior. *Arch Sex Behav.* 2013;42(2):225–236. doi:10.1007/s10508-012-9902-1

11. Hafeez H, Zeshan M, Tahir MA, Jahan N, Naveed S. Health care disparities among lesbian, gay, bisexual, and transgender youth: A literature review. *Cureus.* 2017;9(4):e1184. doi:10.7759/cureus.1184. PMID: 28638747; PMCID: PMC5478215.

12. Casey LS, Reisner SL, Findling MG, et al. Discrimination in the United States: Experiences of lesbian, gay, bisexual, transgender, and queer Americans. *Health Serv Res.* 2019;54 (Suppl 2):1454–1466. doi:10.1111/1475-6773.13229

13. Institute of Medicine. *The Health of Lesbian, Gay, Bisexual, and Transgender People Building a Foundation for Better Understanding.* Washington, DC: The National Academies Press; 2011. https://doi.org/10.17226/13128.

14. *14-556 Obergefell v. Hodges.* US no 14-576. Supreme Court of the United States. 2015. Available at https://www.supremecourt.gov/opinions/14pdf/14-556_3204.pdf

15. *17-1618 Bostock v. Clayton County.* US no 17-1618. Supreme Court of the United States. 2020. Available at https://www.supremecourt.gov/opinions/19pdf/17-1618_hfci.pdf

16. Haviland K, Burrows Walters C, Newman S. Barriers to palliative care in sexual and gender minority patients with cancer: A scoping review of the literature. *Health Soc Care Community.* 2020;1–14. doi:10.1111/hsc.13126

17. Drescher J. Queer diagnoses revisited: The past and future of homosexuality and gender diagnoses in DSM and ICD. *Int Rev Psychiatry.* 2015;27(5):386–395. doi:10.3109/09540261.2015.1053847

18. Department of Health and Human Services. Departmental appeals board: Appellate Division. NDC 140.3, Transsexual Surgery. Docket No A-13-87. Decision No 2576. May 30, 2014. https://www.hhs.gov/sites/default/files/static/dab/decisions/board-decisions/2014/dab2576.pdf

19. Dorsen C, Devanter NV. Open arms, conflicted hearts: Nurse-practitioner's attitudes towards working with lesbian, gay and bisexual patients. *J Clin Nurs.* 2016;25(23–24):3716–3727. doi:10.1111/jocn.13464

20. Bjarnadottir RI, Bockting W, Trifilio M, Dowding DW. Assessing sexual orientation and gender identity in home health care: Perceptions and attitudes of nurses. *LGBT Health.* 2019;6(8):409–416. doi:10.1089/lgbt.2019.0030

21. Higgins A, Hynes G. Meeting the needs of people who identify as lesbian, gay, bisexual, transgender, and queer in palliative care settings. *J Hosp Palliat Nurs.* 2019;21(4):286–290. doi:10.1097/NJH.0000000000000525

22. Fish J, Williamson I, Brown J. Disclosure in lesbian, gay and bisexual cancer care: Towards a salutogenic healthcare environment. *BMC Cancer.* 2019;19(1):678. doi:10.1186/s12885-019-5895-7

23. Caceres BA, Ancheta AJ, Dorsen C, Newlin-Lew K, Edmondson D, Hughes TL. A population-based study of the intersection of sexual identity and race/ethnicity on physiological risk factors for CVD among US adults (ages 18–59). *Ethn Health.* 2020;0(0):1–22. doi:10.1080/13557858.2020.1740174

24. Perrin PB, Sutter ME, Trujillo MA, Henry RS, Pugh M. The minority strengths model: Development and initial path analytic validation in racially/ethnically diverse LGBTQ individuals. *J Clinical Psych.* 2020;76(1):118–136. doi:10.1002/jclp.22850

25. Margolies L, Brown CG. Increasing cultural competence with LGBTQ patients. *Nursing.* 2019;49(6):34–40. doi:10.1097/01.NURSE.0000558088.77604.24

26. Scheer JR, Pachankis JE. Psychosocial syndemic risks surrounding physical health conditions among sexual and gender minority individuals. *LGBT Health.* 2019;6(8):377–385. doi:10.1089/lgbt.2019.0025

27. Gonzales G, Przedworski J, Henning-Smith C. Comparison of health and health risk factors between lesbian, gay, and bisexual adults and heterosexual adults in the United States: Results from the National Health Interview Survey. *JAMA Intern Med.* 2016;176(9):1344–1351. doi:10.1001/jamainternmed.2016.3432

28. Schuler MS, Prince DM, Breslau J, Collins RL. Substance use disparities at the intersection of sexual identity and race/ethnicity: Results from the 2015–2018 National Survey on Drug Use and Health. *LGBT Health.* 2020;7(6):283–291. doi:10.1089/lgbt.2019.0352

29. Nguyen KH, Trivedi AN, Shireman TI. Lesbian, gay, and bisexual adults report continued problems affording care despite coverage gains. *Health Aff.* 2018;37(8):1306–1312. doi:10.1377/hlthaff.2018.0281

30. Valenti KG, Jen S, Parajuli J, Arbogast A, Jacobsen AL, Kunkel S. Experiences of palliative and end-of-life care among older LGBTQ women: A review of current literature. *J Palliat Med.* 2020;23(11):1532–1539. doi:10.1089/jpm.2019.0639

31. Fraser B, Pierse N, Chisholm E, Cook H. LGBTIQ+ homelessness: A review of the literature. *Int J Environ Res Public Health.* 2019;16(15):2677. Published 2019 Jul 26. doi:10.3390/ijerph16152677

32. Centers for Disease Control and Prevention. *HIV Surveillance Report, 2018 (Updated)*; vol. 31. Published May 2020. https://www.cdc.gov/hiv/pdf/library/reports/surveillance/cdc-hiv-surveillance-report-2018-updated-vol-31.pdf

33. Yang HY, Beymer MR, Suen S. Chronic disease onset among people living with HIV and AIDS in a large private insurance claims dataset. *Sci Rep.* 2019;9(1):18514. doi:10.1038/s41598-019-54969-3

34. Gonzales G, Zinone R. Cancer diagnoses among lesbian, gay, and bisexual adults: Results from the 2013–2016 National Health Interview Survey. *Cancer Causes Control.* 2018;29(9):845–854. doi:10.1007/s10552-018-1060-x

35. Haviland KS, Swette S, Kelechi T, Mueller M. Barriers and facilitators to cancer screening among LGBTQ individuals with cancer. *Oncol Nurs Forum*. 2020;47(1):44–55. doi:10.1188/20.ONF.44-55

36. Kelly D, Sakellariou D, Fry S, Vougioukalou S. Heteronormativity and prostate cancer: A discursive paper. *J Clin Nurs*. 2018;27(1–2):461–467. doi:10.1111/jocn.13844

37. Cathcart-Rake EJ, Breitkopf CR, Kaur J, O'Connor J, Ridgeway JL, Jatoi A. Teaching health-care providers to query patients with cancer about sexual and gender minority (SGM) status and sexual health. *Am J Hosp Palliat Care*. 2019;36(6):533–537. doi:10.1177/1049909118820874

38. Seay J, Mitteldorf D, Yankie A, Pirl WF, Kobetz E, Schlumbrecht M. Survivorship care needs among LGBT cancer survivors. *J Psychosoc Oncol*. 2018;36(4):393–405. doi:10.1080/07347332.2018.1447528

39. Peitzmeier SM, Bernstein IM, McDowell MJ, et al. Enacting power and constructing gender in cervical cancer screening encounters between transmasculine patients and health care providers. *Cult Health Sex*. 2020;22(12):1315–1332. doi:10.1080/13691058.2019.1677942

40. National Center for Transgender Equality. Resources. Understanding Drag. April 28, 2017. https://transequality.org/issues/resources/understanding-drag

41. Boehmer U, Gereige J, Winter M, Ozonoff A, Scout N. Transgender individuals' cancer survivorship: Results of a cross-sectional study. *Cancer*. 2020;126(12):2829–2836. doi:10.1002/cncr.32784

42. Shiu C, Muraco A, Fredriksen-Goldsen K. Invisible care: Friend and partner care among older lesbian, gay, bisexual, and transgender (LGBT) adults. *J Soc Social Work Res*. 2016;7(3):527–546. doi:10.1086/687325

43. *Gen Silent*. 2010. The Clowder Group. Available at https://www.theclowdergroup.com/gensilent

44. Bloemen EM, Rosen T, LoFaso VM, et al. Lesbian, gay, bisexual, and transgender older adults' experiences with elder abuse and neglect. *J Am Geriatr Soc*. 2019;67(11):2338–2345. doi:10.1111/jgs.16101

45. Cloyes KG, Hull W, Davis A. Palliative and end-of-life care for lesbian, gay, bisexual, and transgender (LGBT) cancer patients and their caregivers. *Semin Oncol Nurs*. 2018;34(1):60–71. doi:10.1016/j.soncn.2017.12.003

46. Escher C, Gomez R, Paulraj S, et al. Relations of religion with depression and loneliness in older sexual and gender minority adults. *Clin Gerontol*. 2019;42(2):150–161. doi:10.1080/07317115.2018.1514341

47. Bristowe K, Marshall S, Harding R. The bereavement experiences of lesbian, gay, bisexual and/or trans* people who have lost a partner: A systematic review, thematic synthesis and modelling of the literature. *Palliat Med*. 2016;30(8):730–744. doi:10.1177/0269216316634601

48. Kuzma EK, Pardee M, Darling-Fisher CS. Lesbian, gay, bisexual, and transgender health: Creating safe spaces and caring for patients with cultural humility. *J Am Assoc Nurse Pract*. 2019;31(3):167–174. doi:10.1097/JXX.0000000000000131

49. Acquaviva KD. *LGBTQ-Inclusive Hospice and Palliative Care: A Practical Guide to Transforming Professional Practice*. New York: Harrington Park Press; 2017.

50. Bonvicini KA. LGBT healthcare disparities: What progress have we made? *Patient Educ Couns*. 2017;100(12):2357–2361. doi:10.1016/j.pec.2017.06.003

51. Cloyes KG, Tay DL, Iacob E, Jones M, Reblin M, Ellington L. Hospice interdisciplinary team providers' attitudes toward sexual and gender minority patients and caregivers. *Patient Educ Couns*. 2020;103(10):2185–2191. doi:10.1016/j.pec.2020.07.004

52. Human Rights Campaign. Resources. Glossary of terms. 2021. Available at https://www.hrc.org/resources/glossary-of-terms

53. Lambda Legal. Making the Case for Equality. Home page. 2021. Available at https://www.lambdalegal.org/node/24885

54. LGBT HealthLink Health Equity Network. Cancer best practices. 2021. https://www.lgbthealthlink.org/Cancer-Best-Practices

55. National LGBT Cancer Network. Website. 2021. Available at https://cancer-network.org/

56. National LGBTQIA+ Health Education Center A program of the Fenway Institute. 2021. Available at https://www.lgbtqiahealtheducation.org

57. SAGE Advocacy and Services for LGBT Seniors. Home page. 2021. Available at https://www.sageusa.org/

58. Substance Abuse and Mental Health Services Administration. Lesbian, gay, bisexual, and transgender (LGBT). Last Update July 30, 2021. https://www.samhsa.gov/behavioral-health-equity/lgbt

59. University of California San Francisco Prevention Science. Center of Excellence for Transgender Health. Mission and Vision. 2021. https://prevention.ucsf.edu/transhealth

60. Patterson JG, Jabson Tree JM, Kamen C. Cultural competency and microaggressions in the provision of care to LGBT patients in rural and Appalachian Tennessee. *Patient Educ Couns*. 2019;102(11):2081–2090. doi:10.1016/j.pec.2019.06.003

61. Stein GL, Berkman C, O'Mahony S, Godfrey D, Javier NM, Maingi S. Experiences of lesbian, gay, bisexual, and transgender patients and families in hospice and palliative care: Perspectives of the palliative care team. *J Palliat Med*. 2020;23(6):817–824. doi:10.1089/jpm.2019.0542

62. Kamen CS, Alpert A, Margolies L, et al. "Treat us with dignity": A qualitative study of the experiences and recommendations of lesbian, gay, bisexual, transgender, and queer (LGBTQ) patients with cancer. *Support Care Cancer*. 2019;27(7):2525–2532. doi:10.1007/s00520-018-4535-0

23.

CARE OF VETERANS WITH PALLIATIVE CARE NEEDS

Alice C. Foy, Robert David Rice, and Joseph Albert Melocoton

KEY POINTS

- Veterans are a unique population. Knowledge and understanding of the veteran experience, whether during conflict or peacetime, is essential.

- Only a quarter of veterans receive care within veterans' programs. Numerous veterans receive care in communities across all geographies in the United States. Therefore, the palliative advanced practice registered nurse (APRN) must assess for military service and identify local and regional resources.

- Subpopulations of often marginalized veterans deserve special attention and include women veterans, LGBTQ+ veterans, veterans experiencing homelessness, veterans with mental health diagnoses, and veterans with substance use disorder, as well as veterans with both dual diagnoses of mental health and substance use disorders. These veterans may well have especially nuanced needs at end of life given the intersectionality these identities will impose on what may already be challenged coping and adapting skills.

- Within the Veterans Health Administration, there are exceptional resources to care for veterans in all phases of acute and chronic care, including end-of-life care, to guide the delivery of quality, veteran-focused palliative care.

CASE STUDY: PALLIATIVE CARE FOR A VETERAN

Eddie was a 71-year-old Vietnam War veteran with Stage IV pancreatic cancer. Because his cancer responded poorly to treatment and he was not a candidate for additional treatment, he was referred to an outpatient palliative care consultation service by his oncologist. His past medical history was complex including hepatitis C, type 2 diabetes, significant alcohol use history (4–5 beers per day), a brief history of intravenous drug 10 years prior, depression, and generalized anxiety disorder (GAD). The oncologist shared Eddie's history of homelessness; but Eddie had lived in low-income housing for 2 years. She noted that he was reluctant to trust providers, that his follow-up had been sporadic, with a history of leaving hospitalizations against medical advice. She mentioned his brief military service and its effect on his actions and behaviors. Eddie's prognosis was less than 6 months, and the oncologist worried about his poor social supports, his inability to care for himself, and her fear of him falling through the cracks.

At his appointment, the palliative advanced practice registered nurse (APRN), Kim, who was educated about trauma-informed care, applied several principles during their encounter. Kim asked if he would like to meet with the door open or closed, explained in detail all aspects of her physical exam, and asked for permission before each step. Kim took extra time to listen and did not push him when he seemed hesitant. Initially he was withdrawn and stoic, but he slowly began to open up regarding his goals and concerns. He shared his knowledge of his advanced disease but wanted to live as long as possible because he felt guilty about his past life and had many relationships to mend. He shared that he pushed away most people in his life and now worried about dying alone and not having anyone to care for him when he became weaker. He expressed fear of what dying might feel like. He noted that he felt people doubted his pain and thought he was drug seeking due to his past history with drugs and alcohol. Although his pain had been controlled so far, he has been waking up more at night and "remembering bad things I saw during the Vietnam War."

The palliative APRN reassured him that his pain management will be diligent, with sensitivity to his history. They discussed how hospice would manage his increasing pain needs and reviewed options for extreme or unmanaged pain at the end of life, such as palliative sedation. He agreed to a posttraumatic stress disorder (PTSD) screening, which was positive. He demonstrated signs of worsening chronic depression, and Kim suspected possible moral injury related to some of his shame-based statements about his war experience. Kim reached out to the Veteran's Administration (VA) PTSD consultation program and was able to speak with a specialist who recommended starting a selective serotonin reuptake inhibitor (SSRI). They also offered virtual counseling services for the veteran, and Eddie expressed interest in this program.

The palliative APRN requested the social worker to notify the local VA palliative care service to assist the veteran with accessing his VA-related hospice benefits. The social worker also initiated reassuring conversations with him about resources, including home assistance and placement options when his care needs began to escalate. The palliative APRN referred him to a local hospice that participates in the *We Honor Veterans* Program. These hospice professionals had extra training in caring for veterans as well as a volunteer program staffed with other veterans who might provide needed visitation and support. Kim informed Eddie that the hospice social worker would begin to guide him in locating the lost family he hoped to make amends with and could also assist him with legacy work. Kim knew the chaplain would provide needed support for his experience of moral injury.

The palliative APRN thanked Eddie for trusting her with the painful parts of his life and expressed gratitude for the service he gave to the country and the burdens he has carried afterward. In completing her consult, Kim assessed for depression and suicidal ideation, which was negative. Kim scheduled follow-up telephone appointments for a symptom check and medication management, as well as oncology, and ensured the coordination of hospice.

INTRODUCTION

Veterans represent a unique cultural group and a complex population. Title 38 of the *Code of Federal Regulations* defines a veteran as "a person who served in the active military, naval, or air service and who was discharged or released under conditions other than dishonorable."[1] A *military veteran* is a person who has served in one or more branches of the military and is no longer in active service. Veterans who have served directly in combat are considered *war veterans*. *Active service* refers to full-time service as a member of the Army, Navy, Marine Corps, Air Force, Coast Guard, National Guard, or Reserves, or as a commissioned officer of the Public Health Service or the National Oceanic and Atmospheric Administration.[2]

There are approximately 20.3 million living military veterans in the United States and, approximately 15.7 million veterans served in wartime.[3] Fifty-five percent of living veterans are 60 years of age or older. Twenty-four percent are between the ages of 65 and 74, and 23% are between the ages of 75 and 85 and over.[3] Women only represent about 10% of veterans.[3]

While World War II and the Korean War veterans are the oldest of the veteran population, the demographics of the Vietnam War veterans present an aging population with physical and mental health comorbidities which put them at risk. There are an estimated 6.4 million Vietnam era veterans ranging in age from 60 to 102 years old (born between 1918 and 1960).[4] Most notably now because of issues of aging, serious illness, and end-of-life care is the generation of veterans from the Vietnam War. Seventy-five percent of these veterans are older than 65.[4]

The 2.8 million all-voluntary post-9/11 veterans include those in US-led conflicts in Afghanistan and Iraq (Operation Enduring Freedom [OEF], Afghanistan; Operation Iraqi Freedom [OIF], Iraq; and Operation New Dawn [OND], Afghanistan). They are more often younger, male, and White.[4] Service-related disabilities, at 35.9%, are nearly two times as high compared to veterans of previous wars. This is in part due to the survivability of modern-day warfare compared to past combat. Interestingly, a lower percentage of post-9/11 veterans are enrolled in Veteran's Health Administration healthcare under Veterans Affairs (VA) than all other veterans, at only 20.7%.[4]

Nearly half, 9.8 of 20.3 million, of all US veterans used at least one VA service or benefit in fiscal year 2017.[5] All enrolled veterans are eligible for hospice care if they meet the clinical criteria for hospice care.[6] Care, including hospice care, may be delivered in VA medical centers. Of note, 4.7 million veterans live in rural areas: 2.7 million of these veterans are enrolled in VA care and 55% of veterans in rural areas are 65 years and older.[7] Much of the health and medical care services for veterans, including outpatient primary and specialty clinic services, home care, pharmacy, and palliative and hospice care, may be delivered by community providers. Given the unique needs of veterans at end of life, palliative APRNs play a critical role in delivering quality care that addresses the veteran's specific needs, values, and preferences.[8] While many of those needs are similar to the general population, such as symptom management, grief counseling, psychological coping, and seeking closure, care of veterans will have nuances unique to the worldview and life experiences of the veteran.

While veterans, particularly those having served in combat, share unique experiences, it is disingenuous to assume that they all share common experiences. Wars and conflicts each have their place in history. The veteran's service experience will have a profound effect on how they face serious illness and death, including their age and own history. These experiences will be linked to the generation in which the veteran served and encountered them, as well as the life course framework in which the veteran finds themself at the time of the serious illness.[9] The oldest veterans, those from World War II and the Korean War eras, will have a different life perspective than much younger men from the more recent conflicts in the Southwest Asia (the United States has between 60,000 and 70,000 troops stationed in numerous countries in the region).[10]

Men soldiers and women nurses from the earlier wars may have experienced severe, debilitating injuries, particularly if they were prisoners of war (POW). Frostbitten body parts may have portended long-standing cold sensitivity, neuropathic pain, and even the development of skin cancers.[11] Veterans who participated in what is known as "radiation-risk activities" may have developed, subsequent to ionizing radiation exposure, any number of solid tumor cancers and hematologic malignancies such as leukemia, aggressive non-Hodgkin lymphomas, and multiple myeloma.[12]

Hepatitis C (HCV) infection is a chronic health condition. It is particularly prevalent in the general population born between 1945 and 1965, as well as in the Vietnam veteran population which overlaps this era.[13] Chronic and acute HCV infection can cause liver failure, liver cancer, and cirrhosis. With the advent of direct-acting antiviral (DAA) HCV therapy beginning in 2014, the VA has treated more than 92,000 HCV-infected veterans, with cure rates exceeding 90%.[13] Given the preponderance of risk, the chronicity and latency of HCV infection, and therapies that can cure the disease, palliative APRNs should presumptively test for HCV infection in this population.

Vietnam War veterans who had potential exposure to Agent Orange, a tactical herbicide used by the US military to control vegetation, may experience a variety of health conditions such as soft tissue sarcomas, lymphomas, respiratory cancers, blood disorders, and acute peripheral neuropathy.[14] Gulf War veterans had potential exposure to pesticides; oil well fires; heat injuries; chemical and biological weapon exposure; sand, dust, and particulate exposure; noise exposure;

infectious disease exposure; and more. A prominent, chronic, multisymptom illness is described by Gulf War veterans and is being followed closely in a multiyear health survey. These symptom clusters, which are largely otherwise medically unexplained, include dizziness, breathing disorders, insomnia, fatigue, headaches, myalgias, indigestion, and memory issues.[15] Amyotrophic lateral sclerosis (ALS) has been found to disproportionately affect veterans regardless of military branch or service era. As a result, the VA has established service-connected benefits for this population. When a palliative care patient has a diagnosis of ALS and a history of military service, helping them connect to the VA can provide much-needed financial and medical support including home care services, adaptive devices and home modifications, and specialized ALS medical care provided at facilities throughout the country.[16,17]

The phenomenon of PTSD is described in relation to all wars. In the US Civil War, it was called "soldier's heart"; in World War I, "shell shock"; and in World War II, "combat fatigue."[18] PTSD became formalized as a psychiatric diagnostic criterion after extensive experience with Vietnam War veterans. The DSM-5 diagnostic criteria for PTSD can be found at this reference and there will be further discussion of the condition later in the chapter.[19]

To better serve veterans, the palliative APRN should be familiar with these generational and situational specificities of wartime veterans (and peacetime veterans). An excellent web-based resource, sponsored by the National Hospice and Palliative Care Organization (NHPCO), is called *We Honor Veterans* and can be found at https://www.wehonorveterans.org/.[20]

MILITARY CULTURE

Hallmarks of military culture are commitment to the mission and a number of espoused values. These values include honor, duty, courage, commitment, respect, integrity, selfless service (service before self), and personal courage, to name a few (shared among branches) (Table 23.1).

The integration of a shared military ethos begins with basic training—or boot camp—where men and women of diverse backgrounds, geographies, socioeconomic status, religious and political backgrounds, ethnicities, and races undergo intensive training, field exercises, and classroom time. Spurred on by strong military purpose and survival instincts, the inductees gain skills and experiences intended to support responsibility, purpose, discipline, technical and

Table 23.1 SERVICE BRANCHES OF THE US MILITARY

MAIN MILITARY SERVICE BRANCHES	FUNCTION	MOTTO
Army	The Army defends the land mass of the United States, its territories, commonwealths, and possessions. It does so through providing forces and capabilities for sustained combat and stability operations on land. The Army also provides logistics and support to other branches. The Army is the largest and oldest branch of the military.	This We'll Defend[21]
Marine Corps	The Marine Corps maintains ready expeditionary forces, sea-based and integrated air-ground units for contingency and combat operations, and the means to stabilize or contain international disturbance. The Marine Corps is an immediate response force that can be used to overwhelm the enemy.[22]	*Semper Fidelis* "Always Faithful"[21]
Navy	The Navy maintains, trains, and equips combat-ready maritime forces capable of winning wars, deterring aggression, and maintaining freedom of the seas. The Navy is America's forward deployed force and is a major deterrent to aggression around the world.[22]	*Semper Fortis* "Always Courageous"[21]
Air Force	The Air Force provides a rapid, flexible, and, when necessary, lethal air and space capability that can deliver forces anywhere in the world in less than 48 hours. It routinely participates in peacekeeping, humanitarian, and aeromedical evacuation missions. Air Force crews annually fly missions into all but five nations of the world.[22]	"Aim High . . . Fly-Fight-Win"[21]
Space Force	The US Space Force (USSF) is the newest branch of the Armed Forces, established December 20, 2019. The USSF was established within the Department of the Air Force, meaning that the Secretary of the Air Force has overall responsibility for the USSF, under the guidance and direction of the Secretary of Defense.[23]	*Semper Supra* "Always Above"[24]
Coast Guard	The Coast Guard provides law and maritime safety enforcement, marine and environmental protection, and military naval support. Activities can include patrolling our shores, performing emergency rescue operations, containing and cleaning up oil spills, and keeping illegal drugs from entering American communities.[22]	*Semper Paratus* "Always Ready"[21]

tactical proficiency (often leading to occupational specialty training), maturity, strength and resiliency, coping, and pride. The dedication to service over self leads to teamwork and cooperation, protecting the welfare of the team and creating deep friendships.[25]

When service men and women return to civilian life, though, they may drift from the loss of the military community. In dealing with the rigors of military life and combat, veterans may have developed a self-defense mechanism of *stoicism*, which, in challenging times, can be quite helpful. However, in post-military life this may result in a steeling against physical, emotional, and psychological challenges. The idea of self-sufficiency takes precedence over the threat, be it external (such as an attack) or internal (such as cancer-related pain). The "can-do" mentality minimizes the effect of adverse events. The mind overconstructs and imposes this burden on the soldier, and, as a result, the soldier becomes traumatized and may not be able to resolve the bad event.[26]

TRAUMA-INFORMED CARE

When working with veterans, it is essential to let their individual experience guide a thoughtful approach to care planning to promote a culture of empathy and support. *Trauma-informed care* focuses on treating the individual where they are. The palliative APRN must acknowledge that the veteran may have experienced a traumatic event (or multiple traumatic events) and understand the comprehensive picture of how past traumas and subsequent coping mechanisms influence health behaviors and the veteran's response to illness and treatment. This approach to care recognizes the potential impact and consequences of military experience in one's life and informs an evidence-based plan of care that focuses on both physical and psychological needs while ensuring emotional safety.[27] Understanding the effects of trauma can enable a more successful experience in managing and supporting symptoms and other needs, whether the goal is prolonging life or ensuring a peaceful death.

Supporting the complex needs and experience of veterans in the community can be daunting. When veterans are formally enrolled in the VA system, many programs exist to assist both veterans and the palliative APRNs in accessing the delivery of entitlements and resources, including mental health support and palliative care, which are available in person and through telemedicine. Reaching out and partnering with the palliative care providers at local VA centers can assist the community-based palliative APRN with managing the veteran with complex end-of-life issues. A comprehensive care planning guide and free training resources can be found at *We Honor Veterans*–Trauma-Informed Care.[28]

Important initial steps in trauma-focused care are recognizing and screening for common issues such as PTSD, suicidal ideation, and moral injury. It is important to ask patients (or their caregiver) if they have ever served in the military and if they are willing to discuss their service, including possibly completing a military history checklist. Central to providing meaningful trauma-informed care is a thorough understanding of military culture, the uniqueness of each era in which a veteran has served, and how it might have determined their individual experience. Specific groups, including those who have experienced interpersonal violence such as military sexual trauma (MST), will have additional considerations.[29] Women who experienced sexual trauma generally have sexual dysfunction and lower sexual satisfaction. They may have co-morbid mental health issues with the sexual dysfunction.[30] One study found that while most women veterans felt welcome at the VA (85%), a significant percentage (26%) -had "stories about feeling uncomfortable or harassed in the VA."[31] The opportunities for further inquiry and research based on the experience of women veterans are numerous.

POSTTRAUMATIC STRESS DISORDER

PTSD is experienced by up to 7% of the US population at some point during their lifetime, with the highest incidence being in women. In recent studies, 10.6% of veterans being cared for at the VA had a diagnosis of PTSD, and, in the population that served in Iraq or Afghanistan, 27.6% have received the diagnosis.[32] Individuals with PTSD can have an extra layer of complexity to their symptoms and end-of-life experience. PTSD may increase distress and amplify symptoms, particularly pain. Avoidance behaviors may undermine the ability to establish trust and interfere with continuity of medical care and following medical advice. Life-long behaviors related to trauma, including social isolation and avoidance, may result in diminished relationships, which are often a vital source of caregiving and support at end of life.[33]

Assessing and diagnosing PTSD can be critical to providing good end-of-life care and can start with a military history checklist and further exploring any history of trauma.[34] Family, when available, can also be an important source of history. The VA has specific screening resources available on their website via the PTSD Consultation Program. The Primary Care PTSD Screen (available at www.ptsd.va.gov) is a five-item tool that identifies exposure to trauma and its effects on life and is developed for use in a primary care setting.[35]

Treatment for PTSD includes both psychotherapy and pharmacotherapy. Examples of evidence-based therapies are detailed in the Table 23.2. Current guidelines favor trauma-focused psychotherapy as the first-line treatment for PTSD over pharmacotherapy. However, pharmacotherapy may be a preferred approach for some veterans, and medications may be essential in the instance of psychiatric comorbidity.[40] Current VA and Department of Defense (DoD) recommended pharmacotherapy approaches are detailed in Table 23.3.

In selecting the best approach to treatment, estimated prognosis as well as physical and emotional energy available to devote to interventions should be considered. A stepwise approach includes addressing immediate discomfort while ensuring social supports, enhancing coping skills, and later focusing on trauma-specific issues.[42] Strategies for the palliative APRN to support the veteran with PTSD include therapeutic presence. This allows veterans to express emotion and

Table 23.2 THERAPIES FOR POSTTRAUMATIC STRESS DISORDER (PTSD)

PROCEDURE	COGNITIVE PROCESSING THERAPY (CPT)[36]	PROLONGED EXPOSURE THERAPY (PE)[37]	EYE MOVEMENT AND DESENSITIZATION AND REPROCESSING (EDMR)[38]	WRITTEN EXPOSURE THERAPY (WET)[39]
Evidence	Well-studied	Well-studied	Highly studied in civilian populations with strong recommendation as effective treatment.	Increasingly studied and found to be effective. Notable for low attrition rates.
Model and Process	Helps identify how trauma has altered both thoughts and feelings and reorganizes information to provide new interpretation of the experience.	Involves repeated exposure to fears, such as talking about the trauma, over and over, in a safe environment until the impact begins to diminish and emotions and fears are reduced in response to stimuli.	Goal is to change the reaction to memories of trauma by focusing on new learning being assimilated separately from existing memory pathways. Often involves focusing on external stimuli while recalling traumatic events (back-and-forth eye movements or sound).	Experiences of trauma, including thoughts and emotions, are explored through structured writing sessions which include ongoing support and feedback.
Application	Given in both individual and group settings. Helpful in patients with comorbid conditions (such as depression and personality disorders).	Useful in patients with comorbid psychological conditions.	Not studied in comorbid populations. Shorter treatment duration and easier training of providers may make this a useful intervention for hospice teams.	Can be given in both individual and group settings.

Table 23.3 COMMON MEDICATIONS USED FOR POSTTRAUMATIC STRESS DISORDER (PTSD)

THERAPEUTIC CATEGORY	INITIAL DOSE	DOSE RANGE	CLINICAL CONSIDERATIONS: COMORBIDITIES AND SAFETY
Antidepressants *Monotherapy* Fluoxetine[a] Paroxetine[a] Sertraline[a] Venlafaxine[a]	10–20 mg daily 10–20 mg daily 25–60 mg daily IR: 25 mg 2 or 3 times a day XR: 37.5 mg once daily	20–80 mg daily 20–50 mg daily 50–200 mg daily 75–375 mg in 2–3 divided doses of 75–225 mg once daily	Avoid abrupt discontinuation; withdrawal symptoms with sudden discontinuation of SSRIs and SNRIs, paroxetine and venlafaxine in particular Paroxetine and sertraline have FDA label indications for treating PTSD Common adverse effects of the SSRIs and SNRIs include nausea, headache, diarrhea, anxiety, nervousness, sexual dysfunction, agitation, dizziness, hyponatremia or SIADH, and serotonin syndrome Venlafaxine can elevate blood pressure; caution advised with patients with hypertension
Nefazodone[b]	25–100 mg 2 times daily	150–600 mg in 2 divided doses	Nefazodone is associated with life-threatening hepatic failure; monitor for signs and symptoms including LFTs; avoid if active liver disease; do not re-challenge Nefazodone is subject to many drug interactions, particularly those involving CYP3A4 and glycoprotein
Imipramine[b]	25–75 mg daily	100–300 mg in 1 or 2 divided doses	Avoid TCAs within 3 months of an acute MI TCAs are relatively contraindicated in patients with coronary artery disease or prostatic enlargement TCAs side effects include dry mouth, dry eyes, constipation, orthostatic hypotension, tachycardia, ventricular arrhythmias, weight gain, and drowsiness Photosensitivity may occur
Phenelzine[b]	15 mg 3 times daily	15 mg daily; 90 mg in divided doses	Phenelzine considerations include drug-drug and drug-food interactions, risk of hypertensive crisis, hypotension, and anticholinergic effects

Reprinted with permission

FDA, Food and Drug Administration; IR, immediate release; LFT, liver function tests; mg, milligram; MI, myocardial infarction; PTSD, posttraumatic stress disorder; SIADH, syndrome of inappropriate anti-diuretic hormone; SIT, Stress Inoculation Training; SNRI, serotonin-norepinephrine reuptake inhibitor; SSRI, serotonin reuptake inhibitors; TCA, tricyclic antidepressant; XR, extended release.

[a] Strong recommendation.

[b] Weak recommendation.

Adapted with permission from The Management of Posttraumatic Stress Disorder Work Group, Department of Veterans Affairs & Department of Defense.[41]

validate painful or traumatic events, and it helps them to feel in control and to focus on strengths and resilience and avoid triggers.[43]

The VA recognizes the complexity and challenges of treating this condition, including the need to be able to access the latest assessment and diagnostic tools and receive guidance in evolving medication strategies. Individual guidance for the palliative APRN, as well as clinical management tools and resources that can be given to the veteran, are readily available through the free PTSD Consultation Program (www. ptsd.va.gov/consult or 866-948-7880). In addition to war- and military-related trauma, additional guidance and education is available around contemporary issues faced by many veterans, including PTSD and concomitant minority stress among LGBTQ+ individuals, racism-related stress and trauma, and experiences related to the COVID-19 pandemic.[3,44]

MORAL INJURY

PTSD is not the singular form of emotional suffering that veterans face following military service. Often they carry deeper wounds, sometimes described as spiritual, existential, or "soul wounds" that do not respond to standard treatments. This is an increasingly common experience of shame- and guilt-based disturbances that some combat veterans experience after engaging in wartime acts of commission (such as killing), omission (such as failing to prevent atrocities), or simply acts felt to be transgressive and in violation of the goodness perceived in self or others. This experience in the "affliction of conscience" is felt to be the fallout of "morally injurious experiences: Perpetrating, failing to prevent, bearing witness to, or learning about acts that transgress deeply held moral beliefs and expectations."[45 (p.700)] These experiences cause *moral injury* which is known to intensify relational problems, social anxiety, isolation, depression, and suicide. The experience of shame "amplifies the impact of trauma across every category."[46 (p. 56)]

Veterans struggling with moral injury at the end of life may have particular sets of issues that can complicate illness and decline. The life review may reopen unresolved emotional and spiritual wounds. Seriously ill veterans may be unable to forgive themselves or be forgiven by others. They may not trust anyone enough to open up about their negative experiences. They may fear that they are not worthy of redemption and may experience enhanced despair due to loss of life meaning and purpose.[47] To support the veteran with suspected or known moral injury, a coordinated approach to care will include hospice chaplains, social workers, and mental health providers in addition to a compassionate and understanding nurse practitioner. A toolkit of techniques called Stress First Aid is available to support these caregivers.[48]

LGBTQ+ VETERANS

Despite the fact that the Department of Veterans Affairs is presumed to be the largest provider of healthcare for LGBTQ+ (lesbian, gay, bisexual, transgender, queer and questioning, and related identities) veterans, research on end-of-life needs for this population is scant. Many of these veterans have likely faced homophobia, stigma, harassment, and discrimination during their military service, often based on military policy. These acts may have significant long-term effects on their health and well-being. The LGBTQ+ population already has higher risks for depression and suicide, amplified by multiple chronic medical conditions and poor health outcomes.[49] A lifetime of coping with these issues impacts the dying process. Negative experiences may also erode trust and prevent a veteran or their family from seeking much-needed support or resources through the VA.[50] It is essential that the palliative APRN be skilled in communication with LGBTQ+ veterans. Having a relationship of trust and openness with their provider can be an important protective factor [50,51] (see Chapter 22, "LGBTQ+ Inclusive Palliative Care").

To address and support the unique needs of this vulnerable population, most VA facilities have LGBTQ+ websites. All facilities also have an LGBTQ+ Veteran Care Coordinator who can assist veterans with finding culturally competent caregivers comfortable with caring for them.[52] Veteran-based programs and resources that are often essential during terminal illness require a connection through discharge status. For LGBTQ+ veterans, that status may have been undermined by previous policies that forced involuntary separation from the military due to sexual orientation, designating their discharge as "undesirable" or "dishonorable." The *Bay Area Reporter* estimates that 114,000 veterans were "involuntarily separated from the military due to their sexual orientation between the end of World War II and the repeal in 2011 of the homophobic 'Don't Ask, Don't Tell' policy that barred LGBTQ+ individuals from serving openly in the military."[53,54] The acceptance of LGBTQ+ service members remains an active political issue. In 2011, the Obama administration reversed the "Don't Ask Don't Tell" policy and removed restrictions on transgender individuals serving in the military in 2016. This was reversed by Trump administration in 2017. In 2021, the Biden administrative again allowed transgendered service members to openly serve.

Even though veterans can upgrade or correct their discharges, many do not choose to do this because of the time and often substantial effort required to do so. The VA now lends assistance through its website to veterans who have a less than honorable discharge related to issues such as PTSD, sexual orientation (including Don't Ask, Don't Tell), MST, and traumatic brain injury (TBI). The VA provides guidance on discharge upgrades and valuable links to local Veteran Service Organizations, which have specialized claims agents and attorneys who can assist and advocate for veterans when navigating this process.[55] The website also provides guidance to pursue a discharge status upgrade, which may be useful for the veteran not only in terms of resources and benefits, but may also bring end-of-life closure to an experience of trauma, shame, or victimization experienced during their military service and ensure that they are recognized with the honor they are due.

SUBSTANCE USE DISORDERS AND PAIN MANAGEMENT

Management of pain is central to the care of veterans, especially at the end of life. The VA offers comprehensive pain management that is typically provided by an interdisciplinary collaborative team using multimodal approaches (pharmacological and nonpharmacological therapies). Veterans' experiences during their service, stoicism, psychological trauma, chronic disorders, and sociocultural factors (to name a few) can complicate and contribute to suboptimal pain management. Substance use disorder (SUD) remains a significant problem among veterans, and there is an increased risk of suicide associated with SUD for both male and female veterans.[56] (See Chapter 47, "Patients with Substance Use Disorder and Dual Diagnoses.")

Opioid prescription carries inherent risks and dangers for adverse outcomes such as overdose and death. The Comprehensive Addiction and Recovery Act of 2016 mandated the VA to designate a pain management team (PMT) to expand the Opioid Safety Initiative (OSI) and complementary and integrative medicine (CIM) and establish safe opioid prescribing practices such as the use of prescription drug monitoring programs (PDMPs) and the Opioid Overdose Education and Naloxone Distribution (OEND) Program.[57] Harm-reduction strategies, pain resources, and clinical automated decision support tools to assess for risk of adverse events are also available, such as the Stratification Tool for Opioid Risk Mitigation (STORM; a predictive model that estimates the likelihood of drug overdose or suicide-related events) along with the Opioid Therapy Risk Report (OTTR; a primary care panel report showing data or variables about risks, latest urine drug test results, etc.).

In a study by Davis et al. (2018), approximately 9% of veterans in the United States reported past-year cannabis use.[58] While cannabis is legal in many states for recreational and/or medical use, its use is illegal under federal law. A VA systematic review of the benefits and harm of cannabis for chronic pain and PTSD showed little benefit for either condition. While it may alleviate neuropathic pain, there was limited evidence in other pain or PTSD veteran populations and little generalizable evidence about the long-term effects of cannabis use.[59]

COVID-19 AND VETERANS

The COVID-19 pandemic has affected in-person clinic visits and it is anticipated that the future of healthcare delivery will continue to evolve. To meet the demands in servicing geographically diverse and remotely located veterans, virtual technology consultations and the Specialty Care Access Network Extension for Community Healthcare Outcomes (SCAN-ECHO; a clinical videoconferencing from multiple specialty providers at the outpatient clinic nearest to the veteran's home) provide ways to maintain healthcare access. When transitioning to telehealth, palliative providers must deal with the complexities of intimate goals discussions and end-of-life

planning using technology versus usual care. When family members and loved ones cannot be present at the bedside of their dying loved ones due to restrictive visitation policies, palliative providers may use technology to allow those not present physically to participate virtually. COVID-19 has significantly impacted all health delivery, including home hospice, both in terms of demand for services, as well as in agency staff affected by COVID-19 infection. There is also the concern of patients and families, who fear that outsiders coming into the home may pose a risk of infection transmission.

Thus far during this pandemic, there was a 1,470% increase in virtual care telehealth visits (between March 1 and September 26, 2020) and 453,516 prescription refill requests (between September 27 and October 3, 2020) throughout the entire VA.[60] At the onset of the pandemic, geriatric healthcare providers at the VA also outlined proper education and containment strategies and recommended approaches to COVID-19 mitigation in long-term care facilities.[61]

HOMELESSNESS

Homelessness is a significant problem in the United States, with more than a half million people experiencing homelessness according to a 2017 point-in-time estimate.[62] There are challenges to providing palliative and end-of-life care to homeless veterans from personal, clinical, and structural views. Unstable housing and the risks noted earlier can impact care access and follow-through, particularly for a veteran who has declining functional status and symptom burden, possibly in the context of substance use and behavioral mental health issues.[63] The palliative APRN has several roles: clinical responsibility for pain and symptom management, advocate and care coordinator for the veteran experiencing homelessness, and care manager collaborating with social work services and the hospice agencies to maintain seamless care.

At-risk veterans or veterans experiencing homelessness should be referred to their local VA medical center or call 1-877-424-3838 (1-877-4AID-VET) to access supportive services, which can include housing, aid to employment, medical care, and justice outreach (see Table 23.4). The US Department of Veterans Affairs,[64] Centers for Disease Control and Prevention,[65] the National Alliance to End Homelessness,[66] and other local and national organizations provide resources to support homeless people (see Chapter 21, "Economically Challenged Urban Dwellers").

AN EXEMPLAR PROGRAM

The VA Greater Los Angeles Healthcare System (VAGLAHS) has established support for homeless veterans under the Homeless Veteran Program: Community Engagement and Reintegration Services (CERS). This is the largest VA homeless program in the country, with more than 600 staff and resources to house 10,000 homeless veterans through emergency, transitional, and permanent housing. The CERS care

Table 23.4 HOME- AND COMMUNITY-BASED SERVICES AND SURVIVOR BENEFITS HOME- AND COMMUNITY-BASED SERVICES

Homemaker and Home Health Care Aide[a,b]
- Assistance with ADLs and personal care.
- Provided through a VA-contracted agency to allow vets to remain at home.

Skilled Home Health Care[b]
- Skilled transitional care (e.g., physical therapy, occupational therapy, speech therapy, wound care, etc.; short-term or ongoing).

Veteran-Directed Care
- Budget for private workers for personal care services and ADL assistance, managed by the veteran or their representative.

Home-Based Primary Care[b]
- In-home longitudinal support for those with complex health care needs (e.g., severe illness, difficulty with clinic visits).
- Provided by an interdisciplinary team led by the physician.

Adult Day Health Care[b]
- Provides daytime social activities, peer support, companionship, and recreation through VA medical centers, State Veterans Homes, community organizations.

Caregiver Support Program (see updates from the VA Mission Act website)
- Program of General Caregiver Support Services (PCGSS)
  - Provides education, resources, and support to caregivers of veterans (does not need to have a service-connected condition).
- **Program of Comprehensive Assistance for Family Caregivers (PCAFC)**
  - For eligible veterans who have incurred or aggravated a serious injury in the line of duty on or after September 11, 2001. This program provides caregivers with resources, education, support, a financial stipend, health insurance, and beneficiary travel (if eligible).

Respite Care
Pays for short-term care to allow family/caregivers a break.[a,b]
- Home respite care pays for a person to come to the home.
- Nursing home respite care: Short-term nursing home placement (maximum 30 days).

Remote Monitoring Care
- Allows remote follow-up of health measurements with a care coordinator through a home monitoring equipment.

Home Telehealth
- Designed to give ready access to a care coordinator by using technology (e.g., telephone, computers) at home.
- Enhances and extends care management to caregiver and may include education and training or online and telephone support groups).

Services vary by locations and the local VA Medical Centers will have more information on the programs available.

ADL, activities of daily living.

[a]Can be combined with other home and community-based services.

[b]Services vary by location

Weblink Resource for further information:

https://www.va.gov/GERIATRICS/pages/Home_and_Community_Based_Services.asp

SURVIVOR BENEFITS

Health Insurance
Civilian Health and Medical Program at VA (CHAMPVA)
Provides reimbursement for most medical expenses. The person cannot be eligible for TRICARE and must be one of the following:
- Spouse or child of a permanently rated and totally disabled veteran due to a service-connected (SC) disability.
- Surviving spouse or child of a vet who died from a VA-rated service-connected disability or who, at the time of death, was rated permanently and totally disabled.
- Surviving spouse or child of a veteran who died on active duty service and in the line of duty not due to misconduct (in most cases, these family members are eligible for Tricare).

Note: SC disability is an injury or illness that was incurred or aggravated during active military service; ranges from 0–100% and may qualify for disability compensation per regulation.
* CHAMPVA discontinues when a surviving spouse under 55 remarries.
* For those with Medicare entitlement, CHAMPVA becomes the secondary payer.
* Services can be provided under the CHAMP VA in-house Treatment Initiative Program (CITI).
* Coverage of services depends on the CHAMPVA benefit coverage.

TRICARE
Health program for Uniformed service members, National Guard/Reserve members and their families, survivors, former spouses, medal of honor recipients, and others registered in the Defense Enrollment Eligibility Reporting System (DEERS).
https://www.tricare.mil/Plans/Eligibility

Dependency and Indemnity Compensation (DIC)
- Payment to spouse for a veteran's death from a disease or injury incurred or aggravated while on active duty, active duty training, inactive duty training, or a service-connected illness or injury.

* DIC may be paid to certain survivors of veterans who were totally disabled from service-connected conditions at the time of death, even if their service-connected disabilities did not cause their deaths (please visit the VA website for further details/eligibility/payment rates).
* Veteran's discharge must have been under conditions other than dishonorable.

www.va.gov/burials-memorials/dependency-indemnity-compensation

American Battle Monuments Commission
- No-fee passports may be available to family members who want to visit their loved one's grave at an American military cemetery on international soil.

www.abmc.gov

Table 23.4 CONTINUED

Bereavement Counseling
- Provided through VA Vet Centers for families of service members who die while on active duty (including federally activated members of the National Guard and reserve components).
- Available to all family members of veterans who die unexpectedly at a VA medical center or while under VA hospice or similar programs.

Education Benefits
- Dependents' Education Assistance
- Marine Gunnery Sergeant John David Fry Scholarship
- For children and spouses of members who died in the line of duty after 9/10/2001.
- *Education Benefits for Persons with Special Needs*

Montgomery GI Bill (MGIB) Death Benefit
- For educational assistance to designated survivors in the event of a service-connected death of members on active duty or within 1 year after discharge or release.

For more information, please visit www.gibill.va.gov

Burial and Memorial Benefits
- For veterans discharged from active duty under conditions other than dishonorable
- Burial in a VA cemetery (for eligible veterans, their spouses, and dependents): Includes gravesite, grave liner, opening and closing of the grave, headstones/markers, and perpetual care. Specifically, for veterans, it includes a burial flag, Presidential Memorial Certificate (PMC; if requested), military funeral honor, medallions in lieu of government headstone.
- VA operates 136 national cemeteries; for more information please visit www.cem.va.gov.

Death Pension
- For low-income surviving spouses and unmarried children of deceased veterans with wartime service.

Department of Defense Death Gratuity: One-time tax-free payment of $100,000 to beneficiaries of service-members whose death is a result of hostile actions (through a designated combat operation/zone or while training for combat).

Life Insurance Through Veterans Group Life Insurance & Servicemembers Group Life Insurance (VGLI/SGLI)
- Voluntary life insurance products offered to veterans and active-duty personnel. Not all surviving family members may file a claim on this benefit.

VA Home Loan Guaranty
- For a spouse of a veteran or service member who died from a service-related disability.
- May be available to an unmarried spouse, surviving spouse who remarried at or after age 57, or a spouse of veteran or service member officially listed for more than 90 days as missing in action or currently a prisoner of war.

VA Burial Allowances
- Flat rate monetary benefits to cover burial and funeral costs.
- Service-connected death (on or after September 21, 2001): Maximum burial allowance is $2,000 ($1,500 for those who died before 9/21/2001).
- Non-service-connected death (payable if the veteran was VA-hospitalized at the time of death): $300 burial allowance and $780 for a plot (if death occurred on or after 10/1/2018).
- Cremation: VA does not pay for cremation directly, but families may be entitled to a burial allowance as above.

www.benefits.va.gov/compensation/claims-special-burial.asp

This list is not all-inclusive; further details can be obtained from the VA Office of Survivors Assistance (OSA) at www.va.gov/survivors.

Other useful weblinks:

Directory of Veterans Service Organizations: www.va.gov/vso

We Honor Veterans: https://www.wehonorveterans.org/benefits/survivor-benefits/

Tables compiled by Joseph Albert Melocoton, RN, MSN, NP-C, AOCNS, Palliative Care Advanced Practice Provider at VA Greater Los Angeles Healthcare System.

line includes seven distinct programs which provide services including walk-in centers, justice diversion and jail outreach, employment, short-term treatment programs, and primary and mental health care.

On any given night, there are an estimated 3,500 veterans experiencing homelessness in Greater Los Angeles's service area.[67] In fiscal year 2019, VAGLAHS provided services to almost 16,000 homeless veterans. During this time, GLA placed almost 1,830 veterans into their own apartments. Currently, the West Los Angeles campus has helped veterans with mental health issues and living in tents along the campus edge to move to platformed tents on the great lawn. These spaces provide up to 100 tents to house veterans with mental health issues. A building on campus has been repurposed to provide a recuperative and isolation ward for homeless veterans testing positive for COVID-19. A bridge home provides 100 emergency shelter beds in a large, prefabricated, structure. The master building plan for the organization includes the addition of up to 1,200 occupancy units in the next 2–3 years. These efforts have the

shared goal of keeping veterans safe and moving them to transitional and permanent housing and treatment programs.

The treatment programs include the Homeless Patient Aligned Care Team (medical home) which serves 3,000 veterans annually. This program provides high-intensity, interprofessional, team-based care to homeless veterans and prioritizes open-access, high-quality primary care, mental health care, and social work services. The Housing and Urban Development– VA Supported Housing (HUD-VASH) program is the largest in the country, with 7,440 vouchers assigned and case managing 5,100 formerly homeless veterans in their apartments. The Domiciliary Residential Rehabilitation Treatment Program is a 151-bed residential treatment facility where veterans participate in therapeutic programming each day, 7 days a week. The length of stay is typically between 60 and 90 days. These are just a few of the several integrated programs which make up the larger effort to support homeless veterans and help them transition to a more stable living environment, a healthy lifestyle, and better quality of life (unpublished VA report, on file).

SUICIDE

It is not unusual for individuals with serious illness to consider hastening death. A study that examined the experience of advanced cancer patients found depression and hopelessness to be strongest drivers of this desire.[68] Robinson et al. noted a relationship between poor quality of life and the desire to hasten death that is mediated by depression, loss of meaning and purpose, loss of control, and low self-worth.[69] Suicide is especially common in veteran populations, and certain variables are known to increase its probability including being male, depression, manic-depressive disorder, and alcohol abuse disorders. Because most veterans are seen outside of the VA in community settings, "providers should vigilantly assess suicide risk in their patients who are Veterans."[70 (p. 711)] The palliative APRN should be aware of issues that might contribute to suicidal thinking and initiate additional screening and precautions when indicated. Information should always be provided to the veteran for the Veterans Crisis Line (800-273-8255). Preventing suicide in this vulnerable population may require enhanced support at every level. Comprehensive screening, assessment, and treatment tools to assist the APRN in navigating the veteran's needs can be readily accessed at https://www.mentalhealth.va.gov/healthcare-providers/suicide-prevention.asp.[71,72]

PHYSICIAN-ASSISTED DEATH

Within the VA healthcare system, physician assisted death (PAD) is strictly prohibited. Legislation forbids the direct or indirect use of any funds in PAD-related practices. Although veterans have the right and may choose to seek help outside of the VA system for this purpose, APRNs and physicians within the VA may not assist with medical workups, prognostication, referrals, or collaboration with the intent to facilitate or support this practice. The VA is also prohibited from contracting with hospices or agencies that offer this service under 38 US Code § 1725 and 38 US Code § 1728 (Reimbursement for emergency treatment and Reimbursement of certain medical expenses).[73,74]

CONCURRENT CARE

Palliative care is offered at the diagnosis of a serious illness. Hospice, however, is for patients with a prognosis of 6 months or less. Hospice services, when added as an adjunct program to standard care treatment models in end-stage disease, such as Stage IV lung cancer, often improve quality of life, both physically and psychologically. This approach to "concurrent care," or the ability to simultaneously access these sometimes mutually exclusive approaches to disease management, has also been shown to be more cost effective, with patients choosing hospitalization and aggressive life support measures less frequently.[75]

Unfortunately, under the current medical model, enrollment in hospice care focuses on comfort with the discontinuation of many life-sustaining treatments, including palliative chemotherapy, immunotherapies, and radiation treatments, even though they may benefit the individual in terms of symptom management and quality of life. Continuing active treatment and concurrently providing hospice services will minimize the symptom burden on patient and families and provide emotional support as well as the important work of preparing for the end-of-life transition. The VA recognizes the value of both active treatment and hospice care and enables veterans to receive the full array of services through the VA under their funding model. This approach is receiving new appreciation in the private sector as well.[76]

VA HOSPICE AND PALLIATIVE APRNS

The hospice and palliative APRN is an integral part of the VA workforce, serving veterans and their families. The APRN's role has evolved throughout the system and plays a vital role in carrying out the mission of the VA to provide a continuum of care for veterans and their loved ones. The Veterans Health Administration (VHA) serves at least 9 million enrolled veterans yearly with 170 medical centers across the country and 1,074 outpatient clinics.[77] Only veterans with an honorable discharge status are eligible to receive VHA healthcare. However, veterans may challenge to upgrade their discharge status, as noted earlier.

To honor veterans' preferences and promote veteran-centric, quality end-of-life care, the VA was one of the first healthcare institutions to mandate and embed hospice and palliative care services across its infrastructure (acute care consults, outpatient clinic, inpatient palliative/hospice units). The Comprehensive End-of-Life Care (CEC) initiative launched in 2009 paved the way for the concurrent care model, a unique policy which allowed veterans to enroll in hospice while undergoing cancer-directed or disease-modifying treatments. This commendable and concerted effort from the VA was associated with less aggressive medical treatment and significantly lower medical costs.[78] This initiative provides integrated care and bridges the separation between curative and palliative services, giving seriously ill patients a broader range of options for care instead of an either-or decision.

At the VA, palliative and hospice care are provided across care settings such as the home or the community, outpatient care, long-term care facilities, and inpatient units or through the inpatient consult service. Palliative APRNs serve essential roles in the healthcare system, from providing primary care to palliative and end-of-life care. The APRN is an integral part of the palliative care interdisciplinary team (along with physicians, pain pharmacists, chaplains, psychologists, and social workers) providing comprehensive symptom management to address the psychosocial needs of patients and families. The APRN plays a significant role in the day-to-day operations of the palliative care and hospice service to manage pain and other symptoms through interdisciplinary care, focusing on whole-person care, family support, and transitional care as indicated. Palliative care and hospice are part of every enrolled veterans' benefit package. Dual-eligible veterans (with both VA and Medicare benefits) may choose to have hospice services covered under the Medicare Hospice Benefit (thus retaining eligibility for VA care and benefits). If inpatient hospice service is needed, care can be provided through a VA facility (acute care or community living center [CLC]) or a VA-contracted community nursing home.

The military experience and culture create a unique set of care needs requiring distinct and specialized care approaches. Palliative care consultations allow for frank and realistic conversations about goals of care, encourage the initiation of timely discussions between patients and their loved ones/surrogates, and provide veterans with a better understanding of their medical conditions and prognosis. Too often, goals-of-care conversations occur late or happen during a crisis situation. This could be very challenging for such a highly vulnerable population. It may be even more challenging for veterans with few or no friends, family, or social support and those with no surrogate decision-makers. Palliative care consultations can assist in the process of advance care planning and in identifying surrogate decision-makers.

When consulted by a palliative care team, veterans and their families receive better emotional support and care planning.[79] Timely consults at the VA are associated with greater family satisfaction with care (outcomes from the Bereaved Family Survey [BFS]).[79] The impact of palliative care consultations on VA Standardized Mortality Ratio (SMR) and Strategic Analytics for Improvement and Learning (SAIL) indicators represent areas of future research.

A significant portion of veterans die outside the VA healthcare system, in places where their military experience or service-related conditions could be underappreciated or underevaluated.[5] This poses a barrier to accessing veteran-specific care and resources and could severely impact veterans' overall quality of life, including their families and support systems.

EDUCATIONAL PREPARATION AND TRAINING FOR HOSPICE AND PALLIATIVE CARE AT THE VHA

Both general and specialized training and education in palliative/hospice care can be obtained from curricula such as the End-of-Life Nursing Education Consortium for Veterans (ELNEC–for Veterans) and ELNEC for APRNs.[8,80] Free palliative care and hospice care educational services are also available through the VA Training Management System (TMS).

The VHA is one of only a handful of institutions that offer a Hospice and Palliative Care Nurse Practitioner fellowship program.[81] By undergoing postgraduate palliative APRN training, the resident embarks on a year-long skills and development training to enhance competencies for entry-level specialty palliative/hospice care practice. Specifically, the curriculum provides training in pain and symptom management and communication skills along with interprofessional educational training and team-based care through a variety of formats such as supervised clinical experiences, face-to-face, and online, and in a variety of settings (either VHA-based, in

inpatient palliative care units, outpatient clinics, hospice care units at CLCs, pain clinics, hematology and oncology services, etc.; or non–VHA-based at community hospice agency networks). The APRN is a key factor in the selection, orientation, supervision, training, education, promotion of self-care, and role and professional development of the nurse practitioner fellows. APRNs also serve as faculty for VHA Palliative Care and Hospice Medicine fellowships and interdisciplinary hospice/palliative care fellowship programs such as social work, etc.

APRN FULL PRACTICE AUTHORITY

In 2017, the VA granted full practice authority to APRNs (for certified nurse practitioners, certified nurse-midwives, and clinical nurse specialists) to act within the full scope of their employment consistently throughout the VA system, regardless of the state in which they practiced.[82] These APRNs are recognized as licensed independent practitioners (LIP). The VA defined the processes for credentialing, privileging, reappraisal, re-privileging, and adverse privileging actions. Most importantly, it removed APRN practice barriers, and this has been monumental step in improving and maintaining veteran-centric quality care. This directive aimed to increase the pool of qualified healthcare providers, expand access to VHA healthcare (especially primary care in medically underserved areas), and reduce wait times for VHA medical appointments.

These APRNs have the practice authority to conduct goals-of-care conversations, write life-sustaining treatment plans and life-sustaining treatment orders (clear instructions regarding medical goals of care that do not expire unless goals change and that are portable across all VA settings), including do-not-attempt-resuscitation (DNAR)/do-not-resuscitate (DNR) and DNR-with-exception orders. APRNs are in the forefront of supporting and fostering patient-centered communication, engagement, and facilitation, and in documenting timely goals-of-care plan conversations and assisting in clarifying ambiguities to allow a common understanding of the veteran's goals, values, and wishes.

VARIOUS ROLES OF THE HOSPICE AND PALLIATIVE APRN AT THE VHA

The hospice and palliative APRN serves in a variety of roles as educator, advocate, direct clinical management, and healthcare system navigator, and assists with case management and team support. APRNs may be responsible for ensuring that policies and procedures are in place to facilitate the delivery of patient-centered care and for guiding and improving clinical and professional practice. They identify the educational needs and assist with role development of staff (also updating staff competencies) within the service and impacted service areas. They provide expert guidance, act as a consultant in an advisory capacity, and serve locally and nationally to support professional practice and development. They facilitate and are actively involved in quality and performance improvement, evidence-based practice, and formal research to further health outcomes and improve practice. The APRN actively participates in implementing national initiatives and policies.

SYSTEM EDUCATION

In 2017, the VHA, led by the National Center for Ethics, launched a national quality improvement project, the Life-Sustaining Treatment Decisions Initiative (LSTDI). The aim was to promote a more proactive, personalized, patient-centered approach to eliciting, documenting, and honoring medical care preferences for veterans with serious illness.[83] LSTDI standardized practice and approaches to life-sustaining treatment decisions including staff education, training, and resources, as well as monitoring within VHA facilities. It established guidance on naturally administered nutrition and hydration, conflict resolution, and conscientious objection and also explained the prohibition on assisted suicide and euthanasia at the VHA.

VETERANS AFFAIRS MISSION ACT OF 2018

The passing of the VA *Maintaining Internal Systems and Strengthening Integrated Outside Networks* (MISSION) *Act* in 2018 paved the way for the consolidation and redesign of community care programs at the VHA, thus impacting the quality of healthcare delivery for veterans.[84] It created new community care eligibility criteria, provided a new urgent care benefit, modernized information technology, established a new Community Care Network (CCN), innovated service-delivery, expanded the Caregiver Support Program (CSP), and provided timely community provider payments.[85] It also allowed veterans to receive or have more access to care in the private sector for services that are not available within the VHA or when they meet certain eligibility criteria and in consideration of their circumstances (remote living with extended drive time or prolonged appointment wait time at their local VHA facility, etc.). Despite its implementation, challenges remain, particularly as it relates to the continuity, cost, and quality of healthcare that veterans will receive from the community. By opening access to the private sector and partnering care with the local community (e.g., specialty care access such as palliative care), Community Care aims to add more service choices, prevent appointment delays, and accommodate the needs of veterans, particularly those living in remote rural areas.

COMPLEMENTARY AND INTEGRATIVE HEALTH

Patients with life-limiting or serious illnesses may experience a variety of symptoms that affect biopsychosocial well-being and overall quality of life. Relief may be derived not just from pharmacologic approaches, but from other therapeutic interventions aimed at reducing symptom burden while also reducing or avoiding medication side effects. As the nation's largest integrated healthcare system, the VHA has invested in research in, staff training in, and access to a variety of evidence-based integrative and complementary therapies to provide a whole-health system approach to care and also offer nonpharmacologic pain management strategies to combat the opioid crisis. These approaches (acupuncture, biofeedback, clinical hypnosis, guided imagery, massage therapy, meditation, tai chi, and yoga) could not be more relevant and impactful than in the hospice and palliative care population. Ongoing complementary and integrative health provider skills training is available through the VHA, and, thus far, the VHA has trained more than 4,600 providers in Battlefield Acupuncture (protocolized auricular acupuncture for pain), 88 in Battlefield Acupressure, 2,370 in health coaching, and 124 in mindfulness facilitation.[86]

SUMMARY

Florence Nightingale once walked tirelessly through military hospital tents at night, guided by her lamp, giving comfort to wounded and dying soldiers. American Red Cross founder Clara Barton cared for sick and injured Civil War combatants who were starving, without supplies, and often lost and separated from loved ones. On the battlefield, these nurses found conditions unacceptable, and they became activists, scientists, and humanitarians who fundamentally changed entire healthcare systems and built the foundations of modern nursing.

More than a century later, wars are still here and soldiers still suffer. Consistent with the legacy of early nursing, contemporary APRNs now have the autonomy and resources to continue to revolutionize care and improve the lives and conditions of military men and women. Today's veterans are a large group with diverse experiences and complex health challenges and are at increased risk for a multitude of problems such as PTSD, moral injury, and suicide. The APRN ultimately recognizes that those who served often carry both physical and mental wounds for a lifetime and knows how to mobilize a vast array of services to ensure that veterans experience comfort and appreciation during the end of their lives for all they have sacrificed to defend our freedoms. Nightingale shone a light on the pain and suffering of dying soldiers, and her examples of bedside compassion, activism, and fierce advocacy continue to exemplify the greatest callings of the nursing profession.

DISCLAIMER

The views expressed in this chapter do not express the views of the Department of Veterans Affairs or the US government.

REFERENCES

1. 115th Congress. VA claims and appeals modernization. Federal Register. [LLI] 38 CFR § 3.1—Definitions. January 18, 2019. https://www.federalregister.gov/documents/2019/01/18/2018-28350/va-claims-and-appeals-modernization

2. Social Security Administration. Code of federal regulations. Members of the uniformed services. Available at https://www.ssa.gov/OP_Home/cfr20/404/404-1330.htm

3. U.S Department of Veteran's Affairs. National Center for Veterans Analysis and Statistics. Veteran population. Last update April 14, 2021. https://www.va.gov/vetdata/veteran_population.asp

4. U.S Department of Veteran's Affairs. National Center for Veterans Analysis and Statistics. Profile of post-9/11 veterans: 2016. March 2018. https://www.va.gov/vetdata/docs/SpecialReports/Post_911_Veterans_Profile_2016.pdf

5. U.S Department of Veteran's Affairs. National Center for Veterans Analysis and Statistics.VA utilization profile FY 2017.May 2020. https://www.va.gov/vetdata/docs/QuickFacts/VA_Utilization_Profile_2017.PDF

6. US Department of Veterans Affairs. Geriatrics and extended care: Hospice care. Last updated April 2020. https://www.va.gov/GERIATRICS/pages/Hospice_Care.asp

7. US Department of Veterans. Veterans Health Administration. Office of Rural Health. America's veterans thrive in rural communities. ORH Strategic Plan 2020-2024. Available at https://www.ruralhealth.va.gov/docs/ORH_2020-2024_Strategic-Plan_FINAL.PDF

8. Gabriel MS, Malloy P, Wilson LR, Virani R, Jones DH, Luhrs CA, Shreve ST. End-of-Life Nursing Education Consortium (ELNEC)—For veterans: An educational project to improve care for all veterans with serious, complex illness. *J Hosp Pall Nurs.* 2015;17(1):40–47. doi:10.1097/NJH.0000000000000121

9. Elder G. The life course as developmental theory. *Child Dev.* 1998;69(1):1–12. https://doi.org/10.2307/1132065

10. Graphic News. US troop numbers in the Middle East. October 23, 2019. Available at https://www.graphicnews.com/ar/pages/39633/military-us-presence-in-the-middle-east

11. US Department of Veterans Affairs. Health care, public health. Cold injuries. 2021. Available at https://www.publichealth.va.gov/exposures/cold-injuries/index.asp

12. US Department of Veterans Affairs. VA Health Care, Public Health. Disease associated with ionizing radiation exposure. 2021. Available at https://www.publichealth.va.gov/exposures/radiation/diseases.asp

13. Belperio P, Chartier M, Ross DB, Alaigh P, Sulkin D. Curing hepatitis C virus infection: Best practices from the US Department of Veterans Affairs. *Ann Intern Med.* 2017;167(7):499–504. https://doi.org/10.7326/M17-1073

14. US Department of Veterans Affairs. VA Health Care. Public health. Agent Orange. 2021. Available https://www.publichealth.va.gov/exposures/agentorange/index.asp

15. US Department of Veterans Affairs. VA Health Care. Public health. Gulf War veterans' illnesses. 2021. https://www.publichealth.va.gov/exposures/gulfwar/medically-unexplained-illness.asp

16. Weisskopf MG, Cudkowicz ME, Johnson N. Military service and amyotrophic lateral sclerosis in a population-based cohort. *Epidemiology.* 2015;26(6):831–838. doi:10.1097/EDE.0000000000000376

17. Institute of Medicine. *Amyotrophic Lateral Sclerosis in Veterans: Review of the Scientific Literature.* Washington, DC: National Academies Press; 2006. https://doi.org/10.17226/11757

18. Frontline. "Soldier's heart" and "shell shock:" Past names for PTSD. Posted March 1, 2005. https://www.pbs.org/wgbh/pages/frontline/shows/heart/themes/shellshock.html

19. Center for Substance Abuse Treatment (US). Trauma-Informed Care in Behavioral Health Services. Rockville (MD): Substance Abuse and Mental Health Services Administration (US). 2014. (Treatment Improvement Protocol (TIP) Series, No. 57.) Exhibit 1.3-4, DSM-5 Diagnostic Criteria for PTSD. https://www.ncbi.nlm.nih.gov/books/NBK207191/box/part1_ch3.box16/

20. We Honor Veterans. A program of the NHPCO. 2021. Available at www.wehonorveterans.org

21. VA Community Provider Toolkit. https://www.mentalhealth.va.gov/communityproviders/docs/values.pdf

22. US Department of Veterans Affairs. Veterans Employment Toolkit. Structure and branches. Last updated September 2, 2015. https://www.va.gov/vetsinworkplace/docs/em_structureBranches.asp#:~:text=The%20US%20military%20has%20five,%2C%20Marines%2C%20and%20Coast%20Guard

23. The United States Space Force. About the United States Space Force. 2021. Available at https://www.spaceforce.mil/About-Us/About-Space-Force/

24. Richardson, J. About the United States Space logo and motto. The United States Space Force. July 22 2020. Available at https://www.spaceforce.mil/News/Article/2282948/the-us-space-force-logo-and-motto/

25. Today's Military. Ways to serve. 2021. https://www.todaysmilitary.com/ways-to-serve

26. Team RW B. Dr. Nancy Sherman on philosophy, stoicism, the military mindset and living a life of action. May 22, 2017. Available at https://www.teamrwb.org/dr-nancy-sherman-philosophy-stoicism-military-mindset-living-life-action/

27. Kelly U, Boyd M A, Valente SM, Czekanski E. Trauma-informed care: Keeping mental health settings safe for veterans. *Issues Ment Health Nurs.* 2014;35(6):413–419. doi:10.3109/01612840.2014.881941

28. We Honor Veterans. Trauma-informed care for Veterans and Hospice Initials Survey. May 2021. https://www.wehonorveterans.org/trauma-informed-care/

29. Gerber M, ed. *Trauma-Informed Healthcare Approaches: A Guide for Primary Care.* Cham, CH: Springer; 2019.

30. Pulverman CS, Christy AY, Kelly UA. Military sexual trauma and sexual health in women veterans: A systematic review. *Sex Med Rev.* 2019;7(3):393–407. doi:10.1016/j.sxmr.2019.03.002

31. Moreau J, Dyer KE, Hamilton AB, et al. Women veterans' perspectives on how to make Veterans Affairs healthcare settings more welcoming to women. *Womens Health Issues.* 2020;30(4):299–305. doi:10.1016/j.whi.2020.03.004

32. Ostacher MJ, Cifu AS. Management of posttraumatic stress disorder. *JAMA.* 2019;321(2):200–201. doi:10.1001/jama.2018.19290

33. Glick DM, Cook JM, Moye J, Kaiser AP. Assessment and treatment considerations for post traumatic stress disorder at end of life. *Am J Hosp Palliat Care.* 2018;35(8):1133–1139. doi:10.1177/1049909118756656

34. We Honor Veterans. Military history checklist. 2020. Available at https://www.wehonorveterans.org/wp-content/uploads/2020/02/MHC_FactSheet.pdf

35. Prins A, Bovin MJ, Smolenski DJ, et al. The primary care PTSD screen for DSM-5 (PC-PTSD-5): Development and evaluation within a veteran primary care sample. *J Gen Intern Med.* 2016;31(10):1206–1211. doi:10.1007/s11606-016-3703-5

36. Galovski TE, Norman SB, Hamblen JL. Cognitive processing therapy for PTSD. US Department of Veterans Affairs. PTSD: National Center for PTSD. 2019. https://www.ptsd.va.gov/professional/treat/txessentials/cpt_for_ptsd_pro.asp

37. McSweeney LB, Rauch SAM, Norman SB, Hamblen JL. Prolonged exposure for PTSD. US Department of Veterans Affairs. PTSD: National Center for PTSD. 2019. https://www.ptsd.va.gov/professional/treat/txessentials/prolonged_exposure_pro.asp#one

38. Beauvais D, McCarthy E, Norman S, Hamblen JL. Eye movement desensitization and reprocessing (EMDR) for PTSD. US Department of Veterans Affairs. PTSD: National Center for PTSD. 2019. https://www.ptsd.va.gov/professional/treat/txessentials/emdr_pro.asp

39. Sloan D, Marx BP. Written exposure therapy: US Department of Veterans Affairs. PTSD: National Center for PTSD. 2019. https://www.ptsd.va.gov/professional/treat/txessentials/written_exposure_therapy.asp

40. Jeffreys M. Clinician's guide to medications for PTSD. US Department of Veterans Affairs. PTSD: National Center for PTSD. 2017. https://www.ptsd.va.gov/professional/treat/txessentials/clinician_guide_meds.asp

41. The Management of Posttraumatic Stress Disorder Work Group, Department of Veterans Affairs and Department of Defense. VA/DoD clinical practice guideline for the management of posttraumatic stress disorder and acute stress disorder. Version 3.0. 2017. https://www.healthquality.va.gov/guidelines/MH/ptsd/VADoDPTSDCPGFinal.pdf

42. Bernardy N, Bruce L, Haloway-Paulino M, et al. Community hospices: Posttraumatic stress disorder in Vietnam veterans. We Honor Veterans. Available at https://www.wehonorveterans.org/wp-content/uploads/2020/02/Vietnam_Veterans_PTSD_Slides.pdf

43. US Department of Veterans Affairs. PTSD: National Center for PTSD. PTSD Consultation Program. Updated May 20, 2021. https://www.ptsd.va.gov/professional/consult/index.asp

44. Frankfurt S, Frazier P. A review of research on moral injury in combat veterans. *Military Psychology*. 2016;28(5):318–330. https://doi.org/10.1037/mil0000132

45. Litz BT, Stein N, Delaney E, et al. Moral injury and moral repair in war veterans: A preliminary model and intervention strategy. *Clin Psychol Rev*. 2009;29(8):695–706. doi:10.1016/j.cpr.2009.07.003

46. Gaudet CM, Sowers KM, Nugent WR, Boriskin JA. A review of PTSD and shame in military veterans. *J Hum Behav Soc Enviro*. 2016;26(1):56–68. doi: 10.1080/10911359.2015.1059168

47. Griffin BJ, Purcell N, Burkman K, et al. Moral Injury: An Integrative Review. *J Trauma Stress*. 2019;32(3):350–362. doi:10.1002/jts.22362

48. Blackstone K, Dinescu A, Laramie J, Morgan R, Pandey S, Ramsey-Lucas C, Watson P. Healing Vietnam veterans' moral injury: A stress first aid toolkit for hospice teams. We Honor Veterans. April 18, 2020. https://www.wehonorveterans.org/wp-content/uploads/Healing-Vietnam-Veterans-and-Moral-InjuryBlackstoneFINALrevised7-16-203pm-1.pdf

49. US Department of Veterans Affairs. Office of Health Equity. Health disparities among LGBT veterans. Last updated July 21, 2020. https://www.va.gov/HEALTHEQUITY/Health_Disparities_Among_LGBT_Veterans.asp

50. Hinrichs KLM, Christie KM. Focus on the family: A case example of end-of-life care for an older LGBT veteran. *Clin Gerontol*. 2019;42(2):204–211. doi: 10.1080/07317115.2018.1504848

51. Ruben MA, Livingston NA, Berke DS, Matza AR, Shipherd JC. Lesbian, gay, bisexual, and transgender veterans' experiences of discrimination in health care and their relation to health outcomes: A pilot study examining the moderating role of provider communication. *Health Equity*. 2019;3(1):480–488. doi: 10.1089/heq.2019.0069

52. US Department of Veterans Affairs. VA facilities with LGBT program websites. Last updated July 1, 2021. https://www.patientcare.va.gov/LGBT/VAFacilities.asp

53. Bajko M. Vets kicked out for being gay can upgrade their discharges. *Bay Area Reporter*. February 19, 2020. https://www.ebar.com/news/news//288378

54. Burks DJ. Lesbian, gay, and bisexual victimization in the military: An unintended consequence of "Don't Ask, Don't Tell"? *Am Psychol*. 2011;66(7):604–613. doi:10.1037/a0024609

55. US Department of Veterans Affairs. How to apply for a discharge upgrade. 2021. Available at https://www.va.gov/discharge-upgrade-instructions/

56. Bohnert KM, Ilgen MA, Louzon S, McCarthy JF, Katz IR. Substance use disorders and the risk of suicide mortality among men and women in the US Veterans Health Administration. *Addiction*. 2017;112(7):1193–1201 doi: 10.1111/add.13774

57. Congress.gov. S. 524 - Comprehensive Addiction and Recovery Act of 2016 (2015-2016) CARA Act, 42, USC., § 201. 114th Congress. 2016. Available at https://www.congress.gov/bill/114th-congress/senate-bill/524

58. Davis AK, Lin LA, Ilgen MA, Bohnert KM. Recent cannabis use among veterans in the United States: Results from a national sample. *Addict Behav*. 2018;76:223–228. doi:10.1016/j.addbeh.2017.08.010

59. Kansagara D, O'Neil M, Nugent S, et al. *Benefits and Harms of Cannabis in Chronic Pain or Post-traumatic Stress Disorder: A Systematic Review*. Washington, DC: Department of Veterans Affairs. August 2017. https://pubmed.ncbi.nlm.nih.gov/29369568/

60. US Department of Veterans Affairs. COVID-19 pandemic response weekly report: September 4-10, 2021. https://www.va.gov/health/docs/VA_COVID_Response.pdf

61. D'Adamo H, Yoshikawa T, Ouslander JG. Coronavirus Disease 2019 in geriatrics and long-term care: The ABCDs of COVID-19. *J Am Geriatr Soc*. 2020;68(5):912–917. doi.org/10.1111/jgs.16445

62. U.S. Department of Housing and Urban Development. 2017 AHAR: Part 1 – PIT Estimates of Homelessness in the U.S. December 17, 2021. Washington, DC: HUD. https://www.hudexchange.info/resource/5639/2017-ahar-part-1-pit-estimates-of-homelessness-in-the-us/

63. Hutt E, Albright K, Dischinger H, Weber M, Jones J, O'Toole TP. Addressing the challenges of palliative care for homeless veterans. *Am J Hospice Palliat Med*. 2018;35(3):448–455. doi.org/10.1177/1049909117722383

64. US Department of Veterans Affairs. VA homelessness Programs. Last updated September 14, 2021. https://www.va.gov/homeless/

65. Centers for Disease Control and Prevention. CDC.gov. COVID-19. Interim guidance on people experiencing unsheltered homelessness and local officials. Updated July 8, 2021. https://www.cdc.gov/coronavirus/2019-ncov/community/homeless-shelters/unsheltered-homelessness.html

66. The Framework for an Equitable COVID-19 Homelessness response. 2020. Available at https://housingequityframework.org/

67. Los Angeles Homeless Services Authority. HC2019 Veterans data summary. Available at https://www.lahsa.org/documents?id=4011-hc2019-veterans-data-summary

68. Breitbart W, Rosenfeld B, Pessin H, et al. Depression, hopelessness, and desire for hastened death in terminally ill patients with cancer. *JAMA*. 2000;284(22):2907–2911. doi:10.1001/jama.284.22.2907

69. Robinson S, Kissane DW, Brooker J, Hempton C, Burney S. The relationship between poor quality of life and desire to hasten death: A multiple mediation model examining the contributions of depression, demoralization, loss of control, and low self-worth. *J Pain Symptom Manage*. 2017;53(2):243–249. doi:10.1016/j.jpainsymman.2016.08.013

70. Way D, Ersek M, Montagnini M, et al. Top ten tips palliative care providers should know about caring for veterans. *J Palliat Med*. 2019 Jun;22(6):708–713. doi:10.1089/jpm.2019.0190.

71. US Department of Veterans Affairs. Community provider toolkit: Serving veterans through partnership. 2021. Available at https://www.mentalhealth.va.gov/communityproviders/index.asp

72. US Department of Veterans Affairs. Mental health. Suicide prevention. Last updated July 22, 2021. https://www.mentalhealth.va.gov/suicide_prevention/community-providers.asp

73. 38 US Code § 1725.United States Code 2018. Title 38 Veterans Benefits. Part II General Benefits. Reimbursement for Emergency Treatment. Available at https://www.govinfo.gov/content/pkg/USCODE-2018-title38/html/USCODE-2018-title38-partII-chap17-subchapIII-sec1725.htm

74. 38 US Code § 1728, United States Code 2018. Title 38 Veterans Benefits. Part II General Benefits. Reimbursement of Certain Medical Benefits. Available at https://www.govinfo.gov/content/pkg/USCODE-2018-title38/html/USCODE-2018-title38-partII-chap17-subchapIII-sec1728.htm

75. Mor V, Wagner TH, Levy C, et al. Association of expanded VA hospice care with aggressive care and cost for veterans with advanced lung cancer. *JAMA Oncol*. 2019;5(6):810–816. doi:10.1001/jamaoncol.2019.0292

76. Smith TJ, Chung V, Hughes MT, et al. A randomized trial of a palliative care intervention for patients on phase I studies. *J Clin Oncol*. 2020;38(15 suppl):12001–12001. http://clinicaltrials.gov/show/NCT01828775

77. US Department of Veterans Affairs. Veterans Health Administration. Last updated July 12, 2021. Available at https://www.va.gov/health/

78. Manthri S, Simmons C, Cepeda OA. Outcomes of palliative care consults with hospitalized veterans. *Fed Pract.* 2018;35(9):44–47. PMID: 30766386

79. Carpenter JG, McDarby M, Smith D, Johnson M, Thorpe J, Ersek M. Associations between timing of palliative care consults and family evaluation of care for veterans who die in a hospice/palliative care unit. *J Palliat Med.* 2017;20(7):745–751. doi:10.1089/jpm.2016.0477

80. Dahlin C, Coyne PJ, Paice J, Malloy P, Thaxton CA, Haskamp A. ELNEC-APRN: Meeting the needs of advanced practice nurses through education. *J Hospice Palliat Nurs.* 2017;19(3):261–265. doi:10.1097/NJH.0000000000000340

81. Dahlin C. Re-envisioning palliative care APRN education: Developing specialty palliative APRN practice. Hospice and Palliative Nurse Association Webinar Series. 2019. https://advancingexpertcare.org/ItemDetail?iProductCode=APRN1219

82. US Department of Veterans Affairs. Veterans Health Administration (VHA) Health Directive 1350. Advanced practice registered nurse full practice authority. Washington, DC: Veterans Health Administration. September 13, 2017. https://www.va.gov/vhapublications/ViewPublication.asp?pub_ID=5464

83. US Department of Veterans Affairs. Life-sustaining treatment decisions: Eliciting, documenting and honoring patients' values, goals and preferences. VHA Handbook 1004.03(2). Transmittal Sheet. January 11, 2017. Amended May 10, 2021. https://www.ethics.va.gov/docs/policy/VHA_Handbook_1004_03_LST.pdf

84. S.2372, VA Mission Act of 2018 (2017–2018). Maintaining Internal Systems and Strengthening Integrated Outside Networks Act, 38, USC., § 101. 115th Congress. Available at https://www.congress.gov/bill/115th-congress/senate-bill/2372

85. US Department of Veterans Affairs. Community care. Community care overview. Last updated February 2, 2021.https://www.va.gov/COMMUNITYCARE/index.asp

86. Kligler B. Integrative health in the Veterans Health Administration. *Med Acupunct.* 2017;29(4):187–188. doi:10.1089/acu.2017.29055.bkl

24.

RECURRENT DISEASE AND LONG-TERM SURVIVORSHIP

Denice Economou and Brittany Bradford

KEY POINTS

- Cancer survivors experience different trajectories from diagnosis to survivorship and potential recurrence.

- Integrating palliative care with survivorship care can provide more effective and efficient management of survivors' needs while conserving costs and sharing resources.

- Palliative advanced practice registered nurses (APRNs) provide essential care in care coordination and transitions of care.

CASE STUDY 1: PALLIATIVE CARE FOR SURVIVORS

Mrs. P was a 76-year-old woman who presented with a second colon cancer as a new primary 6 years after her initial diagnosis. She had a rare hereditary syndrome, a subtype of hereditary nonpolyposis colorectal cancer (HNPCC) known as *Lynch syndrome,* which predisposed her to colon, gyno-urinary, and skin lesions. She had experienced multiple sebaceous tumors on her face and chest. Mrs. P's genetic findings (HNPCC/Lynch syndrome) put her at a very high risk for recurrence and second cancers. Her risk for developing additional cancers was high and caused her great distress.

Over the past 14 years, she has undergone multiple surgeries, starting with endometrial cancer, followed by her first colon cancer resection. She has had a recent laparoscopic colon resection with anastomosis. As a result, she experienced moderate bowel issues with diarrhea, gas, and minimal incontinence of stool. She lived with her 80-year-old husband of 55 years, who became her primary caregiver. Previously, Mrs. P had been physically challenged due to scoliosis and suffered from neuropathy in her feet. The lack of feeling in the soles of her feet necessitated the use of a walker at home.

Mrs. P was referred to survivorship to help with quality of life. Because Mrs. P was a geriatric oncology patient, maintaining functional mobility was essential for independence. The advanced practice registered nurse (APRN) planned a thorough assessment. In preparation for her planned initial survivorship telehealth encounter, the survivorship APRN asked Mrs. P to complete an Edmonton Symptom Assessment System and Patient Health Questionnaire 9 (PHQ-9). The APRN completed a Geriatric Assessment and the Blessed Memory Test.[1,2] Although the virtual visit did not allow a timed up-and-go

(TUG) review of mobility, the Eastern Cooperative Oncology Group (ECOG) rating and assessment of instrumental activities of daily living and activities of daily living (IADL/ADL) is helpful to establish the baseline independence of this patient to anticipate risk of falls and potential supportive care needs.[3] Mrs. P reported concerns about pain, diarrhea, gas, a history of neuropathy, and distress.

INTRODUCTION

Although survivorship care is defined as care beginning at diagnosis and continuing until death, most survivorship care services focus on the post-treatment care phase and extended survivorship Long-term cancer survivors experience a variety of symptoms related to their disease type, treatment regimens, age, and comorbidities.[4] When these patients have recurrent disease, as in the case study, multiple issues occur at the same time. Therefore, advanced practice registered nurses (APRNs) will provide important coordination of necessary care. The survivorship APRN must determine whether the patient is at risk for increased symptoms and additional cancers and develop a plan of care to manage these symptoms. Unless there are long-standing problems from their cancer treatment, most survivors ultimately return to their primary care physician for standard, annual recommended care, depending on their disease or treatment.

Recurrent disease in long-term survivors illustrates the partnership between the survivorship clinic and palliative care that may be necessary and how the APRN coordinates care between the two services as appropriate. Frequently, palliative APRNs manage patients in the oncology clinic through initial diagnosis—often at late stage—through treatment. These patients then stabilize, and the palliative APRN refers them to the survivorship program to meet their needs at that time. Survivors may deal with multiple long-term and late effects of their cancer and its treatment over time. Aging and other comorbidities may also complicate their management. APRNs with palliative care expertise are essential providers to meet the coordination and transitions of care needed in this population as they transition between survivor and recurrence.

The goal of survivorship care is to improve the quality of life for patients, their caregivers, and their families from the time their cancer is diagnosed through their life span. Integrating palliative care into survivorship care can improve the cancer survivor's quality of life and relieve his or her suffering.[4–6] Transitioning care between end of treatment and survivorship requires coordination of care across multiple cancer specialists and primary care providers.[6] The estimated number of survivors who will be alive by January 2030 will be 22.1 million.[7] People 65 years or older account for 64% of survivors. One in ten are 50 years or younger.[7] Although survival rates are growing, cancer remains our country's leading cause of death. Survivor-focused care includes prevention, detection, surveillance, coordination and communication of care, and interventions to relieve symptoms and suffering, with a focus on improving quality of life and health promotion. Overlapping survivorship care with the domains of palliative care provides a framework for the coordinated management strategies needed for this population. Figure 24.1 illustrates the overlap of survivorship care and palliative care.

In Figure 24.1, the four domains of the quality of life model provide the core framework, while the eight domains of the National Consensus Project for Quality Palliative Care (NCP) *Clinical Practice Guidelines* define the palliative care actions.[5,8] Domain 1: Structure and Processes of Care, encompasses all of the domains and allows for the multidisciplinary assessment of patient and family. Domain 2: Physical Aspects of Care, covers the physical well-being of the quality of life model providing evidenced-based symptom management. Domain 3: Psychological and Psychiatric Aspects of Care, is included in the Psychological Well-Being of Survivorship quality of life model. This area includes anxiety, depression, distress, and fear of cancer recurrence. Domains 4, 6, and 8, the Social, Cultural, and Ethical/Legal Aspects of Care, fall under Social Well-Being in the quality of life domain. Domain 5: The Spiritual, Religious, and Existential Aspects

of Care, relates to the spiritual well-being of survivor's quality of life model. Finally, Domain 7: Care of the Patient Nearing the End of Life, can be recognized from any domain in palliative care as caring for cancer survivors with recurrent disease; long-term survivors may transition to this level of care at any time. APRNs are essential in providing and overseeing this level of care due to their expertise and coordination skills. The key aspect of these models of care is that they both focus on care aimed at improving quality of life and minimizing or alleviating suffering.[4,8]

As people with cancer complete primary treatment, challenges exist as they transition to long-term survivorship. In 2020, the National Coalition for Cancer Survivorship (NCCS) completed a State of Cancer Survivorship Survey, representing a broad range of cancer diagnoses and different stages of survivorship.[9] A total of 1,319 survivors provided self-reported data between April 15 and May 1, 2020, with only 17% reported receiving a survivorship care plan post-treatment.[9] They identified key side effects they were experiencing, which included fatigue (49%), depression and/or anxiety (30%), loss of appetite and/or taste (28%), muscle or joint pain (27%), and nausea/vomiting or diarrhea (27%). People who identified a greater number of post-treatment concerns were African Americans, Hispanics, women, and younger survivors and those who had received chemotherapy as part of their treatment regimens.[9]

Recognizing that symptoms vary depending on type of cancer, age and stage at diagnosis, types of treatments, and socioeconomic status, planning care to meet the needs of this population requires comprehensive and coordinated management. Improved survival has brought the benefits of living longer but also the challenges related to long-term and late

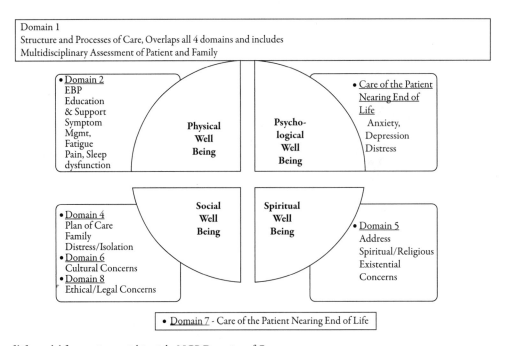

Figure 24.1 Quality of life model for survivors within eight NCP Domains of Care.

Adapted from Institute of Medicine. *From Cancer Patient to Cancer Survivor: Lost in Transition.* Washington DC: National Academies Press; 2006[5]; and National Consensus Project for Quality Palliative Care. *Clinical Practice Guidelines for Quality Palliative Care.* 4th ed. Richmond, VA: National Coalition for Hospice and Palliative Care; 2018.[8]

effects; many survivors are living with cancer as a chronic illness.[10-14]

Cancer survivorship occurs over phases from diagnosis to treatment, the immediate post-treatment stage, long-term survivorship for 5 years or longer to end-of-life care.[15] Cancer survivors may experience multiple symptoms and long-term effects during these phases of survivorship, which begin during treatment and continue into post-treatment, long-term survivorship, and possible recurrence.[15] These late effects include fatigue, chemotherapy-induced peripheral neuropathy (CIPN), sleep dysfunction, and psychosocial problems, such as depression and anxiety.[6,7,13] Late effects associated with cancer survivorship start after treatment completion and include cardiovascular disease related to anthracyclines, osteopenia, and hyperlipidemia. Additional effects include sexual dysfunction, infertility, lymphedema, urinary and bowel dysfunction, psychological symptoms, depression, and cognitive changes. Table 24.1 describes common late-stage recurrence symptoms associated with the top five cancers of both male and female survivors.

These patients may experience cycles of remission, recurrence, and remission; returning for palliative care support is likely, underscoring the importance of integrating survivorship care with palliative care. These effects vary depending on disease, type of treatments, stage of disease, age, culture-related disparities, and other comorbidities. Secondary symptoms may accompany primary symptoms, including weight gain, hyperlipidemia, and the development of hypertension.[6] The potential for multiple symptoms shows how complicated the long-term management of cancer survivors can become.[4] Extended cancer treatments, including endocrine therapy, targeted therapy, and hormone therapy, may cause problems in delineating cancer survivors but clearly influence their needs for combined survivorship and palliative care.[16]

RELATIONSHIP BETWEEN SURVIVORSHIP AND PALLIATIVE CARE

The goal of palliative care is to relieve suffering for the patient and family and improve quality of life.[8] Cancer survivorship care is focused not only on treating symptoms associated with late and long-term effects of cancer and its treatment, but also on providing detection, prevention, and surveillance for recurrent or new disease.[5] Communication and education are essential for both cancer survivorship and palliative models of care. Both palliative and survivorship care are focused on relieving suffering and improving quality of life, and the APRN plays an important role in providing both. Where the APRN roles overlap in these two models of care, integration and communication of the multidiscipline team is essential. Integrated care allows for a shared-care model and the benefit of effective and efficient management of recurrent disease. In the integrated model of care, multidisciplinary experts can help manage the patient's symptoms, coordinate surveillance needs, and plan the patient's goals of care.[6,17,18]

THE ROLES OF THE APRN

APRNs are the essential providers in the interdisciplinary models of both palliative and survivorship care. The coordination and handling of a patient's needs may vary depending on the different disciplines that make up the palliative care team. Nonetheless, the responsibilities of the APRN within the multidisciplinary team remain the same: promoting ethical decisions, providing collaboration and consultation, and providing evidence-based interventions for direct patient care.

About one in six cancer survivors will experience recurrence and advanced disease,[8] most commonly individuals with a history of prostate and breast cancer. Patients whose disease returns in an advanced stage may experience symptoms treated more effectively by the palliative care team. Oncology and palliative APRNs may have discharged these patients into long-term survivorship care and now will be faced with readmitting them to the palliative care service with new or recurrent symptoms related to advanced disease. The survivorship APRN performs a comprehensive assessment of the patient's needs and establishes or re-establishes a therapeutic relationship with the patient and family. Health outcomes depend on six core functions of the patient and provider: these include exchanging information, making decisions, fostering healing relationships, enabling patient self-management, managing uncertainty, and responding to emotions.[19] The level of trust and communication that an APRN establishes serves as the foundation for meeting the comprehensive needs of the patient population experiencing recurrence of disease and approaching the end of life.[20,21] The APRN provides survivorship care that meets the patient's needs, creates a therapeutic relationship, and employs research-based interventions to meet the challenges that these complicated patients present.

PALLIATIVE CARE IN PATIENTS WITH RECURRENT DISEASE

Similar to all health specialties, the COVID-19 pandemic has required survivorship clinics to provide care via telehealth. Although this has long been a model of rural healthcare, it is a new experience for many oncology and survivorship providers. There are many provider tools and applications that can facilitate a quality survivor clinic visit, although the completion of physical exams that include cardiac and pulmonary evaluations may require special telehealth equipment. When necessary, tools to aid physical assessment, such as stethoscopes and dermascopes, can be used but require the patient to be present at a telehealth site. There, a registered nurse assists in those exams and conveys valuable information to the survivorship APRN. Survivorship APRNs can provide an algorithm for the staff registered nurse to follow that is within their scope of practice and supports a shared-care model.

Table 24.1 DISEASE SITE (% SURVIVORS) AND COMMON LATE-STAGE RECURRENCE SYMPTOMS

	MALE		FEMALE
CANCER	SYMPTOMS ASSOCIATED WITH LATE RECURRENCE	CANCER	SYMPTOMS ASSOCIATED WITH LATE RECURRENCE
Prostate (45%)	Pain Osteoporosis/fracture Urinary and bowel dysfunction Sexual dysfunction Increased cardiovascular disease risk Risk of diabetes Sleep dysfunction Depression	Breast (44%)	Pain Osteoporosis/fractures Cardiovascular disease Arthralgias/myalgias Risk of diabetes Peripheral neuropathy Lymphedema Sleep dysfunction Cognitive impairment Psychological late effects
Colorectal (10%)	Bowel dysfunction (diarrhea, constipation, obstruction) Bladder dysfunction Peripheral neuropathy Depression	Uterine corpus (9%)	Osteoporosis Lymphedema lower extremities Infertility Sleep dysfunction Sexual dysfunction
Melanoma (8%)	Pain Depends on where melanoma arises Cutaneous melanoma or mucosal melanoma: Fungating wounds Brain melanoma: Headache, fall risk, weakness, numbness, somnolence, behavioral changes Lung metastasis: Shortness of breath, cough Lymphedema Cord compression: Incontinence, paralysis Immunotherapy and targeted treatment side effects	Colorectal (9%)	Bowel dysfunction (diarrhea, constipation, obstruction) Bladder dysfunction Peripheral neuropathy Depression
Urinary bladder (8%)	Bladder dysfunction: reduced volume, unable to eliminate; failure of neo-bladder; frequency	Melanoma (8%)	Pain Depends on where melanoma arises Cutaneous melanoma or mucosal melanoma: Fungating wounds Brain melanoma: Headache, fall risk, weakness, numbness, somnolence, behavioral changes Lung metastases: shortness of breath, cough Lymphedema Cord compression: Incontinence, paralysis Immunotherapy and targeted treatment side effects
Non-Hodgkin's lymphoma (5%)	Radiation and monoclonal antibody effects Skin changes Stem cell transplant effects Recurrent infections; decreased blood counts	Thyroid (8%)	Thyroglobulin levels changing and difficult to maintain Potential for distant metastasis Symptoms depend on location and extent of tumor. Damage to nerves and voice changes Dry mouth and dental caries

From American Cancer Society.[7]

Other survivorship smart apps allow individualization of a care plan, care reminders, symptom review, and visual patient check-ins.[22] These provide opportunities to enhance care to focus on patients' and families' individual needs in a cost-effective manner and limit exposure to infections. Although one size never fits all, with good risk stratification, telehealth visits can meet the palliative/survivor care needs of this special population of people with advanced cancer who are living with chronic disease or who face recurrence.[22–24]

ASSESSMENT

Initially, the APRN evaluates the patient's areas of concern, focusing on the four domains of quality-of-life which overlap with the eight domains of palliative care, as illustrated in Figure 24.1.

Many long-term cancer survivors are older and the onset of common geriatric syndromes put them in need of complex interventions.[17] In a 2020 national survey done by

Fitch et al. in Canada of 1,655 adults 75 years and older, 68.2% frequently described physical concerns as their number one challenge.[18]

PHYSICAL WELL-BEING-NCP DOMAIN 2: PHYSICAL ASPECTS OF CARE

CASE STUDY 1: PALLIATIVE CARE FOR SURVIVORS (CONTINUED)

The meeting took place at 10 AM because Mrs. P said she was not an early riser. She participated with her husband, who addressed questions about medications and his observations as a caregiver. She was dressed, her hair was combed, and she wore makeup. She claimed to have dressed herself, at which her husband smiled. Mrs. P complained primarily of pain in her back and neuropathy. Using a numeric rating scale, the patient stated her pain at 6–7, which for her was moderate pain. She was currently using a combination pill of oxycodone 5 mg/acetaminophen 325 mg for pain prescribed as 1–2 tablets twice every 6 hours. Her last dose was 4 hours prior, and she stated she would take another dose at 1 PM. Listening to her complaint of a deep pain at the base of her back, her husband explained it as being related to her scoliosis, where her "right hip meets her spine off center." Additionally, when she was engaged in the conversation, Ms. P closed her eyes and admitted to being sleepy.

A primary symptom associated with advanced disease is pain.[25] The goal of the palliative APRN is the relief of the patient's suffering, primarily by focusing on pain sources that are difficult to manage with standard approaches or that require difficult titrations or alternative routes (see Chapter 43 on pain management). In Mrs. P's case, the palliative APRN must establish the patient's pain management history and evaluate the current medication plan for effectiveness and complications. Pain assessment and listening to the patient's self-report are most important.[26]

It is known that in the United States more than 60% of cancer survivors are 65 years or older.[27] Assessing pain in the older adult has been validated using a Verbal Descriptor Scale, the Numeric Rating Scale, and the Faces Pain Scale.[28] Assessing how patients describe the pain is essential to understanding the source of pain. A "deep pain," as Mrs. P describes, is often associated with bone pain. The neuropathy she describes in her feet may be related to spinal instability from scoliosis and possible stenosis related to aging.[29] Neuropathy is associated with motor, sensory, or autonomic dysfunction.[28] It would not be uncommon for long-term survivors who are older to experience non–cancer related pain such as arthritis or osteoporosis overlaying pain associated with their cancer or its treatment.[25] Because Mrs. P's colon cancer was managed both times with a surgical resection and anastomosis, she did not undergo chemotherapy. The APRN differential diagnosis is that Mrs. P's pain is related to both her cancer surgery and arthritic or spinal stenosis pain.

Pain with advanced or metastatic disease occurs in 64% of all cancer survivors.[25] Chronic pain syndromes related to surgery, chemotherapy, or radiation therapy may occur. Patients who have received certain chemotherapy drugs may experience peripheral neuropathy, as well as weakness and numbness. Situations where a tumor impinges on bone or nerves or causes a stretching of the viscera surrounding organs can cause the most pain for survivors.

Managing pain in geriatric survivor population requires coordination to manage symptoms and the secondary effects of pain medicines. Mrs. P's sedation is possibly related to her pain medications. This is a safety issue because sedation can contribute to mobility issues or falls that could severely jeopardize her well-being. The combined product of hydrocodone and acetaminophen is not recommended for the older adult. Rather, the medications should be prescribed separately. It is recommended to use a short-acting opioid for moderate to severe pain and have separate acetaminophen dosing. In addition, nonpharmacologic interventions should be used when possible. Palliative care pain guidelines promote anticipating, preventing, and treating predictable side effects or the risk for adverse events.[30] A systematic review of the effectiveness and sustainability of nonpharmacological methods of managing pain in community-dwelling older adults found that non-pharmacologic methods such as acupressure, acupuncture, guided imagery, qigong, and periosteal stimulation reduced pain levels.[31] Other interventions, such as cognitive behavioral interventions like relaxation and strategies to improve coping have been shown to be beneficial for cancer pain management.[32] Using both pharmacologic and nonpharmacologic approaches in the management of pain in the older patient with cancer promotes better outcomes. Cognitive status may impact the use of behavioral interventions. A patient with minimal cognitive impairment may tolerate acupuncture, for instance, if the patient is prepared carefully for the procedure. Reimbursement remains a challenge for nonpharmacologic approaches. Many integrative therapies are not covered by many insurers or require larger co-payments. Medicare currently covers acupuncture for back pain and possibly soon for migraines, but coverage varies depending on the state where the patient receives care. Additional resources for pain management in the older adult can be found at the American Geriatrics Society website (www.AmericanGeriatric.org) and Geriatrics at Your Fingertips (GeriatricsCareOnline.org).[29,33]

Assessing for the secondary effects of unrelieved pain is important as well. Older patients with unrelieved pain may be experiencing depression, fatigue, and sleep deprivation, which will increase sedation, cause lower energy, and further impact mobility for these patients.[28] Depression has been shown to be present in 25% of elderly cancer patients.[34] Antidepressants may be beneficial in helping with sleep and elevating mood.[30]

Fatigue remains a concern in long-term cancer survivors.[35] Fatigue is associated with progressing disease, pro-inflammatory cytokines, and psychosocial issues like anxiety, depression, and unrelieved pain.[36] Unmanaged or prolonged stressors increase the risk to patients by reducing their immune system function and raising the potential for fatigue and depressive symptoms.[37] Management strategies include understanding fatigue's potential sources, such as stress hormones, anxiety and distress over the risk of recurrence or new cancers, unrelieved pain, physical deconditioning, causing loss of mobility, and sleep dysfunction and attempting to minimize these through coordination with multidisciplinary teams that can assist in managing these multiple symptoms (e.g., occupational therapy, cancer physical therapy, and rehabilitation).

PSYCHOLOGICAL WELL-BEING-NCP DOMAIN 3: PSYCHOLOGICAL AND PSYCHIATRIC ASPECTS OF CARE

Psychological symptoms may fluctuate from diagnosis to long-term survival, and, with recurrence, such symptoms may fluctuate again. Depressive symptoms, anxiety, distress, and posttraumatic stress disorder (PTSD) are associated with recurrence in long-term cancer survivors.[38] Dealing with recurrence may result in PTSD, and the rate of PTSD may be as high as 32% in cancer survivors.[39] In addition, survivors may live with long-term treatment-induced residual cognitive disorders. Both of these conditions affect one's ability to cope with a new and unexpected diagnosis.

The burden that the diagnosis and treatment of cancer puts on a patient and family, the resources available to them, and additional indicators, such as culture, educational level, and economic status, all contribute to the psychological effects in a cancer patient throughout the course of disease.[38] The PHQ-9 Assessment Scale can help identify a major depressive disorder.[38]

Mrs. P and her family required psychosocial support; this is an area that has been historically undermanaged in cancer survivors.[40] Assessment and coordination of support to manage these psychological symptoms can help reduce distress and promote quality of life.

Age and uncertainty related to the patient's increased risk for another cancer recurrence impacts the distress and anxiety they experience.[41] The APRN must provide education where necessary to be sure the patient has accurate information and understands their prognosis. Assessing fears and maintaining communication is essential to help the patient cope with distress.[19,42] Using telehealth visits to support self-management by providing education and goal development to guide the care specific to the patients' needs has been shown to be effective in managing pain, psychological distress, fatigue, and sleep disorders.[24]

SOCIAL WELL-BEING-NCP DOMAINS 4, 6, AND 8

This domain of social well-being encompasses many issues that affect quality of life in cancer survivors after diagnosis. The quality-of-life model related to cancer survivors includes affection and sexual function, body image issues, family roles and relationships, social isolation, and ability to find joy.[5] Social concerns in the cancer survivor include cultural awareness, family concerns, work-related issues, and financial debt.[43] Recurrence brings many of these concerns back to the forefront in cancer survivors' lives. It is important to assess culture-related concerns by thoughtful discussions that can build trust and may be more helpful than standardized tools.[44]

For a patient like Mrs. P, living with the fear of recurrent cancer saddened both her and her husband. The APRN's role of assessment, with a focus on the patient's social/emotional response to the change in health status, is essential. In addition, caregiver distress is important. The palliative APRN in the case study inquired about family distress to develop a plan of care. Posing the question itself can be therapeutic: it allows Mrs. P and her husband to discuss their concerns about their ability to continue to manage care at home "down the road" and their anxieties about healthcare costs and overall social worries of long-term survival in an environment of uncertainty. Voicing and discussing this areas reduces distress. Moreover, it assisted the palliative APRN in coordinating appropriate resources and making them available as part of the interdisciplinary palliative care service.

SPIRITUAL WELL-BEING-NCP DOMAIN 5: SPIRITUAL, RELIGIOUS, EXISTENTIAL ASPECTS OF CARE

Spirituality in cancer survivors may lead to hopefulness and better coping.[45] Studies demonstrate that cancer survivors experiencing psychological and social late effects describe multiple spiritual/religious or existential concerns.[46] Spiritual, religious, or existential concerns are an important part of whole-person care, and yet this is rarely part of a routine assessment.[47]

Because there is a population of advanced disease survivors living with cancer, it is important to recognize that survivorship is relative to the understanding of their disease status. For those who have experienced recurrent disease, even though stable and being followed as survivors, it represents a loss of the future and an opportunity to question the meaning and purpose of life.[47,48] Mrs. P discussed her spiritual beliefs with the palliative APRN. The APRN elicited spirituality concerns when discussing goals of care. As stated by Cormack et al., "spirituality is the essence of every human being."[44 (p. 475)] Providing spiritual and/or religious support to the patient and caregiver as needed is a key component of good palliative and end-of-life care.[48] There will be moments of reappraisal of beliefs and transcendence or changes in what the patient believes that affects how they feel about themselves and what the meaning or purpose of their life has been.[48]

The APRN's role in providing spiritual care begins with respecting the patient's beliefs and recognizing that the APRN is more of a guide, with the goal of relieving suffering as patients try to make sense of their recurrent diagnosis and the loss of the life they expected. The APRN's role is to collaborate with chaplaincy to assist patients through this moment and help them move forward in preparing for end of life. Asking Mrs. P and her husband about their beliefs, values, and desires is essential to help define the goals of care and identify goals that provide them with peace. Compassionate listening displays the respect necessary to build the nurse-patient relationship and provides a supportive environment. Prayer, meditation, guided imagery, and breathing techniques may be meaningful interventions for patients. The role of the APRN in helping these challenging patients can be difficult and draining to one's own spirituality and meaning. Being present necessitates strategies for clinician support.[49]

Ms. P and her husband, although not religious, had spiritual discussions about what was important to them both. They valued time with their children and grandchildren and maintaining the highest quality of life for as long as possible. They accepted their stage of life and did not have expectations of living many years longer. They wanted to focus on pain relief, optimizing mobility, and enjoying what life was left, while being aware of possible new cancers so they could be identified early. For survivors, the provision of a tailored plan specific to the needs of patients living with chronic cancer or recurrence is helpful to coordinate providers to meet their needs and categorize their risks and goals.[4,50,51] In the case study, the multidisciplinary team of palliative care working with the survivorship APRN provided the framework for meeting this complicated patient's needs.

PALLIATIVE CARE IN LONG-TERM SURVIVORS

CASE STUDY 2: SECONDARY CANCER IN SURVIVORSHIP

Ms. D was a 70-year-old-Asian woman with a history of right-sided breast cancer; she was 19 years out from her original diagnosis. She had been followed in the breast cancer survivorship clinic for more than 5 years. Her original cancer was Stage IIIA, estrogen-receptor positive, progesterone-receptor positive, and Her-2/neu negative. She was treated with a right mastectomy and lymph node dissection; 12/15 positive lymph nodes were involved at that time. She underwent high-dose chemotherapy under a clinical trial and had a stem cell transplant, following which she received radiation and endocrine therapy.

Due to the lymph node dissection within her surgery, she has dealt with chronic lymphedema. The APRN assessed her right arm and referred her to occupational therapy for lymphedema manual massage and drainage. The therapists also fit her for a compression sleeve.

When Ms. D presented for her annual follow-up in the survivorship clinic, she had her usual mammogram and ultrasound, with both yielding normal results and no evidence of malignancy. She discussed with her APRN that she had been experiencing worsening fatigue, nausea, and just generally feeling unwell. Lab work revealed macrocytic anemia. Her hemoglobin was not substantially low, but low enough that the decision was made by the APRN to send her for a hematology evaluation.

Ms. D was seen by a hematologist; a bone marrow biopsy and aspiration was done. The hematologist had offered a potential diagnosis of myelodysplastic syndrome (MDS) as a result of

her breast cancer treatment. Ms. D was extremely anxious as she awaited the results of her biopsy. It has been 19 years since her breast cancer, and the thought of developing a secondary cancer as a side effect of her treatment had barely crossed her mind. Indeed, MDS was the diagnosis.

It was difficult for Ms. D to think about going through another cancer diagnosis and treatment alone. Ms. D's husband had passed away from lung cancer 2 years prior. She had a church community that was a source of strength for her. Her survivorship APRN sent a referral to social work to help the patient with coping mechanisms and with logistics, such as determining which transportation services were available. The APRN spoke with the social worker and, based on the social workers assessment, Ms. D was referred to psychiatry.

PHYSICAL WELL-BEING

The APRN evaluated Ms. D using the four domains of quality care, recognizing that it is important to care for the whole person. Initially, the patient's physical well-being was assessed. She felt generally unwell, nauseated, and was experiencing a flare-up in her lymphedema. The APRN used her knowledge of the patient's disease to make educated steps toward getting to the cause of the patients' symptoms.

The majority of hormone-negative breast cancer recurrences occur during the first 5 years after diagnosis, but for hormone-positive breast cancer, as in Ms. D, later recurrences are often seen.[52] Knowing that this was a possibility for Ms. D, it was important to evaluate the patient's mammogram and ultrasound, which was done and yielded benign findings.

The majority of breast cancer survivors have a good quality of life, but it is known that there are long-term effects from breast cancer–related therapy including fatigue, cognitive decline, lymphedema, pain, menopause symptoms, anxiety, and depression.[53] Ms. D expressed that she felt fatigue. This is known to be a long-term survivorship effect; however, she was experiencing worsening fatigue. Ms. D was a cancer survivor of 19 years, thus her description of worsening fatigue seemed to be a new symptom and not her baseline. The APRN evaluated this further by having a complete blood count (CBC) drawn, noticed that she had anemia, and ultimately consulted the hematology service for a bone marrow biopsy. The APRN also had the knowledge that, as a breast cancer survivor, Ms. D was at risk for a secondary cancer such as MDS; in those treated with chemotherapy, this risk is around 1%.[54] Other secondary cancers can be seen following radiation therapy or other chemotherapies.

Ms. D had also complained about lymphedema to the APRN. Breast cancer and its associated treatments are one of the leading causes of lymphedema. One study showed the occurrence of lymphedema in breast cancer survivors to be 17%.[55,56] The main risk factors for breast cancer–related lymphedema include surgery with lymph node removal, invasive breast cancer, and radiation.[55,56] It is important to rule out other causes of upper extremity swelling, in particular if the onset is sudden, as is seen in the occurrence of a thrombosis. In this case, Ms. D had dealt with chronic lymphedema since her surgery, so referring her to occupational therapy for further management was the reasonable next step. Occupational therapists trained in lymphedema management can perform manual massage to drain the lymphatic fluid and ultimately improve the patient's symptom. Ms. D was also fitted for a sleeve and taught exercises that she could do at home to prevent her lymphedema from worsening.

PSYCHOLOGICAL WELL-BEING/SOCIAL WELL-BEING-NCP DOMAINS 3, 4, 6, AND 8

Many cancer patients affirm that once they have been through a cancer diagnosis, the thought of having a cancer recurrence is often in the back of one's mind. Fear of recurrence is a form of anxiety, and anxiety levels have been reported to be higher in patients with a history of cancer.[57] Risk factors for anxiety in cancer survivors include living alone, being a female survivor, and social isolation. The APRN recognized that Ms. D had many risk factors for anxiety and made a prompt referral to social work. Ms. D was in a difficult situation in that she was anxious regarding her own possibility of a second cancer, but was also still grieving the loss of her husband and the loss of her support system. The APRN referred her to social work and psychiatry because she recognized that the patient had unmet psychosocial needs. If she did have a secondary cancer, such as MDS, she would need to be aware of the resources available at the hospital to help her, since she was living alone. Social workers are wonderful resources, and in the case study, they connected Ms. D to transportation services, mentorship programs, and a support group that could help her navigate a new cancer diagnosis. The psychologist helped with cognitive behavioral interventions that have been shown to reduce anxiety over fear of progression.[58]

SPIRITUAL WELL-BEING: DOMAIN 5: SPIRITUAL, RELIGIOUS, EXISTENTIAL

People often search for "meaning" or purpose from their catastrophic illnesses. A serious illness like cancer, or being the caregiver of someone with cancer, can often cause patients or caregivers to have doubts about their own spiritual beliefs. Some may feel they are being punished by God or may have a loss of faith after going through this experience. This is known as *spiritual distress* and is a normal response. Ms. D has been both caregiver and patient, so paying attention to her spiritual needs was an important aspect of her care. Ms. D did mention to the APRN that she attended church and that it was a source of strength and hope for her. Religion/spirituality has been shown to have a positive association with better health outcomes and quality of life.[46] The patient's church was also helpful in providing her support for feelings of loneliness and lack of community.[59] Many religious organizations can provide practical support such as meals, rides to and from appointments, and a sense of community. The APRN discussed these concerns with Ms. D to learn more about what her beliefs were and how she could facilitate and encourage her in this area. Many hospital and cancer facilities have chaplains or spiritual counseling available, and many patients find this helpful.

SUMMARY

The role of the palliative APRN includes evaluating the educational needs of patients and families, promoting the palliative model of care, providing evidence-based practice, promoting organizational ethical values, organizing staffing, and providing economic oversight.[60] The APRN's overall advocacy for patients provides leadership to improve the quality of care. The APRN plays a significant role as a clinical consultant to ensure communication among physicians, the palliative care team, support staff, patients, and families.[61] As the ultimate patient advocate and as part of providing whole-person care, the APRN coordinates the care of patients with recurrence of advanced disease and is committed to recognizing and dealing with the health disparities affecting palliative and end-of-life care. By providing care focused on meeting the quality-of-life needs of the cancer survivor with recurrence, integrating the principles of palliative care, and demonstrating expert symptom management, APRNs offer the comprehensive care necessary to manage this complicated patient population, despite the drop in numbers of the workforce of oncologists and primary care providers.[12,61]

REFERENCES

1. Kroenke K, Spitzer RL, Williams JB. The PHQ-9: Validity of a brief depression severity measure. *J Gen Intern Med.* 2001;16:606–613. doi:10.1046/j.1525-1497.2001.016009606.x
2. Hurria A, Gupta S, Zauderer M, et al. Developing a cancer-specific geriatric assessment: A feasibility study. *Cancer.* 2005;104(9):1998–2005. doi:10.1002/cncr.21422
3. Groessl EJ, Kaplan RM, Rejeski WJ, et al. Physical activity and performance impact long-term quality of life in older adults at risk for major mobility disability. *Am J Prev Med.* 2019;56(1):141–146. doi:10.1016/j.amepre.2018.09.006
4. Dy SM, Isenberg SR, Al Hamayel NA. Palliative care for cancer survivors. *Med Clin North Am.* 2017;101(6):1181–1196. doi:10.1016/j.mcna.2017.06.009
5. Institute of Medicine. *From Cancer Patient to Cancer Survivor: Lost in Transition.* Washington DC: National Academies Press; 2006. https://www.nap.edu/catalog/11468/from-cancer-patient-to-cancer-survivor-lost-in-transition
6. Choi Y. Care coordination and transitions of care. *Med Clin North Am.* 2017;101(6):1041–1051. doi:10.1016/j.mcna.2017.06.001
7. American Cancer Society. *Cancer treatment and survivorship, facts & figures 2019–2021.* Atlanta, GA: American Cancer Society. 2019. https://www.cancer.org/content/dam/cancer-org/research/cancer-facts-and-statistics/cancer-treatment-and-survivorship-facts-and-figures/cancer-treatment-and-survivorship-facts-and-figures-2019-2021.pdf

8. National Consensus Project for Quality Palliative Care. *Clinical Practice Guidelines for Quality Palliative Care.* 4th ed. Richmond, VA: National Coalition for Hospice and Palliative Care; 2018. https://www.nationalcoalitionhpc.org/wp-content/uploads/2018/10/NCHPC-NCPGuidelines_4thED_web_FINAL.pdf

9. National Coalition for Cancer Survivorship (NCCS). State of cancer survivorship survey. August 2020. Arlington, VA: NCCN. https://canceradvocacy.org/policy/2020-state-of-cancer-survivorship-survey/

10. Lobb EA, Lacey J, Kearsley J, Liauw W, White L, Hosie A. Living with advanced cancer and an uncertain disease trajectory: An emerging patient population in palliative care? *BMJ Support Palliat Care.* 2015;5(4):352–357. doi:10.1136/bmjspcare-2012-000381

11. Jacobs LA, Shulman LN. Follow-up care of cancer survivors: Challenges and solutions. *Lancet Oncol.* 2017;18(1):e19–e29. doi:10.1016/S1470-2045(16)30386-2

12. Denlinger CS, Sanft T, Moslehi JJ, et al. NCCN Guidelines Insights: Survivorship, Version 2.2020. *J Natl Compr Canc Netw* 2020;18(8):1016–1023. doi:10.6004/jnccn.2020.0037

13. Ang WHD, Lau Y, Ngo LPE, Siew AL, Ang NKE, Lopez V. Path analysis of survivorship care needs, symptom experience, and quality of life among multiethnic cancer survivors. *Support Care Cancer.* 2020. doi:10.1007/s00520-020-05631-6

14. Ferrell BR, Dow KH, Grant M. Measurement of the quality of life in cancer survivors. *Qual Life Res.* 1995;4(6):523–531. doi:10.1007/BF00634747

15. Economou D. Palliative care needs of cancer survivors. *Semin Oncol Nurs.* 2014;30(4):262–267. doi:10.1016/j.soncn.2014.08.008

16. Jacobsen PB, Nipp RD, Ganz PA. Addressing the survivorship care needs of patients receiving extended cancer treatment. *Am Soc Clin Oncol Educ Book.* 2017;37:674–683. doi:10.14694/EDBK_175673 10.1200/EDBK_175673

17. Bellury LM, Ellington L, Beck SL, Stein K, Pett M, Clark J. Elderly cancer survivorship: An integrative review and conceptual framework. *Eur J Oncol Nurs.* 2011;15(3):233–242. doi:10.1016/j.ejon.2011.03.008

18. Fitch MI, Nicoll I, Lockwood G, Strohschein FJ, Newton L. Main challenges in survivorship transitions: Perspectives of older adults with cancer. *J Geriatr Oncol.* 2020. doi:10.1016/j.jgo.2020.09.024

19. Economou D, Reb A. Communication concerns when transitioning to cancer survivorship care. *Semin Oncol Nurs.* 2017;33(5):526–535. doi:10.1016/j.soncn.2017.10.001

20. Dahlin C, Coyne PJ, Cassel JB. The advanced practice registered nurses palliative care externship: A model for primary palliative care education. *J Palliat Med.* 2016;19(7):753–759. doi:10.1089/jpm.2015.0491

21. Pawlow P, Dahlin C, Doherty CL, Ersek M. The hospice and palliative care advanced practice registered nurse workforce: Results of a national survey. *J Hospice Palliat Nurs.* 2018;20(4):349–357. doi:10.1097/NJH.0000000000000449

22. Bonsignore L, Bloom N, Steinhauser K, et al. Evaluating the feasibility and acceptability of a telehealth program in a rural palliative care population: TapCloud for palliative care. *J Pain Symptom Manage.* 2018;56(1):7–14. doi:10.1016/j.jpainsymman.2018.03.013

23. Chan A, Ashbury F, Fitch MI, Koczwara B, Chan RJ, Group MSS. Cancer survivorship care during COVID-19-perspectives and recommendations from the MASCC survivorship study group. *Support Care Cancer.* 2020;28(8):3485–3488. doi:10.1007/s00520-020-05544-4

24. Cox A, Lucas G, Marcu A, et al. Cancer survivors' experience with telehealth: A systematic review and thematic synthesis. *J Med Internet Res.* 2017;19(1):e11. Published 2017 Jan 9. doi:10.2196/jmir.6575

25. Finnerty D, O'Gara A, Buggy DJ. Managing pain in the older cancer patient. *Curr Oncol Rep.* 2019;21(11):100. doi:10.1007/s11912-019-0854-7

26. Fink R, Gates R, Jeffers K. Pain Assessment. In: Ferrell BR, Paice JA, eds. *Oxford Textbook of Palliative Nursing.* 5th ed. New York: Oxford University Press; 2019: 98–115.

27. Bluethmann SM, Mariotto AB, Rowland JH. Anticipating the "silver tsunami": Prevalence trajectories and comorbidity burden among older cancer survivors in the United States. *Cancer Epidemiol Biomarkers Prev.* 2016;25(7):1029–1036. doi:10.1158/1055-9965.EPI-16-0133

28. Tracy B, Morrison RS. Pain management in older adults. *Clin Therapeut.* 2013;35(11):1659–1668.

29. Reuben D, Herr K, Pacala J, Pollock B, Potter J, Semla T. *Geriatrics at Your Fingertips.* 19th ed. New York: American Geriatrics Society; 2017.

30. Paice J. Pain Management. In: Ferrell BR, Paice JA, eds. *Oxford Textbook of Palliative Nursing.* 5th ed. New York: Oxford University Press; 2019: 116–131.

31. Tang SK, Tse MMY, Leung SF, Fotis T. The effectiveness, suitability, and sustainability of non-pharmacological methods of managing pain in community-dwelling older adults: A systematic review. *BMC Public Health.* 2019;19(1):1488. doi:10.1186/s12889-019-7831-9

32. Syrjala KL, Jensen MP, Mendoza ME, Yi JC, Fisher HM, Keefe FJ. Psychological and behavioral approaches to cancer pain management. *J Clin Oncol.* 2014;32(16):1703–1711. doi:10.1200/JCO.2013.54.4825

33. The American Geriatrics Society. Geriatrics healthcare professionals. Home page. 2021. www.americangeriatrics.org

34. Kua J. The prevalence of psychological and psychiatric sequelae of cancer in the elderly: How much do we know? *Ann Acad Med Singap.* 2005;34(3):250–256. https://www.ncbi.nlm.nih.gov/pubmed/15902346.

35. O'Neil-Page E, Dean G, Anderson P. Fatigue. In: Ferrell BR, Paice JA, eds. *Oxford Textbook of Palliative Nursing.* 5th ed. New York: Oxford University Press; 2019: 132–139.

36. Kessels E, Husson O, Van der Feltz-Cornelis CM. The effect of exercise on cancer-related fatigue in cancer survivors: A systematic review and meta-analysis. *Neuropsychiatric Dis Treat.* 2018;14:479–494. doi:10.2147/NDT.S150464

37. Silva EH, Lawler S, Langbecker D. The effectiveness of mHealth for self-management in improving pain, psychological distress, fatigue, and sleep in cancer survivors: A systematic review. *J Cancer Surviv.* 2019;13(1):97–107. doi:10.1007/s11764-018-0730-8

38. Lie HC, Hjermstad MJ, Fayers P, et al. Depression in advanced cancer--assessment challenges and associations with disease load. *J Affect Disord.* 2015;173:176–184. doi:10.1016/j.jad.2014.11.006

39. Marziliano A, Tuman M, Moyer A. The relationship between post-traumatic stress and post-traumatic growth in cancer patients and survivors: A systematic review and meta-analysis. *Psychooncology.* 2020;29(4):604–616. doi:10.1002/pon.5314

40. Lisy K, Langdon L, Piper A, Jefford M. Identifying the most prevalent unmet needs of cancer survivors in Australia: A systematic review. *Asia Pac J Clin Oncol.* 2019;15(5):e68–e78. doi:10.1111/ajco.13176

41. Fischer IC, Cripe LD, Rand KL. Predicting symptoms of anxiety and depression in patients living with advanced cancer: The differential roles of hope and optimism. *Support Care Cancer.* 2018;26(10):3471–3477. doi:10.1007/s00520-018-4215-0

42. Chawla N, Blanch-Hartigan D, Virgo KS, et al. Quality of patient-provider communication among cancer survivors: Findings from a nationally representative sample. *J Oncol Pract.* 2016;12(12):e964–e973. doi:10.1200/JOP.2015.006999

43. Ness S, Kokal J, Fee-Schroeder K, Novotny P, Satele D, Barton D. Concerns across the survivorship trajectory: Results from a survey of cancer survivors. *Oncol Nurs Forum.* 2013;40(1):35–42. doi:10.1188/13.ONF.35-42

44. Cormack C, Mazanec P, Panke J. Cultural considerations in palliative care. In: Ferrell BR, Paice JA, eds. *Oxford Textbook of Palliative Nursing.* 5 ed. New York: Oxford University Press; 2019: 469–482.

45. Clay KS, Talley C, Young KB. Exploring spiritual well-being among survivors of colorectal and lung cancer. *J Relig Spiritual Soc Work.* 2010;29(1):14–32. doi:10.1080/15426430903479247

46. Hvidt NC, Mikkelsen TB, Zwisler AD, Tofte JB, Assing Hvidt E. Spiritual, religious, and existential concerns of cancer survivors in

a secular country with focus on age, gender, and emotional challenges. *Support Care Cancer.* 2019;27(12):4713–4721. doi:10.1007/s00520-019-04775-4

47. Rosa W. Spiritual care intervention. In: Ferrell BR, Paice JA, eds. *Textbook of Palliative Nursing.* 5th ed. New York: Oxford University Press; 2019: 447–455.

48. Taylor EJ. Spiritual screening, history, and assessment. In: Ferrell BR, Paice JA, eds. *Oxford Textbook of Palliative Nursing.* 5th ed. New York: Oxford University Press; 2019: 432–446.

49. Borneman T, Brown-Saltzman K. Meaning in illness. In: Ferrell BR, Paice JA, eds. *Oxford Textbook of Palliative Nursing.* 5th ed. New York: Oxford University Press; 2019: 456–466.

50. Mayer DK, Green M, Check DK, et al. Is there a role for survivorship care plans in advanced cancer? *Support Care Cancer.* 2015;23(8):2225–2230. doi:10.1007/s00520-014-2586-4

51. Nekhlyudov L, Ganz PA, Arora NK, Rowland JH. Going beyond being lost in transition: A decade of progress in cancer survivorship. *J Clin Oncol.* 2017;35(18):1978–1981. doi:10.1200/JCO.2016.72.1373

52. Richman J, Dowsett M. Beyond 5 years: Enduring risk of recurrence in oestrogen receptor-positive breast cancer. *Nat Rev Clin Oncol.* 2019;16(5):296–311. doi:10.1038/s41571-018-0145-5

53. Lovelace DL, McDaniel LR, Golden D. Long-term effects of breast cancer surgery, treatment, and survivor care. *J Midwifery Womens Health.* 2019;64(6):713–724. doi:10.1111/jmwh.13012

54. Wolff AC, Blackford AL, Visvanathan K, et al. Risk of marrow neoplasms after adjuvant breast cancer therapy: The national comprehensive cancer network experience. *J Clin Oncol.* 2015;33(4):340–348. doi:10.1200/JCO.2013.54.6119

55. DiSipio T, Rye S, Newman B, Hayes S. Incidence of unilateral arm lymphoedema after breast cancer: A systematic review and meta-analysis. *Lancet Oncol.* 2013;14(6):500–515. doi:10.1016/S1470-2045(13)70076-7

56. Rockson SG. Lymphedema after breast cancer treatment. *N Engl J Med.* 2018;379(20):1937–1944. doi:10.1056/NEJMcp1803290

57. Gotze H, Friedrich M, Taubenheim S, Dietz A, Lordick F, Mehnert A. Depression and anxiety in long-term survivors 5 and 10 years after cancer diagnosis. *Support Care Cancer.* 2020;28(1):211–220. doi:10.1007/s00520-019-04805-1

58. Butow P, Sharpe L, Thewes B, Turner J, Gilchrist J, Beith J. Fear of cancer recurrence: A practical guide for clinicians. *Oncology (Williston Park).* 2018;32(1):32–38. https://www.ncbi.nlm.nih.gov/pubmed/29447419.

59. Sherman AC, Merluzzi TV, Pustejovsky JE, et al. A meta-analytic review of religious or spiritual involvement and social health among cancer patients. *Cancer.* 2015;121(21):3779–3788. doi:10.1002/cncr.29352

60. Wiencek C, Wolf A. The advanced practice registered nurse. In: Ferrell BR, Paice JA, eds. *Oxford Textbook of Palliative Nursing.* 5th ed. New York: Oxford University Press; 2019: 809–816.

61. McCanney J, Winckworth-Prejsnar K, Schatz AA, et al. Addressing survivorship in cancer care. *J Natl Compr Canc Netw.* 2018;16(7):801–806. doi:10.6004/jnccn.2018.7054

SECTION V

PEDIATRIC PALLIATIVE CARE

25.

THE PEDIATRIC PALLIATIVE APRN

Cheryl Ann Thaxton and Nicole Sartor

KEY POINTS

- The pediatric palliative advanced practice registered nurse shares many of the same roles and competencies as the adult palliative APRN, with additional expertise in pediatrics.

- The pediatric palliative APRN combines in-depth knowledge of pharmacologic and nonpharmacologic therapies, communication techniques, familiarity with ethical and cultural issues, and ongoing access to grief and bereavement resources for children and their family members.

- Delivery of patient- and family-centered care involves collaboration across several disciplines; the APRN is often the interdisciplinary communication leader in pediatric palliative care (PPC).

- Advocacy for the PPC population may require the APRN to take on innovative roles, such as clinical expert, educator, entrepreneur, business marketing champion, and transformational leader.

CASE STUDY: PEDIATRIC PALLIATIVE CARE

King was a 5-year-old boy diagnosed with Beare-Stevenson cutis gyrata syndrome, epilepsy, hydrocephalus, cranial stenosis, ischemic encephalopathy, and chronic lung disease. King had a tracheostomy, gastrostomy tube, shunted hydrocephalus, history of cranial stenosis repair, history of repaired scoliosis, and was debilitated by spasticity, myoclonus, dystonia, and hypertonicity. The pediatric palliative advanced practice registered nurse provided care for King upon his transfer from a community hospital to the children's hospital with fever, increased secretions, and respiratory insufficiency. The pediatric intensive care unit (PICU) physician consulted the pediatric palliative care (PPC) team to help King and his family with goals of care, advance care planning, and family support. It was King's fifth admission within a 6-month period due to complications related to scoliosis repair and subsequent respiratory infections.

Upon initial examination, the pediatric palliative APRN found King in acute distress with apparent myoclonus in his right leg and dystonia. On examination, he had severe clonus in his upper and lower extremities, worsening dystonia, and agitation with noticeable tears. King was diaphoretic, flushed, and had vital sign variability. His gaze was fixed, and he was not interactive. He had copious clear secretions on his face and mouth, and

his tracheostomy required nearly constant suction as reported by the bedside nurses. Additionally, King had multiple areas of skin breakdown.

King's mother, Saisha, was not at the visit because she was unable to visit the hospital regularly due to limited childcare options for King's siblings and the cold and flu restrictions prohibiting visitors under the age of 13. After completing the assessment, the pediatric palliative APRN called Saisha to introduce the pediatric palliative team. Saisha later stated, "When I first heard about palliative care, I was not sure what it was. I was scared. I thought that it meant 'the end' for my child. The APRN educated me about palliative care and answered all of my questions. I knew that palliative care was the best option for my son. I understood that working with palliative care would give King the best chance to be at home, where he was most comfortable. King loves being around his family! I think that is what helps children thrive, being in their setting, and around their family."

The pediatric palliative APRN discussed King's physical examination with his mother and learned that his symptoms were not new; however, they were getting worse over time and with each episode of acute illness. The pediatric palliative APRN worked with King's mother to treat his pain and neurologic symptoms, thus preventing rapid response events and frequent transfers from the floor to the PICU. His mother further expressed that "King's symptom management has truly improved his quality of life. When King is in pain his heart rate will increase, his oxygen saturation will decrease, and he will cry. He cannot say where he is hurting because he is nonverbal. The symptom management plan that the PPC team put together has allowed us to relieve King's pain and uncontrollable neurologic symptoms. Sometimes King can work himself up, and it can be so hard to get him to calm down. I have found that having this symptom management plan in place allows us to anticipate distressing symptoms and control the symptoms before they get out of control and lead us back to the hospital." The pediatric palliative APRN arranged for community support and a discharge plan to monitor those symptoms.

PEDIATRIC PALLIATIVE NURSING

Many children have chronic, debilitating, and serious illness; although the numbers are lower than for adults. Pediatric palliative care (PPC) focuses on optimizing the quality of life of children; maximizing their function; exquisitely managing physical, psychological, social, or spiritual care needs;

and enhancing support at home. While the nursing process is the same no matter what the population, the care and management must be tailored to the unique needs of a population (see Chapter 26, "The Pediatric Palliative APRN in the Acute Care Setting"; Chapter 27, "The Pediatric Palliative APRN in Perinatal and Neonatal Care"; Chapter 28, "The Pediatric Palliative APRN in the Clinic"; Chapter 29, "The Pediatric Palliative APRN in Oncology"; and Chapter 30, "The Pediatric Palliative APRN in the Community").

Pediatric palliative nursing is different from adult palliative care in that there are often lower caseloads, a wider scope of care members, more continuity across care continuums, and more access to resources, particularly philanthropy. The care provided to children must be age-, developmentally, and functionally appropriate. The necessity for the pediatric palliative advanced practice registered nurse (APRN) to be familiar with conditions and diseases specific to infants, children, and adolescents, as well as their trajectories, is essential. This includes pharmacological and nonpharmacological treatment options. In addition to impeccable assessment and treatment techniques, the pediatric palliative must have expertise in age- and developmentally appropriate communication skills for children and adolescents with serious illness and their families (see Chapter 31, "Communication in Pediatric Palliative Care"). Using skills in collaboration, the pediatric palliative APRN must identify and access community resources to support the infant, child, and adolescent and their family as well as the appropriate educational resources for the family. All aspects of PPC are aimed at keeping the child, parent, guardian, or family at the center of care for all decision-making, thus ensuring a patient- and family-centered approach.

HISTORY OF THE APRN ROLE IN PEDIATRIC PALLIATIVE NURSING

The role of the pediatric palliative APRN emerged based on the need to expand care across the life span, which initially correlated with the role of the palliative APRN (see Chapter 1, "Palliative APRN Practice and Leadership"). It is difficult to establish a definitive timeline for the development of PPC because the subspeciality has developed from multiple avenues: the establishment of the adult hospice and palliative care movement, the acknowledgment that children die, the emergence of family-centered care, the fact that children with chronic complex conditions are living longer,[1] and the grassroots movement of healthcare professionals and parents to promote better care for children. Early on, PPC struggled with care that can be described as being an "inch wide and a mile deep." Programs and clinicians often fought for credibility and acceptance as well as access to patients.[2] The history of the pediatric palliative APRN role extends back to the 1970s and 1980s, with the initial focus of care related to hospice and to specific medical conditions, such as pediatric cancer (Box 25.1).

PPC has experienced rapid growth since 2000. A cross-sectional national survey revealed that many children's hospitals in the United States have PPC programs; however, a majority of these programs were understaffed.[5] Of the 162 hospitals that responded to the survey, the mean full-time FTE for APRNs was 0.4, with a range of 0–3, and 54.5% of the programs employed no APRNs.[6] According to the World Health Organization,[7] people younger than 20 years compromise 25% of the global population and 40% of the global population of least-developed nations; there is an estimated 21 million neonates, infants, children, and adolescents who need PPC each year. Despite this apparent need, there is no clear data about the extent of PPC services internationally.

THE ROLE OF THE PEDIATRIC PALLIATIVE APRN

The expansion of PPC programs brought many significant advancements to the role of the pediatric palliative APRN. More attention is being focused on using PPC measures during the early stages of life-limiting illness for children receiving aggressive therapies for cancer, sickle cell disease, cystic fibrosis, and muscular dystrophy. Currently, around 69% of children's hospitals offer PPC services, and 41% employ dedicated pediatric staff; only 10–20% of dying children receive hospice at the end of life.[8] The trend in transitioning from pediatric to adult chronic illness calls for APRN skills that reflect the unique needs of children. Many communities do not have enough children with life-threatening medical conditions to support sufficient pediatric palliative APRN clinical expertise. Without enough exposure to care in the community, it is difficult to develop and maintain sufficient clinical acumen in assessment, evaluation, and management from diagnosis to end-of-life care. Thus, children with seriously illness and their families often travel far from home for treatment at academic medical centers.[9]

Palliative care coexists with treatment and is important from the time of diagnosis, throughout a child's illness, and beyond. The pediatric palliative APRN is often a consistent team member for children and their families as they navigate inpatient to outpatient settings. APRNs are in ideal roles to provide PPC at the bedside because they spend the most time with children and their families.[10] Pediatric palliative APRNs are often long-standing members of the team, individuals who have pioneered new programs.[11] These APRNs often serve as informal leaders without titles, garnering the respect of others through their longevity of team membership, an open mentoring process, or a nurturing style. The pediatric palliative APRN's role in PPC is multifaceted and involves "wearing many hats."

The pediatric palliative APRN contributes to the dynamic organizational infrastructure of PPC programs. The opening case study offered the story of a mother whose child had been through years of symptom distress related to a life-limiting illness. The pediatric palliative APRN assessed the level of suffering within the family, worked with the family to establish goals of care, and supported them through the illness trajectory. The overall growth rate of PPC programs across the

Box 25.1 HISTORY OF PEDIATRIC PALLIATIVE CARE (1955–2021)

1955	Bozeman, Sutherland, and Orbach published one of the earliest psychological studies of dying children.[4]
1972	Professor Ida Martinson, from the Department of Nursing at the University of Minnesota, recognized the need for pediatric homecare and received a 4-year grant from the National Cancer Institute for researching homecare of the dying child.
1978	Dr. W. Allan Hogge and Mrs. Hogge asked their Presbyterian Church for help in caring for their son with a serious, progressive neurological condition. They established Edmarc Children's Hospice in Suffolk, Virginia.
1978	Professor Myra Blubond-Langer, an anthropologist, published *The Private World of Dying Children*, a book based on her observations of hospitalized children with leukemia.
1979	Dr. L. Joseph Butterfield established a neonatal hospice program in Denver, Colorado.
1983	Ann Armstrong-Dailey established Children's Hospice International (CHI). Her advocacy work contributed to the Children's Program for All-inclusive Coordinated Care (ChiPACC) program in 1999.
1984	St. Mary's Hospital in New York established the first pediatric palliative care department in the United States.
1998	The World Health Organization published *Guidelines on Cancer Pain Relief and Palliative Care for Children*.
2000	Dr. Joanne Wolfe et al. published the seminal article "Symptoms and Suffering at the End of Life in Children with Cancer."
2000	American Academy of Pediatrics (AAP) published first policy statement on pediatric palliative care; it was updated in November 2013.
2004	End of Life Nursing Education Consortium (ELNEC), Pediatric Version, was developed as part of the comprehensive palliative nursing educational initiative with Dr. Betty Ferrell as principal investigator. As of 2022, more than 1 million nurses and other professionals have received ELNEC training in all the versions: Core, Geriatrics, Critical Care, Oncology, APRN, and Pediatrics. The Institute of Medicine (IOM) report, *When Children Die*, brought awareness to the need for clinical expertise, research, and program development.
2010	Education in Palliative and End-of-Life Care (EPEC) Pediatric is developed as part a comprehensive pediatric palliative care curriculum with Dr. Stefan Friedrichsdorf as primary investigator
2013	National Consensus Project for Quality Palliative Care *Clinical Practice Guidelines* (3rd ed.) includes broader pediatric palliative care content, which expanded in 2018 in the fourth edition.
2021	*Palliative Nursing: Scope and Standards of Practice* (6th ed.) was released by the Hospice and Palliative Nurses Association (HPNA); it includes pediatric content.

From Sisk et al.[3]

United States has led to the recognition of this subspecialty by several national organizations.

GENERAL PRINCIPLES OF PEDIATRIC PALLIATIVE CARE

Since its inception, the National Consensus Project Clinical for Quality Palliative Care (NCP) *Clinical Practice Guidelines* support the belief that palliative care is inclusive of all people with serious illness, regardless of setting, diagnosis, prognosis, or age.[12] The NCP *Clinical Practice Guidelines* delineate eight domains of palliative care: Structure and Processes of Care, Physical Aspects of Care, Psychological and Psychiatric Aspects of Care, Social Aspects of Care, Cultural Aspects of Care, Spiritual and Existential Aspects of Care, Care Nearing End of Life, and Ethical and Legal Aspects of Care. Timely integration of palliative care is the responsibility of all clinicians and disciplines caring for infants and children with serious illnesses including primary care practices, specialist care practices (e.g., oncology or neurology), hospitalists, nursing home staff, and palliative care specialist teams such as hospice, hospital, and community-based palliative care teams.[13,14]

The fundamental principle of PPC is that the child and the family, as a unit of care, are the central focus. Moreover, the child's participation in the care—based on age, developmental, cognitive, and functional abilities—should be encouraged. The reinforcement of quality initiatives supports best practices in palliative care and serves as the foundation for promoting evidence-based principles. The pediatric palliative APRN must keep abreast of these guidelines and ensure that the team is empowered to implement them throughout the evolution of the program. Practicing within the scope of care for the pediatric palliative APRN has historically involved the ability to incorporate a physical, biopsychosocial, and spiritual multimodal approach to caring for children and their families. As the role has evolved, the pediatric palliative APRN continues to be the role model for persistent child and family advocacy within institutions and community settings.

ROLE DESCRIPTION AND QUALIFICATIONS

Pediatric palliative APRNs come from a variety of educational and training backgrounds. APRNs employed as providers in PPC programs may be trained as family nurse practitioners, family or pediatric clinical nurse specialists, neonatal nurse practitioners, or pediatric nurse practitioners. A few programs across the United States offer palliative nursing fellowships; many of these offer adult palliative care clinical rotations and may not have extensive access to PPC patients (see Chapter 2, "Fundamental Skills and Education for the Generalist and Specialist Palliative APRN"). Therefore, the pediatric palliative APRN is often the catalyst to establishing a structure for orientation and onboarding of roles in many health settings. The job description of the pediatric palliative APRN incorporates education, research utilization, consultation, and professional leadership and development (Box 25.2).

The role development for the pediatric palliative APRN should be clearly aligned with the job descriptions and incorporate key competencies. The Hospice and Palliative Nurses Association (HPNA)'s 2021 publication *Competencies for the Palliative and Hospice APRN*, delineates eight competencies of specialty palliative nursing practice; these include clinical judgment, advocacy and moral agency, caring practices, collaboration, systems thinking, response to diversity, facilitation

---

Box 25.2 SAMPLE PEDIATRIC PALLIATIVE APRN JOB DESCRIPTION

Position summary

The Pediatric Palliative APRN provides direct patient care services and performs medical care under in collaboration with physician (or supervision of physician as per state APRN statutes). Provides palliative care to perinatal, neonatal, pediatric, adolescent, and young adult patients requiring pain/symptom management, palliative care, and care at end of life. The APRN collects a health history; performs physical exams, collects, and documents data; conducts diagnostic and therapeutic procedures; orders and schedules laboratory studies and professional consultations; analyses and interprets data; prescribes appropriate pharmacotherapeutics and non-pharmacological strategies; conducts and participates in research; provides teaching, education, and provides leadership in the organization.

Position requirements

Education:
　APRN: Work requires completion of accredited graduate nursing NP or CNS program.
Licensure:
　APRN: Current licensure as a Registered Nurse (RN) and NP or CNS in the state of X.
Certification:
　NP: National certification as an NP or CNS in Pediatrics (may consider Family Nurse Practitioner depending on level of experience).
Experience:
　Master's degree required with a preference for a minimum of __ years' experience in the clinical care of patients with complex medical problems facing end-of-life issues. Position requires demonstrated competency in pain, stress, and other symptom management. Strongly prefer candidate with at least one year of experience as an NP or CNS. Acute care experience preferred.
Life support:
- Basic Life Support (BLS)
- Pediatric Advanced Life Support (PALS)
- Advanced Cardiac Life Support (ACLS)
- Neonatal Resuscitation Program (NPR)

Job Responsibilities

Clinical Expert:

- In collaboration with the pediatric palliative care attending physicians and/or residents, round daily on patients to assess, diagnose, plan treatment, set priorities and realistic outcomes, and evaluate the effectiveness and cost efficiency of patient care.

- Provide and coordinate clinical care for service specific patients through established protocols and under the supervising physician or back up physician, who is either on site or virtually.

- Collaborate with the chief resident, residents, fellows, attendings, other APRNs, patient resource managers, chaplains, clinical social workers, and other healthcare providers to formulate treatment plans and monitor patient progress.

- Perform procedures specific to the work environment after demonstrated competency and within the guidelines of scope of practice of advanced practice nursing per the American Nurses Association, APRN credentialing protocols per the National Council of State Boards of Nursing; and palliative practice per the National Consensus Project for Quality Palliative Care, *Clinical Practice Guidelines for Quality Palliative Care*

- Assess patients for change in status and institute appropriate interventions.

- Develop patient care pathways, protocols, algorithms, and guidelines for the management of specific problems in conjunction with the palliative interdisciplinary team of medicine, nursing, social work, chaplaincy, pharmacy and other members of the health care team.

- Analyze and integrate best clinical practice so as to provide the best health care to increase effectiveness, efficiency, and best outcomes.

- Assesses cultural and spiritual aspects of health to ensure health care is respectful and culturally sensitive.

- Assesses social aspects of care including and social determinants of health to ensure health care meets the needs of the patient and their family.

- Communicate effectively on verbal, non-verbal and written forms pertinent to patient care and information.

- Documents effectively in the patients' health record all relevant data including but not limited to results of diagnostic tests; laboratory results; patients' condition and response to therapies/interventions; communications with supervising MD.

- Implements a specific plan of palliative care to alleviate suffering and promote the physical, emotional, psychological, and spiritual comfort of the patient and family.

- Utilizes prescriptive privileges for identified patient population, certification, and licensure.

- Utilizes prescriptive authority for prescribing, ordering, and or administering drugs according to the Drug Enforcement Administration (DEA) regulations within the state.

- Role models competence in all APRN advanced skills.

- Provides daily handoff to appropriate attending, APRN, resident and/or intern at the end of the shift.

- Assures effective transitions of care across settings.

Educator:

- Assesses educational needs of the patient-care staff and provides education in format conducive to learning including just in time learning or more formal education as needed.

- Assesses educational needs of the patients and families and provide culturally sensitive patient/family education interventions as indicated. Use non-technical language when educating patients and families. Document all education in patients' electronic medical record.

- Implements and evaluates appropriate educational programs for patient care staff and other healthcare providers as appropriate; utilize evidenced-based curriculums such as the End-of-Life Nursing Education Consortium (ELNEC) to provide ongoing education at least one or twice a year.

- Role models and precepts healthcare learners through contractual agreements.

Research Utilization:

- Utilizes current research and evidence-based decision-making in all clinical practice.

- Analyzes and integrates clinical research findings in the development and implementation of standards of care.

- Supports IRB approved clinical research/trials though a variety of activities including but not limited to obtaining consent; ordering diagnostic tests; recording laboratory & diagnostic results; administering therapeutic interventions; and reporting patient outcomes including toxicities or adverse events.

- Develops and participates in interdisciplinary quality improvement and/or research activities.

- Develops and participates in measuring and documenting outcomes.

Consultant:

- Provides expertise and resource information to other healthcare providers, patients and families, and the community at large related to palliative care measures and care of seriously ill individuals.

- Implements and evaluates appropriate educational programs for referring providers (physicians, physician assistants, nurse practitioners, clinical nurse specialists).

- Develops, implements, and evaluates standards of care/practice guidelines/policies and procedures/care maps/protocols within area of specialization.

Professional Leadership and Development:

- Role models advanced practice nursing professionalism through conduct, communication, dress, leadership, ethical decision-making, critical thinking, and problem-solving skills.

- Participates in organizational committees such as medical pharmacotherapeutics, quality improvement, measurement, governance.

- Participates in professional organization at the regional and national level.

- Advances the palliative care field through written publications, oral presentations, posters, continuing education, etc.

- Maintains all professional requirements for licensure and certification.

REFERENCES

Dahlin, C. Competencies for Palliative and Hospice Advanced Practice Registered Nurse. Pittsburgh, PA: Hospice and Palliative Nurses Association. 2021.
Dahlin, C. The Professional Practice Guide for the Hospice and Palliative APRN. Pittsburgh, PA: Hospice and Palliative Nurses Association. 2017.

of learning, and clinical inquiry.[15] Pediatric oncology APRNs often work with children facing chronic and life-threatening illnesses. Many of these APRNs pursue additional advanced palliative care training. Pediatric palliative APRNs have the unique opportunity to work with several clinical teams as part of their role in developing collaborations; these include but are not limited to oncology, cardiology, pulmonology, neurology, genetics, rheumatology, neonatology, and neuromuscular disorders. In addition, opportunities exist for APRNs to serve as pioneers for developing PPC programs within institutions that do not have formal PPC teams or sufficient team support. In terms of qualifications for the role, pediatric palliative APRNs may have a background in critical care nursing, oncology, hospice, or variations of chronic disease management (e.g., cardiac, pulmonary, neurology, etc.).

National nursing certification is the recognition of expertise in a specific area. Certification in palliative nursing palliative acknowledges the role of the pediatric APRN. The Hospice and Palliative Credentialing Center (HPCC) is the only organization that offers specialty certification to the hospice and palliative nursing team. More than 15,500 nurses at all levels of practice hold HPCC credentials that establish a professional commitment to safe, ethical, and evidence-based care.[16] The pediatric palliative APRN can pursue palliative nursing certification by four means: (1) the advanced certified hospice and palliative nursing (ACHPN) examination (for the nurse practitioner or clinical nurse specialist), (2) the certified hospice and palliative pediatric nurse (CHPPN) examination, (3) the certified hospice and palliative nursing (CHPN) examination, and (4) the certified in perinatal loss care (CPLC) examination. Certification examination review courses are held across the United States and online.

THE PEDIATRIC PALLIATIVE APRN AS CLINICAL EXPERT

Pediatric palliative APRNs are clinical experts who collaborate with their interdisciplinary team to alleviate the suffering of children with serious illness, their families, and colleagues in the health professions.[17] The pediatric palliative APRN role has evolved over the past 10 years, moving outside of large academic medical centers and into clinics and communities where APRNs practice primary and specialty PPC.[18] As stated by the American Nurses Association (ANA) and HPNA, all APRNs have primary palliative nursing skills and some specialize in palliative care, with a focus on pediatrics.[19] Pediatric APRNs such as family nurse practitioners, clinical nurse specialists, and/or pediatric nurse practitioners must have the clinical expertise to care for PPC patients if they are to work in the role of the pediatric palliative APRN.

Primary PPC focuses on understanding serious illness in the pediatric population, common diseases, important indicators of decision-making for parents, the basics of pain and symptoms management with common medications such as morphine and oxycodone, advance care planning, and the difference between hospice and palliative care. Specialty palliative care is expertise in pediatric diagnoses and their trajectories, communication regarding goals of care and advanced illness, complex pain and symptom management, and a clear understanding of community resources and coverage of hospice, home health, and concurrent care. There can be various ranges of expertise in caring for neonatal, pediatric, adolescent, and young adult patients.

The pediatric palliative APRN cares for children with a wide range of conditions that include accidental and nonaccidental traumas, congenital malformations, chromosomal abnormalities, metabolic disorders, neuromuscular disorders, malignancies, and heart disease. In collaboration with the PPC attending physicians, fellows, residents, social workers, chaplains, child-life specialists, and other members of the team, the pediatric palliative APRN should regularly round on children to assess, diagnose, plan treatment, set priorities, and evaluate outcomes, in addition to assessing the effectiveness and cost-efficiency of patient care. As described in the *Palliative Nursing: Scope and Standards of Practice* and the *Competencies for the Palliative and Hospice APRN*, the pediatric palliative APRN collaborates to assess and identify quality-of-life issues that may hinder clinical progression toward a meaningful recovery for pediatric patients, with a consistent focus on addressing the child's symptom burden. As a liaison for the child, family, and staff, the pediatric palliative APRN provides and coordinates clinical care for children through established protocols.[20]

General pain management policies that are not specific to pediatrics can be reviewed by the pediatric palliative APRN and further developed to support the unique needs of children receiving care for serious illness. Children with chronic pain are best cared for with interdisciplinary assessment and management, and this requires a combination of medicine, psychology, and rehabilitation services for all pediatric patients referred for assessment and management of chronic pain.[21] As a clinical expert in chronic pain, the pediatric palliative APRN collaborates to develop plans that promote pain relief for children with illnesses like juvenile rheumatoid arthritis, sickle cell disease, Crohn's disease, and many other chronic debilitating infirmities.

A major focus in PPC is pain at the end of a child's life. Pain management at end of life requires expert nursing process, including a history, an assessment, and the integration of appropriate therapies. A retrospective cross-sectional survey conducted at two US tertiary care pediatric institutions revealed that unrelieved pain was associated with parents' perspectives of hastening death in children with cancer. This study surveyed 141 parents of children who died of cancer (response rate 64%); only 19 reported that they would have considered hastening their child's death had the child been in uncontrollable pain.[22] This research supports the essential clinical expertise necessary of the pediatric palliative APRNs role to managing pediatric pain, thus eliminating parents feeling that their child suffered.

As stated in the *Palliative Nursing: Scope and Standards of Practice* and the NCP *Clinical Practice Guidelines*, the pediatric palliative APRN should collaborate with palliative APRN and physician colleagues, nurses, case managers, chaplains, child life specialists, clinical social workers, and other healthcare providers to formulate treatment plans and monitor a child's progress. Additional plans for improving and promoting the quality-of-life goals for pediatric patients may involve organizing interdisciplinary team meetings that include respiratory therapists, physical and occupational therapists, pharmacists, nutritionists, home health providers, and hospice teams.

These team meetings help to outline clear pathways to formulate plans that are based on the child's and family's preferences. These gatherings can also help to decrease the chance of implementing treatments that are not aligned with these goals and preferences. The pediatric palliative APRN is often the lead facilitator of interdisciplinary communication. Care coordination by the APRN involves skills to promote safe, quality care (e.g., conduct family care conferences, manage pain and distressing symptoms, provide guidance with advance care planning) while demonstrating competency within state-specific scope of practice and credentialing protocols.

The pediatric palliative APRN should have a job description that sets the parameters of practice. To ensure success, regular performance reviews promote assessment of clinical practice patterns as well as efficient and quality palliative care. The use of prescriptive privileges within the identified pediatric population should reflect expertise and competence. Pediatric palliative APRN documentation in the medical record should incorporate all relevant data. This includes results of diagnostic tests, laboratory results, the child's condition, response to therapies and interventions, and any necessary communication with the supervising physician. Additionally, documentation should include specific recommendations for a child's palliative care plan with the aim of alleviating suffering and optimizing the physical, emotional, psychological, and spiritual comfort of the child and family.

The pediatric palliative APRN partners with other members of the team to address the pain plan and make referrals when necessary. A thorough knowledge of pediatric-specific pharmacological and nonpharmacological measures allows the APRN to provide guidance that helps with transition models for children with chronic illness. For example, the pediatric palliative APRN collaborates with the child life specialist to integrate expressive therapies, pet therapy, or other services available within the institution. Finally, the pediatric palliative APRN promotes continuity by providing daily "handoff" of patient care to appropriate physicians, other APRNs, residents, and/or interns at the end of the shift while ensuring that proper introductions to the child and family have taken place before departing.

THE PEDIATRIC PALLIATIVE APRN AS EDUCATOR

The pediatric palliative APRN assesses the educational needs of the patient care staff for formal and informal education. It is important to understand that education and teaching allow the APRN to role model professionalism. Inherent in each teaching and learning session is consideration of maintaining proper boundaries and being mindful of colleagues' reactions to challenging clinical situations. Pediatric palliative APRNs work to assess the educational needs of children and families as well, providing culturally sensitive educational interventions as indicated. It is essential to use nontechnical language when educating children and families. All education must be documented in the child's medical record. Although is continued growth of PPC programs, there is still limited access to preceptors in the clinical setting; thus, being a resource for new pediatric palliative APRNs is vital.

For APRNs seeking to expand their knowledge base in PPC, several evidence-based curriculums are available for understanding the palliative care needs of children. An End of Life Nursing Education Consortium (ELNEC) curriculum was developed to address the unique needs of APRNs who are starting a palliative care program, leading a hospice/ palliative care team, joining and/or participating in a hospice/

palliative care team, or incorporating palliative care in their role as an APRN.[23] There are nine modules in which participants receive advanced nursing education encompassing an overview of palliative APRN practice, pain assessment and management, symptom assessment and management, communication, and final hours. To assist the APRN with program development, content also includes education about palliative care program development including finances, quality, education, and leadership. Participants can choose one of two tracks—adult- or pediatric-focused care.[24] Further resources are listed in Table 25.1.

Another curriculum, Education in Palliative and End of Life Care (EPEC) Pediatrics is a comprehensive adaptation of the EPEC curriculum designed to address the needs of children, their families, and pediatric oncology providers and other pediatric clinicians.[25] EPEC Pediatrics was developed by and continues to receive input from experts representing several pediatric disciplines as well as parent advocate advisors. It consists of 23 core and 2 elective topics in pain and symptom management in palliative care.[26] Keeping up with current research and trends in clinical practice can help the pediatric palliative APRN

Table 25.1 PEDIATRIC PALLIATIVE APRN RESOURCES

INTENSIVES

NAME	DESCRIPTION	WEBSITE	COST
Palliative Care APP Externship	Week-long in-person training for APRNs and PAs in care to enhance primary palliative care skills through didactic and clinical experiences with pediatric experiences	https://advancingexpertcare.org/aprn-externship	Open to APRNs, PAs, and MDs
Four Seasons Immersion Course	Week-long in-person course that covers extensive palliative care content	https://fourseasonsconsulting.teleioscn.org/education/palliative-care-immersion-course	Open to all members
Harvard Center for Palliative Care- Palliative Care Education and Practice Pediatric Track	Two-week course to enhance communication, teaching, and practice focusing on the unique aspects of caring for children	https://pallcare.hms.harvard.edu/node/126	Application process
CHPPN Review Course	1-day review course for nurses interested in becoming certified in specialty pediatric nursing	https://advancingexpertcare.org/certification-review-courses	Open to all eligible RNs and APRNs

CURRICULA	DESCRIPTION	WEBSITE	AVAILABILITY
End-of-Life Nursing Education Consortium Pediatric Palliative Care Train-the-Trainer (ELNEC-PPC)	Train-the-trainer format pediatric palliative care, both online and in-person curriculum for nurses	http://www.aacn.nche.edu/elnec/trainings/national#PEDIATRIC	Open to all Fee for course In-person and online
Pediatric Pain Masters Class	Education in pharmacological, medical, psychosocial, and integrative therapies for pediatric patient pain management from a holistic and interdisciplinary perspective	http://noneedlesspain.org/ppmc/	Open to all Registration fee
Education in Palliative and End-of-Life Care Program (EPEC)	An annual offering of 23 core and 2 elective topics in pain and symptom management in pediatric palliative care taught as a combination of distance learning modules and in-person conference sessions	epec.net/epec_pediatrics.php	Open to all Registration fee
National Hospice and Palliative Care Organization (NHPO) Pediatric Palliative Care Training (PPCT)	Downloadable symptom control guidelines, palliative care commissioning reports, and patient education pages	http://www.nhpco.org/childrenspediatricschipps/pediatric-palliative-care-training-0	Open to NHPCO members

Table 25.1 CONTINUED

ONLINE RESOURCES

NAME	DESCRIPTION	WEBSITE	COST
Association for Children with Life-Threatening or Terminal Conditions and Their Families (ACT) Professional Resources	Current research and evidence	http://www.togetherforshortlives.org.uk/professionals/resources	Open Access
International Children's Palliative Care Network	Many resources for palliative care	https://www.icpcn.org	Open Access
NINR Palliative Care for Children Palliative Care: Conversations Matter	Many resources for communication	https://www.ninr.nih.gov/newsandinformation/conversationsmatter/palliative-care-for-children#.VY6-pUay4nJ	Open Access
Courageous Parents Network	Conversations with children	https://courageousparentsnetwork.org	Open Access

PRINT RESOURCES

Palliative Nursing

Kobler K, Limbo R. *Conversations in Perinatal, Neonatal, and Pediatric Palliative Care.* Pittsburgh, PA: Hospice & Palliative Nurses Association; 2017.

Santucci G. *Core Curriculum for the Pediatric Hospice & Palliative Nurse.* 2nd ed. Pittsburgh, PA: Hospice & Palliative Nurses Association; 2017

Ferrell B, Paice J. *Oxford Textbook of Palliative Nursing.* New York: Oxford University Press; 2019.

Dahlin C, Coyne PJ. *Advanced Practice Palliative Nursing.* New York: Oxford University Press; 2022.

Program Development Implementation

National Consensus Project for Quality Palliative Care. *Clinical Practice Guidelines.* Henrico, VA: National Coalition of Hospice and Palliative Care; 2018.

World Health Organization. Integrating Palliative Care and Symptom Relief into Paediatrics. Geneva: World Health Organization; 2018.

Clinical Practice and Organizational Guidelines

Center to Advance Palliative Care. *Pediatric Palliative Care Field Guide.* New York: CAPC: 2019.

National Hospice and Palliative Care Organization. *Standards of Practice for Pediatric Palliative Care and Hospice.* Alexandria: NHCPO: 2019.

in developing and implementing standards of care. This includes keeping abreast of the many PPC resources published by palliative care organizations, PPC special interest or focus groups within specialty nursing organizations (e.g., American Association of Critical Nurses, Association of Pediatric Hematology/Oncology Nurses National Association of Pediatric Nurse Practitioners), and palliative care blogs (e.g., BMJ Supportive and Palliative Care Blog, Pallimed). Other activities that promote keeping up to date in PPC development include participating in a palliative care journal club; state hospice and palliative care professional groups; or local, regional, or national HPNA committees, or taking advantage of the Center to Advance Palliative Care (CAPC) offerings and social networks (see Box 25.3).

Analysis of patient care through ongoing case reviews with the interdisciplinary team helps the pediatric palliative APRN to participate in measuring and documenting outcomes. This includes participation in interdisciplinary quality improvement activities, such as chart reviews. Tracking operational data about children seen by pediatric

Box 25.3 LISTING OF PROFESSIONAL ORGANIZATIONS WITH PEDIATRIC FOCUS GROUPS

American Academy of Hospice and Palliative Medicine (AAHPM) – Pediatric Special Interest Group

American Academy of Pediatrics (AAP) – Section on Hospice and Palliative Medicine

Center to Advance Palliative Care (CAPC) – Pediatric Palliative Care Task Force (PPCTF)

Children's Hospice and Palliative Care Services Project (ChiPPS)

Children's International Project on Palliative/Hospice Services Workgroup

Children's Hospice International (CHI)

Hospice and Palliative Nurses' Association (HPNA)

Institute for Patient- and Family-Centered Care (IFCC)

International Children's Palliative Care Network (ICPCN)

National Hospice and Palliative Care Organization (NHPCO)

National Pediatric Hospice and Palliative Care Collaboration (NPHPCC)

Social Work in Hospice and Palliative Care Network (SWHPN)

palliative APRNS and a consultation service (i.e., diagnosis, referring service, reason for consultation, time from referral request to completion of consult, and disposition) is necessary to assess the effectiveness of program outreach, marketing, and education efforts in reaching children in need (not only children with serious illness, but also children who are part of underserved populations) and to plan for program staffing to accommodate a growth in demand for services. In the role of advocate, the pediatric palliative APRN should secure programmatic funding and resources to ensure the sustainability and growth of the PPC program.

As an educator, the pediatric palliative APRN serves as an expert and provides information to other healthcare providers, children, families, and the community at large on palliative care measures and end-of-life care. This effort should include developing, implementing, and evaluating standards of care for pediatric palliative pain and symptom management with the appropriate practice guidelines, policies, and procedures. If there are no clear guidelines for managing distressing symptoms such as dyspnea, insomnia, nausea, or pruritus for children at the end of life, the pediatric palliative APRN works to develop evidence-based plans of care or utilize established guidelines within the field to guide the bedside nurse.

THE PEDIATRIC PALLIATIVE APRN AS CLINICAL LEADER

As a leader, the pediatric palliative APRN serves as a role model of professionalism through conduct, communication, dress, leadership, ethical decision-making, critical thinking, compassion, and problem-solving skills. The pediatric palliative APRN is an advocate for PPC in all settings and ensures access to quality PPC. Advocacy involves speaking at conferences and participating in organization grand rounds or departmental meetings. It includes small-group lunches, learning sessions on a pediatric hospital unit, or an organization's orientation to educate new staff about the services provided by PPC teams. The pediatric palliative APRN also demonstrates responsibility for professional practice by actively participating in professional organizations. Specialty certification also demonstrates professionalism and leadership. The HPCC is the only nursing specialty organization to offer certification to all members of the nursing team (APRN, registered nurse [RN], pediatric RN, licensed practical/vocational nurse [LP/VN], nurse assistant [NA]) as well as hospice and palliative care program administrators and perinatal loss care professionals.[24] The examination measures skills in ethical decision-making, critical thinking, and problem-solving.

The pediatric palliative APRN maintains all professional requirements for licensure and certification (see Chapter 3, "Credentialing, Certification, and Scope of Practice Issues"). Participating in forums about legislative progress and policies surrounding pediatric healthcare initiatives enables the pediatric palliative APRN to talk with colleagues who share similar interests and empowers the APRN to promote

best practices. This is in alignment with advancing expert care. The Hospice and Palliative Nurses Association, the Hospice and Palliative Nurses Foundation, and the HPCC launched an initiative to (1) increase the number of certified hospice and palliative nurses, (2) advance research into best practices of hospice and palliative care, (3) elevate palliative nursing leadership at the local and national levels, and (4) enhance nursing competence through certification.[27] Other professional nursing organizations with palliative care initiatives include the Association of Pediatric Hematology/Oncology Nurses, National Hospice and Palliative Care Organization, National Association of Pediatric Nurse Practitioners, American Association of Colleges of Nursing, American Nurses Association, and National Association of Neonatal Nurses.

Building a PPC program requires qualities like self-motivation, creativity, resourcefulness, assertiveness, and perspicacity. Negotiation skills and flexibility help with navigating challenging cases and assisting in mediating conflict among staff during ethical quandaries. Pediatric palliative APRNs working with a newly developed PPC team may find it helpful to visit a nearby adult palliative APRN or neighboring program. Although many aspects of care are different between adults and children, the experience of rotating with an already established team can provide valuable insights for the APRN as the program moves forward.

THE PEDIATRIC PALLIATIVE APRN AS BUSINESS ADMINISTRATOR

The pediatric palliative APRN must have a business plan for program growth, expansion, and integration of PPC principles within an environment. Many of the palliative professional organizations, such as the Center to Advance Palliative Care, the National Hospice and Palliative Care Organization, and the California Healthcare Foundation, have resources to help develop a plan. In addition, there are several PPC state coalitions across the United States that offer vital resources for the pediatric palliative APRN and help strengthen program recognition through collaboration and partnerships. With the limited resources available in some organizations, pediatric palliative APRNs may need to be creative about marketing the awareness and benefits of PPC. Marketing via team brochures, newsletters, or flyers can help to educate the staff about the "who and what" of the PPC service in a meaningful way. Often parents of children with chronic illness meet several different teams, so a foldable brochure with the details of the services provided by the PPC team can be helpful. The APRN works with the clinical social work team to provide advance care planning services and ensures that bereavement resources and literature are accessible to the family.

Some healthcare providers misperceive that PPC is only appropriate at the end of life. The result is that the pediatric palliative APRN will spend considerable time dispelling myths about PPC. Promoting referrals early in the disease trajectory will enable the pediatric palliative APRN to meet the child and family at a crucial point in the trajectory. APRNs must remain aware that the relationship between the primary team and the child and family is at the forefront of the connection and must not be disregarded. The APRN also partners with the chaplaincy team to support the spiritual needs of the child and family. All members of the team are vital, so the pediatric palliative APRN makes sure that the child and family understand the various roles of those involved in providing care, remaining available to answer questions when necessary.

Individual health teams across the care continuum may have questions about the types of services provided by PPC teams, how teams collaborate, who is responsible for what care issues, and financial aspects of care. To navigate these conversations, the APRN must acquire negotiation skills as well as diplomacy and humility. However, these questions provide the APRN with the opportunity to develop professional relationships and collaborative partnerships.

To increase awareness of PPC services, the pediatric palliative APRN educates teams about PPC by offering to meet with them. Establishing a relationship with the APRN of the referring team promotes partnerships and helps to maintain the relationship through honest feedback from an APRN colleague. The pediatric palliative APRN should solicit feedback about the PPC service including referral process, care delivery, communication, and discharge. This facilitates quality improvement in PPC services. Developing consistent goals for follow-up can be vital to the growth of the program. For example, contacting the hospice agency of the child to discuss transition of care to hospice before and after death is important for the growth of the PPC service and, more importantly, can elicit feedback to review family satisfaction and patient outcomes.

TRANSFORMATIONAL LEADERSHIP

Transformation leadership is an approach that influences change in individuals and social systems. The pediatric palliative APRN must grow and mature as a transformational nurse leader in the midst of an ever-changing healthcare environment, often with limited resources. The APRN develops partnerships that lead to improved access to services for children. Some examples are listed here.

1. Contacting the local hospice agency to educate the nursing staff about managing dyspnea in infants, with

Table 25.2 ROLES OF THE PEDIATRIC PALLIATIVE APRN

ROLE	PROPOSED ACTIONS
Clinical expert	• Maintain advanced clinical skills in pain and symptom management • Acquire knowledge of novel pediatric pharmacological and nonpharmacological therapies • Develop protocols and procedures • Plan interdisciplinary team meetings • Facilitate communication • Provide compassionate care • Document appropriately • Demonstrate competency
Educator	• Provide information to other healthcare providers, children, families, and the community at large • Develop care maps and algorithms for managing distressing symptoms • Precept new pediatric palliative APRNs • Track clinical and/or operational metrics • Participate in quality improvement activities (e.g., chart reviews) • Participate in a journal club
Clinical Leader	• Join a national professional palliative care organization • Participate in hospital grand rounds • Role model professionalism through conduct, communication, dress, leadership, ethical decision making, critical thinking and problem-solving skills • Present during a lunch-and-learn session • Pioneer a new PPC program
Business Administrator	• Develop a business plan to expand services • Create a program brochure, newsletter, or flyer to promote awareness • Follow up regularly with referring teams • Elicit child/family satisfaction through surveys
Transformational Leader	• Contact local home hospice agencies to offer education for the nursing staff • Create a pain management task force • Start a PPC journal club • Promote the use of evidence-based guidelines and protocols for pain and symptom management in PPC • Develop partnerships within and outside of the institution

participation from the community pharmacy based on the evidence.

2. Creating a pain management task force in the pediatric intensive care unit to identify children at risk for having inadequately treated pain, with participation from the pharmacy department.

3. During the implementation of compassionate extubation, the pediatric palliative APRN starts a journal club to promote understanding and best practice organization-wide.

In all these examples, the pediatric palliative APRN seeks to build commitment to children with serious illnesses with the goal of transforming the healthcare environment into a place where all members of the institution are accountable for the care of the pediatric patient.

The pediatric palliative APRN works within the resources of the organization and community, using creativity and expertise to promote the growth and expansion of PPC initiatives. If there are questions about evidence-based guidelines for a procedure, a process of consensus building is initiated. Finally, as a transformational leader in PPC, the pediatric palliative APRN actively engages children, family, and staff throughout the patient care experience. To meet each child's needs, the APRN uses skills as clinical expert, educator, entrepreneur, and administrator, all while considering the available resources. (see Table 25.2).

SUMMARY

There are opportunities and challenges in PPC delivery. The pediatric palliative APRN will need to be adaptable and have a multifaceted skills to create programs that reflect the community, the organization, and available resources. These include clinical expertise, expert communication skills, program development knowledge, leadership skills, and professionalism. Ongoing self-awareness and self-care are vital for the pediatric palliative APRN. Personal goals for the APRN includes improving one's organizational and communication skills. Professional goals may include networking within the field of PPC and assuming a national leadership role in PPC. Finding a mentor within the field may also help tremendously. Ultimately, the goal of the pediatric palliative APRN is to improve the care of children with serious illness and their families by ensuring access to quality PPC.

REFERENCES

1. Feudtner C, Womer J, Augustin R, et al. Pediatric palliative care programs in children's hospitals: A cross-sectional national survey. *Pediatric (Evanston)*. 2013;132(6):1063–1070. doi:10.1542/peds.2013-1286

2. Friebert S. Pediatric palliative care: A specialty comes of age. *Cancer Commons Blog*. October 14. 2019. https://cancercommons.org/latest-insights/pediatric-palliative-care-a-specialty-comes-of-age/

3. Sisk BA, Feudtner C, Bluebond-Langner M, Sourkes B, Hinds PS, Wolfe J. Response to suffering of the seriously ill child: A history of palliative care for children. *Pediatrics (Evanston)*. 2020;145(1):e20191741. doi:10.1542/peds.2019-1741

4. Bozeman MF, Orbach CE, Sutherland AM. Psychological impact of cancer and its treatment. III. The adaptation of mothers to the threatened loss of their children through leukemia: Part I. *Cancer*. 1955;8(1):1–19. doi:10.1002/1097-0142(1955)8:1<1::AID-CNCR2820080102>3.0.CO;2-Y

5. Friedrichsdorf SJ, Bruera E. Delivering pediatric palliative care: From denial, palliphobia, pallilalia to palliactive. *Children (Basel)*. 2018;5(9):120. doi:10.3390/children5090120

6. Negrete TN, Tariman JD. Pediatric Palliative Care: A Literature Review of Best Practices in Oncology Nursing Education Programs. *Clin J Onc Nurs*. 2019;23(6):565–568. doi:10.1188/19.CJON.565-568.

7. World Health Organization. *Integrating Palliative Care and Symptom Relief into Paediatrics: A WHO Guide for Health-Care Planners, Implementers and Managers*. Geneva: World Health Organization; 2018. https://apps.who.int/iris/handle/10665/274561

8. Moody K, McHugh M, Baker R, et al. Providing pediatric palliative care education using problem-based learning. *J Palliat Med*. 2018;21(1):22–27. doi:10.1089/jpm.2017.0154

9. National Hospice and Palliative Care Organization. *Standards of practice for pediatric palliative care*: Professional development and resources series. Alexandria, VA: NHPCO. 2019. https://www.nhpco.org/wp-content/uploads/2019/07/Pediatric_Standards.pdf

10. Akard TF, Hendricks-Ferguson VL, Gilmer MJ. Pediatric palliative care nursing. *Ann Palliat Med*. 2019;8(Suppl 1):S39–S48. doi:10.21037/apm.2018.06.01

11. Dahlin C, Coyne P. The palliative APRN leader. *Ann Palliat Med*. 2019;8(Suppl 1):S30–S38. doi:10.21037/apm.2018.06.03

12. The National Consensus Project for Quality Palliative Care. *Clinical Practice Guidelines*. Pittsburgh, PA: National Consensus Project. 2004. https://www.nationalcoalitionhpc.org/ncp/

13. The National Consensus Project for Quality Palliative Care. *Clinical Practice Guidelines*. 3rd ed. 2013. Pittsburgh, PA: National Consensus Project. https://www.nationalcoalitionhpc.org/ncp/

14. The National Consensus Project for Quality Palliative Care. *Clinical Practice Guidelines*. 4th ed. Richmond, VA: National Coalition of Hospice and Palliative Care. 2018. https://www.nationalcoalitionhpc.org/ncp/

15. Dahlin C. *Competencies for the Palliative and Hospice APRN*. 3rd. ed. Pittsburgh, PA: Hospice and Palliative Nurses Association; 2021.

16. Hospice and Palliative Credentialing Center. Advanced certified hospice and palliative nurse examination webpage. 2021. Available at https://advancingexpertcare.org/HPNA/Certification/Credentials/APRN_ACHPN/HPCC/CertificationWeb/ACHPN.aspx

17. Hagan TL, Xu J, Lopez RP, Bressler T. Nursing's role in leading palliative care: A call to action. *Nurs Education Today*. 2018;61:216–219. http://dx.doi.org/10.1016/j.nedt.2017.11.037. doi:10.1016/j.nedt.2017.11.037

18. Cormack C, Phillips S, McDaniel C. Overcoming Barriers, 1 Child at a Time: An Innovative Approach to Community-Based Pediatric Palliative Care Services. *J Hospice Palliat Nurs*. 2016;18(5):459–463. doi:10.1097/NJH.0000000000000275

19. American Nurses Association, Hospice and Palliative Nurses Association. *Call for Action: Nurses Lead and Transform Palliative Care*. Silver Spring, MD: American Nurses Association; 2017. https://www.nursingworld.org/~497158/globalassets/practiceand-policy/health-policy/palliativecareprofessionalissuespanelcallforaction.pdf

20. Dahlin C. *Palliative Nursing: Scope and Standards of Practice*. 6th ed. Pittsburgh, PA: Hospice and Palliative Nurses Association; 2021.

21. Friedrichsdorf SJ, Goubert L. Pediatric pain treatment and prevention for hospitalized children. *Schmerz (Berlin, Germany)*. 2021;35(3):195–210. doi:10.1007/s00482-020-00519-0

22. Dussel V, Joffe S, Hilden JM, Watterson-Schaeffer J, Weeks JC, Wolfe J. Considerations about hastening death among parents of children who die of cancer. *Arch Pediatr Adolesc Med*. 2010;164(3):231–237. doi:10.1001/archpediatrics.2009.295

23. American Colleges of Nursing, City of Hope. ELNEC Pediatric APRN. 2021. https://www.aacnnursing.org/ELNEC/Courses

24. Dahlin C, Coyne PJ, Paice J, Malloy P, Thaxton CA, Haskamp A. ELNEC-APRN: Meeting the needs of advanced practice nurses through education. *J Hospice Palliat Nurs*. 2017;19(3):261–265. doi:10.1097/NJH.0000000000000340

25. Friedrichsdorf SJ, Remke S, Hauser J, et al. Development of a pediatric palliative care curriculum and dissemination model: Education in Palliative and End-of-Life Care (EPEC) pediatrics. *J Pain Symptom Manage*. 2019;58(4):707–720.e3. doi:10.1016/j.jpainsymman.2019.06.008

26. Hauser JM, Preodor M, Roman E, Jarvis DM, Emanuel LJ. The evolution and dissemination of the education in palliative and end-of-life care program. *Palliat Med*. 2015 Sep;18(9):765–770. doi:10.1089/jpm.2014.0396.PMID: 26302426

27. Hospice and Palliative Credentialing Center. About Certification webpage. 2021. Available at https://advancingexpertcare.org/

26.

THE PEDIATRIC PALLIATIVE APRN IN THE ACUTE CARE SETTING

Faith Kinnear and Gina Santucci

<table>
<tr><td colspan="1">KEY POINTS</td></tr>
</table>

- Pediatric palliative care (PPC) is family-centered care that focuses on a child's and family's quality of life through the prevention and relief of suffering along a physical, psychological, emotional, spiritual, and social continuum.

- Many misconceptions and barriers still exist regarding PPC, including that it signifies death, giving up hope, no further provision of care, and abandonment.

- The number of children living with a variety of life-threatening illnesses is increasing, and families are frequently faced with difficult decisions about what interventions to choose. Pediatric palliative advanced practice registered nurses (PP APRNs) play a key role in guiding conversations about decision-making and goals of care.

- Principles for assessing and managing complex symptoms in children are unique but the PP APRN is well-equipped to take into account the child's developmental, cognitive, and biological factors. Case studies will illustrate a variety of these frequently encountered palliative care symptoms.

- PP APRNs are poised to be knowledgeable in pain and symptom management and advance care planning, to provide clear communication with patients and families, and to assist families with complex medical decision-making, including end-of-life care.

- Aside from patient responsibilities, the PP APRN may play an integral role in staff education, moral support, and well-being.

INTRODUCTION

Care for children living with chronic or life-threatening conditions historically has focused on treatment and cure. Yet, even with our best efforts and expanding scope of knowledge, children continue to experience prolonged courses and many still die from their disease process. Pediatric palliative care (PPC) aims to improve the quality of life for children and their families facing life-threatening illnesses through the prevention and relief of suffering by early identification and treatment of pain and other distressing symptoms, whether physical, psychological, social, or spiritual. PPC is meant to be provided in primary care encounters, tertiary care facilities, community health centers, and children's homes.[1] This chapter focuses on the pediatric palliative advanced practice registered nurses (PP APRNs) in the acute care setting, which focuses on education, collaboration, and coordination.

The delivery of high-quality PPC was promulgated by the landmark 2002 Institute of Medicine (IOM) report *When Children Die*,[2] which challenged all healthcare providers to address the needs of children with complex chronic or life-threatening conditions and their families. Since that time, the field of PPC has continued to grow and healthcare providers now have an obligation to provide high-quality PPC for children with life-threatening conditions and their families, as evidenced by the most recently published IOM report, *Dying in America: Improving Quality and Honoring Individual Preferences Near the End of Life* (2014). More recently, the 2018 edition of National Consensus Project for Quality Palliative Care (NCP) *Clinical Practice Guidelines* emphasizes the needs of children and their families within patient- and family-centered care, such as illness understanding, parental preferences, and family engagement using a developmentally and age-appropriate framework across settings of care.[3]

Figure 26.1 illustrates the complexity of PPC while highlighting the primary goals of (1) prioritization, (2) understanding what is important for the patient and family, and (3) how the PPC team can meet the family's goals.[4] PPC is available and delivered variety of settings. Care along the illness trajectory, from the time of diagnosis to completion of therapy or end of life, can vary greatly in length and is not always linear; goals may shift from care aimed at a cure to care focused on maximizing quality of life and back as patient needs change. This parallel planning or "hoping for the best, preparing for the worst," can be challenging for both providers and families. In pediatrics, prognostic uncertainty continues to be a formidable barrier to exploring the focus of care. Without prognostic certainty, it can be difficult to predict if and when a child's condition may improve or continue to decline or for how long the child will remain stable, which makes parallel planning a necessity.[5] Discussing goals of care during an acute change or crisis may be stressful and emotionally charged for everyone involved, while advance parallel planning may help families express and balance their wants and wishes with their worries.

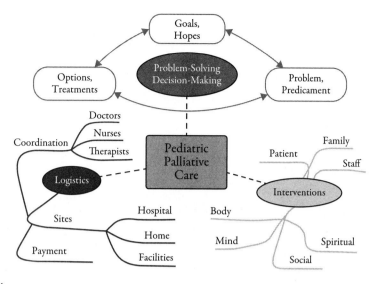

Figure 26.1 Facets of pediatric palliative care.
Reprinted with permission from Committee on Approaching Death: Addressing Key End of Life Issues; Institute of Medicine. *Dying in America: Improving Quality and Honoring Individual Preferences Near the End of Life.* Washington (DC): National Academies Press; 2015 Mar 19.[4]

Another barrier to initiating palliative care alongside cure- or recovery-directed care involves providers' uncertainty or inability to have these discussions, which can lead to their avoidance.[6] Even in cases where providers were able to identify specific physiologic factors or conditions that signaled an appropriate time to involve palliative care, they found that the shift in goals of care was often initiated by parents. Ongoing education about palliative care is important if providers are to partner with families in allowing for ongoing goals-of-care discussions, expectation setting, and parallel planning.[6]

Currently, a great proportion of hospitalized children die in the pediatric intensive care unit (PICU) due to the withdrawal, withholding, or discontinuation of life-sustaining therapies.[7] Research has shown that although pediatric providers in the ICU setting are skilled in providing high-level care, including many primary palliative care skills, most do not have formal training in providing specialized palliative care, and the patient and team may benefit from a specialty consult.[8] The timing for initiating such a consult may be a barrier to connecting the family with palliative care. Inpatient PP APRNs are well-positioned to identify the unique needs of hospitalized children and families when their goals shift more toward palliation and to provide guidance and support to families and the rest of the interdisciplinary team.

ADDRESSING MISCONCEPTIONS AND BARRIERS

"Does palliative care mean that I'm giving up on my child?" is something that a parent shared at the mention of consulting palliative care. This comment illustrates one of many misconceptions and beliefs about PPC. Some believe that PPC signifies impending death, loss of hope, lack of care provision, and abandonment, all misconceptions that serve as barriers to PPC delivery. Other barriers include healthcare providers' lack of understanding and/or training in palliative care and

feelings of inadequacy in offering PPC to families, as well as not knowing when and if it is the right time to make a referral to the palliative care team.[9] The challenge for the PP APRN then becomes not only providing high-quality PPC and staying current on evidenced-based practice but also addressing families' and colleagues' misconceptions about PPC.

One of the most effective methods to address common misconceptions and barriers is through increased PPC education. The pediatric APRN not specifically trained in PPC may wonder when to involve the PPC team: Is it at the time of diagnosis, or only when there are no further options for treatment? Can every child with a specific diagnosis benefit from PPC services? Will families be afraid if the PPC team is introduced too early, and would it signify giving up? Should there be specific time points in the illness trajectory, or should the presentation of specific symptoms warrant a referral to the PPC team, or should PPC be involved at all?[10] The answers to these questions will look different for each patient.

The PP APRN provides PPC education and addresses common questions by "speaking to patients to find out their goals and preferences for treatment and end-of-life care."[10] Currently, patient-centered care in the acute care setting is often perceived as "too little, too late."[10] The pediatric APRN may be able to recommend a palliative care consult, if available, for patient goals that exceed the scope of primary palliative care. The pediatric APRN may also have developed rapport with the family, thus allowing for more open communication to introduce or address PPC benefits for the patient and family. Introducing PPC earlier in the disease trajectory can provide psychosocial support over time and not just at the end of life. The fear that patients and families "are not there yet" is often the worry when providers (and others) equate palliative care with end-of-life care. Educating families and providers about the longitudinal support, assistance with decision-making, and expertise in pain and symptom management of PPC may help alleviate these fears. The benefits of early involvement of PPC are summarized in Box 26.1.

Helping families clarify goals of care as the child's condition changes, assisting with complicated symptom management, and, when needed, providing excellent end-of-life care that honors the child's and family's wishes are pillars of PPC. Pediatric teams are often challenged to "do everything possible" to prolong life—but at what burden? PPC teams can facilitate communication, help with decisions regarding aggressive interventions, acknowledge uncertainty, and offer a space for meaningful conversations regarding prognosis. The American Academy of Pediatrics recommends palliative care consultation upon diagnosis of a serious and or life-limiting illness.[4] Given the diversity of pediatric diagnoses, the pediatric APRN should consider a palliative care consult, when available, if the trajectory of illness is unknown, when there is indecision regarding the right course of action, or when the child's overall quality of life has declined from their baseline, as summarized in Box 26.2.

WHO RECEIVES INPATIENT PEDIATRIC PALLIATIVE CARE?

It is estimated that, in the US, approximately 50,000 children die every year, with some 80% of children dying in a hospital setting.[11] It is estimated that about 25% of these children may have benefited from PPC or hospice services.[12] What about the children who do not die? According to a 2015–2016 National Palliative Care Registry, 52 pediatric programs reported their data, and they represented 40% of the children's hospitals in 27 states and Washington, DC.[12] The age range and top five diagnoses from 75% of children discharged from the hospital are illustrated in Figure 26.2.[13]

IMPACT OF LIFE-THREATENING DISEASE ON PEDIATRIC FAMILY UNITS

Family-centered care can be broadly defined as "a partnership approach to health care decision-making between the family and health care provider."[12] Consensus has been reached about the principles that family-centered care encompasses: (1) information sharing that is "open, objective, and unbiased"; (2) creating relationships with respect for "diversity, culture, linguistic traditions, and care preferences"; (3) decision-making that encompasses the "needs, strengths, values, and abilities of all involved" and includes families "at the level they choose"; and (4) direct medical care and decision-making that reflects children "within the context of their family, home, school, daily activities, and quality of life within the community."[12] One of the most notable attributes of family-centered care is the concept of partnership and providing care that considers "the needs of all family members, not just the child."[14]

PPC is interdisciplinary by nature and includes providing psychological, social, spiritual, and emotional support.[3] This is provided by a team of experts to meet the needs of children and adolescents as well as siblings and parents. This may be delivered by several members of the PPC team, including psychologists/psychiatrists, social workers, child life specialists, integrative therapists, and/or chaplains, in addition to clinicians, such as registered nurses, APRNs, and physicians.[3] PPC involves facilitating "clear, compassionate, and forthright discussions about medical issues and the goals of care" and supporting "families, siblings, and health care staff"[15] because care of a child with a serious illness affects the whole circle of care.

CHILD–FAMILY UNIT

A large component of providing PPC that is family-centered involves providing emotional support.[16] This is especially important because a child living with a life-threatening illness can spend a lot time in the hospital or at various medical appointments, and this affects the entire family unit. Parents, family members, siblings, and the child all suffer throughout the course of an illness, and although this may manifest differently, each person's suffering somehow affects the others.[16]

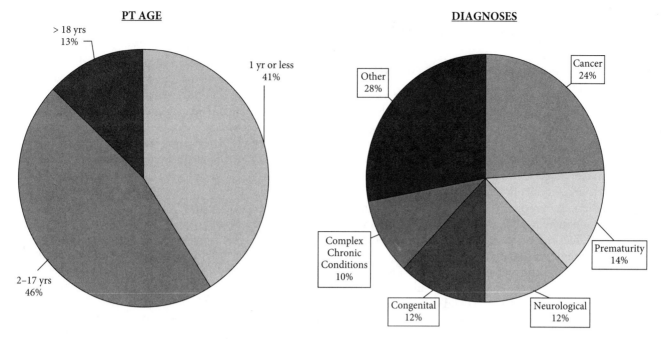

PT AGE

> 18 yrs
13%

1 yr or less
41%

2–17 yrs
46%

DIAGNOSES

Other
28%

Cancer
24%

Complex
Chronic
Conditions
10%

Prematurity
14%

Congenital
12%

Neurological
12%

Figure 26.2 Age distribution and diagnoses of pediatric palliative care patients.
Adapted with data from Rogers M, Kirch R. Spotlight on pediatric palliative care: National landscape of hospital-based programs 2015–2016. CAPC blog. 2017. https://www.capc.org.[13]

Hospitalization is a traumatic and harrowing experience for children and even more so for those who spend time in the ICU.[16] Schedules and daily family routines are interrupted, and parents or caregivers may struggle to find enough time and energy to spend with each other and the ill child's siblings, to transport them to their after-school activities or attend events at school. This burden may be exponentially increased in single-caregiver households. The PP APRN has a distinct role in supporting families by providing education and anticipatory guidance as well as emotional support through a family-centered model of care in the context of primary PPC.

SIBLINGS

Although there is little published evidence to support this hypothesis, it is well-recognized that siblings experience a significant amount of stress when their brothers or sisters face life-threatening illness. "Siblings' needs and suffering continue to be studied, but it has been recognized that they need special attention early on in the course of the disease of another child in the family."[17] It can be difficult, however, for a parent(s) to provide enough support for both the child who is ill and any siblings, and they may unintentionally overlook the needs of their healthy children given that they are overwhelmed by the disease and the needs of the ill child. For this reason, other supports are crucial for siblings, such as school, community, and camp programs, as well as professional counseling and/or support group services that may be available either at the hospital or through an outpatient setting.[17]

Some hospitals offer specific support programs for siblings, such as Sibshops, a program that exists in 10 countries and focuses on meeting the needs of siblings of children living with illness through a mix of unique and developmentally and age-appropriate games, discussions, and friendship.[18] Some

PPC programs may also offer home visits specifically for siblings by social workers, child life specialists, and/or art therapists from the team. Designating a "special person," such as a friend or relative who can take responsibility for each sibling specifically, may be helpful so that siblings get extra attention. The PP APRN can involve child life specialists or art or music therapists who may be beneficial for siblings, depending on the resources available.

EXTENDED FAMILY

Everyone considered part of a child's family, including grandparents, aunts and uncles, cousins, community, and friends, may be affected when a child has a life-threatening illness. The ramifications of life with an ill child can have lasting effects on marriages, partnerships, and relationships including stress, physical, and/or mental health problems. It may also affect finances as well as employment status, create social isolation or disengagement from peer-related activities, and foster a sense of loss, concern for the future, and grief.[19] Grandparents are often very involved in a child's care and feel particularly helpless because of their inability to protect their grandchild from illness or protect their own child (the parent) from any pain and suffering. The PP APRN can assess the greater circle of extended family and their support needs.

Extended family members may wish to be supportive but are often unsure how to do so. It may feel overwhelming to parents to manage others' well-intentioned concerns, inquiries, and attempts to be helpful. The pediatric APRN may be able to anticipate the struggles that families will experience and provide them with anticipatory guidance, tips, and education about diagnoses and treatments. Evidence suggests that clinicians' attention to the needs of family members can enhance their resiliency, but they may need guidance in figuring out new roles and ways in which they can support each other, since everyone copes in his or her own unique way.[19]

SUPPORT FOR FAMILY MEMBERS OUTSIDE THE HOSPITAL SETTING

Caring for the entire family is an essential, especially when care is being provided at home. Family members may have questions about preparation, what changes may occur in the child's physical and mental status, and whom they should call for additional support.[20] An important component of PPC is providing resources to support and involve siblings and other family members. As previously mentioned, some programs offer specific support for siblings, including home visits with child life specialists and art therapists who are trained to help siblings cope with illness and death.

The PP APRN and other members of the team must recognize that every family copes differently and will have an array of grief responses before and after a child dies. Being flexible and keeping communication open is key, as is providing families with ongoing bereavement support following the death. Primary teams should be familiar with local grief resources to which they can refer families. Some PPC teams send cards or make phone calls at regular time intervals and may have a formal bereavement program.

COMMUNITY AND SCHOOL

All families live within a community, and children are often at the epicenter of community-based activities. Within school, place of worship, neighborhood, sports team, or other recreational activities, families develop relationships; when a child becomes ill, the whole community may be affected. Community members can play a tremendous role in providing support to the child and family with hospital visits, support to siblings and family members at home, or helping with everyday tasks like grocery shopping, mowing the lawn, or preparing meals.

CHILD'S VIEW OF ILLNESS AND DEATH

Every child will have their own unique illness experience and may have difficulty expressing it. Children express themselves in different ways; some use words, some draw pictures, some engage in play, some use body language and behavior, and some don't speak at all. The NCP describes the expectation that pediatric teams "ascertain the developmental status and the children or teens' understanding of their disease as well as parental preferences for their child's care at the time of initial consultation,"[3] which should be revisited at each visit. In PPC, the team, including the PP APRN, interprets a child's modes of expression while helping children and families find an appropriate understanding about their illness.

Every child "should be considered as a product of chronological age, developmental stage, medical condition, size, handicap, and cognition."[21] The team must develop a sense of a child's developmental, emotional, and cognitive abilities. Understanding of development stage is essential because "different developmental tasks influence how children perceive and cope with illness and possible death."[21] It is also important to recognize that "children, whose disease trajectory spans more than one developmental stage, require constant reevaluation and adaptation of the delivery of support and care,"[21] because some children with advanced illness may progress or regress in developmental age.[21] Table 26.1 summarizes children's developmental stages and perceptions of death in each stage.

CASE STUDY: A CHILD WITH A CARDIAC CONDITION

MJ was a 16-year-old adolescent with history of coarctation of the aorta repaired during infancy with subsequent biventricular failure requiring a heart transplant at 2 years of age. He was in good health until 3 years prior when he developed transplant-related coronary artery disease and renal insufficiency secondary to his transplant medications. MJ required multiple admissions for complications related to heart failure, including pleural effusions, ascites, fluid overload, and pain. He was evaluated several times for a heart re-transplant but he was deemed not a candidate due in part due to his inability to adhere to medical recommendations and the lack of parental oversight. MJ was known to palliative care from past consultations to assist with symptom management and to discuss his "goals" as they related to treatment options. During one admission to the cardiac care unit, MJ was in moderate respiratory distress due to overwhelming ascites and pleural effusions. A family meeting was planned to discuss potential medical options, acknowledging that MJ was not a re-transplant candidate. The following potential care plans were proposed: (1) frequent admission "tune-ups" to manage symptoms secondary to his heart failure, acknowledging he may have weeks to months to live; (2) placement of a ventricular assist device (VAD) to improve cardiac output, decrease symptom burden, and potentially provide more time with improved quality of life; or (3) minimize hospitalizations and focus on symptom management and maximizing quality of life with the help of hospice. The medical team strongly advocated for a VAD as "destination therapy" with the hopes this therapy would improve MJ's quality of life and potentially give him more time. The team also shared that if MJ demonstrated adherence to VAD therapy and medications he could potentially be re-evaluated for a second transplant.

DESTINATION THERAPY IN PEDIATRICS

Ventricular assist devices (VADs) may be offered in pediatric patients with end-stage heart failure either as (1) a bridge to transplant, (2) a bridge to recovery of myocardial function, (3) a bridge to decision when transplant candidacy has not been determined, or (4) as destination therapy when the child is not a heart transplant candidate.[22] Regardless of the intention, the overriding goal is to reduce symptoms related to cardiac failure and improve the child's quality of life. The

Table 26.1 DEVELOPMENTAL STAGES AND PERCEPTIONS OF DEATH

AGE	BASIC CONFLICT	VIEW OF DEATH	SUGGESTIONS
Birth–18 months	Trust vs. mistrust	No sense of finality and is viewed as continuous with life Reactive to stress	Use simple physical communication and provide comforting and nurturing care.
Early childhood (2–3 years)	Autonomy vs. shame and doubt	Death is seen as reversible and not final May feel death is a punishment May feel responsible for death	Expect regression, clinging, or aggressive behavior. Encourage expression, as the child may be concerned about family function after he or she dies. Use honest and clear language to explain death and dying.
Preschool (3–5 years)	Initiative vs. guilt	Death continues to be understood as temporary May have a literal understanding of death and will respond with curiosity and questioning	Continue to use open communication with clear language. Encourage questions about death and dying.
School age (6–11 years)	Industry vs. inferiority	Death is understood as permanent and that the body ceases to function, with heart and respirations stopping May feel responsible and guilty for the illness May have spiritual ideas about afterlife May not want to discuss feelings	Reassure the child that death is not his or her fault. Strive to maintain as normal a structure as possible. Include the child in afterlife plans (funeral planning, last wishes).
Adolescence (12–18 years)	Identity vs. role confusion	Understands the finality of death and may develop a mature understanding of death May try to take responsibility for adult concerns within the family (such as finances and caretaking) Feelings of anger may be present	Allow time for reflection. Listen to concerns and questions. Support efforts for autonomy and control.

Mandac et al. Reprinted with permission from reference 19.

use of a VAD in children as destination therapy is evolving,[23] providing an important role for the APRN in the delineation of goals of care. These goals-of-care conversations should be initiated upon introduction of the intervention to ensure everyone is on the same page regarding the inherit risks and/or tradeoffs. Prior to the placement of a VAD (similar to other technologies such as pacemakers, implantable cardioverter defibrillator, extracorporeal membrane oxygenation] ECMO], tracheostomy, etc.), there should be an exploration of "what if scenarios" including discontinuation of the therapy if it is found to be no longer beneficial. Possible indications or scenarios for VAD deactivation take into account (1) when quality of life goals are no longer being met, (2) when a child has suffered a neurological insult (i.e., stroke), or (3) parental or patient request.[24] Using parallel planning—hoping for the best while planning for the worst—can be helpful when discussing goals. These conversations can be emotionally and morally charged and may benefit from the institutional support of ethics, leadership, and/or legal teams (see Chapter 53, "Navigating Ethical Conversations"). Advance care planning (ACP) tools can assist practitioners in guiding these discussions prior to an acute crisis. Borrowing language from *Voicing My Choices* or engaging in the card game *Go Wish* can be useful to facilitate conversations or help with prioritizing wishes in the older child or young adult (see Chapter 32, "Advance Care Planning").

CASE STUDY: A CHILD WITH A CARDIAC CONDITION (CONTINUED)

After many discussions, MJ stated he did not want to proceed with a VAD. Although the team worried about decision-making capacity, his parents felt the decision was MJ's to make since "he would have to live attached to a machine." The team was also conflicted if MJ truly understood the ramifications of his decision—that his heart would continue to weaken and he could die within a few months from heart failure—which led to moral distress among the staff. Following consultation with the hospital ethics team, everyone was in agreement to support MJ's decision. MJ was clear that he wanted to go home and live a normal life for as long as possible. Ultimately, a referral was made to hospice and an out-of-hospital do-not-resuscitate (DNR) order was completed. MJ continued to be admitted for "tune-ups" while on hospice but with lessening frequency.

Sometimes, children and families want all potential heart failure treatments even when the risks appear to outweigh the benefits. Healthcare providers should consider only offering interventions that may benefit the patient and are consistent with their goals of care. There are several uses of VAD or ECMO children in heart failure: as a bridge to heart transplantation, as short-term treatment for reversible conditions, or to provide more time to extend or improve the child's quality of life with the "destination therapy" or until death.[25] The term "destination therapy" may be distressing to families, which is why providers may choose to use the term "bridge to decision" instead.[25] Children discharged with a VAD should be followed longitudinally by palliative care providers to ensure goals of care have not changed and that this technology continues to meet their needs.

CASE STUDY: A CHILD WITH A CARDIAC CONDITION (CONTINUED)

MJ's heart failure symptoms were managed at home although he requested to return to the hospital when symptoms, primarily ascites refractory to oral diuretics, were uncomfortable. MJ's hospice nurse provided weekly updates to the PP APRN and cardiology.

Children with congenital heart disease (CHD) are at risk for developing heart failure. The Centers for Disease Control estimates that CHD occurs in 1% of births per year in the United Stated, which accounts for approximately 40,000 birth per year.[26] Approximately 2–3 million children and adults are living with CHD in the United States.[27] Although their mortality rate is decreasing, many are living with increased morbidity and risk of multiorgan complications,[28] often leading to frequent admissions and/or interventions for symptom management.[29] Early involvement of PPC for patient's like MJ can provide psychosocial support over time, which is invaluable when patients and their families may be tasked with complex medical decision-making at various timepoints. Longitudinal support can provide context when discussing changes during acute exacerbations, clarify communication between providers, and help align interventions with goals and wishes.[30,31] The PP APRN plays a major role in collaborating with inpatient and outpatient providers, clarifying communication, assisting with symptom management, and, when appropriate, making a referral to hospice.

MANAGING SYMPTOMS IN HEART FAILURE

MJ's heart failure presented as fatigue, anorexia, dyspnea, abdominal pain, and nausea. In the later stages, patients can also develop hepatic and renal failure, malignant arrhythmias, stroke, or multiple-system organ failure.[32] The hallmark of end-stage heart disease often manifests as low cardiac output, respiratory distress, cachexia, and/or anorexia.[33]

Managing symptoms for heart failure, similar to other life-limiting conditions, should include a plan that offers a multidisciplinary approach including pharmacological, nonpharmacological, and, when appropriate, invasive treatments. Treatment options should ultimately decrease pain, relieve bothersome symptoms, improve functionality, and maximize quality of life. When prescribing medications for children, careful consideration of dosing is necessary due to differences in pharmacokinetics based on the child's age and weight and underlying disease pathophysiology.[34] Table 26.2 illustrates some common symptoms and therapeutic options.

Dosing recommendations for medications can be found in Appendix II.

Dyspnea, or the state of "breathlessness," occurs when the body cannot keep up with oxygenation and ventilation demands. It is a common symptom seen with advanced illness and at the end of life. Dyspnea in children can be difficult to measure, and the use of assessment scales have not been shown to be reliable.[35] Management approaches for dyspnea include addressing and treating underlying reversible causes (anemia, fluid overload, effusion) and using a multimodal approach when possible. Opioids are the first line of treatment, especially at the end of life. In the opioid-naïve pediatric patient, it is recommended to start with 25–50% of the initial dose.[36] MJ's dyspnea was heart failure–related due to overwhelming ascites and pleural effusions. Intermittently, he required admission for intravenous diuretics and fluid drainage via a pleural catheter. Although many hospices have the ability to provide intravenous diuretics, his did not. After several admissions, his inpatient and hospice teams discussed discharging MJ with a pleural catheter for intermittent drainage because hospice had successfully cared for many patients with an implanted catheter at home. The risk-benefit of catheter-related infections and relief of symptoms was discussed with MJ and his family, and, ultimately, the decision was made to proceed with this intervention since infection, leakage at the site, and dislodgement were deemed low risk.[37]

Many patients with advanced heart failure will experience pain secondary to worsening edema or ascites, palpitations, ischemia, or poor perfusion to vital organs. Skin integrity, gut dysmotility, and musculoskeletal pain from immobility are also common. Pain may manifest as visceral or neuropathic in nature.[38] Other symptoms include protein-losing enteropathy, fatigue, insomnia, muscle wasting, and cachexia.[39]

INOTROPIC THERAPY FOR HEART FAILURE FOR INPATIENT OR HOME

Milrinone is a phosphodiesterase-3 inhibitor that has positive inotropic and vasodilator properties and can provide relief in patients with right ventricular heart failure.[42] It requires a hospital admission for central line placement to monitor medication side effects including arrhythmias, thrombocytopenia, and hypotension. In addition, prior to discharge, it is essential for caregivers to receive education on medication safety and maintaining line integrity. Indications for continuous milrinone include short-term management of heart failure either as destination therapy while waiting for a transplant or as a palliative option to improve quality of life. Studies have shown that milrinone has improved cardiac function and quality of life in pediatric patients with heart failure.[43] Discharging a child home with milrinone, as with other treatments and technologies, involves working in partnership with the child's primary care provider, skilled home nursing agency, and, when appropriate, hospice to ensure everyone is up to date with the plan. The PP APRN can assist with care coordination and help bridge information and clarify goals from the inpatient to outpatient settings. The availability of concurrent care for children allows patients

Table 26.2 HEART FAILURE SYMPTOM MANAGEMENT

	POTENTIAL SOURCES	THERAPEUTIC OPTIONS		CONSIDERATIONS
		NONPHARMACOLOGICAL	PHARMACOLOGICAL	
Dyspnea	Anxiety Effusions Anemia Pulmonary embolism Electrolyte disturbances Pneumothorax Rib fracture	Position upright Fan Guided imagery, relaxation techniques Decrease fluids, consider decreasing or discontinuing parenteral fluids Therapeutic trial of supplemental oxygen delivered in least bothersome way Pleural catheter	Low-dose opioids (higher doses may be needed if patient is on chronic opioids) Anxiolytics (short-acting benzodiazepine) Diuretics	Align treatments with goals of care
Ascites, Effusions	Electrolyte disturbances Protein losing enteropathy Malnutrition	Fluid and sodium restriction Drain if aligns with goals of care	Diuretics +/− Albumin	
Pain	Palpitations Organomegaly Inflammation Deconditioning	Physical therapy Heat/cold application Transcutaneous electrical stimulation (TENS) unit Hypnosis	Analgesics Opioids Antispasmodics Tricyclic Antidepressants (TCA) Serotonin norepinephrine reuptake inhibitors (SNRI) Gabapentinoids N-methyl-D-aspartate receptor (NMDA)	Doses may need adjusting in hepatic or renal insufficiency TCA, 5-HT3, and NMDA medications can increase QTc.
Fatigue	Sedation medications Sleep disturbances Deconditioning Depression, anxiety Anemia/Hypoxemia Electrolyte abnormalities Uncontrolled pain Infection	Physical therapy, optimize function Encourage sleep/wake cycle Dietary changes Acupuncture Dietary supplements	Short trial steroids Antidepressants Psychostimulants	Steroids may interfere with sleep

Adapted from references[39, 40, 41]

like MJ access to homecare nursing to monitor vital signs, dosing, and line integrity while continuing hospice support. After several deliberations, MJ decided against milrinone therapy for the same reasons of "not wanting to be hooked up to a machine."

GOALS OF CARE, LIMITATIONS OF CARE, AND DECISION-MAKING

CODE STATUS DISCUSSIONS

Due to advances in medical technology, the number of children living with life-threatening illness continues to rise. Families frequently are faced with difficult decisions about whether to forgo life-sustaining medical treatment and resuscitation. The nomenclature summarized in Table 26.3 and interchangeability by providers can be confusing. "Allow natural death" may be more acceptable from a family standpoint as the result of natural disease progression[44]; however, some cultures think that no death for a young person is natural.

Regardless of the terminology used, discussions regarding resuscitation status can be anxiety-provoking for both family members and providers. It is common for providers to feel pressure to "get the DNR" or to consult the PPC team to accomplish this. Often it becomes the role of the PPC team not only to have discussions with children and family members regarding goals of care as they relate to resuscitation status, but also to provide education and mentoring for other pediatric providers. Commonly, the PPC team's role is to build trusting relationships with families over time and have

Table 26.3 ACRONYMS FOR CODE STATUS DESCRIPTIONS

Do-not-attempt resuscitation (DNAR)	No escalation of care (No ESC)
Do-not-resuscitate (DNR)	Allow natural death (AND)
Do-not-intubate (DNI)	

ongoing discussions about goals of care that are based on both a humanistic and an ethical framework.[45]

Predicting outcomes for children living with life-threatening illness is a complex and difficult task. It is important to recognize that decisions about resuscitation status are usually the result of several conversations between providers and family members about their goals of care and if resuscitation achieves those goals. The role of the PP APRN is to collaborate with the teams involved in these discussions, facilitate family understanding of what interventions may or may not be beneficial to their children (e.g., chest compressions, intubation), and effectively communicate those wishes in the hospital and at home.

DECISION-MAKING AND HONORING WISHES

Decisions about healthcare treatments care are seldom "black and white." Tools to guide decision-making and conversations about goals of care are essential. The NCP *Clinical Practice Guidelines* emphasize that children should be included in age- and developmentally appropriate conversations regarding their goals.[3] Some children may explicitly express their wishes regarding their end-of-life and resuscitation status; other children may not want to address these topics. In some cases, children may feel more comfortable talking with the PPC team or other healthcare providers than talking with their family because they may fear disappointing their family if they choose not to pursue particular interventions. At other times, children and their family may disagree about what the goals of care should be as well as what particular interventions they should receive. Resources are available to help guide the decision-making process and to aid clinicians in navigating conversations with children of all ages and, in some instances, their designated decision-makers, regarding how they want to be treated throughout their illness and at the time of death from a medical, personal, emotional, and spiritual perspective.[46] Helpful documents are reviewed in detail in Chapter 32, "Advance Care Planning."

OUT-OF-HOSPITAL ORDERS FOR LIFE-SUSTAINING TREATMENT

There are two documents that reflect out-of-hospital orders for life-sustaining treatment when children leave the hospital. These are the provider/physician orders for life-sustaining therapies (POLST)/medical orders for life-sustaining therapies (MOLST) and the out-of-hospital DNR (OOHDNR). These documents are state-specific and are a tool for helping to discuss goals of care. As official orders, they are signed by health professionals and the patient or surrogate decision-maker. It should be noted that some states do not allow children to be have a DNR order until they enter hospice care.

The NCP *Clinical Practice Guidelines* state that a child's or adolescent's views and preferences for medical care and treatments, including assent for care (when developmentally appropriate) should be assessed, given weight in decision-making, and documented.[3] Specifically, children and families

deserve to have their wishes honored whether they opt for full resuscitation or elect to forgo potentially life-sustaining treatments. Documentation of desired resuscitation and advance directives is important to limit undesired interventions, such as cardiopulmonary resuscitation (CPR), by first responders.[45] Families are best prepared for emergency situations with proactive discussions before the time of an emergency. Families should be informed that decisions can be changed should there be a change in the child's health status. However, if parents have a strong preference for noninclusion of or nondisclosure to the child in such decisions, the PPC assesses family motivations and values within this decision while simultaneously meeting the needs of the child within these expectations and boundaries.[3]

The PP APRN has a specific role in educating families that a POLST/MOLST is intended to articulate the parent's and child's care preferences and communicate them in a crisis when the parents may not be available. Additional forms that may be helpful to support advance directives in the pediatric population include guardianship documentation and medical power of attorney. The abbreviations, definitions, and intended use are summarized in Table 26.4 (see Chapter 32, "Advance Care Planning," for more details on ACP).

CASE STUDY: PEDIATRIC PULMONARY DISEASE

JH was a 14-year-old girl with end-stage cystic fibrosis (CF), listed for lung transplantation. She was frequently hospitalized for infections, acute CF exacerbations, dyspnea, and worsening lung function. Palliative care was consulted during an admission as part of her lung transplant evaluation to assist with goals of care and medical decision-making. The palliative care team was able to help JH and her family discuss and honor her wishes to not pursue lung transplant due to the risks while providing support and symptom management throughout additional admissions and clinic visits.

Cystic fibrosis (CF) is an autosomal recessive genetic disorder caused by a mutation of the cystic fibrosis transmembrane conductance regulator (CFTR) gene. It is the second most common childhood genetic disorder, with approximately 30,000 people living with the disease in North America.[49] Chronic respiratory infections, inflammation, and pulmonary decline are the primary causes of morbidity and mortality. Other effects of the illness and decline are poor growth, malabsorption, pancreatic insufficiency, diabetes mellitus, hemolytic anemia, and hepatic biliary disease.

Currently, there is no cure for CF but with improvements in technology, aggressive medical management, and supportive care many children are living into adulthood, albeit with an increase in morbidity. Children with CF endure multiple daily therapies and may have frequent hospital stays to manage disease exacerbations. For certain children with advanced disease, lung transplantation may be an option to prolong and improve quality of life.[50] Post lung transplant survival rate is about 80% after 1 year and 50% after 5 years.[51] The decision to proceed with lung transplantation can add new challenges for the patient and their family. Although the new lungs do not

Table 26.4 SUMMARY OF ADVANCE CARE PLANNING TERMS

DNAR, AND, No ESC, DNR	Inpatient code status	Should reflect the family's desires for attempts at resuscitation during the hospital stay
MOLST/POLST/OOHDNR	Outpatient resuscitation	Important to have to respect families desires for EMS or first responders to attempt CPR. Without form present they are required to provide CPR
Advance Directives	Resuscitation and care preferences	These may include inpatient and outpatient resuscitation choices, choice of surrogate decision-maker, end-of-life desires for treatment or interventions, and even funeral planning
Guardianship	Of the patient and/or their estate if the patient does not have mental capacity and is over the age of 18.	May be full, limited to healthcare/financial or other large decisions, or temporary in certain circumstances
Medical Power of Attorney (MPOA)	Person or persons chosen to act on an individual's behalf if incapacitated.	MPOA may be active upon signing or upon the patient's incapacitation. An expiration date can be set. The patient should communicate goals, advanced directives to MPOA(s)

DNAR, do-not-attempt-resuscitation; AND, allow natural death; No ESC, no escalation; DNR, do-not-resuscitate; MOLST, medical orders for life-sustaining treatment; POLST. physician orders for life-sustaining treatment; OOHDNR, out-of-hospital do-not-resuscitate.

Adapted with definitions from Texas Health and Human Services Website [47] and Wikipedia. [48]

have the gene that causes CF, the disease is still present and the ability to fight infection is complicated by the need for continuous immune suppression.

The decision of when to integrate a palliative approach for patients' with chronic conditions like CF can be challenging, given the misconceptions about PPC. Early introduction of palliative care as an additional layer of support during acute CF exacerbations or when a patient is undergoing a transplant evaluation can (1) assist with difficult to manage pain or other bothersome symptoms; (2) help clarify communication among teams, patient, and family; and (3) help align goals of care with treatment options. The PPC team can also be helpful when trying to achieve a balance between aggressive interventions and quality of life (Box 26.3).

Managing progressive symptoms in CF, especially at the end of life, can be challenging. Overwhelmingly, evidence supports the benefits of using very low doses of opioids to treat dyspnea and benzodiazepines to treat associated anxiety. [52] There are some fears and misconceptions that opioids may hasten a child's death, decrease respiratory drive, or that a child may develop an addiction to them. For children with CF, low-dose opioids and nonpharmacologic measures are mainstays to palliate progressive symptoms at the end of life. For example, the patient with worsening dyspnea may benefit from noninvasive positive pressure ventilation (NIPPV), supplemental oxygen, and use of a fan. PPC providers should collaborate with primary CF teams to provide the interdisciplinary support that is needed when caring for children with this progressive, chronic, and life-threatening condition.

CANCER

Curative or palliative treatment for oncological diagnoses may cause increased pain, additional symptom burden, or repeated hospitalizations. There is agreement among oncologists and pediatric oncology nurses that early endorsement of PPC is beneficial to the child and family, improves their quality of life, [52] helps with refractory pain and symptom management, and clarifies communication regarding prognosis. [53–55] Parents have expressed that consultation with a palliative care team was a positive experience, although it was still equated with

Box 26.3 COLLABORATIVE BENEFIT OF PALLIATIVE CARE SERVICES IN CHILDREN WITH CYSTIC FIBROSIS WITH OR WITHOUT LUNG TRANSPLANTATION

- Collaborate with the team to develop strategies to reduce parental grief when given the news their child has a life-threatening disease.

- Support the team during admissions, provide strategies to decrease stress, and offer help with pain and symptom management as needed.

- As the disease progresses, collaborate with the team and family on treating bothersome pain and symptoms, answering difficult questions, addressing the "what ifs" and use of aggressive technologies, developing approaches to facilitate discussions related to transplantation, providing support to siblings, and suggesting care settings, including hospice.

- Support advance care planning discussions, including documenting patient preferences, medical power of attorney in accordance with state law, patient goals of care, and desired site of death.

- Develop a plan to address support for family and medical providers at the time of death, including community services to provide ongoing bereavement services.

Adapted from Dellon, et al. [49]

end-of-life care[56] (see Chapter 29, "The Pediatric Palliative APRN in Oncology").

MANAGING THE MEDICALLY COMPLEX PEDIATRIC PATIENT

CASE STUDY: THE MEDICALLY COMPLEX PATIENT

JJ was a 6-year-old 28-week premature baby with spastic quadriplegia, who was dependent on bilevel positive airway pressure (BiPAP), a gastrostomy tube (G-tube), and a jejunostomy tube (J-tube). JJ had several chronic medical conditions including obstructive sleep apnea (OSA), feeding intolerance of unclear etiology, and spasticity, and he was dependent on caregivers for all activities of daily living. JJ had been in and out of the hospital at least yearly. Over the past 2 years, his feeding intolerance has progressed so that only medications are administered through the G-tube and J-tube. He relies on total parenteral nutrition (TPN) through a central line for the remainder of his nutrition although there were two admission for central line bacteremia. JJ has been admitted to the ICU for 2 weeks with electrolyte abnormalities related to feeding intolerance. He was intubated, then extubated, and he tolerated his home BiPAP regimen. He was followed by multiple subspecialists. We will use JJ's story to illustrate the palliative care topics covered in the next sections of this chapter.

GASTROINTESTINAL DYSMOTILITY/ FEEDING INTOLERANCE

Causes of feeding intolerance or gastrointestinal (GI) dysmotility vary in children. Some may have an extensive history of intestinal surgeries or colitis in infancy, while others may experience a progressive decline following an acute abdominal surgery for obstruction or volvulus.[57] The PP APRN needs to thoughtfully research what has already been tried, trial medications one at a time, and discontinue medications that are not helpful to avoid side effects and polypharmacy. It is also important to partner with the patient's surgeon, dietician, gastroenterologist, and primary care provider to consider pharmacologic and nonpharmacologic management. Table 26.5 lists a table of recommendations from Hauer.[58]

CASE STUDY: THE MEDICALLY COMPLEX PATIENT (CONTINUED)

JJ was trialed on cyproheptadine twice daily, which decreased his retching and secretions significantly. Gabapentin was added for presumed visceral pain; this was rotated to intravenous methadone when JJ could no longer tolerate any oral medications. When he could no longer tolerate medications by G-tube, J-tube, buccal, or rectal routes, intravenous medications were administered.

Table 26.5 MANAGEMENT OF ABDOMINAL DISCOMFORT

CAUSE	MANAGEMENT OPTIONS	COMMENTS
Constipation	Polyethylene glycol Lactulose Milk of Magnesia Senna	Colonic distention from constipation can trigger pain symptoms due to visceral hyperalgesia and central neuropathic pain
GERD, motility disorders	H-2 blockers and PPIs Protective barrier: sucralfate Promotility drugs: erythromycin, metoclopramide Jejunostomy feeding tube	Motility disorders can be a result of impaired input from the CNS to the enteric nervous system Suggested by bloating, distension, retching, vomiting, discomfort Other problems can contribute, including constipation and pain
Vomiting reflex	Medications that block the 5HT-2, 5HT-3, H-1 Arch and D-2 receptors Cyproheptadine (5HT-2, H-1, Arch Ondansetron (5HT-3)	Suggested by retching, forceful vomiting, and associated symptoms of sweating, pale skin, and appearing distressed
Visceral hyperalgesia, central neuropathic pain	Gabapentin Pregabalin Tricyclic antidepressants	Suggested by pain, retching, and emesis associated with feeding, intestinal gas, flatus, and bowel movements
Autonomic dysfunction	Gabapentin Pregabalin Clonidine	Suggested by pain and emesis associated with tachycardia, hyperthermia, diaphoresis, and skin flushing
Pseudo-obstruction	Conservative management Erythromycin Neostigmine or pyridostigmine	Suggested by recurrent episodes of abdominal distension, pain, emesis, and severe constipation, in the absence of mechanical obstruction

Ach: acetylcholine; CNS: central nervous system; D: dopamine; H: histamine; 5HT: serotonin; GERD: gastroesophageal reflux disease; PPI: proton pump inhibitor

Reprinted with permission from Hauer J. Feeding intolerance in children with severe impairment of the central nervous system: Strategies for treatment and prevention. Children (Basel). 2017;5(1):1. doi:10.3390/children5010001.[58]

PAIN MANAGEMENT CONSIDERATIONS IN SPECIAL POPULATIONS

Children with advanced disease deserve optimal pain control. The same guiding principles used for managing pain in adults can be applied to children, with additional considerations. The child's developmental age, cognitive ability, weight, the impact of pain on the child and family, and the maturity of the patient's renal and hepatic systems affect medication choices and dosing in pediatric pain management. (See Appendix II for pharmacological and nonpharmacological management). Palliative care teams, in consultation with the primary team caring for the child, should develop plans in conjunction with patients and families. A good pain management plan includes a thorough assessment using age- and behavior-appropriate tools, clarification of the goals of treatment, a description of expected side effects, a discussion of how increased pain will be addressed, and the incorporation of nonpharmacologic therapies (e.g., distraction, relaxation techniques, acupuncture, guided imagery, and play).[59]

Special attention must be given to children who are nonverbal and have intellectual disabilities. This is a vulnerable group, and their inability to self-report pain can result in erroneous and inappropriate management.[60] It can be challenging to recognize pain in children, especially children who cannot express their pain, which is why so many with advanced illness do not have adequate pain control.[61] Table 26.6 summarizes some pain behaviors by age groups.

The World Health Organization (WHO), the American Academy of Pediatrics (AAP), and the National Coalition for Hospice and Palliative Care (NCHPC) offer guidance on the initiation and titration of pain medications in children. The WHO step ladder is a universally accepted first-line approach to pain management.[62] The key concepts are listed here.

- Provide medications at scheduled times, rather than just as needed.

- Offer medications by the most appropriate route.

- Use oral dosing whenever possible.

The pathophysiology of pain is complex, and often a multimodal approach incorporating pharmacological and nonpharmacological methods work best. Pain medication should be given via the most effective and least traumatic route, at regularly scheduled intervals, with a plan for breakthrough pain. There is no standard dosing for opioids; rather "the right dose is the dose that works." However, there are consideration for opioid-naïve children versus those children who have had opioids in the past. For the opioid-naïve, start with the lowest dose based on weight and consideration of renal and hepatic effect. For children with prior opioid use, start with the medication and dose that was previously safe and effective. At the end of life, gut perfusion and/or absorption may be affected, requiring the APRN to investigate other routes (i.e., sublingual, subcutaneous, or intravenous routes).

Patient-controlled analgesia (PCA), an infusion pump that can be programmed to deliver intravenous medications at continuous prescribed doses, allows the patient (or parent) to deliver boluses of medication as needed. Children as young as 3 or 4 years can be taught how to "press the button" to deliver pain medications. PCA should be considered in the following situations: (1) pain is uncontrolled with increasing doses of oral or transdermal medication, (2) pain is uncontrolled on adequate doses of around-the-clock intravenous opioids, (3) pain is expected to escalate quickly, (4) routine care causes significant pain and may require additional dosing before activity, or (5) more control is desired over pain management by the child or the provider. The two main disadvantages of PCA are a child's unwillingness to use it and the need for intravenous or subcutaneous access. Morphine and hydromorphone are the common PCA opioids utilized, although circumstances may necessitate the use of fentanyl. Depending on the goals of care and resuscitation status, a bag-valve mask, supplemental oxygen, and continuous pulse oximetry may be needed for the first 24 hours on PCA and with subsequent dose increases to counterbalance respiratory depression.

SPASTICITY/DYSTONIA

Children with neurologic impairment can suffer from *dystonia*, abnormal involuntary movements that can lead to uncomfortable positions or postures like extreme back arching,[63] or *spasticity*, which is best characterized as increased tone in the affected body part.[63] While the conditions are different, the therapies may overlap and often require trial and error. It is also important to check for inciting factors

Table 26.6 **PAIN BEHAVIORS IN CHILDREN**

Infancy (1–12 months)	Inconsolability Feeding/sleeping difficulty Grimacing Change in activity level High-pitched cry Frequent yawning Tachycardia/tachypnea
Toddler (1–4 years)	Lost interest in play Moaning Irritability Loss of appetite Difficulty sleeping or excessive sleeping Overly clingy Guarding
School-age and adolescent (5–17 years)	Change in activity level Overly quiet or subdued Irritable or angry Mismatched cues Difficulty sleeping

Adapted from reference [61]

Table 26.7 POTENTIAL SOURCES OF DISCOMFORT IN CHILDREN WHO ARE NONVERBAL

INCITING FACTOR	WHAT TO LOOK FOR
Belly	Constipation, urinary retention, mechanical obstruction, pain
Brain	Change in level of alertness from baseline, sleep behaviors, seizure activity, changes in vital signs, developmental regression, stimulation
Breathing	Secretions; if on positive pressure or ventilator, does the child need more support or oxygen, has the look of the breathing changed?
Bugs	Fever, signs of infection
Bones	Grimacing or crying with diaper changes, episodes occur in certain position or while using certain equipment

that may exacerbate spasticity and dystonia; one approach is listed in Table 26.7. A list of interventions and the indications, as well as their potential drawbacks, is listed in Table 26.8. Patient JJ did well for a period of time with physical therapy, a clonidine patch, and gabapentin. As-needed diazepam for muscle spasms was added to his last hospital discharge.

NEUROIRRITABILITY

A child who has bouts of crying, flushed facies, tachycardia, teeth grinding, or self-injurious behaviors may suffer from neuroirritability. The exact cause is not well understood because these patients are often nonverbal, but the assessment is similar to that for dystonia or spasticity, as shown in Box 26.8. Interventions are directed at potential causes and may include changing positions, giving acetaminophen or ibuprofen to see if the irritability is pain related, venting gastric tubes, relieving a full bladder, decreasing stimulation, or trialing medications. Gabapentin is often first-line treatment if the preceding interventions are not successful because it is generally well-tolerated with minimal side effects.[64] Gabapentin may provide multiple benefits for neuroirritability, visceral or bone pain, and dystonia or spasticity in the neurologically impaired child.[58]

DELIRIUM

When children like JJ are admitted to the hospital, they face a loss of daily routines and familiarity. During one admission, palliative care was informed that JJ was not focusing on his family, could not sleep for more than 20 minutes, and seemed disinterested in a favorite video show that made him smile. Bedside assessment determined that he was likely delirious, and risperidone was initiated.

Pediatric delirium, a disruption in brain function, has become more apparent as children with complex medical conditions are living longer. Those experiencing prolonged

Table 26.8 MANAGEMENT STRATEGIES FOR SPASTICITY AND/OR DYSTONIA

Intervention	Indication for dystonia (D), spasticity (S), or both (B)	Considerations
Nonpharmacologic therapies	B	
Positioning devices, braces, equipment	B	Equipment may need to be reordered as child grows
Targeted therapies		
Botox, ethanol, phenol injections	B	Will likely require repeat treatments
Oral medications		
Baclofen	B	Max doses
Benzodiazepines: Diazepam, clonazepam, lorazepam	B	Can be sedating
Clonidine	B	Hypotension, sedation; has patch form
Gabapentin	B	May exacerbate sedation
Tizanidine	S	Limited pediatric data
Levodopa	D	Limited pediatric data
Trihexyphenidyl	D	Drug interactions, anticholinergic effects
Tetrabenazine	D	Insomnia, mood changes, drug interactions
Surgical		
Intrathecal baclofen pump	B	Refills required, pump failure plan needed
Selective rhizotomy	S	
Orthopedic: Tendons, joint dislocations, scoliosis	B	
Deep brain stimulation	D	

Adapted from information in Graham et al.[63]

hospitalizations have a higher risk of delirium in intensive care settings due to illness severity, medications, and underlying neurologic impairment.[65] The validated screening tools for pediatric delirium are the *Pediatric Confusion Assessment Method for the ICU* (pCAM-ICU), the *Preschool Confusion Assessment Method for the ICU* (psCAM-ICU), and the *Cornell Assessment of Pediatric Delirium* (CAPD).[65] Patients receiving medications that alter alertness or awareness, especially benzodiazepines, can have an increased risk for delirium.[65] Nonpharmacological interventions include clustering care, promoting sleep hygiene, avoiding sedatives when able, using newer agents like dexmedetomidine in place of benzodiazepines, adding melatonin to promote sleep/wake regulation, and using antipsychotic medication like quetiapine, risperidone, and olanzapine, if necessary. Risperidone comes in oral and oral dissolving tablet (ODT) formulations, and quetiapine has the lowest risk for undesirable hepatic effects.[66] See Appendix II for management of delirium.

ADVANCE CARE PLANNING FOR THE CHILD WITH NEUROLOGICAL IMPAIRMENT

As mentioned previously, ACP is a frequent reason for palliative care consultation. Many children are unable to use pediatric-appropriate ACP tools due to developmental abilities. Moreover, no tool specifically assists families of children with neurological impairment to express their desires for life-sustaining technology, extent of medical intervention, or desired location if death is inevitable, and to allow for funeral planning. An alternative option may be to utilize an ACP tool and reframe the questions to ascertain and record the family's wishes as well as the patient's code status. As always, such discussions should be documented and accessible to all health team members. A standardized template specific to an organization promotes consistency of practice.

TRACHEOSTOMY DECISION-MAKING

Patient JJ developed progressive weakness that led to increased respiratory effort and inability to clear his secretions. The option for tracheostomy was presented to the family and palliative care was asked to help with the medical decision regarding tracheostomy. Child tracheostomy decision guides are available on the internet, and some institutions may have their own pamphlets and processes. Regardless if there is a formal process, families should have a good understanding of why the tracheostomy is recommended; the requirements for taking their child home with a tracheostomy; the risks and benefits of the tracheostomy; expectations for speech, oral intake, and chance for decannulation; and what other options may be available.[67] This information is essential for families to make decisions best suited to meet their goals for their child.

END OF LIFE: DYING, PALLIATIVE SEDATION, AND WITHDRAWAL OF LIFE-SUSTAINING THERAPIES

Over 2 months JJ continued to worsen. His family made the decision not to pursue tracheostomy and to focus on his comfort. He was not a candidate for additional interventions as his renal failure progressed and his family made the decision to compassionately extubate him in a withdrawal of life sustaining therapies (WOLST). Given his underlying comorbidities, the team also made a plan for palliative sedation if needed. *Palliative sedation* is best defined as "the use of sedative medications to relieve intractable and refractory distress."[68] Palliative sedation in pediatrics may raise ethical concerns and therefore it is best discussed ahead of time, ideally with experienced providers making the recommendations (see Chapter 57, "Palliative Sedation," and Chapter for "Discontinuation of Other Life Sustaining Therapies" for further discussion).

The decision to discontinue life-sustaining therapies is made over time. It occurs after discussion of the family's goals of care, emphasizes the potential for a peaceful and dignified death, and promotes legacy building for the child and family.[69] A WOLST is a delicate and unique procedure for each child. It is essential that the family is provided a detailed explanation of the procedure, including anticipatory guidance about what to expect, especially in circumstances where the child may live for hours or days. This includes which team members will be involved, medications to be administered and who will administer them, and the timing for removal of equipment like a ventilator, the ECMO circuit, dialysis equipment, etc. The plan should be communicated to all parties involved in the child's care while being sensitive to the family's needs and grief. The same end-of-life care memory-making and legacy-building while providing a good death for any child in the hospital should also be included in the WOLST plan. Box 26.4 is an example of WOLST preparation documentation.

END-OF-LIFE CONSIDERATIONS

While some families may want to keep their child in the hospital for IV medications, the familiarity of providers, or because the child may be too sick to go home, an increasing number of families are choosing to keep their children at home for their death. This is a very personal choice for families and is based on a variety of factors such as honoring their child's wishes, cultural beliefs, availability of resources and support, who lives at home, and the family's past experiences with death. Families must be assured that there is no right or wrong choice about keeping their child in the hospital or taking them home. As with any comprehensive PPC plan, a home care plan should include careful assessment of the child's physical and emotional needs as well as their developmental level and ability to complete developmental tasks. Practical factors such as finances, living situation, social support, and religious or spiritual/existential beliefs and practices should also be considered.[70,71]

The medical team met to discuss the care of JJ. Considering that the patient's disease process is irreversible, it is appropriate to pursue withdrawal of life-sustaining therapies (WOLST) and focus on comfort measures at the end-of-life. This is consistent with the parent's wishes and is in the best interest of the child.

The following members were present for the interdisciplinary team meeting:

The following teams were also notified: ***

Current location:

Planned location for WOLST:

Anticipated time for WOLST:

DNR code status documented in chart:

Autopsy has been presented:

Organ Procurement Agency notified:

Bereavement Plans

Social Needs

Social Work, Child Life, Chaplain contacted:

Family would also like:

Current management and plan for:

Respiratory support   Oral and Airway Secretions

Dyspnea   Pain

Agitation/Anxiety   Delirium

Nausea/Vomiting

Other Medications:

Neuromuscular blockade

Pressors

Oral & inhaled medications

Nutrition & Hydration

Access Lines:

Will remove these lines and tubes:

All other lines and tubes will remain in place.

Adapted from Texas Children's Hospital Palliative Care Team guidelines.

Facilitating a smooth transition from inpatient care to home requires frequent communication between the inpatient teams and the outpatient and home care providers. The role of the PP APRN, along with the other members of the interdisciplinary PPC team, can ensure that families have their physical, emotional, and social needs met whether they choose to remain in the hospital or transition to home. Points to consider prior to a discharge to home are listed in Box 26.5.[72]

HOSPICE CARE

One of the most beneficial resources for the home care of a child is the addition of hospice services. The terms "palliative" and "hospice care" are often used interchangeably due to their similar philosophical approaches to care. However, palliative care can be provided at any time during the disease, whereas

Clarifying expectations of team, family, and home care providers

Instructions for pain and symptom management. Ensure home care equipment and medications can be delivered prior to discharge.

Verify the contact number of medical provider and/or home care agency.

Discuss having an out-of-hospital do-not-resuscitate order if appropriate.

hospice care is traditionally introduced if the patient could die during the next 6 months.[72] The PP APRN should be familiar with the distinct ways in which pediatric hospice care differs from adult hospice care, but especially the issues found in the *Concurrent Care for Children Requirement* section of the *Affordable Care Act*, which allows children to jointly receive curative treatments alongside hospice services. The pediatric APRN is well-suited to serve as the direct liaison with hospices teams prior to discharge. In some instances, the hospital PPC team will direct the care for a child at home with hospice by working directly with hospice providers to adjust medications and care plans to maintain the child's comfort and to support the family while at home. A few guidelines to consider when making a hospice referral are listed in Box 26.6.

Aside from resources like hospice and home care nursing, there are several practical aspects for the PP APRN to arrange for the child's care at home. Effective communication and an organized plan must be established to avoid errors while ensuring that pain and other symptoms are well managed.

Identify child who would benefit from hospice.

Communicate potential referral with primary team and care coordinators.

Determine eligibility of a prognosis of 6 months or less.

- Use the surprise question: "Would I be surprised if the child dies within the next 6 months?" If no, the child is likely eligible.
- Remember the child is not required to have a do-not-resuscitate (DNR) order to enroll in hospice.

Check insurance coverage of the child and discuss with parents.

- Most children with Medicaid may receive concurrent care.
- Many commercial payers may need to negotiate care.

Make referral to hospice program with required demographics and pertinent clinical information.

Contact hospice agency to arrange for meeting with liaison prior to discharge and provide any additional information.

Communicate discharge date and help with logistics of discharge as requested.

Adapted from Texas Children's Hospital Pediatric Advanced Care Team Guidelines.

SUMMARY

PPC is family-centered care by nature and focuses on addressing not only the needs of children living with life-threatening illness, but the needs of their family as well. It continues to evolve as an integral and multifactorial area of healthcare because more children are living with chronic and potentially life-threatening illnesses. As with all individuals with serious illness, children and their families deserve optimal quality of life tailored to pediatric principles of care. PPC is often initiated as the goals of care shift from a focus on cure to a focus on optimizing quality of life.

Access to a PPC interdisciplinary team of professionals promotes quality care; however, these teams are not always available outside of large academic settings. PP APRNs are vital in initiating and providing high-quality primary PPC by adequately addressing and anticipating children's and families' needs, allowing for ongoing discussions about goals of care, collaborating with other providers to provide comprehensive care, and thoroughly assessing and treating pain and other distressing symptoms.

REFERENCES

1. World Health Organization. Palliative care. Key Facts. August 5, 2020. https://www.who.int/news-room/fact-sheets/detail/palliative-care
2. Committee on Palliative and End-of-Life Care for Children and Their Families. *When Children Die: Improving Palliative and End-of-Life Care for Children and Their Families*. Washington, DC: The National Academies Press. 2003. doi:10.17226/10390
3. National Consensus Project for Quality Palliative Care. *Clinical Practice Guidelines for Quality Palliative Care*, 4th ed. Richmond, VA: National Coalition for Hospice and Palliative Care; 2018. https://www.nationalcoalitionhpc.org/ncp
4. Committee on Approaching Death: Addressing Key End of Life Issues; Institute of Medicine. *Dying in America: Improving Quality and Honoring Individual Preferences Near the End of Life*. Washington (DC): National Academies Press; 2015 Mar 19. https://www.ncbi.nlm.nih.gov/books/NBK285681/doi: 10.17226/18748
5. Sidgwick P, Fraser J, Fortune PM, McCulloch R. Parallel planning and the paediatric critical care patient. *Arch Dis Child*. 2019;104(10):994–997. doi:10.1136/archdischild-2018-315222
6. Haines ER, Frost AC, Kane HL, Rokoske FS. Barriers to accessing palliative care for pediatric patients with cancer: A review of the literature. *Cancer*. 2018;124(11):2278–2288. doi:10.1002/cncr.31265. Epub 2018 Feb 16.
7. Trowbridge A, Walter JK, McConathey E, Morrison W, Feudtner C. Modes of death within a children's hospital. *Pediatrics*. 2018;142(4):e20174182. doi:10.1542/peds.2017-4182
8. Morrison WE, Gauvin F, Johnson E, Hwang J. Integrating palliative care into the ICU: From core competency to consultative expertise. *Pediatr Crit Care Med*. 2018;19(8S Suppl 2):S86–S91. doi:10.1097/PCC.0000000000001465
9. Friedrichsdorf SJ, Bruera E. Delivering pediatric palliative care: From denial, palliphobia, pallilalia to palliative. *Children (Basel)*. 2018;5(9):120. doi:10.3390/children5090120
10. Maher K, Mitchell G. Panel discussion summary: When is palliative care everyone's business and when are specialists needed?. *Int J Palliat Nurs*. 2013;19(9):421–422. doi:10.12968/ijpn.2013.19.9.421
11. Keele L, Keenan H, Sheetz J, Bratton SL. Differences in characteristics of dying children who receive and do not receive palliative care. *Pediatrics*. 2013;132(1):72–81. doi:10.1542/peds.2013-0470

12. Friebert S, Williams C. NHPCO's fact and figures: Pediatric palliative & hospice care in America 2015 Edition. National Hospice and Palliative Care Organization. 2015. https://www.nhpco.org/wp-content/uploads/2019/04/Pediatric_Facts-Figures-1.pdf
13. Rogers M, Kirch R. Spotlight on pediatric palliative care: National landscape of hospital-based programs 2015–2016. Center to Advance Palliative Care Blog. Updated March 15, 2019. Available at https://www.capc.org/blog/palliative-pulse-palliative-pulse-july-2017-spotlight-pediatric-palliative-care-national-landscape-hospital-based-programs-2015-2016/
14. Kuo D, Houtrow AJ, Arango P, et al. Family-centered care: Current applications and future directions in pediatric health care. *Matern Child Health J*. 2012;16(2):297–305. doi:10.1007/s10995-011-0751-7
15. Section on Hospice and Palliative Medicine and Committee on Hospital Care. Pediatric palliative care and hospice care commitments, guidelines, and recommendations. *Pediatrics*. 2013;132(5):966–972. doi:10.1542/peds.2013-2731
16. Gerritsen RT, Hartog CS, Curtis JR. New developments in the provision of family-centered care in the intensive care unit. *Intensive Care Med*. 2017;43(4):550–553. doi:10.1007/s00134-017-4684-5
17. Bergstraesser E. Pediatric palliative care: When quality of life becomes the main focus of treatment. *Eur J Pediatr*. 2013;172(2):139–150. doi:10.1007/s00431-012-1710-z
18. Sibling Support Project. Sibshops. 2021. http://www.siblingsupport.org/sibshops
19. Jone B, Contro N, Koch KK. The duty of the physician to care for the family in pediatric palliative care: Context, communication, and caring. *Pediatrics*. 2014;133(S1):S8–15. doi:10.1542/peds.2013-3608C
20. Marsac ML, Kindler C, Weiss D, Ragsdale L. Let's talk about it: Supporting family communication during end-of-life care of pediatric patients. *J Palliat Med*. 2018;21(6):862–878. doi:10.1089/jpm.2017.0307
21. Mandac C, Battista V. Contributions of palliative care to pediatric patient care. *Semin Oncol Nurs*. 2014;30(4): 1–15. doi:10.1016/j.soncn.2014.08.003
22. Kirklin JK, Pagani FD, Kormos RL, et al. Eighth annual INTERMACS report: Special focus on framing the impact of adverse events. *J Heart Lung Transplant*. 2017;36(10):1080–1086. doi:10.1016/j.healun.2017.07.005
23. Tunuguntla H, Conway J, Villa C, Rapoport A, Jeewa A. Destination-therapy ventricular assist device in children: "The future is now." *Can J Cardiol*. 2020;36(2):216–222. doi:10.1016/j.cjca.2019.10.033
24. Kaufman BD, Hollander SA, Zhang Y, et al. Compassionate deactivation of ventricular assist devices in children: A survey of pediatric ventricular assist device clinicians' perspectives and practices. *Pediatr Transplant*. 2019;23(3):e13359. doi:10.1111/petr.13359
25. Rosenthal DN, Almond CS, Jaquiss RD, et al. Adverse events in children implanted with ventricular assist devices in the United States: Data from the Pediatric Interagency Registry for Mechanical Circulatory Support (PediMACS). *J Heart Lung Transplant*. 2016;35(5):569–77. doi:10.1016/j.healun.2016.03.005
26. Knoll C, Kaufman B, Chen S, et al. Palliative care engagement for pediatric ventricular assist device patients: A single-center experience. *ASAIO J*. 2020;66(8):929–932. doi:10.1097/mat.0000000000001092
26. Marelli A, Gatzoulis MW, Webb G. Adults with congenital heart disease: A growing population. In Gatzouliz M, Webb G, Daubeney, eds., *Diagnosis and Management of Adult Congenital Heart Disease*. 3rd ed. Amsterdam: Elsevier; 2018: 2–8.
28. Mazwi ML, Henner N, Kirsch R. The role of palliative care in critical congenital heart disease. *Semin Perinatol*. Mar 2017;41(2):128–132. doi:10.1053/j.semperi.2016.11.006
29. Masarone D, Valente F, Rubino M, et al. Pediatric heart failure: A practical guide to diagnosis and management. *Pediatr Neonatol*. 2017;58(4):303–312. doi:10.1016/j.pedneo.2017.01.001
30. Teitel D. Recognition of undiagnosed neonatal heart disease. *Clin Perinatol*. 2016;43(1):81–98. doi:10.1016/j.clp.2015.11.006

31. Price JF. Congestive heart failure in children. *Pediatr Rev.* 2019;40(2):60–70. doi:10.1542/pir.2016-0168

32. Hinton RB, Ware SM. Heart failure in pediatric patients with congenital heart disease. *Circ Res.* 2017;120(6):978–994. doi:10.1161/CIRCRESAHA.116.308996

33. Morrison WE, Gauvin F, Johnson E, Hwang J. Integrating palliative care into the ICU: From core competency to consultative expertise. *Pediatr Crit Care Med.* 2018;19(8S Suppl 2):S86–s91. doi:10.1097/PCC.0000000000001465

34. LeMond L, Goodlin SJ. Management of heart failure in patients nearing the end of life: There is so much more to do. *Card Fail Rev.* 2015;1(1):31–34. doi:10.15420/cfr.2015.01.01.31

35. Eggink H, Brand P, Reimink R, Bekhof J. Clinical scores for dyspnoea severity in children: A prospective validation study. *PLoS One.* 2016;11(7):e0157724. doi:10.1371/journal.pone.0157724

36. Patel A, Joong A, Lelkes E, Gossett JG. Should physicians offer a ventricular assist device to a pediatric oncology patient with a poor prognosis? *AMA J Ethics.* 2019;21(5):E380–386. doi:10.1001/amajethics.2019.380

37. Narayanan G, Pezeshkmehr A, Venkat S, Guerrero G, Barbery K. Safety and efficacy of the PleurX catheter for the treatment of malignant ascites. *J Palliat Med.* 2014;17(8):906–12. doi:10.1089/jpm.2013.0427

38. Evangelista LS, Sackett E, Dracup K. Pain and heart failure: Unrecognized and untreated. *Eur J Cardiovasc Nurs.* 2009;8(3):169–73. doi:10.1016/j.ejcnurse.2008.11.003

39. P Bharadwaj, A Chandra, D Stevens E, Schwarz. Palliative care for heart failure patients: Practical tips for home based programs. National Hospice and Palliative Care Organization. Palliative Care Resource Series. 2015. https://www.nhpco.org/wp-content/uploads/2019/04/PALLIATIVECARE_Heart_Failure_Patients.pdf

40. Reisfield, G., Wilson, G.: #144 Palliative Care Issues in Heart Failure. *Palliative Care Network of Wisconsin* Revised July 2015. https://www.mypcnow.org/fast-fact/palliative-care-issues-in-heart-failure/

41. Komatz K, Carter B. Pain and Symptom Management in Pediatric Palliative Care. *Pediatr Rev.* 2015;36(12):527–534. doi:10.1542/pir.36-12-527

42. Curley M, Liebers J, Maynard R. Continuous intravenous milrinone therapy in pediatric outpatients. *J Infus Nurs.* 2017;40(2):92–96. doi:10.1097/NAN.0000000000000214

43. DeCastro J. Pediatric home milrinone use while awaiting heart transplant. *Pediatric Nursing.* 2020;46(3):115–118. https://insights.ovid.com/pediatric-nursing/pednu/2020/05/000/pediatric-home-milrinone-use-awaiting-heart/3/01217119

44. Levin TT, Coyle N. A communication training perspective on AND versus DNR directives. *Palliat Support Care.* 2015;13(2):385–387. doi:10.1017/S147895151400039X

45. Dombrowksi D. Care of the patient and family. In: Santucci G ed. *Core Curriculum for the Pediatric Hospice and Palliative Nurse.* 2nd ed. Pittsburgh, PA: Hospice and Palliative Nurse Association; 2017: 109–122.

46. Aging with Dignity. Home page website. 2021. http://www.agingwithdignity.org/index.php.

47. Texas Health and Human Services 2016-2021. Advanced Directives Tab. https://www.hhs.texas.gov/laws-regulations/forms/advance-directives/form-livingwill-directive-physicians-family-or-surrogates

48. Wikipedia. Advanced Healthcare Directive. 2021. https://en.wikipedia.org/wiki/Advance_healthcare_directive

49. Dellon E, Goldfarb SB, Hayes D, Jr., Sawicki GS, Wolfe J, Boyer D. Pediatric lung transplantation and end of life care in cystic fibrosis: Barriers and successful strategies. *Pediatr Pulmonol.* 2017;52(S48):S61–s68. doi:10.1002/ppul.23748

50. Goldfarb SB, Hayes D, Jr., Levvey BJ, et al. The International Thoracic Organ Transplant Registry of the International Society for Heart and Lung Transplantation: Twenty-first pediatric lung and heart–lung transplantation report-2018. Focus theme: Multiorgan transplantation. *J Heart Lung Transplant.* 2018;37(10):1196–1206. doi:10.1016/j.healun.2018.07.021

51. Dalberg T, McNinch NL, Friebert S. Perceptions of barriers and facilitators to early integration of pediatric palliative care: A national survey of pediatric oncology providers. *Pediatr Blood Cancer.* 2018;65(6):e26996. doi:10.1002/pbc.26996

52. Levine DR, Mandrell BN, Sykes A, et al. Patients' and parents' needs, attitudes, and perceptions about early palliative care integration in pediatric oncology. *JAMA Oncol.* 2017;3(9):1214–1220. doi:10.1001/jamaoncol.2017.0368

53. Sisk BA, Friedrich AB, DuBois J, Mack JW. Emotional communication in advanced pediatric cancer conversations. *J Pain Symptom Manage.* 2020;59(4):808–817.e2. doi:10.1016/j.jpainsymman.2019.11.005

54. Kaye EC, Friebert S, Baker JN. Early integration of palliative care for children with high-risk cancer and their families. *Pediatr Blood Cancer.* 2016;63(4):593–597. doi:10.1002/pbc.25848

55. Zawistowski CA, Black C, Spruill TM, Granowetter L. Parental knowledge and opinions on palliative care for children. *Pediatrics.* 2018;141(1 Meeting Abstract):385. doi:https://doi.org/10.1542/peds.141.1_MeetingAbstract.385

56. Santucci G, Obrien J. Pain management for children with life-limiting conditions and at the end of life. In Santucci G, ed. *Core Curriculum for the Pediatric Hospice and Palliative Nurse,* 2nd ed. Pittsburgh, PA: Hospice and Palliative Nurses Association; 2017: 53–72.

57. Rybak A, Sethuraman A, Nikaki K, Koeglmeier J, Lindley K, Borrelli O. Gastroesophageal reflux disease and foregut dysmotility in children with intestinal failure. *Nutrients.* 2020;12(11):3536. doi:10.3390/nu12113536

58. Hauer J. Feeding intolerance in children with severe impairment of the central nervous system: Strategies for treatment and prevention. *Children (Basel).* 2017;5(1):1. doi:10.3390/children5010001

59. Herr K, Coyne PJ, Ely E, Gélinas C, Manworren RCB. Pain assessment in the patient unable to self-report: Clinical practice recommendations in support of the ASPMN 2019 Position Statement. *Pain Manag Nurs.* 2019;20(5):404–417. doi:10.1016/j.pmn.2019.07.005

60. Riquelme I, Pades Jiménez A, Montoya P. Parents and physiotherapists recognition of non-verbal communication of pain in individuals with cerebral palsy. *Health Commun.* 2018;33(12):1448–1453. doi:10.1080/10410236.2017.1358243

61. Friedrichsdorf SJ, Kang TI. The management of pain in children with life-limiting illnesses. *Pediatr Clin North Am.* 2007;54(5):645–672. doi:10.1016/j.pcl.2007.07.007

62. World Health Organization. WHO revision of pain management guidelines. August 27, 2019. https://www.who.int/news/item/27-08-2019-who-revision-of-pain-management-guidelines

63. Graham D, Paget SP, Wimalasundera N. Current thinking in the health care management of children with cerebral palsy. *Med J Aust.* 2019;210(3):129–135. doi:10.5694/mja2.12106

64. Collins A, Mannion R, Broderick A, Hussey S, Devins M, Bourke B. Gabapentin for the treatment of pain manifestations in children with severe neurological impairment: A single-centre retrospective review. *BMJ Paediatr Open.* 2019;3(1):e000467. doi:10.1136/bmjpo-2019-000467

65. Silver GH, Kearney JA, Bora S, et al. A Clinical pathway to standardize care of children with delirium in pediatric inpatient settings. *Hosp Pediatr.* 2019;9(11):909–916. doi:10.1542/hpeds.2019-0115

66. Turkel SB. Pediatric delirium: Recognition, management, and outcome. *Curr Psychiatry Rep.* 2017;19(12):101. doi:10.1007/s11920-017-0851-1

67. G: Edwards JD, Panitch HB, George M, et al. Development and validation of a novel informational booklet for pediatric long-term ventilation decision support [published online ahead of print, 2020 Dec 11]. *Pediatr Pulmonol.* 2020. doi:10.1002/ppul.25221

68. Henderson CM, FitzGerald M, Hoehn KS, Weidner N. Pediatrician ambiguity in understanding palliative sedation at the end of life. *Am J Hosp Palliat Care.* 2017;34(1):5–19. doi:10.1177/1049909115609294

69. Dryden-Palmer K, Haut C, Murphy S, Moloney-Harmon P. Logistics of withdrawal of life-sustaining therapies in PICU. *Pediatr Crit Care Med.* 2018;19(8S Suppl 2):S19–S25. doi:10.1097/PCC.0000000000001621

70. Wiener L, McConnell DG, Latella L, Ludi E. Cultural and religious considerations in pediatric palliative care. *Palliat Support Care.* 2013;11(1):47–67. doi:10.1017/S1478951511001027

71. Mherekumombe MF. From inpatient to clinic to home to hospice and back: Using the "pop up" pediatric palliative model of care. *Children (Basel).* 2018;5(55):1–6. doi:10.3390/children5050055

72. National Hospice and Palliative Care Organization. Hospice standards of practice for hospice programs. Updated 2018. Alexandria, VA: NHPCO. https://www.nhpco.org/hospice-care-overview/

THE PEDIATRIC PALLIATIVE APRN IN PERINATAL AND NEONATAL PALLIATIVE CARE

Maggie C. Root and Mallory Fossa

KEY POINTS

- The pediatric palliative advanced practice registered nurse (PP APRN) serves as a touchpoint for families along their journey, from diagnosis of a serious illness (prenatal or after birth) through transitions in care settings and goals of care, on to survivorship or bereavement.

- The PP APRN assesses, manages, and/or provides consultative service regarding pain and other physical symptoms that infant can experience.

- It is critical to attend to the emotional, psychological, practical, spiritual, educational, and developmental challenges that are faced by the parents, infants, and the extended family.

- The PP APRN is in an ideal position to assess the parents' understanding of the diagnosis, prognosis, and treatment options as well as the cultural and spiritual beliefs and views on what defines quality of life for their infant.

- Communication between family and healthcare providers can be coordinated by the PP APRN to reduce burden on the family and prevent clinician misunderstandings.

CASE STUDY 1: A BABY WITH MANY CONGENITAL ANOMALIES

Kristen (35 years old) and Antonio (32 years old) had been together for 8 years and were the parents of a 2-year-old daughter. Kristen was 32 weeks pregnant with a son with multiple congenital anomalies, including cystic kidney disease and cardiac defects, when she presented at a tertiary referral children's hospital. A perinatal palliative care consult was initiated by the maternal fetal medicine team supervising Kristen's care because their team thought Kristen and Antonio could benefit from added support during and after the pregnancy. In the initial perinatal palliative care consultation, Kristen and Antonio shared that it was important to them to continue to carry the pregnancy, even though their obstetrician had recommended termination. They expressed how it felt helpful to create a birth plan that acknowledged their values. Of primary importance was that they wanted to be present with their son as much as possible while also desiring support from life-prolonging medical technology. They hoped that the medical interventions would provide time to better understand the extent of their son's conditions and how

these may affect his future quality of life. The palliative care team discussed how the birth plan would be a modifiable communication tool and that, despite our best planning, changes were likely to occur over time.

The birth plan for the baby included a vaginal delivery with intubation at delivery if needed. However, the goal would be to protect him from the harm of cardiopulmonary resuscitation (CPR) if his heart were to stop. His parents remained hopeful that his condition would not be as severe as anticipated. They shared a desire for their daughter to meet their son in the hospital if possible. Kristen went into labor at 36 weeks and delivered vaginally. Antonio was present when their son Charlie was born. In the delivery room, the neonatal ICU (NICU) team noted Charlie was dusky with minimal respiratory drive. He was stabilized with noninvasive positive pressure ventilation (NIPPV) and Kirsten experienced skin-to-skin time with him before transfer to the NICU. Confirmatory diagnostic testing including echocardiogram, abdominal ultrasound, and head ultrasounds were performed. Charlie was found to have an atrial-septal defect that would likely require cardiac surgery in the first year of life. His single cystic kidney was confirmed. Charlie was also diagnosed with syndactyly, imperforate anus, and vertebral anomalies suggestive of a VACTERL-like syndrome with life-limiting prognosis.

During a family meeting, diagnostic information was shared and colostomy was recommended. Kristen and Antonio continued to share how it was important for them to follow Charlie's lead, especially since he was otherwise stable and had been weaned to 2L oxygen. Charlie underwent the recommended surgery without complication but developed kidney failure within a few days. A second family meeting where peritoneal dialysis was presented as a potential bridge to hemodialysis or renal transplant, with Charlie likely to require hospitalization until his transplant (which was expected to be more than a year away). Charlie's parents requested more time to consider the benefits and burdens of the procedure.

In follow-up visit with the palliative care team at Charlie's bedside, Kristen and Antonio described the importance of Charlie being able to run and play with his friends as he got older, hopes that they grieved as they saw a different reality. They worried about his quality of life, with frequent medical appointments, surgeries, procedures, and pain. The palliative team acknowledged Kristen and Antonio's love and support and courage in considering Charlie's experience. The palliative care team shared that some loving parents would decide not to pursue dialysis and focus care on Charlie's comfort. The team shared that without dialysis, Charlie's prognosis was days to weeks. Kristen and Antonio shared that they had been wanting to avoid dialysis but were concerned that the medical teams would not approve. After the meeting, the pediatric palliative advanced practice registered nurse (PP APRN) discussed the conversation with the neonatology providers. A do-not-resuscitate (DNR) order was placed, and the palliative care team made recommendations on streamlining Charlie's care to focus on comfort. Education was provided to the bedside nurses regarding the plan of care and anticipated needs for Charlie and his family.

At this point, Kristen stopped visiting the hospital, which distressed the nursing staff. In discussion with Antonio, he revealed he was trying to shoulder the burden of grief and protect Kristen from the heartbreak of their child dying. The palliative care team addressed their fears of grief and normalized the worries regarding watching their child decline. Charlie was moved into a private room where Kristen and Antonio were able to spend time as a family. Both Charlie's sister and his grandparents were able to meet him. The PP APRN supported the family and educated them about signs and symptoms of dying and ensuring comfort. Charlie showed very little discomfort and was weaned to room air. Per Kristin and Antonio's wishes, a chaplain performed a blessing in the presence of extended family. The family engaged in memory- and legacy-making activities with a child life specialist. Ten days later, Charlie died in Kristen's arms with Antonio by their side.

INTRODUCTION

When considering the care of a pregnant person, one must also consider the care for the unborn child. (Within the obstetrics and midwifery communities the inclusive terms "pregnant person" and "birthing person" are becoming more common. This acknowledges that not all people who give birth identify as women [i.e., men and nonbinary people] and not all people who give birth identify as parents [i.e.,

settings of adoption]. This inclusive language is becoming more widely used in the obstetrics and midwifery communities.) If a fetus is prenatally diagnosed with a life-limiting condition, the birthing person will be faced with multiple decisions along the trajectory of care for themselves and the fetus.[1] Palliative care in the setting of a pregnancy and birth straddles two areas: perinatal and neonatal palliative care. Often these two subspecialites are practiced by different providers, but they are presented together in this chapter because some families may cross the perinatal to neonatal path and because neonatal palliative care providers must be mindful of the prenatal journey that families have faced. Figure 27.1 demonstrates how in a perinatal consult differs from a neonatal palliative care consultation.

This chapter illustrates how the pediatric palliative advanced practice registered nurse (PP APRN) uses evidence-based practice to better support parents and infants. Pregnancy and parenting are deeply personal, and each APRN should attempt to limit projections onto the birthing person and family as they navigate these decisions within the context of their own values. It is important to keep in mind that one should maintain a lens of self-reflection and consider how one's own values may impact clinical assumptions and judgments. Therefore, the PP APRN must critically analyze their own values and beliefs regarding quality of life, when life begins, suffering, treatment, and disability. Moreover, one must be mindful of implicit bias around cultural ethnicity, gender identity, and family structure. Awareness allows us to recognize when we feel pulled to make recommendations or judgments based on our own perspectives and values, when, instead, as palliative care providers our role is to support the family in making decisions based on their own values and cultural constructs.[2]

PERINATAL PALLIATIVE CARE
History of Perinatal Palliative Care

This early identification of high-risk pregnancies has allowed for the earlier integration of perinatal

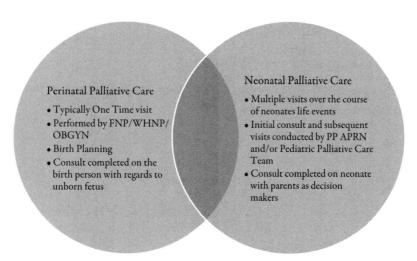

Figure 27.1 Perinatal versus neonatal palliative care.

palliative care.[3] Prior to the creation of hospital-based perinatal palliative care programs, services primarily involved community-based psychosocial supportive services for pregnant persons carrying a fetus with a fatal condition. Perinatal hospice services have grown over the past three decades to include a range of services.[4] Greater uncertainty in prognostication, driven by technological advances, has led to the evolution of perinatal hospice into perinatal palliative care. Perinatal palliative care is a new area of specialization within palliative care and encompasses the journey of pregnancy regardless of the fetal outcomes or decisions around termination. Services may be provided in the home, clinic, or hospital setting and may extend through bereavement.[5]

CURRENT STATE OF PERINATAL PALLIATIVE CARE

Across the country, although perinatal palliative care is growing, most perinatal palliative care programs are relatively young. Therefore, access to services has historically been limited and varied in scope.[5] This puts PP APRNs in a unique position to improve the care of these vulnerable families and their infants. Many perinatal palliative care programs do not meet established guidelines for the provision of comprehensive palliative care, with most lacking formal training palliative care training for all team members.[5] Hospital-based programs are becoming more common.[5] Often, perinatal palliative care clinics and services are provided in addition to subspecialist's primary clinics, and staffing may be difficult and varied based on institution.[6] Frequently it is a nurse coordinator or APRN who will help to coordinate the care of the multiple specialists (including obstetrics, maternal-fetal medicine, neonatology, and pediatric subspecialists) in meeting the needs of the birthing person.[1]

A prenatal palliative care consultation is performed by an interdisciplinary team[2] and may include unique participants, including maternal-fetal medicine specialists, obstetricians, fetal surgeons, and genetic counselors. Consultation emphasizes assistance with shared decision-making, birth planning, sibling support, and the provision of psychoemotional support throughout pregnancy, extending through birth and/or bereavement.[2,6,7] Consistent with the National Consensus Project for Quality Palliative Care (NCP) *Clinical Practice Guidelines*, the provision of perinatal palliative care covers the domains of physical, psychological, social, spiritual, and cultural care of patients.[2] This section highlights the role of the PP APRN in supporting family decision-making, facilitating discussions of goals of care through understanding family values, and addressing the ways families make meaning, balance hopes and worries, and face uncertainty while carrying a fetus with a serious condition.[8] Second, this section highlights the role of the PP APRN in developing a birth plan that covers each of the NCP *Clinical Practice Guidelines* domains. Finally, the role of the PP APRN in supporting other healthcare workers will be discussed (Table 27.1).

Table 27.1 CONDITIONS WHERE PERINATAL AND/OR NEONATAL PALLIATIVE CARE MAY BE APPROPRIATE

Cardiac conditions	*Neurologic conditions*
Acardia	Anencephaly/acrania
Complex congenital heart defects	Intraventricular hemorrhage (Grade IV)
Pentalogy of Cantrell	Periventricular leukomalacia
Patients requiring extracorporeal membrane oxygenation (ECMO) Support	Holoprosencephaly
Heart transplant candidates	Congenital severe hydrocephalus with absent or minimal brain growth
	Neurodegenerative diseases (spinal muscular atrophy)
	Spinal muscular atrophy
	Severe seizure disorders (i.e., Ohtahara Syndrome)
	Severe neurologic impairment
Gastrointestinal conditions	*Pulmonary conditions*
Necrotizing enterocolitis requiring surgical resection	Severe congenital diaphragmatic hernia
Total parenteral nutrition (TPN) dependence	Cystic fibrosis
Short gut	Pulmonary hypertension
Severe gastroschisis	Severe pulmonary hypoplasia
Liver failure	Ventilator dependent respiratory failure
Biliary atresia	Consideration of tracheostomy
	Consideration of lung transplant
Genetic conditions	*Renal conditions*
Trisomy 13, 15, or 18	Oligo/anhydramnios with pulmonary hypoplasia
Triploidy	Potter syndrome
Thanatophoric dwarfism	Renal agenesis
Lethal inborn errors of metabolism	Bilateral multicystic/dysplastic kidneys
Osteogenesis imperfecta, Type II or III	Polycystic kidney disease
Epidermolysis bullosa	
Mitochondrial or metabolic disorders	

Table 27.2 PERINATAL PALLIATIVE CARE ASSESSMENT AREAS

Physical	Consider how the physical experience of birth may guide the plan of care for the fetus or infant; symptom management for a live-born infant, regardless of goals of care.
Psychological	Address the emotional needs of the pregnant parent during the prenatal and post-partum periods.
Social	Consider normal developmental standards of the infant (i.e., first smile) and birth person (i.e., infant bonding, skin-to-skin contact) within a cultural context (i.e., importance of introducing the fetus or infant to family members).
Spiritual	Attend to the spiritual experience of the pregnant parent, their support persons, and family. Consider any the spiritual or religious values placed on birth (such as rituals, baptism, circumcision) may influence the plan of care.
Cultural	Ask the meaning of pregnancy in the pregnant person's culture. What are culturally normative childbirth experiences? What are the cultural reflections on fetal or infant loss (i.e., normal, shameful, meaningful)?
End-of-Life	Consider death of infant. Perinatal palliative care is for both live and non-live births when an infant's death is not imminently expected, as in the case where life-sustaining interventions are planned to address a serious condition.

From Carter.[9]

CASE STUDY 2: FACILITATING A BIRTH PLAN DISCUSSION

Meg, a PP APRN provided an initial perinatal consultation with June, a single woman who was 26 weeks pregnant. June's fetus was recently diagnosed with Trisomy 18. Meg dreaded the consult because she heard that June wanted to continue with her pregnancy. Before the consultation, Meg recognized that her feelings of despair emanated from her worry that June would be alone in caring for an infant with medical complexity. Meg's recognition of her own perceptions of parental burdens and quality of life allowed her to create space to better understand June's values in the consultation. This space allowed Meg to reflect on the families of children with Trisomy 18 who find tremendous joy in their children's continued life. Meg was reminded that this is not her pregnancy but June's and that June is making choices in the best interest of herself and her fetus.

SUPPORT SHARED DECISION-MAKING AND ESTABLISHING GOALS OF CARE

ADDRESSING PRIOR HEALTHCARE EXPERIENCES

The PP APRN holds a unique role in addressing the grief, conflict, and abandonment families may feel from prior healthcare experiences related to a pregnancy (Table 27.2). The PP APRN must acknowledge a journey prior to this point. In receiving a life-limiting, life-threatening diagnosis[9] for their child, parents have already experienced the loss of future-oriented hopes. It is common that, prior to a palliative care consultation, parents have been offered termination of the pregnancy (from an obstetric or specialist provider) if significant anomalies have been diagnosed.[10]

SUPPORTING UNDERSTANDING OF ILLNESS AND FAMILY VALUES

Parents should be given the opportunity to understand their child's diagnosis from the diagnosing specialists, preferably in the context of a family meeting. Unlike adult palliative care teams that frequently break bad news to patients, perinatal palliative care consultants are more frequently consulted after a family has already heard bad news. The palliative care team should arrange a meeting with the parents to further explore their understanding of this new diagnostic and prognostic information. Specifically, the palliative care team acknowledges parents' understanding of what has been told to them by other healthcare providers and asks them reflective questions such as "Based on this, what worries you the most?" and "What are you hoping for?"[8]

To provide perinatal palliative care, it is essential to understand the family system and values. It is well understood that even first-time parents have an internal sense of guiding principles to define a "good parent," which informs their decision-making and sense of parenthood.[11] These principles frame how parents perceive their unborn child's or infant's best interests. The PP APRN should ask open-ended questions such as "I have worked with many parents and have learned they often have a sense of what they need to do to be a good parent. What does being a good parent look like to you?"[11] Providing a silent presence can allow for parents to reflect and elaborate. These value-based questions can give the PP APRN a better understanding of what is important to parents. They should be used throughout the trajectory of care because goals and values are dynamic. Responses to these questions may change with parental experiences over time, redefining what it means to be a good parent and/or evolving in how they see their child.[10,11]

ELICITING WHAT DEFINES QUALITY OF LIFE

Similarly to understanding a parents' definition of "good parent," understanding their definition of a "good life" or quality of life is a critical component of supporting medical decision-making. While parents may have an understanding of what their child's life could look like in the future, parents do not find this as helpful when making decisions about quality of life.[12] The PP APRN should guide the conversation from functional limitation and disease burden to a more holistic understanding of quality of life, as appropriate.[12] This is achieved through open-ended questions such as "What does a good life mean to you?" or "What's most important in thinking about the future for your child?" In thinking about Charlie, initially Kristen and Antonio shared that it was important that Charlie have a more thorough postnatal evaluation to better understand his condition. As his parents learned more how his medical complexities would affect him over time, including the likely need for dialysis and multiple surgeries, they felt this was not consistent with their values of freedom from technology and thus not a good life for their child.

RESPECT FOR THE PARENT

Parents of a fetus or infant with a life-threatening condition face complex decisions throughout the pregnancy and after delivery. It is important to respect the birthing person, partner, and infant as each having value per the family system.[13] Decision-making in the setting of a life-limiting fetal condition has been shown to be influenced by many factors, including religion,[14] culture, severity of the fetal condition,[15] perception of suffering,[16] maternal age and education,[17] if a birthing person has other children,[18] and the level of prognostic certainty.[14] The time course for decision-making may be longer in the setting of early prenatal diagnosis or abbreviated if the diagnosis is made close to birth. The PP APRN should provide anticipatory guidance regarding the birth process and potential interventions and procedures while relating these to alignment with the family's goals of care. It is the role of the PP APRN to encourage a parental sense of control while highlighting how the birth person and partner are good parents who make decisions in their child/fetus's best interest.

SHARED DECISION-MAKING

The transition from a paternalistic model of healthcare to one that emphasizes shared decision-making shifts the focus away from providing objective information and toward supporting the infant's parents in making decisions based on their family's values.[19] The PP APRN supports the family in discerning treatment pathways. In addition to supporting the family, the PP APRN should help the primary care team to better understand how their own biases and values impact the guidance they give to families through modeling a reflective practice and facilitating proactive discussion among clinicians.

MEANING-MAKING

Parents of infants with life-limiting conditions have identified that they find value in continuing a pregnancy because it offers time to develop as a parent and bond with the fetus.[20-22] The process of becoming and identifying as a parent includes multiple steps that should be supported by the PP APRN. Use of the language that identifies the fetus or the fetus's condition as incompatible with life is strongly discouraged[3] as this invalidates the positive or growth-focused parental experiences of pregnancy and the lived experience of the family. Parents may derive meaning and add to their sense of being a parent through becoming informed about their child's condition, adjusting goals of the pregnancy, maximizing the quality of the pregnancy experience, including the unborn child in legacy-making, planning for birth, and serving as the child's advocate before and after birth.[20] This process of becoming a parent to the individual child may reduce feelings of parental regret.[20]

HOPES AND WORRIES

Parents can hold simultaneous hopes and worries that, on face value, may appear in conflict.[23] As with other populations, in perinatal palliative care it is important to assess the multiple hopes that birthing persons and families may hold.[2] As in Charlie's case, parents may have simultaneous worries about their child experiencing pain, being hospitalized, and having a complex medical condition while also hoping for time with the child and/or survival.[21] Parents may hope to connect with families who have had a child with a similar condition. They may also hope that the child be born alive, may be able to go home from the hospital, and/or have what the family determines to be a good life.[21]

UNCERTAINTY

Given the uncertainty in perinatal diagnostics and medical prognostication, children with conditions previously considered fatal may survive beyond the neonatal period.[24] Families report these children as being happy with a good quality of life, despite clinician judgment that the child's disease would be fatal.[24] Uncertainty may underlie much of decision-making for both birthing persons and clinicians. Because of this significant uncertainty, it is critical that families be informed of the range of medically and ethically permissible treatment aims, from termination through life-prolonging or curative-intent therapies.[3] Failing to disclose the range of possibilities fosters distrust between family and providers because parents inevitably will find this information elsewhere.[24] Parents report using community or online sources to find more information regarding others who have faced similar situations.[3,24] Additionally, parents find value and meaning in having choice in the care of the infant, even when that means the choice of pursuing comfort-directed treatments.[25]

Prenatally diagnosed conditions may have additional uncertainty because of limited diagnostic techniques in utero. Families may have received conflicting information from healthcare providers and are likely to have seen multiple specialists who provide organ-specific information. For example, the parent of a fetus with a prenatal diagnosis of anencephaly may have seen a primary obstetrician, who referred them to a maternal-fetal medicine specialist, pediatric geneticist, genetic counselor, pediatric neurologist, etc. It is the role of the PP APRN to synthesize information from these providers and elicit the family's understanding of the conditions. A birth plan may include postnatal diagnostic confirmation using imaging (such as echocardiogram or magnetic resonance imaging) or genetic testing (such as whole-genome sequencing or targeted genetic tests).[12] This information may further inform decision-making and treatment options. While waiting for confirmatory diagnostic results, a time-limited trial of life-prolonging interventions may be appropriate based on family goals of care.

THE BIRTH PLAN

Birth plans are a communication tool for families and clinicians for all types of births, whether a live birth or non-live birth. While there is some overlap in content, a perinatal palliative care birth plan is distinct and more complex than popular birth plans for healthy infants. As such, they are evolving documents that may change as families gain new perspectives on the pregnancy, child, quality of life, and illness. The development of a birth plan is grounded in the individual family's values. Birth plans may reflect goals of care that are focused primarily on comfort, emphasize life-sustaining or disease-directed treatments, or anything in between.[21] Birth plans are also appropriate when a non-live fetus is delivered, whether as a result of termination, miscarriage, or fetal demise. There is significant variation in birth plans among institutions, states, and regions reflecting local culture and legislation regarding the care of fetuses and infants. Birth plans should address five key content areas including identification, communication preferences, labor and delivery plan, postpartum care, and postmortem care. A nonexhaustive sample of birth plan elements is shown in Box 27.1.

DEVELOPMENT OF A BIRTH PLAN

Developing a birth plan incorporates family values, understanding of illness, and goals of care.[10] Birth plans emphasize family-centered care and bring the family voice to the forefront.[10] There is no one "right" plan; rather a plan must match the unique needs of the parents. Given the emotional nature of the content and the potential need for significant education, the process of birth planning can be lengthy and it may change as healthcare issues arise. General topics may include the birthing person's support companion, pain management during labor, comfort measures during labor, and important cultural rituals. When possible, avoid creating a birth plan in one sitting or treating the birth plan as a checklist. Forcing parents to make a decision on every topic or going down a list offering each intervention may be burdensome and run counter to the role of the PP APRN in aligning with the family and understanding the nuances of conversations. Instead, individualize the plan for each family. Not every topic may be appropriate for each family. Offering an "all or nothing" framework may place undue burden on the parents without providing the needed support found in shared decision-making. Many families choose a path that is not all one way or another, and they should be supported just the same by the PP APRN.

CHANGES IN BIRTH PLAN

In the setting of great prognostic and psychoemotional uncertainty, changes are inevitable. Changes to the birth plan may originate from the family, care team, or from the fetus's

Box 27.1 BIRTH PLAN COMPONENTS

- Identification
  - Chosen name of the fetus
  - Preferred terminology of the unborn (fetus, infant, child, baby)
  - Parental desire to know the sex of the fetus

- Communication preferences
  - Language
  - Written, verbal or auditory
  - Desire to know all details or limit content
  - Siblings: Who will communicate with them, and what has been communicated

- Labor & Delivery plan
  - Support person/attendant for the birthing person
  - Preference for vaginal or cesarian delivery
    - Use of cesarian for fetal distress?
  - Fetal monitoring
  - Pain management for birthing person
  - Physical environment (Music, lighting)
  - Does family wish to be informed if loss of heartbeat occurs during labor?
  - Who will cut the umbilical cord?
  - Resuscitative measures/warming plan
  - Parental bonding including skin to skin contact
  - Procedures

- Post-Partum
  - Location of infant care (Room-in, nursery, NICU)
  - Confirmatory diagnostic testing
  - Preferences for visitors/staff presence
  - Feeding and nutrition plan
  - Spiritual or religious preferences and rituals
  - Keepsakes

- Postmortem
  - Organ donation
  - Discussion of autopsy
  - Prior discussions of funeral arrangements (if appropriate)

From Perinatal Palliative Care: ACOG COMMITTEE OPINION, Number 786[6]; Cortez et al.[10]; Garten et al.[32]

presentation. It is important to have ongoing discussions with the parents regarding the potential for changes in the plan of care, especially if the postnatal diagnosis is not equivalent to the prenatal predictions. The multiple hopes and worries that families hold may shift over time[26] as parents may learn more about their child or the illness.

It is an important responsibility of the PP APRN to regularly reassess parental goals as these may change over the course of a pregnancy and/or after birth. The burden of reassessing goals should not lay solely with the parent. Families should be reassured that changes in hopes or goals are common and reflect the parental strength that comes with careful consideration of options.

COMPONENTS OF THE BIRTH PLAN

There are several components of birth plans including identification, communication preferences, labor and delivery plan, postpartum care, and postmortem care. Each birth plan should be customized to the family.

Identification

The PP APRN should elicit information on how the family would like the fetus to be addressed, such as by a specific name; as a child, son, or daughter; or as a fetus. Since birthing persons may or may not want to be identified as "mother" or "father," the APRN should ask the family how they wish to be addressed by the healthcare team. In some pregnancies, the sex of the fetus may be a surprise. The APRN should assess if the family wishes to know the expected sex of the fetus and if the family wishes not to know, care should be taken to protect that knowledge.

Communication

The PP APRN should address the family's preferred mode of communication (written, verbal, auditory) and language. Furthermore, the APRN should assess the extent to which the family would like information shared, whom information can be shared with, and if there are preferred members of the healthcare team whom the family sees as trusted. Siblings may have unique needs regarding communication of the pregnancy and birth (see further discussion later in the chapter).

Labor and Delivery Plan

Labor plans may include a discussion of medical interventions found in typical healthy birth plans, such as mode of delivery, location of labor (home, hospital room, operating room), fetal monitoring (intermittent, continuous, external, invasive), preferred method of pain management (including nonpharmacologic support), and an ideal physical birthing environment (lights dimmed, music choice, visitors in room). Unique components include whether the birthing person wishes to be informed of fetal demise if there is a loss of heartbeat during labor. As part of birth planning, the APRN should provide anticipatory guidance regarding what the infant may look like after birth, such as physical anomalies, color differences, or temperature changes. Care can be taken to cover areas of the child's body with hats, clothing or blankets if the parent desires.

Postpartum Care

This birth plan area may include logistical needs, condition-specific procedures, a plan for breastmilk production and feeding, addressing spiritual needs, and legacy-making. Location of care options based on the medical plan of care should be reviewed (room-in, well-baby nursery, NICU). Routine post-birth care provided to healthy infants may or may not be appropriate for each birth plan. This includes length/weight measurements, vitamin K injection, erythromycin eye drops, and blood glucose testing. Families may choose to focus on the comfort of the infant and forgoing life-sustaining interventions. Therefore, maximizing family time with the child in the parents' arms may dictate what "routine care" elements are continued. Respect for the infant and birthing person should be maintained regardless of whether the infant is born alive or deceased.

Condition-specific procedures may include confirmatory diagnostic or genetic testing,[6] life-sustaining interventions (such as intubation in the setting of congenital diaphragmatic hernia with lung hypoplasia), or a trial of therapies to assess the infant's response (bag-mask ventilation for an infant with Trisomy 13 and apnea at birth).

Lactation consultants are helpful to provide additional support to the birthing person. They may assist with milk production, suppression, pain from engorgement, and milk storage or donation.[27] The PP APRN should coordinate with lactation consultants regarding the evolving clinical scenario and importance of providing ongoing grief support because an inability to feed one's child may be a source of distress for the birthing person.[27]

Feeding one's child may hold emotional, spiritual, or cultural meaning to parents of a seriously ill infant.[28] Feeding strategies need to be targeted to the infant depending on complexity of medical conditions and the family's values and goals of care. There are a range of feeding options for seriously ill infants depending on the physiologic feeding ability, severity of the illness, goals of care, and local and state regulations regarding initiating, withholding, or discontinuing medically prescribed nutrition. In the immediate postpartum period, breast or chest feeding may be offered if congruent with the family goals of care. However, it may not be appropriate if medical resuscitation is anticipated at birth (i.e., if intubation is planned at delivery). Some infants (such as those with significant neurologic injury or craniofacial conditions) may not be able to latch and suck. Consultation with speech therapy may support the infant in engaging in feeding. Medically administered nutrition and hydration (MANH) may meet a variety of goals including providing comfort or life prolongation, and may be included as part of a birth plan. (See the later section on end-of-life care for additional information on feeding in actively dying children and withdrawal of MANH.)

Postmortem Care

Birth plans may address any discussions regarding autopsy (family education, family preferences, family concerns) and organ donation. As appropriate, the plans regarding funeral or memorial services may also be included (such as preferred funeral home or religious needs regarding care of the body).

CASE STUDY 3: LISTENING TO THE INFANT'S BODY

Parents Lisa and Lindsay were counseled that their son, Brad, had a severe cardiac defect that was likely to lead to death shortly after birth. Given his cardiac physiology, the cardiac surgery team felt he was not a surgical candidate and would unlikely tolerate enteral feeds. His mothers felt it important to allow Brad to lead them in decision-making and also wanted to introduce him to his extended family if possible. They felt pursuing cardiac surgery was not in his best interest. The PP APRN prepared Lisa and Lindsay that Brad may not have the strength to breastfeed due to heart failure. Lisa gave birth to Brad at term, and an echocardiogram confirmed the prenatal cardiac diagnosis. Shortly after birth, Brad surprisingly showed interest in breastfeeding. With assistance from a lactation consultant, Brad latched and ate from the breast several times in his first 24 hours. He surprised the medical team and was discharged to home with hospice supports, continuing to breastfeed on demand.

Legacy-Making Activities

Legacy-making activities have been shown to provide benefit to families who experience fetal or infant loss.[3,13] These may include keeping mementos such as lock of hair, identification band, crib card, and clothing and bedding. Parents may wish to take pictures of ultrasound findings, keep a monitoring strip from labor, or record the fetal or infant heartbeat. Some routine care elements may be adjusted to serve the palliative needs of the family. For example, taking length and head circumference measurements at the bedside may be a legacy-building activity with the measuring tape saved as a keepsake. Child life specialists may assist with mold-making of hands or feet, song-making, or recording memories of the pregnancy and infant in a journal.[29] Professional photography may also benefit parents as they grieve fetal or infant loss.[30] Organizations such as Now I Lay Me Down to Sleep (https://www.nowilaymedowntosleep.org/) offer these services through volunteer networks across the United States and internationally.[31]

Sibling Services

There are unique developmental considerations for siblings who are anticipating the birth of a brother or sister. The birth plan should include documentation of discussions regarding if siblings are expected to be present during or after a birth,[32] what information the sibling has received,[10] and context regarding their developmental and learning needs. The PP APRN should address logistical considerations, such as which adult will remain with the child and where they can safely eat and play during a hospitalization. Coordination with child life specialists, art therapists, or music therapists may be helpful in creating space for the sibling(s) to express

their feelings regarding the birth, regardless of the birth outcome and goals of care.[2]

COMMUNICATING THE BIRTH PLAN

The birth plan serves as a planning and communication tool. Each discussion regarding of the birth plan may start with a brief synopsis of the family's understanding of illness/prognosis and their overarching values and goals of care. This helps to frame the decisions contained within the birth plan. It is important that the PP APRN ensure the birth plan has been shared with the involved delivery team and with supportive service providers (spiritual care providers, child life specialists, decedent affairs/patient relations) as appropriate. While birth plans for a planned healthy delivery are often written by parents, birth plans in the context of perinatal palliative care are most often written by healthcare providers to summarize discussions that occur with the family. Depending on the institution, this may be either documented in the medical record via a note or scanned in the electronic health record (EHR), where it can be referenced by all clinicians. Like any advance care plan, decision-makers can choose to deviate from this plan as the pregnancy and birth evolve.

SUPPORT OF HEALTHCARE PROVIDERS

A key role of the PP APRN is to provide both education and emotional support to other healthcare providers.[2,33] Because of the evolving nature of perinatal palliative care and the variety of settings in which it is provided, many clinicians who encounter families may have unharnessed primary palliative care skills. The PP APRN should target education to obstetric, maternal fetal medicine, and neonatal clinicians including nurses, APRNs, and physicians. Providing educational offerings for other clinicians may also increase referrals to palliative care services and improve the care provided to families.[34]

NEONATAL PALLIATIVE CARE

HISTORY

In 2003, the Institute of Medicine released the seminal report *When Children Die: Improving Palliative and End-of-Life Care for Children and Their Families*. This challenged healthcare providers to develop and implement practice guidelines for palliative, end-of-life, and bereavement care for infants, children, and their families.[35] From this report, the field of pediatric palliative care (including neonates) has dramatically evolved. Educational curriculum for APRNs has expanded to include pediatric APRN-specific End-of-Life Nursing Education Consortium (ELNEC) training[36] and specific certifications for perinatal/neonatal loss and pediatric palliative care.[37,38] As the community of pediatric palliative care clinicians has grown, the needs of pediatric patients is more prominent in national discussions and policy documents regarding palliative care. The NCP *Clinical Practice Guidelines* provide standards of care for all patients receiving palliative care including infants.[2]

CURRENT STATE

Despite advances in neonatal healthcare, about one-half of the deaths in children in the United States occur during the first year of life. In 2018, the infant mortality rate was 5.7 out of every 1,000 live births, resulting in more than 21,000 infant deaths.[39] The three leading causes of death in children under the age of 1 year include congenital malformations, low birth weight, and maternal complications.[39] Infants born prior to 32 weeks gestation have higher rates of morbidity and mortality, while those born very preterm (prior to 28 weeks gestation) have the highest rate of mortality, with a risk 186 times greater than an infant born full term.[40] Research demonstrates that palliative care consultation in the NICU increases psychosocial support for families and reduces the use of advanced life-prolonging technology at end of life.[41] However, infants receive specialty palliative care consultation at very low rates despite comprising a large portion of deaths within children's hospitals.[42]

CONSULT ETIQUETTE IN THE NICU

Despite improved outcomes for patients and acceptance by families, the role of palliative care in the NICU continues to be misunderstood in many institutions.[43] Some institutions have high rates of coordination, embedded NICU-specific palliative care teams, or clinicians dually trained in neonatology and palliative care. Other hospitals may have an adult palliative care service that occasionally consults in a community NICU. Because of the wide range of practices, the PP APRN needs to ensure humility as part of the consult process. Consult etiquette[44,45] is of the utmost importance to growing the field of palliative care within the NICU setting. The scope of practice for palliative care in the NICU may be on a consultative basis, where recommendations are provided to the primary service. Unlike many adult ICU settings, even at end of life the primary NICU team may manage all medications and remain the conduit for information for the family. The PP APRN needs to carefully assess the institutional and unit-based norms regarding palliative care services and implement a "low and slow" approach to providing support in the NICU setting. The PP APRN should allow extra time to introduce themselves and the palliative care team to the primary NICU providers, including bedside nurses. This allows the APRN to establish rapport and trust with the NICU team and gather additional subjective information regarding the infant and family.

CARE OF THE INFANT

Much of symptom management for infants is similar in approach to children. Highlights of differences and areas of emerging emphasis in the neonatal population are noted. Please refer to Chapter 26, "The Pediatric Palliative APRN in the Acute Care Setting," for additional symptom management guidance.

Assessment

Careful assessment of infant experience is critical and should include pain,[46] dyspnea, delirium,[47] constipation, and vomiting.[48] The use of validated and reliable screening tools is strongly encouraged.[2] The infant's neurologic status, gestational age, and sedation status should be considered when selecting an appropriate measure because tools may be validated for different clinical scenarios. A list of symptom-specific tools is provided in the NCP *Clinical Practice Guidelines*, pediatric nursing textbooks, and herein.[2,46,49]

Obtaining a history from the infant's caregivers, including parents, respiratory therapists, child life specialists, nurses, and physicians, is very important.[2] Consider the infant's patterns and rhythms during day and night when assessing symptoms. Knowledge of nap times, feeding times, and fussy times may provide insight into potential areas where quality of life may be improved. Infants may find comfort from familiar faces, voices, sounds, smells, and toys/stuffed animals. The PP APRN assesses which of these provides comfort to the infant and can implement comfort measures such wrapping the infant in a blanket that has a parent's scent. Conversely, an overstimulating environment may cause infant distress. The PP APRN introduces neurologically appropriate environment (i.e., stimulation should match the infant's developmental needs) and provides education to the family and care team regarding the importance of sleep, rest, and routine. When assessing the infant for symptoms, observe the facial expressions, level of attention to faces, and responses to familiar sounds/voices as signs of behavior change.

Symptom Assessment and Management

Pain Assessment

The notion that infants do not feel pain has been proved incorrect.[50] Infants may experience pain throughout their lives, not just at end of life.[51,52] Surviving infants who are repeatedly exposed to painful procedures in the NICU demonstrate hypersensitivity to pain in childhood. When caring and assessing for pain in the neonate, the APRN should be mindful of potential pain sources including procedures (e.g., needle sticks or endotracheal suctioning) and underlying conditions (e.g., central/neuropathic pain in severe neurologic impairment).[53,54] The PP APRN should observe the infant's behaviors and assess the parental and bedside nursing's perceptions of pain.[53] Pain behaviors in infants include facial grimace, hiccupping, yawning, furrowed brow, difficulty sucking or latching, inconsolability, irritability, alterations in level of activity, and crying.[46] Pain report by proxy, such as from a parent or nurse, can help in assessing the infant's comfort. Many parents become expert at interpreting their infant's cries and differentiating between cries of hunger versus discomfort.[55]

An observational pain assessment tool that is validated in the specific neonatal or infant population should be utilized.

Many of these tools are multimodal assessments that take into account the infant's facial expressions, vital signs, and behavioral components.[56-58] While hospitals and palliative care organizations may use specific tools in varying settings of care, it is important that the APRN not use a child or adult pain tool as these may under- or over-capture pain levels. In addition, some scales are validated in certain gestational ages (preterm vs. term infants) or based on pain types (acute pain vs. chronic pain vs. postoperative pain).[58] Examples of these tools include N-PASS,[59,60] NIPS, COMFORT,[59] CRIES,[61] FLACC,[53] and the Revised FLACC.[46,55,62]

Pain Management

It is important to consider nonpharmacologic interventions with or without pharmacologic interventions.[56] Nonpharmacologic interventions should be continued even after pharmacologic interventions are initiated. Nonpharmacologic strategies can increase the parent–child bond and support normal infant development. Trial and error can be used to control the environment of care by reducing noxious stimuli (bright lights, noise, unnecessary touch).[46,57] Audio recordings can be played of a parent's voice or favorite lullaby even when the family is not present at the infant's bedside. Swaddling, massage, breast-feeding, and non-nutritive sucking are interventions that may reduce the experience of pain in infants.[62] Skin-to-skin care is now routinely offered in NICU settings as it has been shown to reduce pain in infants.[63] Parents also report that, at the end of life, holding their child skin-to-skin can be a positive experience for both infant and parent. The PP APRN should advocate for opportunities for parent–child bonding at end of life should the family desire.[56,64] Of note, not all families desire to hold their child at end of life. The PP APRN should assess for educational needs (i.e., parental fear of hurting their child or hastening their child's death) and cultural considerations. Families should not be forced to hold their infants at end of life.

When considering pharmacological inteventions for pain, dosing is important (see Appendix II for suggested medication dosing). Of note, opioids can be safely used in the neonatal population for the management of both pain and dyspnea. Due to their immature metabolism, neonates and infants are at higher risk for respiratory depression from opioids.[65] Therefore, opioids are dosed much lower in this population than for children. Starting morphine doses for pain are typically 25–35% of pediatric dosing, with longer dosing intervals due to delayed elimination and significantly prolonged half-life compared to children and adults.[65,66] Depending on the severity of symptoms, either intermittent dosing or continuous infusions can be reasonable for administration.[56] Often morphine is the chosen opioid given its longer half-life than fentanyl.[56]

Dyspnea

Prevalence and Assessment

Subjective assessment by proxy (parent or clinician report) can assist in the identification of dyspnea. Infants experiencing breathlessness may appear restless, have paradoxical breathing, grunting, bob their head, have asynchronous breaths over

a ventilator, nasal flaring, or exhibit facial expressions that imply distress.[67] Vital sign changes including tachycardia and tachypnea should also be considered. While there are currently no valid and reliable measures of dyspnea in the neonatal population, a modified version of the Respiratory Distress Observation Scale is under development for infants.[67]

Management

The PP APRN should assess for dyspnea in all neonates given the high rates of pulmonary compromise in this population. Extra attention should be given to frequent assessment in the neonate at end of life.[56] Decreasing intravenous or enteral fluid supplementation may be considered as a way to reduce dyspnea caused by fluid overload at end of life. In the neonate, even seemingly miniscule fluid volumes can add to symptom burden. Depending on institutional pharmacy offerings, some intravenous medications can be prepared in more concentrated forms to allow for smaller volumes of fluid to be administered. Additional nonpharmacologic therapies include positioning for comfort (sidelying or elevated head of isolate) or having a fan or blow-by humidified air on the face. In addition to the management of pain, opioids can be used to treat dyspnea in the neonate at 25–50% of the dose used for pain.[65] While benzodiazepines can be used to mitigate agitation, it should be noted that they alone do not treat dyspnea.[56]

Delirium

Delirium is the acute change in sensorium with changes to level of consciousness and ability to sustain attention. In the neonatal population this may manifest as psychomotor agitation or retardation.[47] In recent years the acknowledgment of delirium in infants has been more widely recognized. Among all hospitalized children, those under 2 years, critically ill, or requiring mechanical ventilation are at highest risk to develop delirium.[47,68] Since many NICU patients meet all three of these high-risk criteria, the PP APRN should be alert to the possible emergence of delirium.

Assessment

For delirium in infants, it is important that the PP APRN interview both parents and caregivers (nursing, respiratory therapists, physicians, child life specialists, physical therapists) to identify patterns of behavior, preferred activities, and agitation triggers. The Cornell Assessment of Pediatric Delirium (CAPD) has been validated for infants and incorporates longitudinal measurements of behaviors and interactions over an 8- to 12-hour period.[47,68] The Preschool Confusion Assessment Method for the ICU (psCAM-ICU) is also validated in this population.[69] In addition to the use of standardized tools, the APRN should personally assess the child, including watching for ventilatory synchrony, as delirium can be precipitated by dyspnea from uncomfortable vent settings.

Management

Nonpharmacologic management focuses on environmental changes and evaluation of precipitating factors. The PP

APRN should ensure that the infant has a warm, comfortable environment with reduction in overstimulating noise. Daily routines should be developed in consultation with the family, bedside nursing, and child life specialists. These routines may include feedings, nap time, play time, and bath time. Lighting should be used to help cue the infant to day–night differentiation. Clutter in the infant's crib and room should be reduced, and blinking lights or monitor noises minimized as possible.[55] The PP APRN should educate the NICU team regarding the importance of routine and consider posting signs with the infant's schedule at the bedside. Effective treatment of delirium also includes addressing the potential root causes, including uncontrolled pain or infection.[68] The pneumonic "I WATCH DEATH"[70,71] can be used to recall the conditions that may precipitate delirium: infection, withdrawal from substances, acute metabolic conditions, trauma, central nervous system etiology, hypoxia, deficiencies of vitamins or hormones, endocrinopathies, acute vascular changes, toxicities, and heavy metals.[70,71]

While concurrently addressing and assessing the cause, the PP APRN should consider pharmacological interventions for which the literature supports using antipsychotics as first-line pharmacological management. Second-generation antipsychotics can be used effectively in infants.[47] Refer to Appendix I "Pediatric Pain and Symptom Management" for dosing guidelines.

CARE OF THE FAMILY

In addition to the strategies described in Chapter 26, "The Pediatric Palliative APRN in the Acute Care Setting," there are unique psychoemotional considerations for families with a baby in the NICU. Postpartum birthing persons may need additional support. The PP APRN must use language that supports the developing infant–parent relationship because many have difficulty bonding with their ill infant as a result of anxiety or depression.[72] Coordination with social work, chaplaincy, obstetrics, psychology, and psychiatry is indicated as needed for assessment and treatment of postpartum mood disorders. Routine meetings between the family, palliative care team, and primary team are encouraged to establish and maintain collaborative communication.

LEGACY-MAKING IN THE NICU

Legacy-making may be an integrated component of family life for the infant with a prolonged NICU stay or those with life-threatening illness. Normal developmental milestones may be celebrated by the family and care team. Research shows that legacy projects, such as digital story-telling, hand/foot molds, and photography, are acceptable to many parents during the course of the NICU stay.[73] The PP APRN can encourage these activities regardless of goals of care. Allowing parents the opportunity to engage in memory-making, whether it is photography, dressing their infant in a special outfit, or making handprints/molds allows parents to feel more connected to their child while alive and after

death.[74] The PP APRN should work with other members of the healthcare team (social work, child life, nursing) to facilitate this legacy work. Coordinating the visits of extended family and siblings may be important. In the case study about Charlie, Kristen and Antonio initially did not wish for their daughter to meet Charlie. Once he was born, they later felt it was important and appreciated their time together as a family unit.

SIBLING SUPPORT

Siblings of NICU patients have unique needs related to developmental processing, grief, and bereavement. Visiting the baby in the NICU before death should be encouraged because this is associated with reduced anxiety and depression among surviving siblings.[75] Consultation with child life specialists and hospital-based school teachers, when available within the organization, are encouraged. See Chapter 38, "Grief and Bereavement," for additional guidance on developmentally appropriate responses to grief in children.

COMMUNITY RESOURCES

In addition to sibling support and coordinating legacy work, the PP APRN should offer and coordinate referrals to community resources. Some organizations, such as Courageous Parents Network, may be appropriate for referral early in an illness or hospitalization. Courageous Parents Network was created by bereaved parents with the support of pediatric palliative care professionals to provide information on medical decision-making and life in the NICU.[76] Other resources may include a local March of Dimes chapter, disease-specific advocacy and support groups, or local parent networks.

CARE OF THE NICU TEAM

Because no infant remains in the NICU, transitions are a natural part of caring for critically ill neonates. Transitions include transfer to another unit (such as pediatric ICU or long-term ventilator unit), discharge to a skilled pediatric nursing facility, discharge to home (with or without home-based palliative supports), and death.

The PP APRN has a unique viewpoint on caring for children across care settings. It is important that future planning is integrated into the care plan by encouraging the primary healthcare team to anticipate future care needs, complications, or outcomes. The PP APRN can hold the "big picture," allowing the primary care team to navigate the day-to-day illness management. Transitions may be challenging for NICU providers who may feel that transferring an infant equates to professional failure. Providers may also believe the infant or family needs to stay in the NICU because another care setting would not meet the same quality standards. Rarely are such decisions simple or clear-cut. The PP APRN should acknowledge and support the anticipatory grief and loss experienced by parents and the healthcare team prior to the actual transition of care.

MORAL INJURY AND BURNOUT

Moral distress and burnout are common among NICU nurses and physicians.[77] The PP APRN role includes identifying and addressing sources of distress for the care team. This distress may extend to custodial staff, unit clerks, and food service workers who have frequent interactions with the families of seriously ill infants. Skills used by the PP APRN with patients and families (such as active listening and attending to grief experiences) may also be employed to address staff distress and burnout.[33]

Disagreements regarding goals of care and decisions along the treatment course may be a source of distress for parents and clinicians alike. When disagreement occurs, the PP APRN should facilitate a discussion of thoughts and feelings while holding space for grief among all stakeholders. Clinicians need to be aware of how their personal values and opinions can influence how they are providing care for others. The PP APRN should model critical self-reflection for other clinicians and help create a space where psychological safety is the norm. See Chapter 53, "Navigating Ethical Discussions" for additional content.

END-OF-LIFE CARE

FEEDING

Feeding by mouth at end of life may include breast feeding or feeding by bottle with formula or expressed milk. A dropper of expressed breast milk may also be used to moisten an infant's mouth. For infants able to feed orally, feeding the infant may provide comfort to both child and family, especially when included in skin-to-skin care. The PP APRN should continue to assess for symptoms at end of life related to oral feeding such as gagging, dyspnea, vomiting, and constipation.

MEDICALLY ADMINISTERED NUTRITION AND HYDRATION

In rare situations, withdrawal of MANH may best align with goals of care and improve the infant's comfort. The PP APRN should proactively facilitate consultation with pediatric bioethicists regarding the use of MANH at end of life, with the goal of supporting parental decision-making and educating the clinical team on ethically and legally permissible actions. Current ethical guidance from the American Academy of Pediatrics Committee on Bioethics indicates there are limited circumstances in which discontinuation of MANH may be ethically permissible in the care of infants.[78] It is important that the PP APRN be familiar with and adhere to local, state, and institutional laws and policies pertaining to the initiation, withholding, and discontinuing of MANH in infants and children.[79]

Of note, parents of infants and children who died after withdrawal of MANH have reported satisfaction with their decision.[80] Furthermore, parents may feel that their children received good quality end-of-life care, with time to hold their child and make memories together.[41] Infants may live days to weeks after withdrawal of MANH, with one observational study finding an infant lived 37 days.[81] Special attention should be provided to the infant's skin during this time as pressure sores may occur over bony prominences due to limited subcutaneous fat. It is imperative that the PP APRN develop a plan to consistently support the family and healthcare staff during the time after withdrawal of MANH, as this time period can be a source of moral distress for some.

ROLE OF THE PEDIATRIC PALLIATIVE APRN IN END-OF-LIFE CARE

Provide Assessment, Diagnosis, and Management of Symptoms

A primary role of the PP APRN when caring for an infant at end of life is to assess and diagnose symptoms. As discussed in the preceding section on "Consult Etiquette in the NICU," the PP APRN may or may not directly manage medications depending on institutional policies and unit culture. The PP APRN may instead provide recommendations to the NICU service.

Family Counseling

When an infant is nearing end of life, the PP APRN should consider the educational and psychosocial needs of the family. Bereaved parents have shared that their child experiencing symptoms at the end-of-life was very distressing to them, especially after decisions around withdrawal of life-sustaining therapies were made.[74,82] Parents have shared that their most distressing symptoms witnessed in their infant were respiratory distress, agitation, and pain.[82] PP APRNs should provide education to the family on the anticipated course of the dying process and how the family can play an active role in providing care. For example, parents who elected to focus on their child's comfort have shared their appreciation for the opportunity to provide skin-to-skin care and feedings.[57,83,84]

The PP APRN supports parents by providing anticipatory guidance of the signs and symptoms of dying, how their child may appear, and the management of distressing symptoms. This helps to ensure parents that all measures are being taken to ensure the infant's comfort.[82] While counseling on symptom management and physiologic changes are important to discuss with parents, parents have also shared the importance of support for legacy work and bereavement during and after the infant has died.[74,85] The PP APRN can provide guidance to the family regarding ways to create memories in the time left and how the family can anticipate being supported after the death. The PP APRN should work with the NICU team to address which team members will provided education to the family to avoid the family from being overwhelmed by repetitive information. In some cases, the NICU team may want to be present while the PP APRN provides end-of-life counseling to the family.

Coordinating with the Nursing Team

During the time that an infant may be dying, it is crucial to partner with the infant's bedside nursing team. The bedside nurse can help to facilitate nonpharmacologic measures as well as pharmacologic measures to ensure the child's comfort. The role of the PP APRN includes supporting the bedside nurses and nursing leadership. This may include creating a safe space for the nurses to ask questions regarding end-of-life care or addressing concerns around how the family has made decisions regarding goals of care. As part of capacity-building in the NICU, the PP APRN should identify NICU nurse "champions" who are interested and experienced in providing palliative care. These nurses can be advocates for palliative care in the unit[9] and provide additional support to more novice nurses. The PP APRN should round frequently on the nursing staff to reinforce the plan of care and offer additional grief support as needed.[33]

Coordinating Location of Death

In addition to symptom management, parents have shared that the environment in which they are in can be very important. Offering parents the ability to be in a private room may change their experience of their child's death. If parents would like to be at home, the palliative care team can coordinate with hospices to provide end-of-life care in the home when possible.[74] Before this is offered to the family, the PP APRN should consult with local hospices to assess their prior experiences in with caring for an infant at end of life as not all hospices accept infants into their care. Infants with complex symptom management needs (including intravenous medications) or receiving concurrent care may be challenging to place with a home hospice agency if there are no nurses with infant or pediatric experience available. The PP APRN should review all planned treatments, medications, and care instructions with the hospice prior to discharge to ensure that the hospice has a full picture of the family's needs.

Educating and Supporting NICU Team

A significant amount of time may be spent by the PP APRN providing education and support to the NICU team. NICU providers may have curiosity about the pathophysiology of the dying process, concerns regarding the range of parental decision-making, and questions about bereavement support for the family. The PP APRN should elicit and anticipate opportunities to provide just-in-time education to the NICU team. Other support of the NICU team should include assessing the grief and anticipatory bereavement needs of the staff. Clinicians may feel shame or guilt that their patient won't survive and may feel a sense of loss and grief while observing an infant at end of life. The PP APRN should normalize these feelings, create a safe space for clinicians to express vulnerability, and provide grief support to the NICU clinicians.

BEREAVEMENT

Bereavement care is a core component of palliative care, and is discussed in depth in Chapter 38, "Grief and Bereavement."[2] Parents have shared the importance of connecting with bereavement support both prior to the loss of their child and thereafter. This is accomplished by a follow-up phone call by any member of the team because it allows parents to feel connected to their team and may help to prevent any sense of abandonment that bereaved parents have experienced.[85] Sending a bereavement card, sharing memories of the child, and communicating to parents that their child was not forgotten is generally welcomed.[64,74] The PP APRN should provide bereavement support to the family and refer them to hospital- or community-based bereavement services.[2] This may include grief and loss counselors, hospice-based bereavement programs, support groups for parents of children with special needs, and camps for parents or siblings who have had a loss.

SUMMARY

Families facing the birth, life, or death of their fetus or infant have unique needs and require expert support from the PP APRN. Care of the whole family, from diagnosis onward, may occur in multiple care settings and with a variety of healthcare providers. The PP APRN is in a unique position to support the family across this trajectory, holding the family narrative, values, and goals as the pregnancy and infant evolve. It is also imperative that the PP APRN provide support to other healthcare providers who may experience moral distress as a result of facing scenarios that may be emotionally triggering or challenge one's personal beliefs.

REFERENCES

1. Limbo R, Brandon D, Côté-Arsenault D, Kavanaugh K, Kuebelbeck A, Wool C. Perinatal palliative care as an essential element of childbearing choices. *Nursing Outlook*. 2017;65(1):123–125. doi:10.1016/j.outlook.2016.12.003
2. National Concensus Project for Quality Palliative Care. *Clinical Practice Guidelines for Quality Palliative Care*. 4th ed. Richmond, VA: National Coalition for Hospice and Palliative Care; 2018. https://www.nationalcoalitionhpc.org/ncp/.
3. Kamrath HJ, Osterholm E, Stover-Haney R, George T, O'Connor-Von S, Needle J. Lasting legacy: Maternal perspectives of perinatal palliative care. *J Palliat Med*. 2019;22(3):310–315. doi:10.1089/jpm.2018.0303
4. Hoeldtke NJ, Calhoun BC. Perinatal hospice. *Am J Obstet Gynecol*. 2001;185(3):525–529. doi:10.1067/mob.2001.116093
5. Wool C, Côté-Arsenault D, Perry Black B, Denney-Koelsch E, Kim S, Kavanaugh K. Provision of services in perinatal palliative care: A multicenter survey in the United States. *J Palliat Med*. 2016;19(3):279–285. doi:10.1089/jpm.2015.0266
6. ACOG. Perinatal Palliative Care: ACOG COMMITTEE OPINION, Number 786. *Obstet Gynecol*. 2019;134(3):e84–e89. doi:10.1097/aog.0000000000003425

7. Cole JCM, Moldenhauer JS, Jones TR, et al. A proposed model for perinatal palliative care. *J Obstet Gynecol Neonatal Nurs.* 2017;46(6):904–911. doi:10.1016/j.jogn.2017.01.014

8. Kobler K, Limbo R, eds. *Conversations in Perinatal, Neonatal, and Pediatric Palliative Care.* Pittsburgh, PA: Hospice & Palliative Nurses Association; 2017.

9. Carter BS. Pediatric palliative care in infants and neonates. *Children (Basel).* 2018;5(2). doi:10.3390/children5020021

10. Cortezzo DE, Ellis K, Schlegel A. Perinatal palliative care birth planning as advance care planning. *Front Pediatr.* 2020;8(556). Published 2020 Sep 8. doi:10.3389/fped.2020.00556

11. Weaver MS, October T, Feudtner C, Hinds PS. "Good-parent beliefs": Research, concept, and clinical practice. *Pediatrics.* 2020;145(6):e20194018. doi:10.1542/peds.2019-4018

12. Ferrand A, Gorgos A, Ali N, Payot A. Resilience rather than medical factors: How parents predict quality of life of their sick newborn. *J Pediatr.* 2018;200:64–70.e5. doi:10.1016/j.jpeds.2018.05.025

13. Kuchemba-Hunter J. Compassion and community in perinatal palliative care: Understanding the necessity of the patient perspective through narrative illustration. *J Palliat Care.* 2019;34(3):160–163. doi:10.1177/0825859719827020

14. Redlinger-Grosse K, Bernhardt BA, Berg K, Muenke M, Biesecker BB. The decision to continue: The experiences and needs of parents who receive a prenatal diagnosis of holoprosencephaly. *Am J Med Genet.* 2002;112(4):369–378. doi:10.1002/ajmg.10657

15. Chenni N, Lacroze V, Pouet C, et al. Fetal heart disease and interruption of pregnancy: Factors influencing the parental decision-making process. *Prenat Diagn.* 2012;32(2):168–172. doi:10.1002/pd.2923

16. Fortney CA, Baughcum AE, Moscato EL, Winning AM, Keim MC, Gerhardt CA. Bereaved parents' perceptions of infant suffering in the NICU. *J Pain Symptom Manage.* 2020;59(5):1001–1008. doi:10.1016/j.jpainsymman.2019.12.007

17. Schechtman KB, Gray DL, Baty JD, Rothman SM. Decision-making for termination of pregnancies with fetal anomalies: Analysis of 53,000 pregnancies. *Obstet Gynecol.* 2002;99(2):216–222. doi:10.1016/s0029-7844(01)01673-8

18. Michalik A, Preis K. Demographic factors determining termination of pregnancy following the detection of lethal fetal malignancy. *J Matern Fetal Neonatal Med.* 2014;27(13):1301–1304. doi:10.3109/14767058.2013.856411

19. Lantos JD. Ethical problems in decision-making in the neonatal ICU. *N Engl J Med.* 2018;379(19):1851–1860. doi:10.1056/NEJMra1801063

20. Côté-Arsenault D, Denney-Koelsch E. "Have no regrets:" Parents' experiences and developmental tasks in pregnancy with a lethal fetal diagnosis. *Soc Sci Med.* 2016;154:100–109. doi:10.1016/j.socscimed.2016.02.033

21. Janvier A, Farlow B, Barrington KJ. Parental hopes, interventions, and survival of neonates with trisomy 13 and trisomy 18. *Am J Med Genet C Semin Med Genet.* 2016;172(3):279–287. doi:10.1002/ajmg.c.31526

22. O'Connell O, Meaney S, O'Donoghue K. Anencephaly; the maternal experience of continuing with the pregnancy: Incompatible with life but not with love. *Midwifery.* 2019;71:12–18. doi:10.1016/j.midw.2018.12.016

23. Hill DL, Miller VA, Hexem KR, et al. Problems and hopes perceived by mothers, fathers and physicians of children receiving palliative care. *Health Expect.* 2015;18(5):1052–1065. doi:10.1111/hex.12078

24. Janvier A, Farlow B, Barrington KJ, Bourque CJ, Brazg T, Wilfond B. Building trust and improving communication with parents of children with Trisomy 13 and 18: A mixed-methods study. *Palliat Med.* 2020;34(3):262–271. doi:10.1177/0269216319860662

25. Moore BS, Carter BS, Beaven B, House K, House J. Anticipation, accompaniment, and a good death in perinatal care. *Yale J Biol Med.* 2019;92(4):741–745.

26. Hill DL, Nathanson PG, Carroll KW, Schall TE, Miller VA, Feudtner C. Changes in parental hopes for seriously ill children. *Pediatrics.* 2018;141(4). doi:10.1542/peds.2017-3549

27. Warr DL. After the loss of an infant: Suppression of breast milk supply. *Neonatal Netw.* 2019;38(4):226–228. doi:10.1891/0730-0832.38.4.226

28. Chichester M, Wool C. The meaning of food and multicultural implications for perinatal palliative care. *Nurs Womens Health.* 2015;19(3):224–235. doi:10.1111/1751-486x.12204

29. Foster TL, Dietrich MS, Friedman DL, Gordon JE, Gilmer MJ. National survey of children's hospitals on legacy-making activities. *J Palliat Med.* 2012;15(5):573–578. doi:10.1089/jpm.2011.0447

30. Ramirez FD, Bogetz JF, Kufeld M, Yee LM. Professional bereavement photography in the setting of perinatal loss: A qualitative analysis. *Glob Pediatr Health.* 2019;6:2333794X19854941. doi:10.1177/2333794X19854941

31. Now I Lay Me Down to Sleep. Home page. 2021. https://www.nowilaymedowntosleep.org/

32. Garten L, von der Hude K, Strahleck T, Krones T. Extending the concept of advance care planning to the perinatal period. *Klin Padiatr.* 2020;232(5):249–256. doi:10.1055/a-1179-0530

33. Jonas DF, Bogetz JF. Identifying the deliberate prevention and intervention strategies of pediatric palliative care teams supporting providers during times of staff distress. *J Palliat Med.* 2016;19(6):679–683. doi:10.1089/jpm.2015.0425

34. Edlynn ES, Derrington S, Morgan H, Murray J, Ornelas B, Cucchiaro G. Developing a pediatric palliative care service in a large urban hospital: Challenges, lessons, and successes. *J Palliat Med.* 2013;16(4):342–348. doi:10.1089/jpm.2012.0187

35. Field MJ, Behrman RE, Institute of Medicine (US). Committee on Palliative and End-of-Life Care for Children and Their Families. *When Children Die: Improving Palliative and End-of-Life Care for Children and Their Families.* Washington, DC: National Academy Press; 2003. doi:10.17226/10390. https://pubmed.ncbi.nlm.nih.gov/25057608/

36. American Association of Colleges of Nursing. ELNEC Curricula. 2021. https://www.aacnnursing.org/ELNEC/About/ELNEC-Curricula

37. Hospice and Palliative Credentialing Center. Certified in perinatal loss care examination. 2021. https://advancingexpertcare.org/cplc/

38. Hospice & Palliative Credentialing Center. Certified hospice and palliative pediatric nurse examination. 2021. https://advancingexpertcare.org/chppn/

39. Centers for Disease Control and Prevention. Infant mortality 2018. September 20, 2020. https://www.cdc.gov/reproductivehealth/maternalinfanthealth/infantmortality.htm

40. Ely D, Driscoll A. Infant mortality in the United States, 2018: Data from the period linked birth/infant death file. *Nat Vital Stat Rep.* 2020;69(7):1–17. July 16, 2020. https://www.cdc.gov/nchs/data/nvsr/nvsr69/NVSR-69-7-508.pdf

41. Pierucci RL, Kirby RS, Leuthner SR. End-of-life care for neonates and infants: The experience and effects of a palliative care consultation service. *Pediatrics.* 2001;108(3):653–660. doi:10.1542/peds.108.3.653

42. Keele L, Keenan HT, Sheetz J, Bratton SL. Differences in characteristics of dying children who receive and do not receive palliative care. *Pediatrics.* 2013;132(1):72–78. doi:10.1542/peds.2013-0470

43. Niehaus JZ, Palmer MM, Slaven J, Hatton A, Scanlon C, Hill AB. Neonatal palliative care: Perception differences between providers. *J Perinatol.* 2020;40(12):1802–1808. doi:10.1038/s41372-020-0714-1

44. Meier DE, Beresford L. Consultation etiquette challenges palliative care to be on its best behavior. *J Palliat Med.* 2007;10(1):7–11. doi:10.1089/jpm.2006.9997

45. von Gunten CF, Weissman DE. Fast facts and concepts #266: Consultation etiquette in palliative care. Appleton, WI: Palliative Care Network of Wisconsin. 2015. https://www.mypcnow.org/wp-content/uploads/2019/03/FF-266-palliative-consultation-etiquette.-3rd-Ed.pdf

46. O'Brien JH, Root MC. Pediatric pain: Knowing the child before you. In: Ferrell B, Paice JA, eds. *Oxford Textbook of Palliative Nursing.* 5th ed. New York: Oxford University Press; 2019: 773–782.

47. Malas N, Brahmbhatt K, McDermott C, Smith A, Ortiz-Aguayo R, Turkel S. Pediatric delirium: Evaluation, management, and special considerations. *Curr Psychiatry Rep.* 2017;19(9):65. doi:10.1007/s11920-017-0817-3

48. Vandenplas Y, Alarcon P, Alliet P, et al. Algorithms for managing infant constipation, colic, regurgitation and cow's milk allergy in formula-fed infants. *Acta Paediatr.* 2015;104(5):449–457. doi:10.1111/apa.12962

49. Santucci G, ed. *Core Curriculum for the Pediatric Hospice & Palliative Nurse.* 2nd ed. Pittsburgh, PA: Hospice & Palliative Nurses Association; 2017.

50. Goksan S, Hartley C, Emery F, et al. fMRI reveals neural activity overlap between adult and infant pain. *Elife.* 2015;4. doi:10.7554/eLife.06356

51. Anand KJ, Hickey PR. Pain and its effects in the human neonate and fetus. *N Engl J Med.* 1987;317(21):1321–1329. doi:10.1056/nejm198711193172105

52. Perry M, Tan Z, Chen J, Weidig T, Xu W, Cong XS. Neonatal pain: Perceptions and current practice. *Crit Care Nurs Clin North Am.* 2018;30(4):549–561. doi:10.1016/j.cnc.2018.07.013

53. Herr K, Coyne PJ, Ely E, Gélinas C, Manworren RCB. Pain assessment in the patient unable to self-report: Clinical practice recommendations in support of the ASPMN 2019 Position Statement. *Pain Manag Nurs.* 2019;20(5):404–417. doi:10.1016/j.pmn.2019.07.00554

54. Hauer J, Houtrow AJ, Section on Hospice and Palliative Medicine, Council on Children with Disabilities. Pain assessment and treatment in children with significant impairment of the central nervous system. *Pediatrics.* 2017;139(6):e20171002. doi:10.1542/peds.2017-1002. PMID: 28562301.

55. Root MC. Care of the pediatric patient. In: Dahlin C, Moreines LT, Root MC, eds. *Core Curriculum for the Advanced Practice Hospice and Palliative Registered Nurse.* 3rd ed. Pittsburgh, PA: Hospice and Palliative Nurses Association; 2020: 131–158.

56. Carter BS, Brunkhorst J. Neonatal pain management. *Semin Perinatol.* 2017;41(2):111–116. doi:10.1053/j.semperi.2016.11.001

57. Parravicini E. Neonatal palliative care. *Curr Opin Pediatr.* 2017;29(2):135–140. doi:10.1097/mop.0000000000000464

58. Giordano V, Edobor J, Deindl P, et al. Pain and sedation scales for neonatal and pediatric patients in a preverbal stage of development: A systematic review. *JAMA Pediatr.* 2019. doi:10.1001/jamapediatrics.2019.3351

59. Hummel P, Lawlor-Klean P, Weiss MG. Validity and reliability of the N-PASS assessment tool with acute pain. *J Perinatol.* 2010;30(7):474–478. doi:10.1038/jp.2009.185

60. Pasero C. Pain assessment in patients who cannot self-report. In: Pasero C, McCaffery M, eds. *Pain Assessment and Pharmacologic Management.* St. Louis, MO: Elsevier/Mosby; 2011: 123–131.

61. Collins JC, Berde CB, Frost JA. Pain assessment and management. In: Wolfe J, Hinds PS, Sourkes BM, eds. *Textbook of Interdisciplinary Pediatric Palliative Care.* Philadelphia, PA: Elsevier/Saunders; 2011.

62. Malviya S, Voepel-Lewis T, Burke C, Merkel S, Tait AR. The revised FLACC observational pain tool: Improved reliability and validity for pain assessment in children with cognitive impairment. *Paediatr Anaesth.* 2006;16(3):258–265. doi:10.1111/j.1460-9592.2005.01773.x

63. Johnston C, Campbell-Yeo M, Fernandes A, Inglis D, Streiner D, Zee R. Skin-to-skin care for procedural pain in neonates. *Cochrane Database Syst Rev.* 2014 Jan 23;(1):CD008435. doi:10.1002/14651858.CD008435.pub2. Update in: Cochrane Database Syst Rev. 2017 Feb 16;2:CD008435. PMID: 24459000.

64. Catlin A, Carter B. Creation of a neonatal end-of-life palliative care protocol. *J Perinatol.* 2002;22(3):184–195. doi:10.1038/sj.jp.7210687

65. Hunt MON, Protus BM, Winters JP, Parker DC. *Pediatric Palliative Care Consultant: Guidelines for Effective Management of Symptoms.* Montgomery, AL: HospiScript; 2014.

66. Thigpen JC, Odle BL, Harirforoosh S. Opioids: A review of pharmacokinetics and pharmacodynamics in neonates, infants, and children. *Eur J Drug Metab Pharmacokinet.* 2019;44(5):591–609. doi:10.1007/s13318-019-00552-0

67. Fortney C, Campbell ML. Development and content validity of a respiratory distress observation scale-infant. *J Palliat Med.* 2020;23(6):838–841. doi:10.1089/jpm.2019.0212

68. Norris S, Minkowitz S, Scharbach K. Pediatric palliative care. *Prim Care.* 2019;46(3):461–473. doi:10.1016/j.pop.2019.05.010

69. Smith HA, Gangopadhyay M, Goben CM, et al. The preschool confusion assessment method for the ICU: Valid and reliable delirium monitoring for critically ill infants and children. *Crit Care Med.* 2016;44(3):592–600. doi:10.1097/CCM.0000000000001428

70. Schieveld JNM, Ista E, Knoester H, Molag ML. Pediatric delirium: A practical approach. In: Rey J, ed. *IACAPAP e-Textbook of Child and Adolescent Mental Health.* Geneva: International Association for Child and Adolescent Psychiatry and Allied Professions; 2015. https://iacapap.org/content/uploads/I.5-DELIRIUM-2015.pdf

71. DeWitt M, Tune L. Delirium. In: Arciniegas D, Yudofsky S, Hales R eds. *Textbook of Neuropsychiatry.* 6th ed. Washington, DC: American Psychiatric Press; 2018: 185–202.

72. Hancock HS, Pituch K, Uzark K, et al. A randomised trial of early palliative care for maternal stress in infants prenatally diagnosed with single-ventricle heart disease. *Cardiol Young.* 2018;28(4):561–570. doi:10.1017/s1047951117002761

73. Akard TF, Duffy M, Hord A, et al. Bereaved mothers' and fathers' perceptions of a legacy intervention for parents of infants in the NICU. *J Neonatal Perinatal Med.* 2018;11(1):21–28. doi:10.3233/npm-181732

74. Baughcum AE, Fortney CA, Winning AM, et al. Perspectives from bereaved parents on improving end of life care in the NICU. *Clin Pract Ped Psych.* 2017;5(4):392–403. doi:10.1037/cpp0000221

75. Youngblut JM, Brooten D, Del-Moral T, Cantwell GP, Totapally B, Yoo C. Black, White, and Hispanic children's health and function 2-13 months after sibling intensive care unit death. *J Pediatr.* 2019;210:184–193. doi:10.1016/j.jpeds.2019.03.017

76. Courageous Parents Network. Home page. 2021. https://courageousparentsnetwork.org/

77. Tawfik DS, Phibbs CS, Sexton JB, et al. Factors associated with provider burnout in the NICU. *Pediatrics.* 2017;139(5):e20164134. doi:10.1542/peds.2016-4134

78. Diekema DS, Botkin JR. Forgoing medically provided nutrition and hydration in children. *Pediatrics.* 2009;124(2):813–822. doi:10.1542/peds.2009-1299 Reaffirmed January 2014.

79. Hospice and Palliative Nurses Association. Position statement: Medically administered nutrition and hydration. Pittsburgh, PA: HPNA. 2020. https://advancingexpertcare.org/position-statements

80. Rapoport A, Shaheed J, Newman C, Rugg M, Steele R. Parental perceptions of forgoing artificial nutrition and hydration during end-of-life care. *Pediatrics.* 2013;131(5):861–869. doi:10.1542/peds.2012-1916

81. Hellmann J, Williams C, Ives-Baine L, Shah PS. Withdrawal of artificial nutrition and hydration in the neonatal intensive care unit: Parental perspectives. *Arch Dis Child Fetal Neonatal Ed.* 2013;98(1):F21–25. doi:10.1136/fetalneonatal-2012-301658

82. Shultz EL, Switala M, Winning AM, et al. Multiple perspectives of symptoms and suffering at end of life in the NICU. *Adv Neonatal Care.* 2017;17(3):175–183. doi:10.1097/anc.0000000000000385

83. Armentrout D, Cates LA. Informing parents about the actual or impending death of their infant in a newborn intensive care unit. *J Perinat Neonatal Nurs.* 2011;25(3):261–267. doi:10.1097/JPN.0b013e3182259943

84. Parravicini E, Lorenz JM. Neonatal outcomes of fetuses diagnosed with life-limiting conditions when individualized comfort measures are proposed. *J Perinatol.* 2014;34(6):483–487. doi:10.1038/jp.2014.40

85. Cortezzo DE, Sanders MR, Brownell EA, Moss K. End-of-life care in the neonatal intensive care unit: Experiences of staff and parents. *Am J Perinatol.* 2015;32(8):713–724. doi:10.1055/s-0034-1395475

28.

THE PEDIATRIC PALLIATIVE APRN IN THE CLINIC

Alice Bass and Vanessa Battista

KEY POINTS

- Pediatric palliative care (PPC) should exist in multiple care settings to provide continuity and support to children and adolescents and their families.

- Three main models exist for delivering PPC in the outpatient setting: consultative, co-management (embedded), and primary care (medical home).

- The pediatric palliative advanced practice registered nurse (PP APRN) plays a vital role in promoting, modeling, and providing PPC in the ambulatory setting in collaboration with other care teams.

- Specialty pediatric providers face unique challenges in the management of distressing symptoms for specific disease subsets as well as communication around goals of care and medical decision-making, particularly with advancing technology.

- Specialized PPC in outpatient clinic settings widens access to physical, psychosocial, and spiritual support for children suffering from serious illness and their families.

- Similar to inpatient programs, common barriers to ambulatory PPC include misperceptions about PPC only being appropriate at end of life, fears of "giving up" or abandonment, and discomfort around pediatric advance care planning or goals of care discussions.

CASE STUDY: PROGRESSIVE DECLINE IN A PEDIATRIC PATIENT

Meg was a 7-year-old girl who was diagnosed 18 months prior at an outside hospital with pre-B acute lymphoblastic leukemia. Six months following her initial diagnosis, Meg began to show signs of progressive encephalopathy and neurologic decline of unclear etiology. Her parents noticed behavioral changes that progressed to changes in speech and memory. Later, these progressed to difficulty swallowing and regression of fine motor skills. Repeat magnetic resonance imaging of the brain showed worsening global infarcts. Extensive infectious and diagnostic workup was negative or otherwise inconclusive.

In the following months, Meg continued to have worsening symptoms, and her family transitioned care to another institution in hopes of getting better answers about the cause of her symptoms. A referral was made by Meg's new oncologist to the pediatric palliative care (PPC) team to introduce services and follow-along for support, symptom management, and goals-of-care discussions. The pediatric palliative advanced practice registered nurse (PP APRN), Ted, discussed Meg who was concerned for overall very poor prognosis, specifically due to concern for evident neurological deterioration.

Ted met with Meg's mother during a routine oncology clinic appointment. He introduced with the concept of palliative care as an additional support for Meg and the family. He discussed how PPC helped with pain and symptom management and care coordination. The PPC team could assist with defining goals of care to ensure they matched the family's values and definition of a good quality of life. Meg's mother was receptive and easy to engage, processing initial events leading up to Meg's current clinical state. She described how the disease has impacted the family's grief because Meg was a little girl who loved to play with her older sister and enjoyed family dinners and travel. The mother openly processed feelings around all of the barriers that Meg was up against and discussed feelings about suffering and how "perhaps Meg would suffer less if she would die suddenly," rather than how they now found themselves in a situation where they must watch her slowly decline. Meg's mother was able to recognize the value of having discussions around advance care planning, and a plan was made to continue to follow Meg at future clinic appointments.

INTRODUCTION

Pediatric palliative care (PPC) is a unique holistic approach to caring for children and adolescents living with life-threatening illnesses and their families. PPC is aimed at improving quality of life. Because the needs of children and adolescents differ in some ways from those of adults receiving palliative care, the definition of PPC reflects these principles. (*Note*: For simplicity, the term "child" will be used to include both children and adolescents.) The World Health Organization (WHO) defines PPC as "the active total care of the child's body, mind, and spirit, and also involves giving support to the family."[1] It ideally begins at the time of diagnosis yet is appropriate at any stage in a serious illness based on children's needs and not their prognosis.[1,2] PPC includes the evaluation and alleviation of physical, psychological, social, and spiritual distress whether or not a child receives disease-directed treatment.[1,2] PPC requires an interdisciplinary approach, includes the use of community resources, and is designed to be provided in multiple settings including hospitals, tertiary care centers, community health centers, and children's homes.[2]

The National Consensus Project for Quality Palliative Care (NCP) *Clinical Practice Guidelines* state that palliative care principles and practices can be integrated into any healthcare setting and delivered by all interdisciplinary clinicians and specialists with the appropriate professional qualifications, education, training, and support required to deliver optimal patient- and family-centered care.[2] For children, PPC should be tailored to their developmental status and disease understanding, as well as parental or familiar preferences for care, which should be assessed at the initial visit and revisited continually throughout the trajectory of care.[2] The NCP *Clinical Practice Guidelines* support the delivery of palliative care in multiple settings including acute and long-term care hospitals and facilities, rehabilitation centers (which includes settings for children as well), clinic settings, inpatient hospice settings, homes, correctional facilities, and homeless shelters.[2] The focus of this chapter is on the unique aspects of delivering high-quality PPC in ambulatory clinic settings.

THE ROLE OF THE PPC APRN

The pediatric palliative advanced practice registered nurse (PP APRN) plays a vital role in promoting, modeling, and providing PPC for children facing acute or chronic life-threatening illness in the outpatient or clinic setting, working closely with trusted members of the primary team caring for the child or adolescent. The PP APRN conducts visits independently or together with other specialty providers, recommends and/or prescribes medications to promote comfort and quality of life, and communicates compassionately with families regarding prognosis, treatment decisions, and advance care planning (ACP).[3] These discussions are often difficult for not only families but also providers due to prognostic uncertainty, emotional or moral distress, lack of comfort, and lack of confidence or preparedness for having these discussions.[4] PP APRNs are trained in effective verbal and nonverbal communication strategies and prepared to utilize best practice communication tools to promote open and empathic communication between other providers and families.[5] Their understanding of children's views of illness and perceptions of death is a crucial concept for providing high-quality PPC. PP APRNs' knowledge not only directly impacts the children and families for whom they care, but also influences existing knowledge gaps or barriers through education about palliative care principles and skills for interdisciplinary colleagues. Involvement of specialized PPC providers has revealed improved communication and decision-making, which both enhances the care provided to families and reduces moral distress in healthcare providers.[6]

In addition to engaging in communication, the PP APRN actively manages distressing symptoms for children receiving PPC and supports families in navigating the complex path beginning at diagnosis, through treatment, amid shifts in goals of care, to end of life and beyond.[3] Support has different meanings for children and families in various stages of care. Therefore, the PP APRN is skilled in supporting the unique needs of children and families, each in their individual journeys. They develop and advocate for patient-centered

and family-focused goals and promoting family-defined quality of life.[2] An essential skill is the assessment, diagnoses, and management of burdensome physical and psychological symptoms to promote optimal comfort. In collaboration with families and interdisciplinary colleagues, PP APRNs provide decision-making support when families are faced with challenging choices. They facilitate communication between families and care teams, eliciting treatment goals and coordinating care across the scale.[3] Because children receiving PPC in the ambulatory setting may be hospitalized, the PP APRN serves as continuity for families and providers between ambulatory clinic and inpatient settings. Box 28.1 summarizes the role of the PP APRN in the ambulatory clinic setting.

THE NEED FOR PPC IN AMBULATORY SETTINGS

The American Academy of Pediatrics' Section on Hospice and Palliative Medicine advocates for PPC providers to work toward ensuring care that is high quality, readily accessible, and equitable across all settings.[7] Most PPC services occur within the inpatient setting, with only about 60% of these programs offering services in some type of ambulatory setting.[8] In concordance with the philosophy of palliative care, PPC delivery should traverse care settings to ensure support to families throughout the child's life span. This includes ambulatory clinics, in which children and families receive comprehensive care and longitudinal support through follow-up visits and crucial conversations. Outpatient teams specializing in pediatric oncology, cardiology, pulmonology, neonatology, genetics, neurology, and other specialties encounter children experiencing disease progression, with pain and other distressing symptoms, who need of specialized management. Lack of education and training is a consistent barrier to provision of high-quality PPC for children and families.[9,10] The PP APRN's presence in ambulatory clinics, in collaboration with primary teams, bridges these gaps to promote quality of life for children and their families. The ambulatory PP APRN in a clinical setting incorporates PPC principles to assess, diagnose, and manage symptoms; collaborate in defining children's and families' goals of care; and coordinate with interdisciplinary care teams and services to meet these unique needs holistically.

SPECIAL POPULATIONS

To determine which children may benefit most from PPC, *A Guide to the Development of Children's Palliative Care Services*, a 2009 sentinel report, is used to classify disease categories within broad definitions and classification.[11] The PP APRN is mindful of the unique characteristics of these disease classifications and specific clinic populations when approaching primary teams and families. The first category includes children or adolescents with a diagnosis or condition where cure is possible, but there is a risk for failure (e.g., cancer, congenital heart disease, or reversible organ failure).[11] The second category includes children with a near certain premature death, but for whom treatments exist to considerably prolong life and improve quality of life (e.g., cystic fibrosis or Duchenne muscular dystrophy).[11] It should be noted, however, that the landscape is changing dramatically for some of these diagnoses with the advent of technology and treatment since the report was published.[11] The third category is children with progressive disorders for which there is no cure or disease-directed therapy available.[11] Within this group, interventions are largely focused on management of sequelae rather than attempts to reverse or halt progression (e.g., Batten's disease or spinal muscular atrophy).[11] Diseases that once easily fell into this category are slowly shifting into the second category with new available therapies (including gene replacement therapy) aimed at slowing or halting disease

progression.[12] The fourth and final category involves children with neurological conditions whose underlying injuries are not expected to progress; however, their conditions result in significant medical complexities and leave them at very high risk for acute or unexpected life-threatening episodes (e.g., hypoxic ischemic encephalopathy or cerebral dysgenesis).[11,12] See Table 28.1 for a summary of illness categories that may warrant the need for PPC. Clinical acumen is vital, as is a working knowledge of the special challenges that clinicians and families may face when discussing goals of care within each disease category. Table 28.2 summarizes some specialty areas where PPC referrals may be beneficial in the ambulatory setting, as well as some of the common symptoms to consider.

CARDIOLOGY

A variety of cardiac anomalies inherently warrant the philosophy of PPC as part of disease management, including routine PPC involvement in the ambulatory setting. Single ventricle congenital heart defects (SVCHD) occur when a lower cardiac chamber or valve of the heart is underdeveloped or missing.[13] The highest risk of early mortality occurs within the first year of life, but risk remains present throughout the life span, with only 70% of children with SVCHD surviving to age 20 despite surgical palliation. It is recommended that PPC be introduced to these children and families early and routinely so that there is opportunity to establish a therapeutic relationship and provide continuity of support through the journey.[13] For SVCHD, children are followed closely in cardiology clinic settings during interstage periods and beyond, and there are opportunities for the PP APRN to provide symptom management, anticipatory grief support, and discussions around ACP.

Another area where PPC may be helpful in the ambulatory setting is for children with progressive heart failure and those being evaluated for heart transplantation. Centers for Medicare and Medicaid Services (CMS) and the Joint Commission (TJC) require inclusion of palliative care for those patients pursuing ventricular assist device (VAD) as

Table 28.1 SUMMARY OF ILLNESS CATEGORIES THAT TRIGGER PEDIATRIC PALLIATIVE CARE INVOLVEMENT

CATEGORY	DESCRIPTION	EXAMPLE DIAGNOSES/DISEASE CATEGORIES
1	Cure is possible, but there is significant risk of failure	Cancer
2	Premature death is expected, but treatments exist to considerably prolong life and increase quality of life	Cystic fibrosis, Duchenne muscular dystrophy
3	Progressive disorders without available disease directed therapy or cure with interventions largely focused on management of sequelae	Infantile Tay Sach's disease, Aicardi syndrome
4	Neurological conditions whose underlying injuries are not necessarily progressive but remain static. However, their conditions result in significant medical complexities and leave them at very high risk for acute or unexpected life-threatening episodes	Hypoxic ischemic encephalopathy, cerebral dysgenesis

From Chambers et al.[11]

POPULATION	SPECIAL CONSIDERATIONS IN ASSESSMENT

Cardiology	Symptom management
	  Anorexia/Cachexia
	  Cough
	  Dyspnea
	  Nausea/vomiting
	  Feeding intolerance due to gut ischemia
	  Fluid overload
	Pain management
	  Chronic
	  Procedural
	Decision-making support
	  Bridge therapies
	  Transplant
	Advance care planning

Complex care	Symptom management
	  Agitation
	  Dyspnea
	  Feeding intolerance
	  Musculoskeletal pain due to weakness and contractures
	  Neuroirritability
	Pain management
	  Neuropathic
	  Procedural
	  Visceral
	Advance care planning
	Anticipatory grief
	Decision-making support

Neurology	Symptom management
	  Agitation
	  Attention deficit/Hyperactivity
	  Anxiety
	  Constipation
	  Dyspnea/Respiratory failure
	  Musculoskeletal pain due to weakness and contractures
	  Neuroirritability
	  Weight gain or loss
	Pain management
	  Neuropathic
	  Procedural
	  Visceral
	Advance care planning
	Anticipatory grief
	Decision-making support

Oncology	Symptom management
	  Anorexia/Cachexia
	  Anxiety
	  Bone pain
	  Chemotherapy toxicity
	  Constipation
	  Depression
	  Dyspnea
	  Graft versus host disease (GVHD)
	Pain management
	  Neuropathic
	  Procedural
	  Visceral
	Advance care planning
	Decision-making support
	  Disease-specific
	  Treatment-/procedure-related

POPULATION	SPECIAL CONSIDERATIONS IN ASSESSMENT

Pulmonary	Symptom management
	  Anorexia/Cachexia
	  Cough
	  Dyspnea
	  Nausea/vomiting
	  Fluid overload
	  Morning headaches
	  Respiratory failure
	  Shortness of breath
	Pain management
	  Chronic
	  Procedural
	Advance care planning
	Decision-making support
	  Noninvasive positive pressure ventilation (NIPPV) (e.g., BiPAP, CPAP)
	  Tracheostomy and/or ventilation

destination therapy or bridge-to-transplant.[14] Some PPC programs have incorporated automatic "trigger" PPC consultation into their standard of care for transplant workup,[15,16] and, in many cases, evaluation occurs in the ambulatory setting. The PP APRN not only participates in meeting these children and families to assess their understanding of illness trajectory and elicit goals of care, but also provides continuity throughout their course regardless of outcome.

Management of children with cardiac conditions should always include assessment for ischemia and fluid overload issues, which are common and may negatively impact quality of life, as do anorexia, cachexia, cough, dyspnea, nausea, vomiting, and feeding intolerance (Table 28.2). Treatment plans should be approached in an interdisciplinary fashion, consistent with the family's goals of care, focused on alleviation of symptoms or addressing the underlying disease. Pharmacological management of many of these symptoms can be found in the tables of Appendix II.

COMPLEX CARE

Children cared for in the complex care setting strongly benefit from a team of providers who are well-versed in complex, chronic conditions, and these children often require a high degree of care coordination to ensure that care fragmentation is minimized. Communication is a priority as multiple specialties are often involved to address a variety of issues and body systems. A primary care provider specializing in complex healthcare may serve as the child's medical home and should include a multidisciplinary approach to care. The work of PPC is valuable in this arena and often overlaps with complex healthcare services as an adjunct to the coordinated family-centered care that already exists. The PPC assists with symptom management and ensures that families' goals and values are at the forefront of decision-making conversations around treatment options and quality of life.

The population of children often seen in this setting are those who have a condition secondary to static encephalopathy such as hypoxic ischemic injury or congenital brain dysgenesis. While their underlying condition may not be expected to worsen, they are extremely medically fragile and vulnerable to severe complications.[12] The PP APRN provides expertise in pain and symptom management, which commonly focuses on musculoskeletal pain due to weakness and contractures. Procedural, visceral, and neuropathic pain are also common in this population.[12] Challenges to treating symptoms in this population may be related to chronic underlying issues that often require long-standing pain management; assessment of pain and response to interventions is also more challenging due to a large portion of this population being nonverbal or neurologically impaired.[12] Other concerning symptoms involve respiratory issues such as dyspnea or airway obstruction, secretion management, seizures, temperature instability, and/or feeding intolerance.[12]

ONCOLOGY

Given that PPC was initially rooted in oncology, palliative care may be considered more routine in oncologic disease management, especially with certain diagnoses such as bone marrow transplant, certain brain tumors, and rhabdomyosarcoma. The role of the PP APRN in the ambulatory oncology setting is paramount to managing symptoms and navigating goals-of-care conversations during visits as well as longitudinally between visits. The PP APRN frequently partners with the oncology APRN or oncologist to provide maximal support to children and families. For more detailed information on providing PPC in oncology settings, see Chapter 29, "The Pediatric Palliative APRN in Oncology."

PERINATAL

Perinatal palliative care consultation occurs most often in the ambulatory setting, and special consideration should be paid to this population. The PP APRN helps expecting parents develop a palliative birth plan to convey their wishes for their child's birth and the care they want their child to receive. It is important to ensure that appropriate supports are in place for the expectant family, birthing parent, and fetus. Early integration of palliative care in the antenatal period can contribute to parental understanding of the disease trajectory, expected outcomes, care options, and associated benefits versus burdens. This ensures that APRNs caring for the birthing parent and fetal dyad best understand the goals, hopes, worries, and definitions of unique acceptable outcomes for each family.[17] Assessment of cultural and spiritual needs before birth may help clinicians and families better formulate a birth plan that meets families' goals in a manner that extends beyond the physical care of the newborn.[17] For more detailed information on providing PPC in perinatal populations, see Chapter 27, "The Pediatric Palliative APRN in Perinatal and Neonatal Care."

Optimal PPC spans the continuum of care settings and should include primary care, hospitals, and the community.[18] Pediatric primary care providers play an important role near end of life. More than 90% of children in the United States have a primary care provider, and thus they can be a key referral source in identifying PPC needs in children with serious illness.[19] Many primary palliative care needs can be met by primary care providers who have the right tools and knowledge to provide this approach to care. As defined in the NCP guidelines, primary palliative care is "Palliative care that is delivered by health care professionals who are not palliative care specialists, such as primary care clinicians; physicians who are disease-oriented specialists (such as oncologists and cardiologists); and nurses, social workers, pharmacists, chaplains, and others who care for this population but are not certified in palliative care."[2] The primary care provider often has built a foundation of trust, support, and guidance with a child and the family and thus often fosters an ideal space in which to incorporate PPC principles. Primary care providers are not only a source of continuity for a family, but also a space where bereft parents may return for the care of other children or for bereavement support.[20] With the growing demand for PPC and a shortage of specialty PPC providers, pediatric primary care providers can fill primary PPC needs that cannot always be met by specialty PPC providers.

The NCP *Clinical Practice Guidelines* describe how all providers should promote effective transitions of care between settings.[2] There is benefit to improving and maintaining lines of communication between PPC providers and pediatric primary care providers because children may rely on their primary care providers following a life-altering hospitalization or diagnosis; in practice, however, inpatient PPC communication with primary care providers is often lacking.[21] Recommendations exist to improve communication between PPC teams and primary care providers with the transmission of written PPC plans to primary care providers following hospitalizations.[21] When feasible, delivering PPC within the primary care setting can help to directly bridge communication gaps, identify outpatient needs, and provide greater continuity of PPC. Not only are follow-up primary care provider visits after inpatient PPC services appropriate, but primary care providers may place new referrals to PPC for children with more refractory symptoms or who require complex decision-making that calls upon the expertise of specialty providers such as the PP APRN.[20]

Evidence also suggests that primary care providers might not be as likely to discuss the changing landscape of children's medical needs with progression, have less experience in pediatric ACP (pACP) conversations, and may not be as knowledgeable about home-based palliative or hospice resources in the community compared to providers who deliver primary care across the life span.[19] Integration of PPC can serve to enhance the family's medical home as well as encourage and augment primary palliative care skills for the primary care provider.

CLINIC COMPONENTS

REFERRALS

Referrals to ambulatory PPC involve several organizational considerations, including who can make referrals, clinic space, workflow, availability of PPC providers, and specialty care or institutional psychosocial supports. If the PPC clinic is part of a hospital system, the PPC team may be subdivided into two teams: one that responds to inpatient referrals and another that responds to outpatient, ambulatory, or clinic referrals. Creating a referral base for ambulatory clinics requires time and effort on the part of the PPC team. The PP APRN develops relationships with referring providers by offering to provide primary PPC education to clinic providers and staff as well as participate in interdisciplinary clinic rounds. There should be collaboration between PPC teams and referring clinic teams to help identify children and families that would be served best by a PPC presence in the ambulatory setting.[22]

Referrals for ambulatory PPC may be requested for a number of reasons. Referring teams may seek PPC expertise related to decision-making, pain or symptom management, anticipatory grief support, and ACP, as well as information around community-based supports (i.e., home-based palliative programs or hospice). Thus, the first task is to determine the purpose or reason for the consult. It is imperative that communication occurs between the referring team and PPC team so that there is understanding of the focus of the visit based on the clinical situation and the options presented to the child/family,[22] especially if there are constraints on the time or physical space in which the visit can occur.

Another consideration for ambulatory PPC is the desired timeliness of the referral to meet both the children's and families' needs as well as those of the referring team. Common issues for palliative care prioritization of visit timeliness exist for children and adults alike.[22] For example, does the child need to be seen in clinic that very day, or is the preference to meet the family at their clinic visit next month? Does the child or family want a separate visit or one coordinated with a scheduled visit with the primary team? Would the PPC team need to arrange a time to meet the child and family independent of the referring team or set up a time to do telehealth? Last, it is important to ensure that the family is made aware by the primary referring team that a referral is being made to the PPC team and to understand how the referral is explained.

The introduction of palliative care services is often a delicate task because families may confuse the term with hospice or interpret involvement as abandonment on the part of the referring team.[22] Ensuring that families are aware that a referral to PPC is being made as well as the purpose of the visit is essential. This can be challenging if left to an appointment scheduler or a member of the primary team who may not fully understand the role of the PPC team. Members of the primary team must be taught to understand the role of the PPC and use appropriate language to describe it such as, "PPC cares for children with serious illness alongside the primary team as an additional layer of support to promote enhanced communication, symptom management, and decision-making."

ASSESSMENT

The PP APRN's physical assessment includes a thorough history and screening of symptoms using validated pediatric tools as well as assessing their impact on quality of life and function.[2] Symptoms commonly addressed in the PPC clinic visit include pain, nausea, vomiting, dyspnea, anxiety, mood, fatigue, delirium, agitation, anorexia, bowel issues, sleep, and feeding intolerance. Often, more than one issue may present itself, and the PP APRN addresses each issue using a combination of both pharmacological and nonpharmacological treatment options that best align with families' goals, values, and available resources.[23] Assessment should be performed in the child's and family's preferred language, using a qualified medical interpreter to promote effective communication.[2] While the parent's or caregiver's report of symptoms is extremely valuable, the child's report is the gold standard, when possible.[24] Using developmentally and age-appropriate language and techniques is important when assessing the child for symptoms of discomfort. To assess children with cognitive impairment, mental status changes, or developmental delay, the PP APRN should pay particular attention to physical signs and symptoms as well as caregiver reports.[24]

Palliative care assessment of children involves a thorough physical exam, but also a good understanding of the child's culture, language, faith, and psychosocial stressors (finances, transportation, etc.) so that the PP APRN can adequately identify potential barriers to treatment, care, and follow-up. When available, the APRN should collaborate with other members of the child's interdisciplinary team to support families as well to provide developmental and culturally competent care.[2] In pediatrics, the child's role in the family must be considered to best understand what and how information is relayed to the child.[2,23] Additionally, to adequately address goals of care of ACP, it is essential to elicit the child's understanding of their illness, their prognosis, and perception of death. The parents' decision-making framework and communication preferences are helpful to assess using value-based questions, such as asking parent "How do you define being a good parent?" or "How best do you receive information?" These types of questions provide insight into how best to support a family's goals of care and are generally welcomed by parents because they are role-affirming and can serve as a source of guidance.[23,25] As expected, goals and values may change over time, and thus assessment should be continued across the child's illness trajectory and in all care settings.

PEDIATRIC ADVANCE CARE PLANNING

pACP involves furthering discussions around plans of care and clarifying children's and families' long- and short-term goals and treatment preferences. pACP is recommended internationally not only to better inform practitioners but also, more importantly, to support families' abilities to anticipate challenging decisions, seek support, reduce unnecessary suffering, and promote feelings of control and peace of mind in difficult situations.[26] Barriers to initiating and continuing discussions include uncertain prognosis, provider difficulties in initiating discussions, lack of care coordination, concerns regarding parental burden, and challenges in identifying children's wishes.[27] As a result, many pACP conversations occur late, or even after an acute crisis. This is despite recommendations that effective pACP occurs in a timely and continuous manner, soon after diagnosis (based on family's readiness), after a change in care setting (e.g., discharge from hospital), or before acute admission to an ICU setting.[27]

Clinic settings serve as an optimal place in which to initiate or continue pACP discussions. The PP APRN is poised to facilitate communication around pACP, navigating thoughtful conversations around goals of care in a family-centered manner that incorporates both the children's views of illness and death (when appropriate) as well as the parents' values, hopes, and worries around suffering and quality of life. Tools such as the Pediatric Conversation Starter Kit, *Voicing My Choices*, *My Wishes*, and *Five Wishes* may assist the PPC APRN in discussing pACP with families because they may provide more concrete examples and questions that families may wish to consider around care planning.[28,29] Additionally, the PP APRN serves as an educator and collaborator, addressing barriers that exist in certain outpatient settings by promoting education in communication, palliative care skills, and knowledge of ACP[27] (see Chapter 32 for more information).

DEVELOPING A PLAN OF CARE

Effective palliative care requires careful thought about resources that are available to and needed by families. In addition to being part of the PP APRN's assessment, other social determinants of health (SDOH) such as health literacy, access to reliable transportation, insurance coverage, and availability of local resources and support help to determine the appropriate plan of care[2] (see Chapter 20, "Health Disparities in Palliative Care and Social Determinants of Health"). For example, if a pACP discussion is about preferred location of death, it would be important to know what home-based palliative care or hospices would be available to support the family at home because some programs may not be staffed to appropriately support pediatric patients. Similarly, some insurance plans do not cover home-based palliative care encounters nor provide concurrent care coverage (please see Chapters 26 and 30 for information on concurrent care) and so knowledge of community providers and insurance options must be obtained prior to the encounter if the plan involves discussion of home-based services.

Follow-up planning involves a good understanding of transportation barriers, and, when possible, visits should be coordinated with other appointments. This is particularly true if a child is medically complex and getting him or her out of the home requires overcoming multiple hurdles with regards to timing, symptoms, reliable means of transport, and caregiver assistance. There has been increasing use of virtual or telehealth services, and, when available and appropriate, these may be valuable in addressing disparities in access to services.[30] Thus, telehealth follow-up may be a wonderful option

in these cases as well to help both ease the burden on the child and family and allow for continuity of care.[30]

For the older pediatric population, the concept of assent is worth mentioning. Most children under 18 years of age do not have legal decision-making rights but may have the capacity to agree or object to a plan of care put forth by the treatment team and parents.[2] Children with complex or chronic illness often have a greater understanding than what one may assume based on age alone.[2] As such, the PP APRN should, when developmentally and culturally appropriate, make efforts to include the child in decision-making, taking assent or dissent into consideration when practicing family-centered care.[31]

RESPONSIBLE PRESCRIBING

Expertise in symptom management is an important skill in providing high-quality PPC to children and their families. PPC delivery in the ambulatory setting involves participating in the prevention and management of distressing symptoms mentioned previously in this chapter. However with this type of support comes a duty and responsibility to provide safe prescribing of medications that can pose a risk for misuse. The adolescent and young adult (AYA) population has been shown to be susceptible to use of prescription medications for nonmedical use, with peak risk at age 16 years.[32] The principles of safe prescribing and universal precautions in opioid prescribing apply to children (see Chapter 43, "Pain," for comprehensive management of pain syndromes, and Chapter 47, "Patients with Substance Use Disorder and Dual Diagnose," for further information).

OPIOID USE IN CHILDREN

The opioid crisis in the United States remains a significant problem, even in hospice and palliative care, and prescription drug abuse is a national issue worthy of careful thought and discussion for any healthcare provider.[33] While much of the controversy around opioids focuses on adults, the opioid epidemic facing children and adolescents should not go unnoticed. Opioid prescribing to children and adolescents has significantly increased in the past two decades, and, in 2016, 891,000 children in the United States between the ages of 12 and 17 reported nonmedical use of opioids. Adolescents who misuse opioids can be generally described as those who self-treat or use these medications for the sensation it provides.[34] Few pediatric studies exist that examine the risk of opioid abuse or diversion, and recommendations for management are lacking.[35] The PP APRN treating children in the ambulatory setting must maintain vigilance of potential risk factors for opioid misuse when determining an appropriate treatment course by implementing the guidelines from the US Centers for Disease Control and Prevention (CDC) on universal precautions for opioids and risk stratification for opioid prescribing. One PPC program documented the implementation of an "opioid bundle" to risk stratify all children for whom pain was managed in the ambulatory setting. This included a prescription drug monitoring report, urine drug screen (UDS), screening questionnaire for history of drug abuse or mental health disorders, and pill count.[35] Other institutions are adopting similar measures to promote safer prescribing practices both to increase awareness and promote more rapid intervention for those believed to be victims of misuse or diversion, in turn minimizing serious risks to both the individual as well as the prescribing clinician.

Responsible prescribing on the part of the PP APRN also involves taking into consideration other factors that may impact adherence to and thus efficacy of a treatment plan. One significant factor is cost. For example, a decision to transition a child from scheduled oxycodone to long-acting oxycodone for ease of administration and to provide a reasonably long-acting alternative may be appropriate for a child able to swallow pills, but if not covered by the family's insurance, the medication can be cost-prohibitive. This author experienced a parents' struggle with being asked by a pharmacy to pay $760 for a 30-day supply when ordered by their primary care provider. In this situation, this author advocated for transition to long-acting morphine for a fraction of the cost as covered by insurance.

CLINIC CARE MODELS

Providing ambulatory PPC often involves three clinical models: consultative, co-management (embedded), and primary care (a medical home in which PPC assumes the primary care role).[22] Please see Table 28.3 for examples of each of the three clinical models. In a consultative model, the PP APRN may perform a visit within the "host clinic" or referring/primary team's clinic, address the reason for consultation, and provide recommendations to the child and family or referring provider[22] who can choose to accept, decline, or modify them; medication management typically falls to the referrer.

Under the consultative model, the PPC service may not provide ongoing care, although sometimes an initial consult may lead to the identification of further needs necessitating follow-up care. In the co-management or embedded model, the most common ambulatory model of PPC delivery, PPC teams work closely with referring providers in shared clinic settings, co-managing children's care plans[22]; recommendations are provided and care is coordinated over longer periods of time. This model allows referring providers to focus on other aspects of care related to the child's underlying disease if goals remain curative or disease-directed, and families often appreciate the enhanced communication and collaboration that occurs between the PPC and primary team.[36]

The primary care or medical home model is one in which the PPC team cares for children in a setting independent of a referring provider or "host clinic"[22] operating under the medical home philosophy of care in which "a practice-based care team takes collective responsibility for the patient's ongoing care."[37] The PP APRN assumes a more direct role in the child's care, and in some instances, the PP APRN may assume the role of primary care provider when other resources are less available or when the family's goals shift toward less disease-modifying treatments and optimization of the child's health. This model is more time- and resource-intensive because it involves primary medication management, including writing prescriptions and refills and managing medication adjustments and side effects as well as providing off-hours coverage.[38]

OPPORTUNITIES AND CHALLENGES OF AMBULATORY PPC

The PP APRN faces a unique set of challenges when providing PPC in the ambulatory clinic setting. In addition to

Table 28.3 MODELS OF CLINIC-BASED PEDIATRIC PALLIATIVE CARE (PPC)

	EXAMPLES OF PPC MODELS IN THE CLINIC SETTING
Consultative (collaborative) model	The renal team consults the PPC team to consult on a 15-year-old adolescent with end-stage renal disease due to presence of potential delirium as he is picking repeatedly at his skin. The PP APRN evaluates the adolescent in the renal clinic and recommends haloperidol to the primary team. The PP APRN discusses the recommendation with the patient and family, at the primary team's request, but the nephrologist will prescribe the haloperidol and contact the PPC team if further advice is needed.
Co-management (embedded) model	The oncology team consults PPC team on a 4 year-old girl with neuroblastoma who is having some pain. The PP APRN meets meet the girl and her family in the oncology clinic. The APRN evaluates the child, does a pain assessment, and begins discussions on goals of care with the family. The PP APRN creates a pain regimen, discusses the recommendations for pain management with the family and the primary oncologist, and then writes the prescriptions. The APRN plans to see the patient again at her next visit, along with the primary oncologist.
Medical home model (primary care)	The PP APRN schedules a meeting with a 3-month-old with complex congenital heart disease and her parents in the PPC clinic. During the visit with the family, the PP APRN performs a comprehensive history and assessment, including a psychosocial and spiritual assessment. The APRN makes a plan for pain management and discusses signs and symptoms of fluid overload with the parents. The APRN begins to address goals of care with the parents and suggests a possible future referral to hospice. The APRN also suggests meeting with the PPC chaplain and child life specialist for sibling support at the infant's next visit. The PP APRN gives the parents the 24/7 on-call number for the PPC team and plans to follow-up with the family by phone in 2 days and to see them again in 2 weeks.

From Davies, Broglio.[22]

the general barriers to PPC, such as buy-in and misconception from providers, misperceptions about the role of PPC for children and families, and fears around the notion of "giving up,"[39,40] logistical challenges exist. Not all PPC programs have their own dedicated outpatient clinic space and often operate in embedded clinics, which involves coordination with a multitude of other specialty clinics in which to introduce services or deliver care.

While the advantage of embedding PPC within a "host clinic" is closer collaboration with the referring provider and more streamlined communication,[41] the PP APRN is often at the mercy of clinic workflow in terms of timing and space. A busy clinic may lead to unpredictable wait times or interfere with the ability to have longer discussions if an exam room needs to be turned over shortly after the host clinician's visit. Children and families may also be overwhelmed with seeing many providers in one day, and so it may be difficult to add on a visit with the PP APRN, thereby adding an additional 30 or 60 minutes to the total clinic time. In contrast, this may be an advantage for families if it prevents them from having to come to the hospital or clinic setting for an additional visit and spend more time at a healthcare facility. In the current landscape, if physical access is an issue, telehealth visits may also be another viable option for the APRN and other members of the PPC team to meet with children and families while they remain in the comfort of their own home[30] (see Chapter 17, "The Palliative APRN in Telehealth").

An additional "benefit versus burden" point regarding successful integration of ambulatory PPC is the issue of staffing. PPC programs are growing in both size and number in children's hospitals,[8,42] and PPC has become a new standard of practice in children's hospitals. The presence of PPC programs within an institution is now a key criterion in how hospitals nationwide are evaluated.[8] However, the need for PPC services appears to be growing incongruent to PPC teams' abilities to adequately staff consultations or referrals to meet

this demand, depending on widely variable staffing models. This remains an issue within the inpatient consultation realm and raises similar concerns in the ambulatory setting as teams without adequate interdisciplinary PPC staffing to meet inpatient demands find similar challenges to providing care. This can be a significant challenge for PP APRNs when there are only one or two of them working on a very busy PPC team covering inpatient, ambulatory, and home care settings simultaneously. Most pediatric care occurs outside of the hospital, and this charges PPC programs with the task of developing "robust services across all settings, including home-based care and clinic services"[8]

It is important to consider variations in timing for when palliative care may be introduced along a child's illness trajectory (Figure 28.1, Table 28.4). It is widely recommended that PPC ideally be introduced to families at the time of diagnosis, when cure may not be feasible.[43-45] Additionally, parents have reported that the preferred time for PPC discussions is around the time of diagnosis or when their child is medically stable.[46] However, introduction of PPC services often occurs later in the family's journey—during an acute life-threatening hospitalization or following news of disease progression or relapse. PPC involvement in the ambulatory setting may address this gap in preferred versus actual timing of PPC delivery, particularly for those children with disorders with slow or predictable progression who are not hospitalized frequently and have exacerbating symptoms that necessitate a series of outpatient visits with primary providers instead of acute presentations to an emergency department or inpatient admissions. Children with slowly progressive illnesses and their families may find themselves incrementally tackling non-urgent issue after non-urgent issue before realizing they are faced with a burden of care that seemed distant at the time of diagnosis. Additionally, children are often the most medically stable during routine ambulatory follow-up visits, which may also be the time when families are told about a new life-threatening

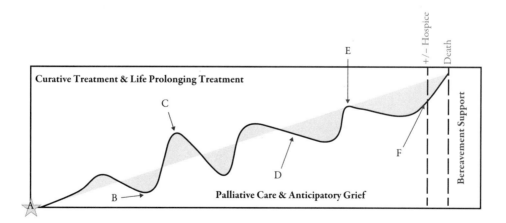

Figure 28.1 Potential healthcare events that may prompt introduction of pediatric palliative care (PPC) services (see Table 28.5 for the key to "The rollercoaster"). A general visualization of the extent of PPC involvement for a child diagnosed with a potentially life-limiting illness. PPC integration may occur at any time along a child's illness trajectory, with multiple cases that can occur in the inpatient, clinic, or home setting. Table 28.2 lists examples of PPC introduced along many points in a child's illness trajectory, from diagnosis to near end of life. Multiple opportunities exist along the continuum, in a variety of possible care settings, for the PP APRN to partner with primary providers in support of family goals and to enhance quality of life.

Table 28.4 KEY TO "THE ROLLERCOASTER"

EVENT KEY	SAMPLE DESCRIPTION OF EVENTS SURROUNDING INTRODUCTION OF PEDIATRIC PALLIATIVE CARE (PPC) SERVICES
A	At the time of diagnosis; the recommended ideal time to introduce PPC[43–45] even with curative options available and driving a family's journey. The PPC can initially play a small role getting to know the family and their unique values and goals.
B	Following a particularly challenging or unexpected acute episode/hospitalization to establish rapport and provide support around grief themes, goals; the child may be medically stable, but family could benefit from initial conversations around pediatric advance care planning (pACP).
C	In the midst of a period where symptom management is a priority alongside curative or life-prolonging interventions, where PPC may assist not only with goal setting but also pain or other signs of physical distress.
D	PPC is sometimes introduced during a prolonged hospitalization where it may be important to address goals of care/pACP, assist with symptoms, facilitate communication, or coordinate care to ensure medical decisions remain in line with family goals.
E	As curative or life-prolonging treatment options begin to fail, or the child endures repeated life-threatening events, there is a clinic visit with news of relapse or progression, or there is concern that future options may negatively impact quality of life, PPC may be introduced to discuss advance care planning around the "what ifs," including the family's critical illness treatment preferences.
F	Parents and family elect to redirect goals toward aggressive comfort measures or child begins showing signs of active decline despite interventions and PPC is introduced to facilitate goals, discuss possible home-based resources (including hospice), and involvement is heavy from the start.

diagnosis or given knowledge of disease progression. Thus, the clinic setting may provide an ideal environment for these conversations to start or continue and the opportunity for the PP APRN to be present, support the child and family, and provide resources as needed.

CASE STUDY: PROGRESSIVE DECLINE IN A PEDIATRIC PATIENT (CONTINUED)

In the 6 months that followed, the PP APRN followed Meg and her family at least monthly in various clinic settings, coordinating closely with her oncologist, neurologist, psychiatrist, complex care, and physical medicine provider. Ted advocated for the involvement of the institution's complex healthcare program and psychology to help optimize Meg's care and provide her mother with resources to promote comfort at home. The PPC social worker worked together with Ted to identify and coordinate a referral to a hospice team local to the family's home. The challenge was finding a program that honored Medicaid Concurrent Care benefits, in which Meg could receive comprehensive support at home and continue oral chemotherapy for her leukemia per the parents' goals. Goals of care were discussed over continued visits and ultimately resulted in her parents' agreement to complete an out-of-hospital do-not-resuscitate form in hopes of keeping comfort at the forefront of Meg's care. Meg's parents stated that if Meg declined to the point of imminent death, they wished her to be at home and surrounded by family.

As Meg's function and interactivity continued to decline, her mother grew concerned about increasing spasticity making diaper changes more difficult. Pain had increased, as had constipation and feeding intolerance. With each visit, Ted performed a thorough assessment and collaborated with multiple members of Meg's care team to implement the following symptom plan after various multiple medication trials and adjustments:

- Pain: Scheduled methadone and PRN oxycodone

- Spasticity: Clonazepam and Botox injections, scheduled Baclofen

- Constipation: Senna and polyethylene glycol

- Feeding intolerance: Intermittent venting, reduction of feeding rate

- Agitation: Quetiapine (scheduled and PRN), Clonidine (scheduled and PRN), clonazepam

While Meg's hospice was providing support in home two or three times a week, they were primarily an adult provider open to accepting occasional pediatric patients. Thus, Ted and the PPC team provided consultation, guidance, and support to the home hospice team at the mother's and hospice's request. Upon further discussion regarding goals of care, her parents recognized continued decline and sought to minimize suffering. Meg ultimately could no longer tolerate enteral feeds and grew increasingly agitated with any movement. At that time, her parents elected to forego further follow-up visits in clinic, discontinue feeds, and continue aggressive comfort measures. Meg ultimately died peacefully at home, in the arms of her mother with her father at her side. At the request of her parents, Ted coordinated with hospice and her institution's pathology department to help arrange the transport of Meg's body to the hospital's pathology department for autopsy and tissue donation. This honored Meg's legacy and their quest to continue to seek answers around the ultimate cause of her neurologically progressive disease.

SUMMARY

PPC in the ambulatory setting provides maximal support to children and adolescents and their families throughout the life span. The PP APRN is uniquely poised to offer pain and symptom management, decision-making support, ACP, and longitudinal support for children and their families, all principles that are the bedrock of high-quality PPC. Different models exist for the delivery of PPC in tertiary care settings, with the collaborative model being most common, where visits are conducted in shared clinic settings to promote close collaboration and communication between primary providers and the PP APRN. Successful presence of PPC in ambulatory settings requires a PP APRN who has expertise in outpatient care and the etiquette of consultation. Program development includes building referral sources, timing, staffing, and dosing of palliative care, all of which may differ from traditional inpatient models. Access to PPC within the pediatric clinic setting can extend longitudinal care and support for families navigating a complex health system, which not only reduces family stress but also improves family-centered care and quality of life for the child with life-limiting illness.[20]

REFERENCES

1. World Health Organization. Palliative care website. 2021. Available at https://www.who.int/health-topics/palliative-care
2. National Consensus Project for Quality Palliative Care. *Clinical Practice Guidelines for Quality Palliative Care.* 4th ed. Richmond, VA: National Hospice and Palliative Care Coalition; 2018. https://www.nationalcoalitionhpc.org/ncp/
3. Thaxton C. The role of the pediatric palliative advanced practice nurse. In: Dahlin C, Coyne P, Ferrell B, eds. *Advanced Practice Palliative Nursing.* New York: Oxford University Press; 2016: 545–550.
4. Battista V, Santucci G. Pediatric palliative care across the continuum. In: Dahlin C, Coyne P, Ferrell B, eds. *Advanced Practice Palliative Nursing.* New York: Oxford University Press; 2016: 551–562.
5. Akard TF, Hendricks-Ferguson VL, Gilmer MJ. Pediatric palliative care nursing. *Ann Palliat Med.* 2018, Feb 1;8(Suppl 1):S39–S48. doi:10.21037/apm.2018.06.01
6. Streuli JC, Widger K, Medeiros C, Zuniga-Villanueva G, Trenholm M. Impact of specialized pediatric palliative care programs on communication and decision-making. *Patient Educ Couns.* 2019;102(8):1404–1412. doi:10.1016/j.pec.2019.02.011
7. Section on Hospice and Palliative Medicine and Committee on Hospital Care. Pediatric palliative care and hospice care commitments, guidelines, and recommendations. *Pediatrics.* 2013;132(5):966–972. doi:10.1542/peds.2013-2731
8. Feudtner C, Womer J, Augustin R, et al. Pediatric palliative care programs in children's hospitals: A cross-sectional national survey. *Pediatrics.* 2013;132(6):1063–1070. doi:10.1542/peds.2013-1286
9. Khaneja S, Milrod B. Educational needs among pediatricians regarding caring for terminally ill children. *Arch Pediatr Adolesc Med.* 1998;152(9):909–914. doi:10.1001/archpedi.152.9.909
10. Davies B, Sehring SA, Partridge JC, et al. Barriers to palliative care for children: Perceptions of pediatric health care providers. *Pediatrics.* 2008;121(2):282–288. doi:10.1542/peds.2006-3153
11. Chambers L, Dodd W, McCulloch R, McNamara-Goodger K, Thompson A, Widdas DA, Johnson M. *A Guide to the Development of Children's Palliative Care Services.* Bristol: Association for Children's Palliative Care; 2009.
12. Siden H. Pediatric palliative care for children with progressive non-malignant diseases. *Children.* 2018;5(2):28. doi:10.3390/children502002
13. Davis JA, Bass A, Humphrey L, Texter K, Garee A. Early integration of palliative care in families of children with single ventricle congenital heart defects: A quality improvement project to enhance family support. *Pediatr Cardiol.* 2020;41(1):114–122. doi:10.1007/s00246-019-02231-y
14. Kavalieratos D, Gelfman LP, Tycon LE, et al. Palliative care in heart failure: Rationale, evidence, and future priorities. *J Am Coll Cardiol.* 2017;70(15):1919–1930. doi:10.1016/j.jacc.2017.08.036
15. Morell E, Moynihan K, Wolfe J, Blume ED. Palliative care and paediatric cardiology: Current evidence and future directions. *Lancet Child Adolesc Health.* 2019;3(7): 502–510. doi:10.1016/S2352-4642(19)30121-X
16. Tremonti N. Palliative Care and the heart transplant team: Offering perspectives and augmenting care. *Pediatrics.* 2018;142(1). 1 MeetingAbstract. 644. doi: 10.1542/peds.142.1_MeetingAbstract.644
17. Carter BS. Advance care planning: Outpatient antenatal palliative care consultation. *Arch Dis Child Fetal Neonatal Ed.* 2017;102(1):F3–F4. doi:10.1136/archdischild-2016-311669
18. Goldhagen J, Fafard M, Komatz K, Eason T, Livingood WC. Community-based pediatric palliative care for health related quality of life, hospital utilization and costs lessons learned from a pilot study [published correction appears in BMC Palliat Care. 2016;15(1):82]. *BMC Palliat Care.* 2016;15:73. doi:10.1186/s12904-016-0138-z
19. Lindley LC, Nageswaran S. Pediatric primary care involvement in end-of-life care for children. *Am J Hosp Palliat Care.* 2017;34(2):135–141. doi:10.1177/1049909115609589
20. Sreedhar SS, Kraft C, Friebert S. Primary palliative care: Skills for all clinicians. *Curr Probl Pediatr Adolesc Health Care.* 2020;50(6):100814. doi:10.1016/j.cppeds.2020.100814
21. Ernst KF, Humphrey L, Rossfeld Z. Improving pediatric palliative care communication with primary care providers: Development and implementation of a discharge letter writing system and palliative care plan. *Pediatrics.* 2019;144(2):2. Meeting Abstract 445. doi:10.1542/peds.144.2_MeetingAbstract.445
22. Davies PS, Broglio K. Palliative care nursing in the outpatient setting. In: Ferrell BR, Paice J. eds. *Oxford Textbook of Palliative Nursing.* 5th ed. New York: Oxford University Press, 2019: 639–651.
23. Root M. Care of the pediatric patient. In: Dahlin C, Tycon-Moreines L, Root M, eds *Core Curriculum for the Hospice and Palliative APRN,* 3rd ed. Pittsburgh, PA: Hospice and Palliative Nurses Association; 2021: 131–158.
24. City of Hope and American Association of Colleges of Nursing. End-of-Life Nursing Education Consortium (ELNEC). 2021. ELNEC-Pediatrics. https://www.aacnnursing.org/ELNEC/About/ELNEC-Curricula
25. Weaver MS, October T, Feudtner C, Hinds PS. "Good-parent beliefs": Research, concept, and clinical practice. *Pediatrics.* 2020;145(6):e20194018. doi:10.1542/peds.2019-4018
26. Lotz JD, Daxer M, Jox RJ, Borasio GD, Führer M. "Hope for the best, prepare for the worst": A qualitative interview study on

parents' needs and fears in pediatric advance care planning. *Palliat Med.* 2017;31(8):764–771. doi:10.1177/0269216316679913

27. Lotz JD, Jox RJ, Borasio GD, Führer M. Pediatric advance care planning from the perspective of health care professionals: A qualitative interview study. *Palliat Med.* 2015;29(3):212–222. doi:10.1177/0269216314552091

28. The Conversation Project. Helping People share their wishes for care through the end of life. Institute for Health Improvement. 2021. https://theconversationproject.org/

29. Five Wishes. Voicing My Choices. Aging with dignity. 2021. https://fivewishes.org/shop/order/product/voicing-my-choices

30. Winegard B, Miller EG, Slamon NB. Use of telehealth in pediatric palliative care. *Telemed J E Health.* 2017;23(11):938–940. doi:10.1089/tmj.2016.0251

31. National Hospice and Palliative Care Organization. *Standards of Practice for Pediatric Palliative Care: Professional Development and Resource Series.* Alexandria, VA: National Hospice and Palliative Care Organization; 2019. https://www.nhpco.org/wp-content/uploads/2019/07/Pediatric_Standards.pdf

32. Nationwide Children's. Pain Treatment Therapy Options. Opioid Safety. 2020. https://www.nationwidechildrens.org/specialties/comprehensive-pain-management-clinic/pain-treatment-therapy-options/opioid-safety

33. Gabbard J, Jordan A, Mitchell J, Corbett M, White P, Childers J. Dying on hospice in the midst of an opioid crisis: What should we do now? *Am J Hosp Palliat Care.* 2019;36(4):273–281. doi:10.1177/1049909118806664

34. Groenewald CB. Opioid prescribing patterns for pediatric patients in the USA. *Clin J Pain.* 2019;35(6):515. doi:10.1097/AJP.0000000000000707

35. Thienprayoon R, Porter K, Tate M, Ashby M, Meyer M. Risk stratification for opioid misuse in children, adolescents, and young adults: A quality improvement project. *Pediatrics.* 2017;139(1):e20160258. doi:10.1542/peds.2016-0258

36. Brock KE, Wolfe J, Ullrich C. From the child's word to clinical intervention: Novel, new, and innovative approaches to symptoms in pediatric palliative care. *Children.* 2018;5(4):45. doi:10.3390/children5040045

37. Medical Home Initiatives for Children with Special Needs Project Advisory Committee. American Academy of Pediatrics. The medical home. *Pediatrics.* 2002;110(1): 184–186.

38. Finlay E, Rabow MW, Buss MK. Filling the gap: Creating an outpatient palliative care program in your institution. *Am Soc Clin Oncol Educ Book.* 2018;38:111–121. doi:10.1200/EDBK_200775

39. J Friedrichsdorf S. Contemporary pediatric palliative care: Myths and barriers to integration into clinical care. *Curr Pediatr Rev.* 2017;13(1):8–12. doi:10.2174/1573396313666161116101518

40. Levine DR, Mandrell BN, Sykes A, et al. Patients' and parents' needs, attitudes, and perceptions about early palliative care integration in pediatric oncology. *JAMA Oncol.* 2017;3(9):1214–1220. doi:10.1001/jamaoncol.2017.0368

41. Brock KE, Snaman JM, Kaye EC, et al. Models of pediatric palliative oncology outpatient care: Benefits, challenges, and opportunities. *J Oncol Pract.* 2019;15(9):476–487. doi:10.1200/JOP.19.00100

42. Mahoney DP, Brook I, Fossa M, Kang T. Attempting to define clinical productivity metrics among pediatric palliative care services at academic children's hospitals. *J Palliat Med.* 2020;23(3):397–400. doi:10.1089/jpm.2019.0164

43. Weaver MS, Rosenberg AR, Tager J, Wichman CS, Wiener L. A summary of pediatric palliative care team structure and services as reported by centers caring for children with cancer. *J Palliat Med.* 2018;21(4):452–462. doi:10.1089/jpm.2017.0405\

44. Thompson LA, Knapp C, Madden V, Shenkman E. Pediatricians' perceptions of and preferred timing for pediatric palliative care. *Pediatrics.* 2009;123(5):e777–e782. doi:10.1542/peds.2008-2721

45. Hauer J. Pediatric palliative care. In: Poplack DG, ed. *UpToDate.* Waltham, MA: UpToDate; Last updated August 19, 2019. https://www.uptodate.com/contents/pediatric-palliative-care.

46. Kaplan N, Kowk C, Alenjandro RE, Berlin H. Rehabilitation of the child with brain and spinal cord cancer. In: Cristian A, ed. *Central Nervous System Cancer Rehabilitation.* Philadelphia, PA: Elsevier; 2019: 107–120.

29.

THE PEDIATRIC PALLIATIVE APRN IN ONCOLOGY

Amy Corey Haskamp and Joanne M. Greene

KEY POINTS

- Early integration of palliative care may mitigate suffering and fosters improved coping throughout the trajectory of the underlying disease.

- The pediatric palliative advanced practice registered nurse (PP APRN) must appreciate that children with a cancer or blood disease often suffer from a multitude of symptoms threatening the intactness and quality of life of the child and family.

- The pediatric palliative APRN can initiate therapies with curative intent concurrently with those that ease suffering and maximize quality of life.

- While the context of hope may change over time, it is an essential component of the well-being of the patient and family faced with a terminal illness.

CASE STUDY

A 13-year-old boy from Puerto Rico, Forest was diagnosed with high-risk pre-B cell acute lymphocytic leukemia. With treatment, he achieved remission and finished therapy approximately 2 years later. Due to his treatment, he developed painful avascular necrosis (AVN) of the right knee.

Prior to his 18th birthday, Forest relapsed and underwent additional chemotherapy. During therapy, he developed a disseminated candida infection and sepsis, and chemotherapy was stopped. Unfortunately, Forest had no access to palliative care services. His mother felt his treatment-related side effects had been poorly managed, resulting in physical and emotional suffering, decreased quality of life, and increased stress and anxiety for their family.

With mounting fears related to suffering and potential relapse, Forest's mother transferred him to another treatment facility. There, Forest was enrolled on a clinical trial and introduced to the pediatric palliative care (PPC) team. Goals of care were discussed, and Forest and his mother desired aggressive treatment therapies working toward a goal of cure. The pediatric palliative advanced practice registered nurse (PP APRN) addressed physical symptoms of painful AVN of the knee, mucositis, nausea, abdominal pain with appetite disturbance, diarrhea, sleep disturbance, and fatigue. A PPC plan was developed which addressed his social and cultural isolation related to relocation to a new city for treatment, anxiety and mood disturbance, and spiritual discord. Pharmacologic and nonpharmacologic interventions as well as integrative and complementary strategies were implemented. Although Forest was 18 years old, he felt ill-equipped to make his own treatment decisions, thus placing a heavy burden on his mother. His mother continued to direct all care decisions, with Forest agreeing or acquiescing to his mother's direction.

Forest received a chimeric antigen receptor T-cellular (CAR-T) infusion with several complications. Three months later, a bone marrow aspiration confirmed another relapse. The PP APRN facilitated many interdisciplinary team, staff, and family meetings to discuss Forest's care, including disease trajectory, goals of care, advance care planning (ACP), and ethical questions to ameliorate moral distress and compassion fatigue. Forest and his mother continued to request aggressive therapies which were non-beneficial nor effective. He suffered from neutropenic enterocolitis, respiratory failure requiring intubation, and sepsis. During this medically complex time, Forest and his mother maintained their desire to seek treatments with a curative intent despite a worsening prognosis. As a bridge to hemopoietic stem cell transplantation (HSCT), Forest received another CAR-T cell infusion. However, additional complications ensued including acute kidney injury (AKI) requiring continuous renal replacement therapy (CRRT), heart failure, and respiratory insufficiency which ultimately resolved. Forest then proceeded to HSCT, where he again required respiratory support. In the weeks leading up to his death, the PP APRN utilized tools such as *Voicing My Choices* to help with reframing goals of care and creating an end-of-life care plan to ensure a good death. Unfortunately, 2 months after his HSCT, Forest was compassionately extubated and died secondary to severe HSCT-related complications and multisystem organ failure with his family and staff at his bedside.

INTRODUCTION

The coordination of care between the primary pediatric oncology team and the pediatric palliative advanced practice registered nurse (PP APRN) is vital to the outcomes of patients and families. Pediatric oncology patients frequently report pain and other physical and psychological symptoms before, during, and after treatment for cancer. The PP APRN, with an interdisciplinary team, utilizes high-quality communication to assess and manage physical and psychological symptoms and facilitate discussions about goals of care and the end of life.

Cancer is much less common in children than in adults. Medical approaches to the management of pediatric cancer have made significant strides over the past decade. The overall incidence of pediatric cancer is 18.2 cases per 100,000 children in the United States and has increased by an average of 0.7% per year from 2000 to 2017.[1] While the 5-year survival rate for children and young adults 20 years old and younger with cancer improved from 58.8% in 1975 to 84.5% in 2012,[2] pediatric cancers remain the second leading cause of death in children aged 5–14 years.[3] There are approximately 375,000 survivors of childhood and adolescent cancer living in the United States.[4] In addition to those with a cancer diagnosis, the PP APRN can provide benefit to children with hematological disorders such as sickle cell disease, aplastic anemia, or hemophagocytic lymphohistiocytosis.

At diagnosis, patients frequently report cancer-related symptoms caused by the invasion or compression of vital structures of the body. Psychological or social distress may be caused by the uncertainty of the diagnosis, prognosis, or diagnostic testing. Cancer-directive therapies focused on a curative intent for highly aggressive cancers, hematopoietic stem cell transplantation, and chimeric antigen receptor T-cellular (CAR-T) therapy are often intensive in terms of time and high side-effect and symptom burden.

While many of the treatments for childhood cancers are administered with a curative intent, more than 12% of children with cancer will die from their illness.[4] Approximately 60% of childhood cancer survivors will experience late effects from their cancer diagnosis and treatment, including infertility, muscular deficiencies, neurocognitive impairments, organ dysfunction, and secondary malignancies.[5] A substantial effort is needed to minimize suffering experienced at the end of life. While survival rates have improved, each child and family faces prognostic uncertainty. The PP APRN can help children with cancer and their families cope with this uncertainty and the physical, psychological, social, and spiritual burdens of cancer and its treatment,[6] thereby increasing quality of life throughout the trajectory of the cancer journey.

EARLY INTEGRATION OF PALLIATIVE CARE

As delineated for all persons with serious illness, palliative care for children with cancer is most beneficial when implemented soon after diagnosis. The physical, psychological, social, spiritual, and/or cultural suffering associated with pediatric cancer begins at diagnosis and continues throughout the child's and family's cancer journey. Unfortunately, children with cancer are often referred to pediatric palliative care (PPC) late in their treatment or close to the time of the child's death.[7] Developing a relationship with the PP APRN at end of life, when physical and psychosocial suffering is acute, limits the benefits palliative care can provide children with cancer and their families.[8]

The American Society of Clinical Oncology (ASCO) recommends any patient with advanced cancer receive palliative care services at time of diagnosis along with active treatment.

Position statements from the American Academy of Pediatrics (AAP), the American Society of Pediatric Hematology/Oncology (ASPHO), and the International Society of Paediatric Oncology (ISPO) each advocate for early integration of pediatric palliative care services in the United States and internationally.[9,10] PPC expands the center of supportive care to include the child's parents, grandparents, siblings, and others who have been integral in the growth and development of the child. Palliative care can enhance pain and symptom management thus enriching a child's quality of life, lead to fewer emergency room visits and shorter hospitalizations, and, in some cases, improve survival outcomes.[11]

The benefits of PPC cannot be overemphasized because of the continual evolution of technology and medical advances to potentially prolong life in the pediatric population. Families without palliative care early in their treatment are less likely to have goals-of-care discussions, which may limit full participation in medical decision-making.[12] This results in a lack of opportunity to provide a detailed review of risks and benefits of proposed interventions which creates the foundation from which the patient/family can make informed shared decisions with the medical team. The PP APRN facilitates more opportunities for discussions related to the patient's and family's wishes surrounding end-of-life care, earlier documentation of advance directives, and fewer interventions at end of life as well as increased admissions to hospice.[6]

PP APRNs are in a unique position to coordinate care, help the child and family identify goals of care over time as the illness trajectory changes, facilitate difficult conversations, and support end-of-life care, death, and bereavement. Finally, there is a growing number of children who survive their cancer and require the expertise of a pediatric palliative team to manage late physical and psychosocial effects of cancer therapies.

INTRODUCING PALLIATIVE CARE INTO PEDIATRIC ONCOLOGY TREATMENT

Introducing palliative care as an integral part of the comprehensive management of children with cancer can be challenging. Families may have strong emotions related to palliative care based on past experiences with adult palliative care and hospice, including preconceived ideas about the implications of palliative care for their child. In addition, families may not fully understand the difference between palliative care and hospice and therefore focus on end-of-life care. It is important for the PP APRN to validate family concerns while articulating the mission of pediatric palliative and hospice care.

The importance of PPC services for children with life-threatening illnesses is supported by an abundance of research, but only 54% of pediatric oncology patients receive palliative care prior to their death.[13] Although the policy statements published by the AAP demonstrate advocacy for referral to palliative care, pediatric oncology providers may be influenced by their own feelings and thoughts about introducing palliative care to patients and families.[14] The rationale underlying the lack of referrals from primary oncology teams to palliative care is most likely multifactorial but may result from the provider's belief that they are providing sufficient supportive care or that a referral will not provide any additional benefit to the current care.[5] Reluctance on the part of the primary oncology provider to consult the palliative care team may also stem from a provider's concern that the family may feel that the oncology team is abandoning a curative approach to care or that the family may not be ready or open to including palliative care in their child's regime.[5,15] Despite recommendations and evidence of improved quality of life and increasing availability of services, a gap continues between knowledge and provider's practice of referral to PPC.[16]

Late referral of children with cancer to palliative care can increase suffering. In a cohort review at a pediatric cancer center, more than one-third of children who died during a 4-year time frame were treated on an experimental protocol, with half of those treated on a Phase I clinical trial.[17] In the same cohort, 51% of the children participating in clinical trials were admitted to the intensive care unit at least once during their treatment.[17] The nature of Phase I and even Phase II clinical trials does not include a curative or therapeutic intent.

Only children who have not achieved success from conventional treatment options are eligible for participation in a Phase I trial. These children often may have a heavy symptom burden prior to participation and are very likely to not survive their cancer. A palliative care consultation prior to enrolling on a Phase I trial can allow families to hold onto the hope that a trial drug will provide a therapeutic benefit while balancing discussions centered around the child's goals and how one wishes to spend time on meaningful and important activities.[18] Similarly, children undergoing hemopoietic stem cell transplantation (HSCT) often have exhausted all other treatment options. They may experience a variety of symptoms throughout their transplant and have a high rate of morbidity and mortality. The PP APRN can assist with treating the side effects of high-dose chemotherapy and/or radiation, symptoms caused by graft versus host disease, and psychosocial distress experienced by those receiving a HSCT.[5] These novel therapies can result in complex and multisystem side effects and associated suffering, as highlighted in the case study.

PP APRNs should initiate conversations with primary oncology teams to identify barriers to referring patients to a PPC service. Providing education on palliative care to primary provider services has shown to improve the incidence of referrals to PPC.[19] Identifying care objectives for management of treatment-related symptoms, the provision of quality care, excellent communication between families and providers, coordination of care between subspecialties, and family and provider shared decision-making will help to pave a pathway for increased referrals.

SETTINGS FOR PALLIATIVE CARE

Access to palliative care services should be available for children with cancer in all care settings. Identification of high-risk children and families without access to palliative care services is important to allow for the physical and psychosocial support necessary to maximize quality of life. Rural areas are less likely to have specialty palliative care services for children than are urban areas, resulting in physical barriers to care.[20] Evolving telemedicine can help to bridge palliative care service gaps but insufficient family financial resources required for computers and smartphones may continue to create barriers. While the number of formal PPC programs has increased over the past decade, a deficit of available programs exists.[21] There is an insufficient number of healthcare providers who have the formal training and knowledge or experience necessary to practice palliative care.[21] Adult home health and hospice teams often provide services to pediatric and adolescent and young adult patients/families but may not have the education and training specific to addressing the needs of these unique populations. Family-specific elements, such as limited financial resources, educational level, race, or culture can influence the circumstances surrounding the family's ability to obtain PPC services.[20]

PP APRNs can create opportunities for providing PPC in settings that best suits the family's individual needs. Generally, the preponderance of cancer care for children is managed in the outpatient setting.[22] Outpatient palliative care increases opportunities to address distressing symptoms, implement psychosocial interventions, and initiate ACP discussions while the child is generally less acutely ill.[22] Pediatric inpatient clinical areas continue to be the place in which most PPC programs reside. Children with cancer admitted to the hospital may have complex symptom burdens, higher acuity, and worsening prognosis or progress toward end of life or be experiencing intense family stress requiring multiple medical decisions.[23] The inpatient setting facilitates close collaboration with the primary oncology team and consulting services like child psychology, social work, child life, spiritual care, and integrative medicine. Inpatient PP APRNs can communicate with hospice to ease the transition to home hospice. Pediatric hospice provides all aspects of PPC in the home setting. Although there are limited data specific to where children and their families prefer to die, it appears that those with childhood cancer prefer to die at home, making hospice a vital setting for PPC.[24]

SYMPTOM MANAGEMENT

Symptom management may be challenging in childhood cancer. A multitude of symptoms have been described in the literature by those undergoing treatment for cancer, childhood cancer survivors, and those at the end of life.[25-28] Successful management of symptoms helps to build trust with the child and family and restores quality of life.[27]

CONSTIPATION

Acute constipation has been identified in as many as 57% of children in active treatment for cancer.[28] Constipation in this population is defined as absence of a bowel movement in a 48-hour period.[28] Most common risk factors include inactivity, dehydration, electrolyte imbalance (e.g., hypercalcemia, hypo-kalemia), bowel compression caused by an abdominal tumor, spinal cord compression, and medications (e.g., opioids, neu-rotoxic chemotherapy agents such as vincristine). Receiving vincristine and/or opioids has been shown to be a significant risk factor due to decreased intestinal motility.[28] Patients with a preexisting history of constipation are at increased risk for developing constipation during treatment. Constipation may impact quality of life due to its physical impact (pain, abdom-inal distension, nausea and vomiting, decreased appetite) as well as the psychological impact caused from the embarrass-ment or social avoidance[28] (for more detail, see Chapter 40, "Bowel Symptoms").

Since older children and adolescents are often embar-rassed when talking about bowel habits, these symptoms may be underreported. Therefore, the PP APRN must assess for risk factors critical to constipation. The APRN should speak honestly with the child about the distress caused by constipa-tion and develop a treatment plan. Some adolescents under-stand the medical management and can be responsible for self-monitoring and treatment without the embarrassment of discussing these issues with their parents. The PP APRN should assess the character and frequency of stools; duration of symptoms; presence of blood or intermittent watery diar-rhea; presence and character of bowel sounds; presence of abdominal, pelvic, or rectal pain; and presence of abdominal distention and palpable fecal masses.[28,29] A rectal assessment for hemorrhoids, fissures, tears, or fistulas may be warranted, but a digital exam should be performed only when necessary and with caution. An abdominal x-ray may be warranted to assess the presence of stool in the bowel.

Prevention and prompt treatment are important to con-stipation management.[28] The PP APRN should provide edu-cation on prevention, including diet, hydration, and activity. Education to prevent constipation should include the impor-tance of a high-fiber diet, which includes fruits, vegetables, grains, and non-dairy fluids. Ensuring privacy for bowel elimination and encouraging increased mobility are other nonpharmacologic strategies. If the child has difficulty with mobility, it may be important to obtain a bedside commode or bedpan. Passive range-of-motion exercises and frequent changing of body position to aid in gastric motility are impor-tant for the inactive child.

Prophylactic medications should be initiated when appro-priate, with a goal of one soft stool every other day.[29] Unlike other side effects of opioids, opioid-induced constipation does not subside with ongoing use. Therefore, patients being pre-scribed opioids should be prescribed both a stool softener and stimulant to prevent constipation. Stool softeners alone have limited efficacy but have been shown to minimize pain associ-ated with hard stools.[29] Initiating senna has been identified as an effective prophylactic agent in children with cancer.[29] Stool softeners such as polyethylene glycol can be very effective. Softeners are more effective when the child is well-hydrated, so increased fluid intake should be encouraged. If softeners and laxatives are ineffective at treating constipation, other agents, such as lactulose, glycerin suppositories, or enemas, may be required[28,29] (see Appendix II, Table II.3). Consider

the risks before using suppositories or enemas in patients with pancytopenia. Methylnaltrexone, a selective inhibitor of mu receptors located in the gastrointestinal tract, has been used in the management of opioid-induced constipation.[28–30]

NAUSEA AND VOMITING

Nausea and vomiting are often among the most distressing symptoms described by children undergoing cancer ther-apy. They have been reported to occur in 35–80% of these patients.[8,25,31] Nausea has been more commonly reported in those with multiday chemotherapy regimens and appears to be more prevalent in adolescents than in younger children.[32] Chemotherapy-induced nausea and vomiting (CINV) may occur in two phases: the acute phase, which occurs within the first 24 hours after chemotherapy is administered, and the delayed phase, which may linger for up to a week or more after administration is complete. Improved control of acute CINV has been associated with control of delayed CINV.[32] Prolonged nausea and vomiting may lead to the development of anticipatory nausea.

Nausea may occur with or without vomiting, but vomit-ing typically is associated with nausea. Many factors may con-tribute to the presence of nausea and vomiting: side effects of medications (e.g., antimicrobials, chemotherapy agents, and opioids), biliary or intestinal obstruction or tumor invasion, central nervous system tumors, decreased gastric motility, constipation, metabolic disturbances (e.g., hypercalcemia, hyponatremia, and adrenocortical insufficiency), primary renal or hepatic failure, abdominal irradiation, and increased intracranial pressure (for more detail, see Chapter 42, "Nausea and Vomiting").

Nausea and vomiting may result in fatigue, dehydration, electrolyte imbalances, pain, anorexia, and decreased quality of life. Children find it difficult to attend school and perform schoolwork when nauseated. Nausea and vomiting have a negative impact on both the physical and psychological well-being of the child.[28]

The PP APRN should assess for risk factors, triggers, frequency and duration, character of bowel sounds, pal-pable masses, hydration status, and associated neurological sequelae (e.g., headache, ataxia, or changes in consciousness). Electrolytes and kidney and liver function should be monitored, and abdominal radiography may be needed.[33] Treatment is aimed at removing triggers, if possible; alleviat-ing symptoms; and relieving the psychological distress caused by nausea and vomiting. Management should include both a nonpharmacologic and pharmacologic approach. Parents should encourage small, frequent meals selected by the child, avoiding fatty or greasy foods. Oral care after meals and eme-sis is also recommended. It is important to eliminate strong smells or those that are unpleasant to the child to eliminate any environmental triggers. Anxiety can often provoke or potenti-ate nausea. Relaxation exercises, guided imagery, distraction, acupressure, and acupuncture are integrative approaches to reduce nausea and vomiting.[28,34] In severe nausea and vomit-ing due to gastroparesis, the placement of a nasogastric tube can be helpful.

Choosing the appropriate pharmacologic prophylactic management for the management of CINV is critical. 5-HT$_3$-receptor antagonists (ondansetron and granisetron) have been shown to be appropriate for the treatment of CINV.[28,32–34] Given concomitantly with an NK$_1$-receptor antagonist (aprepitant), they have been shown to be highly effective in managing acute CINV.[32,34] If indicated, adding dexamethasone to this combination has shown greater efficacy than if these agents are used alone.[28,32,34,35] Adding olanzapine to the standard antiemetic regimen of those patients who have experienced poor CINV control during previous cycles has been shown to help children achieve better nausea control.[34,36] Scopolamine, an ACh$_m$-receptor antagonist, can be applied as a transdermal patch and is useful when children are too nauseated to take oral medications and obtaining line access is difficult. Benzodiazepines or alprazolam can be beneficial for those with anticipatory nausea.[34] If gastric irritation is suspected, an H$_2$ blocker or proton pump inhibitor would be warranted.[33] Cannabinoid receptor agonists (dronabinol) may be considered for refractory CINV.[33,35,37] Families may also seek the use of medical cannabis for relief of CINV. While medical cannabis may be a potential treatment, it remains controversial due to its side effects and lack of evidence on a suggested route, schedule, or dose for maximal efficacy and safety.[33,35] Access to medical cannabis depends on the location of the patient and legality within the patient's state of residence. (See Appendix II, Table II.5 for pharmacologic management of nausea and vomiting.)

ANOREXIA AND CACHEXIA

Anorexia is a decreased appetite and decreased consumption of food. *Cachexia* is the involuntary loss of more than 10% of a patient's weight, or muscle wasting, whereby the body breaks down skeletal and adipose tissue (see Chapter 39, "Anorexia and Cachexia").

These conditions generally lead to weakness and fatigue, decreased resistance to infections, shortened survival, body image changes in older children and adolescents, and psychological distress for patients and families, and they significantly impact a child's quality of life.[28,38] Loss of appetite has been shown to occur in 50–75% of patients undergoing cancer treatment[8,25,28] and nearly 100% of children dying of cancer.[28]

Physical factors that contribute to anorexia are uncontrolled pain or other symptoms and feeding or swallowing problems like mucositis, nausea and vomiting, constipation, delayed gastric emptying, and changes in taste. Psychological factors include depression and anxiety.[39] Researchers believe that inflammation plays a role in cachexia. Inflammation is a result of the body's immune response to the tumor, resulting in cytokine production. Cytokines can aid in killing tumor cells, but they also increase the body's metabolism, resulting in a breakdown of muscle and fat.[28,39]

The PP APRN should assess the pattern and timing of weight loss, daily caloric intake, changes in taste or smell, and presence of dysphagia, mucositis, nausea, constipation, or pain.[39] Laboratory tests to assess for nutritional depletion may prove beneficial. Serum albumin decreases as nutritional status declines and has a half-life of 20 days, therefore is less affected by daily intake.[39] Assessing prognosis and goals of care is necessary to develop a care plan.

Treatment should be aimed at reversing contributing factors while focusing on the patient's comfort and minimizing distress caused by the anorexia and weight loss. Due to the multifactorial components that lead to anorexia and cachexia, its management may combine a variety of approaches, including treating secondary causes of anorexia, nutritional support, enteral or parenteral nutrition, pharmacological management, and psychosocial support.[39] Treating secondary causes of anorexia or weight loss include management of those potentially correctible contributing factors such as pain, nausea, fatigue, or depression. Nutritional support includes encouraging small, frequent meals of high-calorie foods and fluids, with as much choice as possible to maximize caloric intake and limit the focus on eating. The choice of when and what to eat allows the child some amount of control. Consulting a dietician may aid in providing education and recommendations for appropriate supplements. If required, enteral nutrition is favored over parenteral nutrition due to the side effects (e.g., infection, thrombosis, and electrolyte abnormalities) of parenteral nutrition, despite the need for placement of a nasogastric or gastrostomy tube. Enteral nutrition allows for continued stimulation of the intestine, making the transition to oral feedings much more tolerable. Many pediatric cancer patients have central venous access during the last phase of their life, and parents may wish to utilize this to provide their child with parenteral nutrition. However, given the associated risks, the APRN must provide education, and parenteral nutrition should be carefully considered in light of the patient and family's goals.[28,39] Research findings on appetite stimulants is varied, showing some improvement in anorexia, but only minimal weight gain, no improvement in muscle mass or quality of life, and side effects.[28,39,40]

Megestrol acetate improves appetite but appears to increase weight by increased adipose tissue rather than skeletal muscle.[40] Glucocorticoids also increase appetite but should be used judiciously due to side effects. Cannabinoids, such as dronabinol, are approved for appetite stimulation but lack consistent evidence on effectiveness in pediatric patients.[28] Dronabinol has shown an increase in appetite without weight gain.[39,40] Medical cannabis or CBD oil is not recommended for cancer-related anorexia/cachexia given the lack of evidence supporting its use and potentially distressing side effects; in addition, it is not legally or financially available for all patients.[28,40] See Appendix II, Table II.7 for pharmacological management of anorexia.

In terminal cancer, the metabolic demands of the tumor may exceed any nutritional supplements provided. As previously stated, these interventions have generally shown no improvement in weight gain, length of survival, or quality of life and may lead to increased suffering and decreased quality of life.[28,39,40] Electing to forgo nutritional support is a difficult decision for many families because offering food is generally associated with comfort and plays a significant role in a family's culture. Therefore, the choice to withhold nutrition creates many personal and ethical dilemmas for families.

FATIGUE

Cancer-related fatigue is a subjective, distressing side effect of cancer or its treatments. The physical, emotional, or cognitive tiredness or exhaustion is not proportional to the patient's activity level and interferes with daily function and quality of life.[28] Fatigue is one of the most commonly reported symptoms in children with cancer and is reported in 50% of those undergoing cancer treatments, at end-of-life, and in childhood cancer survivors.[25,28,41]

There are multiple etiologies of cancer-related fatigue. It may be due to the cancer itself, treatments, or emotional factors. Cancer therapies have been identified as the primary cause, but other factors, such as pain, anemia, sleep/wake disturbances, metabolic abnormalities, nutritional deficiencies, emotional distress, reduced activity, deconditioning, and side effects of medications, may contribute (see Chapter 41, "Fatigue").

Physical and psychological factors may develop. The child may be too tired to eat, leading to anorexia. For adolescents, fatigue may lead to a lack of desire to attend school or interact socially with friends, leading to social isolation and depression. Adolescents may also find it difficult to perform age-appropriate tasks due to fatigue, leading to an increased dependence on others and further decreasing their quality of life.[28]

Fatigue's multifactorial etiology necessitates a multidimensional approach to assessment. The PP APRN should ask if the child feels tired or lacks energy. Then the onset, duration, aggravating and alleviating factors, and its effect on the child's ability to go to school, play, or sleep should be assessed. Validated tools to evaluate fatigue are available, such as the Pediatric Quality of Life Inventory, the Childhood Fatigue Scale, and the Patient Fatigue Scale.[42] Objective assessment includes evaluating vital signs, muscle strength, the presence of anxiety or depression, and hemoglobin levels to assess for anemia.

An interdisciplinary approach to the management of fatigue is most effective. Medical management may include blood transfusions for the treatment of anemia and/or medications, such as psychostimulants, antidepressants, sleep agents, or other agents, to combat the cause of the fatigue (e.g., nausea and vomiting, poor nutrition). While little evidence exists for the use of psychostimulants in fatigue management for children, based on the results of adult oncology studies and its frequent use in children for behavioral management, methylphenidate is commonly used for management of fatigue in children with cancer.[42] Nursing interventions include minimizing sleep disturbances and developing a schedule and routine for each day. Child life specialists or psychotherapists can teach techniques for stress management, guided imagery, and other skills to promote relaxation or allow the child to discuss feelings associated with fatigue. Nutritionists can teach families proper nutrition to promote energy. Finally, physical and/or occupational therapy can implement a low-intensity exercise program and age-appropriate activities to minimize

boredom and social isolation. Increased physical activity may decrease the severity of cancer-related fatigue.[42] Encouraging good sleep hygiene is also important in managing sleep/wake disturbances. Appendix II, Table II.6 highlights pharmacological management for fatigue.

PAIN

Pain has been reported in nearly half of all children with cancer,[25,28,43] with nearly 75% of parents reporting pain in the first month of cancer therapy[8] and as many as 62% at the end of life.[25,28] Pain is one of the most frightening and anxiety-provoking components of cancer therapy. The presence of pain in children with cancer has been identified as a symptom associated with a decreased quality of life.[38,43] In those with sickle cell disease, one-third reported experiencing pain by the age of 1 year, two-thirds by the age of 2 years, and more than 90% by the age of 6 years, with up to one-third of patients reporting pain daily.[44]

Pain associated with cancer therapy (e.g., chemotherapy, radiation, medication, and/or surgery) was the most frequently reported source of pain for those undergoing cancer treatments.[43] Common causes of cancer therapy pain include surgical interventions and side effects of chemotherapy and radiation therapy (e.g., oral mucositis, peripheral neuropathy, skin burns, perirectal breakdown). Pain caused from medical procedures was the second most common source of pain (e.g., bone marrow aspiration/biopsy, lumbar punctures, venipuncture, dressing changes, injections). Vaso-occlusive crises are the most common cause of pain in children with sickle cell disease. Previous pain episodes as well as developmental, environmental, cultural, and psychosocial factors affect the pain experience (see Chapter 43, "Pain").

The child may report nociceptive and/or neuropathic pain and acute and/or chronic pain (Appendix II, Box II.2). Untreated pain can lead to a multitude of other complaints, such as depression, anxiety, sleep disturbance, fatigue, loss of appetite, increased pain sensitivity, limitation of social activities, and loss of trust in the healthcare team.[28,43] Likewise, many of these symptoms can exacerbate pain, and generally all symptoms must be treated to achieve successful management.

To properly assess pain, the PP APRN must acknowledge that pain is a subjective experience, and the pain experience is unique to each patient. A history of the child's pain is essential, along with its potential causes or sources. Pain may go underreported in children with cancer if they fear it indicates progression or return of the disease. The PP APRN should learn the language the child uses to report pain. A self-report represents the gold standard, but behavioral observational scales may be required for a nonverbal patient.[45] It is important to use a developmentally appropriate and evidence-based pain assessment tool. Education of parents and children should include how to use the appropriate pain scale to ensure consistent measurement of pain. Parents should also be taught to maintain a daily log of the child's pain, what treatment or intervention was provided, and the effects of that intervention. Parents' confidence in their ability to manage their child's pain has been shown to be associated with how much pain they perceived their child to have and whether they administered pain medications to their child.[43] Therefore, educating and empowering parents about their child's pain and available tools for pain management may improve a parent's confidence and thereby improve their child's overall pain and quality of life.[43]

Assessment of pain includes pain score, location, characteristics, intensity, quality, pattern, alleviating/aggravating factors, duration, and the impact of pain. Behavioral indicators of pain should be observed (restlessness or agitation, grimacing, guarding, or moaning). Vital sign changes are generally not seen in those with chronic pain or in children who have learned to cope with pain in other ways.

The primary goal of pain management is to eliminate or reduce pain with the fewest side effects possible to restore quality of life. Acute pain should be treated based on the two-step analgesic ladder approach recommended by the World Health Organization (WHO). See Chapter 43, "Pain," for more information, and Appendix II, Table 11.1 for pediatric dosing recommendations. Pediatric dosing of sustained-release medications can be difficult, particularly if the child cannot swallow pills. Available dosage forms of many long-acting opioids may not be appropriate for smaller children. Methadone is available in a liquid form; it can be easily titrated for pediatric dosing and provides long-acting pain relief.

A multimodal approach to managing cancer pain, including a combination of pharmacological, physical, and psychosocial strategies, is recommended for best outcomes.[43,46,47] Complementary nonpharmacologic methods can augment opioid administration (Appendix, II, Box II.1). Psychotherapists can introduce cognitive-behavioral therapy to teach the child ways to relax and to learn to think about something other than pain. Physical therapy can be helpful to show the patient ways to move that are less painful or even stretching techniques that reduce pain.

PSYCHOSOCIAL DISTRESS

The diagnosis and treatment associated with pediatric cancer results in substantial psychosocial distress for the child and family and impacts the quality of life of the child.[6,25,38,48–51] Psychological distress is defined by the National Comprehensive Cancer Network as a "multifactorial, unpleasant, emotional experience of a psychological (feelings, worries, thoughts, behavior), social and spiritual nature that may interfere with the ability to cope with cancer, its physical symptoms (and side effects) and treatment."[49] Although the majority of those psychologically affected during treatment will adjust over time, approximately 10–30% of cancer survivors or family members will have long-term severe psychological distress.[6,48,49,51] Parents or caregivers of children with cancer are at higher risk for developing posttraumatic stress symptoms than are the patients themselves—as many as 50% of caregivers.[6,51] Delayed introduction of routine psychosocial services has been linked to increased suffering.[6,48,49,51,52] *The Psychosocial Standards of Care Project for Childhood Cancer* (PSCPCC), published in 2015, standardized the delivery of psychosocial care of children with cancer and their

family members.[48,50] Early integration of routine psychosocial assessments by clinicians as well as an interdisciplinary palliative care team have been recommended to reduce immediate and long-term adverse psychosocial effects.[6,48,49,51,52]

Psychosocial distress in children during therapy may manifest as image issues, difficulty concentrating, worrying, sadness, nervousness, sleep disturbance, and irritability. It has been reported in 15–40% of those undergoing cancer treatments, occurring at similar rates at end of life.[25] Psychological distress has been reported higher in girls than boys and for those children with brain tumors.[25]

It is important for the PP APRN to ensure an early psychological screening and assessment using valid and reliable tools to identify and address individual and family strengths, resources, and challenges.[26,49,53] Screening should then occur at regular intervals throughout the cancer trajectory, particularly during significant treatment milestones.[49]

Implementing psychosocial interventions with those higher risk patients and families has shown to decrease depressive and anxiety symptoms in patients and have an impact on longer-term psychological outcomes.[5] Encouraging psychosocial support of the child, siblings, and caregivers can serve as a protective factor against negative psychosocial outcomes; however, these interventions should be tailored to the individual patient and family.[6] Hospital or online support groups or camps for children with cancer or their siblings may be beneficial to decrease the social isolation experienced by these patients.[6] Expressive therapies, such as art, play, music, dance, and pet, may be helpful for expressing feelings and reducing distress during cancer treatments.[49] Referral to pediatric psychology for further assessment and integration of cognitive-behavioral therapy and counseling may be beneficial.[6,49,51]

CARE OF ADOLESCENT AND YOUNG ADULTS

Adolescent and young adult (AYA) oncology as a subspecialty which developed from of the Adolescent and Young Adult Oncology Progress Review Group held in 2006.[54] There are approximately 70,000 individuals between the ages of 15 and 39 years diagnosed with cancer each year.[55] Eighty percent of those AYAs will achieve 10-year survival.[56] Psychosocial maturation and movement toward adulthood for the AYA is the developmental priority, compared to the focus of physical growth in the earlier childhood years. Emotional and financial independence, maturing body image, social connections outside the family, and work identity and future roles become paramount.[7] A cancer diagnosis can and often does negatively interfere with the AYA's maturation process and their ability to meet age-appropriate developmental milestones.[57] Coping with all the factors related to living with a life-threatening illness, AYAs with cancer are commonly affected by delayed or arrested emotional maturity, mood disorders, and priorities that conflict with oncology treatment plans.[58] AYAs commonly are not prepared for a life-changing diagnosis and may have inadequate or no health insurance. Individuals without adequate financial means to pay for healthcare are known to have increased disease- and treatment-related complications, worse survival outcomes, and higher mortality rates than populations with adequate access to care and medical insurance.[59] Even when AYAs have access to healthcare, adherence to oncology management plans is a significant concern in this age group.[60]

The AYA, family caregivers, and clinicians must be educated on the impact that cancer and associated therapies can have on the normal growth and development of AYAs. Early implementation of a comprehensive palliative care plan will help to mitigate challenges related to the AYA's age and developmental stage. Concerns commonly shared by this age group include worries about romantic relationships and social connections, symptom management, and late effects of treatment which may interfere with life goals after cure and well into survivorship.[61] For the AYA population, APRNs must be prepared to assess and manage distress surrounding finances, post high school vocational training or education, employment, fertility and family planning, and family disagreements about goals of care. Coordination of care involving complex treatment plans and multiple psychosocial services is the foundation of the supportive care plan for the AYA.

By meeting AYAs where they are developmentally, APRNs help to facilitate and support the their participation in their own medical decision-making. Engaging AYAs in conversations aimed at helping them shape a picture of quality of life is a vital palliative care intervention. Every AYA has their own level of cognitive understanding and emotional maturity, psychologic strengths and weakness, and thoughts about their own goals of care. Assessing and understanding those factors will allow the APRN to help AYAs communicate their wishes while advocating for themselves throughout the cancer journey.[62] "Facilitating an AYA's concept of living well may be an empowering intervention, which initiates information sharing between AYAs and clinicians, thereby supporting their engagement in care across a disease trajectory."[63]

GOALS OF CARE AND DECISION-MAKING

ACP is the process by which, through discussion, healthcare providers can begin to understand what an individual wants with respect to medical care in the future and at end of life (see Chapter 32, "Advance Care Planning"). As a part of ACP for children, shared decision-making and the development of goals of care build on some of the same principles used in adult practice although these are often viewed as much more difficult in pediatrics. Healthcare providers may be reluctant to initiate conversations with parents to discuss those medical interventions they may want for their child because the provider fears the conversation will be upsetting for the family and potentially undermine hope.[64] In a recent study, 56% of bereaved parents stated they wished they had developed an advance care plan prior to their child's death.[65]

The process of shared decision-making between pediatric patients, their families, and healthcare teams must be approached as a fluid process. Healthcare decisions and goal development in pediatric oncology are generally not concluded after one or two discussions. Instead these conversations happen along the care continuum. In addition, the roles that the child and families take in this process may change over time. A child's age, developmental level, acute or chronic issues, and understanding of their disease trajectory will impact how these conversations occur. Children at a variety of ages, including those possibly considered too young for decision-making, may be very involved in discussions about their care. Shared decision-making in pediatric oncology must be based on an assessment of each child's individual ability to understand and respond to information regardless of their chronologic age.[66]

A parent's will to care for their child, protect them from unfavorable outcomes, guilt related to their child's illness, and their desire to ensure their child has the opportunity to grow and experience life may impact decision-making and goal-setting.[66] The PP APRN must recognize and address parental fears and concerns; they must be respectful of the child or parent whose goals of care may differ from those of the medical team and facilitate movement toward mutual understanding and agreement. Understanding what the child and family truly comprehend about the illness, treatment options, risks, and benefits related to interventions and potential short- and long-term outcomes will facilitate the family's ability to make informed decisions. Helping the child and family clarify supportive and palliative interventions, set goals for the present, and consider options should the child's disease progress or bring them closer to end of life is vital to medical decision-making in pediatrics and is known as *parallel planning*.[67] With each situation, making sure the desired care is congruent with parent and child values and preferences is the most important outcome.[68]

REFRAMING GOALS OF CARE

Goals-of-care discussions are always a challenge when a child, adolescent, or young adult is the focus of the discussion. Goals of care may change many times during the cancer journey. At diagnosis, goals are often more cure-oriented, including the use of aggressive, life-sustaining therapies. At relapse, the focus may change to prolonging life and balancing the benefits of treatment against symptom distress. Goals for survivorship may include optimizing functionality, quality of life, and sense of well-being in all domains.

When it becomes evident that cure is no longer a possibility, helping the patient and family reframe their goals can be very difficult in that the family's mindset of ongoing treatment routines and potential cure is suddenly disrupted. Having a solid framework from which to initiate reframing a goals-of-care discussion helps to bring organization to a difficult conversation. REMAP (Reframe, Expect Emotion, Map out patient goals, Align with goals and Propose a plan) is a framework developed to help providers have conversations in which reframing of goals of care is necessary.[69] REMAP provides an organized process of sharing the changing or poor prognosis, responding to the emotions that the family will express, discussing family values, and supporting shared decision-making when creating plans for medical care going forward, and this ultimately results in better care at end of life.[69] Reframing of patient and family goals at end of life should be used as a time for focusing on the child and family and what unmet needs they wish to address and less about making the right medical decisions. It is important to recognize that grief and bereavement start before the child's death, and reframing goals to support that process should be the focus. Finally, viewing the process as a healing one may dampen the moral distress often seen in those caring for a dying child.[70]

ESSENTIAL ROLE OF HOPE

Hope is a very common emotion expressed by children and families in pediatric oncology. Hope is a valuable tool humans use as a protective factor directly impacting health and well-being.[71,72] Hope serves as a mechanism by which people are able to express and attain their goals and achieve positive outcomes, particularly during times of uncertainty or stress.[71] Hope can be an effective coping strategy and can provide the family a reason for placing one foot in front of the other and continuing with daily routines.

Hope has often been linked to an expectation of a favorable prognosis or cure.[71,73–75] Given this belief that hope is connected to a positive outcome, clinicians often perceive giving bad or difficult news about a child's cancer diagnosis as being in opposition to a family's hope or taking away hope.[73,74] The clinician may, therefore, find it difficult to give them full prognostic information. One example is relapsed or refractory cancer. Families may elect to take part in a Phase I study without understanding that these studies are designed to test the safety profile of a new agent with little known benefit. Clinicians may inadvertently intensify the family's hopes by overestimating the outcomes of the clinical trial. While the medical team is aware that the treatment may be of little benefit to the child, the family may elect to focus their discussions on the hope that the treatment will cure their child's cancer. Led by their own hopes for a cure, the survival of the child and a desire to support what they believe is the family's only hope, oncologists may sidestep disclosing the likely outcome of the trial to avoid further distress for the family. Yet parents are able to both hope for a cure and acknowledge realistic expectations for their child's future with an incurable cancer.[73–75] Parents reported other hopes centered on their child's well-being, such as an improved quality of life, minimal suffering, for the child to feel loved, and for better treatments of future children with cancer.[73,74] Open and honest dialogue regarding a child's prognosis has been shown to encourage patient and family autonomy and allow for personal choices for end-of-life care.[73]

Two categories of hope have been identified in parents of children with cancer: future-oriented hope and present-oriented hope.[74] *Future-oriented hope* involves hope for a cure and treatment success, hope for the child's future, hope for a miracle, and hope for more quality time with the child.

Present-oriented hope involves hope for each day and each moment, hope for no pain and suffering, and hope for no complications.[74] Many parents recognize that their hope for a cure may differ from their expectations of what is likely to occur.[73] However, if clinicians assume a family's only hope is for a cure and do not assess or identify the patient or family's more achievable, present-oriented hopes (i.e., minimize suffering, being home, improving quality of life), these may never be achieved. It is important for the PP APRN to assess the patient's and family's future-oriented hopes, their expectations, and "what else are you hoping for" to identify those more achievable hopes in order to develop an effective plan of care for the child.[73,74]

Hope expressed by families often vacillates over time depending on the presence of uncontrolled symptoms (i.e., pain, fatigue, dyspnea) and how the child is responding to therapy.[71,75] The presence of anxiety or depression also appears to have an effect on hope.[72] Children with clinical levels of anxiety and depressive symptoms have been shown to have significantly lower hope scores compared to those without clinical levels of anxiety and depressive symptoms.[72] Likewise, improvements in quality of life are associated with improvements in one's hope.[71] The PP APRN can enrich the family's hope by enhancing the child's quality of life by relieving suffering and optimizing function.

Patients and families will struggle if they have no hope or goals to work toward. Developing realistic goals can provide a sense of hope for something they can achieve. Families may need guidance with identifying realistic goals to provide for a new sense of hope when faced with a child with terminal cancer. Even though the plan of care may not involve a longer life, developing realistic goals can help children and families work on psychological healing and in achieving other milestones for closure. This produces more positive emotions in those with terminal illness and their families.

EMERGING THERAPIES

When a child has exhausted standard treatment options, the family may seek additional available therapies. In recent years, new and evolving biologic and immunotherapies have rapidly altered the landscape of cancer-directed therapy for children with advanced cancer.[76] Prior to these advances, when a child with cancer had not found success on an open Phase I clinical trial, few options for additional treatments were available.

However, currently, there are more potential therapies, generally without a curative intent. Occasionally these treatments may provide little symptom burden, can be done at home, and may meet the goals of the family to continue treatment for the child's cancer. Occasionally some of these therapies result in burdensome side effects, negatively impact the child's quality of life, and may require hospitalization or assessments away from their primary institution, their home state, and support systems.[76,77] In addition, healthcare payment models may not allow for concurrent care (i.e., cancer-directed therapy received simultaneously with hospice).[76] Besides ensuring the child's symptoms are properly addressed, delaying hospice enrollment may prevent the child from dying in their preferred location and also result in lack of preparation for the child's end of life.[78]

The PP APRN must ensure open, honest communication with the patient and family to explore hopes, worries, goals, and perspectives to assist in guiding the family through informed decision-making. Through this process, the PP APRN serves as an advocate for the patient and family, collaborating with the oncologist, local healthcare systems, and the patient's payer source to ensure sound treatment options that meet the child's and family's goals.[76]

SUMMARY

The diagnosis of cancer in a child is difficult for both families and medical teams. Recent advancements in pediatric cancer-directed therapies, particularly for advanced cancers, can pose additional interesting challenges for the APRN. Palliative care may relieve suffering and promote improved coping and a sense of hope for the family and healthcare teams. Assessment and management of symptoms and reevaluation of goals are paramount throughout the illness trajectory. Early integration of palliative care in this setting can allow relationships and trust to develop over time and can allow an improved understanding of the patient's and family's wishes. The PP APRN has an essential role in care of the child with cancer.

REFERENCES

1. US Department of Health and Human Services. National Cancer Institute. Surveillance, epidemiology, and end results (SEER) program. Recent trends in SEER age-adjusted incidence rates, 2000-2018. By sex, all races, ages < 20, observed rates. 2021. https://seer.cancer.gov/explorer/application.html?site=1&data_type=1&graph_type=2&compareBy=age_range&chk_age_range_15=15&rate_type=1&sex=1&race=1&hdn_stage=101&advopt_precision=1&advopt_show_ci=on&advopt_display=2

2. US Department of Health and Human Services. National Cancer Institute. Surveillance, epidemiology, and end results (SEER) program. 5-year relative survival rates, 2010-2016 all stages by age, both sexes, all races. 2021. https://seer.cancer.gov/explorer/application.html?site=1&data_type=4&graph_type=5&compareBy=sex&chk_sex_3=3&chk_sex_2=2&series=9&race=1&age_range=15&hdn_stage=101&advopt_precision=1#tableWrap.

3. Centers for Disease Control and Prevention. Child health: Leading causes of death children aged 5–14 years. Last Updated August 3, 2021. https://www.cdc.gov/nchs/fastats/child-health.htm.

4. Cure Search. Childhood cancer statistics. 2020. www.curesearch.org.

5. Spruit JL, Prince-Paul M. Palliative care services in pediatric oncology. *Ann Palliat Med.* 2019;8(Suppl 1):S49–S57. doi:10.21037/apm.2018.05.04

6. Snaman J, McCarthy S, Wiener L, Wolfe J. Pediatric palliative care in oncology. *J Clin Oncol.* 2020;38(9):954–963. doi:10.1200/JCO.18.02331

7. Hill DL, Walter JK, Casas JA, DiDomenico C, Szymczak JE, Feudtner C. The codesign of an interdisciplinary team-based intervention regarding initiating palliative care in pediatric oncology. *Support Care Cancer.* 2018;26(9):3249–3256. doi:10.1007/s00520-018-4190-5

8. Levine D, Mandrell B, Sykes A, et al. Patients' and parents' needs, attitudes, and perceptions about early palliative care integration in pediatric oncology. *JAMA Oncol.* 2017;3(9):1214–1220. doi:10.1001/jamaoncol.2017.0368

9. Kaye EC, Friebert S, Baker JN. Early integration of palliative care for children with high-risk cancer and their families. *Pediatr Blood Cancer.* 2016;63(4):593–597. doi:10.1002/pbc.25848

10. Liberman D, Song E, Radbill L, Pham P, Derrington S. Early introduction of palliative care and advanced care planning for children with complex chronic medical conditions: A pilot study. *Child Care Heal Dev.* 2016;42(3):439–449. doi:10.1111/cch.12332

11. Ferrell BR, Temel JS, Temin S, et al. Integration of palliative care into standard oncology care: American society of clinical oncology clinical practice guideline update. *J Clin Oncol.* 2017;35(1):96–112. doi:10.1200/JCO.2016.70.1474

12. Friedrichsdorf S, Bruera E. Delivering pediatric palliative care: From denial, palliphobia, pallilalia to palliactive. *Children.* 2018;5(9):120. doi:10.3390/children5090120

13. Cuviello A, Raisanen JC, Donohue PK, Wiener L, Boss RD. Defining the boundaries of palliative care in pediatric oncology. *J Pain Symptom Manage.* 2020;59(5):1033–1042. doi:10.1016/j.jpainsymman.2019.11.022

14. Feudtner C, Friebert S, Jewell J. Pediatric palliative care and hospice care commitments, guidelines, and recommendations. *Pediatrics.* 2013;132(5):966–972. doi:10.1542/peds.2013-2731

15. Cheng BT, Rost M, De Clercq E, Arnold L, Elger BS, Wangmo T. Palliative care initiation in pediatric oncology patients: A systematic review. *Cancer Med.* 2019;8(1):3–12. doi:10.1002/cam4.1907

16. Walter JK, Hill DL, Didomenico C, Parikh S, Feudtner C. A conceptual model of barriers and facilitators to primary clinical teams requesting pediatric palliative care consultation based upon a narrative review. *BMC Palliat Care.* 2019;18(1):116. doi:10.1186/s12904-019-0504-8

17. Kaye EC, Gushue CA, DeMarsh S, et al. Illness and end-of-life experiences of children with cancer who receive palliative care. *Pediatr Blood Cancer.* 2018;65(4):1–11. doi:10.1002/pbc.26895

18. Lord S, Weingarten K, Rapoport A. Palliative care consultation should be routine for all children who enroll in a phase I trial. *J Clin Oncol.* 2018;36(11):1062–1063. doi:10.1200/JCO.2017.76.3938

19. Newton K, Sebbens D. The impact of provider education on pediatric palliative care referral. *J Pediatr Heal Care.* 2020;34(2):99–108. doi:10.1016/j.pedhc.2019.07.007

20. Currie ER, McPeters SL, Mack JW. Closing the gap on pediatric palliative oncology disparities. *Semin Oncol Nurs.* 2018;34(3):294–302. doi:10.1016/j.soncn.2018.06.010

21. Haines ER, Frost AC, Kane HL, Rokoske FS. Barriers to accessing palliative care for pediatric patients with cancer: A review of the literature. *Cancer.* 2018;124(11):2278–2288. doi:10.1002/cncr.31265

22. Brock K, Allen K, Falk E, et al. Association of a pediatric palliative oncology clinic on palliative care access, timing and location of care for children with cancer. *Supportive Care in Cancer.* doi:10.1007/s00520-020-05671-y

23. Drake R. Palliative care for children in hospital: Essential roles. *Children.* 2018;5(2):26. doi:10.3390/children5020026

24. Johnston EE, Martinez I, Currie E, Brock KE, Wolfe J. Hospital or home? Where should children die and how do we make that a reality? *J Pain Symptom Manage.* 2020;60(1):106–115. doi:10.1016/j.jpainsymman.2019.12.370

25. Wolfe J, Orellana L, Ullrich C, et al. Symptoms and distress in children with advanced cancer: Prospective patient-reported outcomes from the PediQUEST study. *J Clin Oncol.* 2015;33(17):1928–1925. doi:10.1200/JCO.2014.59.1222

26. Snaman J, Kaye E, Baker J, Wolfe J. Pediatric palliative oncology: The state of the science and art of caring for children with cancer. *Curr Opin Pediatr.* 2018;30(1):40–48. doi:10.1097/MOP.0000000000000573

27. Ameringer S, MacPherson C, Jibb L. Symptom science in pediatric oncology. In: Hinds P, Linder L, eds. *Pediatric Oncology Nursing:*

Defining Care Through Science. Cham, Switzerland: Springer; 2020: 79–93. doi:10.1007/978-3-030-25804-7

28. Postovsky S, Lehavi A, Attias O, Hershman E. Easing of physical distress in pediatric cancer. In: Wolfe J, Jones B, Kreicbergs U, Jankovic M, eds. *Palliative Care in Pediatric Oncology*. Cham, Switzerland: Springer; 2018: 119–157. doi:10.1007/978-3-319-61391-8

29. Winegard B. The lack of movement. In: Ragsdale L, Miller E, eds. *Pediatric Palliative Care*. New York: Oxford University Press; 2020: 157–164. ISBN:9780190051853

30. Lexicomp. Lexi-Drugs. 2021. www.online.lexi.com

31. Evans A, Vingelen M, Yu C, Baird J, Murray P, Bryant P. Nausea in numbers: Electronic medical record nausea and vomiting assessment for children with cancer. *J Pediatr Oncol Nurs*. 2020;37(3):195–203. doi:10.1177/1043454219900467

32. Dupuis L, Tomlinson G, Pong A, Sung L, Bickham K. Factors associated with chemotherapy-induced vomiting control in pediatric patients receiving moderately or highly emetogenic chemotherapy: A pooled analysis. *J Clin Oncol*. 20AD;38(22):2499–2509. doi:10.1200/JCO.20.00134

33. Levy C, Dickerman M. She won't stop vomiting. In: Ragsdale L, Miller E, eds. *Pediatric Palliative Care*. New York: Oxford University Press; 2020: 123–133. ISBN:9780190051853

34. Hesketh P. In: Drews RE, eds. Prevention and treatment of chemotherapy-induced nausea and vomiting in adults. UpToDate. Waltham, MA; Uptodate. Last updated July 27, 2021. https://www.uptodate.com/contents/prevention-and-treatment-of-chemotherapy-induced-nausea-and-vomiting-in-adults.

35. Phillips R, Friend A, Gibson F, et al. Antiemetic medication for prevention and treatment of chemotherapy-induced nausea and vomiting in childhood. *Cochrane Database Syst Rev*. 2016;2:1–95. doi:10.1002/14651858.CD007786.pub3

36. Flank J, Thackray J, Nielson D, et al. Olanzaprine for treatment and prevention of acute chemotherapy-induced vomiting in children: A retrospective, multi-center review. *Pediatr Blood Cancer*. 2015;62(3):496–501. doi:10.1002/pbc.25286

37. Wong S, Wilens T. Medical cannabinoids in children and adolescents: A systematic review. *Pediatrics*. 2017;140(5):1–16. doi:10.1542/peds.2017-1818

38. Rosenberg A, Orellana L, Ullrich C, et al. Quality of life in children with advanced cancer: A report from the PEDIQUEST study. *J Pain Symptom Manage*. 2016;52(2):243–253. doi:10.1002/cncr.31668

39. Schack E, Wholihan D. Anorexia and cachexia. In: Ferrell B, Paice J, eds. *Oxford Textbook of Palliative Nursing*. 5th ed. New York: Oxford University Press; 2019: 140–148. ISBN: 9780190862374

40. Loprinzi C, Jatoi A. In: Hesketh PJ, ed. Management of cancer anorexia/cachexia. *UpToDate*. Waltham, MA: Uptodate. Last updated August 17, 2021. https://www.uptodate.com/contents/management-of-cancer-anorexia-cachexia.

41. Karimi M, Cox A, White S, Karlson C. Fatigue, physical and functional mobility, and obesity in pediatric cancer survivors. *Cancer Nurs*. 2020;43(4):E239–245. doi:10.1097/NCC.0000000000000712

42. Moore D, Marty C. Teenage "bleh." In: Ragsdale L, Miller E, eds. *Pediatric Palliative Care*. New York: Oxford University Press; 2020: 165–170.

43. Tutelman P, Chambers C, Stinson J, et al. Pain in children with cancer: Prevalence, characteristics, and parent management. *Clin J Pain*. 2018;34(3):198–206. doi:10.1097/AJP.0000000000000531

44. Vichinsky E. In: DeBaun MR, eds. Overview of the clinical manifestations of sickle cell disease. UpToDate. Waltham, MA: UpTodate. Last updated December 14, 2020. https://www.uptodate.com/contents/overview-of-the-clinical-manifestations-of-sickle-cell-disease.

45. Herr K, Coyne P, Ely E, Gelinas C, Manworren R. Pain assessment in the patient unable to self-report: Clinical practice recommendations in support of the ASPMN 2019 position statement. *Pain Manag Nurs*. 2019;20(5):404–417. doi:10.1016/j.pmn.2019.07.005

46. Hauer J, Jones B. In: Poplack, DG, ed. Evaluation and management of pain in children. UpToDate. Waltham, MA: UpTodate. Last updated February 5, 2020. https://www.uptodate.com/contents/evaluation-and-management-of-pain-in-children.

47. Friedrichsdorf S. From tramadol to methadone: Opioids in the treatment of pain and dyspnea in pediatric palliative care. *Clin J Pain*. 2019;35(6):501–508. doi:10.1097/AJP.0000000000000704

48. Jones B, Currin-McCulloch J, Pelletier W, Sardi-Brown V, Brown P, Wiener L. Psychosocial standards of care for children with cancer and their families: A national survey of pediatric oncology social workers. *Soc Work Heal Care*. 2018;57(4):221–249. doi:10.1080/00981389.2018.1441212

49. Barrera M, Rapoport A, Daniel K. Easing psychological distress in pediatric cancer. In: Wolfe J, Jones B, Kreicbergs U, Jankovic M, eds. *Palliative Care in Pediatric Oncology*. Cham, Switzerland: Springer; 2018: 159–187. doi:10.1007/978-3-319-61391-8

50. Mattie Miracle Cancer Foundation. Home page. 2020. https://www.mattiemiracle.com

51. Steele A, Mullins L, Mullins A, Muriel A. Psychosocial interventions and therapeutic support as a standard of care in pediatric oncology. *Pediatr Blood Cancer*. 2015;62(S5):S585–S618. doi:10.1002/pbc.25701

52. Weaver M, Heinze K, Kelly K, et al. Palliative care as a standard of care in pediatric oncology. *Pediatr Blood Cancer*. 2015;62(S5):S829–833. doi:10.1002/pbc.25695

53. Kazak A, Abrams A, Banks J, et al. Psychosocial assessment as a standard of care in pediatric cancer. *Pediatr Blood Cancer*. 2015;62(S5):S426–S459. doi:10.1002/pbc.25730

54. Shaw PH, Reed DR, Yeager N, Zebrack B, Castellino SM, Bleyer A. Adolescent and young adult (AYA) oncology in the United States: A specialty in its late adolescence. *J Pediatr Hematol Oncol*. 2015;37(3):161–169. doi:10.1097/MPH.0000000000000318

55. Pyke-Grimm KA, Franck LS, Patterson Kelly K, et al. Treatment decision-making involvement in adolescents and young adults with cancer. *Oncol Nurs Forum*. 2019;46(1):E22–E37. doi:10.1188/19.ONF.E22-E37

56. Sender A, Friedrich M, Leuteritz K, et al. Unmet supportive care needs in young adult cancer patients: Associations and changes over time. Results from the AYA-Leipzig study. *J Cancer Surviv*. 2019;13(4):611–619. doi:10.1007/s11764-019-00780-y

57. Barnett M, McDonnell G, DeRosa A, et al. Psychosocial outcomes and interventions among cancer survivors diagnosed during adolescence and young adulthood (AYA): A systematic review. *J Cancer Surviv*. 2016;10(5):814–831. doi:10.1007/s11764-016-0527-6

58. Pinkerton R, Donovan L, Herbert A. Palliative care in adolescents and young adults with cancer: Why do adolescents need special attention? *Cancer J (United States)*. 2018;24(6):336–341. doi:10.1097/PPO.0000000000000341

59. Close AG, Dreyzin A, Miller KD, Seynnaeve BKN, Rapkin LB. Adolescent and young adult oncology: Past, present, and future. *CA Cancer J Clin*. 2019;69(6):485–496. doi:10.3322/caac.21585

60. Coccia PF, Pappo AS, Beaupin L, et al. Adolescent and young adult oncology, version 2.2018: Clinical practice guidelines in oncology. *J Natl Compr Cancer Netw*. 2018;16(1):66–97. doi:10.6004/jnccn.2018.0001

61. Graetz D, Fasciano K, Rodriguez-Galindo C, Block S, Mack J. Things that matter: Adolescent and young adult patients' priorities during cancer care. *Pediatr Blood Cancer*. 2019;66(9):1–8. doi:10.1002/pbc.27883

62. Sisk BA, Canavera K, Sharma A, Baker JN, Johnson LM. Ethical issues in the care of adolescent and young adult oncology patients. *Pediatr Blood Cancer*. 2019;66(5):1–9. doi:10.1002/pbc.27608

63. Schreiner K, Grossoehme DH, Friebert S, Baker JN, Needle J, Lyon ME. "Living life as if I never had cancer": A study of the meaning of living well in adolescents and young adults who have experienced cancer. *Pediatr Blood Cancer*. doi:10.1002/pbc.28599

64. Lotz JD, Daxer M, Jox RJ, Borasio GD, Führer M. "Hope for the best, prepare for the worst": A qualitative interview study on parents' needs and fears in pediatric advance care planning. *Palliat Med*. 2017;31(8):764–771. doi:10.1177/0269216316679913

65. DeCourcey D, Silverman M, Oladunjoye A, Wolfe J. Advance care planning and parent-reported end-of-life outcomes in children, adolescents, and young adults with complex chronic conditions. *Crit Care Med.* 2019;47(1):101–108. doi:10.1097/CCM.0000000000003472

66. Kon A, Morrison W. Shared decision-making in pediatric practice: A broad view. *Pediatrics.* 2018;142(3):S129–S132. doi:10.1542/peds.2018-0516B

67. Jack BA, Mitchell TK, O'Brien MR, Silverio SA, Knighting K. A qualitative study of health care professionals' views and experiences of paediatric advance care planning. *BMC Palliat Care.* 2018;17(1):93. doi:10.1186/s12904-018-0347-8

68. Myers J, Cosby R, Gzik D, et al. Provider tools for advance care planning and goals of care discussions: A systematic review. *Am J Hosp Palliat Care.* 2018;35(8):1123–1132. doi:10.1177/1049909118760303

69. Childers JW, Back AL, Tulsky JA, Arnold RM. REMAP: A framework for goals of care conversations. *J Oncol Pract.* 2017;13(10):e844–850. doi:10.1200/JOP.2016.018796

70. Brown A. Reconceiving decisions at the end of life in pediatrics: Decision-making as a form of ritual. *Perspect Biol Med.* 2019;62(2):301–318. doi:10.1353/pbm.2019.0015

71. Conway M, Pantaleao A, Popp J. Parents' experience of hope when their child has cancer: Perceived meaning and the influence of health care professionals. *J Pediatr Oncol Nurs.* 2017;34(6):427–434. doi:10.1177/1043454217713454

72. Germann J, Leonard D, Stuenzi T, Pop R, Stewart S, Leavey P. Hoping is coping: A guiding theoretical framework for promoting coping and adjustment following pediatric cancer diagnosis. *J Pediatr Psychol.* 2015;40(9):846–855. doi:10.1093/jpepsy/jsv027

73. Kamihara J, Nyborn J, Olcese M, Nickerson T, Mack J. Parental hope for children with advanced cancer. *Pediatrics.* 2015;135:868–874. doi:10.1542/peds.2014-2855

74. Sisk B, Kang T, Mack J. Sources of parental hope in pediatric oncology. *Pediatr Blood Cancer.* 2018;65(6):1–7. doi:10.1002/pbc.26981

75. Cotter V, Foxwell A. The meaning of hope in the dying. In: Ferrell B, Paice J, eds. *Oxford Textbook of Palliative Nursing.* 5th ed. New York: Oxford University Press; 2019: 379–389.

76. Feraco A, Manfredini L, Jankovic M, Wolfe J. Considerations for cancer-directed therapy in advanced childhood cancer. In: Wolfe J, Jones B, Kreicbergs U, Jankovic M, eds. *Palliative Care in Pediatric Oncology.* Cham, Switzerland: Springer; 2018: 95–101. doi:10.1007/978-3-319-61391-8

77. Cuviello A, Boss R, Shah N, Battles H, Beri A, Wiener L. Utilization of palliative care consultations in pediatric oncology phase I clinical trials. *Pediatr Blood Cancer.* 2019;66(8):1–4. doi:10.1002/pbc.27771

78. Neha C, Vivek K. Challenges to palliative care in pediatric patients. *J Palliat Care Med.* 2016;6(3):1–3. doi:10.4172/2165-7386.1000256

30.

THE PEDIATRIC PALLIATIVE APRN IN THE COMMUNITY

Joan "Jody" Chrastek and Jaime Hensel

KEY POINTS

- The family is the unit of care. All interventions must be culturally sensitive, holistic, and evidence-based, addressing the physical, psychosocial, emotional, and spiritual needs of the child and family.

- As guide, ally, and advocate, the community-based pediatric palliative advanced practice registered nurse (CBPP APRN) collaborates with the child and their family in their own setting to ensure a culturally appropriate, equitable, practical, and realistic plan of care.

- No PP APRN works alone; team support and excellent professional boundaries are a must to provide best care and to protect the child and family and the professionals caring for them.

- There is a need for more widespread pediatric palliative care in the community; experienced providers of adult hospice and palliative care can help meet this need.

- Adult hospices unfamiliar with the care of children should access pediatric-specific resources to assure quality care.

CASE STUDY 1: INITIAL DIAGNOSIS OF A CHILD

Amir was 3 years old when his mother, Zara, noticed that his belly had enlarged over the span of a couple of weeks. During a diaper change, his mother found a firm abdominal mass. Amir was taken to his primary care pediatric nurse practitioner, who did a workup. Based on the concerning results, Amir was admitted to the hospital for an oncology workup which revealed a Wilms tumor of his right kidney.

Amir's initial hospital stay was difficult, for both Amir and Zara. Amir had difficult-to-control pain after his tumor resection. He developed nausea and constipation caused by the pain medications and itching secondary to an allergic reaction to the adhesive in one of his bandages. As a single working mother, Zara often felt guilty that she couldn't be at the hospital during the day. Amir's oncologist consulted inpatient pediatric palliative care for family support and symptom management.

Amir improved significantly with the implementation of the pediatric palliative care recommendations. Oncology made plans for Amir's outpatient chemotherapeutic regimen. As discharge planning started, Zara asked if there was any community-based palliative care available. A referral was placed to outpatient community-based pediatric palliative care.

INTRODUCTION

Community-based palliative care services have increased rapidly in the past couple of decades in the United States.[1] However pediatric services may be difficult to access because programs serving adults may not accept children.[2] Often, palliative care professionals who are competent to care for adults are unfamiliar with the care of children and may feel unprepared or even refuse to provide care for children.[3] The adage "children are not little adults" may be used as a justification. Although this is both a truism and a guiding principle in pediatric care, professionals with palliative care skills should be reassured that they still have much to offer when caring for pediatric patients. Most adult palliative care interventions and techniques carry over to children, but some attributes make the provision of community pediatric palliative care (PPC) unique.[2]

The underlying principle of PPC is its fundamental grounding in a family-centered approach. The majority of children are neither their own decision-makers nor their own caretakers, although older adolescents may sometimes assume more of these responsibilities.[4] Caregiving is, however, the natural role and privilege of parents or parental surrogates, whatever the health status of the child. The fact that family values, preferences, and goals serve as the basis for PPC cannot be overestimated.[5–7] Most children eligible for palliative care, especially those who live past the neonatal stage, spend the majority of their lives at home. Research suggests that home is often the preferred location of death for children, according to both children and their families.[3,8–10]

Sometimes the best comfort measure for a child is to facilitate a safe transition of care from the hospital to home. Managing a medically fragile child at home may be intimidating for families, particularly as the child nears end of life. Excellent education, support, and 24-hour availability of professionals allows families to remain at home through a child's disease process, their decline, and even death.[3] Creative use of technology and collaborative alliances with existing providers often facilitate the provision of care, particularly for those patients who live in rural or underserved areas.[11–13]

It is essential that palliative care is delivered with respect, compassion, and collaboration. A home is the family's space, and it is the team's privilege to be allowed to enter as a visitor. It is important to honor and respect the family's customs and rules. To be successful in providing excellent palliative care at home, the team must listen closely to the family and seek to understand their point of view, values, and beliefs to engage them as partners. The intimate nature of home-based care requires cultural sensitivity for all healthcare professionals involved and a comprehensive view of the care of family which includes siblings, extended family, and the community.[11,12]

To ensure holistic and collaborative care, the community-based pediatric palliative advanced practice registered nurse (CBPP APRN) often needs to engage diverse partners such as schools, community nursing agencies, summer camps, primary pediatricians, faith communities, and hospices. The CBPP APRN is a combination of clinician, supportive counselor, care coordinator, patient and family advocate, and educator. These roles may vary widely depending on the child's diagnosis, where the child lives, who comprises the interdisciplinary team, and the needs and preferences of the family, along with myriad other factors. The strength of palliative APRNs lies in their flexibility, adaptability, and the patient- and family-centered approach that is at the heart of palliative care.

ENTRY INTO PEDIATRIC COMMUNITY-BASED PALLIATIVE CARE

A thorough community assessment is critically important to providing comprehensive community palliative care, especially for APRNs new to community-based PPC or new to a healthcare community. Resources vary widely from one community to another; therefore, knowledge about social services and provider agencies may dramatically impact the way care is provided.[11,14,15]

The initiation of community-based PPC varies widely. While children are most often referred from hospitals, they are also referred by primary care providers, parents, social services, home nursing agencies, or even other palliative or hospice organizations. Children with serious illness admitted to community-based palliative care may have an estimated prognosis of years or may be admitted to home hospice with an anticipated death within days or months.

Prior to admission to community palliative or hospice care, the primary care provider must have a goals-of-care conversation with the family (and the child if appropriate).[16] PPC is a big tent that encompasses a wide breadth of care plans and treatment goals, from long-term symptom management to end-of-life care.[17] It is important to listen to the family's understanding of their child's condition and what are their hopes and wishes.[18]

There may be times where a family's understanding is different from that of the medical team. In these situations, the team should gently attempt to align the family's understanding of their child's medical prognosis with the team's understanding. The team should also educate about the anticipated course of the illness and the likely symptoms the child may experience. Clinicians must be thoughtful about leaving room for differing cultural and religious beliefs, as well as leaving space for participation by the child if the child is able and the family permits this.[18,19]

Once the family–clinician dyad forms a common understanding, then a shared plan of care can be developed. Faced with similar situations, each family chooses a different path. One family with a child diagnosed with widely metastatic cancer may prioritize time spent out of the hospital and desire a hospice plan of care. Another family, faced with a child with a similar diagnosis, may prioritize seeking additional treatment. The ability to have a kind, compassionate, culturally sensitive goals-of-care conversation is a necessary skill for all hospice and palliative APRNs.[20,21] Box 30.1 offers selected resources about pediatric goals of care conversations.

Most states have forms that communicate preferences for life-sustaining treatments to community providers and

---

Box 30.1 SELECTED RESOURCES FOR GOALS-OF-CARE CONVERSATIONS

Organizations

- National Institute of Nursing Research (NINR)

  Palliative Care: Conversations Matter
  https://www.ninr.nih.gov/newsandinformation/
  conversationsmatter/about-conversations-matter

- Hospice and Palliative Nurses Association: Pediatric topics

  www.advancingexpertcare.org

- National Hospice and Palliative Care Organization:

  ChIPPs E-Journal. Pediatric Palliative and Hospice Care. Communicating with children and their parents. 2016;44.
  https://www.nhpco.org/wp-content/uploads/2019/04/
  ChiPPS_e-journal_Issue-44.pdf

- Courageous Parents Network: Videos of conversations with parents and children

  https://courageousparentsnetwork.org

- Providence Institute for Human Caring: Resources

  www.instituteforhumancaring.org

Talking with Children

- VitalTalk: Effective communication; app, website, and classes

  www.vitaltalk.org

- Five Wishes, Voicing My Choices: Advance care planning

  www.fivewishes.org

- Ariadne Lab–Serious Illness Project–*The Serious Illness Conversation Guide*: Pediatric adaptations described in the two articles below

1) DeCourcey DD, Partin L, Revette A, Bernacki R, Wolfe J. Development of a stakeholder driven serious illness communication program for advance care planning in children, adolescents, and young adults with serious illness. *J Pediatr.* 2020 Sep 16. PMID: 32949579; 2) van Breemen C, Johnston J, Carwana M, Louie P. Serious illness conversations in pediatrics: A case review. *Children (Basel).* 2020;7(8):102. doi:10.3390/children7080102

emergency medical personnel, generically known as out-of-hospital orders for life-sustaining treatment. Many states refer to this document as a *provider/physician orders for life sustaining treatment* (POLST). The completion of such documents requires a family meeting about what the form means and does not mean. Its completion offers families peace of mind and some reassurance that their wishes for their child will be followed in the community setting (see Chapter 32, "Advance Care Planning").

The specific name and statutes for the completion of these documents may vary from state to state. In some states, APRNs may sign them; in other states it is the sole purview of physicians.[22] In some locations families are required to co-sign the document on behalf of their child, while in other states this is not required. In some locations the document may be legally binding for adults but not for children. CBPP APRNs must understand the rules of POLST documents in the communities in which they practice, as well as the portability of POLST documents from one state to another. Of note, while a POLST is meant to simply express the wishes of the family, some hospices do require a POLST (with "do not resuscitate" selected) as a condition of admission. Even more confusing is that some states do not allow children to have a no-code status. A do-not-resuscitate (DNR) code status is not a requirement for hospice under the Centers for Medicare and Medicaid Services (CMS) Medicare Hospice Benefit Conditions of Participation (COPs). Thus, CBPP APRNs should understand the eligibility requirements of the hospices and states they work with.

Once goals are determined and documented, referral to a pediatric hospice is a formal process, requiring a physician to complete a form certifying terminal illness. Quality transitions of care include a handoff conversation between the referring provider and the receiving program to confirm the appropriateness of enrollment; provide additional information, such as a brief synopsis of relevant medical and social information; and to communicate the patient/family goals of care.[23] It should be noted that the primary or referring team often remains involved in the child's care through the child's end of life.

To enroll in hospice, the CMS Medicare Hospice Benefit COPs require certification of a terminal illness, specifically that an individual is in the last 6 months of life.[24] For adult patients, the decision to elect hospice is predicated on whether a patient is willing to forgo curative, disease-directed treatments to focus solely on comfort and quality of life.[25] While there are eligibility criteria for adults relating to common terminal conditions in adults, such as cancer, heart or liver failure, and dementia to name a few, there are no similarly standard criteria for pediatric patients.[24,25] This is because children, in general, die of different diseases than adults. Genetics, for instance, plays a much larger role in pediatric end of life.[26] Children with conditions commonly found in the adult population, such as liver failure, often have a different underlying illness.[26] Moreover, children are more likely to have advanced medical support, such as total parental nutrition (TPN) dependence or gastrostomy (G-tube) feeding access, as part of their daily life.[26] Therefore, determination of hospice eligibility in children is based on clinician best judgment.

Although it is hard to talk about the financial cost of caring for seriously ill and dying children, it is a responsibility of the CBPP APRN to do so. Many children with life-limiting illnesses are covered under state Medicaid insurance or Children's Health Insurance Program (CHIP),[27] while others are covered under their parents' major commercial insurances. *Concurrent care* allows children to receive hospice care while remaining enrolled in other services, including disease-directed therapies and life-prolonging interventions[28] Although a provision of the *Affordable Care Act*, passed in 2010, requires that Medicaid allow for a concurrent care model, this is not uniformly enacted in each state. While the *Concurrent Care for Children Requirement* (CCCR) is mandated on the federal level, the ways in which individual states have implemented and supplemented the CCCR differ because it is covered under Medicaid.[29] Many commercial insurance companies do honor concurrent care, but some do not, so clarity about insurance coverage is essential. These payer source differences have implications for financial aspects of care, and families must be informed about what a child's insurance benefits will cover and what costs the families will incur when they consider individual treatment plans. The CBPP APRN needs to tailor plans to the finances and resources of the family. However, unlike adults, there is more often philanthropy available to support the care of children with financial hardship.

Community palliative care programs working with children must also work to be fiscally responsible. The Center to Advance Palliative Care collated data to demonstrate how palliative care can improve satisfaction and reduce costs.[30] The complexity of the healthcare reimbursement system in the United States has made demonstrating these metrics difficult because regulations can vary from state to state. But research has found that the provision of home-based palliative care across the country shows cost savings as well as improved quality of life for children with life-limiting illnesses.[31-34] California (which has a state mandate for palliative care) and Washington have both implemented programs that have reduced costs and improved satisfaction,[35] and other states are following suit.[31] As part of doing a community assessment, the CBPP APRN should gain a thorough understanding of the health landscape in their own region in order to best serve and guide children and their families. The National Hospice and Palliative Care Organization has a webpage that offers resources about pediatric care (https://www.nhpco.org/pediatrics/).

Prior to admission to the home-based organization, the CBPP APRN should perform a verbal home assessment, where the family is queried about the physical home itself. The APRN should ask questions about whether the house has running water, electricity, heat and cooling systems; the number of stairs into the home; whether the home has adequate outlets to plug in necessary equipment; and if there are adequate cooking facilities and food storage areas. Furthermore, the CBPP APRN should be proactive about care in potential emergencies: Is the house accessible by emergency services in the snow? Can the power company be notified that, if there is a power loss they should try to restore service to the patient's house more quickly? What is the plan should there be a natural disaster? The CBPP APRN should allow the parents to take the lead in addressing perceived barriers to care and be flexible in what solutions are considered acceptable while still formulating a safe and secure plan.

The home assessment continues throughout the time the child is under the home services. Once services have been initiated, the CBPP APRN or other members of the team can assess the child and family in their own environment. They may notice minor hazards such as loose carpet fringe, or major hazards such as hoarding, indoor smoking, or unsecured firearms. If a concern is noted, the CBPP APRN should find ways to sensitively and diplomatically express their concern and work with the family to find an acceptable remedy. The home care team should also be vigilant about the possibility of abuse. While most children are lovingly cared for, it is important to know that children with disabilities are considerably more likely than their peers without disability to experience physical, mental, and sexual abuse. As always, CBPP APRNs remain mandated reporters. See Box 30.2 for additional home assessment considerations.

Not all palliative care visits have to be conducted in person to be effective. Video visits have increased in healthcare and can be of great benefit for some PPC patients, such as those who have difficulty leaving the house or those who live in remote areas.[37] With the appropriate introduction, technology allows the CBPP APRN to visualize where the child lives, interact with the child and their family, and partner in care provision. Once barriers to utilization, such as acquisition of appropriate hardware and adequate internet bandwidth, are overcome, virtual palliative care home visits and consultations have generally been shown to be beneficial and acceptable to many families.[37,38] One drawback of telehealth visits is the limited physical exam. However, additional technology in the form of biometric trackers, smart devices, and apps may be a way to provide remotely some of the information usually gathered in a physical exam.[39]

CARE PROVISION IN THE HOME

Continuity of care or "seamless care" is a common goal in today's healthcare world for providers and patients alike. Continuity, guided by patients and families along with the healthcare team, is often highly complex.[40] Continuity of care

---

Box 30.2 SELECT HOME ASSESSMENT TOPICS

Caregiver considerations: Are there enough willing caregivers in the home? Are there back-up caregivers? Do the caregivers have the necessary training?

Abuse considerations: Is there concern for illicit substance use in the home? Does the child or any family member seem fearful, neglected, or show signs of physical abuse?

Safety considerations:
  Neighborhood: Is the neighborhood safe? If not, what steps need to be taken to ensure visiting staff are safe?
  Dwelling: Are there smoke detectors and carbon monoxide detectors? Is there a safe and useable emergency evacuation route available for the child? Are there pets in the home that might harm the child (or the nurse)? Are medications stored securely so that other children and pets don't accidently ingest them? Are there guns in the house, and, if so, are they safely stored? Are there fringed rugs? Is there a cigarette, cigar, or pipe smoker in the home?

Transportation: How far does the family and child live from regular medical care? Does the family and child have a reliable way to get to and from appointments? Can the family and afford the transportation?

Medical equipment considerations: Does the child need a specialized bed or mobility devices? Does the child need a lift? Is oxygen delivery available in the area? Where will other supplies, such as bed pads or syringes, come from? Will the child's insurance cover all the costs and supplies? Is there a limit to how many disposable supplies the insurance will pay for?

Emergency medical services (EMS): Does the child live in an area covered by EMS? Is EMS aware of the child's medical condition (if the family would like them to be)? How far is the nearest emergency room? What is the back-up plan for the child in the event of an emergency or loss of power?

Building considerations: Are there steps into the home? Does the home have adequate lighting? Are the doorways wide enough? Are the bathrooms equipped for the child's use? Will deep pile rugs interfere with mobility devices? Is there an elevator?

Utility considerations: Does the house have an adequate and reliable power supply for the child to safely live at home? What is the plan if a power outage occurs? Will the new equipment increase utility bills, and, if so, can the family afford this increase?

Finance considerations: Is the family able to pay their bills? Does the family have enough food?

Community resources: Is the family connected to community resources? Is there access to grocery stores and pharmacies?

Cultural and language issues: Does the family have hold cultural beliefs that may influence how the care is provided and who the caregivers are? Is an interpreter needed for home visits? Is an interpreter available for on-call or urgent needs?

Housekeeping considerations: Is the house clean enough for care delivery? Is there is specialized medical waste (such as sharps)? What is the plan to dispose of medical waste safely?

is described as the continuous relationship between a provider or team of providers and a patient, as well as the coordination and sharing of information between providers' practices.[41,42] This can be a particular challenge in PPC due to the large number of specialists involved in the care. It is here that the CBPP APRN is an important bridge between silos of care.[43] The need for collaboration extends even further beyond the hospital into all aspects of the child's life. For example, home-based services, nursing, physiotherapy, academic programs or other school-based therapies, outpatient clinics, and hospitals may all be part of a child's care team but may not share electronic medical records. With such a large and diverse team, communication often is incomplete, leaving providers and families frustrated and exhausted trying to fit the pieces together.[43]

As discussed earlier, when a child comes home for hospice or palliative care, it is essential for the CBPP APRN to discuss the situation, including the social, emotional, physical, spiritual, and cultural aspects of care, with the referring team. Attention should be paid to reducing any health disparities. The child may live in a foster home, a group home, or move between the homes of divorced parents. The referring team can provide helpful context to the home-based team, including any concerns they may have regarding family coping, mental health issues, or substance abuse potential. In these situations, the CBPP APRN and team can develop a care plan in concert with the managing team to provide the best and safest care for the child and family and work to make the transition as smooth as possible.

Communication is essential for good palliative care. Once the child is at home, this means reaching out to many different parts of the child's life. See Box 30.3 for an example of the

---

Box 30.3 POTENTIAL PEDIATRIC COMMUNITY TEAM MEMBERS

Primary care physician

Neurologist and office care coordinator

Gastroenterologist and office care coordinator

Pulmonologist and office care coordinator

Physical medicine and rehabilitation, hospital- and home-based

Pediatric palliative care team: Physician, speech and language pathologist (SLP), occupational therapist (OP), physical therapist (PT), and registered nurse: hospital- and community-based

Social worker: Hospital-based social worker, disability social worker, and county social worker

School home-based services: Physiotherapist, teacher, social worker, and speech and language pathologist

Nursing agency: Home health nurses and home health aides

Insurance company personnel

Medical equipment company personnel and pharmacy

Pediatric palliative APRN, palliative care and hospice team, Social worker, spiritual care, music therapist, volunteer hospice aide

Extended family

Religious community

---

larger community team that may interact with the child and family. It is important to ensure that communication aligns with the parents' wishes, especially with regards to confidentiality. As the CBPP APRN meets with the parents or caregivers in the home, the family is the center of all decisions: everything must be coordinated with them. Not all families are traditionally structured, nor do they make choices in the same way. The CBPP APRN can explore with the family who is involved in decision-making, how decisions are made, and what role culture and religion play in the care of the child.

Parents often have a close relationship with their child's primary medical provider or specialist, and that relationship continues to be very important even as care becomes more home-based. The CBPP APRN should collaborate with the family and involved teams to ensure clarity on who is managing which pieces of the child's care. The CBPP APRN may serve as the key point of communication among all of the teams.

When resources are scarce, the CBPP APRN collaborates with the family to access all available local resources. For instance, a palliative care team may not have a child life specialist, but they may be able to recruit the child's teacher to help guide the team in how best to work with the child and siblings on an appropriate developmental level. Telehealth can be a wonderful tool for collaboration and continuity, especially in areas where a specific specialist does not exist (see Chapter 17, "The Palliative APRN in Telehealth"). Parents have expressed decreased anxiety when a specialist is involved in their child's care,[29,44] and video visits are one way to bring specialists to the child and family in underserved and rural areas. The CBPP APRN is often the coordinator of these types of collaborations, working to develop a comprehensive and cohesive team.

The CBPP APRN often takes the role of organizer and team lead on behalf of the child. They must use expert communication, provide attentive listening, build collaborative relationships, and share information. This can be quite stressful for the palliative APRN who lacks formal education in community-based pediatric palliative care.[45,46] However, a CBPP APRN has a deep toolbox from which to draw in the roles of clinician, consultant, educator, leader, and researcher in service of their pediatric patients.

Families live in communities with friends and neighbors, many of whom may want information about the child or to offer assistance. At times this can be helpful, but at other times it may feel awkward and invasive. The home-based team can discuss child and family preferences and concerns in this area, specifically who they want as part of their inner circle of support and how much they want to share, if at all, outside that circle. Families often need assistance in creating pat answers for those times they do not wish to share. For example, a casual acquaintance may ask, "So how is the little darling?" and the parents can be coached to respond, "We are happy to have her home" and leave it at that. Each family will, of course, decide what phrases work best for them and their situation. However, it is helpful to have a plan in mind because often inquiries about the child's health come paired with unwanted advice and judgments.

Visitors to the home may also be helpful or burdensome. Some families may want private time at home without visitors but feel rude turning well-meaning friends or caregivers away. In such cases, the CBPP APRN can offer to set up guidelines of the family's choosing that can then become the "provider rules." In this manner, the APRN helps the family set boundaries and relieves the family of the burden of saying no to visitors. For example, a family may let people know that "hospice has set visiting hours" for the child or limited the length of visits. Communicating closely with families can assure that the team is helping them make the most of their time at home with their child and keeping a keen focus on quality of life.

All children have wishes and desires: those children under palliative care or hospice are no different. The home-based palliative APRN can work with the team and family to investigate how to grant some of those wishes. For some children and their families, a last trip to a special place is extremely important. The palliative care team can help identify resources such as community or national organizations that may have funding to make these trips possible. The team can support these efforts by taking care of the medical logistics, which may include close collaboration with professionals at the trip destination. Some places, such as theme parks, are very familiar with hosting children with medical complexities, while other destinations are not. It is important to put together a travel packet that includes an official letter from the managing clinician with the child's diagnosis, history, code status, and medications, as well as contact information for the palliative team. Copies of other important documents related to the child's care should also be included. Pre-identifying hospitals on the way and at the destination can be helpful. Local hospices near the destination may be willing to contract to provide care if needed.

There are also camps for children with palliative care and hospice needs. The child may already be connected with one or may benefit from a referral. These camps tend to be well-organized and suited to provide both excellent medical care and a fun experience for the child. The forms and requirements are unique to each setting but are usually straightforward.

HOME DEATHS

CASE STUDY 2: INFANT DEATH AT HOME

Jenna was born with trisomy 13, with fatal renal and cardiac complications. Her parents, Ravi and Andrea, when informed about the diagnosis prenatally, requested comfort care only at birth. They asked for discharge home as soon as possible with hospice. They especially wanted their 4-year-old son David to have a chance to meet Jenna. Andrea had explained to David that Jenna would "just be a visitor and not stay very long," but reassured him that they themselves would not leave.

Jenna was born on a Monday evening and was stable. An early discharge was planned, and the hospice team visited the same day. The family was sent home from the hospital with emergency comfort medications (sublingual morphine for dyspnea, lorazepam for agitation, and atropine drops to reduce secretions) because they are not always easy to obtain quickly in the community.

The inpatient PP APRN also sent home a completed provider/physician orders for life-sustaining treatment (POLST).

Jenna and her parents arrived home to a family birthday party for Jenna arranged by her grandparents. The hospice APRN and the social worker arrived shortly after the family and were invited to enjoy a piece of cake. David was shy at first, but quickly warmed up to the hospice team, which had brought him some crayons and a coloring book to keep him occupied while they talked to his parents.

The hospice team listened to the parents' story and concerns and asked how much information on what to expect they would like. Andrea wanted to know everything but Ravi wanted just the minimum and said that Andrea could fill him in later. He wanted to just enjoy his new daughter.

As Andrea had never seen anyone die—or even been to a funeral—it was important to review the expected physiological changes, as well as medications and nonmedication interventions that could bring Jenna comfort. A step-by-step explanation was provided verbally and via a written symptom management guide. The team let Andrea know that Jenna would be registered as an expected death at home, so likely there would not be police involvement. Therefore, they emphasized, it was important at the time of death to call hospice and not 911.

Later that night, Jenna started to have apnea spells and some cyanosis. Andrea quickly called hospice and gave the morphine as instructed. It helped and Jenna fell asleep; her parents did not. The next morning, the hospice nurse found Jenna was declining quickly with 30- to 45-second apneic spells and cool, blue extremities. The nurse gently informed the parents death was close. Her grandparents were called and came to be there for David. Andrea and Ravi lay down in bed on either side of Jenna, while the hospice nurse gave them privacy and spent time playing with David. He said, "I found a dead bird in the garden—my mom said Jenna was going to die." This allowed the hospice nurse to engage in an age-appropriate conversation about death with him.

Twenty minutes later, the nurse heard Andrea calling for her. She told the nurse that Jenna had not breathed for 3 minutes, and she thought she had died. The nurse listened and found that her heart was still beating, just as Jenna took another breath. The nurse did a little bit of education about apnea at end of life, and let them know death was still close. Jenna died peacefully when both parents had dozed off, about an hour later. Initially Andrea and Ravi felt bad that they had missed the moment but were comforted by the nurse's reassurance that it was OK. The hospice nurse said, "Sometimes it seems that those who are loved as much as Jenna was can only die when their loved ones are asleep or not totally focusing on them. She knew she was surrounded by your love." The hospice nurse allowed them private time, called the medical examiner to report the expected death at home, then answered the family's questions about the experience.

CASE STUDY 3: DEATH OF CHRONICALLY ILL CHILD

Rosie, an only child, was diagnosed with a slow neurodegenerative condition when she was 5 years old, after an astute pediatrician noticed her increasing difficulty walking. Over the years as her disease progressed, her parents became her nurses, case managers, advocates, and assumed many other roles on her behalf. Rosie's parents knew her condition was inevitably fatal, but their lives revolved around her. In addition to her parents, Rosie had a dedicated team of personal care attendants (PCA) who had cared for her for years. Rosie had been also referred to palliative care at the time of her diagnosis.

Rosie saw the palliative team infrequently for many years while her symptom needs were relatively low. With the slow progression of her condition, palliative care was there mainly to build rapport and to assist in decision-making. For instance, as a young child, Rosie loved to eat, but over time her swallowing became ineffective. The palliative care team helped facilitate a meeting with a gastroenterology consult to decide whether advanced nutrition support would be right for Rosie. Ultimately, a gastrostomy tube was placed and was used for many years.

Rosie's condition declined quickly when her respiratory system became more involved. When she started to have difficulty breathing, palliative care became more intensively involved in her care, and, not long after, hospice was initiated. Six months into her respiratory decline, Rosie was actively dying. Her parents were desperate to keep her at home but were also profoundly exhausted. They had good social support but found they needed help to organize all the willing volunteers. The palliative social worker was helpful in identifying community resources that allowed the family some relief.

Rosie began to show signs of feeding intolerance, vomiting, and cramping when she was given her medically administered nutrition. Hospice staff had discussed that this might occur, but the gastrostomy tube had become much so much a part of who Rosie was that it was very difficult for the family to even think about stopping. The team tried many different interventions to see if Rosie could tolerate the feeds, but eventually realized that her body could no longer process food and it was causing her pain. Her parents listened to the silent message Rosie was giving them and made the loving decision to stop the medically administered nutrition. It was clear her comfort improved even as she was dying. The hospice APRN met with the PCAs as they struggled to accept and support the family's decisions.

The hospice APRN and social worker met with the family regularly to talk about their wishes for Rosie, to keep her comfort at the center of her care, and even to help them plan the funeral. The parents had been thinking about Rosie's death for many years, but had done no concrete planning and appreciated the support to do so.

In the last month of Rosie's life, the hospice team reviewed with Rosie's parents and caregivers what Rosie's death might look like while cautioning them that every death is unique. Not long after the conversation, Rosie became very agitated, with frightening hallucinations and confusion. After multiple interventions failed, she needed significant sedation to be comfortable. Even the medical team was surprised at the amount of medication she needed, but they were able to titrate to an appropriate dose for comfort. The sedation decreased Rosie's agitation and induced relaxation, allowing her parents to concentrate on just spending time with her. It was a precious but difficult time, lasting 3 weeks. The long trajectory of her dying process was very difficult for the family. They expressed feeling like they were hanging on a cliff with their fingernails. Although they did not want the death to happen, they found the stress of waiting for the inevitable was excruciating.

Rosie died peacefully one afternoon when everyone was in the kitchen making dinner. Her parents were sad, but also relieved that her suffering was over. They were confident that Rosie had known she was surrounded by love.

MEDICATIONS

When a family transitions home with a child who is expected to die in a short time, it is important to send them home with comfort medications, not just prescriptions. Some commonly used comfort medications may not be easily available in the community. Although many hospices have standing orders for their adult hospice patients, these standing orders may not be appropriate for children and young adults. Standing orders, if used at all, should be reviewed and individualized to the unique needs of that child. This process assures that the team has a customized comfort plan in place for each child.

It is expedient to give families a small supply of end-of-life comfort medications to have available if urgently needed prior to hospice's arrival and subsequent medication delivery. Usually this is a sublingual liquid opioid for pain and dyspnea, a benzodiazepine for anxiety, and an anticholinergic to help with secretions. (See Appendix II for pediatric pain and symptom management medications and dosages.) At times, intranasal medications such as midazolam or fentanyl may be the drug and route of choice due to their rapid action. Rectal and transdermal medications may also be utilized. Instructions on the use of all medications must be provided verbally and in writing, in a language the family understands and can read. If the family is not health or language literate, the CBPP APRN needs to help the family develop a way to ensure appropriate dosages and medications are given using pictures, color coding, or another similar tactic. A medical interpreter may also be needed.

INFORMATION

Families need to be provided information about what they might expect to see as the child moves toward death and the child's body shuts down in the dying process. It can be helpful to emphasize that every death is unique, just like every birth is unique. Death can come quickly, or it may take much longer than expected. The parents should be reassured that, whatever happens, the team has many strategies to keep the child comfortable.

Due to culture, ethnicity, or religion, some families are deeply uncomfortable or even refuse to talk about the upcoming death. This should be assessed by the CBPP APRN. However, it is very important that the main caregivers of a child at home know how to care for their dying child. In such situations, the use of hypothetical situations and stories can be useful. For example the nurse may say, "Of course we never know exactly what will happen in the future, but I want to tell you a story about a similar child and how the parents took such good care of her." This tactic provides an avenue to talk about how that (real or imagined) other family saw various changes that alerted them that their child was nearing death, gave the various prescribed medications, and what other helpful actions they took to ensure their child was comfortable and well cared for.[47,48] There may be parents who refuse even oblique mentions of death and are offended that it is even mentioned. In these cases, in the home setting, the hospice team must continue to gently offer the family information but should not force conversations. It is the family's prerogative whether to receive information or not.

It is essential that the hospice team be aware of any cultural traditions that the family observes around death and dying.[47,48] For example, in some cultures, a dying child must be clothed in a specific garment, facing a certain direction, or have restrictions on who can touch the body after death. Impending death may also require rituals, such as baptism or other religious ceremonies, which require the presence of a clergy person. Families may rely on the APRN's expertise in knowing when a child has transitioned to actively dying to ensure the rituals take place.

Funeral planning can be a terribly difficult thing for families to do, but when it is done prior to the death it can make it a little less awful since it can relieve the burden of decision-making in the immediate aftermath of a child's death. The home hospice staff can help guide the family in the process if they are open to it. Often some funeral information is also provided in the standard written information from the home-based hospice team.

Some families may want to keep their child's body at home for a prolonged period of time or even have a home funeral. In this case, pre-planning—either with the funeral home in mind or in collaboration with a home funeral group—is important to ensuring a smooth process. For instance, if the body is not kept properly cooled, rigor mortis sets in and the body starts to change colors. The length of time that it takes to set in depends on many factors, including the ambient temperature, but rigor mortis generally appears rapidly in children.[49] Advance planning makes a significant difference to the experience families have and ensures sure they have the right resources on hand to care for their child. Websites such as the Home Funeral Alliance can be helpful (https://www.homefuneralalliance.org).

SIBLINGS OR OTHER CHILDREN

It is helpful to talk to the parents about their plans for siblings when a child dies. Often siblings are left out as death nears, but children are perceptive and will feel the increased tension in the house as their sibling moves closer to dying. If the parents allow, it is important for the CBPP APRN or other members of the team to pay attention to the other children in a dying child's life.[50] Families differ in their comfort of allowing the sibling or other children to be present during the dying process. A family member or a close friend may be willing to be the buddy for the sibling if they are present. Regardless of where the siblings are at the time of death, parents should be strongly encouraged to provide age-appropriate truthful information to their other children. Otherwise, there is a real danger that siblings will use their vivid imaginations to construct their own narratives about what is happening, and these ideas may be much worse than reality.[51]

THE EXTENDED TEAM

PPC, especially end-of-life care for children, is commonly seen as a very stressful position for care providers,[45,50] not only because of the child's situation but also because of the close relationships that frequently develop between caregivers and the family in the community setting. Extended-hours (private duty) nurses or personal care attendants may themselves need the support of the hospice team. Some of these individuals may have cared for the child for many years and may have strong attachments to the child and family. This closeness, born of being at home with the family for long periods of time, can make it challenging for caregivers to maintain professional boundaries.[37] Even the family may begin to experience the visits as personal as well as professional.[51] However, the relationship between the family and the nursing team is a professional one and differs from their personal friendships. It is not a relationship where both parties can share confidences equally. Rather, it is a relationship where families may share confidences in ways that a professional cannot. Healthy boundaries protect the patient, family, and the professional, and if boundaries are not maintained it can result in unfortunate consequences.[45,50] Being aware of this possible facet of end-of-life care for children with an extended team is an important function of the CBPP APRN. Moreover, the pediatric palliative APRN may help facilitate anticipatory grief support for extended teams.

THE TIME OF DEATH

Most often, the CBPP APRN will not be present at the exact time of a child's death. Therefore, the family will need clear instructions on who to call to report that the child has died. Most often this is the hospice provider, but the family may instinctively call one of their child's physicians, who should then call hospice. A registered nurse will perform a home visit to verify the death and report it to the medical examiner. The medical examiner may ask a list of standard questions. See Box 30.4 for common medical examiner's office questions. Depending on local laws and statutes, in some cases, a formal investigation may need to take place. Families should be prepared for this possibility and the prerogative of the medical examiner to initiate it at the time of death. However, families should be reassured that for most preregistered expected deaths at home there is not a police investigation. A formal investigation is much more likely if the death is due to a previous nonaccidental injury, a vehicle accident, suspicious circumstances, or other unique situations.

A plan should be in place for care of the child's body after death. The home hospice agency may or may not have a set protocol regarding care of the child's body. If there is not a protocol, the CBPP APRN can gently ask the parents if they would like the nurse to wash the body, remove any tubes or medical paraphernalia, or dress the child in a special outfit. If the family has not planned on a home funeral, the funeral director will ultimately prepare the body and put on the final outfit, but some families prefer to wash or perform special rituals before the body is taken away.

After death, some families want their child's body removed quickly from the house, while others may want to keep the body at home for some time. If the family plans to keep the body at home for more than a few hours, the nurse should educate them about the changes they may see as rigor mortis sets in and about the skin color changes that may happen.

Families may also appreciate information about how the child's body will be picked up. Most commonly the funeral home will send two representatives to remove the body, but will come only after ensuring the family is ready. The vehicle used will depend on the funeral home. For infants and young children, they may simply come in a car. However, some funeral homes will always use a hearse. Once the vehicle arrives, some families prefer to carry the child's body out to the car if the child is small enough. For older children and young adults, the funeral home representatives will usually come with a stretcher, similar to an ambulance transfer. In some states, the family is allowed to transport the body themselves in a personal vehicle. It is important for the CBPP APRN to investigate local regulations before the child dies in order to provide families with accurate information.

MEDICATIONS AND SUPPLIES

The disposition of medications can be tricky. The issue of safe disposal should be discussed. With the enactment of the 2018 *Substance Use–Disorder Prevention that Promotes Opioid Recovery and Treatment (SUPPORT) for Patients and Communities Act*,[51] medications ordered when a child is under hospice care can be disposed of by certain hospice personnel in states where laws allow it. A common disposal procedure is to empty all the medications into a sealable container with an inert substance such as flour, coffee grounds, or kitty litter; add water to make a slurry; and then place the whole container in the garbage.[51,52] The home care and hospice nurse should use their agency's guidelines and have the signature of a witness. A nurse cannot take the medications out of the home to destroy them—this must occur on site.[52]

The family may also ask what they should do with the child's durable medical equipment and remaining disposable supplies, such as wheelchairs, diapers, or cans of nutrition. While the family is obviously welcome to keep these supplies, many families wish to help others by donating them. The hospice or home health agency may have a list of local agencies that accept donations. Each agency will have its own guidelines regarding what it will accept.

AFTER THE CHILD'S DEATH

It can be very meaningful for many families when healthcare professionals attend a wake or a funeral for a child, especially if the relationship has been long or close. It is also usual for hospice clinicians to make a specific bereavement visit in the period after the child's death and funeral. On this visit, the hospice and palliative APRN should gently assess for any concerning signs of complicated grief that may lead to mental health issues (see Chapter 38, "Grief and Bereavement"). The bereavement care for the family may be taken over by the bereavement team, or the hospice team many provide that service for the next 13 months.

COMMUNITY PROVIDER SUPPORT

The CBPP APRN's role as educator and mentor cannot be overemphasized. While the APRN may provide formal and structured educational offerings, much of the time the APRN teaches by role-modeling excellent care and provides "just in time" education. This type of education is done at the point of care. With adult learners, this format is often more effective and lasting than a formal educational intervention. "Just in time" education is a common need for community-based service providers who have little or no prior experience in the provision of palliative or hospice care to children.

Excellent access and 24-hour availability of palliative care professionals can provide needed support to hospice staff who may not have pediatric experience and any private duty or extended-hours staff in the home and therefore help support families in staying at home through a child's decline and death.[1] Many of the nurses in a child's care will have worked in the home for years and have a long-standing relationship with the child and family. Yet it is also common for nurses or other team members to have very little or no palliative care training or experience, resulting in fears and misunderstandings about palliative care.[45] In these situations, the CBPP APRN can provide technical clinical instruction, such how to flush a particular line or care for a wound. But the APRN also may give emotional and psychosocial support to help the home care nurse deal with personal fears concerning caring for a dying child or a child with a life-limiting condition. The intimate nature of home-based care may require particular cultural sensitivity on the part of providers and a comprehensive view of care that includes other clinicians and family members.[11,12] Creative use of technology and collaborative alliances with existing providers may facilitate the provision of this support, particularly for those practicing in rural or underserved areas.[54,55]

It is helpful for all team members to realize that palliative care is characterized by continuous learning for the whole team.[11] This education should include providing resources such as the national consensus guidelines. The National Consensus Project for Quality Palliative Care (NCP) *Clinical Practice Guidelines*[56] and the Center to Advance Palliative Care (CAPC) pediatric toolkit[57] are both valuable resources for those providing PPC.

WELL-BEING AND RESILIENCY FOR THE COMMUNITY-BASED PEDIATRIC PALLIATIVE APRN AND THE PEDIATRIC PALLIATIVE CARE TEAM

Caring for children who are dying or have life-limiting conditions can be emotionally taxing for the staff as well as for the family.[5,58,59] Domain 1 of the NCP *Clinical Practice Guidelines* states that creating support for staff and including strategies for team well-being are part of quality care.[57] The concept of well-being has been a focus for all healthcare professionals in the past few years, as evidenced by initiatives from the National Academy of Medicine (Clinician Wellbeing), the Institute of Health Improvement (Joy at Work), and more recently the American Nurses Association (Wellbeing Initiative).[60,61] To be sustainable, a PPC team must incorporate support mechanisms into regular practice and even have support as a focus of their strategic plan.[62] Even while working as part of a community-based PPC team, clinicians and nurses often do their day-to-day rounds individually and thus lack the easy "curbside" check-ins available to hospital- or clinic-based practice. Therefore, it is essential for each community-based team member to develop a personalized plan to manage the inherent stress and emotional toll of PPC work. When this is ignored, it is to the detriment of not only the individual but also the functioning of the team and, ultimately, to the child and family.[59]

Some programs require every team member to complete a personalized self-care plan and ask each person to choose other team members as accountability partners to help maintain adherence. Individuals should select supportive and renewing activities that best suit their lifestyle and personality. The plan serves as a guide to remind individuals and the team of the importance of self-care so they can continue sustainably in this challenging but rewarding field of work. Supporting families through difficult times can be challenging but is a skill that all those who work in palliative care must build, particularly less-experienced nurses and clinicians. There are many different ways that well-being is accomplished: the important thing is that it *is* achieved.[62,63]

One very important aspect of support that is often neglected is the skill of listening. Listening and caring for each team member is essential and is a shared responsibility between the team members and the organizations to which they belong. In the words of Julian of Norwich (1342–1416),

> The sorrowing, the sick, the unwanted, the lonely, both young and old, rich and poor, all come to my window. No one listens, they tell me, and so I listen and tell them what they have just told me. And, I sit in silence, listening, letting them grieve. "Julian, you are wise," they say, "You have been gifted with understanding." All I did was listen. For I believe full surely that God's spirit is in us all, giving light, wisdom, understanding, speaking words in us when we cannot speak, showing us gently what we would not see; what we are afraid to see; so that we may show pity, mercy, forgiveness.

SUMMARY

This chapter has highlighted a few ways in which pediatric community palliative and hospice care differs from adult care or from PPC in other settings. However, the general shape of pediatric community palliative care should feel familiar. APRNs with primary palliative skills should find that their expertise forms a solid foundation from which to learn and adapt. Learning the local landscape of laws and resources, partnering with and educating diverse allies, and a strong emphasis on coordination will help ensure seamless care for children and their families.

While there are unique challenges, many CBPP APRNs find that providing community-based PPC is a privilege. Relationships formed with children and their families over the course of days, weeks, months, or years are especially intimate due to the location and style of care. Special consideration must be taken to partner with families and provide culturally sensitive and individually tailored support. In addition to the benefit to the family, the coordination of care can build stronger community ties among hospitals, schools, primary care practices, state agencies, hospice organizations, religious communities, and even utility companies. Community-based PPC is deeply necessary. There is currently considerable unmet need in many areas of the country. In addition to building community alliances in the service of patients, CBPP APRNs should be deliberate about finding support for themselves and their own practice. Well-being is a necessity in building a sustainable career in PPC. A sustainable career in community PPC can be extraordinary: helping children and families to remain in their homes and facilitating lives outside of hospitals is immensely rewarding.

REFERENCES

1. Lindley LC, Shaw SL. Who are the children using hospice care? *J Spec Pediatr Nurs.* 2014;19(4):308–315. doi:10.1111/jspn.12085

2. Vesel T, Beveridge C. From fear to confidence: Changing providers' attitudes about pediatric palliative and hospice care. *J Pain Symptom Manage.* 2018;56(2):205–212.e3. doi:10.1016/j.jpainsymman.2018.03.019

3. Castor C, Hallstrom I, Hansson H, Landgren K. Home care services for sick children: Healthcare professionals' conceptions of challenges and facilitators. *J Clin Nurs.* 2017;26(17–18):2784–2793. doi:10.1111/jocn.13821

4. Kon AA, Morrison W. Shared decision-making in pediatric practice: A broad view. *Pediatrics.* 2018;142(Suppl 3):S129–S132. doi:10.1542/peds.2018-0516B

5. Thienprayoon R, Grossoehme D, Humphrey L, et al. "There's just no way to help, and they did": Parents name compassionate care as a new domain of quality in pediatric home-based hospice and palliative care. *J Palliat Med.* 2020;23(6):767–776. doi:10.1089/jpm.2019.0418

6. Madrigal VN, Kelly KP. Supporting family decision-making for a child who is seriously ill: Creating synchrony and connection. *Pediatrics.* 2018;142(Suppl 3):S170–S177. doi:10.1542/peds.2018-0516H

7. Boyden JY, Ersek M, Deatrick JA, et al. What do parents value regarding pediatric palliative and hospice care in the home setting? *J Pain Symptom Manage.* 2020;60(1):12–13. doi:10.1016/j.jpainsymman.2020.07.024

8. Kaye EC, DeMarsh S, Gushue CA, et al. Predictors of location of death for children with cancer enrolled on a palliative care service. *Oncologist.* 2018;23(12):1525–1532. doi:10.1634/theoncologist.2017-0650

9. Bender HU, Riester MB, Borasio GD, Fuhrer M. "Let's bring her home first": Patient characteristics and place of death in specialized pediatric palliative home care. *J Pain Symptom Manage.* 2017;54(2):159–166. doi:10.1016/j.jpainsymman.2017.04.006

10. Friedrichsdorf SJ, Bruera E. Delivering pediatric palliative care: From denial, palliphobia, pallilalia to palliactive. *Children (Basel).* 2018;5(9):120. doi:10.3390/children5090120

11. Koch A, Grier K. Communication and cultural sensitivity for families and children with life-limiting diseases: An informed decision-making ethical case in community-based palliative care. *J Hosp Palliat Nurs.* 2020;22(4):270–275. doi:10.1097/NJH.0000000000000654

12. Kirby E, Lwin Z, Kenny K, Broom A, Birman H, Good P. "It doesn't exist": Negotiating palliative care from a culturally and linguistically diverse patient and caregiver perspective. *BMC Palliat Care.* 2018;17(1):90. doi:10.1186/s12904-018-0343-z

13. Weaver MS, Neumann ML, Navaneethan H, Robinson JE, Hinds PS. Human touch via touchscreen: Rural nurses' experiential perspectives on telehealth use in pediatric hospice care. *J Pain Symptom Manage.* 2020;60(5):1027–1033. doi: 10.1016/j.jpainsymman.2020.06.003

14. Lindley LC, Edwards SL. Geographic access to hospice care for children with cancer in Tennessee, 2009 to 2011. *Am J Hosp Palliat Care.* 2015;32(8):849–854. doi: 10.1177/1049909114543641

15. Lindley LC, Oyana TJ. Geographic variation in mortality among children and adolescents diagnosed with cancer in Tennessee: Does race matter? *J Pediatr Oncol Nurs.* 2016;33(2):129–136. doi:10.1177/1043454215600155

16. Rubenstein J, Klick J. Pediatric palliative care: Focusing on helping patients live best life. August 2, 2019. American Academy of Pediatrics News. https://www.aappublications.org/news/2019/08/02/focus080219

17. Dahlin C. *Palliative Nursing: Scope and Standards of Practice.* 6th ed. Pittsburgh, PA: Hospice and Palliative Nurses Association; 2021.

18. van Breemen C, Johnston J, Carwana M, Louie P. Serious illness conversations in pediatrics: A case review. *Children (Basel).* 2020;7(8):102. Published 2020 Aug 18. doi:10.3390/children7080102

19. Lotz JD, Jox RJ, Borasio GD, Führer M. Pediatric advance care planning from the perspective of health care professionals: A qualitative interview study. *Palliat Med.* 2015;29(3):212–222. doi:10.1177/0269216314552091

20. Sanderson A, Hall AM, Wolfe J. Advance care discussions: Pediatric clinician preparedness and practices. *J Pain Symptom Manage.* 2016;51(3):520–528. doi:10.1016/j.jpainsymman.2015.10.014

21. Postier A, Catrine K, Remke S. Interdisciplinary pediatric palliative care team involvement in compassionate extubation at home: From shared decision-making to bereavement. *Children (Basel).* 2018;5(3):37. Published 2018 Mar 7. doi:10.3390/children5030037

22. National POLST Paradigm. Signature requirements for a valid POLST form by state. Last update June 1, 2018. http://polst.org/wp-content/uploads/2018/06/2018.06.01-Signature-Requirements-by-State.pdf

23. Izumi S, Noble BN, Candrian CB, et al. Health care worker perceptions of gaps and opportunities to improve hospital-to-hospice transitions. *J Palliat Med.* 2020;23(7):900–906. doi:10.1089/jpm.2019.0513

24. Teoli D, Bhardwaj A. Hospice appropriate diagnoses. [Updated 2021 Aug 7]. In: StatPearls [Internet]. Treasure Island (FL): StatPearls Publishing; 2021 Jan. https://www.ncbi.nlm.nih.gov/books/NBK538196/

25. National Hospice and Palliative Care Organization. *Standards of Practice For Pediatric Palliative Care: Professional Development and Resource Series.* Alexandria, VA: National Coalition for Hospice and Palliative Care; 2019. https://www.nhpco.org/wp-content/uploads/2019/07/Pediatric_Standards.pdf

26. Wojcik MH, Schwartz TS, Yamin I, et al. Genetic disorders and mortality in infancy and early childhood: Delayed diagnoses and missed opportunities. *Genet Med.* 2018;20(11):1396–1404. doi:10.1038/gim.2018.17

27. Musumeci M, Chidambaram O. Medicaid's role for children with special health care needs: A look at eligibility, services, and spending. Kaiser Family Foundation. June 12, 2019. https://www.kff.org/medicaid/issue-brief/medicaids-role-for-children-with-special-health-care-needs-a-look-at-eligibility-services-and-spending/

28. Keim-Malpass J, Hart TG, Miller JR. Coverage of palliative and hospice care for pediatric patients with a life-limiting illness: A policy brief. *J Pediatr Health Care.* 2013;27(6):511–516. doi:10.1016/j.pedhc.2013.07.011

29. Dingfield L, Bender L, Harris P, et al. Comparison of pediatric and adult hospice patients using electronic medical record data from nine hospices in the United States, 2008–2012. *J Palliat Med.* 2015;18(2):120–126. doi:10.1089/jpm.2014.0195

30. Meier D, Silvers A. *Serious Illness Strategies for Health Systems, Health Plans, and ACOs.* New York: Center to Advance Palliative Care; 2021. https://www.capc.org/strategies/

31. Gans D, Hadler MW, Chen X, et al. Cost analysis and policy implications of a pediatric palliative care program. *J Pain Symptom Manage.* 2016;52(3):329–335. doi:10.1016/j.jpainsymman.2016.02.020

32. Chirico J, Donnelly JP, Gupton A, et al. Costs of care and location of death in community-based pediatric palliative care. *J Palliat Med.* 2019;22(5):517–521. doi:10.1089/jpm.2018.0276

33. Goldhagen J, Fafard M, Komatz K, Eason T, Livingood WC. Community-based pediatric palliative care for health related quality of life, hospital utilization and costs lessons learned from a pilot study. *BMC Palliat Care.* 2016;15:73. doi:10.1186/s12904-016-0138-z

34. Bogetz JF, Friebert S. Defining success in pediatric palliative care while tackling the quadruple aim. *J Palliat Med.* 2017;20(2):116–119. doi:10.1089/jpm.2016.0389

35. Lustbader D, Mudra M, Romano C, et al. The impact of a home-based palliative care program in an accountable care organization. *J Palliat Med.* 2017;20(1):23–28. doi:10.1089/jpm.2016.0265

36. Lori A. Legano, Larry W. Desch, Stephen A. Messner, et al. Maltreatment of Children With Disabilities. Pediatrics May 2021; 147 (5): e2021050920. 10.1542/peds.2021-050920

37. Wang T, Lund B. Categories of information need expressed by parents of individuals with rare genetic disorders in a Facebook community group: A case study with implications for information professionals. *J Consumer Health Internet.* 2020;24(1):20–34. doi:10.1080/15398285.2020.1713700

38. Holmen H, Riiser K, Winger A. Home-based pediatric palliative care and electronic health: Systematic mixed methods review. *J Med Internet Res.* 2020;22(2):e16248. doi:10.2196/16248

39. Vaughn J, Gollarahalli S, Shaw RJ, et al. Mobile health technology for pediatric symptom monitoring: A feasibility study. *Nurs Res.* 2020;69(2):142–148. doi:10.1097/NNR.0000000000000403

40. Bosch A, Wager J, Zernikow B, et al. Life-limiting conditions at a university pediatric tertiary care center: A cross-sectional study. *J Palliat Med.* 2018;21(2):169–176. doi:10.1089/jpm.2017.0020

41. Arthur KC, Mangione-Smith R, Burkhart Q, et al. Quality of care for children with medical complexity: An analysis of continuity of care as a potential quality indicator. *Acad Pediatr.* 2018;18(6):669–676. doi:10.1016/j.acap.2018.04.009

42. Kaye EC, Snaman JM, Baker JN. Pediatric palliative oncology: Bridging silos of care through an embedded model. *J Clin Oncol.* 2017;35(24):2740–2744. doi:10.1200/JCO.2017.73.1356

43. Kerr AM, Harrington NG, Scott AM. Communication and the appraisal of uncertainty: Exploring parents' communication with credible authorities in the context of chronic childhood illness. *Health Commun.* 2019;34(2):201–211. doi:10.1080/10410236.2017.1399508

44. Weaver MS, Robinson JE, Shostrom VK, Hinds PS. Telehealth acceptability for children, family, and adult hospice nurses when integrating the pediatric palliative inpatient provider during sequential rural home hospice visits. *J Palliat Med.* 2020;23(5):641–649. doi:10.1089/jpm.2019.0450

45. Kaye EC, Gattas M, Kiefer A, et al. Provision of palliative and hospice care to children in the community: A population study of hospice nurses. *J Pain Symptom Manage.* 2019;57(2):241–250. doi:10.1016/j.jpainsymman.2018.10.509

46. Kaye EC, Abramson ZR, Snaman JM, Friebert SE, Baker JN. Productivity in pediatric palliative care: Measuring and monitoring an elusive metric. *J Pain Symptom Manage.* 2017;53(5):952–961. doi:10.1016/j.jpainsymman.2016.12.326

47. Cochran D, Saleem S, Khowaja-Punjwani S, Lantos JD. Cross-cultural differences in communication about a dying child. *Pediatrics.* Nov 2017;140(5):e20170690. doi:10.1542/peds.2017-0690

48. Shedge R, Krishan K, Warrier V, et al. Postmortem changes. [Updated 2020 Jul 27]. In: StatPearls [Internet]. Treasure Island (FL): StatPearls Publishing; 2021 Jan. https://www.ncbi.nlm.nih.gov/books/NBK539741/

49. Battista V, LaRoigione V. Pediatric hospice and palliative care. In: Ferrell B, Paice J. ed. *Oxford Textbook of Palliative Nursing.* 5th ed. New York: Oxford University Press; 2019: 708–727.

50. Brimble MJ, Anstey S, Davies J. Long-term nurse-parent relationships in paediatric palliative care: A narrative literature review. *Int J Palliat Nurs.* 2019;25(11):542–550. doi:10.12968/ijpn.2019.25.11.542

51. USA House of Representatives. Text—H.R.5041—115th Congress (2017-2018): Safe Disposal of Unused Medication Act. Congress. gov. Library of Congress. HR 5041. Washington DC. 2017–2018. https://www.congress.gov/bill/115th-congress/house-bill/5041

52. Medication Safety in Hospice and Palliative Care Settings. *J Hosp Palliat Nurs.* 2019;21(4):E24–E27. doi:10.1097/NJH.0000000000000582

53. Weingarten K, Macapagal F, Parker D. Virtual reality: Endless potential in pediatric palliative care: A case report. *J Palliat Med.* 2020;23(1):147–149. doi:10.1089/jpm.2019.0207

54. Weaver MS, Neumann ML, Navaneethan H, Robinson JE, Hinds PS. Human touch via touchscreen: Rural nurses' experiential perspectives on telehealth use in pediatric hospice care. *J Pain Symptom Manage.* 2020;60(5):1027–1033. doi:10.1016/j.jpainsymman.2020.06.003

55. National Consensus Project for Quality Palliative Care. *Clinical Practice Guidelines for Quality Palliative Care.* 4th ed. Richmond, VA: National Hospice and Palliative Care Coalition; 2018. https://www.nationalcoalitionhpc.org/ncp/.

56. Center to Advance Palliative Care. *Pediatric Palliative Care: Field Guide.* A Catalog of tools and Training to Promote Innovation, Development and Growth New York: Center to Advance Palliative Care; 2019.

57. Cacciatore J, Thieleman K, Lieber AS, Blood C, Goldman R. The long road to farewell: The needs of families with dying children. *Omega (Westport).* 2019;78(4):404–420. doi:10.1177/0030222817697418

58. Jalmsell L, Kontio T, Stein M, Henter JI, Kreicbergs U. On the child's own initiative: Parents communicate with their dying child about death. *Death Stud.* 2015;39(1–5):111–117. doi:10.1080/07481187.2014.913086

59. Perlo J, Balik B, Swensen S, Kabcenell A, Landsman J, Feeley D. *IHI Framework for Improving Joy in Work.* IHI White Paper. Cambridge, MA: Institute for Healthcare Improvement; 2017. http://www.ihi.org/resources/Pages/IHIWhitePapers/Framework-Improving-Joy-in-Work.aspx

60. National Academy of Medicine (NAM). *Action Collaborative Knowledge Hub and Resources: Action Collaborative on Clinician Well-Being and Resilience.* Washington, DC: NAM; 2019. https://nam.edu/initiatives/clinician-resilience-and-well-being/.

61. Altilio T, Dahlin C, Remke SS, Tucker R, Weissman D. *Strategies for Maximizing the Health/Function of Palliative Care Teams: A Resource Monograph.* New York: Center to Advance Palliative Care; 2014.

62. Donohue PK, Williams EP, Wright-Sexton L, Boss RD. "It's relentless": Providers' experience of pediatric chronic critical illness. *J Palliat Med.* 2018;21(7):940–946. doi:10.1089/jpm.2017.0397

63. Il bel far niente. Blog. Julian of Norwich. https://ilbelfarniente.wordpress.com/tag/julian-of-norwich/

31.

COMMUNICATION IN PEDIATRIC PALLIATIVE CARE

Mallory Fossa, Julia McBee, and Rachel Rusch

KEY POINTS

- Expert communication skills are essential for the pediatric palliative advanced practice registered nurse (PP APRN) to navigate the myriad of pediatric healthcare experiences.

- As a part of the interdisciplinary palliative care team, the PP APRN is integral to eliciting goals and values with families from consult, through end-of-life, and into bereavement.

- Building on the foundation of nursing, the PP APRN is in an ideal position to bridge the medical and psychosocial aspects of pediatric care.

Only through communication can human life hold meaning.
    Paulo Freire

CASE STUDY 1: INVESTMENT VISIT OVER TIME

Allison was a 5-month-old infant girl born prematurely at 30 weeks gestational age with tetrasomy 22q11 and progressive maxillomandibular syngnathia and tracheobronchomalacia. After an emergent tracheostomy placement at her local, rural out-of-state hospital, she was transferred to the Children's Hospital neonatal intensive care unit (NICU) for craniofacial surgical reconstruction. The surgery was considered "elective" with the hope that reconstruction could eventually improve her quality of life. The pediatric palliative advanced practice registered nurse (PP APRN) and pediatric palliative care (PPC) team were introduced to Allison and her mother, Jill, early in her admission for support, given the anticipated lengthy and complicated hospital stay.

Allison's NICU course was initially stable and the PPC team visited 2–3 times a week, building strong rapport and addressing quality-of-life issues which were small but impactful. Since Allison and Jill were out of state, they were alone in the city, with limited psychosocial supports. One intervention was to obtain Jill some "comfort food" and guide her to a local prayer group.

In one of the early visits, Jill shared her worries surrounding Allison's requirement for postoperative opioids after revealing her partner's death from a heroin overdose 3 years prior. The PP APRN validated and normalized these fears and provided anticipatory guidance about the safety and benefits of adequate analgesia and pain management with opioids.

After a month in the NICU, Allison underwent a craniofacial surgical reconstruction. Unfortunately, Allison developed two bilateral middle cerebral artery strokes and evolving herniation with a poor prognosis and profound neurological impairment even if she survived. Jill was devastated and requested meeting with the PPC team to discuss next steps and options for care. The PP APRN and PPC team supported Jill and the NICU team through their difficult decision to discontinue life-sustaining therapy and allow for a natural death. The PP APRN worked alongside the NICU team to optimize Allison's symptom management at end of life. The PP APRN and social worker followed Jill and her extended family into bereavement and coordinated the transport of Allison's ashes back to their hometown.

INTRODUCTION

Empathetic and effective communication is essential to providing high-quality palliative care to children with life-threatening and serious illnesses in both inpatient and outpatient settings. Recommendations and standards of practice provided within the *Palliative Nursing: Scope and Standards of Practice* and by the American Academy of Pediatrics, the National Consensus Project, Center to Advance Palliative Care, and the National Hospice and Palliative Care Organization underscore the necessity of developmentally appropriate communication for the child, and family.[1-5] One of the main tasks of the pediatric palliative advanced practice registered nurse (PP APRN) within the interdisciplinary team (IDT) is to align with the child and family, build trust, and create an individualized and goal-concordant plan of care. Along with dedicated psychosocial providers, PP APRNs often serve as the continuity members of the team, providing longitudinal support as other clinicians rotate on and off service. PP APRNs are educated to practice expert and efficient communication throughout a child's illness trajectory.[6] As continuity providers, PP APRNs act as communication liaisons in a variety of situations, including but not limited to the following:

- Eliciting goals of care and assessing a family's and child's understanding of illness and prognostic awareness.

- Respecting the family's and child's communication preferences for receiving and sharing information.

- Assessing and honoring the family's cultural and spiritual preferences surrounding experience with illness.

- Providing pharmacological and nonpharmacological interventions focused on the child's physical, emotional, psychosocial, and spiritual well-being consistent with goals of care.

- Ensuring collaborative communication among care teams.

- Leading open and honest communication across care settings between the family and the team members: primary care providers, pediatric subspecialists, psychosocial clinicians, community palliative providers, community hospice providers, therapists, and school professionals.

- Communicating changes in illness trajectory and prognosis, especially as the child approaches end of life.

- Supporting the child's and family's voice in medical decision-making and advance care planning.[1,3]

This chapter aims to elucidate the role of the PP APRN in providing high-quality pediatric palliative care (PPC) and provide strategies to develop and improve communication throughout the child's experience with illness, their death, and the family's bereavement.

COMMUNICATING WITH CHILDREN, ADOLESCENTS, AND YOUNG ADULTS AND THEIR FAMILIES

UNIQUE COMMUNICATION NEEDS OF THE PEDIATRIC PATIENT

The World Health Organization defines palliative care as "the prevention and relief of suffering of adult and pediatric patients and their families facing the problems associated with life-threatening illness. These problems include the physical, psychological, social and spiritual suffering of patients, and psychological, social and spiritual suffering of family members."[7] In order to achieve the goals of PPC for the mind body and spirit, communication is essential. PP APRNs draws on their experiences at the bedside to provide holistic and humanistic care synonymous with the ethos of palliative nursing practice.[6,8] A major aspect of palliative nursing is communication. To achieve this, the PP APRN utilizes both verbal and nonverbal communication techniques: establishing eye contact with the patient and family, listening carefully, pausing for moments of silence, and staying present and engaged when working with children and their families.[6,9,10]

Children vary from adults in that their ability to understand concepts depends on their age and development. Providers, including APRNs, should familiarize themselves with developmental concepts when working with children, adolescents, and their families.[3] While some parents and clinicians may be uncomfortable with it, children are able to provide insight into how they experience their own health and care.[11] Table 32.2 demonstrates general principles of childhood development and the understanding of death and illness for the typically developing child. When communicating with children and their families, it is important to give clear, honest, and consistent information.[12–14]

Because there are developmental differences between children and adults, decision-making and communication varies from that with adult because with children, discussions occur with the parents. Parents have shared the importance of feeling partnered with the child's medical team.[15] This is defined as shared decision-making, where together the parents and the medical team make decisions for the child with their best interest in mind and which are consistent with the family's

Table 31.1 FIVE DOMAINS OF CHILD AND FAMILY ASSESSMENT

DOMAIN	FOCUS	QUESTIONS TO ASK
1. Who is the child?	Learning who the child is as a person	Tell me about (child's name). How would your friends describe you? What does a good day look like for (child's name)? How do they show you when they are happy? What does a difficult day look like for (child's name)? How do they show you they are upset or in pain?
2. Assessing decision-maker understanding of the illness	Eliciting the decision-maker's insight of the illness	What is your understanding of your child's illness? Tell me about your medical journey . . . What have your doctors told you about your child's name condition?
3. Eliciting hopes	Eliciting hopes and dreams for the future	What are you hoping for? Given what the doctors have told you, what are you most hopeful for?
4. Eliciting worries and fears	Assessing how they are coping	What are you most worried about? Are their other things you are worried about? What keeps you up at night?
5. Strengths and Support	Evaluating how they finding strength and support	Where do you draw your strength? Who is supporting you? Do you belong to a faith community? Do faith or spiritually provide support to you?

From Waldman, Levine[16]; Feudtner et al.[17]; and Waldman, Wolfe.[18]

values and beliefs.[3,15,19] Parents are often granted the ability to make decisions on the behalf of their child, including adolescents. Decision-making can fall on a spectrum. Children and adolescents who demonstrate understanding of information relevant to their choice and express reason and rationally may be capable of making certain decisions.[3,19]

INITIAL CONSULT OF THE PEDIATRIC PATIENT

INTRODUCING THE TEAM

When meeting a patient and their family for the first time, it is important for the PP APRN be aware of how or what the family may have been told about PPC. This can be simply be done by asking the family or young adult what they were told when first meeting them. The Center to Advance Palliative Care (CAPC) has developed key phrases and messaging identified through interviews and focus groups with patients and caregivers, including the following descriptions of palliative care:

- Palliative care provides an extra layer of support for families and children with serious illness.

- Palliative care can help provide the best quality of life for children and families.

- Palliative care is a partnership between the child, family, and all medical specialists.

- Palliative care can help children and families manage pain, symptoms, and the stress of serious illness.

- Palliative care is appropriate at any age and stage of serious illness and can be provided concurrently with curative treatment.[4]

Families report valuing sincere communication and genuine relationships with providers.[20] The PP APRN is frequently the first team member to clarify the role of the palliative care team, often utilizing language to destigmatize any associations the child or family may have with the term "palliative care." Patient-centered language should be employed and modeled by the PP APRN when describing the role of palliative care. The PP APRN can use an array of these examples when introducing the team and the services provided before setting up the conversation for the initial consult.[13] The APRN should also assess the nonverbal cues of the patient and family and/or ask if it is a convenient time to meet with the family. If it is not, the APRN can arrange a time to return to complete the consult.[10]

THE PEDIATRIC PALLIATIVE CARE CONSULT

When establishing a relationship with the child or family, the PP APRN can promote an understanding of what is important and how the patient and family perceive the care they are receiving. Fostering this communication begins with an assessment of the child's current status and the patient or

family's daily experience. In a PPC consult, there are generally five domains to explore with the child and/or family: (1) learning who the child is as a person, (2) assessing the decision-maker's understanding of illness, (3) eliciting hopes and worries in the context of their life, (4) assessing how they are coping, and (5) determining how are they finding strength and support[16] (Table 31.1). The five domains are helpful across the spectrum of the relationship and trajectory of illness, from initial consultation to end of life, and are dynamic and evolving. While conducting this initial conversation, the single biggest intervention that the PP APRN will do is to listen.[10,12] It is important to remember that listening is being fully present; physically, emotionally, and mentally.[10]

Establishing a trusting and safe environment is critical to communication and this conversation.[10,16] By taking the time to learn about the child's or young adult's identity or personhood, the APRN can foster a deeply meaningful moment within the chaos of the medical situation.[16] It models to the child, adolescent, or young adult and their family that knowing who they are outside of their medical condition is important to care delivery.[3] This information, given either by the child or the family, can provide the PP APRN with insight to how the parents view the child and/or what makes the individual the person they are.[16] Table 31.1 illustrates examples of questions or statements that can be made to help elicit this information.

Once the PP APRN has identified key components of the child's personhood, the conversation can lead to assessing the

Table 31.2 CHILDHOOD DEVELOPMENT AND DEATH UNDERSTANDING

AGE	CONCEPT
Infants and Toddlers (0-2 years old)	Infants experience loss through their environment as they learn object permanence
	Death is experienced as separation or abandonment
	No cognitive understanding of death
Early Childhood (2–6 years old)	Magical thinking occurs in that unconnected actions or behaviors may have caused the death of sibling or family member
	Death is thought to be reversible or temporary
	Death may be seen as a punishment
School Age (6–11 years old)	Gradual awareness that death is final cessation of life
	May believe only happens to elderly, animals, or pets
	Concrete reasoning allowing understanding of cause and effect
	May ask direct questions about death
Adolescents/ Young Adults (>11 years old)	Understand death is finite and universal
	All people and self will die, though latter is far off
	Comprehend physical and biological process of death
	Abstract and philosophical reasoning

From Crozier, Handcock[13]; Jonas et al.[14]

patient's and family's understanding of the medical condition. The information gleaned from questions around a parent's or child's understanding allows the clinical team to help tailor information in the future or identify areas where further information is necessary for future decision-making.[12,16] This can also aid the PP APRN in advocating for the child and family based on what is shared in the conversation.[3]

Parents encounter frequent decision points as they navigate the care for their child with a serious illness. Often, they are attempting to find a path which will result in full recovery or a return to previous baseline. Sometimes it can be difficult for parents or decision-makers to determine whether treatment decisions are leading them toward their desired goal or not.[17] Research has revealed that "parents have deeply held, diverse beliefs about their principal duties for their children."[21] By eliciting these beliefs, the PP APRN can better understand the framework within which parents are making decisions and how they are thinking about what is important for their child. A few questions include, "What do you think is most important for you to focus on?" or "What do you feel you most need to do to be, in your own judgment, a good parent?"[22] As the illness journey proceeds, how parents consider the five domains changes along with their definition of "a good parent." It is therefore important to regularly explore these values with parents, especially as their child's illness progresses.[16,17,21,22] While it may sound counterintuitive to ask about what a parent or a young person hopes for, doing so offers a useful baseline assessment. When the disease progresses, the recognition that the prior hope for a cure is now likely unattainable facilitates the exploration of other hopes that may be important to the young person and family.[16]

It is important to be aware that parents may be holding worries in their mind and heart yet choose not to say them out loud. They report that it is difficult to share these feelings with family, friends, and the healthcare team. Some parents of children with serious illness prefer to convey a positive outward expression, holding their true feelings close.[17] Parents, especially mothers, often experience judgment by others, including family, friends, and community, for their decisions and behaviors.[17,23] The result may be emotional miscues and consequent miscommunication with the healthcare team.

The PP APRN must be mindful to evaluate communication effectiveness during each family encounter, assessing and shifting strategies as necessary. It may take multiple encounters before a parent can verbalize a deep concern. When members of the child's healthcare team comment that "the parents don't get it," the PP APRN advocates for the parents in conveying they "do get it," they just choose carefully when and to whom to acknowledge their understanding, fears, and worries.[19] Connecting with the consulting team or provider before the visit can provide an opportunity for the PP APRN to potentially focus on eliciting certain concerns, thus better evaluating a family's understanding.[3]

An essential component of a consultation is the assessment of the psychosocial support system in place for this child and family.[16] This is a cultural assessment that includes the community resources in place and sources of strength and support. Additionally, a brief spirituality screening should be completed.[3,16] While the goal is not to directly engage in a theological discussion, the PP APRN should identify spiritual distress as well as spiritual care needs and, when necessary, refer or offer spiritual care services.[3,16]

In closing the visit, the PP APRN should acknowledge and thank the child or adolescent and family for the information shared. Discussion then shifts to next steps in the relationship and how the palliative care team will support them.[16]

When discussing the consult with the consulting team, either in the hospital or in the outpatient setting, it is most respectful to use a person-centered approach. This presentation includes the child's name, history, and diagnosis versus labeling the child by their disease process. For example: "Jane is a 5-year-old girl with a history of AML, admitted for initiation of chemotherapy in the setting of progressive disease" versus "a 5-year-old leukemic admitted for chemo after failing multiple therapies." PP APRNs can model care directed at the whole patient, not just the disease process, by focusing on the physical, social, emotional, and spiritual needs of child and family.[24] Table 31.3 provides examples of how to rephrase language when communicating with patients and families.

ESTABLISHING RAPPORT AND INVESTMENT VISITS OVER TIME

Building trust, taking a big picture view of the patient and family, and understanding their unique narrative in times of both health and illness is imperative to providing high-quality palliative care. Unlike the adult population, children receiving palliative care may live for more than a year after the initial inpatient palliative care consultation. This may allow for more time to establish rapport and invest in longitudinal relationships.[25] The nature of PPC consultations vary by setting. In the inpatient setting, consult requests are most often for assistance with symptom management, followed by facilitating communication, assistance in decision-making, discharge planning, and, less often, discussions regarding resuscitation status.[26] Outpatient consults are generally for establishing goals of care in the medically complex patient and symptom management.

After the initial consultation, even when a substantial role for PPC is not immediately apparent, the PP APRN and PPC team can engage in "investment visits" with the child and family. Investment visits are otherwise known as "holding the space" or "showing up." Although these visits can appear like idle "chit chat," in reality they can aid in rapport building with patients and families and encourage self-care and coping for caretakers and patients. Moreover, these visits allow for development of connections with the family and the entire care team, which fosters improved collaboration and family support at times of unexpected crisis. Frequent visits in times of stability help families associate the PPC team with moments of positivity and hope.[27] Use of an IDT is critical because it provides continuity of care among all team members.

The story of Allison and Jill highlights the importance of communication among care teams and the investment in future relationships with primary and consulting providers. It highlights the importance of investment visits as a key element to providing high-quality palliative care to an infant

Table 31.3 PEDIATRIC PALLIATIVE CARE COMMUNICATION FAUX-PAS AND TIPS

TOPIC	COMMON RESPONSE	UNINTENDED MESSAGE	ALTERNATIVE WORDING
Discussion about pain management	"We can best treat your pain by using narcotics."	"And you may become a drug addict."	"We can best treat your pain by using opioid or pain medications...."
Discussion about defining goals of care	"What would you like us to do if...?"	Implies that the patient/family can choose from a menu of options.	Use open-ended questions to define treatment goals: "What's most important to you/for your child right now?"
Discussion of disease-directed therapy	"We can use this experimental agent or we can do nothing."	"If we don't opt for medical management, we are 'giving up.'"	"Whether or not we continue with disease-directed therapy, we will care for you and do our best to manage symptoms and optimize your quality of life."
Discussion about medically administered nutrition and hydration	"We could stop the TPN/G-tube feeds."	Discontinuing supplemental nutrition means starving the patient to death.	"Our recommendation is that your child's body is at a point where medically administered nutrition is not going to be of benefit. In fact, it may cause harm and/or suffering."
Discussion about resuscitation	"Do you want us to do everything?"	What would a "good parent" do?	"You have made the best decisions possible and done everything to help your child survive. There are no more medical therapies we know of that will change the disease course. Based on our conversations we would recommend limiting attempts at resuscitation."

From Levetown.[71]

and mother in the NICU. This case not only elucidates the necessity for holistic, patient- and family-focused care but also underscores the multifaceted role of the palliative care APRN across the child's illness trajectory.

CULTURAL SENSITIVITY, HUMILITY, AND ATTUNEMENT IN PPC COMMUNICATION

Culture frames one's understanding and responses to illness or death.[3,29] Personal, familial, and community culture offers structure for daily living, influencing how emotions are experienced and communicated. Learning about a child's and family's experience of living with serious illness from a cultural perspective can provide profound insight into their values, expectations, and hopes that may guide future care-planning discussions. The following questions may be helpful in clarifying the family's understanding of the child's condition as influenced by their cultural or spiritual beliefs and values.[16,30]

QUESTIONS IN SUPPORT OF EXPLORING PERSONAL AND FAMILY CULTURE

What is happening (has happened) to your child from your perspective?

What do you think is causing (caused) this to happen?

How is your family being affected (have you and your family been affected) by what has happened?

Has your family experienced anything similar to this before?

What meaning does this experience have for you and your family?

Health professionals must approach each patient and family system with an intention toward cultural humility and sensitivity.[31] Cultural humility and cultural sensitivity call on the PP APRN to be humble and aware of their own deficiencies in knowledge of other cultures; it requires continued education and the investigation of implicit and explicit bias.[32] PP APRNs may be an important voice in aligning and speaking thoughtfully to a family's individual value system, especially when it may differ from that of the personal perspectives of a primary medical team.[3] Continued education, in partnership with psychosocial colleagues when possible, will aid in providing culturally respectful and supportive communication, particularly for marginalized populations. Please refer to Chapter 20, "Health Disparities in Palliative Care and Social Determinants of Health," for additional information and guidance.

The PP APRN, in partnership with IDT members when possible, may also assess for culturally influenced communication cues by watching how family members interact with each other and the medical team, noticing personal space or boundaries, eye contact, or the extent of physical touch. These observations can then be communicated to the team as the partnership between the patient, family, and PPC team continues.

Noticing a parent's nonverbal behavior can provide opportunity to glean important insights about how best to provide culturally respectful communication. For example, the PP APRN observed a father's distraught behavior after participating in his daughter's family-centered PICU rounds. The PP APRN remarked, "I'm noticing that something is troubling you." To which the father responded in a heightened tone, "All of these medical details are keeping me from my real duty, praying for my daughter's healing." The father then shared his beliefs about healing as a practicing Christian Scientist. While the father desired PICU medical interventions for his daughter—something that he mentioned was not supported by his church elders—the daily rounding information conflicted with his deeply felt responsibility to pray for healing. The PP APRN helped the parents and PICU team to determine a rounding schedule that created a supported environment for the father to remain in prayer when needed.

Medical interpreters should be used whenever English is not the family's primary language. In one study exploring the experiences of Mexican American and Chinese American families, parents described more anger, distress, and sadness during their child's illness when interpreters were absent because trust eroded when parents felt they were provided insufficient information.[33] In preparation, clinicians should inform the medical interpreter about the nature of the planned discussion and then debrief accordingly, especially if interpretation involves delivering difficult or sad news.

Even though PP APRNs must do their best to understand a family's cultural lenses, they can never fully understand another's perception. As an example, one PP APRN entered a baby's room with the goal of learning her family's progress in decision-making for a potential surgery. The grandmother was weeping as she rocked her granddaughter. The anguish on her face was evident, prompting the APRN to say, "Your tears reflect much emotion." The grandmother replied, "I weep because I have not received a call today from my family in Syria. They usually call each day, so that I can know they are safe from the violence happening in our country. Children are being murdered there by the minute! Here, I safely hold my granddaughter in my arms, knowing your team will do everything to save her life. Yet back home, life is being wasted, thrown away. How . . . how do I make sense of all of this?" The APRN sat quietly with the grandmother as she rocked and wept, recognizing through this exchange that this family was holding more on their minds than the PPC team could ever comprehend. The PP APRN demonstrated cultural sensitivity as well as created space and acknowledgment of the situation by listening and remaining silent, showing that she understood the significance of what was said.[10,12]

SPIRITUALITY AND COMMUNICATION

Patients and family members may share their spiritual and/or religious beliefs when reflecting on their ongoing coping and their hopes for the future. When possible, partnership with spiritual care providers and chaplains ensures comprehensive support around one's individual and familial spiritual needs. In this way, the PP APRN respects the expertise found within collaboration with chaplain colleagues and maintains appropriate therapeutic boundaries when engaging in communication around one's religious and spiritual beliefs.[34]

At times, a family may share their hope for a miracle or for divine intervention to cure their child of their illness. This may be seen by some clinicians as a distressing expression of denial, ending further supportive and productive communication. The PP APRN, in partnership with the interdisciplinary PPC team, may see this as an opportunity for further assessment and learning about a family's expressions of hope.[35] After thoughtful and supportive assessment to assure that the family has an appropriate understanding of their child's condition, the PP APRN may discover that the hope for a miracle may be a space of helpful coping for a family because it may be too difficult to live in the space of worry around a child's death in every moment. Utilizing this language to communicate that hope and worry can exist side by side for parents, the PP APRN can provide a safe and supportive place to reflect on both. Some helpful language can be provided through VitalTalk's proposed NURSE statements[10,36] listed here.

Naming: Name the child's and family's expressed emotion.

Understanding: Empathize with and acknowledge the child's and family's emotional response.

Respecting: Praise the child and family for their expert role in their child's care.

Supporting: Demonstrate support of the family's needs and/or decisions.

Exploring: Ask the child and family to elaborate their feelings, concerns, or hopes.

Some examples of potential language to use when engaging families around themes of hope include the following:

What I hear you saying is that you are worried for your child's future and also want to hold your hope for their survival.

What would a miracle look like to you and your family?

Hope and worry can exist side by side. I deeply admire and appreciate your openness in sharing this with us.

What else do you hope for?

We hope so, too. And we are worried.

CHILDREN'S VOICES, FAMILIES, AND DECISION-MAKING

CASE STUDY 2: ADVANCE CARE PLANNING WITH THE ADOLESCENT OR YOUNG ADULT

Jamilla, a 17-year-old girl, first learned of her diagnosis of rhabdomyosarcoma in the pediatric ICU. She had been admitted for respiratory failure due to pleural effusions from her metastatic lung disease. Jamilla shared with her nurses that she was scared of treatment, "If I'm going to die anyway, what is the point?" Due to her presentation, palliative care was consulted shortly after diagnosis. Jamilla revealed feeling scared about the side effects of treatment, specifically the pain. She wanted to maintain her identity and independence. While she felt uncertain about pursuing treatment, she acknowledged that she would move forward with disease-directed therapy, mostly for her family. It was important for Jamilla to have assurance that her team would manage her symptoms and have open and honest communication with her and her family. Although her parents understood that Jamilla's cancer was very aggressive and that there was a high likelihood she would relapse from her disease, they remained very hopeful for a cure. Together, they all agreed to pursue disease-directed therapy.

It became clear that Jamilla was thinking about her mortality and wanted a place to share what was important to her. The PP APRN introduced Jamilla and her family to *Five Wishes*. Among the things she documented was her desire to die at home, her desire to have her hair washed by her mother, and her wish for people to pray for her "because my parents would want it." Jamilla even added a list of songs she wanted played at her memorial service in the margins of the Five Wishes document. When her cancer recurred, Jamilla agreed to second-line treatment although she was uncertain if she would pursue further chemotherapy. Her mother was tearful and supportive, recognizing Jamilla's individual experience of her disease and her mortality. Jamilla shared how she worried about letting her oncologist down by stopping treatment. The PP APRN acknowledged Jamilla's bravery and thoughtfulness, advocating for her with her oncologist. The PP APRN coordinated Jamilla's admission to hospice to honor her wishes of being at home with her family and for her symptoms to be managed as her cancer progressed.

Listening carefully to the child or young adult's experience of living with serious illness represents the heart of PPC. The child's voice is best heard through the combined skills and expertise of the IDT. The PP APRN collaborates with a variety of expressive therapies, including art, music, play, pet, and bibliotherapy, to connect with children, helping them to communicate their experiences at their own pace. As play is the language of children, play therapists, child life specialists, or psychologists trust the child's inner direction to lead play and conversation, allowing them to express their fears, hopes, and perceptions of the situation.[10,36] When children or young adults are diagnosed with a life-limiting illness, they may worry about the loved ones they may be leaving behind or of being forgotten.[12] Engaging in legacy activities have helped these young people communicate and strengthen bonds even after death.[12,37,38] By partnering with other members of the IDT, different age-appropriate activities can be offered to the patient, including but not limited to storytelling, song-writing, creating a digital storyboard, or simply drawing pictures.[12,39]

As the PP APRN builds a trusting and open relationship with the child or adolescent and family, it is important to explore the child's own understanding of their illness or prognosis. These conversations are often delicate, and the PP APRN should be aware of the patient's nonverbal cues.[10,40] Using or modifying the five domain questions can help the team understand what the young person is thinking of or worried about.[16,41] Identifying the patient's personal goals, beliefs, and values as they relate to quality of life is the initial and essential element to advance care planning conversations.[12,41] When the palliative care team worked with Jamilla, they first worked to establish her understanding of her disease as well as the treatment plan. They were able to learn that it was important for Jamilla to maintain her own sense of "personhood," which helped to establish the framework by which they worked with Jamilla and her family. While families may discuss future issues without the help of a skilled facilitator, having a clinician for more challenging conversations, such as those around advance care planning, may allow for improved communication between all parties.[42] Box 31.1 identifies tools across the age spectrum that can be used to evoke the child patient's voice.

Although a child may possess a mature understanding of their serious illness, they may choose to refrain from sharing this knowledge with others. In addition, families may engage in a phenomenon of mutual care. The child and parent(s) experience similar concerns yet attempt to protect one another from their sorrow and negative emotions or the possibility of negative outcomes by avoiding open discussion with each other.[19,43,44] Just as parents take seriously their role to protect and nurture, children want to please and live up to the expectations of parents, possibly resulting in crucial

---

Box 31.1 SUGGESTED RESOURCES TO ELICIT CONVERSATIONS WITH CHILDREN ABOUT FEELINGS AND GOALS

For School-Aged Children

My Wishes available from https://fivewishes.org/five-wishes/individuals-families/individuals-and-families/children-and-adolescents
The Invisible String, by Patrice Karst
When Someone Has a Very Serious Illness: Children Can Learn to Cope with Loss and Change, by Marge Heegaard
When the Wind Stops, by Charlotte Zolotow
How Are You Peeling, by Saxton Freymann
In My Heart, by Jo Witek

For Teens and Young Adults

5 Wishes available from www.agingwithdignity.org
Voicing My Choices available from www.agingwithdignity.org
Stanford Letter Project available from https://med.stanford.edu/letter.html
Digging Deep, a Journal for Young People Facing Health Challenges, by Rose Offner and Sheri Brisson
In My World, by Bonnie Byers Crawford and Linda Lazar (available from Center Corporation)
Stuff that Sucks: A Teen's Guide to Accepting What You Can't Change and Committing to What You Can, by Ben Sedley
When You Know You're Dying: 12 Thoughts to Guide You Through the Days Ahead, by James E. Miller

conversations left unspoken. Other times, parents recognize, understand, and wish to honor their child's cues to not speak out loud of dying but rather to focus on living.[45] When parents share their worries with the PP APRN around disclosing prognostic information with their child or adolescent, the APRN may provide examples of how often the child is already thinking about the changes in their body and that disclosure allows adequate time for them to process their illness, thus decreasing fear and anxiety of the unknown.[38,45]

COMMUNICATING WITH ADOLESCENTS AND YOUNG ADULTS

Establishing communication preferences with adolescents and young adults (AYAs) is paramount to the development of rapport as well as partnership in advance care planning. This population has described the need for honest and respectful communication as key components of relationship building, and this communication has been shown to affect the young person's perception of healthcare.[46,47] When meeting initially with the AYA patient, the PP APRN can ask questions around communication preferences including, "How do you like to hear medical information? With your family/support person? By yourself?" Acknowledging that there may be information they do not wish to hear and taking their lead shows respect for their sense of personhood. Some may wish for this information at a later date, so remaining flexible is key to communication with the AYA population.[40,48] Additionally, it is important to explore with this population from whom they would like to hear the information. Most AYAs prefer information to come from their clinicians, while others may want to hear it from their parents[40,47] When Jamilla shared with the PP APRN that she preferred to hear information from her doctors, with her parents, and ultimately made her own decisions about her care, this was communicated with the other members of the care team.

DISCLOSURE OF DIAGNOSIS AND PROGNOSIS: CHALLENGES IN THE PEDIATRIC POPULATION

Parents often worry about delivering bad news to children in an effort to protect them.[48,50] This basic parental instinct should not be overlooked or misunderstood as poor prognostic awareness. Families experience profound grief when hearing their child has a life-threatening illness, which is compounded by the idea of disclosing the diagnosis. A mother of a teen with a newly diagnosed diffuse intrinsic pontine glioma (DIPG) once tearfully stated, "I can barely comprehend what lies ahead; it makes me sick to imagine telling my son he has a year to live." Families agonize over what information should be shared and by whom. Barriers to parents disclosing a poor prognosis to their child (as described through self-report) include emotional distress and information overload, inadequate knowledge on how to disclose, and worry over burdening their children with bad news.[45,50] A father of a 10-year-old girl with metastatic osteosarcoma explained, "she should be playing soccer with her friends, not thinking about what a prosthetic leg will feel like."

There is an extensive history of clinicians also feeling uncomfortable engaging in difficult discussions regarding diagnosis and prognosis for fear of taking away hope and causing distress.[43,51] For physicians, this fear frequently comes from a lack of training in medical schools and residency programs on how to communicate difficult news.[43] For pediatric APRNs, there is a similar fear from lack of training or mentorship in delivering difficult news. The hesitancy of APRNs to discuss a poor prognosis can lead to patients misjudging their chance of cure or life prolongation, which may impact their decision-making.[43,52] In an effort to avoid openly discussing a poor prognosis, APRNs often use optimistic language and frequently wait for patients and families to ask specific questions directed at prognosis.[53]

A recent study of AYAs with cystic fibrosis (CF) revealed that patients with CF want their parents to be involved in discussions regarding prognosis and believe that their provider should be the one to initiate such disclosures.[47] Approximately one-third of the study participants reported learning of their prognosis and clinical trajectory from their CF healthcare providers, one-third deduced the progressive nature of CF from their own health decline, and the rest gleaned this knowledge from their parents or from online sources.[47] The patient participants often felt that prognosis was "sugar coated" by whomever disclosed the information, be it providers or parents. Interestingly, when patients learned of their prognosis, 62% reported no impact on future CF treatments and 38% reported a positive impact on their attitude. None of the study participants reported that disclosure had a negative impact on their emotional state or adherence to treatment regimens. The majority (77%) of patients reported that learning of their prognosis had no effect on their overall goals of care and life plans, and, if it did, it was positive.[47]

Although the evidence supports developmentally appropriate, open, and honest disclosure of diagnosis and prognosis, the matter is complex and case dependent.[43] In the field of PPC (and pediatrics in general), it is imperative to view the child as part of a larger family infrastructure influenced by history, values, culture, and religion. In particular, culture and religion may weigh heavily on a parent's willingness to disclose diagnosis and prognosis.[3,43,45] In some cases, parents may instruct medical personnel to omit facts regarding a diagnosis and, in rare cases, to even lie. In these cases, clinicians can offer a "compromise" that strikes a balance between upholding their code of ethics as clinicians and respecting a family's wishes and maintaining trust and alliance.[19,45] Helpful phrasing may include "We will honor your communication preferences with your adolescent; however, if they ask us direct questions regarding their disease and prognosis, we cannot lie."[3] Unfortunately, these instances are often fraught with distress for the interdisciplinary healthcare team, especially in cases involving adolescents.

Every family system functions differently and has its own unique communication preferences.[43,45] To build trust and rapport, clinicians must respect the framework and preferences of the family first and foremost. After receiving permission from the family to disclose a diagnosis, medical information, and prognosis, finding the right time, environment, IDT members, and developmentally appropriate language is imperative for effective communication.[10,54] Once the stage is set, it is crucial to address the child's goals, hopes, worries, understanding of illness, and coping mechanisms.

Sometimes, there may be a conflict between the culture of healthcare and the culture of the child and family. In these instances, it is helpful to further explore the family's culture, values, and belief systems.[43] It may be culturally inappropriate for some discussions to occur, or there may be the need for spiritual providers or community leaders to be part of the conversations. Discussions with parents and children regarding prognosis may evolve and shift over time as an illness progresses.[43] Repetitive attempts at forced conversations with family systems who decline communication and prognostication can cause undue distress to the child and family and border on harassment. In these cases, the risk of negatively impacting a family's experience with illness and grief and disrespecting their culture outweighs the benefit of total disclosure. Maintaining the treatment alliance and trust, openness to compromise when required, and honesty when questions are posed directly are all of paramount importance.[19,50,53]

ADVANCE CARE PLANNING

Ultimately, when eliciting the child's voice or hearing parents values, the PP APRN is initiating pediatric advance care planning conversations.[41] As a child's or AYA's disease advances, it may be helpful to have more discrete conversations around the topic of end of life. It is important to recognize that parents or patients may be reticent to engage in these difficult conversations.[52] However, those who do acknowledge that it gives them a sense of control, empowers parents to make good decisions aligned with their definition of being a good parent, and facilitates coping.[41,42,44,55] To facilitate advance care planning discussions, the PP APRN may wish to access the *Decision-Making Tool* (DMT) developed by the Pediatric Advance Care team at Seattle Children's Hospital. Similar to other tools, the DMT provides a flexible structure that addresses the medical, psychosocial, and spiritual concerns of the decision-maker.[56] Or the PP APRN may use one of the advance planning tools available from Aging with Dignity.[57] My Wishes is a child-focused tool which allows for younger, school-aged children to draw or write their responses. *Voicing My Choices* and *Five Wishes* are for AYAs. While some healthcare providers may choose to allow the AYA to work independently, working together can provide a chance to further strengthen the patient–clinician relationship.[41] When completed and signed before witnesses or notarized, *Five Wishes* is recognized in many states as a legal advance directive for persons over the age of 18.[57] When participating in these discussions with parents and young persons, the PP APRN should remain mindful of the desire to maintain hope while promoting the important conversations across the illness trajectory, even when death approaches.[41] Once the tools are completed

by the child and family, the PP APRN plays a key role in disseminating the desired plan to the entire team.

As advance care planning conversations occur, they should be documented in the chart as either an advance directive, delineation of code status, or an out-of-hospital order for life-sustaining treatment. When the health of the child appears to be declining, clinicians and parents may choose to engage in conversations around limiting interventions and the placement of do-not-resuscitate (DNR)/do-not-intubate (DNI) orders as well as other limitations to medical interventions or technology.[17,55] It should be noted that holding hope for a cure does not prohibit parents or young adults from reaching agreement on DNR/DNI orders. In fact, establishment of patient and family preferences at end of life has shown to empower decision-making and provide peace of mind.[55] Although difficult, these conversations have been documented to reduce stress, depression, and anxiety in the bereaved.[42,45] It is also important to reframe these decisions as loving decisions that minimize suffering or undue distress[58] (see Chapter 32, "Advance Care Planning").

WHEN EXPECTATIONS OF CARE BETWEEN FAMILIES AND PRACTITIONERS DIFFER

Conflict may occur when the healthcare team perceives that the child is suffering while parents are saying, "We want everything done." Often, the hope is that the PP APRN or PPC team will step in and resolve the conflict. PP APRNs play a key role in holding conversations about care choices should the child's condition deteriorate. Strong external reactions by parents or team members are often rooted in equally strong internal beliefs of wanting the best for the child. Using phrases like "I'm curious," or "Help me understand" and consciously using "and" instead of "but" are useful in drawing out the differing perspectives of the parties.[10,59]

The PP APRN can help parents consider limiting treatments or shifting the treatment focus from high-tech, invasive medical interventions to less invasive yet still intensive caring or comfort-focused measures.[22] Parents' expression of "wanting everything" done for their child is often a reflection of their fear and anticipatory grief. It is this grief that translates the parents' plea into the following sentiments, "Care for us," "Care about us," "Don't abandon us," and "We are terrified to think that our child will die."[60] In this situation, the burden of decision-making should *not* be placed on the shoulders of families with phrases that reflect an abdication of responsibility such as "You (the child/family) need to decide what you want us to do if. . . ." Rather, the APRN should partner with families, making honest recommendations for next steps in the child's care based on the team's combined medical expertise while honoring the child's and family's expertise about their values as they intertwine with the child's declining physical reality. The PP APRN can take the lead in understanding what "doing everything" means to the parents, providing affirmation of both the parents' love for the child and the team's ongoing commitment.[60,61] Table 31.3 offers language for conversations that may lead to unintended miscommunication.

CONTINUITY OF CARE: COMMUNICATION ACROSS SETTINGS

The PP APRN is in a unique position to provide continuity of care as patients and families make transitions between the community and the hospital.[62] Parents of seriously ill children have shared that it can be burdensome to reshare experiences to additional providers. While this may not be completely avoided, the PP APRN may make attempts to coordinate and collaborate with the child's caregivers when changes occur, whether in the hospital or in an outpatient setting.[62,63] By fostering communication between community providers and hospital providers, a more seamless experience may allow for improved patient and family care.

Palliative care teams may have their own home-based programs or collaborate with those in the community. Pediatrics is unique in that children under 21 qualify for concurrent care while under hospice care.[62] Even when patients qualify for home hospice, concurrent care allows pediatric patients to receive the hospice benefit while continuing with disease-directed therapies and interventions.[62,64,65] This may mean that a patient moves between acute care and the home hospice setting.[62] PP APRNs are often the bridge for communication with hospice staff to learn about ongoing conversations occurring at home regarding goals of care as well as any changes in symptom management needs. The same communication can prove beneficial as a model for home-based palliative care when available or provided by a hospice agency.[62]

When children are not on hospice and for whom ongoing communication in the outpatient setting is required, the PP APRN may provide assistance in psychosocial support as well as symptom management. Creating open lines of communication between the child and family and the PP APRN allows for this ongoing communication no matter the location of the child (home or hospital).[3] Phone calls and email can be productive and helpful ways to ensure continued comprehensive care is provided. When available, clinic visits can also be a useful space in which to reflect on a family's values and speak to future times when more acute goals-of-care discussions may arise. Access to palliative care through telehealth is changing the way palliative care teams can support families. In areas where access to palliative care may be limited, telehealth may provide the bridge for continuity of care.[66,67] Whether it is through telehealth, regular outpatient appointments, or home-based palliative care, conversations that may be emotionally heavy that occur in the less acute setting can provide a rich opportunity for exploration and support.[62,66]

COMMUNICATION AS DEATH APPROACHES

As the child nears the end of their life, communication with the patient and family becomes incredibly crucial. As with advance care planning, preparing families for the death experience is paramount.[3,58] Unless it is asked, the PP APRN and team will not know whether it is helpful for the child or family to engage in explicit conversations about end of life. Bereaved parents have shared how important it is to work with providers who provide honest and compassionate information.[3,63] Additionally, the NCP *Clinical Practice Guidelines* recommend a bereavement assessment be conducted.[3] When possible, the PP APRN should explore with families where they would prefer to be at the time of their child's death. For some this may be at home, while others have shared that it feels better to be admitted to the hospital, receiving care from the nurses and doctors who have been caring for them throughout the illness.[56] It can be helpful to provide information about the dying process, allowing caregivers to prepare and consider how to spend the time they have with their child.[3,19,58]

It may feel unimaginable for a parent to consider having conversations with their child about death and their wishes should they die. Often, this communication is initiated by the child.[49] A child may also ask the question: "Am I going to die?" or "Where do I go after I die?" which may catch the clinician or parent off guard. Just as it is recommended that other care providers provide honest communication, it is important to provide this counseling to parents.[58,63] A parent's instinct may be to provide reassurance or redirection by answering, "No, we are going to keep fighting." The PP APRN can often model this language by asking the child or the parent, "Why are you asking me this right now?" or asking for further clarification with the statement, "Tell me more."[58] Children should not be told that they or their sibling will "go to sleep" or other language around sleep when discussing death. A teenage patient with a brain tumor shared they were told this by their neuro-oncologist, and they then set hourly alarms to wake up in hopes that this would prevent them from dying. Children may express their worries about the changes they feel in their bodies and fear of the unknown. Parents and providers can respond with these phrases.

Your body is starting to shut down and you may die soon.

You will never be alone.

We will help you feel as comfortable as possible.

You are very sick right now.

The team is worried you won't get better and you may die. But you aren't dying right now.

Is that something you want to know in the future, when time may be limited?

The PP APRN should offer frequent guidance and support to parents and other providers surrounding these difficult conversations.

STAFF COMMUNICATION AND SUPPORT

While the primary focus when caring for children with serious illness or those nearing the end of their life is the patient and family, the PP APRN should consider the team caring for the patient and family. The staff who care for these children may experience their own sense of grief, which can impact them both personally and professionally.[68] The palliative care team should be aware of and recognize potential staff distress and be prepared to support them. Encouraging debriefings, regular group discussions, and self-care practices following challenging situations may be helpful to all care providers.[68,69] Providing a safe space for staff to process their own experience may prevent provider burnout and allow for continuation of high-quality care.[69]

BEREAVEMENT SUPPORT

It is a responsibility of the PPC team to provide bereavement support and assist the family in accessing community supports when needed. Initially, a member of the PPC IDT may aid in guiding the family in regard to funeral arrangements, identifying support for siblings, and providing opportunity to express initial experiences of grief. The PP APRN collaborates and coordinates with the PPC social worker or other team members in calling on a family, which can provide the opportunity for continued connection and processing. Mailing bereavement cards signed by team members and filled with handwritten words may provide the opportunity to reiterate the ongoing connection and availability of continued support to a grieving family. Inserting specific language related to the deceased child and their family creates a card that is personal and thoughtful in its communication. Listed here are some examples of helpful language to include when writing such cards or sending mailings that include additional resources.

I am thinking of (child's name) and your family so much.

I will never forget how (child's name) loved Legos and playing with their sister.

(Child's name) smile always lit up the room.

You are such remarkable parents. Your love for (child's name) is profound.

It was an honor and a privilege to be a part of caring for (child's name).

Our team is here for you and your family; we continue to think of you and offer our ongoing support.

Parents often say they would like to connect and learn from parents who have gone through similar losses. Offering a bereavement group for the families of children treated at the same institution, although with a variety of diagnoses, has been successful.[70] The PP APRN can partner with PPC social workers and spiritual care providers to form such support groups, offering parents a way to form new communities and healing bonds. The PP APRN can also make referrals for individual or family counseling, transitioning the family to community providers who will continue to offer comprehensive, supportive bereavement care.

After a child's death, the parents may ask the PP APRN or social worker to arrange bereavement visits with primary providers so they can reconnect, ask lingering questions, or review autopsy results. Such parent–clinician conferences allow the parents to review events around the child's death, provide feedback to staff on the family's experience, and receive emotional support.[71]

SUMMARY

High-quality, expert communication with children and families is central to the delivery of excellent palliative care across the illness trajectory. As valued continuity members of the team, PP APRNs are poised to make a difference with their voice, their touch, and their perseverance in showing up and staying present in moments of both unimaginable suffering and joy. They honor these children, their parents, and their extended families throughout the process and recognize the power of love in birth, life, and death.

REFERENCES

1. Dahlin C. *Palliative Nursing: Scope and Standards of Practice*. 6th ed. Pittsburgh, PA: Hospice and Palliative Nurses Association; 2021.
2. Section on Hospice and Palliative Medicine and Committee on Hospital Care. Pediatric palliative care and hospice care commitments, guidelines, and recommendations. *Pediatrics*. 2013;132(5):966–972. doi:10.1542/peds.2013-2731
3. National Consensus Project for Quality Palliative Care. *Clinical Practice Guidelines*. 4th ed. Alexandria, VA: National Coalition for Hospice and Palliative Care; 2018. https://www.nationalcoalitionhpc.org/ncp
4. Center to Advance Palliative Care. Pediatric palliative care field guide. Updated February 3, 2019. New York, NY: CAPC. https://www.capc.org/documents/257/
5. National Hospice and Palliative Care Organization. *Standards of Practice For Pediatric Palliative Care: Professional Development and Resource Series*. Alexandria, VA: National Hospice and Palliative Care Organization; 2019. https://www.nhpco.org/wp-content/uploads/2019/07/Pediatric_Standards.pdf
6. França J, Costa S, Lopes M, Nóbrega M, França I. The importance of communication in pediatric oncology palliative care: Focus on humanistic nursing theory. *Rev Lat Am Enfermagem*. 2013;21(3):780–786. doi:10.1590/S0104-11692013000300018
7. World Health Organization. Integrating palliative care and symptom relief into paediatrics: A who guide for healthcare planners, implementers and managers. Geneva, CH: WHO. August 8, 2018. https://www.who.int/publications/i/item/integrating-palliative-care-and-symptom-relief-into-paediatrics
8. Wu H-L, Volker DL. Humanistic nursing theory: Application to hospice and palliative care. *J Adv Nurs*. 2012;68(2):471–479. doi:10.1111/j.1365-2648.2011.05770.x
9. City of Hope, American Association of Colleges of Nursing. End of Life Nursing Education Consortium (ELNEC) Communication Curriculum. 2021 Available at https://www.aacnnursing.org/ELNEC/About/ELNEC-Curricula
10. City of Hope, American Association of Colleges of Nursing. End of Life Nursing Education Consortium (ELNEC). APRN Curriculum. 2021. Available at https://www.aacnnursing.org/ELNEC/About/ELNEC-Curricula
11. Wyatt KD, List B, Brinkman WB, et al. Shared decision-making in pediatrics: A systematic review and meta-analysis. *Acad Pediatr*. 2015;15(6):573–583. doi:10.1016/j.acap.2015.03.011
12. Akard TF, Hendricks-Ferguson VL, Gilmer MJ. Pediatric palliative care nursing. *Ann Palliat Med*. 2019;8(S1):S39–S48. doi:10.21037/apm.2018.06.01

13. Crozier F, Hancock L. Pediatric palliative care: Beyond the end of life. *Pediatr Nurs.* 2012;38(4):198–203.

14. Jonas D, Scanlon C, Rusch R, Ito J, Joselow M. Bereavement after a child's death. *Child Adolesc Psychiatr Clin N Am.* 2018;27(4):579–590. doi:10.1016/j.chc.2018.05.010

15. Norris S, Minkowitz S, Scharbach K. Pediatric palliative care. *Prim Care.* 46(3):461–473. doi:10.1016/j.pop.2019.05.010

16. Waldman ED, Levine JM. The day two talk: Early integration of palliative care principles in pediatric oncology. *J Clin Oncol.* 2016;34(34):4068–4070. doi:10.1200/JCO.2016.69.3739

17. Feudtner C, Schall T, Hill D. Parental personal sense of duty as a foundation of pediatric medical decision-making. *Pediatrics.* 2018;142(Suppl 3):S133–S141. doi:10.1542/peds.2018-0516C

18. Waldman E, Wolfe J. Palliative care for children with cancer. *Nat Rev Clin Oncol.* 2013;10(2):100–107. doi:10.1038/nrclinonc.2012.238

19. Barone S, Unguru Y. Ethical issues around pediatric death. *Child Adolesc Psychiatr Clin N Am.* 2018;27(4):539–550. doi:10.1016/j.chc.2018.05.009

20. Melin-Johansson C, Axelsson I, Jonsson Grundberg M, Hallqvist F. When a child dies: Parents' experiences of palliative care: An integrative literature review. *J Pediatr Nurs.* 2014;29(6):660–669. doi:10.1016/j.pedn.2014.06.009

21. Feudtner C, Walter JK, Faerber JA, et al. Good-parent beliefs of parents of seriously ill children. *JAMA Pediatr.* 2015;169(1):39. doi:10.1001/jamapediatrics.2014.2341

22. Hill DL, Miller V, Walter JK, et al. Regoaling: A conceptual model of how parents of children with serious illness change medical care goals. *BMC Palliat Care.* 2014;13(1):9. doi:10.1186/1472-684X-13-9

23. Woodgate RL, Edwards M, Ripat JD, Borton B, Rempel G. Intense parenting: A qualitative study detailing the experiences of parenting children with complex care needs. *BMC Pediatr.* 2015;15(1):197. doi:10.1186/s12887-015-0514-5

24. Jasemi M, Valizadeh L, Zamanzadeh V, Keogh B. A concept analysis of holistic care by hybrid model. *Indian J Palliat Care.* 2017;23(1):71. doi:10.4103/0973-1075.197960

25. Feudtner C, Kang TI, Hexem KR, et al. Pediatric palliative care patients: A prospective multicenter cohort study. *Pediatrics.* 2011;127(6):1094–1101. doi:10.1542/peds.2010-3225

26. Berry JG. Hospital utilization and characteristics of patients experiencing recurrent readmissions within children's hospitals. *JAMA.* 2011;305(7):682. doi:10.1001/jama.2011.122

27. den Herder-van der Eerden M, Hasselaar J, Payne S, et al. How continuity of care is experienced within the context of integrated palliative care: A qualitative study with patients and family caregivers in five European countries. *Palliat Med.* 2017;31(10):946–955. doi:10.1177/0269216317697898

28. Levetown M. Communicating with children and families: From everyday interactions to skill in conveying distressing information. *Pediatrics.* 2008;121(5):e1441–e1460. doi:10.1542/peds.2008-0565

29. Cormack C, Mazanec P, Panke J. Cultural considerations in palliative care. In: Ferrell B, Paice J, eds. *Oxford Textbook of Palliative Nursing.* 5th ed. New York: Oxford University Press; 2019:469–482.

30. Koch A, Grier K. Communication and cultural sensitivity for families and children with life-limiting diseases: An informed decision-making ethical case in community-based palliative care. *J Hosp Palliat Nurs.* 2020;22(4):270–275. doi:10.1097/NJH.0000000000000654

31. Mosher DK, Hook JN, Farrell JE, Watkins Jr. CE, Davis DE. Cultural humility. In: Washington E, Davis D, Hook J. eds. *Handbook of Humility: Theory, Research, and Applications.* New York: Routledge/Taylor & Francis Group; 2017: 91–104.

32. Foronda C, Baptiste D-L, Reinholdt MM, Ousman K. Cultural humility: A concept analysis. *J Transcult Nurs.* 2016;27(3):210–217. doi:10.1177/1043659615592677

33. Davies B, Contro N, Larson J, Widger K. Culturally-sensitive information-sharing in pediatric palliative care. *Pediatrics.* 2010;125(4):e859. doi:10.1542/peds.2009-0722

34. Shirado A, Morita T, Akazawa T, et al. Both maintaining hope and preparing for death: Effects of physicians' and nurses' behaviors from bereaved family members' perspectives. *J Pain Symptom Manage.* 2013;45(5):848–858. doi:10.1016/j.jpainsymman.2012.05.014

35. Ferrell B, Wittenberg E, Battista V, Walker G. Nurses' experiences of spiritual communication with seriously ill children. *J Palliat Med.* 2016;19(11):1166–1170. doi:10.1089/jpm.2016.0138

36. October TW, Dizon ZB, Arnold RM, Rosenberg AR. Characteristics of physician empathetic statements during pediatric intensive care conferences with family members: A qualitative study. *JAMA Netw Open.* 2018;1(3):e180351. doi:10.1001/jamanetworkopen.2018.0351

37. Boucher S, Downing J, Shemilt R. The role of play in children's palliative care. *Children.* 2014;1(3):302–317. doi:10.3390/children1030302

38. Akard TF, Gilmer MJ, Friedman DL, Given B, Hendricks-Ferguson VL, Hinds PS. From qualitative work to intervention development in pediatric oncology palliative care research. *J Pediatr Oncol Nurs.* 2013;30(3):153–160. doi:10.1177/1043454213487434

39. Akard TF, Dietrich MS, Friedman DL, et al. Randomized clinical trial of a legacy intervention for quality of life in children with advanced cancer. *J Palliat Med.* 2021;24(5):680–688. doi:10.1089/jpm.2020.0139

40. Brand SR, Fasciano K, Mack JW. Communication preferences of pediatric cancer patients: Talking about prognosis and their future life. *Support Care Cancer.* 2017;25(3):769–774. doi:10.1007/s00520-016-3458-x

41. Zadeh S, Pao M, Wiener L. Opening end-of-life discussions: How to introduce voicing my choicestm, an advance care planning guide for adolescents and young adults. *Palliat Support Care.* 2015;13(3):591–599. doi:10.1017/S1478951514000054

42. Lotz JD, Jox RJ, Borasio GD, Fuhrer M. Pediatric advance care planning: A systematic review. *Pediatrics.* 2013;131(3):e873–e880. doi:10.1542/peds.2012-2394

43. Sisk BA, Bluebond-Langner M, Wiener L, Mack J, Wolfe J. Prognostic disclosures to children: A historical perspective. *Pediatrics.* 2016;138(3):e20161278–e20161278. doi:10.1542/peds.2016-1278

44. Weaver MS, Heinze KE, Kelly KP, et al. Palliative care as a standard of care in pediatric oncology: Palliative care as a standard of care. *Pediatr Blood Cancer.* 2015;62(S5):S829–S833. doi:10.1002/pbc.25695

45. Gaab EM, Owens RG, MacLeod RD. Primary caregivers' decisions around communicating about death with children involved in pediatric palliative care: *J Hosp Palliat Nurs.* 2013;15(6):322–329. doi:10.1097/NJH.0b013e318293dc20

46. Weaver MS, Heinze KE, Bell CJ, et al. Establishing psychosocial palliative care standards for children and adolescents with cancer and their families: An integrative review. *Palliat Med.* 2016;30(3):212–223. doi:10.1177/0269216315583446

47. Farber JG, Prieur MG, Roach C, et al. Difficult conversations: Discussing prognosis with children with cystic fibrosis. *Pediatr Pulmonol.* 2018;53(5):592–598. doi:10.1002/ppul.23975

48. Mack JW, Fasciano KM, Block SD. Adolescent and young adult cancer patients' experiences with treatment decision-making. *Pediatrics.* 2019;143(5):e20182800. doi:10.1542/peds.2018-2800

49. Jalmsell L, Kontio T, Stein M, Henter J-I, Kreicbergs U. On the child's own initiative: Parents communicate with their dying child about death. *Death Stud.* 2015;39(2):111–117. doi:10.1080/07481187.2014.913086

50. Badarau DO, Wangmo T, Ruhe KM, et al. Parents' challenges and physicians' tasks in disclosing cancer to children. A qualitative interview study and reflections on professional duties in pediatric oncology: Challenges in disclosing cancer to children. *Pediatr Blood Cancer.* 2015;62(12):2177–2182. doi:10.1002/pbc.25680

51. Mack JW, Fasciano KM, Block SD. Communication about prognosis with adolescent and young adult patients with cancer: Information needs, prognostic awareness, and outcomes of disclosure. *J Clin Oncol*. 2018;36(18):1861–1867. doi:10.1200/JCO.2018.78.2128

52. Ewing KB. Improving nurses' understanding of pediatric-focused advance directives. *Pediatr Nurs*. Jan/Feb 2020;46(1):9. http://www.pediatricnursing.net/issues/20janfeb/abstr2.html

53. Mack JW, Joffe S. Communicating about prognosis: Ethical responsibilities of pediatricians and parents. *Pediatrics*. 2014;133(Suppl):S24–S30. doi:10.1542/peds.2013-3608E

54. Olszewski AE, Goldkind SF. The default position: Optimizing pediatric participation in medical decision-making. *Am J Bioeth*. 2018;18(3):4–9. doi:10.1080/15265161.2017.1418921

55. Lotz JD, Daxer M, Jox RJ, Borasio GD, Führer M. "Hope for the best, prepare for the worst": A qualitative interview study on parents' needs and fears in pediatric advance care planning. *Palliat Med*. 2017;31(8):764–771. doi:10.1177/0269216316679913

56. Hays RM, Valentine J, Haynes G, et al. The Seattle pediatric palliative care project: Effects on family satisfaction and health-related quality of life. *J Palliat Med*. 2006;9(3):716–728. doi:10.1089/jpm.2006.9.716

57. Five Wishes. Empowering your child to express his or her own wishes. 2020. Available at https://fivewishes.org/five-wishes/individuals-families/individuals-and-families/children-and-adolescents

58. Lockwood B, Humphrey L. Supporting children and families at a child's end of life. *Child Adolesc Psychiatr Clin N Am*. 2018;27(4):527–537. doi:10.1016/j.chc.2018.05.003

59. Feudtner C. Collaborative communication in pediatric palliative care: A foundation for problem-solving and decision-making. *Pediatr Clin North Am*. 2007;54(5):583–607. doi:10.1016/j.pcl.2007.07.008

60. Gillis J. "We want everything done." *Arch Dis Child*. 2008;93(3):192. doi:10.1136/adc.2007.120568

61. Mitchell S, Spry JL, Hill E, Coad J, Dale J, Plunkett A. Parental experiences of end of life care decision-making for children with life-limiting conditions in the paediatric intensive care unit: A qualitative interview study. *BMJ Open*. 2019;9(5):e028548. doi:10.1136/bmjopen-2018-028548

62. Kaye EC, Rubenstein J, Levine D, Baker JN, Dabbs D, Friebert SE. Pediatric palliative care in the community: Community pediatric palliative care. *CA Cancer J Clin*. 2015;65(4):315–333. doi:10.3322/caac.21280

63. Cacciatore J, Thieleman K, Lieber AS, Blood C, Goldman R. The long road to farewell: The needs of families with dying children. *Omega—J Death Dying*. 2019;78(4):404–420. doi:10.1177/0030222817697418

64. Pediatric concurrent care. Mary J. Labyak Institute for Innovation. Alexandria, VA: National Hospice and Palliative Care Organization, 2012. https://www.nhpco.org/wp-content/uploads/2019/04/Continuum_Briefing.pdf

65. Lindley LC, Keim-Malpass J, Svynarenko R, Cozad MJ, Mack JW, Hinds PS. Pediatric concurrent hospice care: A scoping review and directions for future nursing research. *J Hosp Palliat Nurs*. 2020;22(3):238–245. doi:10.1097/NJH.0000000000000648

66. Bradford N, Armfield NR, Young J, Smith AC. The case for home based telehealth in pediatric palliative care: A systematic review. *BMC Palliat Care*. 2013;12(1):4. doi:10.1186/1472-684X-12-4

67. Weaver MS, Robinson JE, Shostrom VK, Hinds PS. Telehealth acceptability for children, family, and adult hospice nurses when integrating the pediatric palliative inpatient provider during sequential rural home hospice visits. *J Palliat Med*. 2020;23(5):641–649. doi:10.1089/jpm.2019.0450

68. McConnell T, Scott D, Porter S. Healthcare staff's experience in providing end-of-life care to children: A mixed-method review. *Palliat Med*. 2016;30(10):905–919. doi:10.1177/0269216316647611

69. Jonas DF, Bogetz JF. Identifying the deliberate prevention and intervention strategies of pediatric palliative care teams supporting providers during times of staff distress. *J Palliat Med*. 2016;19(6):679–683. doi:10.1089/jpm.2015.0425

70. Morris SE, Dole OR, Joselow M, Duncan J, Renaud K, Branowicki P. The development of a hospital-wide bereavement program: Ensuring bereavement care for all families of pediatric patients. *J Pediatr Healthcare*. 2017;31(1):88–95. doi:10.1016/j.pedhc.2016.04.013

71. Meert KL, Eggly S, Berg RA, et al. Feasibility and perceived benefits of a framework for physician-parent follow-up meetings after a child's death in the PICU. *Crit Care Med*. 2014;42(1):148–157. doi:10.1097/CCM.0b013e3182a26ff3

SECTION VI

COMMUNICATION IN PALLIATIVE CARE

32.

ADVANCE CARE PLANNING
ADVANCE DIRECTIVES, MEDICAL ORDER SETS,
AND SURROGATE DECISION-MAKING

Hannah N. Farfour

KEY POINTS

- Advance care planning (ACP) is a process through which individuals can use their values, goals, and preferences to outline medical care consistent with their wishes.

- Advanced practice registered nurses (APRNs) should understand opportunities and barriers in ACP and advocate for and engage in effective ACP in diverse populations.

- APRNs should support patients, surrogates, and family members as they participate in ACP and make decisions regarding treatment preferences.

- Preferences for medical care should be documented in legal documents as well as within the medical record.

- Billing codes have been created to support ACP conversations and documentation.

CASE STUDY: ADVANCE CARE PLANNING

Ms. W was a 62-year-old retired schoolteacher who identified as African American. She was unmarried, had a long-time partner, Joan, with whom she lived. She was recently diagnosed with Stage IV triple-negative breast cancer after presenting to an emergency department with shortness of breath, where she found to have a malignant pleural effusion and sepsis secondary to a urinary tract infection. The inpatient palliative care team was consulted to assist in goals-of-care delineation and symptom management; however, over the past 2 days, the patient declined the team's attempts to visit. The primary oncology registered nurse (RN) for Ms. Watts called the palliative advanced practice registered nurses (APRN) and shared that she had spent the past several days trying to encourage Ms. W to see the team for help with cancer-associated pain and shortness of breath as she felt like these symptoms were poorly controlled. She shared that Ms. W does not complain but was unable to move/reposition without significant discomfort, and the primary service was focused on cancer diagnosis and management. The APRN reviewed the chart and noted that there was no advance directive or living will within Ms. W's electronic medical record. Her code status

is documented as "full." There were sparse medical records from visits with other health team providers from prior years.

Important things to consider:

1. When is the appropriate time to engage in advance care planning (ACP)?

2. Is there a structure that the APRN can follow for initiating ACP?

3. Are there cultural or spiritual considerations that the APRN should explore prior to engaging in conversation?

4. If information is gained through ACP, where should it be documented?

5. Are there any potential biases or assumptions that either the patient or healthcare team may have?

INTRODUCTION

An understanding of patients' care goals is an essential element of high-quality and patient-centered care. Advance care planning (ACP) is the process that includes communication and documentation that supports this understanding. ACP supports adults at any age or stage in health in understanding and sharing their personal values, life goals, and preferences regarding future medical care, with the goal of helping the individual receive medical treatment consistent with their wishes. High-quality ACP is an individualized and patient-centered process that includes assistance in the appropriate documentation of personal preferences and discussion about preferences with key family members, close friends, and surrogate decision-maker, as well as healthcare providers. Ideally, ACP is an ongoing process among patients, families, and healthcare providers that begins while individuals are healthy and able to communicate their wishes, and these are readdressed at transitions in care.[1] These discussions can serve to prepare the patient and surrogate decision-makers to participate with clinicians in making the best possible "in the moment" decisions as they navigate medical care during serious illness. This process is influenced by legislation and institutional policies, as well as by cultural factors in addition to healthcare provider and patient conversations.[2]

ROLE OF THE PALLIATIVE APRN IN ADVANCE CARE PLANNING

The palliative advanced practice registered nurses (APRN) plays an important role in providing high-quality ACP through expert communication with the patient, family, and/or surrogate decision-maker. Numerous studies have shown that the overall quality of communication between healthcare providers and patients with advance illness is poor. Good communication has been associated with higher patient satisfaction, better patient outcomes, less patient anxiety, better adherence to treatments, and better care at the end of life.[3] However, there are often barriers in initiating this communication such as time, provider/patient discomfort, inability to transfer documentation across continuum of medical care, and a lack of understanding of prognosis or illness trajectory by the patient or healthcare provider.[4,5,6] Studies show that often patients wait for their healthcare providers to initiate these conversations, and, historically, they only happen in a small number of interactions.[3] There have also been many barriers in providing effective ACP in racially and ethnically diverse populations as these individuals may not be aware of community interventions to facilitate ACP or feel uncomfortable in engaging in these conversations. The role, perspective, and training of a palliative APRN allows for crucial and effective conversations to occur that not only elicit preferences in care but ensure that the medical care provided is in alignment with these preferences.

A structured but adaptable approach that is focused on person-centered care is important for effective ACP discussions (see Box 32.1).[7,8] These discussions are appropriate along the continuum of care and may be a short and focused discussion or evolve into a detailed conversation regarding specific medical interventions involving multiple healthcare providers and/or family members. For example, if an individual is healthy, then the initial conversation could serve to discuss documentation of a surrogate decision-maker and to normalize the discussions surrounding preferences in care. ACP conversations can be readdressed at any point along the continuum, but specifically when there is a diagnosis of a life-threatening illness and with each transition in care. Unfortunately, these discussions often occur late in an individual's disease trajectory, resulting in care that does not correlate with care preferences.[3] Furthermore, discussions surrounding ACP information must align with and potentially enhance an individual's readiness stage. These stages range from precontemplation, to preparation, to action, and then to maintenance.[9] Frequently, it is the palliative APRN who initiates the conversation to begin the process. In the precontemplative stage, these conversations may not lead to actionable items but will introduce the concept and value of ACP, and the conversations may evolve over time. As a palliative care specialist, the APRN will also be engaged in more complicated discussions due to medical complexity as well

Helpful phrases:

"I worry that the treatment you are undergoing may not give you what you are hopeful for."

"Is it OK if we talk about time?"

Step 5: Honor emotion

Action:

- Acknowledge that the conversation may have brought up emotion.

- Allow for time to process the information prior to continuation.

Helpful phrases:

"I wish things were different."

"This is hard."

Step 6: Determine values for care and treatment priorities

Action:

- Explore what it means to live well.

- Recognize that there are many influencers of values/beliefs such as race and culture.

- Discuss acceptable disease states and specific scenarios when appropriate.

- Consider a scenario at end of life.

Helpful phrases:

"Given what we have discussed today, what is most important for you to focus on with the remaining time?"

"What are you hopeful for?"

"Some people have thought about how they prefer to be cared for if they should stop breathing due to their serious illness. Some individuals choose attempts of resuscitation and others choose to be made comfortable. Have you ever thought about this situation?"

Step 7: Agree on a plan

Action:

- Offer value-centered recommendations.

- Make specific plans.

- Review that together you will readdress decisions over time to ensure that care continues to be in alignment with preferences.

Helpful phrases:

"Based on what you have shared with me today, I recommend that you elect a do-not-resuscitate status."

"We will continue to address your preferences to ensure that your medical care remains in alignment."

Adapted from Baile WF, Buckman R, Lenzi R, et al. SPIKES: A six-step protocol for delivering bad news- application to the patient with cancer. *Oncologist*.2000;5(4);302–311; and Back, A, Arnold, R., Tulsky, J. *Mastering Conversations with Seriously Ill Patients: Balancing Honesty with Empathy and Hope*. New York: Cambridge University Press; 2009.

as intricate patient and family needs. Therefore, the palliative APRN should be an expert communicator and should role-model a structured approach to engaging in goals of care conversations.

The goal of ACP is to help ensure that individuals receive medical care that is consistent with their preferences and values. Legislation, institutional policies, and cultural factors influence ACP development and growth. There are documented benefits for ACP such as improved communication between patients, surrogates, and clinicians.[9] Patients also have reported a greater source of control and increased quality of life.[10] Surrogate decision-makers have also benefited from reduced stress, anxiety, and depression as surviving family members.[11] Healthcare benefits include a decrease in unwanted intensive medical interventions, hospitalizations, and hospital deaths, as well as earlier palliative care consultations and hospice utilization.[12] Due to the diversity of approaches to ACP and diverse individual needs, it remains difficult to determine through research if ACP actually yields medical care concurrent with preferences.[1] Thus, the role of the palliative APRN is extremely important in facilitating and documenting these discussions along an individual's health trajectory. The impact of this engagement may be felt across the medical system.

BILLING

In an effort to improve healthcare professionals' discussion of ACP with patients, family members, or surrogates, the Centers for Medicare and Medicaid Services (CMS) introduced *Current Procedural Terminology* (CPT) reimbursement codes for ACP visits in January 2016.[13] These codes (99497, first 30 minutes with a minimum of 16 minutes; and 99498, add on for additional 30 minutes) can be used if a healthcare professional provided an explanation and discussion of the advance directive, discussed goals of care, or engaged patients, family member, and/or surrogate decision-makers in discussion as the clinical situation allows.[13,14] Thus far, the use of ACP codes is increasing slightly annually, with older female and White beneficiaries' most frequently receiving an ACP claim.[13] Palliative care professionals are the subset of medical providers using the code the most frequently.[15]

HEALTHCARE DECISION-MAKING

Autonomous individuals are free to hold certain views, make certain choices, and take certain actions based on personal values and beliefs.[16] An individual's ability for self-determination is based on the principle of autonomy and on respect for the individual. Thus, autonomous individuals are free to make personal and variable healthcare decisions. These decisions can range from simple to complex and may change over the course of an illness or injury trajectory. For example, the voluntary choice of an informed person with decision-making capacity determines whether any treatment, including life-sustaining therapies, is initiated, continued, or withdrawn.[17] These decisions are best made when the individual is informed and afforded the time needed to make a decision. Palliative APRNs can be an important part of this process. They can assess whether patients have decision-making capacity, provide the information that patients need to make decisions, and determine whether patients understand the information provided.

The palliative APRN will need to perform an assessment if there are questions regarding decisional capacity. There is not a uniform approach for determining capacity, but a structured interview is recommended.[18] The APRN may find it helpful to assess decision-making capacity by determining if (1) the patient can make and communicate a decision; (2) the patient is able to articulate an understanding of the medical situation and prognosis, the nature of the recommended care, alternative courses of care, and the risks, benefits, and consequences of each alternative; (3) decisions are consistent with the patient's known values and goals; and (4) the patient uses reasoning to make the choice[19] (see Box 32.2). In complex cases, it would be helpful to use a tool such as the MacArthur Competency Tool for Treatment, which allows for a structured interview with good interrater reliability. There is special training available to develop skills in implementing the tool.[20]

A patient's decision-making capacity can change over even a short period of time based on a variety of issues, including, for example, the time of day (the patient may have clear cognition in the morning after a restful night of sleep) and when certain medications are given (especially medications that impair cognition). Palliative APRNs must assess each patient's decision-making capacity and have ongoing discussions with patients about their preferences for care, including end-of-life care.

Box 32.2 HELPFUL QUESTIONS FOR ASSESSING DECISION-MAKING

1. What is your understanding of your health or condition now?

2. What is the therapy/treatment likely to do for you? What are the likely positive and negative outcomes of the therapy/treatment from your perspective?

3. What are you hoping the treatment will do for you?

4. What do you think will happen if you do not have the therapy/treatment?

5. What do you think will happen if you do have the therapy/treatment?

6. How did you decide to accept or refuse the therapy/treatment?

7. What makes the therapy/treatment seem better or worse than the alternatives?[19–30]

ADVANCE DIRECTIVES

The process of ACP gained support, as well as garnered skepticism, with the creation of the *Patient Self-Determination Act* in 1990. This statute required healthcare agencies that received funding from Medicare or Medicaid to provide information about the patient's decision-making rights regarding participation in healthcare decisions, ability to accept/refuse medical treatment, and the right to create an advance healthcare directive to ensure these wishes are communicated to healthcare providers.[20] This legislation did not mandate healthcare providers to have conversations with patients regarding their disease trajectory or prognosis. After this statute, the implementation of the creation of advance care directives had a heterogenous approach with limited success in widespread adoption. Approximately 1 in 3 individuals completes an advance directive, with the majority being older, female, and White.[21] Over the past years, there have been targeted interventions across national, state, and community levels to increase the creation of advance directives. These interventions include national and state databases for the storage of the documentation of advance directives and living wills. There are also websites or smart device applications that provide education in varying platforms, guidance, and forms for the documentation of ACP, with attention given for health literacy, language, and cultural nuances (see Table 32.1). Individuals do not need to have communication with a healthcare professional to create an advance directive. The most common types of advance directives are living wills and durable power of attorney for healthcare documents.

LIVING WILL

A living will is a type of advance directive that outlines patient preferences for treatments like cardiopulmonary resuscitation (CPR), medically administered nutrition and hydration, life-sustaining treatments, and comfort care. A living will takes effect when a patient can no longer speak on his or her own behalf and when the condition discussed in the advance directive is met. For example, a patient's living will may state, "I do not want life-sustaining treatments if I am in a permanent state of unconsciousness or a persistent vegetative state, or my condition is terminal." Each state has different rules about whether a living will or advance directive is recognized.

DURABLE POWER OF ATTORNEY

A durable power of attorney for healthcare might also be referred to as a *healthcare proxy or a surrogate decision maker*. In these legal documents, a person designates the person who will make medical decisions on his or her behalf if something happens in the future and the individual no longer has decision-making capacity. Each state has its own legal form to designate the surrogate decision maker. Some forms are recognized within contiguous states.

Table 32.1 RESOURCES FOR ADVANCE CARE PLANNING

RESOURCE	DESCRIPTION	LINK
ACP Decisions	Written and video resources in over 20 languages	https://www.acp.org
The Conversation Project	Written and video resources in several languages	https://www.theconversationproject.org
Consumer's Toolkit for Healthcare Advance Planning	Written resources for defining values and priorities	https://www.americanbar.org
National POLST	Describes POLST/MOLST documents for each state	https://www.polst.org
PREPARE	Written and video resources including copies of state specific advance directive templates	https://www.prepareforyourcare.org
GoWish	A set of cards that can be used in various settings including with children and individuals with cognitive impairment	https://www.gowish.org

ROLE OF THE PALLIATIVE APRN

Legal requirements and laws related to advance directives vary from state to state. Palliative APRNs need to know the legal requirements in the state where they practice and whether specific living will and healthcare proxy documents are available in their state. It is also important to know if witnesses are needed and if the documents need to be notarized. Palliative APRNs should know if advance directive documents developed in other states can be honored in the state in which they practice.

It is important for palliative APRNs to ask patients if they have written advance directives. If the patient has a living will and/or a durable power of attorney for healthcare, the palliative APRN should review the document(s) with the patient and ask the patient to confirm that his or her wishes are still the same as that written in the document(s). If a patient would like to change the documents, the APRN supports the patient in doing so and offers assistance or direction as needed. The palliative APRN should document all advance directive discussions. If patients do not have advance directives, they should be provided with information regarding why they are important, encouraged to develop them, and helped to do so.

Advance directives should be completed early so that there is a clear understanding of what each patient's preferences are for palliative and end-of-life care. The palliative APRN should review each patient's advance directives periodically because preferences can change. Patients should be encouraged to communicate any changes in treatment preferences or in their healthcare proxy with their healthcare providers. The palliative APRN plays a vital role in ensuring that these changes are documented.

Patients should discuss their treatment preferences not only with clinicians but also with their proxy decision-maker and close family members and friends. Patients should know that if they would like the palliative APRN's support while discussing or sharing advance directives with family members, the APRN will help them to do this.

If the patient has a living will and/or a durable power of attorney for healthcare, copies of the documents should be distributed to key people. A copy can be given to healthcare providers so the documents can be added to the patient's medical record and placed in an area that can be easily accessed. If an electronic medical record system is used, the advance directive documents can be scanned and included in the electronic record.

Patients should also be advised to keep copies of advance directive documents in several places. One copy should be scanned into the healthcare record. The original copy may be kept in a personal safe or safety deposit box. Other copies should be given to the patient's surrogate decision-maker and to other close family members. It is also a good idea to have a card in one's wallet stating that the patient has an advance directive and describing where it is located. An individual may also be able to scan the advance directive and store it in an email, or on a phone, computer, or other smart device so that it can be easily accessed.

MEDICAL ORDER SETS

Out-of-hospital do-not-resuscitate (DNR) orders were historically developed in an effort to honor individuals' wishes to avoid cardiopulmonary resuscitation (CPR) and limit aggressive interventions. They were honored by emergency personnel, but they were often not honored if a patient was admitted to an acute care setting.

Many states have now passed legislation regarding medical order sets. There are state variations, but the order sets are commonly referred to as the medical orders for life-sustaining treatment (MOLST) or the provider/physician orders for life-sustaining treatment (POLST). The MOLST and POLST documents are portable order sets that were developed for patients with serious health problems. The objective was to respect the patient's wishes regardless of the setting. MOLST and POLST documents are honored in the home, acute care, long-term care, palliative care, and hospice settings. Thus, multiple documents are not needed in different settings; the same document follows the patient as he or she moves from setting to setting.

These medical orders are written to ensure that care is provided according to the patient's wishes. The document includes information regarding patient preferences for CPR, medically administered nutrition and hydration, antibiotic use, other life-sustaining therapies, and comfort care. The documents address the entire spectrum of care, from aggressive treatment to comfort care interventions.

A MOLST/POLST differs from an advance directive in that it is a portable medical order. Individuals may have both an advance directive and a MOLST/POLST. The documents should complement each other. Some individuals will have just the MOLST/POLST. MOLST/POLST forms create a legal obligation that medical professionals will honor the individual's treatment preferences.

As with other aspects of ACP, palliative APRNs need to be aware of state legislation related to these medical order sets. The MOLST and POLST forms are signed by the patient's physician or, as allowed in some states, the form can be signed by an APRN or a physician assistant. Depending on the state, the patient and his or her surrogate may sign the document. Orders on the MOLST/POLST form do not expire and can be revised by voiding the form and completing a new one.

As with the living will and durable power of attorney for healthcare documents, it is important that these order sets are completed and reviewed to ensure that care is consistent with the patient's preferences because a recent study shows that MOLST/POLST forms can be inaccurate, undisclosed, or not consistent with patient preferences.[22]

SURROGATE DECISION-MAKING

As individuals become seriously ill or move closer to end of life, they may lose the capacity to make decisions. It then becomes the responsibility of the surrogate decision-maker, either by proxy or by previous selection and documentation as a durable medical power of attorney, to engage in legal decision-making on behalf of the patient. Each state has differing laws about who should serve as a surrogate decision-maker but often members of the family are designated in this role.

As with other ACP documents, the document designating a healthcare proxy should be shared with the individual's healthcare providers. The palliative APRN should ask each patient if the person designated as surrogate decision-maker knows that he or she is aware of this designation. The APRN should also ask the patient if they have reviewed the living will and, if applicable, MOLST/POLST documents with the surrogate decision-maker or healthcare proxy. Engaging in these conversations is an essential part of helping the surrogate decision-maker to fully understand the patient's wishes.

The healthcare proxy or surrogate decision-maker needs to know that they will be involved in the decision-making process if the patient no longer has decision-making capacity. The role of the surrogate decision-maker is to make decisions on the patient's behalf. The surrogate decision-maker will make decisions based on information that the patient wrote in a living will, advance care planning documents, and discussions between the surrogate decision-maker and the patient had about the patient's wishes.

Periodically, when advance directive documents are reviewed, it is important for the palliative APRN to review the healthcare proxy document and confirm that the person designated as healthcare proxy has not been changed. If patients want to make changes, they should be encouraged to develop a new document. A healthcare proxy needs to change if the surrogate dies or if the relationship changes between the patient and the surrogate.

If the patient has not designated a healthcare proxy or surrogate decision-maker, the palliative APRN should discuss this process and provide the patient with information regarding how to do this (see Table 32.2). Selecting the right person is key to successful proxy selection. When selecting a surrogate decision-maker, individuals should consider someone who can be trusted to make sound decisions, is emotionally stable, who would be comfortable asking healthcare providers questions, and is available.

If the time comes that a patient cannot communicate or no longer has decision-making capacity, then the palliative APRN and other members of the healthcare team will turn to the surrogate decision maker if important decisions need to be made. The surrogate decision maker is responsible for making decisions based on what the patient would want done. This supports the patient's previously stated wishes and honors and respects them. If the surrogate decision maker does not know what the patient would want, then they must make decisions based on what they thinks would be in the best interest of the patient. The palliative APRN should acknowledge that serving as a surrogate can be stressful. It is important to educate the healthcare proxy that a blended approach to decision-making that balances the individual's preferences with the surrogate's judgment about what would be best for the patient may lead to better surrogate satisfaction.[23]

If a patient did not designate a healthcare proxy and cannot communicate his or her wishes and is unmarried, the team turns to the family for advice. Decades ago, the President's Commission for the Study of Ethical Problems in Medicine and Biomedical and Behavioral Research recommended that the family is the patient's best advocate if the patient does not have decision-making capacity.[24] The palliative APRN should

Table 32.2 SURROGATE DECISION-MAKER

CHARACTERISTICS	POTENTIAL ACTIONS
18 years of age or older	Choose medical caregivers
Can talk to you about your wishes	Chooses tests, treatments, or medications
Can be there for you when you need them	What happens to body after death
You trust to follow your wishes	Agree to, refuse, or withdraw any life support or treatment

www.prepareforyourcare.org

ask the family if the patient ever stated what he or she would want at the end of life.

Most states have surrogacy laws that specify who can make decisions for a patient. These state laws should be followed when determining which family member has legal authority to make decisions for a patient without decision-making capacity. Legally determined standards are typically set and need to be followed by the palliative APRN. A patient's spouse is typically legally authorized as the primary decision-maker. If the patient's spouse has died or the patient is divorced, the next legal decision-maker might be the eldest adult child. In other states, all adult children need to come together to make a decision. It is important that palliative APRNs know and understand surrogacy laws. In cases of conflict, or where no previously designated surrogate is available, it may be necessary to petition a court to appoint a surrogate.[24] The appointed guardian then serves in the role of surrogate.

If the patient does not have decision-making capacity, then the designated healthcare proxy, surrogate decision-maker, or the family member legally designated to make decisions for the patient does so based on the patient's preferences identified in the living will. If there is no living will, then decisions may be guided by conversations that the surrogate previously had with the patient. If a patient had no living will and did not state what he or she would have wanted at the end of life, *substituted decisions* are made. This is when decisions are made based on what decisions the surrogate decision-maker thinks that the patient would make. If the surrogate decision-maker has no idea what decision the patient would make, a *best interest decision* is made. This decision is based on what might be best for an average person.

Although one person is designated as surrogate decision-maker, multiple family members are often present and involved when a patient nears death. Even though one decision-maker has legal authority for decision-making, it is common for the surrogate decision-maker to include multiple family members in discussions regarding goals of care, especially in the context of end-of-life care.[25] Surrogate decision-makers commonly seek advice and help from other family members when making end-of-life decisions.[26] Families have found advance directives helpful when making end-of-life decisions related to life-sustaining therapies.[27–32]

Making end-of-life decisions on behalf of someone else places a tremendous burden on surrogate decision-makers.[33,34] Some family members may support and some family members may not support the surrogate decision-maker as he or she comes to terms with the decision that needs to be made. It is important for the palliative APRN to help and support the surrogate decision-maker and the patient's family through this process. Once decisions are made, the APRN should ensure that the decisions are respected and honored.

DIVERSE POPULATIONS

There is a significant need to develop interventions to enhance ACP in diverse populations. Rates of ACP among racial and ethnic minority and those with limited health literacy are much lower than in White individuals.[35] For example, African American individuals are less likely to receive end-of-life care aligned with their preferences and are less likely to receive hospice services.[36,37] The completion of ACP in this population remains less than 25%.[32] ACP disparities persist for LGBTQ+, incarcerated, and homeless populations as well.[38–40] Some of the reasons for these disparities include the lack of ACP knowledge, lack of trust, experiences of racism or discrimination, low health literacy, or a preference for others to make medical decisions on their behalf. As this gap has been identified, there is evolving research on systemic interventions to better support ACP in those facing complex barriers. This research varies widely. Some of this research includes using decision aides such as videos and the creation of easy to read documents in a variety of languages.[41] An example of this intervention is *PREPARE for Your Care*, (https://preparefory ourcare.org/welcome) which is a resource that offers videos, simple advance directives, and education in simple terms in a multitude of languages. It remains challenging to create and research scalable interventions to meet the needs of diverse populations.

The palliative APRN is in an important to position to advocate for and employ strategies to engage in effective ACP in special populations. To effectively provide palliative care to all individuals, an APRN should be committed to continually expanding awareness of their own biases and perceptions specific to race, ethnicity, gender identity, gender expression, sexual orientation, immigration status, refugee status, social class, religion, spirituality, physical appearance, and abilities.[19] This is an active process, one that requires personal reflection and awareness. For example, there could be assumptions made, such as a good death is one at home with loving individuals present. Unfortunately, many individuals do not have a safe home and/or caregivers to care for them at end of life. Thus, this assumption could contribute to negative experiences at end of life, although this is not the intention of the healthcare provider. By understanding the complex barriers to ACP in special populations and recognizing that ACP is a highly personalized process, the palliative APRN can help to address the gap between the medical preferences of diverse populations and the medical care received.

WHAT COVID-19 TAUGHT US ABOUT ADVANCE CARE PLANNING

The emergence of the novel coronavirus brought challenges to healthcare systems globally and put the spotlight on ACP in a time of medical uncertainty and in some cases limited resources. COVID-19 highlighted the lack of ACP, the lack of availability of surrogate decision-makers, and put tremendous stress on healthcare providers. Palliative care specialists and organizations supported the frontline by adapting and disseminating communication tools for the intricacies of prognosis sharing and care planning in medical uncertainty. Their challenge was to also support surrogate decision-makers who often were not prepared for the role and whose decision-making was complicated by not being able to see their loved ones due to visitation restrictions. Outpatient palliative care providers were calling patients to readdress preferences and facilitate documentation in a time of much uncertainty. These visits shifted to telehealth as shutdowns and attempts to protect patients and healthcare workers hurtled technology forward. The challenges of this work, whether directly performed or supported, took a toll on everyone. Yet it did move forward discussion and implementation of ACP across the continuum as the effects of poor planning created a significant burden on the medical care teams as well as patients.

On a community level, individuals used tools to create their own advance directives. For example, COVID-19 led West Virginians to call their state center for end-of-life care for forms, urgent desire to initiate ACP, temporary rescindment of treatment-limiting forms, and questions on how to honor patients' wishes in advance directives and medical orders in light of their COVID-19 status.[42] Another study reviewed the monthly rates of completion, completion of number of goal-setting modules, and distributions of preferences for care for care on the free advance care planning website, *OurCareWishes.org*. It showed a 4.9 times increase in advance directive completion as well as more comprehensive completion since the onset of COVID-19. [43] This increase shows that community-facing tools that have been refined through years of implementation can accommodate to large shifts in the completion of ACP documentation necessitated by the COVID-19 pandemic.

SUMMARY

Palliative APRNs play an essential role in the ACP process. They can educate and help patients to develop living wills, designate healthcare proxies, and develop MOLST/POLST documents. Conversations that palliative APRNs have with the patient, surrogate, and family not only help to identify the patient's wishes but also help to ensure that these wishes are honored and respected.

REFERENCES

1. Sudore RL, Lum HD, You JJ, et al. Defining advance care planning for adults: A consensus definition from a multidisciplinary delphi panel. *J Pain Symptom Manage.* 2017;53(5):821–832.e1. doi:10.1016/j.jpainsymman.2016.12.331

2. Jimenez G, Tan WS, Virk AK, et al. Overview of systematic reviews of advance care planning: Summary of evidence and global lessons. *J Pain Symptom Manage.* 2018;56(3):436–459. doi:10.1016/j.jpainsymman.2018.05.016

3. Institute of Medicine. *Dying in America: Improving Quality and Honoring Individual Preferences Near the End of Life.* Washington, DC: National Academies Press; 2015. https://www.nap.edu/catalog/18748/dying-in-america-improving-quality-and-honoring-individual-preferences-near

4. Granek L, Krzyzanowska MK, Tozer R, Mazzotta P. Oncologists' strategies and barriers to effective communication about end of life. *J Oncol Pract.* 2013;9(4):E129–e135. doi:10.1200/JOP.2012.000800

5. Bernacki RE, Block SD, for the American College of Physicians High Value Care Task Force. Communication about serious illness care goals: A review and synthesis of best practices. *JAMA Intern Med.* 2014;174(12):1994–2003. doi:10.1001/jamainternmed.2014.5271

6. Howard M, Bernard C, Klein D, et al. Barriers to and enablers of advance care planning with patients in primary care: Survey of health care providers. *Can Fam Physician.* 2018;64(4):E190–e198.

7. Baile WF, Buckman R, Lenzi R, et al. SPIKES: A six-step protocol for delivering bad news- application to the patient with cancer. *Oncologist.*2000;5(4);302–311.

8. Back A, Arnold R, Tulsky J. *Mastering Conversations with Seriously Ill Patients: Balancing Honesty with Empathy and Hope.* New York: Cambridge University Press; 2009.

9. Walczak A. Butow PN, Bu S, Clayton JM. A systematic review of evidence for end-of-life communication interventions: Who do they target, how are they structured, and do they work? *Patient Educ Couns.* 2016;99(1):3–16. doi:10.1016/j.pec.2015.08.017

10. Murray L, Butow PN. Advance care planning in motor neuron disease: A systematic review. *Palliat Support Care.* 2016;14(4):411–432. doi:10.1017/S1478951515001066

11. Detering KM, Hancock AD, Reade MC, Silvester W. The impact of advance care planning on end of life care in elderly patients: Randomized controlled trial. *BMJ.* 2010;340:c1345. doi:https://doi.org/10.1136/bmj.c1345

12. Wright AA, Zhang B, Ray A, et al. Associations between end-of-life discussions, patient mental health, medical care near death, and caregiver bereavement adjustment. *JAMA.* 2008;200(14):1665–1673. doi:10.1001/jama.300.14.1665

13. Pelland K, Morphis B, Harris D, Gardner R. Assessment of first-year use of Medicare's advance care planning billing codes. *JAMA Intern Med.* 2019;179(6):827–829. doi:10.1001/jamainternmed.2018.8107

14. Centers for Medicare and Medicaid Services. MLN fact sheet: Advance care planning. Baltimore, MD: CMS. October 2020 https://www.cms.gov/Outreach-and-Education/Medicare-Learning-Network-MLN/MLNProducts/Downloads/AdvanceCarePlanning.pdf

15. Gazarian P. Uptake and trends in the use of Medicare advance care planning visits. *Health Serv Res.* 2020:55. Suppl 1):16. doi:10.1111/1475-6773.13344

16. Beauchamp TL, Walters L, Kahn JP, Mastroianni AC. *Contemporary Issues in Bioethics.* 8th ed. Belmont, CA: Wadsworth; 2013.

17. President's Commission for the Study of Ethical Problems in Medicine and Biomedical and Behavioral Research. *Deciding to Forgo Life-Sustaining Treatment: A Report on Ethical, Medical and Legal Issues in Treatment Decisions.* Washington, DC: US Government Printing Office; 1983. https://repository.library.georgetown.edu/bitstream/handle/10822/559344/deciding_to_forego_tx.pdf?sequence=1

18. Shibu J, Rowley J, Bartless K. Assessing patients decision-making capacity in the hospital setting: A literature review. *Aust J Rural Health.* 2020;28(20):141–148. https://doi.org/10.1111/ajr.12592

19. National Consensus Project for Quality Palliative Care. *Clinical Practice Guidelines for Quality Palliative Care.* 4th ed. Richmond, VA: National Coalition for Hospice and Palliative Care; 2018. https://www.nationalcoalitionhpc.org/ncp

20. Congress.gov. H.R. 4449 Patient Self Determination Act of 1990. 1990. https://www.congress.gov/bill/101st-congress/house-bill/4449

21. Yadav KN, Gabler NB, Cooney E, et al. Approximately one in three us adults completes any type of advance directive for end of life care. *Health Aff.* 2017;36(7):1244–1251. doi:10.1377/hlthaff.2017.0175

22. Mirarchi FL, Juhasz K, Cooney TE, et al. Triad XII: Are patients aware of and agree with DNR or POLST orders in their medical records. *J Pat Saf.* 2019;15(3):230–237. doi:10.1097/PTS.0000000000000631

23. Sulmasy D, Hughes MT, Yenokyan G, et al. The trial of ascertaining individual's preferences for loved one's role in end-of-life decisions (tailored) study. A randomized control trial to improve surrogate decision making. *J Pain Symptom Manage.* 2017;54(4):455–465. doi:10.1016/j.jpainsymman.2017.07.004

24. Tilden VP, Tolle SW, Nelson CA, Thompson M, Eggman SC. Family decision making in foregoing life-extending treatments. *J Family Nurs.* 1999;5(4):426–442. https://doi.org/10.1177/107484079900500405

25. Pope TM. Legal fundamentals of surrogate decision making. *Chest.* 2012;141(4):1074–1081. doi: 10.1378/chest.11-2336

26. Kelly B, Rid A, Wendler D. Systematic review: Individuals' goals for surrogate decision-making. *J Am Geriatr Soc.* 2012;60(5):884–895. doi:10.1111/j.1532-5415.2012.03937.x

27. Wiegand DL. In their own time: The family experience during the process of withdrawal of life-sustaining therapy. *J Palliat Med.* 2008;11(8):1115–1121. doi: 10.1089/jpm.2008.0015

28. Hickman RL, Pinto MD. Advance directives lessen the decisional burden of surrogate decision-making for the chronically critically ill. *J Clin Nurs.* 2013;23(5–6):756–765. doi: 10.1111/jocn.12427

29. Jacob DA. Family members' experiences with decision making for incompetent patients in the ICU: A qualitative study. *Am J Crit Care.* 1998;7(1):30–36.

30. Mayer SA, Kossoff SB. Withdrawal of life support in the neurological intensive care unit. *Neurology.* 1999;52(8):1602–1609. doi:10.1212/WNL.52.8.1602

31. O'Callahan JG, Fink C, Pitts LH, Luce JM. Withholding and withdrawing of life support from patients with severe head injury. *Crit Care Med.* 1995;23(9):1567–1575. doi:10.1097/00003246-199509000-00018

32. Swigart V, Lidz C, Butterworth V, Arnold R. Letting go: Family willingness to forgo life support. *Heart Lung.* 1996;25(6):483–494. doi:10.1016/S0147-9563(96)80051-3

33. Fritsch J, Petronio S, Helft PR, Torke A. Making decisions for hospitalized older adults: Ethical factors considered by family surrogates. *J Clin Ethics.* 2013;24(2):125–134. https://www.ncbi.nlm.nih.gov/pmc/articles/PMC3740391/

34. Wengler D, Rid A. Systematic review: The effect on surrogates of making treatment decisions for others. *Ann Intern Med.* 2011;154(5):336–346. doi:10.7326/0003-4819-155-3-201108020-00023

35. Harrison KL, Adrion ER, Ritchie CS, Sudore RI, Smith AK. Low completion and disparities in advance care planning activities among older medicare beneficiaries. *JAMA Intern Med.* 2016;176(12):1872–1875. doi:10.1001/jamainternmed.2016.6751

36. LoPresti MA, Dement F, Gold HT. End-of-life care for people with cancer from ethnic minority groups: A systematic review. *Am J Hosp Palliat Care.* 2016;33(3):291–305. doi:10.1177/1049909114565658

37. Mack JW, Paulk ME, Viswanath K. Prigerson HG. Racial disparities in the outcomes of communication non-medical care received near death. *Arch Intern Med.* 2010;170(17):1533–1540. doi:10.1001/archinternmed.2010.322

38. Hughes M, Cartwright C. Lesbian, gay, bisexual, and transgender people's attitudes to end-of-life decision-making and advance care planning. *Australas J Ageing.* 2015;34(Suppl 2):39–43. doi:10.1111/ajag.12268

39. Kaplan LM, Sudore RL, Cuervo IA, Bainto D, Olsen P, Kushel M. Barriers and solutions to advance care planning among homeless-experienced older adults. *J Palliat Med.* 2020;23(10):1300–1306. doi:10.1089/jpm.2019.0550

40. Ekaireb R, Ahalt C, Sudore R, Metzger L, Williams B. "We take of patients, but we don't advocate for them": Advance care planning in prison or jail. *J Am Geriatri Soc.* 2018;66(12):2382–2388. doi:10.1111/jgs.15624

41. Sudure RL, Sillinger D, Katen BA, et al. Engaging diverse English and Spanish speaking older adults in advance care planning: The PREPARE randomized clinical trial. *JAMA Inter Med.* 2020;178(12):1116–1625. doi:10.1001/jamainternmed.2018.4657

42. Funk DC, Moss AH, Speis MS. How COVID-19 changed advance care planning: Insights from the West Virginia center for end-of-life care. *J Pain Symptom Manage.* 2020;60(6):e5–e9. doi:10.1016/j.jpainsymman.2020.09.021

43. Auriemma CL, Halpern SD, Asch JM, et al. Completion of advance directives and documented care preferences during the coronavirus disease 2019 (COVID-19) pandemic. *JAMA Network Open.* 2020;3(7): E2015762. doi:10.1001/jamanetworkopen.2020.15762

33.

FAMILY MEETINGS

Jennifer Gentry, Kerrith McDowell, and Paula McKinzie

KEY POINTS

- Excellent communication is the foundation for effective family meetings.

- Leading family meetings is a key role for the advanced practice registered nurse (APRN).

- The APRN must prepare for a family meeting.

- When there is conflict, the palliative APRN must address the emotion from the patient and/or the family.

CASE STUDY: CONFLICTING GOALS

Mrs. R was a 55-year-old woman with a history of substance misuse disorder, hypertension, and an anoxic brain injury following an out-of-hospital cardiac arrest 3 months ago. She was admitted to the hospital with worsening myoclonus and an unstageable sacral ulcer. Mrs. R had a tracheostomy and a percutaneous gastrostomy tube (PEG); she was noncommunicative and dependent for all activities of daily living (ADLs). She was cared for at home by her family with assistance from the community palliative care team. The palliative advanced practice registered nurse (APRN) was consulted to assist with clarifying goals of care with Mrs. R's family. A family meeting was arranged after reviewing the medical record, examining the patient, and obtaining information from the care nurse and primary team. The family meeting participants included the palliative APRN, the palliative care social worker, the patient's spouse, Lester, and Mrs. R's son from a previous relationship, Randy. After introductions, the APRN reviewed the issues leading to the hospital stay, purpose of the meeting, and family perception of the illness.

APRN: Would it be OK to talk about Mrs. R's illness and what has been happening with her health so that we can provide the best possible care?

LESTER: Sure . . . I've been so worried about her and I didn't know what else to do.

APRN: Tell me more about what has been worrying you.

LESTER: I was doing everything they [the home palliative care team] told me to do but she kept having twitching and the wound was worse. . . . I didn't want her to suffer so I called 9-1-1. [Lester sighs and appears fatigued.]

APRN: I can only imagine how difficult that this was.

LESTER: It has been really tough, and I feel like I am running out of steam and don't have enough help.

APRN: I hear that this is really difficult and exhausting.

RANDY: She is my mother and you [speaking to Lester] never include me in what is going on. I know she can get better and you are just giving up and calling hospice. [Randy abruptly storms out and slams the conference room door. The palliative social worker leaves the meeting to check on Randy while the APRN continues to speak with Lester.]

LESTER: "I know he [Randy] is having a hard time with all this . . . he had a hard time seeing her this way. The doctor's told us that she is dying and he just can't accept that.

Over subsequent follow-up family meetings and discussions, the decision was made to focus all efforts on aggressive symptom management and comfort. Tube feedings were discontinued, and Mrs. R was transitioned to an inpatient hospice setting to receive continued symptom management and family support.

INTRODUCTION

When a serious illness occurs, patients and their families may find themselves at the mercy of a complex and often unyielding healthcare system with limited insight into their situation and how to proceed. Nonexistent or poorly delivered communication during the course of an illness may result in conflict, confusion, frustration, and mistrust. Thoughtful communication and facilitated family meetings can go far to bridge the communication gap. These can take place in the acute care setting, clinic, home, or long-term care setting. Leading a family meeting is an essential skill for the palliative advanced practice registered nurse (APRN).[1,2] By its nature, palliative care is interdisciplinary and collaborative. As leaders on the interdisciplinary team, palliative APRNs frequently lead formal and informal family meetings, discuss prognosis, clarify goals of care, assist with advance care planning, deliver bad news, and provide care when death is imminent.[2,3]

Communication expertise is a core competency for palliative APRNs and is woven throughout the scope and standards of palliative nursing practice.[1] Principles of good communication include use of open-ended questions, sitting down, maintaining eye contact, being present, listening, use of empathic responses, and attending to emotion.[3–5] Whether practicing in an inpatient acute care setting, an outpatient clinic, or hospice, APRNs lead and participate in complex communication episodes with patients and families.[1,2] Despite having an important role in family meetings, APRNs may feel unprepared to lead them.[6-9] This chapter reviews the literature around family meetings and the process for effective family meetings.

DEFINITION OF FAMILY MEETINGS

While no single definition of a family meeting exists, these meetings may be described as a facilitated, dynamic means of exchanging information about illness, prognosis, and treatment options with the patient, family, and healthcare team. "Family" is described by the patient or, if they are not able to participate, by designated surrogate decision-makers or next of kin. Family meetings, also referred to as *family conferences*, provide a vehicle for two-way communication about the goals, values, concerns, and decisions needed to formulate a plan of care.

Seaman and colleagues have proposed five goals for clinician–family communication which are of key importance in family meetings: establish trusting relationships; providing emotional support; facilitate understanding of diagnosis, prognosis, and treatment options; helping clinicians understand the patient as a person; and creating conditions for deliberation about decisions.[10] Family meetings have been reported to result in improved family perception of empathy and goal-concordant care, and can serve as a way provide interdisciplinary family support.[4,11] Although recommendations exist for routine family meetings, further research is needed to support the most effective manner, timing, and use of family meetings as a communication tool.[12-14]

The family meeting has been called the major "procedure" of the palliative care clinician or the major tool on which to base palliative care interventions.[15,16] For this "procedure" to be effective, the palliative APRN must use excellent communication skills, including active listening, empathy, a nonjudgmental approach, and observation.[7,17,18] Essential elements of communication required during a family meeting include listening, information gathering, imparting information, therapeutic presence, and sensitivity.[7,18] Information must be provided in a manner that is educationally, culturally, and developmentally appropriate without overwhelming the recipients' coping styles.[17,18] To best facilitate these meetings, the APRN must have a working knowledge of common conditions and disease processes and their trajectory and prognoses, as well as potential technology and treatment options, to guide patients and families in making informed decisions about their healthcare.[1,17] APRNs frequently provide palliative care and associated communication in many different settings. Care provided by APRNs is rated highly in terms of satisfaction and the achievement of comfort.[2,19] In a systematic review of outcomes, the care provided by APRNs has been shown to be similar to that provided by physicians.[20,21] Patients rate APRN care delivery as high-quality and highly satisfying.[21] To be the most effective, palliative APRNs should be allowed to function fully within the scope of their education and training. It is within the APRN's scope of practice to lead family meetings and discuss prognosis, disease process, and therapeutic options.[1,2]

Family meetings should not be used only when there is a crisis.[2,9,14,15] Proactive use of family meetings, ensuring adequate preparation, are essential components for success.[15] The APRN addresses potential barriers to family meetings by identifying and setting aside specific times for family meetings, supporting communication skills training for clinicians, and using assistance from members of the interdisciplinary team to help with the logistics of scheduling, coordinating, and finding a location for the meeting.[14,15] It has been suggested that identifying specific indications for family meetings and palliative care consultation may promote the involvement of palliative care and family (Box 33.1). The need for a family meeting could be triggered by clinician assessment of clinical changes, the need for transitions in care, discussion of prognosis, the need to make treatment decisions, or disagreement among family members and clinicians.[15,16] Patients and families may also request family meetings as palliative care moves upstream.

RESEARCH ON FAMILY MEETINGS

Miller and colleagues examined palliative care consultations, mainly provided by APRNs, for patients in skilled nursing facilities.[22] The authors concluded that these palliative care consultations had good patient outcomes because they resulted in lower use of acute care services and lessened the burden of care transitions. Palliative APRNs embedded in an oncology clinic demonstrated improvement in areas requiring complex communication including advance care planning and end-of-life hospice discussions.[23] Nurse-led family meetings have been shown to increase family satisfaction and improve communication in support of shared decision-making.[24] Over the process of developing and employing communication skills in family meetings, nurses have reported increased confidence in communication, improved listening skills, deeper understanding of families, and higher levels of professional satisfaction.[7,25] Appropriate education and mentoring were essential components of the success of nurse-led family meetings.[7,8,24,25]

Despite the importance of communication skills, a lack of emphasis has been placed on communication education and training in nursing programs.[7,8,26,27] Palliative care team members without specific counseling backgrounds, including nurses and physicians, often have not received training in meeting facilitation or conflict resolution. Additionally, advanced practice providers and APRNs may lack an understanding of their role in family meetings or feel unempowered to be active participants.[28,29] Fortunately, like other clinical skills, communication and facilitation skills can be effectively taught using simulated patients, mentoring, expert observation, and feedback.[6,7,18,30]

Regular communication and family meetings may have immediate and long-term benefits for patients and families. A common reason for palliative care consultation is to facilitate communication.[23,31,32] Temel and colleagues noted that for patients with advanced gastrointestinal and lung cancers, early palliative care involvement was associated with improved quality of life and mood, and patients found discussions of prognosis to helpful.[31] Trends in hospital-based palliative care between 2013 and 2017 indicate that a majority of palliative care consultations were obtained to facilitate communication.[32] A mean of 1.3 family meetings per palliative care consultation was identified, and a large number of palliative care consultations were associated with multiple family meetings during one admission.[32] Conclusions from several systematic reviews suggest low-quality evidence for family meetings and identified areas for additional research, such as perspectives of the individual participants, the most effective clinician participants, and timing and frequency of family meetings in inpatient settings.[27,33] In a structured palliative care communication intervention in the intensive care unit (ICU) setting, family-caregiver anxiety and depression did not improve following family meetings facilitated by palliative care providers.[34] The investigators theorized that outcomes may have been impacted by lack of interdisciplinary and ICU team participation in the family meetings, which underscores the importance of collaboration in family meetings.[34] Though nurses are in an ideal position to lead and participate in family meetings, in one study nurses were rarely asked by the family or other healthcare team members to contribute to the discussion.[28] As leaders of family meetings, palliative APRNs have an obligation to include the valuable input of bedside nurses and other interdisciplinary team members in family meetings.[1]

Communication in the context of palliative care consultation has been shown to improve respect for treatment preferences, emotional and spiritual support, and symptom management.[22,23,35,36] Without the information that may be gained in a family meeting, clinicians may struggle to predict patient preferences.[37,38] Evidence has demonstrated that physicians do not accurately assess a patient's quality of life, functioning, or preferences for cardiopulmonary resuscitation (CPR) even if there is a relationship with the patient over time.[39] Palliative care consultation teams have been shown to improve symptom management, quality of life, and processes of care, such as transitions across care settings and documentation of patient goals.[32]

OUTCOMES OF POOR COMMUNICATION

Poor communication has been identified as the greatest source of anxiety and frustration for family members.[9,14,38] Several counterproductive behaviors that clinicians may unintentionally use may result in conflict and suffering in a family meeting (Box 33.2): (1) forcing the discussion, (2) linking relief of suffering with limited life expectancy, (3) pressuring through repeated attempts to persuade, (4) misdiagnosing denial, (5) presenting information out of context, and (6) making treatment recommendations without incorporating the context of the surrogate's perception of the patient's wishes.[40,41]

Poor-quality communication during family meetings may lead to misunderstandings, missed opportunities, and distress for all involved.[16] Medical jargon may not be well understood, and the importance of every single word must be measured. It is not surprising that family members view emotional support provided through empathic communication as critical, and it is associated with better psychological outcomes.[42] When the family is not fluent in the language to be used during a family meeting, the use of an interpreter is best practice.[16,43] Family members should not be used as interpreters during family meetings because it puts them in an awkward situation of both responding to information and having to convey difficult news.[16,43] English terms that may be used in the context of family meetings such as "palliative," "hospice," and "DNAR" (do not attempt resuscitation) may not have a corresponding word in other languages or may be translated into a more negative context.[43] Interpreters may not have had specific training in palliative care related communication such as delivering bad news and can benefit from a pre-meeting to review the medical history, information to be discussed, key participants, and current understanding if known.[43] The

---

Box 33.2 COMMON CLINICIAN COMMUNICATION ERRORS

Proceeding without assessing readiness: Forcing the goals-of-care discussion when the patient or family is not ready.

Linking relief of suffering with demands to accept limited life expectancy: "I'm sorry, but there is nothing else we can do for you. Should we just keep you comfortable now?"

Misdiagnosing denial: Patients and families may have the initial, "This is not happening" response as part of normal grief, self-protection, and coping.

Destructive debates: Repeated attempts to convince the patient and family of a certain viewpoint (e.g., repeated attempts to "get the DNR").

Presenting hypothetical decisions in an impersonal manner without a context: "If your heart and lungs stop, what do you want us to do?"

Making treatment recommendations without incorporating the context of the surrogate's perception of the patient's wishes: "Based on what you know (about the patient) what would be important to them in this situation?"

From Weiner[40], Pecanac[41]

literature supports the use of medical interpreters as "culture brokers" with a knowledge of language and an awareness of cultural nuances so that they can provide information in the most respectful manner.[43]

If family meetings are beneficial, why do they happen late in the course of illness or not at all?[14,44] Recommendations have been made to hold a family meeting in the ICU within 72 hours of admission to promote family satisfaction and communication.[36] The authors of a retrospective study of family meetings in the ICU noted that almost half of the patients had not received a family meeting 5 days following admission and that timely family meetings were highly associated with death during the ICU stay.[14] The authors hypothesized that clinicians may be using family meetings to negotiate discontinuation of life-sustaining technology rather than as a vehicle for family support and patient autonomy.[14]

Several barriers to timely family meetings have been identified (Box 33.3). Wright and colleagues suggest that conversations about difficult things like poor prognosis and end of life are avoided for fear that the patient will "lose hope" or experience distress.[44] Despite the ambivalence that patients and providers may have about difficult discussions, patients with terminal cancer who participated in these discussions were less likely to receive aggressive ICU care, mechanical ventilation, or attempts at resuscitation and did not experience higher rates of depression.[6,16,44] When patients underwent more aggressive medical treatments at the end of life, they experienced a lower quality of life before death, and their caregivers were at a higher risk for depression.[16] Other potential barriers to family meetings include lack of time, resource intensiveness with involvement of multiple providers, lack of provider training in communication and facilitation, cultural differences, lack of space, and provider burnout.[14,33,44–46]

SETTING THE STAGE FOR FAMILY MEETINGS

Several essential components of family meetings have been identified.[16,47] The mnemonic VALUE has been developed and used as a communication strategy to facilitate proactive family meetings for patients dying in the ICU (Box 33.4).[27,47] Proactive family meetings and use of palliative care interventions have been associated with reduction in ICU utilization

at the end of life.[47,48] Additionally, fewer nonbeneficial interventions were done in those who received a proactive family meeting, and there was a lower incidence of depression, anxiety, and posttraumatic stress disorder among survivors in the 3 months following the death of the patient.[12,47] Several models have been proposed for family meetings; these contain four overarching components: (1) conference organization, including the setting, participants, and structure of the meeting; (2) negotiation or building consensus and reaching decisions; (3) personal stance or the attitude and mode of information delivery; and (4) emotional work or use of empathic responses[16,49] (Box 33.5).

THE STEPS OF A FAMILY MEETING

PREPARATION

Identifying the Decision-Maker and Who Should Be Present

Patients with capacity have a right to self-determination and should be included in decisions about their healthcare, per their preference, but the reality is that many deaths occur in the hospital and ICU, where patients are frequently too ill to participate in decision-making.[9,12,50,51] Deaths commonly occur after the decision is made in a family meeting to discontinue life-sustaining measures or limit treatment. Attempts to prepare the family for this outcome should be made by the provider during the family meeting in the acute care setting.[38,52]

Family members often serve as surrogate decision-makers for incapacitated patients.[12,27,38,52] The definition of "family" is very individual, and family members may include anyone who is important to the patient, rather than just a legal or biological relative. A surrogate decision-maker or next-of-kin status is individually defined by the state via statute. Some patients have such an individual designated through written advance directives or a durable power of attorney for health, in the event they are not able to speak for themselves.[53]

The ethical principle of substituted judgment is applied when there is no advance directive and the patient lacks decision-making capacity.[9] Palliative APRNs must be knowledgeable about the laws in their practice location so they can determine the appropriate legal decision-maker. The palliative APRN must also identify other persons important to the patient who should be included in a family meeting. Although the legal surrogate may be authorized to act on behalf of the patient, there may be others who hold great influence in the decision-making process. They may include relatives, close friends, or spiritual care providers who know the patient's wishes and can contribute to the meeting. Even with a written advance directive, surrogate decision-making can be difficult. Surrogate decision-makers' ability to predict what the patient would have wanted in a given situation may be inaccurate, and authorizing overtreatment is a common error.[42,54]

Shared decision-making, a dynamic process in which the responsibility is shared by the treating provider and the patient's family, has been endorsed by numerous professional societies.[52] It is best carried out using a stepwise approach.[52] Family members who are involved in decision-making frequently report feeling overwhelmed and overburdened by the responsibility (Box 33.6).[38,42,55] Exploring the family's preferred role in the decision-making process and the uncertainty about the prognosis is essential and should be reassessed frequently. Some families prefer that the provider make

---

Box 33.6 SAMPLE QUESTIONS TO CLARIFY ROLES IN DECISION-MAKING

"How has your family made decisions in the past?"

"Some families make decisions as a group and others appoint a spokesperson. Can you help me understand how your family makes decisions?"

"I can see how difficult this is for you. Would it help if I make a recommendation?"

"Would it be helpful to include your family in these discussions and decisions?"

From Pecanac[41], Kavalieratos[56]

---

recommendations; others prefer to accept ultimate responsibility for the decisions made.

Participants from the clinical team should be limited to those crucial for information, decision-making, and family support. The patient's care nurse, spiritual care provider, social work, essential consultants, the primary team, and palliative care provider may attend.[16] Having a large number of participants from the clinical team may be overwhelming for a smaller family group. Depending on where the meeting is held, logistics may dictate who may attend in person, but, even in the clinic and home, other providers may participate virtually. For patients and families lacking proficiency in English, a trained medical interpreter should be available by phone or in person.[16,43]

Meeting Place

Finding an appropriate setting and space for the meeting may seem like a simple task, but healthcare facilities are designed for utility and may not provide the patient- and family-friendly space needed for family meetings.[52] However, at home and in residential settings, there are often more private meeting areas. An ideal space would allow for privacy, adequate seating, and use of technology, such as speakerphones and computers to allow for participation of distant family members.[52] While technology can facilitate communication, it may also be a distraction. Clinicians should silence their cellphones and pagers prior to the meeting and may consider asking family members to do the same. Evidence to support the best physical arrangements for family meetings is lacking, but arranging the room and seating to allow good eye contact and observation of participants' nonverbal communication may be helpful.[15,16,52] In some cases, a patient with decision-making capacity may be too ill to move to a separate location, requiring the meeting to be held in the patient's room. The space may not accommodate seating for everyone, but at a minimum the person leading the meeting should be seated.

History and Medical Facts

Another element of preparation includes being knowledgeable about the medical facts in the case.[15,27,52] Prior to a family meeting, the palliative APRN should review the medical history, consult with members of the team knowledgeable about the patient's situation, and become familiar with the patient's psychosocial, spiritual, and family background.[1,2] Key stakeholders and subspecialists to be included or consulted prior to the meeting should be identified prior to the meeting and invited as appropriate.[27] "Who is the health provider you trust the most (on the medical team)?" can be a helpful question to pose ahead of time to patients and families in an effort to identify important stakeholders. If other team members will be attending the meeting, set aside a few minutes to discuss key facts, such as prognosis, treatment options, and concerns, before the meeting. In the pre-meeting conference, everyone attending should be clear on the purpose of the meeting, which team member is leading the meeting, and what role each team member will play.

MEETING STRUCTURE

INTRODUCTIONS

Everyone present in the room should be introduced, and their role and relationship to the patient should be made clear. In large groups, the person leading the meeting or a designee may wish to discreetly jot down this information to refer to later. Consider the role of the interdisciplinary team members, such as social work, to help mitigate complicated family dynamics.[52] Ground rules can often help and include clarifying the legal decision-maker if the patient lacks decision-making capacity and noting that there will be an opportunity for everyone to ask questions and participate during the meeting.

ELICIT UNDERSTANDING AND INFORMATION NEEDS

Beginning the discussion by asking an open-ended question like "What have you heard so far?" or "How do you feel things are going at this point?" provides important information about the patient's and family's perception and allows the APRN to use active listening skills and assess the family's need for information.[50] Using the phrase "What do you understand?" may get at the information needed but should be used cautiously as patients and families may perceive this as condescending or may conclude that the clinician views them as uninformed. While many patients and families want as much information as possible, this is not always the case.[55] The need for information is very individual and should be determined prior to the meeting[27,52,55] The palliative APRN should avoid making assumptions about the type and amount of information that should be disclosed. Culture and health literacy may dictate what and how information is shared.[55]

PROVIDE INFORMATION

Deliver information using an honest and direct manner while continually assessing the response and nonverbal communication.[3] Some families report that statistical data regarding outcomes is helpful in decision-making while others state this is not useful information and can be overwhelming.[55] Checking in about the group's understanding should be done frequently and with tact and diplomacy. A question like "Am I making sense to you so far?" "Does this make sense to you?" or "Sometimes I forget that I use medical jargon. Would you mind sharing what you heard me say, so that I know I am being clear?" puts the responsibility for communication difficulties on the provider and not on the recipient's lack of understanding.

RESPOND TO EMOTION

The palliative APRN should pause after information is delivered and allow the group to process it and express emotion. The natural inclination may be to "fill the space" with words, but the APRN must recognize that silence and presence are vital communication tools.[3,16] Expressions of emotion and distress are common during palliative care consultation.[16] Anxiety and fear were the most frequently encountered emotion, followed by sadness, anger, and frustration.[11] Expressions of distress and emotion should be handled by clinicians with compassion and empathy.[3,4,16,52] Allowing time to speak and express emotion has been correlated with higher levels of satisfaction when patients and families speak more than the clinician.[11] Addressing emotions, while intuitive for some, is a skill that can be learned like any other.[4,7] The NURSE mnemonic has been suggested as a way to remember five different skills for handling emotions (Table 33.1).[50] In some instances, the patient or family members may state how they are feeling, and the palliative APRN can reflect back the emotion; in other instances, it may be helpful for the APRN to name what he or she observes and allow the patient or family to validate or clarify. Although no one can fully appreciate another person's exact situation, the palliative APRN can still convey empathy for what the patient and family are experiencing. Acknowledging and offering respect for the emotions being expressed can go far toward building a trusting and supportive therapeutic relationship. Respect and affirmation can be conveyed through the APRN's body language and facial expression as well as with words.

There may be a point in the conversation where the palliative APRN is unsure where things stand based on a patient's quietness or lack of emotion. Using empathic curiosity is a way of exploring, using an open-ended question such as "Are you able to tell me what you are thinking at this point?" or

Table 33.1 EMOTION-HANDLING SKILLS USING THE NURSE MNEMONIC

EMOTION-HANDLING SKILLS	PHRASES TO USE/QUESTIONS TO ASK
N: Recognizing and naming emotion	"I'm hearing that you are really concerned and upset about this situation." "I wonder if you are feeling angry about this?"
U: Expressing understanding and "normalizing" the emotion	"I can't imagine how difficult that it must be, seeing your loved one go through this." "I wouldn't be surprised if you were feeling really sad."
R: Acknowledging and offering respect	"I really appreciate your commitment to your loved one and all the time that you have spent at the hospital." "I have great respect for the care that you have given your loved one."
S: Offering support and demonstrating commitment to the patient and family	"We will continue to adjust your pain medications until you are comfortable."
E: Explore to gain clarity and insight into the story/experience	"Tell me more about . . ." "I heard you say that you felt confused. Can you say more about this?"

From Martin[50]

"We have been discussing some difficult things. How are you doing with this?"[50]

All of the skills to address emotion ultimately offer patients and families support, but none of them specifically addresses the fear of what may happen in the future. In today's healthcare environment, it is crucial to help families plan for what may be coming next.[52] Assuring patients that they will continue to receive personal care, skilled assessment, and pain and symptom management while attending to psychosocial, spiritual, and emotional needs no matter what happens or what decisions they make will go far to allay this fear. Offering false promises of support that is not possible should be avoided, however. Support can be conveyed by making good handoffs, advocating for the needs of the patient and family, and using words that affirm commitment such as "we will continue to care for you and your loved one."

DEVELOPING THE PLAN

In some cases, the emotion of the situation is so overwhelming that it may be best to summarize, plan another meeting, and adjourn. In other situations, further conversation and goal-setting flow naturally from the conversation. Clarifying goals through open-ended questions like "Given what you have heard, what is most important to you now?" and "What things are you hoping for?" can help the palliative APRN make recommendations based on the values and expectations of the patient.[52]

Realistically, it may take several communication episodes or meetings to fully develop the plan of care. While a "meeting before the meeting" can be helpful for the team, a post-meeting debriefing can be just as useful. Delivering bad news and attending to emotion can be stressful for healthcare providers who may or may not have a long-standing relationship with the patient.[56] Taking time to talk about what went well and areas that could be improved upon and assessing the patient's and family's response can be therapeutic as well as educational.

DOCUMENTATION

Documentation of the family meeting is part of the process of communicating with other members of the team and helps to promote continuity (Box 33.7). Several important pieces of information should be included in the documentation for both communication and billing purposes.[16,27,35] It may be helpful to provide a copy to the patient and family for their review and reference and, with the movement of "open notes" in the electronic medical record, they will be able to more readily access it.

DELIVERING BAD NEWS

In addition to leading family meetings and facilitating communication for patients and families, the palliative APRN may be in the position of delivering bad news. Bad news has been defined as any information that adversely alters one's

---

Box 33.7 KEY ELEMENTS OF DOCUMENTATION FOLLOWING A FAMILY MEETING

1. Date and time and where meeting took place (emergency department, intensive care unit, medical floor, clinic, home) which helps to later understand the context of the meeting
2. Participants including patient, family, and the healthcare team. If the patient was unable to participate, note the reason (e.g., "The patient lacked decision-making capacity and was unable to participate.")
3. Purpose of meeting or necessity for medical decision-making
4. A brief summary of information discussed, including:
   Current state of illness
   Patient and family illness understanding
   Prognosis
   Treatment plan
   Specific discussions of bad news
5. Patient and family response (e.g., "After the current state of illness was discussed Mr. Rose states: 'It has been really tough and I feel like I am running out of steam and don't have enough help'")
6. Specific treatments discussed or decisions made (e.g., advance care planning, resuscitation status, medically administered nutrition and hydration, other life-support measures)
7. Disposition planning, including referral to home health, hospice, skilled nursing facility placement, financial concerns, caregiving concerns
8. Concerns, questions, and areas of disagreement or agreement
9. Plan of care or decisions made
10. Next steps or follow-up plan with the patient and family
11. Time the meeting started and ended

From Widera[16], Singer[27]

---

expectations for the future.[49] When delivering bad news, the APRN must use all the principles of good communication, including active listening, open-ended questions, and attention to emotion, as previously described. Just as with a family meeting, appropriate preparation is essential. Preparation includes familiarity with the medical history, arranging the best physical setting possible, and ensuring that the appropriate team members are present.[36] Beginning with a question to elicit understanding is the best starting place.[49] After hearing from the patient and family, correct misunderstandings or validate accurate information.

Communication experts recommend using a warning phrase, commonly referred to as a "warning shot," to allow the patient and family to prepare—something like, "I have some serious news to share with you." After delivering the news, pause and allow the information to be absorbed.[49] Give the patient and family adequate time to express emotions and use open-ended questions. Continuously assess their nonverbal communication and response to the news. Whether the meeting ends after the bad news is delivered or if a detailed plan of care is developed, the APRN should summarize and clarify plans for follow-up with the patient and family before adjourning.

DISCUSSING PROGNOSIS

Discussions of prognosis are common during family meetings and palliative care consultation.[57] Predictions of survival may weigh heavily in decisions to pursue aggressive treatments or choose a less aggressive plan of care.[58] The palliative APRN must be prepared for these discussions and knowledgeable about both prognostic indicators and limitations in the ability to prognosticate. In several studies, surrogate decision-makers have indicated that (1) avoiding these discussions is an unacceptable way to maintain hope and (2) they wanted to receive more than only bad news.[57] "Hope for the best and prepare for the worst" addresses the challenge of providing an honest prognosis with hope and optimism.

Help families not only hear but see the prognosis. Do not give only prognostic information but also provide education on the disease process using drawings or radiographic images. Showing the evidence of the condition or the effect of treatments helps the APRN put the discussion into the context of the patient's goals. Instead of asking, "Do you have any questions?" the APRN should ask, "What questions do you have?" Although surrogates sometimes want numeric estimates of prognosis, clinicians may be reluctant to provide them for fear of misinterpretation.[55] For example, a 95% estimate of death may be reframed positively by a family as a 5% chance of survival. Given the challenges of providing precise estimates of life expectancy, a common approach is to provide ranges (e.g., hours to days, days to weeks, weeks to months). Performance scales, such as the Palliative Performance Score, may be used to support prognostication.[59]

Communication of prognosis may be an iterative process involving information provided at a family meeting being reinforced over time by various members of the team, including the bedside nurse and social worker. Surrogate decision-makers may employ coping strategies to balance the tension between honesty and hope.

1. *Focusing on minutia*: Small positive changes, such as improvement in urine output or respiratory rate or the patient's level of consciousness, provided both information and hope.[60]

2. *Relying on personal knowledge and beliefs about the patient*: The decision-maker believes he or she can interpret a patient's response that a stranger would not be able to identify or the patient has unique strengths unknown to the medical team For example, the family may believe a facial expression is special communication meant only for them and not the medical team or that the patient is a "fighter."[60]

3. *Seeking information and support from sources outside of the medical team*: The decision-maker may contact friends, family, and others with similar experience or a medical background, as well as online resources.[9]

4. *Avoidance and disbelief*: Some surrogates avoided doctors whom they perceived as pessimistic, or they expressed blatant disbelief.[60]

5. *Optimism grounded in religious beliefs or a worldview different from that of the medical team*: For example: "The doctors do what they need to and God will do the rest.[54] Research has illustrated the limitations of the palliative care clinician's ability to predict life expectancy.[61]

The significance of functional prognosis should not be underestimated. For many persons, loss of cognitive or functional abilities resulting in dependence on others would be in conflict with their goals and values and may directly impact decision-making. Studies have demonstrated that the most common prognostic error among providers, including palliative care clinicians, is overestimating life expectancy.[61]

Predictions of survival for patients with specific diagnoses have also been studied. For example, in cancer patients, functional status is the single greatest prognostic factor.[45,51] The Karnofsky Performance Status (KPS) score, Palliative Performance Scale (PPS) score, and Eastern Cooperative Oncology Group (ECOG) score are commonly used to rate a patient's performance status.[45,62] For patients with a poor functional status (defined as spending more than 50% of their day in bed or chair), a rough estimate of survival is less than 3 months.[45,62] For patients with end-stage renal disease on maintenance hemodialysis, several variables have been independently associated with mortality, including older age, dementia, peripheral vascular disease, decreased albumin, and a negative answer to the "surprise question" ("Would I be surprised if my patient died within the next 6 months?").[63] Predicting survival in disease states like congestive heart failure remains difficult given the increasing use of advanced therapies, such as transplantation and ventricular assist devices (VADs), as well as the risk of sudden death.[64]

Prognosis can include much more than just survival estimates. Medical decisions should not be made in isolation, but rather in context with long-term implications. Together, this may help patients and families make more informed choices. Patients and families need explanation that treatments like feeding tube insertion may lead to other consequences, such as skilled nursing facility placement or use of physical and chemical restraints.[65]

DISCUSSING TECHNOLOGY AND WITHHOLDING, DISCONTINUING, WITHDRAWING TREATMENTS IN FAMILY MEETINGS

Use of aggressive therapies and technology is common in seriously ill patients and those at the end of life.[43] APRNs must be knowledgeable about commonly used technologies and how the use of technology fits into the context of the patient's goals of care[10] (see Chapter 54, "Discontinuation of Cardiac Technology"; Chapter 55, "Discontinuation of Respiratory Technology"; and Chapter 56, "Discontinuation of Other Life-Sustaining Therapies"). In family meetings, use of technology should be closely tied to the patient's values and goals as well as to what is feasible and the long-term implications of particular decisions.[10] Although withholding and discontinuing therapies are viewed as ethically equivalent, they may be perceived very differently.[41,66] Families may feel they are playing a more active role or are the cause of a poor outcome by discontinuing a therapy already in use rather than never initiating it in the first place. Clinicians may also make a moral distinction between withholding and discontinuing and may be more comfortable withholding than discontinuing therapies[66-68] (see Chapter 53, "Navigating Ethical Dilemmas").

The APRN must recognize and support families who are struggling with these painful decisions and help them prepare for outcomes that will include consequences of treatments.[68] Reframing the situation may be helpful. For example, if a decision is made to discontinue ventilator use in a patient with end-stage lung disease based on knowledge of the patient's wishes, the disease is allowed to follow its natural course and is actually the cause of death, not the removal of the ventilator. Words matter greatly in these discussions. Well-intended clinicians may use phrases like "withdrawing care" when they really mean discontinuing a specific treatment.[69] The palliative APRN must communicate that, although specific treatment is no longer to be used, attention to care and comfort will continue. See Section IX of this book, "Ethical Dilemmas," which includes chapters on the discontinuation of cardiac, respiratory, and other interventions.

RESUSCITATION

CPR techniques were developed in the 1960s with the purpose of supporting individuals experiencing a significant out-of-hospital healthcare emergencies, such as a heart attack, drowning, or accident. They were not intended to become part of routine treatment at the time of death from a terminal illness.[70] In our current healthcare system, though, use of CPR is an "opt out" request, and the default assumption is that everyone desires CPR.[70] Many patients and families do not understand the low likelihood of survival in a person with advanced disease and may believe that the chances of a good outcome are much higher.[71] Discussing do-not-resuscitate (DNR) status during a family meeting is best done in the context of the overall goals of care.[72] Making recommendations tied to the ability of resuscitation attempts to meet the patient's goals rather than asking a question is often a more effective approach. Phrases like "If your heart and lungs stop, do you want to us to do everything?" The phrases "Restarting your heart" and "Putting on a breathing machine" convey a false assurance of success and reversibility.[45] Families may worry that if doing everything possible includes CPR, then the opposite is doing nothing. Patients and families may be under the false assumption that "do not resuscitate" is the same as "do not treat" or being abandoned.[73] The APRN should reassure the patient and family that they will continue to be cared for and that treatments that support their goals will continue. The following dialog is a good example of explaining DNR status.

PATIENT: I would never want to be kept alive on machines..."
APRN: You have told me that you would prefer your death to be peaceful and that you want to be at home. I would recommend that we make your wishes clear to the medical team and place a do-not-attempt-resuscitation order in your medical record. We will continue to provide all the appropriate treatments to manage your symptoms and support the quality of life that we have discussed.

IMPLANTABLE CARDIAC DEVICES

Despite the benefits of implantable cardiac devices such as pacemakers, VADs, and defibrillators in terms of improving and lengthening life, all of the patients who receive them will eventually reach the end of their lives[73] (see Chapter 13, "The Palliative APRN in Specialty Cardiology"). As many as 30% of patients with implantable cardiac defibrillators receive shocks as they approach the end of life, which can lead to significant distress for patients and families alike.[73] Ideally, conversations about deactivation should occur when the devices are implanted, and the issue should be readdressed as the underlying heart disease progresses.[73] Decisions about device deactivation should occur in the context of goals of care and resuscitation discussions during a family meeting. The APRN should obtain a history from the patient and family about their past experience with a device (e.g., prior defibrillator activations). Some patients may have little memory; others may describe the episode as being painful or frightening ("being kicked in the chest" or "an explosion"). If a decision is made to deactivate the device, the APRN should prepare those involved for what to expect when the device is deactivated. Patients may incorrectly assume that deactivation is a surgical procedure or that death will occur when the device is turned off. The APRN should assess the patient's and family's understanding and provide appropriate education about the deactivation process and its implications.

VADs are surgically implanted pumps to support damaged left, right, or both ventricles. Discussion related to discontinuation of VAD therapy should be in the context of goals in a family meeting when there are complications or the device no longer supports the desired quality of life. The APRN should advise patients and families that after VAD discontinuation time of survival may range from a few minutes to a few days[74] (see Chapter 54, "Discontinuation of Cardiac Therapies").

MEDICALLY ASSISTED NUTRITION AND HYDRATION

For many patients and families, medically assisted nutrition and hydration are not medical treatments but symbols of love and care. Any suggestion that these elements be withheld or discontinued can be perceived as tantamount to neglect. Current guidelines advise against placement of percutaneous endoscopic gastrostomy tubes (PEG) in patients with advanced dementia, yet many of these tubes are inserted.[65,75] Clinicians may lack knowledge about risks and benefits of these tubes and may feel pressure from families to place them or fear litigation.[75] During a family meeting, it is important for the palliative APRN to help families make the connection between medically assisted nutrition and hydration as a treatment and how it supports or does not support the goals of care. For example, use of medically administered nutrition and hydration in a frail elderly person with advanced dementia will not help the person get stronger, prevent aspiration, reverse the underlying disease, or prolong life.[65] Without the clinician's direction, families may continue to harbor erroneous beliefs about the benefits of medically administered nutrition and hydration. The astute palliative APRN can show the family how they can demonstrate love and care in other ways, such as inviting family participation in careful hand feeding or providing oral or other physical care[65] (see Chapter 56, "Discontinuation of Other Life-Sustaining Therapies").

CRITICAL CARE OR EMERGENCY DEPARTMENT FAMILY MEETINGS

Twenty percent of all deaths in the United States occur in an ICU.[38,55] Decisions to withhold or discontinue specific ICU treatments are often done in the context of a family meeting.[14] Family meetings in the ICU have been associated with higher levels of satisfaction, and guidelines recommend that family meetings occur within 72 hours of an ICU admission.[36] Family meetings in the ICU have been associated with higher mortality rates, which may reflect the increased importance of and attention to communication in end-of-life situations.[14] Improved communication and additional family support in the ICU have been associated with a shorter ICU length of stay.[38,48]

The need for family meetings in the emergency department (ED) may parallel those in the ICU. ED visits may be precipitated by a health crisis in which discussion of prognosis and treatment is of vital importance.[76] (See Chapter 10, "The Palliative APRN in the Emergency Department.") The chaotic ED environment presents significant communication challenges independent of the crisis situation. Palliative care consultation in the ED is a growing area and has been associated with improved quality of life without change in survival.[77] More research is needed to understand the use of family meetings in the ED.

When a person is ill enough to require ICU care, it may be too late to discuss values and wishes with the patient, and the information must be obtained from surrogates.[12,27,38,54] The "U" in the VALUE mnemonic (Box 33.4), understanding the patient as a person, involves engaging surrogate decision-makers by using open-ended questions. The APRN can ask questions such as "Tell me about your loved one," "What things did he/she enjoy doing?," "What was life like for him/her prior to this illness?" to help the family or surrogate decision-maker construct a picture of the patient and what was important to him or her.[5,7,10,12,47] Discussions should point surrogates toward what the patient would have expressed for him- or herself rather than what the surrogate would want, or to determine what is in the best interest of the patient when his or her wishes are not known.[9]

Of all of the ICU technologies, mechanical ventilation is the most common life-support measure to be discontinued.[38] Other ICU technologies that may be discussed during family meetings include continuous renal replacement therapy (CRRT), vasopressors, and extracorporeal membrane oxygenation (ECMO). The APRN should have a basic understanding of these therapies and the implications for their use or discontinuation if they are to be addressed during a family meeting.

DEALING WITH CONFLICT

Conflict in family meetings is to be expected.[58,78,79] Conflict may be defined as a disagreement or difference of opinion on the management of a patient involving more than one individual and requiring a decision or action.[58,78] The conflict may be between family members, within the team, or between the team and the family. Nurses may be the team member most likely to identify conflicts.[58,78] A common area of disagreement between team and family and between family members is around decisions to withhold or discontinue life-sustaining therapies.[58,78,79] Decision-making around life-sustaining therapies may be complicated by uncertainty about the clinical outcomes and prognostic challenges. Conflict often arises when families request more aggressive treatment than the team believes to be appropriate.[58] Other sources of conflict may include the surrogate's inability to make a decision or the lack of available decision-makers.

The burden of decision-making is not insignificant for families who must process complicated information during a time of uncertainty and unprecedented stress. The shift toward autonomy in decision-making has, in some cases, allowed the healthcare team to take a passive approach and avoid the obligation to provide recommendations based on their experience and medical knowledge.[79] Palliative APRNs should be aware of the risk factors for conflict that have been identified.[58,78]

1. An ICU setting where life-sustaining treatment is in use or being considered

2. An unmarried patient

3. A decision-maker (patient or family member) who is medically naïve or views the body in more mechanistic terms

4. A decision-maker (patient or family member) who has underlying cognitive or mental health concerns

5. A prior history of poor coping skills (in patient or family member)

6. A history of substance abuse (in patient or family member)

7. A culture in which the patient or family member is traditionally mistrustful of the medical establishment

8. A belief system of patient or family member that allows for miracles as the sole option

When there is conflict about the goals of care and the reality of the medical situation, recognize and respond to emotion. Grief, anger, mistrust, unfinished personal business, and guilt may lie beneath the more visible conflict.[5] Using emotion-handling skills such as NURSE (see Table 33.1) or "wish statements" can help diffuse conflict.[35] By saying "I wish there was a more effective treatment for your mother's condition," the APRN is entering into the patient's situation empathically but at the same time acknowledging that the situation is not reversible.[5] Empathic responses, especially when there is conflict, will help to foster trust and build a therapeutic relationship.[3–5]

Although lack of information may also precipitate conflict, attempts to convince the family of a certain viewpoint may deepen the divide. Seeking understanding and clarity about the family's position is essential: "I heard you mention that you want everything done for your loved one.[5] Please help me understand what 'everything' means to you." Even when there is disagreement, it is important to seek common ground. It may be that the medical team and family can only agree that they both want what is best for the patient and decide on a time to meet again.

SUMMARY

Family meetings are an essential tool in palliative care. More research is needed to examine the best timing, participants, and methods for use of family meetings. By the nature of their education and expertise, palliative APRNs often lead these meetings. APRNs must be skilled in principles of good communication, including attending to emotion and negotiating conflict, to provide effective care through family meetings. The APRN should pay careful attention to advance preparation and take a "time out" to make sure that everyone is ready before continuing. Above all, proceed with sensitivity, employ empathy, and listen before speaking.

REFERENCES

1. Dahlin C. *Palliative Nursing: Scope and Standards of Practice. 6th ed.* Pittsburgh, PA: Hospice and Palliative Nurses Association; 2021.
2. Dahlin C, Coyne P. The palliative APRN leader. *Ann Palliat Med.* 2019;8(Suppl 1):S30–S38. doi:10.21037/apm.2018.06.03
3. Dahlin C, Wittenberg E. Communication in palliative care In: Ferrell B, Paice J. eds. *Oxford Textbook of Palliative Nursing.* 5th ed. New York: Oxford University Press; 2019: 55–78.
4. Forbat L, François K, O'Callaghan L, Kulikowski J. Family meetings in inpatient specialist palliative care: A mechanism to convey empathy. *J Pain Symptom Manage.* 2018;55(5):1253–1259. doi:10.1016/j.jpainsymman.2018.01.020
5. Derry HM, Epstein AS, Lichtenthal WG, Prigerson HG. Emotions in the room: Common emotional reactions to discussions of poor prognosis and tools to address them. *Expert Rev Anticancer Ther.* 2019;19(8):689–696. doi:10.1080/14737140.2019.1651648
6. Adams A, Mannix T, Harrington A. Nurses' communication with families in the intensive care unit: A literature review. *Nurs Crit Care.* 2017;22(2):70–80. doi:10.1111/nicc.12141
7. Fuoto A, Turner KM. Palliative care nursing communication: An evaluation of the comfort model. *J Hosp Palliat Nurs.* 2019;21(2):124–130. doi:10.1097/NJH.0000000000000493
8. American Nurses Association and Hospice and Palliative Nurses Association. *Call for Action: Nurses Lead and Transform Palliative Care.* Silver Spring, MD: ANA; 2017. https://www.nursingworld.org/~497158/globalassets/practiceandpolicy/health-policy/palliativecareprofessionalissuespanelcallforaction.pdf
9. Izumi S. Advance care planning. *Am J Nurs.* 2017;117(6):56–61. doi:10.1097/01.NAJ.0000520255.65083.35
10. Seaman JB, Arnold RM, Scheunemann LP, White DB. An integrated framework for effective and efficient communication with families in the adult intensive care unit. *Ann Am Thorac Soc.* 2017;14(6):1015–1020. doi:10.1513/AnnalsATS.201612-965OI
11. Curtis JR, Downey L, Back AL, et al. Effect of a patient and clinician communication-priming intervention on patient-reported goals-of-care discussions between patients with serious illness and clinicians: A randomized clinical trial. *JAMA Intern Med.* 2018;178(7):930–940. doi:10.1001/jamainternmed.2018.2317
12. Davidson JE, Aslakson RA, Long AC, et al. Guidelines for family-centered care in the neonatal, pediatric, and adult ICU. *Crit Care Med.* 2017;45(1):103–128. doi:10.1097/CCM.0000000000002169
13. Cahill PJ, Lobb EA, Sanderson C, Phillips JL. What is the evidence for conducting palliative care family meetings? A systematic review. *Palliat Med.* 2017;31(3):197–211. doi:10.1177/0269216316658833
14. Piscitello GM, Parham WM 3rd, Huber MT, Siegler M, Parker WF. The timing of family meetings in the medical intensive care unit. *Am J Hosp Palliat Care.* 2019;36(12):1049–1056. doi:10.1177/1049909119843133
15. Weissman D, Quill T, Arnold R. Palliative care fast facts and concepts #222. *The Family Meeting—Part 1.* Appleton, WI: Palliative Care Network of Wisconsin. 2015. https://www.mypcnow.org/fastfact/the-family-meeting-part-1-preparing/
16. Widera E, Anderson WG, Santhosh L, McKee KY, Smith AK, Frank J. Family meetings on behalf of patients with serious illness. *N Engl J Med.* 2020;383(11):e71. doi:10.1056/NEJMvcm1913056
17. National Consensus Project for Quality Palliative Care. *Clinical Practice Guidelines for Quality Palliative Care.* 4th ed. Richmond, VA: National Coalition for Hospice and Palliative Care; 2018. https://www.nationalcoalitionhpc.org/ncp
18. Wittenberg E, Reb A, Kanter E. Communicating with patients and families around difficult topics in cancer care using the comfort communication curriculum. *Semin Oncol Nurs.* 2018;34(3):264–273. doi:10.1016/j.soncn.2018.06.007
19. Hospice and Palliative Nurses Association. *Position Statement: The Value of the Professional Nurse in Palliative Care.* Pittsburgh, PA: Hospice and Palliative Nurses Association; 2021. https://advancingexpertcare.org/position-statements
20. Martin-Misener R, Harbman P, Donald F, et al. Cost-effectiveness of nurse practitioners in primary and specialised ambulatory care: Systematic review. *BMJ Open.* 2015;5(6):e007167. Published 2015 Jun 8. doi:10.1136/bmjopen-2014-007167
21. Woo BFY, Lee JXY, Tam WWS. The impact of the advanced practice nursing role on quality of care, clinical outcomes, patient satisfaction, and cost in the emergency and critical care settings: A systematic review. *Hum Resour Health.* 2017;15(1):63. Published 2017 Sep 11. doi:10.1186/s12960-017-0237-9
22. Miller SC, Lima JC, Intrator O, Martin E, Bull J, Hanson LC. Palliative care consultations in nursing homes and reductions in acute care use and potentially burdensome end-of-life transitions. *J Am Geriatr Soc.* 2016;64(11):2280–2287. doi:10.1111/jgs.14469
23. Walling AM, D'Ambruoso SF, Malin JL, et al. Effect and efficiency of an embedded palliative care nurse practitioner in an oncology clinic. *J Oncol Pract.* 2017;13(9):e792–e799. doi:10.1200/JOP.2017.020990
24. Wu H, Ren D, Zinsmeister GR, Zewe GE, Tuite PK. Implementation of a nurse-led family meeting in a neuroscience intensive care unit. *Dimens Crit Care Nurs.* 2016;35(5):268–276. doi:10.1097/DCC.0000000000000199
25. Dorell Å, Östlund U, Sundin K. Nurses' perspective of conducting family conversation. *Int J Qual Stud Health Well-Being.* 2016;11:30867. Published 2016 Apr 20. doi:10.3402/qhw.v11.30867

26. Buller H, Virani R, Malloy P, Paice J. End-of-Life Nursing and Education Consortium Communication Curriculum for Nurses. *Journal of Hospice & Palliative Nursing.* 2019;21(2):E5–E12. doi:10.1097/NJH.0000000000000540.

27. Singer AE, Ash T, Ochotorena C, et al. A systematic review of family meeting tools in palliative and intensive care settings. *Am J Hosp Palliat Care.* 2016;33(8):797–806. doi:10.1177/1049909115594353

28. Pecanac K, King B. Nurse-family communication during and after family meetings in the intensive care unit. *J Nurs Scholarsh.* 2019;51(2):129–137. doi:10.1111/jnu.12459

29. Wittenberg E, Ferrell B, Goldsmith J, Buller H, Neiman T. Nurse communication about goals of care. *J Adv Pract Oncol.* 2016;7(2):146–154. doi:10.6004/jadpro.2016.7.2.2

30. Brown CE, Back AL, Ford DW, et al. Self-assessment scores improve after simulation-based palliative care communication skill workshops. *Am J Hosp Palliat Care.* 2018;35(1):45–51. doi:10.1177/1049909116681972

31. Temel JS, Greer JA, El-Jawahri A, et al. Effects of early integrated palliative care in patients with lung and GI cancer: A randomized clinical trial. *J Clin Oncol.* 2017;35(8):834–841. doi:10.1200/JCO.2016.70.5046

32. Schoenherr LA, Bischoff KE, Marks AK, O'Riordan DL, Pantilat SZ. Trends in hospital-based specialty palliative care in the United States from 2013 to 2017. *JAMA Netw Open.* 2019;2(12):e1917043. Published 2019 Dec 2. doi:10.1001/jamanetworkopen.2019.17043

33. Cahill PJ, Lobb EA, Sanderson C, Phillips JL. What is the evidence for conducting palliative care family meetings? A systematic review. *Palliat Med.* 2017;31(3):197–211. doi:10.1177/0269216316658833

34. Carson SS, Cox CE, Wallenstein S, et al. Effect of palliative care-led meetings for families of patients with chronic critical illness: A randomized clinical trial [published correction appears in JAMA. 2017 May 23;317(20):2134]. *JAMA.* 2016;316(1):51–62. doi:10.1001/jama.2016.8474

35. Paladino J, Fromme EK. Preparing for serious illness: A model for better conversations over the continuum of care. *Am Fam Physician.* 2019;99(5):281–284.

36. Walter JK, Arnold RM, Curley MAQ, Feudtner C. Teamwork when conducting family meetings: Concepts, terminology, and the importance of team-team practices. *J Pain Symptom Manage.* 2019;58(2):336–343. doi:10.1016/j.jpainsymman.2019.04.030

37. Institute of Medicine; Committee on Approaching Death: Addressing Key End of Life Issues. *Dying in America: Improving Quality and Honoring Individual Preferences Near the End of Life.* Washington, DC: The National Academies Press; 2015 Mar 19. https://www.ncbi.nlm.nih.gov/books/NBK285681/ doi:10.17226/18748

38. White DB, Angus DC, Shields AM, et al. A randomized trial of a family-support intervention in intensive care units. *N Engl J Med.* 2018;378(25):2365–2375. doi:10.1056/NEJMoa1802637

39. SUPPORT Principal Investigators. A controlled trial to improve care for seriously ill patients: The study to understand prognoses and preferences for outcomes and risks of treatments (support). *JAMA.* 1995;274: 1591–1598.

40. Weiner JS, Roth J. Avoiding iatrogenic harm to patient and family while discussing goals of care near the end of life. *J Palliat Med.* 2006;9: 451–463.

41. Pecanac KE, Brown RL. Decision proposals in the family conference. *Patient Educ Couns.* 2017;100(12):2255–2261. doi:10.1016/j.pec.2017.06.011

42. Torke AM, Callahan CM, Sachs GA, et al. Communication quality predicts psychological well-being and satisfaction in family surrogates of hospitalized older adults: An observational study. *J Gen Intern Med.* 2018;33(3):298–304. doi:10.1007/s11606-017-4222-8

43. Silva MD, Tsai S, Sobota RM, Abel BT, Reid MC, Adelman RD. Missed opportunities when communicating with limited English-proficient patients during end-of-life conversations: Insights from Spanish-speaking and Chinese-speaking medical interpreters. *J Pain Symptom Manage.* 2020;59(3):694–701. doi:10.1016/j.jpainsymman.2019.10.019

44. Wright AA, Zhang B, Ray A, et al. Associations between end-of-life discussions, patient mental health, medical care near death and caregiver bereavement adjustment. *JAMA.* 2008;300: 1665–1673.

45. Weisman D. Palliative Care Fast Facts and Concepts #13. Determining prognosis in advanced cancer. Appleton, WI: Palliative Care Network of Wisconsin. 2015. https://www.mypcnow.org/fast-fact/determining-prognosis-in-advanced-cancer/

46. Wu H, Ren D, Zinsmeister GR, Zewe GE, Tuite PK. Implementation of a nurse-led family meeting in a neuroscience intensive care unit. *Dimens Crit Care Nurs.* 2016;35(5):268–276. doi:10.1097/DCC.0000000000000199

47. Lautrette A, Darmon M, Megarbane B, et al. A communication strategy and brochure for relatives of patients dying the ICU. *N Engl J Med.* 2007;356: 469–478. doi:10.1056/NEJMoa063446

48. Hua M, Lu Y, Ma X, Morrison RS, Li G, Wunsch H. Association between the implementation of hospital-based palliative care and use of intensive care during terminal hospitalizations. *JAMA Netw Open.* 2020;3(1):e1918675. doi:10.1001/jamanetworkopen.2019.18675

49. Baile WF, Buckman R, Lenzi R, Glober G, Beale EA, Kudelka AP. SPIKES: A six-step protocol for delivering bad news: Application to the patient with cancer. *Oncologist.* 2000;5(4):302–311. doi:10.1634/theoncologist.5-4-302

50. Martin EJ, Rich SE, Jones JA, Dharmarajan KV. Communication skill frameworks: Applications in radiation oncology. *Ann Palliat Med.* 2019;8(3):293–304. doi:10.21037/apm.2019.03.03

51. Congress.gov. H. R. 5835. Omnibus budget reconciliation act of 1990. *Patient Self-Determination Act.* 1990 P.L. 101–508. https://www.congress.gov/bill/101st-congress/house-bill/5835

52. Meeker MA, Waldrop DP, Seo JY. Examining family meetings at end of life: The model of practice in a hospice inpatient unit. *Palliat Support Care.* 2015;13(5):1283–1291. doi:10.1017/S1478951514001138

53. Ketterer B, Arnold R. Palliative care fast facts and concepts #378. How to help a patient choose a surrogate decision-maker. Appleton, WI: Palliative Care Network of Wisconsin. 2015. https://www.mypcnow.org/wp-content/uploads/2019/06/FF-378-Choosing-a-Surrogate.docx.pdf

54. Batteux E, Ferguson E, Tunney RJ. A mixed methods investigation of end-of-life surrogate decisions among older adults. *BMC Palliat Care.* 2020;19(1):44. Published 2020 Apr 2. doi:10.1186/s12904-020-00553-w

55. Anderson WG, Cimino JW, Ernecoff NC, et al. A multicenter study of key stakeholders' perspectives on communicating with surrogates about prognosis in intensive care units. *Ann Am Thorac Soc.* 2015;12(2):142–152. doi:10.1513/AnnalsATS.201407-325OC

56. Kavalieratos D, Siconolfi DE, Steinhauser KE, et al. "It is like heart failure. It is chronic . . . and it will kill you": A qualitative analysis of burnout among hospice and palliative care clinicians. *J Pain Symptom Manage.* 2017;53(5):901–910.e1. doi:10.1016/j.jpainsymman.2016.12.337

57. Hui D, Paiva CE, Del Fabbro EG, et al. Prognostication in advanced cancer: Update and directions for future research. *Support Care Cancer.* 2019;27(6):1973–1984. doi:10.1007/s00520-019-04727-y

58. Cifrese L, Rincon F. Futility and patients who insist on medically ineffective therapy. *Semin Neurol.* 2018;38(5):561–568. doi:10.1055/s-0038-1667386

59. Baik D, Russell D, Jordan L, Dooley F, Bowles KH, Masterson Creber RM. Using the palliative performance scale to estimate survival for patients at the end of life: A systematic review of the literature. *J Palliat Med.* 2018;21(11):1651–1661. doi:10.1089/jpm.2018.0141

60. White DB, Ernecoff N, Buddadhumaruk P, et al. Prevalence of and factors related to discordance about prognosis between physicians and surrogate decision-makers of critically ill patients. *JAMA.* 2016;315(19):2086–2094. doi:10.1001/jama.2016.5351

61. Gramling R, Gajary-Coots E, Cimino J, et al. Palliative care clinician overestimation of survival in advanced cancer: Disparities and association with end-of-life care [published correction appears in j pain symptom manage. 2019 Oct;58(4):e19–e20.

J Pain Symptom Manage. 2019;57(2):233–240. doi:10.1016/j.jpainsymman.2018.10.510

62. Wilner LS, Arnold R. Palliative Care Fast Facts and Concepts #125. The Palliative Performance Scale. Appleton, WI: Palliative Care Network of Wisconsin. https://www.mypcnow.org/fast-fact/the-palliative-performance-scale-pps/

63. Cohen LM, Ruthazer R, Moss AH, Germain MJ. Predicting 6-month mortality for patients who are on maintenance hemodialysis. *Clin J Am Soc Nephrol.* 2010;5:72–79. doi:10.2215/CJN.03860609

64. Warraich HJ, Allen LA, Mukamal KJ, Ship A, Kociol RD. Accuracy of physician prognosis in heart failure and lung cancer: Comparison between physician estimates and model predicted survival. *Palliat Med.* 2016;30(7):684–689. doi:10.1177/0269216315626048

65. American Geriatrics Society Ethics Committee and Clinical Practice and Models of Care Committee. American Geriatrics Society feeding tubes in advanced dementia position statement. *J Am Geriatr Soc.* 2014;62(8):1590–1593. doi:10.1111/jgs.12924

66. Hospice and Palliative Nurses Association. *Position Statement: Withholding/Withdrawing Life Sustaining Therapies.* Pittsburgh, PA: Hospice and Palliative Nurses Association; 2016. https://advancingexpertcare.org/position-statements

67. Chung GS, Yoon JD, Rasinski KA, Curlin FA. Us physicians' opinions about distinctions between withdrawing and withholding life-sustaining treatment. *J Relig Health.* 2016;55(5):1596–1606. doi:10.1007/s10943-015-0171-x

68. American Nurses Association. *Code of Ethics.* 2nd ed. Silver Spring, MD: American Nurses Association; 2015.

69. Wentlandt K, Toupin P, Novosedlik N, Le LW, Zimmermann C, Kaya E. Language used by healthcare professionals to describe dying at an acute care hospital. *J Pain Symptom Manage.* 2018;56(3):337–343. doi:10.1016/j.jpainsymman.2018.05.013

70. Fowler R, Chang MP, Idris AH. Evolution and revolution in cardiopulmonary resuscitation. *Curr Opin Crit Care.* 2017;23(3):183–187. doi:10.1097/MCC.0000000000000414

71. Shif Y, Doshi P, Almoosa KF. What CPR means to surrogate decision-makers of ICU patients. *Resuscitation.* 2015;90:73–78. doi:10.1016/j.resuscitation.2015.02.014

72. American Nurses Association. Position Statement: *Nursing Care and Do-Not-Resuscitate (DNR) Decisions.* Silver Spring, MD: American Nurses Association; 2020. https://www.nursingworld.org/~494a87/globalassets/practiceandpolicy/nursing-excellence/ana-position-statements/social-causes-and-health-care/nursing-care-and-do-not-resuscitate-DNR-decisions-final-nursingworld.pdf

73. Thompson JH, Thylén I, Moser DK. Shared decision-making about end-of-life care scenarios compared among implantable cardioverter defibrillator patients: A national cohort study. *Circ Heart Fail.* 2019;12(10):e005619. doi:10.1161/CIRCHEARTFAILURE.118.005619

74. Wordingham SE, McIlvennan CK, Fendler TJ, et al. Palliative care clinicians caring for patients before and after continuous flow-left ventricular assist device. *J Pain Symptom Manage.* 2017;54(4):601–608. doi:10.1016/j.jpainsymman.2017.07.007

75. Gieniusz M, Sinvani L, Kozikowski A, et al. Percutaneous feeding tubes in individuals with advanced dementia: Are physicians "choosing wisely?" *J Am Geriatr Soc.* 2018;66(1):64–69. doi:10.1111/jgs.15125

76. Cooper E, Hutchinson A, Sheikh Z, Taylor P, Townend W, Johnson MJ. Palliative care in the emergency department: A systematic literature qualitative review and thematic synthesis. *Palliat Med.* 2018;32(9):1443–1454. doi:10.1177/0269216318783920

77. Wilson JG, English DP, Owyang CG, et al. End-of-life care, palliative care consultation, and palliative care referral in the emergency department: A systematic review. *J Pain Symptom Manage.* 2020;59(2):372–383.e1. doi:10.1016/j.jpainsymman.2019.09.020

78. Studdert DM, Mello MM, Burns JP, et al. Conflict in the care of patients with prolonged stay in the ICU: Types, sources, and predictors. *Intens Care Med.* 2003;29: 1489–1497. doi:10.1007/s00134-003-1853-5

79. Mehter HM, McCannon JB, Clark JA, Wiener RS. Physician approaches to conflict with families surrounding end-of-life decision-making in the intensive care unit: A qualitative study. *Ann Am Thor Soc.* 2018;15(2):241–249. doi:10.1513/AnnalsATS.201702-105OC

34.

COMMUNICATION AT THE END OF LIFE

Marlene E. McHugh, Penelope R. Buschman, and Susan M. Delisle

---

KEY POINTS

- Communication at the time of death requires sensitivity and compassion.

- The palliative advanced practice registered nurse (APRN) must communicate effectively and compassionately with the patient, family, and healthcare team at the end of life.

- Using a family systems theoretical framework enhances the ability of palliative APRNs to assess and intervene with patients and families at the end of life.

- The COVID 19 pandemic has highlighted unique communication challenges for the palliative APRN.

CASE STUDY 1: FAMILY DECISION-MAKING IN A PATIENT WITH DEMENTIA

Mr. H was a 76-year-old man with a history of hypertension and mild dementia who resided in a skilled nursing facility. He was brought by ambulance to the emergency department (ED) with acute dyspnea and fever.

The ED advanced practice registered nurse (APRN) who assessed him in the ED telephoned Mr. H's healthcare agent, his eldest daughter, to disclose that his clinical picture of respiratory distress, confusion, fever, and hypoxia, along with his chest imaging, were consistent with severe pneumonia, and that intubation, mechanical ventilation, and intensive care unit (ICU)-level care would be required. The APRN advised that even with this manner of invasive support, his overall prognosis was poor given his age and severity of illness. His daughter was then asked to provide consent for treatment. Although she had traveled to the hospital, she was not allowed entry to the ED due to COVID-19 no visitor rules. Her father had not done any advance planning, nor had he ever expressed his thoughts about resuscitative measures. Therefore, she requested a conference call between the medical staff and her other siblings in order to have a fuller discussion regarding what her father would have wanted under the current circumstances. However, she was told that these decisions had to be made quickly, as his condition was deteriorating. She gave verbal consent for intubation, ICU transfer, and specified his code status as full code.

Mr. H spent the subsequent 5 weeks in the ICU with COVID-19 and underwent antiviral treatment and antibiotics for a superimposed bacterial infection. His hypoxia improved, but he remained unable to tolerate ventilator weaning. His family had been unable to communicate with him because he required sedation and paralytics in order to promote ventilator synchrony. In response to the no visitor policy, the ICU team developed an ad hoc position called the "family liaison." The ICU family liaison APRN provided daily medical updates via telephone to the family and utilized a tablet to allow the children to see their father. With the tablet placed by his ear, although he was unresponsive, they could speak to him on a regular basis.

Despite weaning sedation, Mr. H had persistent ventilator dependence, so the team planned a virtual family meeting to discuss options for care, including the indications for tracheostomy placement. The ICU family liaison APRN and ICU social worker coordinated a video conference that included the ICU attending physician, a Spanish translator, and the patient's children. Potential treatment options included compassionate extubation and comfort-focused care or tracheostomy surgery. The team advised that tracheostomy might facilitate ventilator weaning, and the family provided consent for this intervention.

After the tracheostomy and two additional weeks of ventilator support, Mr. H was still unable to tolerate lessening of ventilatory support. In a second virtual family meeting, the hospital team was reassembled to confer with the patient's children because the patient was deemed to continue to lack capacity. The medical team proposed the surgical implantation of a percutaneous gastrostomy tube, which would make him a candidate for discharge to a long-term facility that could accommodate tube feedings and ventilator support. In this discussion, his children collectively felt that tube feedings and indefinite tethering to a ventilator would not be what their father would have wanted.

At the request of the ICU team, a palliative APRN called the patient's daughter and organized a conference call with all the children, allowing the family to express their views on their father's values and what they hoped for him. Interdisciplinary support from palliative care social work and chaplaincy was also provided telephonically. The family elected to transfer Mr. H to the hospice unit for discontinuation of the ventilator and intensive symptom management. In addition, there was the opportunity for in-person goodbyes because the hospice unit was able to accommodate family member visitation at imminent end of life.

INTRODUCTION

Communication across settings at the end of life involves not only the patient and family but also multiple APRNs and other members of the healthcare team. The case study demonstrates two essential teaching points: effective communication skills used by the APRN while caring for patients with serious or life-threatening illnesses and the need for earlier palliative care consultation. The current pandemic highlights various communication challenges that are unique during this time.[1]

The work of palliative nursing is born of the knowledge of family systems theory, communication skill, and bereavement theories, as well as expert assessment and patient/family teaching. It is also made manifest in a delicate dance of unspoken communication between the nurse and the relationships served: the intuitive knowing of nurses as relationships change dramatically, as death approaches, and ultimately in the basic tenet of palliative nursing that our care is family-centered and, if done well, is relationship-centered.[2]

The American Nurses Association (ANA) requires nurses to provide comfort, and this includes expertise in the relief of suffering whether physical, emotional, spiritual, or existential. Increasingly, this means that the nurse's role includes discussing end-of-life choices before a person's death is imminent, being present at the time of death, and providing care to the family dealing with loss.[3] The following sections from the *Code of Ethics for Nurses* serve as support for this position statement.

Provision 1.2
- Nurses establish relationships of trust and provide nursing services according to need, setting aside any bias or prejudice. When planning patient-, family-, and population-centered care, factors such as lifestyle, culture, value system, religious or spiritual beliefs, social support system, and primary language shall be considered. Such considerations must promote health, address problems, and respect patient decisions. The respect for patient decisions does not require the nurse agree with or support all patient choices (p. 1)

Provision 1.4
- Nurses should promote advance care planning conversations and must be knowledgeable about the benefits and limitations of various advance directive documents. (p. 3)

Provision 2.3
- Collaboration intrinsically requires mutual trust, recognition, respect, transparency, shared decision-making, and open communication among all who share concern and responsibility for health outcomes. Nurses assure that all relevant persons, as moral agents, are participatory in patient care decisions. Patients do not always know what questions to ask. Nurses assure informed decision-making by assisting patients to secure the information that they need to make choices consistent with their own values.[4] (p. 6)

In 2016, the ANA underscored the need for nurses to collaborate with other members of the healthcare team to ensure adequate symptom management, optimal support, and expertise in understanding and navigating the ethical issues involved in care. More specifically, nurses are expected to be able to discuss death comfortably with patients and families, encourage their participation in decision-making (including goals of care and advance directives), and also collaborate with care team colleagues to ensure that timely and accurate information is being shared.[3] This position statement provides direction to nurses as they support and advocate for patients and families in preparation for impending death.

In 2017, the ANA in partnership with the Hospice and Palliative Nurses Association (HPNA) published the *Call for Action – Nurses Leading and Transforming Palliative Care*, challenging nurses to be leaders in palliative care and delineating roles for primary and specialty care.[5] Identifying nurses as critical partners in the care of persons and families living with serious and life-limiting illness requires them to develop astute listening and communication skills as they guide patients and families in goals-of-care conversations and care planning discussions.

Effective communication skills are requisite in palliative care. These include the ability to share developmentally appropriate information, practice active listening, encourage the expression of goals and preferences, and assist with medical decision-making. In addition, skill is required in advocating for patients by extending communication to include all members of the healthcare team.[6] The function of communication is to reduce uncertainty and to provide a basis for action. Information conveyed wisely and with sensitivity can improve the patient's and family's ability to act now and in the future and strengthens the patient–nurse relationship. In contrast, ineffective communication can cause harm, "paralyze" action, and destroy the relationship. Nurses must have the skills necessary for these discussions to provide valuable support for patients to achieve their goals at the end of life.[5,6]

COMMUNICATION FOR THE PALLIATIVE APRN

While there is widespread agreement about the importance of effective communication in palliative care and, to that end, the development of myriad tools in the form of protocols, algorithms, and step-wise guides, the approach has been largely pragmatic. While valuable in terms of providing language to guide the APRN into sensitive conversation, these tools have limitations. Ferrell writes, "that true advances in communication in serious illness will only occur through a deeper reflection. Beyond the right words or steps, what are the real human dynamics. . . ? What is the essence of a compassionate conversation?"[7] (p. 304)

Communication in palliative care seen as "compassionate conversation" has the potential to create a deep relational connection between caregiver and patient. It is this form of communication woven through the fabric of care that begins at the time of diagnosis and continues throughout the life of the patient and in bereavement for the family. Communication is beyond information sharing about a disease, its treatment, and the prognosis. It is about establishing a context of trust and truthfulness. Sourkes writes that truth is neither principle nor rule but rather a state in which there can be interaction, astute listening, and deep respect.[8] Trust unpins communication within the partnership among patient, family, and caregiver and is integral to the practice of palliative care.[8]

Nursing theorist Hildegard Peplau's theory of interpersonal relations provides a conceptual framework derived in part from the empirical study of human interactions that is helpful to an understanding of communication. In her seminal work, Peplau describes the nurse–patient relationship as the human connection central in a most fundamental way to the provision of care.[9] Within this relationship, which is largely unscripted, is the potential to connect and overcome separateness, creating the essence of communication, especially at the end of life.[9]

Communication, as a broad construct, includes any behavior or action, intentional or not, that influences the attitudes, ideals, or responses of another human being. Communication is transactional and occurs between and among persons. Yet Levetown notes that, too often, caregivers place emphasis and focus on conveying information, with little regard for feelings, relationships, and continuity in care.[10]

One of the most complex and amazing developments of the first 3 years of life is the transformation of newborns who communicate through body language and vocalizations into children who use multiword utterances to describe their imaginations, emotions, memories, and wishes. While infants can communicate with their caregivers at birth, the reciprocal partnership in which complex symbolic ideas are exchanged, conflicting agendas are negotiated, and feeling states are shared must await a series of developmental advances. These advances depend on both the hardwiring in the child's central nervous system and, over time, the child's experiences within a family. Thus, the factors that support the evolving development of the ability to communicate are found in the family and social environment. Language, one means of communication, is a complex, conventional system of symbols that are combined and used in a rule-governed way. Language is culturally bound and learned initially within the family of origin and later in education systems.[11] Communication occurs in multiple ways and forms, in addition to the written and spoken word, through the medium of movement, expression, music, art, and, of course, play.

Communication in palliative care and especially at the end of life is the focus of this chapter. Understanding communication in its broadest sense, appreciating the significant barriers altering its effectiveness, and developing strategies both personal and in practice ultimately will enhance the work of palliative nursing. Conscious nonverbal communication is rarely practiced, yet it can be as powerful as verbal communication at the end of life.[12]

PALLIATIVE APRN COMMUNICATION AT CRITICAL JUNCTURES

The palliative APRN assesses the patient's and family's communication style, with attention to primary language, culture, religious beliefs, and literacy (in both ability to understand language and health literacy). When English is not the primary language of the patient or family, a translator (not a family member) must be enlisted either in-person, virtually, or telephonically. Understanding cultural diversity and cultural preferences and the need for equity and inclusion must characterize the APRNs palliative care practice. Support and respect for cultural preferences during illness, the illness continuum, and end of life are integral to the delivery of culturally congruent care.[13]

Before the palliative APRN communicates with the patient and family, they must gather essential information. The APRN must understand the patient's past history diagnosis, the underlying pathophysiology of the condition, the current medical treatment and plan for future treatment, any side effects of treatment, whether a treatment is curative or palliative, and where the patient is being treated. It is also important that the palliative APRN understand prognostic scores like Palliative Prognostic Score, the Karnofsky, and Eastern Cooperative Oncology Group scales, which will help determine whether treatment is an option based on the patient's functional status.

Often there is overlap in the roles and functions of palliative interdisciplinary team members. This can be a challenge for palliative APRNs, given their advanced educational preparation and the long-standing relationships that they may have with patients and families. It is important for the palliative APRN to recognize that the characteristic of a well-functioning team is that all members share equal responsibility for care and promote nonhierarchical team structures.

Prior to family meetings, it is best practice that the palliative APRN organize a team pre-meeting. The purpose of the "meeting before the meeting" is to determine which member will lead the meeting and what members of the team will provide information to the patient and family. Various team members should be included in this meeting, with the focus being organized delivery of information (Box 34.1).

Box 34.1 ONGOING COMMUNICATION WITH THE FAMILY

1. Coordinate a meeting with the family, which may be a virtual meeting. Make sure to have an interpreter, if there are language barriers.

2. Offer information about their loved one's care and treatment options.

3. Gain insights as to their understanding about the present situation.

4. Reconfirm for the family the contact information for the treating team, the nursing unit, and the primary nurse.

5. Discuss if care is congruent with the patient's wishes.

6. Acknowledge the psychological and emotional work of trying to make care decisions for a loved one if they are not able to be present.

7. Offer and provide support in family decision-making. This may include an offer of chaplaincy or social work.

8. Always ask if they have any questions regarding the care of their family member.

9. Before ending the meeting, summarize what was discussed and the next steps.

Adapted from End-of-Life Nursing Education Consortium.[1]

COMMUNICATION ACROSS THE TRAJECTORY OF ADVANCING ILLNESS AND AT THE TIME OF DEATH

As illustrated in Figure 34.1, communication with patient and family changes over the course of advancing illness, building on early assessment, a growing trust, and a deepening connection. The focus shifts from advance care planning discussions and settings for care, sharing bad news at the time of diagnosis, to maintaining connection through transitions in illness. The preference for site of death may change based on the patient's wishes, the symptom burden, and the family's resources. Participants in the planning process are palliative care team members, primary care providers, and the ever-changing staff of physicians and nurses on hospital units, as well as home care providers. Flexibility is required as new information and options are offered and changing goals of care are reviewed. Moving across this trajectory provides an opportunity for palliative APRNs to be proactive in anticipating care issues and integrating them with the patient's and family's individual needs. In addition, APRNs provide guidance in the context of a nurtured trust.

Palliative APRNs may have patients who express the desire to die. Van Loon posits that wishes to die expressed close to the end of life have many meanings requiring evaluation. They may reflect the person's wish to end a life in which suffering has become unbearable or burdensome.[15] Palliative APRNs may evaluate patients for depression and suicidal ideation using the PHQ-9 depression scale.[16] Breitbart et al. report that desire for hastened death among terminally ill cancer patients is common and that depression and helplessness are strong predictors of this desire. The authors recommend that interventions including pharmacological and behavioral treatment as well as social support be integrated into palliative care for their patients.[17]

COMMUNICATION WITH FAMILIES ABOUT THE STAGES OF DYING

I've learned that people will forget what you said, people will forget what you did, but people will never forget how you made them feel.

Carl W. Buehner (1971)

The concept of anticipatory guidance is often used by palliative APRNs to prepare a patient and family for a specific developmental milestone or crisis. In working with families whose loved ones are imminently dying, the palliative APRN should expect to discuss the dying trajectory, death itself, and common concerns that they may have and are afraid to ask. Many families will be interested in understanding the process of dying and what they should expect. Communication helps their final planning stages as a unit of care. However, some families will choose not to have information shared with them, and this should be respected. Recognition of the trajectory of imminent death is essential for clinicians in order to provide the most appropriate interventions for the patient and family. Some commonly anticipated questions are listed in Box 34.2.

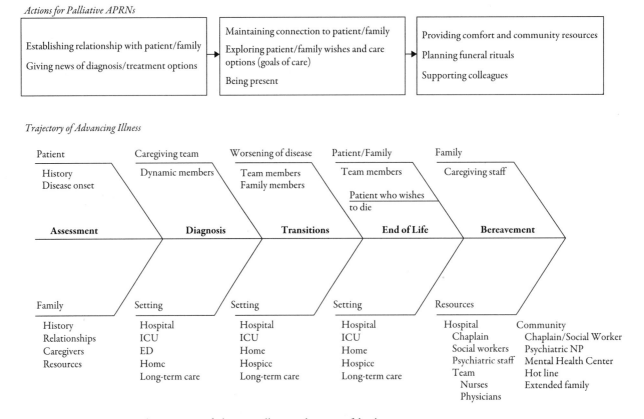

Figure 34.1 Communication across the trajectory of advancing illness and at time of death.
From McHugh ME, Buschman P. Communication at the time of death. In: Dahlin C, Coyne P, Ferrell P, eds. *Advanced Practice Palliative Nursing.* Oxford: Oxford University Press; 2016: 305–404.[14]

The proximal reality of a patient's death is typically very difficult for families. APRNs are often in a position to provide guidance for families observing clinical changes in their loved one. Table 34.1 lists the stages of the dying process that APRNs can discuss with families as they observe the clinical stages of dying.

Without an invitation, families may be reluctant to initiate discussion, fearful of hastening death by speaking of it. The APRN may use the following questions with patient and family to promote planning for an expected death:

1. Have you thought about what it will be like for your family when your loved one dies?

2. Sometimes families find it helpful to discuss planning for rituals after death such as a funeral, memorial service, or some special remembrance for your loved one before they die. Would this be helpful for you?

3. Have you considered how you will include family members, particularly young children, in your family ritual of mourning?

The emphasis of end-of-life communication with the patient is presence, standing with and bearing witness, providing comfort for the family, discussing any wishes for end-of-life rituals and funerals, and making referrals to hospital- and community-based resources. Holmberg describes poignantly in the following passage communication in action between family caregivers and palliative nurses at the time of death. When knowing that no words could make the loss bearable, there was just empathy and compassion to offer.[19]

The nurses made the examinations that are legally required to declare death. Then they and the family all gathered in the kitchen. There was a time to tell about the last hours, there were opportunities to weep, to share hugs. The nurses said they would help out dressing my son and arrange for the rest of the family to say goodbye. His wife changed his clothes and ironed his shirts. One of the nurses and my son's younger brother arranged my son on his bed and lit a candle in the window. The nurses took charge of the practicalities. They arranged for the last transportation. And they stayed as long as the family members wanted them to. There was an atmosphere of respectful silence in the house.[19 (p. 283)]

SUDDEN, UNEXPECTED DEATH: SUICIDE, HOMICIDE, VIOLENCE, ACCIDENTAL INJURY, SUDDEN ONSET, OR WORSENING OF DISEASE

The challenges are significant when a person dies unexpectedly and the family does not have an ongoing connection with a caregiver. Much of the initial communication focuses on events surrounding the death as well as on resources in the community for the family (Figure 34.2). The APRN must remain in the room to answer medical questions and lend a respectful presence. Because of the unexpected nature of the death and lack of preparation, family members may be in shock and require the services of social workers, chaplains, and psychiatric staff. Family members may require assessment for self-harm, harm to others, or damage to the environment.

The palliative APRN meeting the family for the first time will be asked for information and clarification. Accompanying the family to the emergency room or morgue to view the patient's body requires a calm presence and the ability to prepare the family for what they will see, such as changes in skin color or visible injuries. If the family wishes to touch their loved one, they should be prepared for changes in body temperature. Immediately after death, family members may be encouraged to touch the body's core area, rather than the extremities.

In unexpected death, the palliative APRN, in concert with team members, may refer families to community resources for bereavement counseling. Family members who threaten suicide or who may be at risk for suicide may need to be accompanied to a hospital ED by family members or by the APRN for a full psychiatric evaluation.

Table 34.1 STAGES OF THE DYING PROCESS

EARLY	MIDDLE	LATE
• Bedbound • Loss of interest and/or ability to drink/eat • Cognitive changes: increased time spent sleeping and/or delirium	• Further decline in mental status to obtundation (slow to arouse with stimulation; only brief periods of wakefulness) • Terminal secretions—pooled oral sections in the larynx as a result of loss of the swallowing reflex	• Coma • Fever • Altered respiratory pattern—periods of apnea, hyperpnea, or irregular breathing • Mottled extremities

From Weissman.[18]

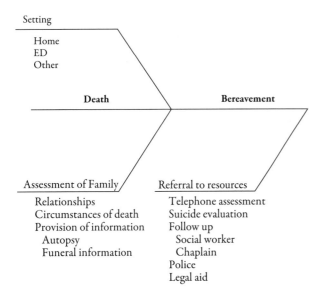

Setting
  Home
  ED
  Other

Death   Bereavement

Assessment of Family   Referral to resources
  Relationships   Telephone assessment
  Circumstances of death   Suicide evaluation
  Provision of information   Follow up
    Autopsy   Social worker
    Funeral information   Chaplain
                                Police
                                Legal aid

Figure 34.2 Communication at the time of death and beyond with family. From McHugh ME, Buschman P. Communication at the time of death. In: Dahlin C, Coyne P, Ferrell P, eds. *Advanced Practice Palliative Nursing*. Oxford: Oxford University Press; 2016: 305–404.[14]

BARRIERS TO COMMUNICATION AT THE END OF LIFE

Perhaps the most obvious and far-reaching barrier to the provision of therapeutic communication at the end of life lies in our failure to teach and model the process. Levetown notes that far more time is spent focusing on facts and descriptions of procedures than on the process of communication. Moreover, efforts to elevate healthcare communication, empathy, and patient- and family-centered care as competencies within education have thus far failed.[10] Clearly, communication across the trajectory of illness and so importantly at the end of life deserves space and time in our curricula and clinical supervision. In specific vulnerable populations of patients, circumstances and conditions impede the communication process and challenge the palliative nurse to find innovative approaches.

GERIATRIC PATIENTS WITH COGNITIVE AND SENSORY DEFICITS

Geriatric patients may lose physiological function and capacity, which serve as more powerful determinants of prognosis than chronological age.[20] Delirium and dementia are the two major cognitive deficits in the elderly population. Both complicate the assessment of pain and symptoms in those with advanced illness and interfere with communication in general. When cognition and language are limited, communication becomes behavioral in nature.[21] Contrary to current thinking, behaviors should be seen as forms of communication, rather than as unpredictable or random events with no meaning. To intervene, the palliative APRN must attempt to identify a message in the behavior.

The visual and hearing impairments common in older adults further limit verbal and nonverbal communication.[20] In addition to these deficits, the presence of multiple comorbidities challenges the palliative nurse's ability to derive goals of care. The APRN should make sure the patient has hearing aids or glasses, if needed, to promote communication.

PATIENTS WITH DEPRESSION, ANXIETY, POSTTRAUMATIC STRESS DISORDER, AND SERIOUS PERSISTENT MENTAL ILLNESS

While the recommended therapeutic response to patients with psychological distress at the end of life is to listen and provide support, patients with serious persistent mental illness pose significant challenges. Here, too, the palliative APRN observes behaviors and mannerisms as means of communication, respecting the need for space and sometimes the inability to tolerate touch. For many of these patients, families are disengaged and not involved in care. This population is underserved and truly vulnerable; they may live in jails or shelters or on the streets, unable to access adequate palliative care. Goldenberg, Holland, and Schachter note that palliative patients with serious mental illness have not been studied and their prevalence is unknown.[22] An appalling lack of articulation between the mental health and other healthcare systems contributes to the lack of palliative and end-of-life care for this population.[23] Baker writes that a combination of factors, including the psychiatric symptoms exhibited by these patients and providers' attitudes and feelings toward the mentally ill, influence planning for end-of-life care (Box 34.3).[24,25] The palliative APRN, in collaboration with

---

Box 34.3 **COMMUNICATION WITH PERSONS WITH COGNITIVE AND DEVELOPMENTAL DISABILITIES**

When caring for a developmentally delayed patient at the end of life, the palliative APRN must engage family members and caregivers in discussion. The following strategies promote more compassionate care.

- Allot extra time.

- Assist parents and/or caregivers to identify unspoken wishes that may be displayed by their developmentally disabled child/adult, such as repeated self-removal of feeding tubes.

- Invite trusted family friends, physicians, and caregivers to assist parents and/or caregivers with decision-making.

- Take time to listen, talk, and develop trust and rapport with the family.

- Introduce the topic of advance directives early. Encourage parents to think about the next potential admission.

- Recognize the differences and similarities between the population of developmentally disabled persons and the general population.[26]

- Provide more opportunities for expressions of grief.[27]

a psychiatric nurse practitioner, can provide compassionate end-of-life care, as illustrated in the second case study.

CASE STUDY 2: CLINICAL DEPRESSION IN A PALLIATIVE CARE PATIENT

Jane was a 36-year-old woman who had been diagnosed as an adolescent with major depressive disorder. She contracted HIV as a young adult and was estranged from her family of origin and her only son. She sought services from an agency providing medical and psychiatric services as well as residential care. Jane was enrolled in a methadone maintenance treatment program in her residence. As her HIV/AIDS worsened, Jane was encouraged by staff and her psychiatric mental health nurse practitioner (PMHNP), Joann, to agree to inpatient hospitalization, where she would be able to receive palliative care. Jane adamantly refused, stating that she wanted to remain at "home" in the residence, where she was known by staff and other residents. Joann agreed to coordinate a home hospice program involving a community-based palliative APRN, Katherine, and a trained aide who would provide 24-hour care to address increasing symptoms.

Jane began to experience periods of confusion, delusional thinking, and neuropathic and nociceptive pain in her lower extremities, which was well controlled by oral methadone 5 mg/mL every 8 hours, prescribed by the APRN. Jane was at the end of life. With Joann, Jane discussed her wish to see her 16-year-old son who had lived with Jane's sister since birth. Jane was ashamed of her diagnosis and the circumstances of her life. Yet, she firmly believed that her son was better off with her sister. However, as Jane faced the end of her life, her only wish was to see, and perhaps reconcile with, her son. Joann contacted Jane's sister, who agreed to accompany the son to visit Jane and say goodbye. Jane died at "home" in her residence. Katherine met with residents and staff who had known and stood by Jane to assess their level of comfort, respond to questions about symptoms, listen to their sadness, and prepare for Jane's death. Joann, in her ongoing therapy with Jane, had explored her values, wishes, and hopes. Both Katherine and Joann offered support and bereavement care to Jane's sister and son after her death.

CONFIRMATION WHEN DEATH HAS OCCURRED

The APRN often confirms that death has occurred by assessing that there is no presence of respirations or heartbeat. In some situations, another clinician is required to verify the patient has died. In other settings, an electrocardiogram must be obtained. In many states, a professional nurse may determine and pronounce the death and even sign the death certificate. APRNs should be familiar with their scope of practice regarding death pronouncement and completion of death certificates.

Communication with families at the time of death includes notification that the death has occurred and what to anticipate when the body is viewed immediately after

Box 34.4 KEY ELEMENTS TO VIRTUAL AND TELEPHONE DEATH NOTIFICATION

1. Make the call as soon as possible after the death.

2. Prepare for the call by talking with a colleague about the deceased to review the events of the last few days.

3. Gather and verify the facts about the patient: name, gender, age, medical record number, religious denomination, and circumstances of death. Have the chart available, if possible, depending on the location where you will take the call.

4. Establish the next of kin to be notified: contact person, full name(s), address(es), relationship to the patient.

5. Arrange for a medical interpreter, if needed.

6. Review with a colleague the context of the call, the history of the care, and what you will say.

7. Take a few moments to collect and prepare oneself—with a mindfulness minute or deep breathing.

8. Find a quiet space in which to make the call.

9. Remember to talk slowly and use simple language.

Making the Call

10. Consider using technology to block personal phone telephone number or computer access such as *67 or Doximity.

11. Initiate call. If call goes to voice mail, do not leave information about the death. Leave your specific contact information such as "Martha Mark, CNS at West Hospital. Please call me back at the following number."

12. Identify yourself and your position at the healthcare facility.

13. Ask to speak to the contact person and verify their relationship to the deceased.

14. Provide a warning shot: "I am afraid I have some serious/difficult news to share." "Are you available to talk now or should I call you back in a few minutes?"

15. Ask if person has anyone with them or if they are driving.

16. Allow them time to get to a room with another person, call another person, or pull over on the road.

17. Check in they are ready to receive the news.

Delivering the News

18. Provide clear and direct language: "I am so sorry to inform you that X has just died." "I am sad to have to tell you X has just died." Do not use euphemism such as "passed on," "expired," or "didn't make it" as you do not want to be ambiguous.

19. Allow time and silence for the family member/friend to take in the information.

20. Be prepared for the expression of emotions.

21. Offer simple details about what happened if the family member/loved one asks.

    a. Explain how the patient was doing earlier and the sudden deterioration.
    b. Explain the possible reasons for the sudden deterioration.

22. Allow the family members to ask additional questions and express feelings.

23. Provide therapeutic listening and support.

From Dahlin.[28]

Box 34.5 CLOSING THE CALL

1. Offer information about next steps in terms of planning for the discharge of the body.

    a. Ability to view the body at the facility
    b. Basic guidance about funeral planning

2. Offer follow-up phone calls by the social worker or chaplaincy to help with memory-making (as resources allow), support, and funeral planning.

3. Provide information about follow-up telephone calls from the hospital, including the release of the body.

4. Offer condolences and a statement for having to receive this information by phone: "Again, my condolences on your loss. I wish I had been able to tell you this in person."

5. Document the call in the chart.

6. Notify the clinical team and the bereavement liaison that the call has been completed.

7. Take a moment to reflect and provide a positive affirmation for providing a difficult call with empathy.

From Dahlin.[28]

---

death. Box 34.4 reviews telephone notification.[28] Families should be aware that muscles are relaxed after death, resulting in passage of stool and urine, and relaxing of the jaw, causing the mouth to open. Presentation and care of the body after death, including cleaning, is an important nursing intervention.

DEATH NOTIFICATION VIA VIRTUAL PLATFORM OR TELEPHONE

Communication with the patient's family a video platform (e.g., Facetime, Zoom, Skype) or by telephone regarding his or her condition, prognosis, and death carries the same responsibilities for the nurse as meeting in person: assessment, listening, and providing concrete medical information (Box 34.4). Performing such calls in a private areas is still fundamental. Additionally, assuring appropriate power for any device, landline, or smart device is critical, as is a stable internet connection. Finally, it is necessary to have the facts of what occurred or is occurring. Communication virtually or over a telephone is challenging in that the clinician cannot assess the family member's safety using nonverbal clues and unsafe living arrangements or privacy. Whether by phone or virtually, the APRN must evaluate the situation and convey empathy, visually with body language and verbally with tone. Not only is conveying the information about the death important, but the APRN also must conduct an assessment of family members' coping abilities. The APRN who believes a family member is at high risk can arrange for follow-up by team members or, if more emergent, summon emergency support using 911.

Boxes 34.4 and 34.5 outline the process and steps for the APRN to follow in calling a family to notify of a loved one's death.[28]

THE ROLE OF TELEHEALTH IN COMMUNICATION DURING SERIOUS ILLNESS AND END-OF-LIFE: IMPACT OF COVID-19

Telehealth is broadly defined as the use of telecommunication technologies to support clinical healthcare. Telehealth technologies include telephone (both wired and wireless communications), remote patient monitoring (e.g., coverage of intensive care units), video conferencing, the internet, and streaming media.[29] Telehealth has been historically used to provide care to those in rural areas and in military health systems with forward-deployed and remote settings. Telehealth has also supported public health during emergencies such as the 2014 water crisis in Flint, Michigan, and the 2016 Zika virus outbreak in Puerto Rico, locations where telehealth clinicians were able to compensate for the inadequate supply of local providers in the affected areas.[30]

The global pandemic caused by the novel SARS-CoV-2 (severe acute respiratory syndrome coronavirus 2), or coronavirus disease 2019 (COVID-19), has caused millions of infections, hundreds of thousands of deaths, and caused international economic contraction. The necessity for lockdowns, quarantines, and social distancing as critical infection control measures has profoundly changed the way healthcare has been provided. The provision of palliative care has been similarly transformed (see Chapter 17, "The Palliative APRN in Telehealth"). While the role of palliative care at end of life remained focused on comfort in dying and providing

palliative care unit in Italy, in which family members in the pre-COVID era had been allowed to stay with the patients "8 days a week," they employed a commercial smartphone video app to allow families to participate in daily clinical rounds.[31] Other centers responded to the sudden and enormous demand for palliative care inpatient consult services by enlisting consultative services from palliative care specialists in other, less impacted geographic areas, utilizing telephone or video communications for goals-of-care discussions.[32,33] Informally, and routinely, bedside providers held up bedside phones or used smartphones to access commercial video platforms to meet the simple and essential request for families to be with their loved ones before death.[34] Outpatient palliative APRNs were able to provide continuity of care with patients at home due to the Centers for Medicare and Medicaid (CMS) liberalization of Medicare reimbursement for telemedicine, allowing substitution of virtual visits for prescribing controlled substances.[35]

While the emergence of COVID-19 accelerated the use of telehealth—under the most urgent of conditions—it is likely that telehealth will remain a prominent component of healthcare delivery. It is incumbent upon hospice and palliative APRNs to participate in optimizing this modality. Research is needed to investigate the most effective communication strategies for telehealth encounters while retaining our current priorities: to share information, identify needs, be fully present, and respond with empathy.[36] Engaging in goals-of-care conversations at end of life, under pandemic conditions, highlighted the importance of APRNs' ongoing efforts to encourage advance care planning (ACP) completion before health crises occur.[37,38] The high volume of cases and the highly charged clinical scenarios favor the incorporation of structured conversations in crisis encounters.[33,39] Aiming for the best possible care that telemedicine can provide mandates that APRNs address social and healthcare disparities, working toward equitable access to telemedicine technologies for vulnerable populations.[40,41]

emotional, psychosocial, and spiritual support for patients and families, delivery models evolved to meet radically changed practice conditions. In this context, telehealth emerged as a critical tool for palliative care providers in communicating with patients and family members.

The no-visitor policies instituted by acute and subacute facilities have presented a formidable challenge to one of the central principles of palliative care at end of life: to facilitate contact between patients and their loved ones. The prohibition on visiting dying patients in their final days has required that palliative care providers find creative ways to foster connection, provide comfort and meaning to patients, and help families in the grieving process. This context of unprecedented physical separation at end of life generated psychosocial, spiritual, and moral distress among patients, loved ones, and providers alike, thus presenting several unique communication challenges (Box 34.6).

Internationally, palliative care providers and other frontline clinicians developed a spectrum of practical applications of telehealth during the pandemic. In an acute supportive/

FAMILIES AND LOSS

Coming to terms with death and loss is the most difficult challenge a family must confront. From a family systems perspective, loss can be viewed as a transactional process involving the dying and deceased with the survivors in a shared life cycle that acknowledges both the finality of death and the continuity of life.[42 (p. 3)]

While palliative APRNs view both the patient and family as the focus of care, the major effort at the end of life is to prepare the patient and family for death. Bereavement care follows acknowledgment of the loss. Missing is a systematic view of the family and the impact of the loss on the family as an interactional system. This theoretical framework provides caregivers the opportunity to see beyond the number of members and roles in order to view the system as a whole in a particular phase of life-cycle development. Rolland describes three major phases in the unfolding of chronic or advanced illness for the family member: initial crisis, chronic phase, and terminal phase.[43]

To respect religious and cultural variations, Rolland recommends helping families during the initial crisis (or time of diagnosis) to establish open and effective disease- and treatment-related communication.[43] Establishing this pattern early on and knowing the ill person's wishes can benefit both patient and family. With advanced disease, where the timing of loss is ambiguous but the inevitable deterioration is not, family members will grieve at each transition. At key periods, families can be encouraged to shift their roles and responsibilities to other members.

In the crisis phase of illness, families will grieve for the loss of family life prior to the diagnosis. Family members in the chronic phase grieve for the ambiguities they must endure over the long term.[43] As the patient enters the terminal phase, the main question asked is how much time there will be to prepare for death and survivorship. Rolland suggests that a family's tasks at this time are as follows:

1. Completing the task of anticipatory grief and unfinished business

2. Supporting the dying member and family survivors to continue their life together for as long as they can

3. Beginning or continuing the family reorganization process[43]

Rolland encourages the palliative care provider to "join with" the family when members are anticipating a final separation. This phase provides an opportunity for some families to experience emotional and relational healing. Relationships in highly dysfunctional families where there is a history of abuse or abandonment may not be mended. Patients who have no families or who are estranged from their families of origin may be content to be surrounded by friends and caregivers. Walsh and McGoldrick describe loss as a powerful nodal event that affects the entire family system and every member.[42] Loss reverberates over time, starting with the threat of death and progressing to the actual approach, the immediate aftermath, and the long-term implications. The authors propose four major tasks that promote immediate and longer-term adaptation for family members and the unit as a whole:

1. Shared acknowledgment of the reality of death

2. Shared experience of loss

3. Reorganization of the family system

4. Reinvestment in other relationships and life pursuits[42]

PALLIATIVE APRN WELL-BEING

The grief that does not speak,
Whispers the o'er fraught heart and bids it break.
William Shakespeare, Macbeth

Palliative APRNs touch the fringes of family grief and are touched deeply by that grief; they must find ways to share with colleagues and peers for sustainability. Feldstein and Gemma surveyed nurses caring for terminally ill adults and found those nurses who did not share their grief with colleagues experienced a chronic, compounded grief that interfered with their personal and professional lives and relationships. The authors posited that protracted exposure to distressing symptoms and suffering in patients and families at end of life generates a high level of stress and dysfunction in APRNs who are not vigilant about caring for themselves.[44] There are many vehicles to promote and support well-being, including sharing their grief (Box 34.7).

SUMMARY

Communication at the end of life is a complex and therapeutic transactional process between and among human beings. No more than at the end of life does it become the relational connection, the empathic link between the person whose life is ending and those who will continue to live. Communication occurs through the spoken word, the listening ear, in silence, and in action. For the palliative APRN, communication is an essential skill to be learned and practiced, to teach, model, and support. This communication, the "compassionate conversation" as a form of authentic human interaction, is not an exact science; it is shaped by the transactional process of the persons engaged in it. Ferrell suggests that palliative APRNs explore more deeply this relational aspect of communication, "What does it really mean to share bad news? Or to hear it? What is it really like to comfort a parent who holds a dying child? What does it mean to invite a patient to share their life regrets or need for forgiveness? Perhaps we have only begun to know what it means to care in serious illness. Perhaps we need deeper reflection."[7 (p. 305)] This becomes the ongoing challenge for the palliative APRN, beyond clinical competency in all aspects of care: the exploration of meaning in relational connection through communication (Box 34.8).

Box 34.7 **SUPPORTING PALLIATIVE APRNS PSYCHOLOGICAL HEALTH**

1. Institutional and administrative recognition of the unique stressors and challenges in caring for COVID-19 patients and families

2. Provision of evidence-based psychological support to:

   - Address psychological and safety needs
   - Engage in support of peers
   - Focus on team support interventions
   - Promote mentoring among APRN staff[45]

3. Supportive workplace activity to help palliative APRNs share grief and find support

   - Discussion groups/workshops
   - Support groups
   - Remembrance services
   - Referral to mental health therapists when indicated[14]

Domain 6: Cultural Aspects of Care

GUIDELINE 6.1 GLOBAL

The IDT delivers care that respects patient and family cultural beliefs, values, traditional practices, language, and communication preferences and builds upon the unique strengths of the patient and family. Members of the IDT work to increase awareness of their own biases and seeks opportunities to learn about the provision of culturally sensitive care. The care team ensures that its environment, policies, procedures, and practices are culturally respectful.

CRITERIA

6.1.1 The IDT asks the patient or surrogate to identify and define family, which may include members of the family of origin, as well as the patient's family of choice.

6.1.7 Communication occurs using verbal, nonverbal, and/or symbolic means appropriate to the patient, with particular attention to cultural and linguistic considerations, cognitive capacity, the presence of learning or developmental disabilities, and the developmental stage across the lifespan.

Domain 7: Caring for the Patient Near the End of Life

GUIDELINE 7.2 SCREENING AND ASSESSMENT

The interdisciplinary team (IDT) assesses physical, psychological, social, and spiritual needs, as well as patient and family preferences for setting of care, treatment decisions, and wishes during and immediately following death. Discussions with the family focus on honoring patient wishes and attending to family fears and concerns about the end of life. The IDT prepares and supports family caregivers throughout the dying process, taking into account the spiritual and cultural background and preferences of the patient and family.

CRITERIA

7.2.1 The IDT:

  a. Reviews advance directives (as applicable) and honors the patient's wishes
  b. Provides information and support to the family and others who are providing care to the patient

7.2.2 For patients who have not accessed hospice, the IDT discusses the benefits of hospice with the patient and family.

7.2.3 Before the patient's death, the IDT discusses autopsy, organ and tissue donation, and anatomical gifts in a culturally sensitive and age-appropriate manner, adhering to applicable organizational policies and laws.

CRITERIA

7.3.1 With the involvement of the patient and family, a plan is developed to meet patient needs during the dying process, as well as the needs of family members before, during, and immediately following the patient's death. Cultural and spiritual preferences of the patient and family are particularly relevant when developing this plan. Reassessment and revision of the plan occurs regularly, with the frequency identified in agency or program policies.

7.3.2 Care of the patient at the end of life is time- and detail-intensive, requiring expert clinical, psychological, social, and spiritual attention to the process as it evolves.

7.3.5 In all care settings, the IDT provides education and instructions to family members and/or caregivers in preparation for the patient's death, with emphasis on whom to notify, and what to expect when symptoms change and after the patient dies.

  a. Education and instructions are provided in accordance with the patient- and family's health literacy levels and cultural preferences.

7.3.6 Family expectations regarding IDT availability during the dying process are identified in advance so that staff can alleviate concerns and communicate realistic expectations.

7.3.7 The IDT elicits and honestly addresses hopes, fears, and expectations about the dying processes in ongoing communications with the patient and their family in a developmentally appropriate and culturally sensitive manner.

7.3.8 The IDT provides anticipatory grief support to the family and caregivers.

GUIDELINE 7.4 TREATMENT DURING THE DYING PROCESS AND IMMEDIATELY AFTER DEATH

During the dying process, patient and family needs are respected and supported. Post-death care is delivered in a manner that honors patient and family cultural and spiritual beliefs, values, and practices.

CRITERIA

7.4.1 The IDT communicates signs and symptoms of imminent death in culturally and developmentally appropriate language, taking into account the cognitive abilities of the patient and family

7.4.4 An IDT member supports the family before and immediately following the patient's death, assisting with cultural or spiritual practices, funeral arrangements, and cremation or burial planning.

GUIDELINE 7.5 BEREAVEMENT

Bereavement support is available to the family and care team, either directly or through referral. The IDT identifies or provides resources, including grief counseling, spiritual support, or peer support, specific to the assessed needs. Prepared in advance of the patient's death, the bereavement care plan is activated after the death of the patient and addresses immediate and longer-term needs.

CRITERIA

7.5.1 The IDT directly, or through referral, provides bereavement services and support to the family.

7.5.7 Grieving children are referred to pediatric grief specialists, programs, and camps based on their age and needs.

7.5.8 The IDT assesses resiliency, cumulative loss, and grief, and offers supports and services to IDT members. Emotional support services are also made available to ancillary team members involved in supporting palliative care patients.

From National Consensus Project for Quality Palliative Care.[13]

REFERENCES

1. American Association of Colleges of Nursing. End-of-Life Nursing Education Consortium. ELNEC Support For Nurses During COVID-19. Communication guide for nurses and others during COVID-19. 2020. https://www.aacnnursing.org/Portals/42/ELNEC/PDF/ELNEC-Communication-Guide-During-COVID-19.pdf
2. Ferrell B. From the editor. *J Hospice Palliat Nurs.* 2012;14(1):1.
3. American Nurses Association. Position statement. Nurses' roles and responsibilities in providing care and support at the end of life. Silver Spring, MD; ANA. 2016. https://www.nursingworld.org/~4af078/globalassets/docs/ana/ethics/endoflife-positionstatement.pdf
4. American Nurses Association. Position statement: Nursing care and do-not-resuscitate (DNR) decisions. Silver Spring, MD: ANA. https://www.nursingworld.org/~494a87/globalassets/practiceandpolicy/nursing-excellence/ana-position-statements/social-causes-and-health-care/nursing-care-and-do-not-resuscitate-dnr-decisions-final-nursingworld.pdf 2020
5. American Nurses Association and Hospice and Palliative Nurses Association. *Call for Action: Nurses Lead and Transform Palliative Care.* Silver Spring, MD: American Nurses Association; 2017. http://www.nursingworld.org/~497158/globalassets/practice-andpolicy/health-policy/palliativecareprofessionalissuespanel-callforaction.pdf
6. Wittenberg E, Buller H, Ferrell B, Koczywas M, Borneman T. Understanding family caregiver communication to provide family-centered cancer care. *Semin Oncol Nurs.* 2017;33(5):507–516. doi:10.1016/j.soncn.2017.09.001
7. Ferrell BR, Buller H. Palliative care communication: On deeper reflection. *J Palliat Med.* 2020;23(3):304–305. doi:10.1089/jpm.2019.0636
8. Sourkes B. *Armfuls of Time: The Psychological Experience of the Child with a Life-Threatening Illness.* Pittsburgh, PA: University of Pittsburgh Press; 1995.
9. Peplau HE. Peplau's theory of interpersonal relations. *Nurs Sci Q.* 1997;10(4):162–167. doi:10.1177/089431849701000407
10. Levetown M. American academy of pediatrics committee on bioethics. Communicating with children and families: From everyday interactions to skill in conveying distressing information. *Pediatrics.* 2008;121(5):e1441–e1460. doi:10.1542/peds.2008-0565
11. Saletta M, Windsor J, Communication disorders in infants and toddlers. In: Zeanah CH, ed. *Handbook of Infant Mental Health.* 4th ed. New York: Guilford; 2019: 345–357.
12. Cook D, Rocker G. Dying with dignity in the intensive care unit. *N Engl J Med.* 2014;370(26):2506–2514. doi:10.1056/NEJMra1208795
13. National Consensus Project for Quality Palliative Care. *Clinical Practice Guidelines for Quality Palliative Care,* 4th ed. Richmond, VA: National Coalition for Hospice and Palliative Care; 2018. https://www.nationalcoalitionhpc.org/ncp.
14. McHugh ME, Buschman P. Communication at the time of death. In: Dahlin C, Coyne P, Ferrell P, eds. *Advanced Practice Palliative Nursing.* Oxford: Oxford University Press; 2016: 305–404.
15. Van Loon RA. Desire to die in terminally ill people: A framework for assessment and intervention. *Health Soc Work.* 1999;24(4):260–268. doi:10.1093/hsw/24.4.260
16. American Psychological Association. Patient health questionnaire (PHQ-9 &PHQ-2). January 2011. Last update June 2020. https://www.apa.org/pi/about/publications/caregivers/practice-settings/assessment/tools/patient-health
17. Breitbart W, Rosenfeld B, Pessin H, et al. Depression, hopelessness, and desire for hastened death in terminally ill patients with cancer. *JAMA.* 2000;284(22):2907–2911. doi:10.1001/jama.284.22.2907
18. Weissman DE. Palliative care fast facts and Concepts #3. Syndrome of imminent death. Appleton, WI: Palliative Care Network of Wisconsin. 2015. https://www.mypcnow.org/wp-content/uploads/2019/01/FF-3-Imminent-Death.-3rd-ed.pdf
19. Holmberg L. Communication in action between family caregivers and a palliative home care team. *J Hosp Palliat Nurs.* 2006;8:276–287. doi:10.1097/00129191-200609000-00013
20. Delgado-Guay MO, De La Cruz MG, Epner DE. "I don't want to burden my family": Handling communication challenges in geriatric oncology. *Ann Oncol.* 2013;24(Suppl 7):vii30–vii35. doi:10.1093/annonc/mdt263
21. Sutor B, Rummans TA, Smith GE. Assessment and management of behavioral disturbances in nursing home patients with dementia. *Mayo Clin Proc.* 2001;76(5):540–550. doi:10.4065/76.5.540
22. Foti M. Palliative care for patients with serious mental illness. In: Chochinov HM, Breitbart W, eds. *Handbook of Psychiatry in Palliative Medicine.* 2nd ed. New York: Oxford University Press; 2009: 113–121.

23. Levinson Miller C, Druss BG, Dombrowski EA, Rosenheck RA. Barriers to primary medical care among patients at a community mental health center. *Psychiatr Serv.* 2003;54(8):1158–1160. doi:10.1176/appi.ps.54.8.1158

24. Baker A. Palliative and end-of-life care in the serious and persistently mentally ill population. *J Am Psychiatric Nurs Assoc.* 2005;11(5):298–303. doi:10.1177/1078390305282209

25. Sheridan AJ. Palliative care for people with serious mental illnesses. *Lancet Public Health.* 2019;4(11):e545–e546. doi:10.1016/S2468-2667(19)30205-1

26. Lindley LC, Colman MB, Meadows JT Jr. Children with intellectual disability and hospice utilization. *J Hosp Palliat Nurs.* 2017;19(1):28–33. doi:10.1097/NJH.0000000000000301

27. Sue K, Mazzotta P, Grier E. Palliative care for patients with communication and cognitive difficulties. *Can Fam Physician.* 2019;65(Suppl 1):S19–S24.

28. Dahlin C. An APRN telephone death notification to family tool. ELNEC COVID-19 Communication Resource Guide. ELNEC Support for Nurses During COVID-19. End-of-Life Nursing Education Consortium. ELNEC. https://www.aacnnursing.org/Portals/42/ELNEC/PDF/APRN-Death-Notification-Resource-Guide.pdf

29. Health Resources and Services Administration (HRSA). Office of the Advancement of Telehealth. Telehealth programs. Last Reviewed January 2021. https://www.hrsa.gov/rural-health/telehealth

30. Lurie N, Carr BG. The role of telehealth in the medical response to disasters. *JAMA Intern Med.* 2018;178(6):745–746. doi:10.1001/jamainternmed.2018.1314

31. Mercadante S, Adile C, Ferrera P, Giuliana F, Terruso L, Piccione T. Palliative care in the time of COVID-19. *J Pain Symptom Manage.* 2020;60(2):e79–e80. doi:10.1016/j.jpainsymman.2020.04.025

32. Israilov S, Krouss M, Zaurova M, et al. National outreach of telepalliative medicine volunteers for a New York city safety net system COVID-19 pandemic response. *J Pain Symptom Manage.* 2020;60(2):e14–e17. doi:10.1016/j.jpainsymman.2020.05.026

33. Nakagawa S, Berlin A, Widera E, Periyakoil VS, Smith AK, Blinderman CD. Pandemic palliative care consultations spanning state and institutional borders. *J Am Geriatr Soc.* 2020;68(8):1683–1685. doi:10.1111/jgs.16643

34. Wakam GK, Montgomery JR, Biesterveld BE, Brown CS. Not dying alone: Modern compassionate care in the COVID-19 pandemic. *N Engl J Med.* 2020;382(24):e88.doi:10.1056/NEJMp2007781

35. Center for Medicare and Medicaid Services (CMS). Medicare telemedicine healthcare provider fact sheet. Mar 17, 2020. CMS.gov. www.cms.gov/newsroom/fact-sheets/medicare-telemedicine-health-care-provider-fact-sheet

36. Cooley L. Fostering human connection in the COVID-19 virtual health care realm. Commentary. *NEJM Catal Innov Care Deliv.* May 202020. doi:10.1056/CAT.20.0166

37. Rao JK, Anderson LA, Lin F, Laux JP. Completion of advance directives among US consumers. *Am J Prev Med.* 2014;46(1):65–70. doi:10.1016/j.amepre.2013.09.008

38. Yadav KN, Gabler NB, Cooney E, et al. Approximately one in three US adults completes any type of advance directive for end-of-life care. *Health Aff (Millwood).* 2017;36(7):1244–1251. doi:10.1377/hlthaff.2017.0175

39. VitalTalk. Covid ready communication playbook. 2021. https://www.vitaltalk.org/guides/COVID-19-communication-skills

40. Webb Hooper M, Nápoles AM, Pérez-Stable EJ. Covid-19 and racial/ethnic disparities. *JAMA.* 2020;323(24):2466–2467. doi:10.1001/jama.2020.8598

41. Holtgrave DR, Barranco MA, Tesoriero JM, Blog DS, Rosenberg ES. Assessing racial and ethnic disparities using a COVID-19 outcomes continuum for New York state. *Ann Epidemiol.* 2020;48:9–14. doi:10.1016/j.annepidem.2020.06.010

42. Walsh F, McGoldrick M. Loss and the family: A systemic perspective. In: Walsh F, McGoldrick M, eds. *Living Beyond Loss: Death in the Family.* 2nd ed. New York: Norton; 2004: 3–14.

43. Rolland JS. Helping families with anticipatory loss and terminal illness. In: Walsh F, McGoldrick M, eds. *Living Beyond Loss: Death in the Family.* New York: Norton; 2004: 213–237.

44. Feldstein MA, Gemma PB. Oncology nurses and chronic compounded grief. *Cancer Nurs.* 1995;18(3):228–236. doi:10.1097/00002820-199506000-00008

45. Maben J, Bridges J. Covid-19: Supporting nurses' psychological and mental health. *J Clin Nurs.* 2020;29(15–16):2742–2750. doi:10.1111/jocn.15307

SECTION VII

PSYCHOSOCIAL, CULTURAL, AND SPIRITUAL ASPECTS OF CARE

35.

CULTURALLY RESPECTFUL PALLIATIVE CARE

Helen Foley and Polly Mazanec

KEY POINTS

- Delivering culturally respectful care is a fundamental principle of nursing.

- Self-reflection on one's own cultural beliefs, values, practices and biases is essential to providing culturally sensitive palliative care.

- The palliative advanced practice registered nurse (APRN) must assess the patient's and family's cultural values, practices, and beliefs and identify their significance in the diagnosis and management of serious illness and at end of life.

- Goals of care must be established in concert with the patient's and family's cultural values, practices, and beliefs.

- Disparities in access and delivery of quality palliative care must be addressed in order to improve care for the most vulnerable.

- Essential components of palliative care, such as communication, including disclosure, prognosis, and medical decision-making; pain and symptom management; end-of-life care; and death, should be considered through a cultural lens.

CASE STUDY 1: IMMIGRATION STATUS

A palliative advanced practice registered nurse (APRN) was consulted to see Mr. S, who was admitted to the hospital for hemoptysis, weight loss, and debilitating pain in his left hip. His son brought him to the emergency room and told the staff that he had been feeling poorly, had lost 20 pounds, and had been coughing up blood for 4 months. Mr. S spoke only Spanish and had delayed seeking healthcare as he did not have US citizenship and feared deportation. Upon admission, he was diagnosed with lung cancer with bone metastasis. The palliative APRN, Mary, found him withdrawn, and the nurses reported he was refusing to take pain medication. Through the use of the hospital's interpreter service, the patient shared his fears about taking pain medication and becoming addicted. Mary ensured that there was a computer-based interpreter service every day for rounds with the patient to promote trust. The palliative APRN coordinated his pain regimen and assisted the oncology team in planning for a short course of outpatient palliative radiation that would allow him to return home with his son.

INTRODUCTION

Culture is dynamic process and its language is a cultural phenomenon subject to changing terminology. Culture influences an individual's perception about health, wellness, death, and dying and is a dominant aspect of palliative care. This chapter discusses the delivery of culturally respectful care and the integration of culture into advanced practice palliative nursing. Culturally respectful care begins with self-reflection about one's own values, practices, beliefs, and biases and their impact on the delivery of culturally respectful, sensitive, or intelligent care. Assessing for primary language and health, numeracy, and technology literacy is essential, along with implementing strategies to overcome any barriers to culturally sensitive care. The palliative advanced practice registered nurse (APRN) must use these communication strategies to elicit the patient's and family's cultural values, practices, and beliefs. Moreover, the palliative APRN must attend to the cultural disparities and racism that exist in healthcare, hospice, and palliative care.

Definitions and terms used in this chapter reflect the healthcare and cultural environment in the United States at the time the chapter was written. The chapter describes special considerations in the delivery of culturally respectful palliative care, such as supporting beliefs regarding disclosure of prognosis and medical decision-making, recognizing cultural implications of pain and symptom management, integrating cultural rituals and practices into clinical care, and dealing with cultural clashes.

OVERVIEW OF CULTURE WITHIN PALLIATIVE NURSING

It is the fabric of nursing practice to attend to culture. This component of practice is identified within the American Nurses Association (ANA) *Code of Ethics*[1] and *Nursing Scope and Standards of Practice*.[2] Standard 8, Culturally Congruent Practice, of the ANA *Nursing Scope and Standards of Practice*, describes the competencies needed to ensure that the nurse practices in a manner that is congruent with cultural diversity and inclusion principles.[2] The Hospice and Palliative Nurses Association (HPNA) emphasizes the importance of culture in *Palliative Nursing: Scope and Standards of Practice*[3] and in its competency statements.[3,4] Standard 8 *Culturally Congruent Care* emphasizes that the palliative registered nurse has the cultural sensitivity to recognize, appreciate, and incorporate the different cultural needs of individuals with serious illness into the provision of care,[3] and HPNA's *Competencies for the Palliative and Hospice Advanced Practice Registered Nurse* define cultural and spiritual competence at that level of clinical practice. Cultural competency for advanced practice palliative nursing focuses on respecting diversity, in particular race and ethnicity, spirituality, religion, gender identity and expression, sexual orientation, immigration and refugee status, social class, physical appearance, and abilities.[4] The *Competencies for the Palliative and Hospice Advanced Practice Nurse*[5] describe behaviors that demonstrate competency in cultural aspects of palliative care and align with the National Consensus Project for Quality Palliative Care (NCP) *Clinical Practice Guidelines for Quality Palliative Care.*[6]

Quality palliative care is clearly defined in the fourth edition of the *Clinical Practice Guidelines for Quality Palliative Care.*[6] Cultural considerations are so essential in quality palliative care that one of the eight domains, Domain 6, is reserved specifically for Cultural Aspects of Care. The clinical implications of this domain emphasize that respecting cultural values, practices, and beliefs is an essential element in the delivery of quality palliative care. Criteria that are identified in the guidelines for palliative care practice and that are emphasized in this chapter are summarized in Box 35.1.

Box 35.1 NCP CLINICAL PRACTICE GUIDELINES FOR QUALITY PALLIATIVE CARE

Domain 6: Cultural Aspects of Care

GUIDELINE 6.1 GLOBAL

The interdisciplinary team (IDT) asks the patient or surrogate to identify and define family, which may include members of the family of origin, as well as the patient's family of choice. The IDT recognizes that:

- Quality palliative care requires an understanding of the patient's and family's culture and how it relates to their decision-making process, and their approach to illness, pain, psychological, social, and spiritual factors, grief, dying, death, and bereavement.

- Each person's self-identified culture includes the intersections of race, ethnicity, gender identity and expression, sexual orientation, immigration and refugee status, social class, religion, spirituality, physical appearance, and abilities.

- Patients and families may have experienced barriers to receiving culturally respectful healthcare, and these prior experiences may result in mistrust of the health care system.

- Culture is a strength that patients and family members bring to their plan of care.

Adapted from National Consensus Project for Quality Palliative Care.[6]

UNDERSTANDING CULTURE

The United States is a multicultural society with increasing diversity. By 2060, minority groups are expected to make up 57% of the US population.[7] Americans have traditionally valued independence and self-reliance with an emphasis on the importance of autonomy and each individual's happiness.[8] However, many minority groups in the diverse United States and the non-Western World value collectivism, interdependence, community, and continuity of the generations.[8] Because of this increasing diversity, the palliative APRN must be aware of and respond to the diversity of customs, norms, beliefs, and languages.[9] Respecting and valuing cultural diversity are key to delivering culturally appropriate palliative care.

Culture is the "learned, shared and transmitted values, beliefs, norms and life ways of a particular group that guide their thinking, decisions, and actions in patterned ways."[10] Culture is shaped over time, during which the beliefs, values, and lifestyle patterns pass from one generation to another.[10] The biopsychosocial and ecological organizing system within which a population of people exists is an adaptive, dynamic system, one designed to ensure survival and well-being.[10] Culture is the way human beings find meaning and purpose in life and make sense out of life events. In times of crisis, culture can be a source of resilience for the individual and the family and therefore should be respected by the healthcare team.[10]

A commonly held misconception is that culture is synonymous only with race and ethnicity. Race and ethnicity are important components of culture because of systemic racism in today's society and subsequent racism and health disparities even in hospice and palliative care.[11-13] It should be noted that race and ethnicity are merely sociopolitical categories determined by the US Office of Management and Budget.[14] When considering culture, the NCP *Clinical Practice Guidelines*[6] have outlined essential components which have major palliative care implications. Table 35.1 identifies key components of culture and considerations regarding the delivery of quality palliative care.[6,15-17]

Even though an individual may belong to a cultural group, he or she may or may not adhere to its cultural norms.[18] Members of cultural groups can be very similar or very diverse. Behaviors of individuals within a cultural group can range from totally adherent to group practices, values, and beliefs to completely nonadherent. It is critical that the palliative APRN not engage in stereotyping, assuming that all persons from one group will behave in a certain way.

Textbooks and respected internet websites with information on certain cultural groups may be helpful in guiding clinical practice, and they may facilitate an understanding of culturally sensitive topics in healthcare and particularly palliative care. While it is important to seek to understand the practices and values of cultural groups commonly seen in one's clinical setting, the palliative APRN must assess the values, practices, and beliefs of each patient as an individual and determine the importance of these values, practices, and beliefs to the patient and family.[6]

Table 35.1 EXAMPLES OF COMPONENTS OF CULTURE AND IMPACT ON PALLIATIVE CARE

CULTURAL COMPONENTS	PALLIATIVE CARE CONSIDERATIONS
Race	Discrimination exists regarding healthcare delivery, treatment options, and palliative and hospice care utilization among minority races when compared to non-Hispanic whites; Racism and implicit bias negatively impact equitable care.
Ethnicity	Currently more than 100 ethnic groups and more than 500 American Indian Nations in the United States; ethnic minorities are less likely to use hospice services than non-Hispanic Whites for numerous reasons including culture.
Age	Age cohorts have their own identity and culture, the very young and very old are considered vulnerable populations. Cultural attitudes of ageism can affect the care of the older adult, who may be seen as frail and unable to make decisions.
Gender identity and expression	Gender disparity in palliative care exists for those identifying as lesbian, gay, bisexual, transsexual, queer, inquiring (LGBTQI+); ethical and legal issues in decision-making and advance care planning depend on documentation of who is "family"; gender minorities have high rates of poverty, food and housing insecurities, and experience discrimination in healthcare settings (i.e., older LGBTQI+ adults in nursing facilities).[17]
Sexual orientation	Respect one's sexual orientation. Use language that is nonjudgmental. Educate patients and families about the importance of appointing a healthcare power of attorney, especially if partners are unmarried.
Immigration or Refugee status	Immigrants may face health literacy deficiencies, insurance barriers, and may lack social and financial resources depending on status. Undocumented immigrants fear deportation, often waiting until serious illness is very advanced to seek healthcare.
Socioeconomic status (measured as a combination of education, occupation, and income)	One's physical and psychological well-being; preferences for hospice and palliative care are shaped by economic condition, healthcare access, insurance, and neighborhoods. Patients of lower socioeconomic status experience disparities across the disease trajectory of serious illness.
Religion	For those practicing a faith tradition, it may be important to integrate community clergy into healthcare team; faith and practice rituals can be a source of support and critically important at end of life.
Spirituality	Spirituality is the essence of every human being, giving life its meaning and purpose; can help transcend suffering in serious illness and at end of life.
Abilities	Those with physical disabilities often feel stigmatized because of their physical appearance. Those who are physically, emotionally, or intellectually challenged are at risk for receiving inferior care, especially if unable to speak for themselves or without an advocate.

From Cormack et al.[15]; Mazanec, Panke[16]; and Barrett, Wholihan.[17]

CULTURAL AWARENESS

Palliative APRNs must be aware of the impact of their own culture on their clinical practice.[6,15,16] To provide culturally sensitive care, APRNs must reflect on their individual values, practices, beliefs, and biases. This self-reflection should occur as a review of the essential components of nursing practice and competencies required of all practicing APRNs. It is recommended that a formal self-reflection be performed and revisited regularly because one's cultural beliefs are ever-changing and are heavily influenced by knowledge, experience, and cultural encounters.[16] Box 35.2 contains an example of a self-reflection exercise that can provide great insight into one's own worldview and how it may influence clinical care.

IMPLICIT BIAS

Within the realm of culture and racism, there is also *implicit bias*. Implicit bias refers to attitudes and beliefs that are in one's subconscious or are part of a person's belief system and that they are unwilling or unable to report because they are inaccessible to one's conscious awareness.[19] Implicit bias is based on interactions and observations from childhood and formed from the ages of 2–5, and influences one's adult actions, and decisions.[19] For example, one may hold negative stereotypes about others based on age, gender orientation, race, or religion without conscious realization, which may unknowingly influence clinical practice later in life.

A collaborative research effort at Harvard University, University of Virginia and the University of Washington offers an online self-administered Implicit Association Test (IAT)[20] that measures implicit attitudes, stereotypes, and biases. The test is somewhat controversial because the test's reliability, validity, and accuracy have been questioned. However, it may give insight into unconscious biases that one is not aware of and which can be unlearned once identified.

Box 35.2 CULTURAL SELF-ASSESSMENT

1. Where were you born? If an immigrant, how long have you lived in this country? How old were you when you came to this country? Where were your grandparents born?

2. What is your ethnic affiliation, and how strong is your ethnic identity?

3. Who are your major support people: family members, friends? Do you live in an ethnic community?

4. How does your culture affect decisions regarding your medical treatment? Who makes decisions—you, your family, or a designated family member? What are the gender issues in your culture and in your family structure?

5. What are your primary and secondary languages? What is your speaking and reading ability?

6. How would you characterize your nonverbal communication style?

7. What is your religion? How important is it in your daily life? What are your current religious practices? Is religion an important source of support and comfort?

8. What are your food preferences and prohibitions?

9. What is your economic situation, and is the income adequate to meet your needs?

10. What are your health and illness beliefs and practices?

11. What are your customs and beliefs surrounding birth, illness, and death? What are your experiences with death and bereavement? What are your beliefs about the afterlife and miracles? What are your beliefs about hope?

12. How have the patient and family encounters you have had over the past year influenced your values, practices, and beliefs?

Adapted from Mazanec, Panke.[16]

CULTURAL HUMILITY

A great deal is written about cultural competence, cultural sensitivity, and cultural humility, and confusion exists among these terms. The concept of *cultural competence* inaccurately assumes that competency is an endpoint or something to be mastered. Those striving for cultural competency recognize it is a dynamic process rather than an outcome.[15,21] *Cultural humility*, a term coined by Trevalon and Murray-Garcia, is a desirable attribute for clinical practice.[22] It is a "process of intercultural exchange, paying attention to clarifying the values and beliefs of provider and of patient and family and incorporating the cultural characteristics of healthcare professionals and individuals into a mutual balanced relationship."[22] Cultural humility requires that one enters into each new encounter with an open mind and open heart. Recognizing that our individual and professional perspective is but one of many perspectives that will be part of the larger context we are encountering, the goal of cultural humility is to create a shared understanding.[23-25] The NCP *Clinical Practice Guidelines* stress that the entire interdisciplinary team practices cultural humility in all clinical encounters.[6]

INTEGRATING CULTURAL ASSESSMENT INTO CLINICAL PRACTICE

Once the palliative APRN recognizes their individual cultural values, practices, and beliefs, the next step in developing a culturally respectful palliative care clinical practice is to gain skill in assessing the cultural backgrounds of patients and families. Performing a thorough cultural assessment is essential to understanding the patient's and family's healthcare preferences, especially in the provision of palliative care. Although many cultural assessment tools are available, some are lengthy and require a great deal of time on the part of the clinician and also the patient and family. These tools are actually long checklists, so administration not only may be burdensome but also may hinder the establishment of a trusting clinical relationship, which is the essence of culturally sensitive care.[15,26]

In the clinical setting, presence, active listening, and strong communication skills are the best tools for assessing cultural considerations in palliative care.[16,23] An understanding of the patient's values and culture is likely to be revealed over time as the APRN establishes a trust relationship with the patient and family. Palliative APRNs should ask the patient and/or the family member to tell about themselves. Listening intently to their stories is the most effective way to gain an understanding of the patient's and family's cultural norms. Box 35.3 provides an example of open-ended assessment questions that can guide the patient and family in sharing their cultural values, practices, and beliefs and what is important to them.

THE IMPACT OF CULTURE ON COMMUNICATION

Communication is the foundation for all encounters among human beings, and this is especially true in the delivery of palliative care. Communication is an interactive, multidimensional process, often dictated by cultural norms, and it provides the mechanism for human interaction and connection.[24] Abiding by general communication principles for quality palliative care in a culturally sensitive manner will ensure the establishment of a trusting relationship between the clinician and the patient and family, regardless of where the interaction takes place (e.g., clinic office, hospital room, skilled care facility). Following these principles will help the APRN and the palliative care team understand patient/family norms for communication style and the giving and receiving of information (Box 35.4).[23-26]

Box 35.3 KEY CULTURAL ASSESSMENT
QUESTIONS

- We want to make sure we respect how you prefer to be addressed:

  What name do you use?
  What sex were you assigned at birth?
  What gender do you identify as now?
  What gender pronouns do you use?

- Whom do you consider to be your family?

  To whom do you go for support (family, friends, community, or religious or community leaders)?

- Where were you born and raised? (If an immigrant, how long have you lived in this country?)

- What language would you prefer to speak?

- Is it easier to write things down, or do you have difficulty with reading and writing?

- I want to be sure I'm giving you all the information you need.

  What do you want to know about your condition?
  To whom should I speak about your care?

- Whom do you want to know about your condition?

- How are decisions about healthcare made in your family?

  Should I speak directly with you, or is there someone else with whom I should be discussing decisions?

- Tell me about your understanding of what has been happening up to this point. What does this illness mean to you?

- We want to work with you to be sure you are getting the best care possible and that we are meeting all your needs.

  Is there anything we should know about any customs or practices that are important to include in your care?
  Are you comfortable having both men and women as healthcare providers?

- Many people have shared that it is very important to include spirituality or religion in their care.

  Is this something that is important for you?
  Would you like me to contact our chaplain or another spiritual provider you would like to be involved in your care?

- Are there any foods you would like or that you should avoid?

- Do you have any concerns about how to pay for care, medications, or other services?

Death Rituals and Practices

- Is there anything we should know about care of the body or about rituals, practices, or ceremonies that should be performed during the dying process or at the time of death?

  Who should be involved in the care of the body immediately after death?
  Are there religious leaders who should be involved?

- What is your belief about what happens after death?

- Is there a way for us to plan for anything you might need both at the time of death and afterward?

- Is there anything we should know about whether or not a man or woman should be caring for the body after death?

- Should the family be involved in care?

Adapted from Cormack et al.[15]

DIFFERING ABILITIES AFFECTING COMMUNICATION

Patients and families who are hearing- or sight-impaired face additional challenges when trying to understand communication related to their palliative care needs. One in six individuals experience impaired hearing, with impairment being more common in the geriatric population.[27] When caring for a patient who is completely deaf and can use sign language, use a healthcare interpreter fluent in sign language. When caring for a hearing-impaired patient, the palliative APRN can facilitate communication by (1) decreasing background noise and distractions during conversations; (2) encouraging the patient to wear eyeglasses or hearing aids during the conversation; (3) ensuring the listener can see the APRN's face; (4) speaking clearly and distinctly, but not shouting; (5) enhancing the discussion with written words and pictures to aid in explanation; and (6) asking the listener to summarize the conversation to ensure understanding.[27] Keep in mind that speech comprehension is more difficult for persons with hearing loss. It can be compounded by the use of protective masking which interferes with both lip movement and nonverbal cues, as became evident in the recent coronavirus pandemic.

Those who have visual impairments are usually very capable of hearing and participating in the verbal part of communication but may be unable to observe nonverbal communication, depending on the severity of the loss of sight. The American Foundation for the Blind[28] offers suggestions to support those with vision impairment. Avoid using nonverbal responses, such as nodding in agreement or shaking your head in disagreement as the visually impaired person may not see these responses. When entering the room, greet the patient verbally first and then offer a handshake or touch the shoulder, if appropriate. If sight is limited but present, offer written materials in large print. When the visit is over, be certain to inform the patient when you are leaving. Seek additional help from experts like the American Association for the Blind for assistance with Braille materials and other resources.[29]

1. Select a setting that is private and as free from interruption as possible.

   - Turn off cellphones and put pagers on vibrate mode.
   - Greet the patient in a respectful, professional manner. Cultural norms related to verbal introduction and nonverbal touch or handshake should be identified early in the initial encounter to avoid making a culturally inappropriate mistake.
   - Determine the dominant language and dialect spoken and the literacy level of both the patient and the family. If there is a language difference between clinician and patient, a professionally trained interpreter of the appropriate gender, if culturally significant, should be contacted prior to proceeding with the visit.
   - Recognize that the professional's message and the understanding of the patient/family can differ, even when they share the same language. When confronted with a life-limiting illness, almost everyone experiences compromise in literacy and difficulties in processing.

2. During the initial interaction, determine how the patient would like to be addressed.

   - Some patients prefer to be called by their last name (e.g., Mr. Jones, Ms. Smith), whereas others may prefer to be called by their first names. Identify the patient's preference for gender pronouns.
   - Document the patient's preference in the medical record so that all members of the healthcare team can respect this preference.
   - Be cognizant of nonverbal communication that may be culturally insensitive.
   - Ask permission to sit down and maintain a respectful distance that does not invade private space but demonstrates empathy.
   - Introduce yourself to all present at the visit.

3. Once introductions have been made, assess patient and family cultural norms for giving and receiving information and for decision-making at the first visit.

   - Share with the patient and family that there will likely be important information about the patient's condition discussed at every visit.
   - Ask the patient with whom they would like healthcare information discussed.
   - If there are people important to the patient who cannot be present, such as a long-distance son or daughter, consider ways to use technology to share information with them and to include them in future visits using telephone or computer conferencing.

4. Find out how much information the patient and family would like to have when decisions need to be made.

   - Normalize the information-gathering process: "Some people like to hear all about the illness, its course, and treatments as well as all labs or scan results. Others prefer that we share the information needed to make decisions and limit the detail on the illness, treatment, and testing. How much information would you like us to share with you?" This may be different for patient and caregiver, and it can be challenging to respect differing needs for information.
   - Understand that accepting the family's usual process of decision-making will be critical to providing culturally respectful palliative care throughout the patient's disease trajectory.

Adapted from Mazanec, Panke.[16]

PREFERRED LANGUAGE, HEALTH LITERACY, HEALTH NUMERACY, AND FINANCIAL LITERACY

The NCP *Clinical Practice Guidelines*[6] emphasize that palliative care providers should tailor communication to the patient's and family's level of literacy, health literacy, numeracy, and financial literacy. This requires attention to the information provided orally and in written formats and consideration of an individual's or group's language preference. When there is not a common preferred language between the APRN and the patient, or when the patient and family have low health literacy and numeracy, the APRN must use culturally sensitive strategies to help them navigate the healthcare system.

PREFERRED LANGUAGE

A 2018 Census Bureau Report identified that 67.3 million people in the United States spoke a language other than English in their home.[30] This number has doubled since 1990 and reflects about 22% of all US residents.[30] The NCP *Clinical Practice Guidelines* Domain 6, Cultural Aspects of Care,[6] defines the current standard in the criteria that outline how palliative care programs should make all reasonable efforts to provide interpreter services and written materials in the preferred language to facilitate patient and family understanding of information.

Individuals facing serious illness must receive information in a format and a language that are easily understood so they can make informed healthcare decisions. Preferred language, health literacy, and health numeracy affect the person's ability to understand complex medical information and treatment options during serious illness. Even things that seem routine and simple to healthcare providers might be confusing to the public. Literacy and language issues may compound the challenge of understanding the medical situation.

The palliative APRN should assess the environment in which they practice; this includes

- Determining the dominant languages and dialects spoken by individuals in your community and the setting where you practice.

  - If the preferred language is not English, a professionally trained interpreter of the appropriate gender to the health issues should be contacted when verbal communication is required. For any interpreters, it is appropriate to ask them if a question is appropriate or how it should be asked. As of 2019, every state and the District of Columbia have enacted multiple laws addressing language access.[31] It is important for APRNs to know the laws in their state of practice. It is important for palliative APRNs to become skilled in using the particular programs available in the setting where they work: home, hospital, clinic, long-term care facility, etc.
  - Language assistive services must be provided by a qualified translator and interpreter and must be free for the patient/family. If a qualified professional interpreter is not available, access a telephone language line to assist in conversations. Examples of language lines that have interpreters for healthcare include Language Line Services,[32] CyraCom International,[33] and Mobile Martti.[34] They offer 24-hour availability, 365 days/year for those with an account. Newer technology services, such as video-remote interpreting (VRI), allow for face-to-face interactions, especially important for those with hearing or speech impairments. Family members should only act as interpreters in an emergency.
  - Family members are often uncomfortable when placed in the interpreter role, especially if sensitive topics are being addressed. Moreover, there may be challenges placed on family members depending on their gender and age for discussing gender-related issues. In some

non-Western cultures, family members have a responsibility to protect the patient from distress or worry. Therefore, family interpreters may selectively choose what and how to translate information. If the APRN is unsure if the family member is sharing accurate information with the patient, it could lead to major misunderstandings.[15,18]

- Assessing the literacy level of the patient and family. Consider the literacy level of both the patient and the family when developing a plan of care.

- Always remaining conscious of your verbal and nonverbal communication when using an interpreter. For example, when speaking, make eye contact with the person you wish information to be directed toward, rather than looking at the interpreter. Consider tone of voice and expressions.

- Ensuring understanding by having the patient explain to you or the interpreter what he or she has heard using his or her own words.

HEALTH LITERACY

The National Academy of Medicine (formerly the Institute of Medicine) Committee on Health Literacy defines *health literacy* as the degree to which individuals can obtain, process, and understand basic health information and services needed to make appropriate health decisions.[35] Only 12% of adults have proficient health literacy, and 14% of adults have below-basic health literacy which negatively impacts health outcomes.[35,36] Patients with low literacy are less likely to manage chronic conditions effectively and are more likely to be hospitalized, which may lead to poorer health outcomes and higher healthcare costs. Several key findings from National Assessment of Adult Literacy (NAAL)[37] underscore how important it is for the APRN to pay attention to the patient's literacy level (Box 35.5).

Box 35.5 BEHAVIORS THAT MAY INDICATE LITERACY CHALLENGES

1. Taking medications incorrectly

2. Offering an excuse when asked to read written materials (e.g., "I forgot my glasses")

3. Identifying medications by shape or color rather than name, or opening medicine bottle rather than reading the label

4. Not looking at written materials or not turning them right side up if handed materials upside down

5. Not being able to fill out simple, age- and language-appropriate forms; providing incorrect information; leaving many items blank

Adapted from Mazanec, Panke.[16]

Recommendations from Healthy People 2030 have added to the current understanding of health literacy by highlighting two definitions: *personal health literacy* (the ability to find and use information for decision-making) and *organizational health literacy* (to what extent the organization is equitably enabling the individual to access this information).[38] The palliative APRN can improve how critical information is equitably delivered, received, and understood by asking two important questions:

1. *Is the information appropriate for the individual?*
   - Identify the intended audience and determine whether materials and messages reflect the age, social and cultural background, and language and literacy skills of that audience.
   - Evaluate each individual's understanding before, during, and after delivery of information.
   - Acknowledge and respect cultural variations. Consider components of culture when developing materials or speaking with individuals (see Table 35.1). Acknowledge and respect individual and group preferences and assess for variations within groups.

2. *Is the information easy to use?*
   - Limit the number of messages being delivered at any given time. In general, no more than four messages should be conveyed.
   - Give specific recommendations and expected actions. Focusing on behavior rather than medical principles or concepts may lead to better understanding and outcomes.
   - Use plain language that is familiar to the audience. Keep it simple, and avoid long sentences and words with many syllables. Avoid acronyms and medical jargon.
   - Offer to call a family member to review instructions with them if the patient is alone and you suspect difficulty in understanding.
   - Use pictures when giving instructions. This can help individuals comprehend complicated instructions related to medical conditions, treatments, medications, and abstract concepts. Pictures should reflect the message and should not be merely decorative additions. An example is for medications: use a picture of sunrise for medications taken in the morning, high sun for medications taken in the day, moon rise for the evening, and moon in the sky for medications taken at night.

Behaviors that may indicate limited health literacy are described in Box 35.5.[39] Resources, instructional materials, and marketing can be made more understandable by following a few simple suggestions from the Department of Health and Human Services: use a simple 12-point font, limit line length to 40–50 characters, use headings and bullets to focus on key points, and leave plenty of white space on the paper.[38]

HEALTH NUMERACY

Patients will receive information that involves numbers, and there is a growing recognition that attention to health numeracy is needed to help individuals who cannot fully comprehend or use the information they are given to make informed decisions about their health. Health numeracy is closely related to health literacy. Health numeracy is the degree to which individuals have the capacity to assess, process, interpret, communicate, and act on numerical, quantitative, graphical, biostatistical, and probabilistic health information to make effective health decisions.[40] Basic numeracy skills are those required to identify numbers and comprehend data without having to manipulate any figures—for example, the ability to read and understand a prescription label. We often ask patients to make treatment decisions based on percentages and averages: these data need to be put in terms that are easy to understand. An example might be saying "one in five people will respond to this treatment" instead of 20%. While more research is needed, studies on numeracy are finding results similar to those on health literacy, in that individuals with lower numeracy skills have poorer health outcomes.

The palliative APRN should be able to assess how numerical information is received and understood by patients and families. If difficulties are uncovered, consider alternative ways of presenting important numerical information. Using pictures and plain language that describe concepts and demonstrate the desired action (e.g., how many morphine pills equal the dose ordered) may improve adherence with medical advice and lead to better outcomes. Pictures can help with the timing of medications. Illustrations of a sunrise may help identify morning medications and a sunset or full moon can signify it is time to take evening medications.

COMMUNICATING IN THE AGE OF TECHNOLOGY

The goals of digital health technology were to improve quality, safety, and efficiency of healthcare while decreasing healthcare disparities. Telehealth allows palliative APRNs to reach those in rural or underserved areas, but only if internet access and the technology is available. Patients and families must also have at least a basic level of technology literacy to be able to engage with healthcare providers. About 31.8 million adults (16% of US adults) are considered digitally illiterate.[41] Those without these skills are more likely to be Black, Latinx, foreign-born, older, and less educated.[42]

The coronavirus pandemic of 2020 has changed the way palliative APRNs and other healthcare professionals communicate with patients and families.[43] In many settings, patients must come alone to their medical visit or hospital stay, which complicates culturally appropriate delivery of medical information, medical decision-making, and advance care planning. For patients and families who value collective decision-making rather than individual decision-making, the family must be able to be "brought into the visit" for

Table 35.2 TECHNOLOGIES FOR VIRTUAL COMMUNICATION

TYPE OF TECHNOLOGY	STRENGTHS	CHALLENGES
FaceTime[44]	Easy to use on any iOS device Can use phone number or email; phone charges may apply depending on the phone service High-quality technology No longer needs wifi	Must have an iOS device; forward-facing camera phone or Mac computer with camera, so not available on Android or Windows
Zoom[45]	Works on Android and iOS Available in 26 countries Offers free 40-minute calls with up to 100 people As of March 2020, the #1 most downloaded app	Has had privacy and security issues; easily hacked
Skype[46]	Easy to use on any device with a Skype app "Meet now" feature allows anyone to link into a host, much like Zoom Calls are free anywhere in the world More than one person can be on the call Can record the call Can share screen if desired	Has had a history of being challenging to use because participants all must have a link; this has been recently resolved

From FaceTime[44]; Zoom[45]; and Microsoft Skype.[46]

these discussions. Video technology, either by smart device, tablet, or computer, can help to accomplish this if the family has the equipment and technology literacy as well as internet access. It is important to make every effort to use technology that allows for face-to-face conversations. Existing commercial platforms such as FaceTime,[44] Zoom,[45] and Skype[46] are examples of useful technologies (Table 35.2). Since more than 70% of communication is nonverbal, it is helpful to be able to read body language as well as verbal responses.[47] Many patients have shown a preference for remote visits, challenging healthcare providers to find a platform that offers ease of use and full assessment and communication with the patient and family.

CASE STUDY 2: TELEHEALTH FAMILY CONFERENCING

During the COVID-19 pandemic, the palliative care team was asked to help with advance care planning and family conferencing for Ms. W. The palliative APRN met Ms. W, a 67-year-old African American woman with diabetes and moderate obesity admitted with respiratory distress after a 6-day history of fevers, nonproductive cough, and arthralgia. Ms. W was the mother of four grown children: three daughters living locally and a son in Mississippi. She was a nursing assistant employed at a local nursing home.

Within 6 hours of admission, she required intubation and sedation. The palliative APRN contacted Ms. W's children and a virtual family meeting was scheduled. Because visitors were not allowed during the pandemic, for the last three days of her illness the family conducted daily virtual meetings with the palliative care team to receive updates on Ms. W's condition. When Ms. W became unstable and the team was concerned that her life was short, the palliative APRN coached the family to say goodbye to their mother virtually. They sang her favorite hymns and

were able to tell her how much they loved her while the APRN held her hand in the room. The palliative APRN promised the family that she would stay with her, manage any symptoms she might have, and would make sure that a team member was with her until her death.

CULTURALLY SENSITIVE PALLIATIVE CARE TOPICS

Numerous palliative care topics (e.g., disclosure or "truth telling"; medical decision-making, including withholding and discontinuing technology; pain and symptom management; and the care of the dying and bereaved) have important cultural implications.[23] Another sensitive topic is the continued disparity in access and delivery of palliative and end-of-life care among racial and ethnic minorities.

RACIAL AND ETHNIC DISPARITIES IN ACCESS TO QUALITY PALLIATIVE CARE

Healthcare disparities in palliative and end-of-life care exist among racial and ethnic minorities. These disparities are shaped by economic conditions, insurance status, structural features of the neighborhood, knowledge, and access to care.[23,48] Although the intention of the *Affordable Care Act* (ACA)[49] was to improve access to healthcare, safety net hospitals serving economically disadvantaged individuals and minorities still struggle with funding.[48] There is inadequate access to palliative care services, hospices, and long-term care facilities for racial and ethnic communities, negatively impacting the treatment options for care during serious illness.[50] Disparities in hospice use are evident in 2018 statistics that reflect that hospice use is less among minority groups

(82% White, 8.2% Black, 6.7% Hispanic, 1.8% Asian, 0.4% Native Americans).[51]

Evidence from the Health and Retirement Study explored racial and ethnic differences in end-of-life care utilization and advance care planning.[52] The study demonstrated that people from minorities are less likely to be informed about end-of-life care options, if available, and are more likely to die in hospitals with a greater intensity of treatment at end of life. The preference for more intensive treatment may be due in part to a strong religious belief that only God can decide life and death, but it may also be due to a history of mistrust with the healthcare system and belief that any type of care other than aggressive care is of lower quality.[52] The study also highlighted disparities in participating in advance care planning, which is known to be important for patient-centered care and cost-effective use of resources.[52] The data from the Health and Retirement study identified that many African Americans believe they would receive poorer-quality care if they completed an advance directive and thus were less likely than Whites to do so.[52] Lack of advance care planning may also be due in part to health literacy issues, language barriers, and mistrust of healthcare providers.[53,54]

Palliative APRNs must address these racial and ethnic disparities in hospice and palliative care. Recommendations by Payne[54] define what is needed to make this happen: (1) acknowledge the negative effects of past and present racism, (2) learn and respect every individual's cultural and religious values, (3) commit to continuous improvement in patient–provider communication, and (4) engage in strategies with community partners to foster trust.[54]

CASE STUDY 3: GOALS-OF-CARE PLANNING

The palliative care team was called in to help manage symptoms of shortness of breath and help with goals-of-care planning for a patient in the cardiac care unit. Ms. A, an African American woman, had been admitted to the cardiac care unit for the fourth time in three months due to worsening heart failure. The cardiology team recommended she transition to hospice care.

During the initial visit with the palliative APRN, Ms. Anderson reported how tired and scared she was. She was concerned about her son, who was increasingly angry about her illness, always questioning if she was getting the best care for her condition.

The palliative APRN set up a goals-of-care conversation with Ms. A and her son. During the discussion, the son became angry and accused the team of not doing everything they could for his mother. He stated, "You are not giving her the best care because she is Black—I know that is the reason." He refused any plan of care other than transfer to intensive care, despite his mother telling him that she just hated being in the ICU and was tired of all the treatment. To calm him, she agreed to ICU care.

The palliative APRN set up a meeting with Ms. A's son. She asked him to talk about his mother's care and inquired about injustices in care that had occurred in the past. They discussed the current course of treatment, her life-limiting illness, and all that could be done to manage her symptoms and provide quality care while still honoring her wishes to not return to the ICU.

DISCLOSURE OF INFORMATION AND PROGNOSIS

The *Patient Self-Determination Act* (PSDA)[55] of 1991, grounded in Western cultural values and beliefs, was written to protect individuals' healthcare preferences.[54] Western cultural preferences include the right to be informed of one's diagnosis and prognosis and the risks and benefits of treatment. *Autonomy*, as the guiding principle, assumes that the individual, rather than the family or other social group, is the appropriate decision-maker. This European-American model of patient autonomy has its origin in the present-day US dominant culture, a predominantly White, middle-class perspective that does not consider diverse cultural perspectives.[23,56]

Some non-Western cultures believe that telling the patient they have a terminal illness strips away any and all hope, causes needless suffering, and may actually hasten death. If disclosing the patient's diagnosis and/or prognosis violates the patient's and family's cultural norms, or if the patient does not wish to receive information, doing so directly violates the patient's right to autonomy. For example, some people from indigenous populations (American Indians and Alaskan Natives) believe talking about the future is taboo.[57] Imposing negative information, such as a prognosis of a life-limiting illness, on the person who is ill is a dangerous violation of traditional Navajo values: those who adhere to Navajo traditions believe that talking about death will actually cause death. In families who adhere to Middle Eastern practices, telling the patient the diagnosis, who is perceived by the family as "vulnerable," is considered culturally unacceptable.[58] The palliative APRN may find the *Prognosis Declaration Form* helpful for assessing patient/family choice in receiving information for persons of any cultural background (Box 35.6).[59]

MEDICAL DECISION-MAKING

The principle of respect for patient autonomy emphasizes the patient's right to participate in decisions about the care he or she receives. The underlying assumption of patient autonomy is that all patients want control over their healthcare decisions, yet this is not always accurate.[56] In some families, patient autonomy may not be viewed as empowering but rather as

---

Box 35.6 PROGNOSIS DECLARATION

- Tell me everything.

- I've not decided what I want to know about my prognosis, so ask me over the course of my treatment.

- I want to participate in my treatment, but I don't want to receive any information on my prognosis.

- I don't wish to know any information about my prognosis but I authorize you to speak with (PERSON) about my case and to answer any questions that this person may have about my likely prognosis and treatment.

From Scheier.[59]

isolating and burdensome for patients who are too sick to make difficult decisions.[60] In fact, depending on patient and family cultural preferences, patient autonomy actually may violate the very principles of dignity and integrity it proposes to uphold.

In many non-Western cultures, the concept of interdependence among family and community members is valued more than individual autonomy.[60] If the palliative APRN is caring for a patient who adheres to this belief, it is culturally sensitive to include, rather than exclude, the family in decision-making. In some religious practices, it is important that the religious leaders also be included in the decision-making. Cultural groups that practice family-centered decision-making may prefer that the family, or perhaps a particular family member, rather than the patient, receive and process information (see Chapter 32, "Advance Care Planning," and Chapter 33, "Family Meetings").

Keep in mind that some individuals prefer to communicate their wishes verbally rather than put them in writing. They may be unwilling to sign advance directive forms because of a lack of trust in the healthcare system or a belief that God is the ultimate decision-maker over life-and-death matters.[48,54]

DISCONTINUATION OF LIFE-PROLONGING THERAPIES

Family members may feel that by agreeing to stop potentially life-prolonging therapies they are, in fact, responsible for the death of their loved one. For families who believe that it is the duty of children to honor, respect, and care for their elders, they may feel obligated to continue futile life-sustaining interventions. Allowing a parent to die may violate the principles of "filial piety."[61]

Religious beliefs may also play a role in decisions about withholding or discontinuing medical interventions. For example, some people from the Middle-East who are practicing Islam believe that potentially curative treatment should continue until the last moment of life.[62] For those practicing Orthodox Judaism, which believes that all life is precious and only God can decide our time to die, agreeing to discontinue life-prolonging therapies may violate their beliefs.[63] In both examples, involving a religious leader from the family's religious community may help the family and the healthcare team integrate religious tenets into a culturally appropriate plan of care.

All healthcare personnel should be acutely aware of the medical jargon and language they use. Many phrases, such as "do not resuscitate" and "withdrawal of life support," have negative connotations. What is standard terminology in healthcare can get lost in translation even if the parties are speaking the same language. "Withdrawal of life support" or "withdrawal of care" may be easily confused with stopping *all* care, which is certainly not the intention. The family may feel as though the team is giving up on the patient and abandoning him or her, resulting in family suffering, isolation, and distress. Instead, use language that conveys the benefits versus the burdens of all therapies, such as discontinuing a specific

therapy and aggressively managing symptoms. Focus on what the team will do to care for the patient rather than what burdensome interventions should be stopped (see Chapter 54, "Discontinuation of Cardiac Therapies"; Chapter 55, "Discontinuation of Respiratory Therapies"; and Chapter 56, "Discontinuation of Life-Sustaining Therapies").

PAIN AND SYMPTOM MANAGEMENT

The experience of pain and other symptoms commonly addressed in palliative care (e.g., anorexia, cachexia, nausea and vomiting, fatigue, dyspnea, and depression) must be appreciated from a cultural perspective. Pain and subjective symptoms demand a self-report of the severity and the meaning associated with them. For some, culturally learned responses to pain and symptoms may influence tolerance and behavior. Persons who have English as a second language are at risk of being unable to express pain and other symptoms.[64] It is important to remember cultural considerations and health literacy when assessing pain and symptoms. Labels like "pain" or "depression" may be culturally unacceptable for patients to self-report, so asking about a "hurt" or "ache" instead of "pain" and "a tired state" instead of "depression" may elicit a more accurate response from the patient.[65]

The meaning of the pain or symptom also influences assessment and treatment.[66,67] Religious and spiritual practices as well as ethnic values and beliefs may influence a patient's willingness to accept treatment. Enduring pain or severe symptoms may be important to a patient who believes that suffering is necessary to achieve a good afterlife.[65,66] Try to find a common understanding of the suffering experience and the value of pain/symptom management using a team approach, possibly including a religious leader. Finally, consider that racial, ethnic, age, or gender biases can hinder good pain and symptom management.[68] Pain is often undertreated in minorities.[69] Pain is underrated in the Latinx and African American populations, and this is associated with inadequate pain management.[70] Women, children, and elderly people are also at risk for inaccurate assessment and poor management[65,70] (see Chapter 43, "Pain").

Additional common signs and symptoms in palliative care that have cultural implications are anorexia and cachexia. For families who are caring for a loved one who is no longer able to eat or no longer interested in eating, anorexia and cachexia can be a source of distress. Food is seen as essential for life in all cultures.[71] It is used in celebrations and rites of passage and as an expression of social relationships and connections with families, friends, and others. The intense meaning attached to food and nutrition can result in cultural and ethical conflicts over providing medically administered nutrition and hydration at the end of life. The palliative APRN must use listening and presence to understand what feeding the patient means to the family and to help the family develop alternative expressions of comfort and love. If the family's health literacy is low, not feeding the patient may be akin to "starving him to death" or abandoning a basic human right of feeding. The APRN should provide a culturally sensitive explanation of the benefits and burdens associated with feeding.

DEATH AND DYING

A conversation about patient and family wishes during the dying process, at the time of death, and immediately after death should take place well in advance, provided it is not culturally unacceptable to discuss prior to death.[26,72,73] In some cultures, important rituals and customs must take place prior to or at the time of death. These practices need to be identified and integrated into the plan of care. For example, those who are of the Hindu tradition may prefer to die at home, lying on the floor, close to the earth, whereas it is important for those who are Muslim that the body should be positioned facing Mecca.[23,72–74] Care of the body after death is also important. In some traditions, it is unacceptable for the body to be cared for by someone of a different gender.[72–74] Beliefs about autopsy or organ donation should be discussed before death. Keep in mind that some cultures and religious communities believe that organ donation and autopsy are disrespectful to the sanctity of the body.[23] The family will hold on to the memory of the patient's final days and death forever, so if cultural practices are not honored, family members may experience complicated grief after the death of their loved one.

GRIEF AND BEREAVEMENT

Grief is an emotional response to a loss with which there was an emotional attachment.[75] The experiences of loss, grief, bereavement, and mourning are guided by cultural traditions, rituals, and beliefs. The expressions of grief can vary significantly among cultures, making it important to assess expressions of grief and individuals' behavior during mourning within a cultural context. Behaviors that are acceptable in non-Western cultures may be misconstrued as inappropriate by others.[72,75] It is important for the APRN to learn from family what are culturally appropriate practices during the mourning period in order to recognize if family members are experiencing complicated grief and need referrals for counseling and support (see Chapter 38, "Grief and Bereavement").

DIVERGENT CULTURAL VALUES AND BELIEFS

The three most common sources of cultural conflict are between the patient and family, among the healthcare team members, and among the healthcare team, patient, and family. In our multicultural society, patients and family members may have different values and beliefs that can result in conflicting opinions regarding healthcare practices. Healthcare providers, too, bring the values and beliefs of their own cultures to the clinical setting. Keep in mind that there also may be generational differences among persons from a particular ethnicity and culture. If one of the parties involved is more assimilated into the Western culture and the other aligns with non-Western values, practices, and beliefs, conflict may occur. When there is conflict over culture norms, the healthcare provider should suspend their personal beliefs and biases and focus on grasping the meaning of the message being sent.[76] APRNs can support all parties by facilitating a family meeting with culturally appropriate discussion around the conflict. The palliative APRN may need to be the advocate for patient and family wishes. An ethics consult and family meeting may help to resolve conflict and reach a shared understanding of the goals of care; see the chapters of Section IX, "Ethical Dilemmas".

SUMMARY

With the increasing cultural diversity of the United States, the APRN must be culturally sensitive to provide quality comprehensive palliative care as delineated by nursing practice as per the ANA *Code of Ethics for Nursing*[1], the ANA *Nursing Scope and Standards of Practice*,[2] and the NCP *Clinical Practice Guidelines*.[6] This requires moving beyond one's own ethnocentric view of the world to appreciate and respect the similarities and differences in others. There are many situations in which the palliative APRN is challenged to come to appreciate and understand an individual's preferences in care based on cultural values, practices, and beliefs. However, by maintaining a sense of cultural humility, caring for each patient and family member as a unique human being with unique needs, and attending to those needs with dignity and respectfulness, the APRN can provide culturally sensitive palliative care.

REFERENCES

1. American Nurses Association. *Code of Ethics for Nurses with Interpretive Statements.* 2nd ed. Silver Spring, MD: American Nurses Association, 2015. https://www.nursingworld.org/practice-policy/nursing-excellence/ethics/code-of-ethics-for-nurses/coe-view-only/

2. American Nurses Association *Nursing: Scope and Standards of Practice.* 4th ed. Silver Spring, MD: Nursesbooks.org; 2021.

3. Dahlin C, ed. *Palliative Nursing: Scope and Standards of Practice.* 6th ed. Pittsburgh, PA: Hospice and Palliative Nurses Association; 2020.

4. Dahlin C. *Competencies for the Palliative and Hospice Advanced Practice Registered Nurse.* 3rd ed. Pittsburgh, PA: Hospice and Palliative Nurses Association; 2020.

5. Dahlin CM, Moreines Tycon L, Root M, eds. *Core Curriculum for the Hospice and Palliative Advanced Practice Registered Nurse.* 4th ed. Pittsburgh, PA: Hospice and Palliative Nurses Association; 2020.

6. National Consensus Project for Quality Palliative Care. *Clinical Practice Guidelines for Quality Palliative Care.* 4th ed. Richmond, VA: National Coalition for Hospice and Palliative Care; 2018.

7. Vespa J, Medina L, Armstrong DM. "Demographic turning points for the United States: Population projections for 2020 to 2060." Current Population Reports, p25-1144, US Census Bureau. Washington, DC, 2020. https://www.census.gov/content/dam/Census/library/publications/2020/demo/p25-1144.pdf

8. Green A, Jerzmanowska N, Thristiawati S, Green M, Lobb EA. Culturally and linguistically diverse palliative care patients' journeys at the end-of-life. *Palliat Support Care.* 2019;17:227–233. https://doi.org/10.1017/S1478951518000147

9. American Association of Colleges of Nursing. *The Essentials: Core Competencies for Professional Nursing Education.* Washington, DC: AACN. April 6, 2021. https://www.aacnnursing.org/Portals/42/AcademicNursing/pdf/Essentials-2021.pdf

10. Leininger M. Quality of life from a transcultural nursing perspective. *Nurs Sci Q*. 1994;7:22–28. doi:10.1177/089431849400700109

11. Wasserman J, Palmer RC, Gomez M, Berzon R, Ibrahim SA, Ayanian JZ. Advancing health services research to eliminate healthcare disparities. *Am J Public Health*. 2019;109:S64–S69. doi:10.2105/AJPH.2018.304922

12. Ornstein KA, Roth DL, Huang J et al. Evaluation of racial disparities in hospice use and end-of-life treatment intensity in the regards cohort. *JAMA Network Open*. 2020;3(8) E2014639. doi:10.1001/jamanetworkopen.2020.14639 (Reprinted

13. Boucher NA Johnson KS. Cultivating cultural competence: How are hospice staff being educated to engage racially and ethnically diverse patients? *Amer J Hosp Palliat Med*. 2020. doi:10.1177/1049909120946729

14. National Institute of Health. Office of Research on Women's Health. Office of Budget and Management (OMB) Standards. 2021. https://orwh.od.nih.gov/toolkit/other-relevant-federal-policies/OMB-standards

15. Cormack C, Mazanec P, Panke JT. Cultural considerations in palliative care. In: Ferrell B, Paice JA, eds. *The Oxford Textbook of Palliative Nursing*. 5th ed. New York: Oxford University Press; 2019: 469–482.

16. Mazanec P, Panke J. Culturally respectful palliative care. In: Dahlin C, Coyne P, Ferrell B, eds. *Advanced Practice Palliative Nursing*. New York: Oxford University Press; 2016: 414–424.

17. Barrett N, Wholihan D. Providing palliative care to LGBTQ patients. *Nurs Clin North Am*. 2016;51(3):501–511. doi:10.1016/j.cnur.2016.05.001

18. Andrews MM. Culturally competent nursing care. In: Andrews MM, Boyle JS, Collins JW, eds. *Transcultural Concepts in Nursing Care*. 8th ed. New York: Wolters Kluwer; 2020: 31–54.

19. Project Implicit, Inc. About Us. Boston, MA. https://www.project-implicit.net/who-we-are/

20. Project Implicit, Inc. Implicit Association Test (IAT). Project Implicit, Inc. https://implicit.harvard.edu/implicit/takeatest.html

21. Campinha-Bacote J. Delivering patient-centered care in the midst of a cultural conflict: The role of cultural competence. *Online J Issues Nurs*. 2011;16(2). Published 2011 May 31.

22. Trevalon M, Murray-Garcia J. Cultural humility versus cultural competence: A critical distinction in defining physician training outcomes in multicultural education. *J Health Care Poor Underserved*. 1998;9: 117–125. doi:10.1353/hpu.2010.0233

23. Carey EC, Sadighian MJ, Koenig BA, Sudore RL. In Arnold RM, eds. Cultural aspects of palliative care. UptoDate. Waltham, MA: UptoDate. Last update March 31, 2021. https://www.uptodate.com/contents/cultural-aspects-of-palliative-care?search=cultural%20aspects%20of%20palliative%20care&source=search_result&selectedTitle=1~150&usage_type=default&display_rank=1

24. Barclay JS, Blackhall LJ, Tulsky JA. Communication strategies and cultural issues in the delivery of bad news. *J Palliat Med*. 2007;10:958–977. doi:10.1089/jpm.2007.9929

25. Wittenberg-Lyles E, Goldsmith J, Ferrell B, Ragan SA. Orientation and opportunity. In: Wittenberg-Lyles E, Goldsmith J, Ferrell B, Ragan SA, eds. *Communication in Palliative Nursing*. New York: Oxford University Press; 2013: 59–92.

26. Palos G. Cultural considerations in palliative care and serious illness. In: Wittenberg E, Ferrell B, Goldsmith, Smith T, Ragen S, Glajchen M, Handzo G, eds. *Textbook of Palliative Care Communication*. New York: Oxford University Press; 2016: 153–160.

27. Hearing Loss Association of America. Guide for effective communication in healthcare. Bethesda, MD: NLSA. 2018. https://www.hearingloss.org/hearing-help/communities/patients/

28. American Foundation for the Blind. Flatten inaccessibility: Healthcare. 2021. https://www.afb.org/research-and-initiatives/flatten-inaccessibility-survey/healthcare

29. Defini, J. Suggestions for the helping professionals who work with individuals with visual impairment. VisionAware – American Publishing House for the Blind. https://visionaware.org/emotional-support/working-with-people-new-to-visual-impairment/offering-support-to-people-who-are-visually-impaired-as-a-helping-professionals/

30. Scamman, K. Limited English proficiency by US state. March 12. 2018. Telelanguage. https://telelanguage.com/limited-English-proficiency-lep-populations-by-u-s-state/

31. Youdelman M. Summary of state law regulations addressing language needs in healthcare. Washington, DC: National Health Law Program. April 29, 2019. https://healthlaw.org/resource/summary-of-state-law-requirements-addressing-language-needs-in-health-care-2/

32. Language Line Solutions. Home page. https://www.languageline.com

33. CyraCom International. Home page. http://interpret.cyracom.com

34. Mobile Martti. Home page. https://www.martti.us

35. U.S. Department of Health and Human Services. National Institute of Health. Definition of health literacy. July 7, 2021. https://www.nih.gov/institutes-nih/nih-office-director/office-communications-public-liaison/clear-communication/health-literacy

36. Sierra M, Cianelli R. Health literacy in relation to health outcomes: A concept analysis. *Nurs Sci Q*. 2019;32(4):299–305. doi:10.1177/0894318419864328

37. Richard RW, Thompson MS, McKinney J, Beauchamp A. Examining health disparities in the US: A third look at the national assessment of adult literacy. *BMC Pub Health*. 2016;16(1):975. Published 2016 Sep 13. doi:10.1186/s12889-016-3621-9

38. US Department of Health and Human Services. Office of Disease Prevention and Health Promotion. October is Health Literacy Month. *October 1, 2-020*. https://health.gov/news/202010/october-health-literacy-month

39. Reisfeld GM, Wilson GR. Palliative Care Fast Facts and Concepts #153: Health literacy in palliative medicine. Appleton, WI: Palliative Care Network of Wisconsin. 2015. https://www.mypcnow.org/?s=health+literacy+in+palliative+medicine&post_type=fast-facts

40. Center for Disease Control and Prevention. Health literacy. Understanding literacy and numeracy. Last review September 1, 2021. https://www.cdc.gov/healthliteracy/learn/UnderstandingLiteracy.html

41. Mamedova S, Pawlowski E. A description of US adults who are not digitally literate. Stats in brief. NCES 2018-161. US. Department of Education. May 2018. https://nces.ed.gov/pubs2018/2018161.pdf

42. deVries K, Bansta E, Dening KH, Ochieng B. Advance care planning for older people: The influence of ethnicity, religiosity, spirituality, and health literacy. *Nurs Ethics*. 2019;26(7–8):1946–1954. doi:10.1177/096973301983313

43. American Association of Colleges of Nursing. ELNEC support for nurses during COVID-19. 2021. https://www.aacnnursing.org/ELNEC/COVID-19

44. Wikipedia. FaceTime. Last edited September 13, 2021. https://en.wikipedia.org/wiki/FaceTime

45. Zoom. Home page. 2021. https://zoom.us

46. Microsoft. Skype. Home page. 2021. https://www.skype.com/en/

47. Hart JC, Courtright KR. Family-centered care during the COVID-19 era. *J Pain Sympt Manage*. 2020;60(20):e93–e97. https://doi.org/10.1016/j.jpainsymman.2020.04.017

48. Cain CL, Surbone A, Elk R, Kagawa-Singer M. Culture and palliative care: Preferences, communication, meaning, and mutual decision making. *J Pain Sympt Manage*. 2018;55:1408–1419. doi.org/10.1016/j.jpainsymman.2018.01.007

49. Health and Human Services (HHS). HHS.gov/ About the Affordable Care Act. Last Washington, DC: HHS. Reviewed March 23, 2021. https://www.hhs.gov/healthcare/about-the-aca/index.html

50. Teriyaki VS, Nery M, Kraemer H. Patient reported barriers to high quality end-of-life care: A multi-ethnic, multi-lingual, mixed methods study. *J Palliat Med*. 2016;19(4):373–381. doi:10.1089/jpm.2015.0403

51. National Hospice and Palliative Care Organization (NHPCO). Facts and figures, 2020 Ed. Alexandria, VA: National Hospice

and Palliative Care Organization. August 20, 2020. https://www.nhpco.org/nhpco-releases-updated-edition-of-hospice-facts-and-figures-report/

52. Rollover M, Smith K, Missiakos E. Racial and ethnic differences in end-of-life care in the United States: Evidence from the Health and Retirement Study (HRS). *Pop Health*. 2019;7:1–8. doi.org/10.1016/j.ssmph.2018.10031

53. Clark MA, Person SD, Gosline A, Gawande AA, Block SD. Racial and ethnic differences in advance care planning: Results of a state-wide population-based survey. *J Palliat Med*. 2018;doi.org/10.1089/jpm.2017.0374

54. Payne R. Racially associated disparities in hospice and palliative care access: Acknowledging the facts while addressing the opportunities to improve. *J Palliat Med*. 2016;19(2):131–133. doi:10.1089/jpm.2015.047

55. Congress.gov. Patient Self Determination Act (PSDA) of 1990. H.R. 4449. Available at https://www.congress.gov/bill/101st-congress/house-bill/4449

56. Perkins HS. Decisions at the end of patients' lives. *A Guide to Psychosocial and Spiritual Care at the End of Life*. New York: Springer; 2016: 35–55.

57. Issacson MJ, Lynch AR. Culturally relevant palliative and end-of-life care for US indigenous populations: An integrative review. *J Transcultural Nurs*. 2018;29(2):180–191. doi:10.1177/1043659617720980

58. Wu J, Wang Y, Jiao X, Wang J, Ye X, Wang B. Differences in practice and preferences associated with truth-telling to cancer patients. *Nurs Ethics*. 2020. doi.org/10.1177/0969733020945754

59. Miller BJ, Berger S. Don't tell me when I am going to die. *New York Times. Opinion Page*. June 22, 2019. https://www.nytimes.com/2019/06/22/opinion/sunday/death-disease-life-expectancy.html

60. Cho HL, Grady C, Tarzian A, Povar G, Manga J, Danis M. Patient and family descriptions of ethical concerns. *Am J Bioethics* 2020;20(6):52–64. doi.org/10.1080/15265161.2020.1754500

61. La S, Lee MC, Hinderer KA, Liu R, Liu M, Fu Y. Palliative care for the Asian American adult population: A scoping review. *Am J Hosp Palliative Care*. 2020;1–13. doi:10.1177/1049909120928063

62. Mendieta M, Buckingham RW. A review of palliative and hospice care in the context of Islam: Dying with faith and family. *J Palliat Med*. 2017;20(11):1284–1290. doi:10.1089/jpm.2017.0340

63. Schweda M, Schicktanz S, Silvers A. Beyond cultural stereotyping: Views on end-of-life decision making among religious and secular persons in the USA, Germany and Israel. *BMC Med Ethics*. 2017;18(1):13. Published 2017 Feb 17. doi:10.1186/s12910-017-0170-4

64. Fink R, Gallagher E. Cancer pain assessment and management. *Sem Onc Nurs*. 2019;35(3):229–234. doi.org/10.1016/j.soncn.2019.04.003

65. Fink R, Gates RA, Jeffers KD. Pain assessment. In: Ferrell B, Paice JA, eds. *The Oxford Textbook of Palliative Nursing*. 5th ed. New York: Oxford University Press; 2019: 98–115.

66. Borneman T, Brown-Saltzman K. Meaning in illness. In: Ferrell B, Paice JA, eds. *The Oxford Textbook of Palliative Nursing*. 5th ed. New York: Oxford University Press; 2019: 456–466.

67. Mitchell A, Jozwiak-Shields C. Cultural perspective and palliative care. *Nurs Palliat Care*. 2017;2(4):1–2. doi:10.15761/npc.1000160

68. Cavalier J, Hampton SB, Langford R, Symes L. The influence of race and gender on nursing care decisions: A pain management intervention. *Pain Manage*. 2018;19(3):238–245. doi:10.1016/j.pmn.2017.10.015

69. Meghani SH, Green C. Disparities in pain and pain care. In: Moore R, ed. *Handbook of Pain and Palliative Care*. Cham: Springer; 2018: 821–834.

70. Robinson-Lane SG, Booker SQ. Culturally responsive pain management for black older adults. *J Geront Nurs*. 2017;43(8):33–41. doi.org/10.3928/00989134-20170224-03

71. Loofs TS, Haubrick K. End-of-life nutrition considerations: Attitudes, beliefs and outcomes. *Am J Hosp Palliat Med*. 2021;38(8):1028–1041. doi.org/10.1177/1049909120960124

72. Partain DK, Strand JJ. Providing appropriate end-of-life care to religious and ethnic minorities. *Mayo Clinic Proc*. 2017;92(1):147–152. doi:10.1016/j.mayocp.2016.08.024

73. Taylor EJ. *Fast Facts About Religion for Nurses: Implications for Patient Care*. New York: Springer Publishing Co; 2019.

74. Gustafson C, Lazenby M. Assessing the unique experiences and needs of Muslim oncology patients receiving palliative and end-of-life care. *J Palliat Care*. 2019;34(1):52–61. doi:10.1177/0825859718800496

75. Corless IB, Meisenhelder JB. Bereavement. In: Ferrell B, Paice JA, eds. *The Oxford Textbook of Palliative Nursing*. 5th ed. New York: Oxford University Press; 2019: 390–404.

76. Ellis-Fletcher SN. When cultures clash. Reflections on nursing leadership. May 19, 2016. Sigma Theta Tau, Int. https://nursingcentered.sigmanursing.org/stories/view/Vol42_2_when-cultures-clash

36.

ENSURING QUALITY SPIRITUAL CARE

Betty Ferrell

KEY POINTS
• Assessment of spiritual needs is a component of comprehensive patient evaluation in palliative care.
• Spirituality encompasses a broad spectrum including religion, purpose and meaning, values, beliefs, and hopes.
• Advanced practice registered nurses (APRNs) provide spiritual care through communication, coordination of care, and responding to spiritual distress.

INTRODUCTION

Spiritual care becomes especially important as patients face any serious illness and at the end of life. Spirituality is closely related to culture and encompasses religious beliefs as well as a broad array of dimensions including meaning, a sense of purpose, hope, and connection.[1-4] As advanced practice registered nurses (APRNs) provide leadership, mentorship, and model expert clinical care, they act as important agents to ensure quality spiritual care. However, as with other aspects of advanced practice, APRNs need knowledge and skill development to deliver the care patients and families need.

This chapter reviews evidence-based guidelines for delivery of spiritual care with discussion of both spiritual assessment and interventions. Case examples are provided to illustrate the role of APRNs in spiritual care. The chapter also reviews spiritual assessment tools for application in advanced practice as well as suggested resources for continued learning.

The National Consensus Project identifies spiritual, religious, and existential care as one of the eight essential domains of quality care.[5] Spiritual care is often led by the specialist member of the team, the chaplain, but all members of the team must be competent in their roles in assessment and prepared to respond to spiritual needs. As with other aspects of care in serious illness, nurses are centrally involved in the provision of this care as the most prevalent discipline across all settings of care.[6]

This textbook is devoted to advanced practice nursing, and, as is the case with areas such as complex pain or symptoms, APRNs need advanced skills in spiritual care. While all palliative nurses should be skilled in basic spiritual assessment and response to spiritual needs,[2-4] palliative APRNs can be a valuable resource for complex spiritual needs. Box 36.1 presents the recommendations for Spiritual Care from the National Consensus Project *Guidelines for*

Quality Palliative Care. Some examples of complex spiritual needs might include

• Conducting a spiritual assessment for patients with less common religious affiliations or whose religious beliefs are creating ethical conflicts in care.

• Working collaboratively with the chaplain to facilitate support of spiritual distress in patients who express a sense of abandonment.

• Expert communication skills to support patients as they conduct life reviews, resolve issues of forgiveness, grasp for miracles, or in those instances when conflicting religious beliefs within families create conflicts in care.

The role of the palliative APRN has been described throughout this text as encompassing many responsibilities including that of expert clinician, educator, manager, and researcher. These roles also apply to the domain of spiritual care. Nurses work collaboratively with chaplains, and together they ensure that patients receive the spiritual care they need (Box 36.2).[7] The APRN serves as a clinical expert in spiritual care, supported by chaplaincy, to model spiritual assessment and care. Knowledge and clinical skills are important competencies for staff education provided by the APRN to new graduates or new staff.

Nurses are also involved in the development of policies and procedures, documentation, and other structures and processes of care. Selection of spiritual care assessment tools and procedures for documenting spiritual needs and care is necessary as palliative care teams are initiated.

As with all other aspects of advanced practice nursing, proficiency in spiritual care requires life-long learning. This is especially true given the increasing diversity of the US population, which includes a vast array of religious traditions and spiritual beliefs that are critical in serious illness. See Table 36.1[4,8-13] for mnemonic tools that may be used to guide APRNs in performing a spiritual assessment. See Table 36.2[14,15] for spiritual care guidelines and implications for the palliative APRN.

SPIRITUAL ASSESSMENT

The importance of spiritual care rests on the foundation of key healthcare concepts such as patient-centered care, respect for the person, and culturally respectful care.[7,10]

Box 36.1 NATIONAL CONSENSUS PROJECT - DOMAIN 5: SPIRITUAL DOMAIN

Domain 5: Spiritual, Religious, and Existential Aspects of Care

Spirituality is recognized as a fundamental aspect of compassionate, patient- and family-centered palliative care. It is a dynamic and intrinsic aspect of humanity through which individuals seek meaning, purpose, and transcendence, and experience relationship to self, family, others, community, society, and the significant or sacred. Spirituality is expressed through beliefs, values, traditions, and practices. Palliative care interdisciplinary teams (IDT) serve each patient and family in a manner that respects their spiritual beliefs and practices. Teams are also respectful when patients and families decline to discuss their beliefs or accept spiritual support.

GUIDELINE 5.1 GLOBAL

CRITERIA

5.1.1 The IDT has clearly defined policies and processes in place to ensure spiritual care is respectful of patient and family age, developmental needs, culture, traditions, and spiritual preferences.

5.1.2 Either directly, through referral, or in collaboration with the professional chaplain, the IDT facilitates spiritual and cultural rituals or practices as desired by the patient and family.

5.1.3 IDT members respect patient and family beliefs and practices, never imposing their individual beliefs on others.

5.1.4 The spiritual needs of family members may differ from those of the patient and are recognized and supported.

5.1.5 Care of children, adolescents, and their family members recognizes that spirituality is integral to coping with serious illness and is provided in a developmentally appropriate manner.

5.1.6 In all settings, the IDT includes professional chaplains who have evidence-based training to assess and address spiritual issues frequently confronted by pediatric and adult patients and families coping with a serious illness.

5.1.7 The professional chaplain is the spiritual care specialist, conducting the assessment and addressing the spiritual aspects of the care plan.

5.1.8 Professional chaplains develop community partnerships to ensure patients have access to spiritual care providers trained and supervised by a professional chaplain. The IDT and community spiritual care providers share information and coordinate service.

5.1.9 The IDT integrates the patient's and/or family's faith community into the care plan when requested.

5.1.10 Led by the professional chaplain, opportunities are provided to engage staff in self-care and self-reflection regarding their own spirituality.

5.1.11 Every member of the IDT is trained in spiritual care and recognizes the importance of the spiritual aspects of care.

5.1.12 Members of the IDT receive training to cultivate an openness to the spirituality of patients and families through empathic listening.

GUIDELINE 5.2 SCREENING AND ASSESSMENT

The spiritual assessment process has three distinct components: spiritual screening, spiritual history, and a full spiritual assessment. The spiritual screening is conducted with every patient and family to identify spiritual needs and/or distress. The history and assessment identify the spiritual background, preferences, and related beliefs, values, rituals, and practices of the patient and family. Symptoms, such as spiritual distress and spiritual strengths and resources, are identified and documented.

CRITERIA

5.2.1 All aspects of the screening, history, and assessment are conducted using standardized tools.

5.2.2 Spiritual screening is completed as part of every clinical assessment to identify spiritual distress and the need for urgent referral to a professional chaplain. Screening is designed to evaluate the presence or absence of spiritual needs and spiritual distress.

5.2.3 IDT members also include a spiritual history as part of the clinical evaluation in the initial assessment process. A spiritual history identifies patient preferences and values that may affect medical decision-making.

5.2.4 A spiritual assessment is triggered based upon the results of the spiritual screening and history. It is an in-depth and ongoing process of evaluation of spiritual needs, results in a plan of care, and is conducted by a professional chaplain as the spiritual care specialist, in collaboration with the faith community, based upon patient wishes.

5.2.5 The spiritual assessment explores spiritual concerns including, but not limited to:
  a. Sources of spiritual strength and support
  b. Existential concerns such as lack of meaning, questions about one's own existence, and questions of meaning and suffering
  c. Concerns about relationship to God, the Holy, or deity, such as anger or abandonment
  d. Struggles related to loss of faith, community of faith, or spiritual practices
  e. Cultural norms and preferences that impact belief systems and spiritual practices
  f. Hopes, values and fears, meaning, and purpose
  g. Concerns about quality of life

h. Concerns or fear of death and dying and beliefs about afterlife
i. Spiritual practices
j. Concerns about relationships
k. Life completion tasks, grief, and bereavement

GUIDELINE 5.3 TREATMENT

The IDT addresses the spiritual needs of the patient and family.

CRITERIA

5.3.1 Spiritual elements of the plan of care are based on needs, goals, and concerns identified by patients and families, recognizing and maximizing patient and family spiritual strengths. The care plan, including religious rituals and other practices, details the expected outcomes of care.

5.3.2 Patient and family spiritual needs are addressed according to established processes, documented in the interdisciplinary care plan, and emphasized during transitions of care, including identification of significant practices which bring strength and comfort to the patient.

5.3.3 Professional and institutional use of symbols and language are inclusive of patient and family cultural and spiritual preferences.

5.3.4 The patient and family are supported and accommodated in their desires to display and use their own spiritual and/or cultural symbols.

5.3.5 Palliative care teams serving pediatric patients have expertise in honoring and meeting the spiritual needs of children and adolescents, including in situations where children or adolescents have differing values, beliefs and needs from their parents or designated decision-makers.

GUIDELINE 5.4 ONGOING CARE

Patient and family spiritual care needs can change as the goals of care change or patients move across settings of care.

CRITERIA

5.4.1 Throughout the trajectory of the patient's illness, the IDT performs spiritual screening to identify new or emergent issues, identifying services and supports to help navigate these transitions. Changes in prognosis and other significant transitions prompt reassessment of spirituality.

5.4.2 The plan of care continues to evolve based upon the changing needs of the patient and family.

Organizations addressing quality in healthcare have recognized the importance of spiritual care even before the development of palliative care. The Joint Commission (TJC), which accredits healthcare organizations, requires spiritual assessment "to determine the patient's denomination, beliefs and what spiritual practices are important."[20] Spiritual assessment is closely aligned with culturally competent care, which is emphasized by many accreditation bodies since religious beliefs are very often central to cultural identity (Box 36.3).[21]

The following case study illustrates the APRN's role in spiritual assessment and how such assessment impacts care and outcomes of that care.

Box 36.2 CHAPLAINCY SERVICES

Areas of chaplaincy assessment
Grief
Concern about death and afterlife
Conflicted or challenged belief systems
Loss of faith
Concern with meaning/purpose of life
Concern about relationship with deity
Isolation from religious community
Guilt
Hopelessness
Conflict between religious beliefs and recommended treatments
Ritual needs

Adapted from Riba et al.[7]; and National Comprehensive Cancer Network. Distress Management (Version 2.2013). http://www.nccn.org/professionals/physicain_gld/f_guidelines.asp

CASE STUDY 1: CONFLICTING RELIGIOUS BELIEF SYSTEMS

Joseph is a nurse practitioner in a 200-bed Catholic hospital. His primary position is in oncology but he is now devoting 20% of his time to the new palliative care service. He has been contacted by the intensive care unit (ICU) to assist in the care of a 70-year-old Iranian man Mr. S who was visiting his brother in the United States when he experienced a cerebral aneurysm. Mr. S is being maintained on a ventilator but is declining, and death is anticipated soon. His wife is extremely distraught, being far away from her family and friends and never having been close to the brother they were visiting. She blames the brother for insisting that her husband come to the United States to work out some family business. The patient and his wife are devout Muslims.

There are two chaplains in the hospital who support the palliative care service, but their time is very stretched between the busy emergency department and trauma center, the large

Table 36.1 MNEMONICS TOOLS TO GUIDE A SPIRITUAL ASSESSMENT

AUTHOR/S	COMPONENTS (MNEMONIC)	ILLUSTRATIVE QUESTIONS
Maugens[8]	• S (spiritual belief system)	• What is your formal religious affiliation?
	• P (personal spirituality)	• Describe the beliefs and practices of your religion or spiritual system that you personally accept. What is the importance of your spirituality/religion in daily life?
	• I (integration with a spiritual community)	• Do you belong to any spiritual or religious group or community? What importance does this group have to you? Does or could this group provide help in dealing with health issues?
	• R (ritualized practices and restrictions)	• Are there specific elements of medical care that you forbid on the basis of religious/spiritual grounds?
	• I (implications for medical care)	• What aspects of your religion/spirituality would you like me to keep in mind, as I care for you? Are there any barriers to our relationship based on religious or spiritual issues?
	• T (terminal events planning)	• As we plan for your care near the end of life, how does your faith impact your decisions?
Anandarajah, Hight[9]	• H (sources of hope)	• What or who is it that gives you hope?
	• O (organized religion)	• Are you a part of an organized faith group? What does this group do for you as a person?
	• P (personal spirituality or spiritual practices)	• What personal spiritual practices, like prayer or meditation, help you?
	• E (effects on medical care and/or end-of-life issues)	• Do you have any beliefs that may affect how the healthcare team cares for you?
Puchalski[4]	• F (faith)	• Do you have a faith belief? What is it that gives your life meaning?
	• I (import or Influence)	• What importance does your faith have In your life? How does your faith belief influence your life?
	• C (community)	• Are you a member of a faith community? How does this support you?
	• A (address)	• How would you like for me to integrate or address these issues in your care?
LaRocca-Pitts[15]	• F (faith)	• What spiritual beliefs are important to you now?
	• A (availability/accessibility/applicability)	• Are you able to find the spiritual nurture that you would like now?
	• C (coping/comfort)	• How comforting/helpful are your spiritual beliefs at this time?
	• T (treatment)	• How can I/we provide spiritual support?
Skalla, McCoy[11,16]	• M (moral authority)	• Where does your sense of what to do come from? What guides you to decide what is right or wrong for you?
	• V (vocational)	• What gives your life purpose? What work is important to you? What mission or role do you feel passionate about?
	• A (aesthetic)	• What brings beauty or pleasure to your life now? How are you able to express your creativity? How do you deal with boredom?
	• S (social)	• What people or faith community do you sense you belong with most? Do you belong to a community that nourishes you spiritually?
	• T (transcendent)	• Who or what controls what happens in life? Who/what supports you when you are ill? • Is there an Ultimate Other (an entity that is sacred, for example)? If so, how do you relate to It?

(continued)

Table 36.1 CONTINUED

AUTHOR/S	COMPONENTS (MNEMONIC)	ILLUSTRATIVE QUESTIONS
McEvoy (pediatric context)[12]	• B (belief system)	• What religious or spiritual beliefs, if any, do members of your family have?
	• E (ethics or values)	
	• L (lifestyle)	• What standards/values/rules for life does your family think important? • What spiritual habits or activities does your family commit to because of spiritual beliefs? (e.g., Any sacred times to observe or diet you keep?)
	• I (involvement in spiritual community)	• How connected to a faith community are you? Would you like us to help you reconnect with this group now?
	• E (education)	• Are you receiving any form of religious education? How can we help you keep up with it?
	• F (near future events of spiritual significance for which to prepare the child)	• Are there any upcoming religious ceremonies that you are getting ready for?

From Johnston-Taylor.[16]

neonatal care unit, and conducting daily Mass. Joseph sees that the ICU nurses are very frustrated by Mr. S's situation. They are frustrated because of the wife's accusations that the nurses and physicians are trying to kill her husband. She refuses to have a visit by the chaplain because he is a Catholic priest. Joseph meets with the staff, communicates with the neurologist and intensivist physicians, and then organizes a family meeting. Joseph is familiar with Muslim beliefs and has arranged an ICU staff education meeting. He discusses the importance of prayer in the Muslim faith, the patient's beliefs prohibiting any discussion of death and code status, and her resistance to a do-not-resuscitate order. He also reviews the care and Muslim spiritual rituals and practices which the staff should provide as the patient dies. The hospital

chaplain connects Joseph with an imam, the Muslim spiritual leader in the community, who arranges a visit. Joseph meets with the imam when he arrives, to explain the patient's condition and plan of care. Joseph works with the ICU manager to look at the schedule for the next few days to assure the availability of a male staff member for postmortem care since only a male will be allowed to touch the body after death. Finally, Joseph collaborates with the palliative care physician and ICU staff to address the patient's symptoms, including his agitation, fevers, respiratory distress, and pain.

This case illustrates the central role of the APRN in a complex situation through proactive management of spiritual, social, and cultural care. Through his varied roles as an APRN, Joseph

Table 36.2 SPIRITUAL CARE GUIDELINES AND IMPLICATIONS FOR THE PALLIATIVE APRN

GUIDELINES REGARDING SPIRITUALITY IN PALLIATIVE CARE	APPLICATION TO APRN ROLES AND RESPONSIBILITIES
All healthcare professionals should be trained to do a spiritual screening or history.	APRN should promote, facilitate, and participate in palliative care team spiritual care education and training. Team should have consensus on which tool team will us, with input and guidance from chaplain/spiritual care provider.
Spiritual background/information should be communicated and documented and shared with interprofessional team.	APRN should assess spirituality and document finding. An appropriate referral should be made to chaplain/spiritual care provider.
Follow-up on spiritual condition changes as part of routine follow-up.	APRN should reassess spirituality as part of routine visits.
Address spiritual concerns related to psychological, physical suffering.	APRN should ensure holistic assessment of all of the domains of care and ensure spiritual interventions are holistic.
Spiritual treatment should include referral to trained spiritual care provider.	APRN should refer patients to trained spiritual care providers congruent with the patient's beliefs and religion. This may be a person on the palliative care team, the organization, or community spiritual leaders.

Adapted from Puchalski C, Ferrell B, Virani R, et al. Improving the quality of spiritual care as a dimension of palliative care: the report of the consensus conference. *J Pall Med.* 2009; 12(10):885–904. http://www.ncbi.nlm.nih.gov/pubmed/19807235; and Wittenberg E, Sun V. Interdisciplinary team collaboration in spiritual care. In: Dahlin C, Coyne P, and Ferrell B., eds. *Advanced Practice Palliative Nursing.* New York: Oxford University Press; 2016.

Spiritual Well-Being

1. How important to you is your participation in *religious activities* such as praying, going to church?

2. How important to you are other *spiritual activities* such as meditation?

3. How much has your *spiritual life* changed as a result of cancer diagnosis?

4. How much *uncertainty* do you feel about your future?

5. To what extent has your illness made *positive changes* in your life?

6. Do you sense a *purpose/mission* for your life or a reason for being alive?

7. How *hopeful* do you feel?

Adapted from City of Hope Quality of Life Instrument.[21]

---

ensures quality care for Mr. S and family, support for the staff, and avoidance of further cultural clash which could make this difficult situation even worse. In addition, this case demonstrates that the care is contingent on an assessment of the beliefs, practices, and values of both the patient and family. Thorough spiritual assessment is an essential aspect of quality palliative care. When cultural clashes or ethical dilemmas arise in palliative care, it is common for spiritual beliefs to be a key contributing factor.[22–25]

SPIRITUAL CARE

The spiritual care provided to patients and families is as widely diverse as the cultures represented in our population. Palliative APRNs contribute to spiritual care provided by palliative care teams in many ways. The following three case studies are intended to illustrate the delivery of spiritual care.

CASE STUDY 2: SPIRITUAL SUFFERING

George was a 70-year-old Hispanic man diagnosed with pancreatic cancer. He was referred by his oncologist to the outpatient palliative care clinic for pain and nausea management. The palliative nurse practitioner, Jim, saw George every 2 weeks for his symptoms through alternating clinic visits with telehealth calls each week. George's symptoms improved, but he seemed very anxious and sad. Jim reviewed the initial assessment completed in the oncology clinic to identify any useful psychosocial information in the medical record. Seeing nothing documented and knowing that George was generally alone for his visits, Jim asked George about his family support and if he was depressed. George

shared that his wife, Anita, had been a cook in a local nursing home, and she had contracted COVID early in the pandemic and died. He shared that he has not attended church since her death and that he was really angry at God because he knew that, soon, his grandchildren will "lose me, too, and have no grandparents left." George told Jim that, in his family and in their close Hispanic culture, grandparents are very important for children.

This case highlights the role of the APRN in advanced disease and the need for nurses to recognize that it is common for symptom management to move beyond pharmacologic interventions and to address suffering.[6] In this case, George is not only a patient, he is also a bereaved family caregiver. The case also illustrates the most important skill for APRNs in spiritual care: listening. Presence and listening are essential to understanding and responding to spiritual needs.

CASE STUDY 3: SPIRITUAL LONELINESS

Mary was an 82-year-old African American woman living in the South in a residential care facility. She experienced multiple symptoms from her end-stage cardiac disease and was referred to palliative care after three hospital urgent care visits over 6 weeks due to dyspnea and edema. She is now preparing for discharge after a hospital admission related to her symptoms. Mary's children live out of state, and she is described as a lonely woman, fiercely independent, and very stoic.

Mary was being seen by a master's prepared nurse, Jean, the clinical nurse specialist in the cardiac care program. Jean did a thorough assessment of Mary, including an assessment of her physical, psychosocial, and spiritual needs. When Jean asked if Mary had a church community that might offer support, Mary angrily replied that she "quit believing in God" as a child, after witnessing common hatred and racial discrimination. When asked about her life before retirement, Mary described her career as a high school science teacher, one of the first African American women to be allowed to teach science in the public school. She said she was proud to have been there at a time "when girls weren't supposed to be smart," and she became calm and proud as she told Jean about the many young women she had inspired to get an education.

Jean collaborated with the cardiology service and the palliative care team in arranging for home-based palliative care because Mary adamantly refused hospice care and insisted on returning home alone. Jean shared with the palliative care service the information she had learned from Mary about her psychosocial and spiritual needs.

This case illustrates an instance where the patient's spiritual journey, from early religious affiliation to movement away from God, becomes expressed in the final phase of life. Nursing assessment helped move beyond the religious aspect to identify positive aspects of spirituality for this patient through the meaning of her life and legacy. The literature and research related to spirituality have emphasized that spiritual care encompasses aspects beyond religious affiliation to also include life meaning, purpose, and existential needs.[23–30]

CASE STUDY 4: SPIRITUAL CONFLICTS

Kim was a nurse practitioner on a hematology service in an urban academic medical center. One of Kim's most challenging patients was a 20-year-old Korean male, Jyen, who was admitted 40 days prior with severe graft versus host disease following stem cell transplant for leukemia. Jyen's large extended family refused to face the seriousness of his illness despite worsening renal and pulmonary complications. Jyen and his family were devout Catholics and believed in miracles. Jyen was a full code, and he and his family refused any discussion of avoiding resuscitation or life support.

Over the past few days, tensions escalated because the family believed the staff had given up on Jyen. They became angry when the nurses interrupted their bedside prayer sessions, which they believe are important for God to see they are awaiting a miracle healing. They refused palliative care. The hematology service was becoming frustrated because they believed Jyen's distress and increasing agitation was caused by his family's distress.

The family developed a good relationship with Kim, who was also Catholic. They believed that she had not given up on Jyen. Kim arranged a meeting with the family, chaplain, and social worker to both better understand the family's beliefs in miracles and their understanding of his declining status.

This case illustrates the challenges often inherent in palliative care related to spirituality. There are times when spiritual beliefs clash with clinical care goals. The APRN can be the link between the healthcare system and preserving the patient's dignity and values. Kim's action now can potentially help to avert worse conflict as Jyen's disease progresses and at the time of death.

SPIRITUAL CARE IN PEDIATRICS

There is a very significant role for nurses in pediatric palliative care to respond to the spiritual needs of children and their families.[34–38] This requires attention to the child's developmental stage, how the serious illness has affected that stage, and the context of religious or spiritual beliefs within the family. APRNs may provide an initial spiritual assessment along with their spiritual colleagues to explore these issues.

Spiritual care in pediatrics is an example of the importance of interdisciplinary care because nurses will need the guidance of chaplaincy to understand the child's and family's religious and spiritual beliefs and practices. A child's understanding of God or a higher power and the meaning of life events is related to their developmental stage. Thus, the APRN's knowledge of childhood development is essential.[34–38] APRNs may often be the primary providers to whom patients, siblings, parents, grandparents, and friends express their emotional responses to spiritual concerns such as anger toward God, guilt, distress, and blame.

McEvoy provides a model for assessment in pediatrics, the BELIEF mnemonic.[12]

B: Belief system (such as participation in religious activities or discussion of an afterlife)

E: Ethics of values

L: Lifestyle (such as rituals or practices related to religion)

I: Involvement in a spiritual community

E: Education to assess religious education in the family

F: Future events, including important rites and the future role of the faith community in the child's care

As stated previously, spirituality is also closely intertwined with culture, which is particularly important in pediatric care because nurses need to assess both the child's as well as the parents' and extended family's spiritual and cultural beliefs. Thus, the APRN can contribute best to the care of seriously ill children through cultural assessment, including cultural meanings of illness, traditions, rituals, and language.

RESOURCES

While the important need for APRN involvement in spiritual care may seem overwhelming, extensive resources exist. In addition to the above-cited guidelines, there are many spiritual assessment tools available for clinical use.[39–52] The CASH tool is an example of a spiritual assessment tool that is brief to use.[52] It includes questions on *Care*: What do I need to know about you to take better care of you; *Assistance/Help*: What has helped you most during the course of your illness; *Stress*: What are the biggest stressors in your life now; and *Hopes/Fears*: What is your biggest fear? What are you hoping for?

There are increasing numbers of textbooks and model projects advancing the domain of spiritual care. Box 36.4,[53–56] Box 36.5,[13] and Box 36.2[14–15] and Table 36.1 summarize many of these resources.

Box 36.4 KEY RESOURCES FOR ADVANCED PRACTICE NURSES FOR SPIRITUAL CARE

- George Washington University Institute for Spirituality in Health http://www.GWISH.org

- Puchalski C, Ferrell, B. *Making Healthcare Whole*. West Conshohocken, PA: Templeton Press; 2010.

- Ferrell B, Coyle N. *The Nature of Suffering and the Goals of Nursing*. New York: Oxford University Press; 2008.

- Johnson-Taylor E. *Religion: A Clinical Guide for Nurses*. New York: Springer; 2012.

- Johnson-Taylor E. *Fast Facts About Religion for Nurses: Implications for Patient Care*. New York: Springer; 2019.[56]

Box 36.5 NURSING SPIRITUAL ASSESSMENT

Dear _____,

Your palliative care team wants to make sure you receive the physical, emotional, and spiritual care and comfort you need.

Typically, persons receiving palliative care find themselves becoming more aware of their spirituality or religion. Please help us to understand what are your spiritual care and comfort needs.

Directions: Place an "X" on the lines to show the answer that comes closest to describing your experience.

1. How important is spirituality and/or religion to you now?

/ _____

Not at all important   Very important

2. *Recently, my spiritis have been . . .*

/ _____

Awful. . . . low. . . .okay. . . .good. . . .great

What can a nurse do to nurture or boost your spirits? (check all that apply)

— pray with me

— allow time and space for my private prayer or meditation

— bring art or music to nurture my spirit

— listen to my thoughts about certain spiritual matters

— provide assistance so I can record my life story

— just be with me

— help me stay connected to my spiritual community by contacting:

- My church/temple/mosque/local faith community's name and Location

_____

- My clergy or spiritual leader's name (any contact information will be helpful)

Is there anything else about your spiritual beliefs or practices that the palliative care team should know about? (e.g., diet or lifestyle proscribed by your religion? Beliefs guiding your preparation for death?) Please write here (or on the back side) or tell your nurse.

From Johnston-Taylor E.[43]

SUMMARY

Palliative care is, by its very definition and existence, based on a foundation of whole-person, comprehensive care. It is incomplete without full attention paid to the spiritual domain. Palliative APRNs contribute to this goal of whole-person care through an assessment of the spiritual needs of the entire family and application of evidence-based guidelines. Through close collaboration with chaplains and other team members, care can be respectful and inclusive of spiritual needs.

REFERENCES

1. Balboni T, Fitchett G, Handzo G et al. State of the science of spirituality and palliative care research part II: Screening, assessment, and interventions. *J Pain Symptom Manage.* 2017;54(3):441–453. doi:10.1016/j.jpainsymman.2017.07.029

2. HealthCare Chaplaincy Network. Spiritual Care: What it means, why it matters in health care. 2016; HealthCare Chaplaincy Network. https://healthcarechaplaincy.org/docs/about/spirituality.pdf Accessed January 21, 2021.

3. Puchalski CM, Vitillo R, Hull SK, Reller N. Improving the spiritual dimension of whole person care: Reaching national and international consensus. *J Palliat Med* 2014;17(6):642–656.

4. Puchalski CM, Ferrell B. Making health care whole: Integrating spirituality into patient care. West Conshohocken: Templeton Press, 2010.

5. National Consensus Project for Quality Palliative Care. *Clinical Practice Guidelines for Quality Palliative Care,* 4th ed. Richmond, VA: National Coalition of Hospice and Palliative Care. 2018. http://www.nationalconsensusproject.org. Accessed January 15, 2021.

6. Ferrell BR, Paice JA. Oxford Textbook of Palliative Nursing, New York, NY: Oxford University Press, 2019.

7. Riba MB, Donovan KA, Andersen B, et al. Distress Management, Version 3. 2019, NCCN Clinical Practice Guidelines in Oncology. *J Natl Compr Canc Netw.* 2019;17(10).

8. Maugans TA. The SPIRITual history. *Arch Fam Med.* 1996;5(1):11-16.

9. Anandarajah G, Hight E. Spirituality and medical practice: using the HOPE questions as a practical tool for spiritual assessment. *Am Fam Physician.* 2001;63(1):81–89.

10. Larocca-Pitts MA. FACT: taking a spiritual history in a clinical setting. *J Health Care Chaplain.* 2008;15(1):1–12.

11. Skalla K, McCoy JP. Spiritual assessment of patients with cancer: the moral authority, vocational, aesthetic, social, and transcendent model. *Oncol Nurs Forum.* 2006;33(4):745–751.

12. McEvoy M. An added dimension to the pediatric health maintenance visit: the spiritual history. *J Pediatr Health Care.* 2000;14(5):216–220.

13. Johnston-Taylor E. Chapter 34: Spiritual screening, history, and assessment. In: Ferrell, B, Paice J, (Eds.) *Textbook of Palliative Nursing.* 5th ed. New York, NY: Oxford University Press. 2019.

14. Puchalski C, Ferrell B, Virani R, et al. Improving the quality of spiritual care as a dimension of palliative care: the report of the Consensus Conference. *J Palliat Med.* 2009;12(10):885–904.

15. Wittenberg E, Sun V. Interdisciplinary team collaboration in spiritual care. In Dahlin C, Coyne P, and Ferrell B. (Eds.) *Advanced Practice Palliative Nursing*. New York, NY: Oxford University Press. 2016.

16. Emanuel L, Handzo G, Grant G, et al. Workings of the human spirit in palliative care situations: A consensus model from the Chaplaincy Research Consortium. *BMC Palliat Care*. 2015;14(1). doi:10.1186/s12904-015-0005-3.

17. Giske T, Cone PH. Discerning the healing path–how nurses assist patient spirituality in diverse health care settings. *J Clin Nurs*. 2015; 24: 2926–2935, doi:10.1111/jocn.12907.

18. Minton ME, Isaacson MJ, Varilek BM, Stadick JL, O'Connell-Persaud S. A willingness to go there: Nurses and spiritual care. *J Clin Nurs* 2018;27(1–2):173–181. doi:10.1111/jocn.13867.

19. Otis-Green S. Integrating spirituality into care at the end of life: Providing person-centered quality care. *Death Stud*. 2015;39(3): 185–187. doi:10.1080/07481187.2014.899425.

20. The Joint Commission. *The Source*. January 2018. Vol. 16, Issue 1. Accessed July 6, 2020. https://www.nacc.org/wp-content/uploads/2018/01/Part-1.-Body-Mind-Spirit-JC-The-Source-Jan.2018-Vol.16.1.pdf Accessed January 15, 2021.

21. City of Hope, Nursing Research and Education. Resources. https://www.cityofhope.org/research/beckman-research-institute/research-departments-and-divisions/population-sciences/nursing-research-and-education/nursing-research-and-education-resources Accessed January 15, 2021.

22. Borneman T, Brown-Saltzman, K. Meaning in Illness. In Ferrell BR, Paice JA (eds), *Oxford Textbook of Palliative Nursing*, 5th ed. New York, NY: Oxford University Press, 2019:456–467.

23. Ellington L, Reblin M, Ferrell B et al. The religion of "I Don't Know". *OMEGA*. 2015;72(1):3–19. doi:10.1177/0030222815574689.

24. Epstein-Peterson ZD, Sullivan AJ, Enzinger AC, et al. Examining Forms of Spiritual Care Provided In The Advanced Cancer Setting. *Am J Hosp Palliat Care*. Nov 2015;32(7):750–757.

25. Fang M, Sixsmith J, Sinclair S, Horst G. A knowledge synthesis of culturally- and spiritually-sensitive end-of-life care: Findings from a scoping review. *BMC Geriatr*. 2016;16(1). doi:10.1186/s12877-016-0282-6.

26. Camargos M, Paiva C, Barroso E, Carneseca E, Paiva B. Understanding the differences between oncology patients and oncology health professionals concerning spirituality/religiosity. *Medicine* (Baltimore). 2015;94(47):e2145. doi:10.1097/md.0000000000002145.

27. Delgado-Guay M, Rodriguez-Nunez A, De la Cruz V et al. Advanced cancer patients' reported wishes at the end of life: a randomized controlled trial. *Support Care Cancer*. 2016;24(10):4273–4281. doi:10.1007/s00520-016-3260-9.

28. Fitchett G, Emanuel L, Handzo G, Boyken L, Wilkie DJ. Care of the human spirit and the role of dignity therapy: a systematic review of dignity therapy research. *BMC Palliat Care* 2015;14:8.

29. George L, Park C. Does spirituality confer meaning in life among heart failure patients and cancer survivors? *Psycholog Relig Spiritual*. 2017;9(1):131–136. doi:10.1037/rel0000103.

30. Gonzalez P, Castañeda SF, Dale J, et al. Spiritual well-being and depressive symptoms among cancer survivors. *Support Care Cancer* 2014;22(9):2393–400.

31. Jim HS, Pustejovsky JE, Park CL, et al. Religion, spirituality, and physical health in cancer patients: A meta-analysis. *Cancer*. Nov 1 2015;121(21):3760–3768.

32. Piderman KM, Kung S, Jenkins SM, et al. Respecting the spiritual side of advanced cancer care: a systematic review. *Curr Oncol Rep* 2015;17:6.

33. Salsman JM, Pustejovsky JE, Jim HS, et al. A meta-analytic approach to examining the correlation between religion/spirituality and mental health in cancer. *Cancer*. Nov 1 2015;121(21):3769–3778.

34. Ferrell B, Wittenberg E, Battista V, Walker G. Nurses' experiences of spiritual communication with seriously ill children. *J Palliat Med*. 2016;19(11):1166–1170. doi:10.1089/jpm.2016.0138.

35. Petersen C, Callahan M, McCarthy D, Hughes R, White-Traut R, Bansal N. An online educational program improves pediatric oncology nurses' knowledge, attitudes, and spiritual care competence. *J Ped Oncol Nurs*. 2017;34(2):130–139. doi:10.1177/1043454216646542.

36. Chrastek J, van Breemen C. Symptom Management in Pediatric Palliative Care, In Ferrell BR, Paice JA (eds), *Oxford Textbook of Palliative Nursing*, 5th ed. New York, NY: Oxford University Press, 2019: 699–707.

37. Battista V, LaRagione G. Pediatric Hospice and Palliative Care, In Ferrell BR, Paice JA (eds), *Oxford Textbook of Palliative Nursing*, 5th ed. New York, NY: Oxford University Press, 2019: 708–726.

38. Alvarenga, Willyane & Carvalho, Emilia & Caldeira, Sílvia & Vieira, Margarida & Nascimento, Lucila. (2017). The possibilities and challenges in providing pediatric spiritual care. *Journal of Child Health Care*. 21. 1367493517737183. 10.1177/1367493517737183.

39. Bennett V, Thompson ML. Teaching spirituality to student nurses. *J Nurs Educ*. 2015;5(2). doi:10.5430/jnep.v5n2p26.

40. Borneman T, Ferrell B, Puchalski CM. Evaluation of the FICA Tool for Spiritual Assessment. *J Pain Symptom Manage*. 2010; 40(2):163–73.

41. Carrion I, Nedjat-Haiem F, Macip-Billbe M, Black R. "I Told Myself to Stay Positive" perceptions of coping among Latinos with a cancer diagnosis living in the United States. *Am J Hosp Palliat Care*. 2016;34(3):233–240. doi:10.1177/1049909115625955.

42. FACIT.org. Functional Assessment of Cancer Therapy - General (FACT-G) https://www.facit.org/measures/FACT-G Accessed January 15, 2021.

43. Gomez-Castillo B, Hirsch R, Groninger H et al. Increasing the number of outpatients receiving spiritual assessment: A pain and palliative care service quality improvement project. *J Pain Symptom Manage*. 2015;50(5):724–729. doi:10.1016/j.jpainsymman.2015.05.012.

44. Harrad R, Cosentino C, Keasley R, Sulla F. Spiritual care in nursing: an overview of the measures used to assess spiritual care provision and related factors amongst nurses. *Acta Biomed*. 2019;90(4-S): 44–55. Published 2019 Mar 28. doi:10.23750/abm.v90i4-S.8300.

45. King S, Fitchett G, Murphy P, Pargament K, Harrison D, Loggers E. Determining best methods to screen for religious/spiritual distress. *Support Care Cancer*. 2016;25(2):471–479. doi:10.1007/s00520-016-3425-6.

46. Rosa W, Spiritual Care Intervention. In Ferrell BR, Paice JA (eds), *Oxford Textbook of Palliative Nursing*, 5th ed. New York, NY: Oxford University Press, 2019: 447–455.

47. Rosa W, Hope Stephanie, Matzo Marianne. Palliative Nursing and Sacred Medicine: A Holistic Stance on Entheogens, Healing, and Spiritual Care, *Journal of Holistic Nursing*, 2018;37(1): 100–106. DOI link: https://doi.org/10.1177/0898010118770302.

48. Sherman AC, Merluzzi TV, Pustejovsky JE, et al. A meta-analytic review of religious or spiritual involvement and social health among cancer patients. *Cancer* 2015;121(21):3779–88. doi: 10.1002/cncr.29352. Epub 2015 Aug 10.

49. Steinhauser K, Fitchett G, Handzo G et al. State of the science of spirituality and palliative care research part I: Definitions, measurement, and outcomes. *J Pain Symptom Manage*. 2017;54(3): 428–440. doi:10.1016/j.jpainsymman.2017.07.028.

50. Timmins F, Caldeira S. Assessing the spiritual needs of patients. *Nurs Stand*. 2017;31(29): 47–53. doi: 10.7748/ns.2017.e10312.

51. Wang CW, Chow AY, Chan CL. The effects of life review interventions on spiritual well-being, psychological distress, and quality of life in patients with terminal or advanced cancer: a systematic review and meta-analysis of randomized controlled trials. *Palliat Med* 2017;31:e883–e894.

52. Alesi ER, Ford TR, Chen CJ et al. Development of the CASH assessment tool to address existential concerns in patients with serious illness. *J Palliat Med* 2015; 18(1):71–75. Doi: 10.1089/jpm.2014.0053.

53. George Washington University Institute for Spirituality in Health. http://www.GWISH.org.

54. Ferrell B, Coyle N. *The Nature of Suffering and the Goals of Nursing*. New York: Oxford University Press; 2008.

55. Johnston-Taylor E. *Religion: A Clinical Guide for Nurses*. New York: Springer; 2012.

56. Johnston-Taylor E. *Fast Facts About Religion for Nurses: Implications for Patient Care*. New York: Springer; 2019

37.

LIFE REVIEW

Jamil Davis, Mimi Jenko, and James C. Pace

KEY POINTS

- Life review has the power to heal and contribute meaning to one's life.

- Life review has its roots in life-span developmental psychology.

- Life review is a structured process that involves analytic self-evaluation.

- Life review can involve a patient/client and/or family member(s).

- Essential components of life review include active listening, a nonjudgmental attitude, superior communication skills, and firm boundaries of the therapeutic relationship.

- Life review is a spiritual intervention that creates a covenantal relationship between parties.

- Three components of life review include recontextualizing, forgiveness, and reclaiming an unlived life.

- Mindful of patient confidentiality and privacy, highlights of life review are incorporated into the electronic medical record, reflecting patient preference, decision-making, and goals of care.

- The palliative advanced practice registered nurse (APRN) works closely within the context of a team; when complex issues arise beyond the APRN's scope of practice, consultation is then requested (e.g., from board certified chaplains, mental health providers, marriage and family counselors).

CASE STUDY 1: THE LIFE WELL-LIVED

Nan was a 67-year-old woman recently lost her husband of 43 years and now is close to death with metastatic pancreatic cancer. During a visit with the palliative advanced practice registered nurse (APRN), she mentioned that all her life was lived through her husband (she "stood in his shadow"). Now she had nothing to show for her life now that it is reaching its conclusion. As the visit evolved, the APRN asked Nan to describe what she did as a young parent, recount where she worked while raising her children, detail her church activities where she served as the Director of the Altar Guild, and describe her hobbies (she loved to do needle-point chair coverings and crosier quilts with multiple color pieces of cloth). Once each topic was fully developed, the APRN summarized the major movements and accomplishments that highlighted a life fully lived. Nan remarked at the visit's conclusion that she had never taken the time to document how her life had made a difference in the lives of so many others.

INTRODUCTION

Life review as a formal concept has its roots in life-span developmental psychology.[1] According to Butler[1] and Erikson,[2] one's development is formed or shaped by the myriad of events and circumstances encountered throughout the entire life span. In his seminal article, Butler[1] (p. 66) conceptualized life review as

> a naturally occurring, universal mental process characterized by the progressive return of consciousness of past experiences, and, particularly, the resurgence of unresolved conflicts. . . . Presumably this process is prompted by the realization of approaching dissolution and death and the inability to maintain one's sense of personal invulnerability.

Life review allows the teller of the story to recast the past in the context of the present.[3] In so doing, one reviews and reexamines one's life and is given various opportunities to solve old problems, make amends, and restore any lost sense of harmony.[4] Any form of life review involves key questions such as "Who am I?" "How did I live my life over time?" "Did I take every advantage that I could to live my life well?"

For many, there is a *distinct* difference between periodic episodes of life reminiscence and life review. Life review is not "a random sharing of pleasurable past events, but rather a structured process containing a component of self-evaluation."[5] (p. 9) A possible end result of such a review is the chance to find new meaning in life, especially when one faces the realities of impending death.[6]

Whether conducted with the patient, the family, or both patient and family together, life review includes the outcomes of increased life satisfaction and accomplishment, the promotion of more peaceful inner feelings, and a renewed state of integrity.[7] Consistent with Erikson's theory of development,[2,8] the final task of ego integrity entails the acceptance of one's life as lived, an awareness of one's place in history, the gradual release of death anxiety, and a greater satisfaction with life overall. Erikson[8] believed that the greater part of adulthood is spent finding creative and meaningful experiences (including one's life work/career) to avoid feeling stagnant; then, during the final stages of living, the person can look back over the years at their accomplishments and feel a sense of pride and satisfaction in the summation of the outcome(s). The alternative, ego-despair, involves the lack of pride in accomplishment, the absence of hope going forward, and the idea of stagnancy in living.[2]

The aforementioned end-of-life issues have sizable practice implications for palliative advanced practice registered nurses (APRNs). By 2030, older adults will outnumber children—creating the so-called "silver tsunami."[9] Despite generational differences between providers and clients, Byock[10] asserts that caring and compassionate healthcare providers are well-positioned to listen and explore patient and family stories during those needed moments, and the outcome is a greater sense of meaning and purpose in life. When the palliative APRN *actively* welcomes and fosters these "critical opportunities," especially in terms of interdisciplinary team interventions, the result is a more compassionate healthcare environment that promotes patient awareness, comfort, ease, and satisfaction with life.

VARIED USES OF LIFE REVIEW

LIFE REVIEW WITH THE INDIVIDUAL PATIENT

According to Jenko, Gonzalez, and Alley,[11] when a person's goals of care shift definitively from cure to comfort, life review provides an evidence-based approach that brings the members of a family together, alleviates suffering, and focuses specific attention on the patient's holistic care. Storytelling is an ageless form of artful human communication. It is interactive, uses both verbal and nonverbal forms of expression, and recounts a story that engages the imagination of the listener.[12] Furthermore, in reviewing one's life "story," the storyteller is given the opportunity to find meaning that is discovered in everyday life problems along with the strengths and the depths of love and devotion that are revealed in and through one's story.[12,13]

Storytelling is also richly explored in the nursing literature; Smith and Liehr[14] proposed a mid-range nursing theory which uses story as the central feature. Story theory assists the palliative APRN in determining what "matters most" to a patient by connecting past incidents and future aspirations to the present health challenge. The health challenge is then addressed using available evidence-based literature, and the stories are integrated into the plan of care. The APRN interprets and reinterprets the story, thereby helping the patient resolve the challenge.[14]

LIFE REVIEW WITH THE FAMILY

Though the process of life review most often involves the exchanges between a patient and the healthcare provider, life review can also involve the family unit. In clinical situations where the patient is incapacitated, life review is conducted

with the family and often involves clarifying goals-of-care and navigating anticipatory grief.[15] In these instances, an understanding of family systems is vital. Families are seen as an organized whole, comprised of both individuals and complex relationships among those individuals. When one member of a family experiences a life-limiting situation, the remaining family members struggle between processing rapidly changing contextual realities and maintaining a sense of cohesion and constancy. Families are grappling with the impending loss of a loved one as well as the realization of new family patterns and relationships.[16] In addition, at the death of a loved one, the family is in a unique place to enter into dialogues about the events of the loved one's life and subsequent death. Telling these stories allows the family to maintain higher levels of emotional functioning, retain or regain hope for the future, and find a renewed passion for living.[17]

The literature supports storytelling as a model for patient coping with difficult and significant life stressors.[18] Additionally, a systematic review conducted by Scarton and colleagues[19] found families also experience emotional and spiritual distress, and the effects of supportive approaches are mostly positive.

CASE STUDY 2: THE FAMILY LIFE REVIEW

A 42-year-old man, Jack, with a large extended family suffered a massive brain injury due to a motorcycle accident. The family had made the agonizing decision to discontinue life support but were sharply divided with regard to organ donation. Their loud, arguing voices had disrupted the trauma intensive care unit, and a stalled treatment plan had prompted a "stat" palliative care consult. To set a less divisive tone, the palliative APRN first established a therapeutic milieu: an empty patient room with chairs formed in a circle. Over the next 90 minutes, the APRN evoked earlier and happier memories gained from a life richly lived. Memories of a "larger-than-life" person arose: romances with multiple women, an infectious laugh, and an adventuresome spirit. Conversations were then gently guided to philanthropic themes. Although Jack did not participate in formal nonprofit work, the family recalled that he always participated in Girl Scout cookie drives, Little League team car washes, and military veterans' events. Then the palliative APRN facilitated family agreement that Jack had a charitable giving spirit toward others; this insight led to a peaceful family consensus for organ donation.

LIFE REVIEW AS A HOLISTIC INTERVENTION

A large amount of information is shared with the provider during any given session of life review. The provider needs the luxury of time, as most patients are invested in telling detailed accounts and remembrances. As a palliative care intervention, life review is about "having conversations in human-scale time, which means you can't do it in five minutes."[20] This careful, unhurried approach is a *critical* element of this intervention. When the provider engages in a session of life review, there is an unspoken covenant relationship that takes place between the patient and the healthcare provider. This notion of entering into a covenantal relationship presupposes that two people come together; they agree on any promises, stipulations, boundaries, and/or responsibilities that are made.[21,22] There is a bond that is being made between two equal parties for therapeutic outcomes. In the case of life review, this covenant relationship incorporates three fundamental nursing assumptions: the individual or patient agrees to enter into such a conversation, there is the promise to listen in a nonjudgmental and therapeutic manner, and there exists an unspoken pledge to intervene and address any issues of suffering that may be called forth.

Life review as a spiritual intervention, with its attending covenant relationship, presents unique opportunities to provide additional information regarding the patient's social, emotional, physical, cultural, religious, and spiritual needs. Life review calls forth the importance of the nursing process as the guide for the provision of holistic care to patients and family members. Particularly with end-of-life care, knowledge of the evolving needs of the patient and family better informs all healthcare directives and assists with advance care planning. End-of-life situations can often trigger spiritual and emotional distress, thus reducing the patient's abilities to cope, communicate, and participate in all care decisions. Knowledge of patient preferences as they evolve in these areas can be incorporated into the plan of care and further communicated to staff and the interdisciplinary healthcare team. These nursing actions help to satisfy The Joint Commission requirements for advancing effective communication, cultural competence, and patient- and family-centered care.[23]

According to Kaufman,[24] there are 23 themes that commonly evolve from the processes of life review (see Table 37.1). With time, the experiences are seen collectively and can be woven into a cohesive whole; when this occurs, the patient's identity is further clarified and meaning-making evolves. A person not only comes to conclusions about a life lived, but is actively present when communicating that life to others.

In terms of process, the palliative APRN may want to take copious notes while listening or simply take brief notes of key topic areas. The APRN may choose to follow a set format that has worked previously for the gathering of key pieces of data as conversations evolve. Or the APRN may choose to listen intently to the patient without paper, pencil, or computer and then summarize key points and conversation trends following the session. In any respect, the analysis of the "data" (information gathered) is extremely important in formulating an in-depth understanding of the person, the development of his or her personality, the significance of certain key life events, and how aging is playing out in terms of health, disease, distress, integrity, and decline. These data will begin to crystalize into social, psychological, historical, spiritual, and cultural life themes. In fact, the life review process shares many commonalities with qualitative research methods in that content analysis of the information gathered is essential. As content themes emerge, the meaning of the information to the patient takes shape, texture, and form. A wide range of experiences is sampled; those that require further analysis and additional work then become a part of the ongoing plan of care.

At any time during the life review process, the healthcare provider may be tipped off to an episode of a life experience needing further exploration. The patient's face may reveal a brief, fleeting glimpse of a pained affect or there may be words *not* spoken or expressed, the silence indicating a sensitive or controversial key event. This is especially true when an unspoken situation may not be socially acceptable or publicly sanctioned.

CASE STUDY 3: THE UNSPOKEN EPISODES IN LIFE REVIEW

Bill, a 41-year-old male had been married to his partner for 4 years. Because his family did not agree with his sexual orientation, the patient had not spoken to his extended family since his marriage. Their last words were harsh and angry: "We hope we never see you again." Several years later, Bill was diagnosed with colon cancer and experienced significant complications, resulting in a lengthy hospitalization. His suffering has caused severe distress to his partner, yet his extended family remained uninformed of his deteriorating state. When Bill was given 2–3 months to live, the oncologist consulted the palliative care team.

While listening to Bill discuss his family, the palliative APRN observed a moment of hesitation in his voice. It was an elusive clue, one that could have been easily dismissed or overlooked. Yet there was something that just was "not right," so the APRN closed the door to Bill's room and said softly, "I could totally be in left field, but I think there is something you want to tell me—something that causes you great pain in the situation." After a long silence, Bill revealed that marriage had alienated his extended family. With only a few months left to live, Bill desired to both offer and receive forgiveness. After speaking with his partner, a phone call was finally arranged. Bill and his extended family had a lengthy conversation, which ultimately resulting in healing for all family members.

As providers will discover, patients often have deeply buried feelings and memories. Once brought to the surface, providers must be prepared to occasionally bear witness to intense affect, deep remorse, and searing personal pain. When facilitating a life review, the provider needs to be prepared to deal with literally anything. In instances of extremely subtle clues of suffering, one might agree with Sir Arthur Conan Doyle:

Table 37.1 MAJOR THEMES THAT EVOLVE FROM LIFE REVIEWS

Affective ties	Service
Financial status	Acquiescence
Marriage	Self determination
Work	Financial security
Social status	Religion
Community service	Disengagement
Self-reliance	Family
Industry	Achievement
Initiative	Orientation
Search for spiritual understanding/ meaning	Creativity
	Need for relationships
Discipline	Selflessness

From Kaufman.[24]

"It has long been an axiom of mine that the little things are infinitely the most important."[25]

LIFE REVIEW: THREE COMPONENTS

As Byock asserts, "Illness is personal; it is not just medical. People need to have services not merely to suppress suffering, but to help them in completing their lives."[26] To achieve this outcome, palliative APRNs need to be aware of three interconnected components to life review[11,27]: recontextualizing, forgiving, and reclaiming unlived life.

Recontextualizing values the worth of accrued life wisdom. Life experiences, no matter what a person's chronological age, contribute to a "store" of wisdom. Recontextualizing enables the patient to recall and perhaps "reframe" self-defined mistakes and failures. Negative life events and/or situations are reframed in ways that can be positively (re)configured.[11] What is assumed in this process is the willingness of the patient to face the past in a different light, especially when reliving painful or unpleasant memories. Recontextualizing asserts that one is not so much a victim of the past but rather is more in control of life's experiences, having the opportunity to recast one's memories based on perceptions of the past.[1] One can reflect on past experiences and then begin the valued reparation process of those relationships and events formerly perceived as being negative. Changed perceptions can change memories, going from a sense of failure to a new-found sense of accomplishment, even success. Recontextualizing asks one to search for the deeper meanings, even to the often-elusive patterns of life events. Recontextualizing assumes that new-found meanings can heal past scars and wounds over time. One does not necessarily change the way that he or she lives, but rather begins to see life through a different filter or lens.

Recasting meanings to past events can give life a new sense of order and changes the way once sees self, others, and the world.[1,28] Regarding the accrual of life wisdom, Baldwin[29] asserts that story connects one's past, present, and future, thus allowing one to live in a generational context. Often a life review serves two purposes: it helps to heal the storyteller and also begins the process of healing future generations.

CASE STUDY 4: GENERATIONAL EFFECTS OF LIFE REVIEW

Jill's life review pondered a deathbed conversation with her mother, Anna. Anna was trying to reconcile *her* parents' divorce in the 1940s and the challenging economic and painful emotional impact of her father's remarriage. Due to her highly unstable childhood, Anna had based her own marriage and childrearing on traditional values and low-risk choices. Jill was able to "connect the dots" of the generational impact and the limited view of life she unconsciously inherited from her mother. Jill verbalized a desire to change her own view of life; she began a new way of seeing life as abundant and filled with possibility. Cultivating additional positive, upbeat, and energizing friends helped to improve the quality of her own life while significantly impacting the lives of her own children.

Forgiveness is a voluntary choice to release retaliation, bitterness, or unfavorable judgments toward a wrongdoer and attempt to respond with a charitable spirit. Forgiveness is not necessarily predicated on reconciliation, and it does not involve minimizing or forgetting the offense. There are at least two types of forgiveness: offense-specific (which involves a particular action) and a general inclination to forgive others (which is true across settings and is stable over time).[30] The process of forgiveness helps to promote reconciliation between self, others, and one's higher power (where applicable).[31] Forgiveness entails the release of anger, resentment, and feelings of being wronged, and entails the pardoning, forgiving, or absolving of the other from a debt, crime, or action.[32]

Forgiveness is a central and potent theme in almost every world religion.[33-35] The world religions can be categorized into three major groups: the *Abrahamic religions* (Christianity, Judaism, and Islam), the *Indic religions* (Buddhism and Hinduism), and *aboriginal beliefs* (tribal beliefs among indigenous groups).[36] The Abrahamic religions usually frame the relationship between God and human as Forgiver–forgiven and regard forgiveness as a consciously developed pattern of living. Of all the Abrahamic religions, Christianity places the strongest emphasis on an unconditional forgiveness of others. Judaism addresses forgiveness of others, yet the offender has an obligation of restitution to the offended in order to earn forgiveness. In Islamic thought, absolute forgiveness is commendable but not required. Within the Indic religions, there is an overarching theme of compassion. In Buddhism, the non-theistic notion of forgiveness is seen as the skillful means of promoting internal harmony, helping to free a person from internal regret and conflict.[33] Both Buddhism and Hinduism believe personal resentments increase suffering, both to the offender and the offended. Thus, forgiveness is a means to a higher level of mindful living for both parties.[36] Within aboriginal/tribal belief systems, life is seen as holistic, without a distinction between the sacred and the secular. A distinct emphasis is placed on restoration of all parties: victims are mended, transgressors are reinstated, and the community can then return to a healthy equilibrium.[36]

Regardless of faith background, obtaining the forgiveness of a higher power is often dependent on or mutually inclusive of the way(s) that human beings first forgive self and others while asking for forgiveness in return. Restoring a sense of personal harmony allows for the quietude of the mind, which helps to foster deeper insights. A careful assessment of the patient's spiritual/religious beliefs and practices better allows the healthcare team to plan for and provide forgiveness-oriented clinical interventions.[31,33]

Several authors[10,36,37] agree that the final stage of life is a cherished chance to express love and gratitude between self, others, and one's higher power. Opportunities to forgive self and others yield important results at end of life. Jealousies, anger, and negativity can be redirected toward more positive thoughts and attitudes; long-standing resentments and sorrows can be released. Byock[10] cautions that forgiving is not about absolving another's responsibilities, but rather provides one with a way to reframe what has been fractured, serving as the beginning steps to unfolding healing processes. The repair work that is a part of life review does not discount the pain or the responsibilities of those involved, but does give one the tools to begin coming to terms with what was painful or unpleasant.

Reclaiming an unlived life involves reflection over one's life experiences, where a multitude of regrets are possible: educational opportunities were ignored, career aspirations and goals went unrealized, healthful living practices were minimized; romances were unfulfilled, relationships were unsuccessful, and personal disappointments seemingly overshadowed any sense of accomplishment in terms of abilities, attitudes, and behaviors. Regrets place sharp boundaries around "what should have been," leaving limitless possibilities and hopes as gradually shattered dreams, never fully realized. Unresolved conflicts can be examined in a new light and through the lens of accumulated life experience that allows for and brings forward new ways of thinking as well as problem-solving. Individual and key events can be placed into the context of one's entire life course and the "value" of the whole can expand one's sense of vision.[11,38]

CASE STUDY 5: REFRAMING LIFE EXPERIENCES

Stephen was a 45-year-old man recently diagnosed with end-stage liver disease, with only months to live. Stephen was divorced twice and was unable to conceive a child during either marriage. Additional life disappointments included the end of a college football career following life-changing injuries after a motor vehicle accident. Upon sharing with the palliative APRN about his life, Stephen's affect was despondent and filled with anguish. Stephen tearfully emphasized his negative feelings toward failed marriages, incompletion of his college education, inability to conceive, and his unhealthy choices of poor diet and substance abuse. Stephen continued to weep while pensively looking through old photos. Using contemplative techniques with Stephen, the palliative APRN encouraged what was previously perceived as failure and disappointment to be reframed, repaired, and/or rebuilt because reparation is always possible. Stephen was able to identify aspects of his life that brought him joy and meaning. This new awareness brought increased peace, despite his lingering regrets about what "could have been."

VARIED ELEMENTS OF LIFE REVIEW

PAIN AND SYMPTOM MANAGEMENT

Before any work can begin in regard to life review, the patient must have adequate pain and symptom management and be in a self-reported state of comfort. Once the patient's comfort is reasonably assured, life review activities can begin. The life review process assumes a therapeutic relationship between patient and provider: all of the major therapeutic elements (see Box 37.1) are present between those engaged in review and the healthcare provider who listens, draws forth, extracts, and further develops chains of thought drawn from the patient's unconscious. The healthcare provider must be comfortable with asking open-ended questions, listening

---

Box 37.1 ELEMENTS OF A THERAPEUTIC RELATIONSHIP

Ensuring confidentiality and privacy of experiences shared, data collected

Establishing trust

Having an open attitude

Possession of a nonjudgmental spirit

Obtaining "consent" before any life review process begins

Being truthful, transparent, authentic

Maintaining boundaries and having a professional demeanor

Clarifying meaning; restating the patient's thoughts; remembering information shared

Watching for key verbal and nonverbal cues

Using open-ended questions

Being comfortable with periods of silence

Not being in a rush to complete a session or move to the next topic

Using self-disclosure and self-expression appropriately

Understanding the meaning and potential importance of being culturally sensitive/humble

Knowing about one's own spiritual and religious development/understanding

Have a genuine sense of caring and compassion for the experiences of another

Adapted from Jenko et al.,[11] and Butler.[3]

---

attentively and actively, being comfortable with periods of silence and reflection, always taking care not to interrupt the patient or to interpret or attempt the completion of another's sentences/thoughts.

Life review for the healthcare provider is grounded in cultural competence, often reconceptualized as cultural humility/awareness.[39–41] The provider is open to all ideas, viewpoints, ways of thinking, conceiving, and integrating life events. The provider remains nonjudgmental. The patient begins with free association, recall, and a personal sense of assessment. Life review has to do with a person's memory and how those memories are organized and retrieved. The patient's (and often the family's) cultural, emotional, social, and spiritual beliefs and feelings are explored and respect is duly shown throughout the entire process.

Typical topics for life review include family and friendships, loves and losses, achievements and disappointments, and adjustments made during the life trajectory. Opening questions to prompt life review can take the form of those found in Box 37.2, balancing both positive and negative aspects of life and living. If a person has difficulty remembering what occurred in the past, various prompts can be used including pictures, music, jewelry, tape-recordings, letters, or familiar personal items from the past. Memory prompting may be especially indicated with the frail elderly who may have mood or memory problems.[42]

There is no single way to initiate a "right" life review. Healthcare providers are adept at finding the perfect teachable, reachable moment in terms of the initiation of the review process (which may take minutes, hours, weekly sessions,

Box 37.2 PROMPTS FOR BEGINNING A
LIFE REVIEW

Tell me when and where you were born.

What was your life like growing up?

What was school like for you?

If you have siblings, tell me about your brothers and sisters.

Tell me about a particularly enjoyable time or place that you experienced or visited.

Tell me about an event in your life that you found to be troubling or challenging.

Tell me something that you particularly remember about your childhood.

Talk to me about some of the things you remember as your grew into your teenage years.

Tell me something unique about your family or a close relationship with someone.

Did you ever marry? If so, tell me about how you met, your courtship, and how you proposed.

Tell me something about your friends, particularly your best ones.

Describe an obstacle in your life, and tell me how you were able to get through it.

Who are the people who have most influenced your life?

What is that one "most important" event you experienced in your life?

What were the most difficult deaths that you had to deal with in your lifetime?

What do you most enjoy right now?

Do you keep in touch with any of your old friends?

How did you feel (or do you feel) about retirement?

What are your thoughts about death, dying, and the possibility of an afterlife?

Who are the people that you most admire in your life?

Describe the way that a person who knows you well would describe you.

What makes you happy now?

Tell me about your work experiences; you career; your business; your vocation.

What do you think that you will really be remembered for best?

What has been the deepest regret or disappointment in your life as a child, young adult, middle or older aged adult?

How do you think you have changed over the course of your life?

What was the hardest thing you had to face as you were growing older?

What is the absolute best thing about being older?

Note: When appropriate, many find intense satisfaction in discussing significant historical/social events including the Great Depression, World Wars, political movements, and shared experiences with a community of friends, family, soldiers, members of a congregation.

Adapted from Jenko et al.[11]; and Butler.[3]

lasting even up to an indefinite end place) and not press for discussions that are too intimate or sensitive for patient/family members. In every sense of the word, the storyteller is always the "hero" of the story; the provider is a nonjudgmental, open, caring, compassionate, active listener.

RELIGIOUS AND SPIRITUAL IMPLICATIONS

Humans are intrinsically spiritual, and spiritual beliefs affect healthcare decision-making and healthcare outcomes. According to the Hospice and Palliative Nurses Association (HPNA) *Position Statement on Spiritual Care*,[43] because human beings are intrinsically spiritual, they are in relationship with self, others, nature, and the significant or sacred. Direct clinical care entails a holistic viewpoint which addresses a cohesive and inclusive view of the patient's overall health experience.[44] APRNs embody a holistic perspective that promotes health and wellness, assists with healing, and helps to prevent or alleviate suffering[44,45]; this practice philosophy often leads the nurse "to greater awareness of the interconnectedness of self, others, nature, spirit and relationship with the global community."[45 (para 1)]

Spirituality may include specific religious beliefs, be completely divorced from same, or have some intermittent combinations depending on the patient's circumstances. Religion involves specific teachings and customs, a structured approach to life, and a certain moral code as understood in or structured according to specific authoritative/holy text(s). Religion is most commonly practiced in community with others, whereas spirituality, characterized by meditation and awareness of a universal consciousness, is more of an inner search to find one's own truth.[46] Spirituality defines those constructs that give a person strength to carry on even in the midst of life's troubles. Spirituality provides comfort, courage, and appreciation. Spirituality encompasses a person's beliefs, values, practices, and rituals and assumes certain spiritual needs: meaning, purpose, life satisfaction, forgiveness, love, and belonging.[43]

It is within the practice of nursing to address the patient's spiritual concerns: a concept of God or higher power, a source of hope and strength, significance of particular rituals or practices, and the correlation between beliefs and health.[47] Appropriate nursing interventions that help to meet the spiritual needs of patients include listening to patient/family concerns, praying with the patient upon request (when the provider feels comfortable in so doing), and reading a patient's favorite religious materials.[47] In fact, giving attention to the spiritual dimension of patient care is one of the Joint Commission (TJC) requirements as it contributes to advanced effective communication, cultural competence, and patient- and family-centered care.[23]

In facilitating life review, a patient may express themes of spiritual distress: the inability to find meaning in life[48]; an impairment in connectedness, inner peace and harmony[49]; or an inability to cope with multiple losses and cumulative grief.[50] Spiritual distress can be seen when a person's spiritual beliefs are threatened through physical and/or emotional symptoms. Spiritual distress is associated with poorer healthcare outcomes including emotional despair, depression, mood disorders, anxiety, suicidal thoughts, and increased substance abuse.[51] Spiritual care necessitates the ability of the healthcare provider to be fully present; identify their own boundaries, barriers, and limitations; listen nonjudgmentally; and appreciate one's own spirituality as a lifelong companion that informs, develops, challenges, and helps with one's personal growth. See Chapter 36 for more information about spiritual assessment.

During the process of life review, the provider seeks to recognize and respond to spiritual distress and help the patient discover deeper meaning in the experience of illness, suffering, grief, and loss.[43] However, spiritual distress can be extremely complicated and detrimental to a patient's overall comfort and satisfaction with life. Because the roots of spiritual distress can be extremely complicated, it is recommended that providers frequently consult with board-certified chaplains who are trained spiritual care specialists.[43]

Holistic nursing embodies the authentic presence of the nurse, which Cumbie[52] views as an essential component of human-to-human interaction. With this viewpoint, human beings are fundamentally good and have an inborn capacity for self-healing.[45] The APRN also recognizes and attends to multiple ways that the environment (including social, physical, financial, emotional, and spiritual aspects) impacts one's health and illness.[44] The palliative APRN strives to assist the patient to find meaning and purpose in one's life so that he or she might better find comfort, peace, and harmony.[44,45] The

palliative APRN is uniquely educated and prepared to help patients and families find relief, support, and meaning in chronic and potentially life-threatening illness, as one's sense of spirituality may be of special concern as health deteriorates. Spiritual care, provided best through an interdisciplinary team approach, entails an assessment and monitoring of the multiple aspects involved with the spiritual dimension of living, including a life review.[43]

The processes of life review address the spiritual components of a person, such as one's hopes, fears, purpose and meaning, guilt and forgiveness, faith community, inner sources of power, and beliefs about the possibilities of an afterlife.[43] Empirical patterns of knowing inform the science of nursing practice through scientific data, yet personal patterns of knowing support the nurse–patient relationship through reflections, listening, and centering. This type of knowing is gathered through autobiographical stories.[53] The construct of life review has often been compared and contrasted with several associated constructs (see Box 37.3) including remembering, storytelling, life-review, life review therapy, and dignity therapy.[42,54,55] The memory of one's life accomplishments, hopes, and goals has a large role in understanding emotional

---

Box 37.3 SELECTED DEFINITIONS RELATED TO LIFE REVIEW

Life Review:
The process of life review is much more structured than simple reminiscence. "Usually covers the entire life-span and is most often performed in a one-to-one format. Rather than simply describing past events (as in simple reminiscence), life-review focuses on the (re-) evaluation of life events and on the integration of positive and negative life events in a coherent life story."[55 (p. 541)] "Life review is the systematic and structured process of recalling past events and memories in an effort to find meaning in and achieve resolution of one's life. Although traditionally used in gerontology, life review is applicable with any person facing the end of life."[11 (p. 159)]

Remembering/Reminiscence Therapy:
A simple form of therapy that "encourages the patient to talk about earlier memories. It's generally offered to people in their later years who have mood or memory problems, or need help dealing with the difficulties that come along with aging . . . this treatment has a small but significant effect on mood, self-care, the ability to communicate and well-being."[42 (p. 1)] The use of life histories—written, oral, or both—to improve psychological well-being.[42]

Reminiscence:
"Unstructured autobiographical storytelling with the goal of communicating and teaching or informing others, remembering positive past events, and enhancing positive feelings."[55 (p. 541)] "The process of thinking or telling someone about past experiences that are personally significant . . . a therapeutic mode for promoting self-acceptance and psychological health."[55 (p. 541)]

Life Review Therapy:
Refers to the use of life review with persons with serious mental health problems, such as depression. It is characterized by linking life review to a clear theory of causal factors of depression or mental illness. . . .It often explicitly applies therapeutic techniques that have been developed in other therapeutic frameworks, such as cognitive therapy, problem-solving therapy, or narrative therapy."[55 (p. 541)]

Storytelling:
According to the National Storytelling Network,[56] storytelling is an ancient art form of human expression that uses words and actions to reveal the content of the story while encouraging the imagination of the listener. Storytelling involves five component parts: (1) interactive communication between the storyteller and the listener, (2) employing the use of words, (3) with the use of actions such as vocalization and physical motions or gestures, (4) that together present a story (narrative), (5) which encourages the imagination of the listener(s). The completed story "happens" in the mind of the listener who "co-creates" the story as seen through personal experiences, beliefs, and understandings.

Dignity Therapy:
A brief, individualized psychotherapeutic intervention designed to address psychosocial and existential distress among terminally ill patients. Such distress has often been linked to the notion of suffering and described in terms of the challenges that threaten the intactness of a person. The intervention is designed to engender a sense of meaning and purpose, thereby reducing reported suffering and distress.[57]

health and well-being, as well as emotional distress and illness.[42] For some people, life review may be painful, stressful, and possibly problematic, indicating the need for further assessment and possible therapy. For others, the process of remembering one's accomplishments, joys, and the achievements that define a life well-lived sets the stage for a peaceful death.

RESEARCH IMPLICATIONS OF LIFE REVIEW

Butler was perhaps the prime mover in the quest to discover the therapeutic effects of life review, particularly in older people.[3] In evolving reviews of gerontological literature and practice, Butler[3] concluded that life review demonstrated the following positive effects: having the time and ability to right old wrongs; reconciling with old enemies; coming to a more peaceful acceptance of one's mortality; and promotion of a sense of serenity, pride in one's accomplishments, and the feeling that one did the best one could in life. Older people who suffered from depression and who participated in life review reported better self-esteem and felt more positively about their life experiences than a similar group who did not participate in life review.[42] In addition, the group who participated in life review had a more favorable view about their past experiences and had greater levels of hope for the future. Also, caregivers who participated in the sessions gained a deeper knowledge of the patient's experiences, which helped to decrease self-reported stress.[42] Despite several limitations across studies, there was a statistically significant effect in all studies indicating that life review is an effective treatment of depressive symptoms in older adults. The effects were comparable to other well-established treatments, including antidepressive and cognitive-behavioral therapy.[58]

Dignity therapy, a variation of life review, is designed to address psychosocial and existential distress in the terminally ill. Pioneered by Max Chochinov, dignity therapy involves a brief, individualized psychotherapeutic intervention that has accumulated a considerable amount of evidence for its utility and success in patients who are facing significant end-of-life concerns.[58-60] Each "session" is designed to engender a sense of meaning and purpose and reduce the amount of suffering that a patient may be experiencing. There are seven dignity themes: generativity, continuity of self, role preservation, maintenance of pride, hopefulness, aftermath concerns, and care tenor.[60] During a session, which typically lasts between 30 and 60 minutes, the patient is asked question(s) from an interview guide based on a dignity model.[61] Sessions are taped and transcribed verbatim, edited for clarity, chronology, and possible psychological harm that may be caused to others who may read the content of any given session. The edited version becomes a "written legacy document that the person shares with others important to him or her" [62 (p. 2)] and ends with an appropriate statement of life closure (a generativity, legacy-making exercise). Several studies reported significant findings where patients reported feeling satisfied or highly satisfied with the intervention and believed that dignity therapy increased their sense of purpose, heightened their sense

of meaning, and helped increase quality of life and feelings of well-being.[58-62]

POSSIBLE "RISKS" OF LIFE REVIEW

When one engages in past remembrances, there are risks to the patient and family, as well as to the healthcare provider who actively listens and then intervenes to improve health and well-being. For the patient, there is the risk that engaging in life review might result in psychopathological outcomes where past experiences become an obsession or in which anxiety, guilt, and/or despair are magnified.[3] Excessive or obsessional "rumination" on a past event, depression, or states of panic lead to increasing rigidity rather than to increased self-awareness and flexibility.[3] Tragic outcomes occur in that rare instance where a person whose increasing (but partial) insight leads to a sense of total waste.[3] In this instance, just before death occurs, the patient concludes that he or she has never truly lived life as hoped and sees this clearly for the first time as he or she is about to die. In the most tragic of circumstances, a severely depressed patient might contemplate suicide.[3] Another group of individuals who are prone to the risks of life review are those for whom their sense of guilt is palpable and who believe that forgiveness and/or redemption are impossible for them.[3]

In particularly difficult and/or vulnerable patient care situations, the APRN may personally be subject to the harmful effects of life review. The provider may feel as if they "caused" any existential angst and/or pain and suffering brought forward. If a patient engaged in this suffering later attempts suicide (successfully or not), the provider may question their role in the situation and may bear terrible feelings of guilt. In these situations, the provider must be aware of the limits of one's professional capabilities and skillsets and be able to refer to others as the need arises. The provider must also have sufficient self-care habits and emotional/physical support systems to be able to reflect, recharge, reevaluate, renew, and resume.

Additionally, the inherent nature of palliative care can create additional risks to the practitioner. In working with the dying, love and compassion are fundamental components.[57] In palliative care, the practitioner develops the ability to "see purely," meaning that one bears witness to the full range of the suffering experienced by the patient while concurrently keeping in mind each person's inherent goodness.[63] One must truly listen to another's story, which gives "our suffering meaning, our dying depth, and our grieving perspective."[64 (p. 66)] Yet all of life is interconnected; when patients suffer, practitioners suffer. To be sustainable in the provision of palliative care, personal well-being is not "an optional indulgence but an absolute necessity."[64 (p. 93)] Practitioners should be mindful of their *literal homes* (an uncluttered physical place that provides refuge) and their *inner homes* (an uncluttered spiritual place that fosters contemplation and reflection).[64]

Viewing one's personal limits as a palliative APRN is vital; compassion fatigue, moral distress, and even burnout are indeed possible. Neglecting care of the self both hurts the self and can lead to potential harm for others.[64] Whether religious or not, several authors[65,66] stress the concept of "sabbath time." In this spiritual practice, either for an entire day or for a portion of a day, one ceases routine, daily activity and consciously takes time off to regroup, meditate, and recharge. During sabbath time, one appreciates the normal rhythms of life—joy and sorrow, death and life, full and empty, acting and waiting. Making time to acknowledge the significant or sacred and seek personal renewal and reflection is a *crucial* life lesson for the palliative APRN, one that promotes sustainability for professional growth and ongoing clinical practice.

LIFE REVIEW AND THE ELECTRONIC HEALTH RECORD

Healthcare professionals are entrusted with the most sensitive and private information in regard to their patients and have a strong ethical responsibility to protect their patients from all types of misuse, fraud, and breaches of confidentiality.[11] The information gained from a life review may involve sensitive information, thus raising the issue of patient and family agreement. The agreement to initiate a life review session is best obtained verbally (rather than implied). The following statement serves as one example to gain verbal consent (or refuse it):

> Based on what I now know, I believe it would be helpful for us to engage in a therapeutic process known as life review (either at that moment in time or scheduled for a later time). Life review looks at how past experiences influence what is happening to you at this moment. This process may involve up to an hour of your time for any given session with the possibility of multiple sessions. There is no charge for this time together; it is a part of your overall care. What we discover together may be very beneficial to your care, and a summary of our discussion may be included in your electronic medical record. Do you have any questions? [Then, after questions are answered] Would you like to engage in this process?

Indeed, the patient's permission to having each and every life review that is shared become a part of their healthcare record is recommended. The healthcare provider will explain that such updates will continue to direct future interventions, actions, team communications, and ways to secure evidence-based outcomes. Additionally, data entered in the electronic health record (EHR) can be constituted of "broad brushstrokes" (e.g., "Patient spoke at length about the estranged relationship with his incarcerated son"), instead of "nitty-gritty" details (e.g., "Patient's son serving a life sentence in the state prison for double homicide of his ex-girlfriend and his male cousin"). It is vital to remind patients and families that all data obtained are considered private and confidential and will be honored as such at all times.

There continue to be several categories that warrant higher degrees of security when it comes to entering data into the EHR.[67] The law affords special protection in regard to patients with mental illness since EHRs contain the patient's innermost personal communications and information. In addition, patients with HIV/AIDS and sexually transmitted illnesses constitute another category with special privacy concerns; sensitive information that may be shared in these areas must be handled cautiously and appropriately. Patients who are experiencing substance abuse and chemical dependency require special considerations over and above the categories previously described. Finally, release of the above-mentioned records to any outside source requires patient consent, and recipients must include a written statement prohibiting redisclosure of said information.

Life Review and COVID-19

Beginning in March 2020 Americans have been struggling with the coronavirus pandemic. In many instances, patients are dying alone in intensive care units or long-term care facilities, creating the possibility of "unfinished business" or incomplete, unexpressed, and/or unresolved relationship issues.[68] Researchers have identified that unfinished business takes multiple forms: *statements of affirmation and value* (such as a missed opportunity to express love or recognize worth), *missed opportunities or intentions* (such as unfulfilled plans and feeling a future absence), or *unresolved confessions and disclosures* (such as corrosive secrets that exist in families and lack of closure). Interventions for practice are varied; these are outlined in Box 37.4. Unfinished business is of particular importance for the palliative APRN, since Neimeyer asserts that "it is a big deal . . . it can account for the lion's share of prolonged grief symptomatology of complicated grief."[68] Practitioners can also use the 28-item Unfinished Business in Bereavement Scale, developed by Holland and colleagues,[70] with prompts such as "I should have been there when ___ died," or "I never got to resolve a breach in our relationship."

SUMMARY

Offering life review to a patient is a spiritual intervention that involves active listening; keen and subtle communication skills; the utmost in attentive behaviors; an open, nonjudgmental, and objective frame of mind; and the luxury of time in order to allow the patient the opportunity to develop their story. It is an incredible opportunity for the patient to reflect on one's life accomplishments, legacies, achievements, and the framing of one's life-course. It allows the reframing of harsh memories and the celebrations of joyous events. As Myss[71] asserts, "Healing does not always mean that the physical body recovers from an illness. Healing can also mean that one's spirit has released long-held fears and negative thoughts toward oneself or others. This kind of spiritual release and healing can occur even though one's body may be dying physically."[(p. 7)] Palliative APRNs are wise to remember this truth.

Box 37.4 GUIDELINES FOR WORKING WITH INDIVIDUALS WHO ARE BEREAVED

1. *Speak the name of the deceased*: Conversations about the loved one avoids a "second death" by falling silent about their life.

2. *Keep a journal*: Express both troubling and inspiring feelings via directive journaling.

3. *Connect with others*: Share your grief either within family or through online communities.

4. *Review photos*: Celebrate both low and high points in a life.

5. *Reconstruct the legacy*: Tell stories to keep memories alive.

6. *Review resilience*: Discover strengths and the possible growth through grief.

7. *Live in the now*: Avoid living in the past so much that the present is overshadowed.

8. *Conduct rituals*: Honor loved ones in symbolic events.[69]

From Doka et al.[68]

Recommended Resources

Classic books

Brussat F, Brussat MA. *Spiritual Literacy: Reading the Sacred in Everyday Life*. New York: Touchstone; 1996.
> A collection of meaningful examples from contemporary books, movies, and life experiences which promote a new way of looking at and "reading" the world. Helps answer the age-old question: "How can I live a spiritual life every day?" Available on Audible and in print.

Callanan M, Kelley P. Final Gifts: *Understanding the Special Awareness, Needs, and Communications of the Dying*. New York: Bantam Books; 1992.
> A classic text that describes a period of time termed "nearing death awareness." During this time, the dying tell stories and attempt communications with friends and family members that are often misunderstood. Learning what to listen for and how to approach various situations allow the reader to respond to the dying in new and authentic ways. Available on Kindle and in print.

Frankl VF. *Man's Search for Meaning*. New York Pocket Books; 1997.
> This classic book was originally published in 1946 and is now translated into more than 24 languages. It recounts psychiatrist Viktor Frankl's personal experience in Nazi concentration camps and his quest to discover meaning in the midst of horrific and sustained suffering. His subsequent theory, called logotherapy, explores how human beings cope with suffering by creating renewed meaning and purpose for life. Available on Audible, on Kindle, and in print.

Websites

Hospice Foundation of America offers a broad array of educational resources (on-demand, live, books, DVDs, and COVID-19 programming). At the time of this publication, many of the COVID-19 resources were free of charge. https://hospicefoundation.org/Education

Association of Death Education and Counselling has a multitude of on-demand continuing education works from prior conferences and webinars. At the time of this publication, many of the COVID-19 and racial injustice resources were free of charge. https://www.adec.org/

Healthy Nurse-Healthy Nation is an initiative by the American Nurses Association.
> Nurses are role models, educators, and advocates, and the well-being of nurses is fundamental to the health of our nation. Palliative care can be a rewarding yet draining profession. Learn how to stay healthy at the individual, organizational, or interpersonal level. https://www.healthynursehealthynation.org/en/about/about-the-hnhn-gc/

Contemporary YouTube Videos

The active phase of dying can last days to weeks. While some patients die gently and tranquilly, others may face inevitable battles. These two videos strive to answer the question: "What would make the final moments of life best for you?"

The Guardian (2019, November 14).

> Before I die: a day with terminally ill patients | Death Land #2 (14:16 minutes)
> https://www.youtube.com/watch?v=aZdDXNmD9wk

> Despite the advances in modern healthcare, aging and death continue to be inevitable. Although modern technologies have assisted us with extending life, it is easy to forget about living the remainder of our time with a higher quality. Dying can mean different things to different people. This video strives to answer the question: "What does being mortal mean to you?"

Frontline PBS. (2020, March 17), Being Mortal (54:02 minutes)
https://www.youtube.com/watch?v=lQhI3Jb7vMg

> This documentary is based on the best-selling book of the same name, written by surgeon Atul Gawande. His reflections include the topics of age-related frailty, serious illness, and mortality. His call to action: the medical community should focus on improving quality of life and well-being, rather than just survival.

REFERENCES

1. Butler RN. The life review: An interpretation of reminiscence in the aged. *Psychiatry*. 1963;26:65–76. doi:10.1080/00332747.1963.11023339

2. Erikson EH, Erikson JM, Kivnick HQ. *Vital Involvement in Old Age*. New York: Norton; 1986.

3. Butler RN. Successful aging and the role of life review. *J Am Geriatr Soc*. 1974;22(12):529–535. doi:10.1111/j.1532-5415.1974.tb04823.x.

4. Lewis MI, Butler RN. Life-review therapy: Putting memories to work in individual and group psychotherapy. *Geriatrics*. 1974;29(11):165–173. PMID: 4417455

5. Black G, Haight BK. Integrality as a holistic framework for the life review process. *Holist Nurs Pract*. 1992;7(1):7–15. doi:10.1097/00004650-199210000-00005

6. Wallace JB. Reconsidering the life review: The social construction of talk about the past. *Gerontologist*. 1992;32(1):120–125. doi:10.1093/geront/32.1.120

7. Burnside I, Haight BK (1992). Reminiscence and life review: Analyzing each concept. *J Adv Nurs.* 1992;17(7):855–862. 10.1111/j.1365-2648.1992.tb02008.x

8. Erikson EH. *Life History and the Historical Moment.* New York: Norton; 1975.

9. Sullivan T. Silver tsunami is coming to healthcare: Time to prepare. Healthcare IT News. March 15, 2019. Available at https://www.healthcareitnews.com/news/silver-tsunami-coming-healthcare-time-prepare

10. Byock I. *Dying Well: Peace and Possibilities at the End of Life.* New York: Berkley; 1997.

11. Jenko M, Gonzalez L, Alley P. Life review in critical care: Possibilities at end-of-life. *Crit Care Nurse.* 2010;30(1):17–28. doi:10.4037/ccn2010122

12. McAdams DP. *The Stories We Live By: Personal Myths and the Making of the Self.* New York: William Morrow; 1993.

13. Bruner J. *Acts of Meaning.* Cambridge, MA: Harvard University Press; 1990.

14. Smith MJ, Liehr P. Story theory to advance nursing practice scholarship. *Holist Nurs Pract.* 2005;19(6):272–276. doi:10.1097/00004650-200511000-00008

15. Jenko M. Life review. In: Neimeyer RA, ed. *Techniques of Grief Therapy: Creative Practices for Counseling the Bereaved.* New York: Routledge; 2012: 181–183.

16. Shapiro ER. *Grief as Family Process: A Developmental Approach to Clinical Practice.* New York: Guilford; 1994.

17. Pennebaker JW. *Opening Up: The Healing Power of Expressing Emotions.* New York: Guilford; 1997.

18. Harvey JH, Carlson HR, Huff TM, Green MA. Embracing their memory: The construction of accounts of loss and hope. In: Neimeyer RA, ed. *Meaning Reconstruction and the Experience of Loss.* Washington, DC: American Psychological Association; 2001: 231–243.

19. Scarton LJ, Boyken L, Lucerno RJ, Fitchett G, Handzo G, Emanuel L, Wilkie DJ. Effects of dignity therapy on family members: A systematic review. *J Hosp Palliat Nurs.* 2018;20(6):542–547. doi:10.1097/NJH.0000000000000469

20. Meier D. Palliative care- the "ah-ha" moment. [YouTube video]. May 29, 2008. *Available at* https://www.youtube.com/watch?v=wunepUqZ0DI&list=PL69C2E181A563759A&feature=c4-overview-vl

21. Coffee S. The nurse patient relationship in cancer care as a shared covenant. A concept analysis. *Adv Nurs Sci.* 2006; 29(4):308–323. doi:10.1097/00012272-200610000-00005

22. O'Brien ME. The nurse patient relationship: A sacred covenant. In: O'Brien ME, ed. *Spirituality in Nursing. Standing on Holy Ground.* 2nd ed. Sudbury, MA: Jones and Bartlett; 2003: 84–117. https://repository.library.georgetown.edu/handle/10822/1005125

23. The Joint Commission. *Advancing Effective Communication, Cultural Competence, and Patient and Family Centered Care: A Roadmap for Hospitals.* Oakbrook Terrace, IL: The Joint Commission; 2010. https://www.jointcommission.org/-/media/tjc/documents/resources/patient-safety-topics/health-equity/aroadmapforhospitalsfinalversion727pdf.pdf?db=web&hash=AC3AC4BED1D973713C2CA6B2E5ACD01B

24. Kaufman SR. *The Ageless Self: Sources of Meaning in Late Life.* Madison, WI: University of Wisconsin Press; 1986.

25. Goodreads. Quotes of Arthur Conan Doyle. 2014. Available at https://www.goodreads.com/author/quotes/2448.Arthur_Conan_Doyle

26. Institute for Human Caring. Illness is personal. Ira Byock Interview. February 28, 2019. Available at https://www.instituteforhumancaring.org/About-Us/Media-Library/Our-Stories.aspx

27. Schachter-Shalomi Z, Miller RS. *From Age-ing to Sage-ing.* New York: Warner Books; 1995.

28. Garland J, Garland C. *Life Review in Health and Social Care.* Philadelphia, PA: Taylor & Francis; 2001.

29. Baldwin C. *Storycatcher: Making Sense of Our Lives Through the Power and Practice of Story.* Novato, CA: New World Library; 2005.

30. Toussaint LL, Owen AD, Cheadle A. Forgive to live: Forgiveness, health, and longevity. *J Behav Med.* 2012;35(4):375–386. doi:10.1007/s10865-011-9362-4

31. Kemp C. Spiritual care interventions. In: Ferrell B, Coyle N, eds. *Textbook of Palliative Nursing.* 2nd ed. New York: Oxford University Press; 2006: 595–604.

32. Gehman HS. *The Westminster Dictionary of the Bible.* Philadelphia: Westminster Press; 1980.

33. Buck G, Lukoff D. Forgiveness III: Spiritual perspectives on forgiveness. Spiritual Competency Resource Center. Available at https://www.ministrymagazine.org/archive/2017/01/The-role-of-forgiveness-in-the-recovery-of-physical-and-mental-health1

34. Rye MS, Pargament KI, Ali MA, et al. Religious perspectives on forgiveness. In: McCullough ME, Pargament KI Thoresen CE, eds. *Forgiveness: Theory, Research, and Practice.* New York: Guilford; 2000: 17–40.

35. Lutjen LJ, Silton NR, Flannelly KJ. Religion, forgiveness, hostility and health: A structural equation analysis. *J Relig Health.* 2012;51(2):468–478. doi:10.1007/s10943-011-9511-7

36. Mullet E, Neto F. Forgiveness and religious tradition. In: Lemming DA, ed. *Encyclopedia of Psychology and Religion.* Berlin: Springer-Verlag; 2016.

37. Byock I. *The Four Things That Matter Most: A Book About Living.* New York: Free Press; 2004.

38. Keeley MP, Yingling JM. *Final Conversations: Helping the Living and the Dying Talk to Each Other.* Acton, MA: VanderWyk and Burnham; 2007.

39. Butler RN, Lewis MI. *Aging and Mental Health.* St. Louis, MO: Mosby; 1982.

40. Lauderdale J. Becoming a culturally competent nurse. Johnson & Johnson Nursing. [YouTube]. December 3, 2018. Available at https://www.youtube.com/watch?v=r62Zp99U67Y

41. Austerlic S. Cultural humility and compassionate presence at the end of life. February 2009. Markkula Center for Applied Ethics at Santa Clara. http://www.scu.edu/ethics/practicing/focusareas/medical/culturally-competent-care/chronic-to-critical-austerlic.html

42. Martinez M, Arantzamendi M, Belar A, Carrasco JM, Carvajal A, Rullán M, Centeno C. "Dignity therapy,: a promising intervention in palliative care: A comprehensive systematic literature review. *Palliat Med.* 2016;31(6):492–509. doi:10.1177/0269216316665562

43. Hospice and Palliative Nurses Association (HPNA). Position statement on spiritual care. Pittsburgh, PA: HPNA. 2021. https://advancingexpertcare.org/position-statements

44. Brown SJ. Direct clinical practice. In: Hamric AB, Spross JA, Hanson CM, eds. *Advanced Practice Nursing: An Integrative Approach.* 3rd ed. St Louis, MO: Elsevier Saunders; 2005: 143–186.

45. American Holistic Nurses Association. What is holistic nursing. 2021. https://www.ahna.org/About-Us/What-is-Holistic-Nursing

46. Shapiro E, Shapiro D. The differences between religion and spirituality. HuffPost Blog. September 20, 2011. Available at http://www.huffingtonpost.com/ed-and-deb-shapiro/religion-and-spirituality_b_967951.html

47. O'Brien ME. *Spirituality in Nursing: Standing on Holy Ground.* 6th ed. Sudbury, MA: Jones and Bartlett; 2018.

48. Burnard P. Spiritual distress and the nursing response: Theoretical considerations and counseling skills. *J Adv Nurs.* 1987;12(3):377–382. doi:10.1111/j.1365-2648.1987.tb01344.x

49. Villagomeza LR. Spiritual distress in adult cancer patients: Toward conceptual clarity. *Holist Nurs Pract.* 2005;19(6):285–294. doi:10.1097/00004650-200511000-00010

50. Boston PH, Mount BM. The caregiver's perspective on existential and spiritual distress in palliative care. *J Pain Symptom Manage.* 2006;32(1):13–26. doi:10.1016/j.jpainsymman.2006.01.009

51. Meraviglia M, Sutter R, Gaskamp CD. Evidence-based guideline: Providing spiritual care to terminally ill older adults. *J Gerontol Nurs.* 2008;34(7):8–14. doi:10.3928/00989134-20080701-0

52. Cumbie SA. The integration of mind-body-soul and the practice of humanistic nursing. *Holist Nurs Pract.* 2001;15(3):56–62. doi:10.1097/00004650-200104000-00010

53. Fawcett J, Watson J, Neuman B, Walker PH, Fitzpatrick JJ. On nursing theories and evidence. *J Nurs Scholarsh*. 2001;33(2):115–119. doi:10.1111/j.1547-5069.2001.00115.x

54. Chochinov HM. Dignity-conserving care: A new model for palliative care: Helping the patient feel valued. *JAMA*. 2002;287(17):2253–2260. doi:10.1001/jama.287.17.2253

55. Pinquart M, Forstmeier S. Effects of reminiscence interventions on psychosocial outcomes: A meta-analysis. *Aging Ment Health*. 2012;16(5):541–558. doi:0.1080/13607863.2011.651434

56. National Storytelling Network. What is storytelling? 2021. https://storynet.org/what-is-storytelling/

57. Chochinov HM, Hack T, Hassard T, Kristjanson LJ, McClement S, Harlos M. Dignity therapy: A novel psychotherapeutic intervention for patients near the end of life. *J Clin Oncol*. 2014;23(24):5520–5525. doi:10.1200/JCO.2005.08.391

58. Bohlmeijer E, Smit F, Cuijpers P. Effects of reminiscence and life review on late-life depression: A meta-analysis. *Int J Geriatr Psychiatry*. 2003;18(12):1088–1094. doi:10.1002/gps.1018

59. Chochinov HM, Hack T, McClement S, et al. Dignity in the terminally ill: A developing empirical model. *Soc Sci Med*. 2002;54(3):433–443. doi:10.1016/s0277-9536(01)00084-3

60. Chochinov HM, Hack T, Hassard T, et al. Dignity in the terminally ill: A cross-sectional cohort study. *Lancet*. 2002;360(9530):2026–2030. doi:10.1016/S0140-6736(02) 12022-8

61. Chochinov HM. Dying, dignity, and new horizons in palliative end-of-life care. *CA Cancer J Clin*. 2006;56(2):84–103. doi:10.3322/canjclin.56.2.84

62. Fitchett G, Emanuel L, Handzo G, Boyken L, Wilkie DL. Care of the human spirit and the role of dignity therapy: A systematic review of dignity therapy research. *BMC Palliat Care*. 2015;14:1–12. doi:10.1186/s12904-015-0007-1

63. Halifax J. Compassion and the true meaning of empathy. [TED Talk]. December 2010. https://www.ted.com/talks/joan_halifax#t-13992

64. Halifax J. *Being with Dying: Cultivating Compassion and Fearlessness in the Presence of Death*. Boston, MA: Shambhala; 2008.

65. Dass R. *Still Here: Embracing Aging, Changing, and Dying*. New York: Riverhead; 2000.

66. Muller W. *Sabbath: Finding Rest, Renewal, and Delight in Our Busy Lives*. New York: Bantam; 1999.

67. Barbera L, Costa T, Engel V, et al. Ensuring security of high-risk information in EHRs. *J AHIMA*. 2008;79(9):67–71.

68. Doka KJ, Neimeyer RA, McDonald L. Complicated grief in the COVID-19 era. [webinar]. Hospice Foundation of America. June 2020. https://hospicefoundation.org/Education/Complicated-Grief-in-the-COVID-19-Era

69. Pace JC, Mobley TS. Rituals at end-of-life. *Nurs Clin North Am*. 2016;51(3):471–487.

70. Holland JM, Klingspon KL, Lithtenthal WG, Neimeyer RA. The unfinished business in bereavement scale (UBBS): Development and psychometric evaluation. *Death Studies*. 2018;44(2):65–77. doi.org/10.1080/07481187.2018.1521101

71. Myss C. *Anatomy of the Spirit: The Seven Stages of Power and Healing*. New York: Crown; 1996.

38.

GRIEF AND BEREAVEMENT

Katharine Adelstein and Elizabeth Archer-Nanda

KEY POINTS

- Grief theories have evolved to reflect a much more nuanced individual experience, dispelling common myths that a specific timeframe exists for recovery from loss and that failing to confront one's feelings always leads to delayed grief.

- Complicated grief is relatively uncommon but left untreated it has serious health consequences.

- Palliative advanced practice registered nurses (APRNs) should pay attention to self-care around grief and bereavement, particularly while working closely with terminally ill individuals and families.

CASE STUDY 1: COMPLICATED GRIEF

Prior to his diagnosis of Parkinson disease, Jim and Louise experienced a strained relationship. Jim had a long history of alcohol use and episodes of emotionally and mentally demeaning behavior toward Louise, which caused them to grow apart rather than closer together during their "golden years." Despite these years of abuse, Louise maintained closeness to Jim and feared life without him. She continued to seek Jim's approval and relied heavily on him for reassurances that were more reflexive than genuine. At the onset of Jim's diagnosis, Louise continued in her usual manner with Jim, deferring to his demands, at times feeling alone and helpless, with periods of worry that she would not be able to care for herself after Jim's death.

Jim and Louise had three children together. Challenges within family dynamics led to strained relationships between Jim, Louise, and their children. Louise struggled to regain her own sense of self, even in the face of Jim's progressive medical illness and end of life. After Jim's death, Louise attempted to shift her focus toward her children. However, injured family relationships made it difficult for Louise to garner the attention and support from her children that she desired.

Although Louise anticipated it would be difficult to move through her grief, she did not foresee the inability to reconnect with her children to the level she had hoped. Although her children attempted to reach out, none could provide the level of validation and support she required. Louise felt socially isolated, empty, and filled with self-doubt. Louise struggled in the months after Jim's death; she had not predicted it would have been so hard for her children to support her in the way she needed. Louise found herself longing for Jim. She seemed to have difficulty recalling the challenging aspects of her relationship with Jim, often romanticizing him, which seemed to push her children further away. She struggled to find other aspects of meaning or purpose and was often numb. At times she believed things would be better if she were the one to have died. Louise slowly lost connection with friends and family. Louise gradually stopped maintaining her home. She developed feelings of guilt that if she had been a better wife and caregiver, Jim may not have died. Louise's symptoms are consistent with *persistent complex bereavement disorder (PCBD)*. Louise would benefit from intervention for her complicated persistent bereavement.

The palliative advanced practice registered nurse (APRN) who cared for Jim at the end of his life discussed Louise's grief with her and helped her to find a referral for a mental health provider who specialized in bereavement. Louise participated in a grief support group, sought individual therapy, and began to rebuild relationships with her children very gradually.

CASE STUDY 2: PREPARING FOR BEREAVEMENT

Ms. J was in the prime of her life at age 50 when she received her new diagnosis of multiple myeloma. A married mother of two, she and her husband were just beginning to enjoy the benefits of an empty nest. At the onset of her diagnosis, she had worked for her employer for more than two decades, enjoyed outdoor activities with her husband, and was hopeful her two adult children would someday gift her with grandchildren. Ms. J initially presented with a spontaneous fracture. She struggled to adjust to changes to her level of independence. Household chores were not up to her usual standard, and she grieved the inability to be active to her previous level of satisfaction. She was devastated that she was no longer able to care for her husband and the household to the level she had previously enjoyed.

Ms J. maintained hope throughout several lines of chemotherapy. Unfortunately, her illness did not respond; despite aggressive intervention, her cancer continued to progress. She enrolled in a clinical trial, maintaining her willingness to have done "everything possible" to "fight" her cancer. Her efforts toward the clinical trial were to ensure that no one in her family was disappointed in her for "giving up." During her treatment trajectory, she required hospitalization on several occasions for chemotherapy. Ms. J experienced difficulties with cognitive acuity during one of her hospitalizations. Treatment with ifosfamide led to an acute episode of delirium that was upsetting for both Ms. J and her family. She also experienced continued difficulty with functional decline, which was perhaps more bothersome because it was an assault on her sense of personhood and created tremendous role strain.

The palliative APRN, Marcy, met with the patient and her husband for an initial consult. In preparing for the visit, the APRN decided to utilize a dignity-conserving approach to explore the patient's and her family's perspective on illness, opportunities for enhancing support, as well as the ways the patient and family can honor their grief while maintaining hope. In assessing the patient's grief, Marcy explored with the patient aspects of loss the patient might be experiencing: physical capabilities; role strain in her roles as mother, wife, employee, daughter, and sister; and challenges to personhood. During the interview, Marcy allowed space for exploration of anticipatory loss through acknowledgment of an anticipated death and the identification of supportive care that would prepare the patient and family for a "good death" that would meet both the patient and her family's goals while reducing caregiver burden. To preserve the patient's autonomy as much as possible and address aftermath concerns and foster legacy, Marcy collaborated with the embedded psychiatric team, expressive therapists, and chaplains.

INTRODUCTION

The World Health Organization (WHO) reports that 56.9 million individuals died worldwide in 2016.[1] Each death is believed to directly affect an average of five individuals.[2] Accordingly, an estimated 284.5 million persons experienced a bereavement in 2016. The WHO views bereavement support, even counseling, for a family as an important aspect of palliative care.[3] Advanced practice registered nurses (APRNs) witness death across the life span, and palliative APRNs are uniquely positioned to encounter complications from the impact of death in their daily practice. Located at the front line of the healthcare system, palliative APRNs meet a broad range of health- and illness-related demands, including grief and bereavement assessment. Like any physical symptom in palliative care, grief and bereavement exist on a continuum and may be easy to identify and manage or may become unrelenting, making optimal relief difficult to achieve. Palliative APRNs will encounter a myriad of grief-related experiences: loss of independence and functioning, role strain or changes, disruption in relationships, and the death of an individual. To expertly manage grief and bereavement in palliative care, the APRN should (1) understand common terms, including loss, grief, and bereavement; (2) understand the application of theories related to human grief to clinical practice; (3) be able to conduct an assessment of a grieving person and distinguish normal grief from complicated bereavement; (4) know when to refer patients for psychiatric services; and (5) employ strategies for self-care.

COMMON TERMS

Common terms for death-related experiences such as grief and bereavement are sometimes used interchangeably, which can lead to confusion.[4] *Grief* is defined as "the primarily emotional/affective process of reacting to the loss of a loved one through death."[5,6] Patients may also experience grief related to losses other loved ones including illness-related losses such a loss of role, loss of independence, and loss of imagined future, as well as material and other significant losses.[7] *Mourning* is defined as "the public display of grief."[5] While the term "grief" focuses more on the personal, internal, and emotional experience of loss, mourning refers to the outward display of grief and can be influenced by personal beliefs, religion, and culture.[5] The broadest death-related term is *bereavement*, defined as "the objective situation one faces after having lost an important person via death."[5,6] Bereavement can be conceptualized as a distinct state of being after a loss (Figure 38.1).[7]

Special consideration is given to different types of grief, including anticipatory, complicated, and disenfranchised. *Anticipatory grief* refers a grief reaction that occurs before an impending loss and can be defined as "the total set of cognitive, affective, cultural, and social reactions to expected death felt by the patient and famliy."[5,8,9] The term "anticipatory grief" is most often used when referring to the families of a dying patient; however, the dying patient can experience anticipatory grief as well.[5] Anticipatory grief is associated with increased distress, pain, and medical complications in the dying patients and increased overall distress in their social networks.[5,10] Anticipatory grief and post-death grief can be regarded as two end of the same grief spectrum for family members and caregivers; thus, assessing and meeting the needs of individuals experiencing anticipatory grief can reduce the likelihood of negative outcomes at the end of life and after death.[11,12]

Complicated grief is an overarching term that refers to various patterns of abnormal grieving including inhibited or absent grief, delayed grief, chronic grief, and distorted grief.[5] Empirical evidence for inhibited, absent, or delayed

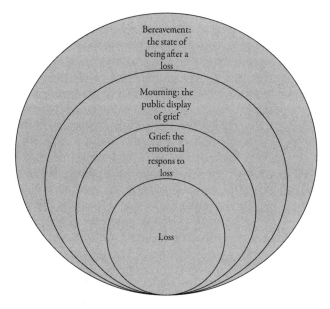

Figure 38.1 Overlay of Grief, Bereavement, Mourning, and Loss

grief reactions is inadequate, and there is significant debate among experts as to whether these patterns can be better described as forms of resilience.[13] Chronic and distorted grief patterns are often referred to as complicated grief, and these patterns of grief are defined as "a chronic, impairing form of grief brought about by interference with the healing process."[4] Complicated grief was not officially recognized in the *Diagnostic and Statistical Manual of Mental Disorders*[14] (DSM) until its most recent edition,[15] when persistent complex bereavement disorder (PCBD) was recognized as a formal diagnosis.

Disenfranchised grief is hidden and socially marginalized such as occurs with family members who died from socially undesirable causes (e.g., suicide).[7] Among worldwide deaths, 800,000 individuals die by suicide each year.[16,17] Complicated grief and depression are more likely to occur in the context of sudden or violent deaths and in those experiencing disenfranchised grief.[18]

LOSS

Further characterization of loss provides an important framework for understanding the nature of loss and its impact on the palliative care patient. One useful description of six major types of loss is found in the pastoral care literature[19] (Box 38.1).

Patients and families may experience some or all of these types of loss with advanced illness. Acknowledging the possibility that patients and families may suffer more than one type of loss related to serious or terminal illness and death can help the palliative APRN support a patient and family as they navigate a new diagnosis or worsening prognosis. Additional consideration of the categorization of loss is based on the nature of the loss: avoidable and unavoidable loss, temporary and permanent loss, actual and imagined loss, anticipated and unanticipated loss, and leaving versus being left.[19]

Box 38.1 MAJOR TYPES OF LOSS

Material loss: Loss of an item or an environment with particular attachment

Relationship loss: The end of opportunities to engage with others

Intrapsychic loss: Loss of an image of oneself or hopes for the future

Functional loss: Loss of control of bodily function

Role loss: Loss of an individual role in a social group

Systemic loss: Loss experienced by a system (e.g., family or workplace)

Adapted from Mitchell, Anderson.[19]

THEORETICAL MODELS

Human grief is a universal experience and has been observed and explored over time through many different disciplinary perspectives. The resulting theories of grief and bereavement act as a set of definitions, constructs, and assumptions that help express a systematic view of grief as a phenomenon.[20] Clinicians can use theories to guide their own understanding of the phenomena they witness in patients and their caregivers in order to provide more holistic grief and bereavement care.[20] A brief review of some of the key models of grief demonstrate that early psychological models, stage theories, and more current nuanced theoretical models contribute to an overall complex conceptual framework of grief and bereavement.

Most historic models of grief and bereavement are based in psychoanalytic theory.[21] Foundational frameworks to our current theoretical models of grief include the ethological theory of Darwin and the psychodynamic theory of Freud.[20] Freud described grief as profound sadness requiring "the work of mourning" to sever ties with a loved one. This work includes a process that eventually returns the person to a fully functional, engaged state.[22] In 1977, Bowlby[23] applied attachment theory to grief as an integrated interpretation of separation distress with his psychoanalytic understanding of child development.[20] Bowlby proposed that children and adults form attachments and that when one experiences a loss, there is constant tension between that attachment and the knowledge that the person is gone. Bowlby also introduced phases of grieving and the concept that early loss influences later loss (e.g., a person experiencing multiple losses in childhood may react more strongly to a loss in adulthood).[23]

The most widely recognized model of grief was developed by Elisabeth Kübler-Ross in 1969.[24] Through a series of interviews with terminally patients, Kübler-Ross identified five stages of grief including denial, anger, bargaining, depression, and acceptance. She conceptualized the stages of grief with task-oriented goals necessary to achieve relief from mourning.[24] Though the stages of grief are well-known and recognized by the public, there is very little empirical support for this model.[25] Major critics of Kübler-Ross's model suggest that the expectation that a bereaved person will or should go through these stages at all, much less in the prescribed order, can be harmful to those who do not.[25] Additionally, concerns regarding the conceptual clarity of the model, the lack of practical utility for development or provision of treatment, and the model's lack of guidance in identifying those at risk for complications in the grieving process have been raised.[25] In 2005, Kübler-Ross reconceptualized the stages of grief to domains of grief and loosened the model to suggest that bereaved persons can move among the domains without expectation of a predefined progression, as implied by the term "stages."[5,26] Other theories developed using an adapted "stages of grief" model have organized grief patterns into four stages including (1) numbness/disbelief, (2) separation distress (yearning, anger, anxiety), (3) depression-mourning, and (4) recovery[5,27]; and (1) shock-numbness, (2) yearning-searching, (3) disorganization-despair, and (4) reorganization.[5,28–31]

Table 38.1 MAJOR GRIEF THEORIES

THEORY	AUTHOR	DATES	MAIN POINTS
Ethological theory	Darwin	1843	Grief is a natural part of having had and lost.
Psychodynamic theory	Freud	1950s	Work is to sever ties with a loved one.
Stages of grief	Kübler-Ross	1969; 2005	Task-oriented approach to achieve relief from mourning. Reconceptualization allowed for more fluidity rather than stepwise approach.
Attachment theory	Bowlby	1977	Integrated interpretation of separation distress. Tension of attachment and loss.
Dual-process model	Stroebe and Schut	1990s	Loss-oriented and restoration-oriented coping.
Meaning reconstruction	Neimeyer	2001	Ascription of meaning to death and reconstructed relationship with the deceased.
Four-component model	Bonanno	2004	Minimization of negative emotion, focus on positive experiences to cope.

References: Neimeyer,[32] Borden & Kurtz Uveges,[33] Bonanno & Kaltman,[34] Strobe & Schut.[35]

More modern theories of grief emphasize that grief is an individual experience that involves integrating the loss while working to cope with negative emotions. Neimeyer's theory of meaning reconstruction[32] conceptualizes bereavement as an active and ongoing process of ascribing meaning to the death and reconstructing a relationship with the deceased. In this sense the process of grief becomes less about progression toward a goal and more about finding a new relationship with the deceased that fits into a consistent life narrative.[32,33] Other more recent models include Bonanno's four-component model[34] and the dual-process model outlined by Stroebe and Schut,[35] both of which describe a process in which the bereaved finds balance between negative and positive emotions and experience with regard to the loss and the ability to integrate and move forward with their grief. Bonanno emphasized minimizing the negative emotions associated with loss and focusing on positive experiences as a way to cope with loss. He also devised a framework of four components of grief that influence how an individual responds to loss: the context of the loss, the subjective meaning of the loss, changes in how one maintains a connection with the loved one over time, and the role of coping.[34] Stroebe and Schut[35] describe two processes—loss-oriented and restoration-oriented coping—that individuals use to adapt to loss. Loss-oriented coping involves the memories of the individual and features the loss itself, whereas restoration-oriented coping focuses on present life events (Table 38.1).

Theories of grief and bereavement have changed over time, moving from a model of psychopathology to a series of stages or tasks undertaken by the bereaved, to a process of loss integration and coping. The history of grief theory has taught us that grief is universal, complex, and difficult to describe. Grief theory draws from many different schools of thought, including neurobiopsychosocial science, social constructionism, and cognitive-behavioralism.[7,36] Further research is needed to continue testing these models in a variety of populations and for varying types of loss.

NORMAL OR COMMON GRIEF

While the aforementioned grief theories guide our understanding that grief is a highly individualized process, it can be useful to look at the experience of acute grief as a common one with some expected findings that may help clinicians differentiate normal grief, depression, and grief complications. Generally, normal or common grief reactions are distinguished by a steady progression toward integration of the loss and maintenance of normal daily activities, though the bereaved can be counseled that daily functioning can be difficult in the early days and weeks following a loss.[5]

About 50–85% of bereaved persons will experience normal or common grief after the loss of a loved one.[37] Common emotional reactions after the loss of a loved one include numbness, shock, and disbelief, with much of the focus of the emotional distress relating to the anxiety of separation from the loved one.[5] This can lead the bereaved to experience intense yearning, searching, preoccupation with the loved one, and sometimes intrusive images of death.[27] Bereaved persons may also experience emotions including anger, guilt, and significant periods of sadness, even despair, in the context of physical symptoms including insomnia, hypersomnia, anorexia, and fatigue.[5] Sometimes bereaved persons even feel physical pain in relation to their loss.[38] The palliative APRN can reassure patients that it also is normal to experience positive emotions such as gratitude, relief, and even joy throughout the timeline of bereavement and sometimes in conjunction with negative or distressing emotions.

A frequent occurrence in bereavement is *grief pangs*, *bursts*, or *waves*, defined has highly intense, time-limited (20 minutes to several hours) period of distress.[5,27] Very often these waves of grief occur in response to triggers or reminders of the deceased, including major holidays, the anniversary of the patient's death or birthday, or specific tasks associated with the aftermath of a death including estate planning, funeral preparations, choosing what to do with the deceased's special possessions, etc.[5] However, very often, these waves of grief may occur without warning or in the context of an unrelated activity. A modern phenomenon in grief and bereavement is the role of social media in both providing support for people going through difficult times and creating a space that can trigger grief and trauma.[39–41]

Over time most grieving people will experience symptoms less often with shorter duration or with somewhat less intensity.[5] While there is no specific time frame for integration of loss, most bereaved person will begin to experience some relief in their symptoms within 6 months to 1 year after their loss with occasional, more intense grief waves occurring indefinitely.[42–44] It is important to note, however, that actual symptom improvement may be on a different time line than the outward expression of grief, which may be influenced by social, religious, or cultural factors.[5]

PROLONGED, PERSISTENT, OR COMPLICATED GRIEF

Those experiencing loss are at risk for complications resulting from grief. Family caregivers experience the burden of caring for the dying individual and are at risk for increased emotional and physical sequelae.[45] Caregivers experiencing loss are at risk for a myriad of negative outcomes, including worsening health, weight loss, and functional impairment.[45,46] Social and emotional decline is also associated with bereavement, as is loneliness and a reduction in well-being.[47] Although most individuals will naturally start to experience a more integrated grief, allowing them to reengage in activities, including those bringing pleasure, some will go on to develop PCBD. The prevalence of PCBD is difficult to determine given that many bereft individuals do not seek help, and the specifics of the diagnosis are debated among experts; however, it is thought that approximately 1 out of every 10 bereaved adults may develop prolonged or complicated grief.[48–50]

Complicated grief differs from normal grief not in the type of symptoms experienced by the bereaved person, but in the intensity of the symptoms and the length of time that symptoms are experienced.[5] According to the DSM-5 and the *International Classification of Disease* (ICD-11), prolonged grief disorder occurs when elevated levels of grief symptoms continue after 6 months post-loss, and PCBD occurs when elevated grief symptoms continue for more than 12 months post-loss in adults and 6 months in children.[5,15]

The hallmark of complicated grief is the level of disability or impairment it causes the bereaved person. Whereas in normal or common grief some difficulty engaging in day-to-day activities can occur immediately following the death of a loved one, those experiencing complicated grief may struggle with ruminative thoughts and extreme, persistent, and pervasive sadness that essentially disables them.[51]

PCBD criteria include experiencing the death of a loved one, persistent symptoms, difficulties in functioning, or a "bereavement reaction [that] is out of proportion to or inconsistent with cultural, religious, or age-appropriate norms."[15 (p. 790)] While symptoms of PCBD can occur as early as the initial months after the death, the onset of full symptoms can appear after several years.[15] Individuals must have a specific number of symptoms, which range from perseverative thoughts of the deceased, rejection or denial of the death, preoccupation with the circumstances of the death, feeling that life is meaningless or empty, profound avoidance of situations where the loss will be felt, and wishing for death themselves to difficulty trusting or connecting with other people, self-blame and guilt, or an inability to make plans.[5,15] Level of impairment is determined by observing clinically significant difficulty in social, occupational, or other important areas of functioning.[5,15]

Risk factors for the development of PCBD include being female, having fewer years of education, preexisting or a history of depression and/or anxiety, poor physical health, and poor or maladaptive coping styles.[52] Additional risk factors include lower perceived social support, family conflict at end of life, and difficulty accepting the death.[52] Studies have shown that the risk for complicated grief is higher in individuals who have suffered the loss of a child or life partner. In such cases, the risk for depressive and anxious disorders is present for up to a decade after the death.[53,54] Individuals with comorbid mood and anxiety disorders are at increased risk to develop PCBD, with associated concern for disability, poor health, and suicidality.[55,56] Additionally, suicide loss survivors are vulnerable to feelings of shame, guilt, and stigmatization, increasing the risk for social distress and complications of grief including PCBD.[17]

Palliative APRNs must have a full understanding of the diagnostic criteria for PCBD so they can differentiate it from other potential diagnoses, including normal grief, depressive disorders, posttraumatic stress disorder (PTSD), and separation anxiety disorder. Shear[4] described a primary difference between acute grief and depression as symptoms occurring *in relation to the deceased*. For example, those with depression may express a general lack of interest in others and activities, but those with acute grief will have those symptoms *because* of the death. Additionally, the DSM-V carefully outlines the hallmarks of normal grief as compared with major depression, including the waves of sadness mixed with positive emotion seen in grief as compared to the constant sadness and negative emotion seen in major depression.[15] Additionally, in grief, self-esteem is usually preserved in the long run, while in major depression feelings of worthlessness are common.[5,15] The palliative APRN should also understand the risk for comorbid major depressive disorder, PTSD, and substance abuse disorders and should refer individuals as appropriate to mental health professionals for ongoing assessment and treatment. Individuals with a history of depression or a vulnerability to depressive disorders may benefit from treatment with an antidepressant.[15]

ASSESSMENT

Palliative APRNs are intimately involved with individuals approaching end-of-life, as well as their caregivers. In 2002, the national practice standards from the National Organization of Nurse Practitioner Faculties (NONPF) called for the expanded capability of nurses to identify grief responses as a health concern and to address these needs.[57] Palliative APRNs are well-positioned to assess patients who are experiencing bereavement and to facilitate the grief process through a grief assessment. A full understanding of the development of PCBD as well as an understanding of normal or common grief provides the foundation for accurate assessment and referral for treatment. Clinicians must also balance cultural, religious, and social considerations in their assessment of grief while evaluating and distinguishing symptoms that are common to both depression and bereavement.[57,58]

For the palliative APRN, assessment of grief begins before death occurs. Anticipatory grief in caregivers is correlated with post-death grief, and significant pre-death symptoms are seen in up to 38.5% of family caregivers.[59] Anticipation of death in family caregivers very often leads to intense emotional distress, specifically separation anxiety; however, these feelings can be fluctuating because of the role of hope and uncertainty near the end of life.[59] In the context of current death-avoidant sociocultural norms, caregivers may be reluctant to think or talk about the reality of impending death in order to sustain hope and the functional capacity to continue caring for their loved one.[59] Pro-active coping with regards to anticipatory grief, however, has been shown to improve post-death outcomes in family caregivers and should be promoted by palliative APRNs.[60-62] The Anticipatory Grief Scale is a tool that may be helpful for palliative APRN's in assessing the severity of symptoms of anticipatory grief in family caregivers.[63]

The bereavement experience is multifaceted, individual, and often occurs along with other medical illnesses, making it difficult to differentiate the symptoms of normal grief, major depression, and PCBD.[64] It is important for palliative APRNs to conceptualize bereavement care as part of their role because the consist presence and relationship-building that occurs during the pre-death period is crucial in evaluating the level of grief in family caregivers post-death.[46] Understanding the risk factors for complicated grief and follow-up care for families is important in identifying patients who may be suffering from PCBD and may need referral to mental health resources.[36] Individuals who suffer from persistent bereavement are at risk for a number of comorbidities, including cardiovascular disease, cancer, depressive disorders, anxiety disorders, post-traumatic stress, and sleep impairment.[28] Therefore follow-up care from a trusted palliative care clinician can have an immediate impact on the health of bereaved family caregivers. Additionally, safety assessments should be conducted in individuals with higher levels of bereavement and other risk factors for suicide.

Bereavement-related stressors may be comorbid with other psychiatric disorders and can trigger major depression, post-traumatic stress, or substance use disorders.[28] Bereavement with comorbid depressive and anxiety disorders is associated with negative physical and mental health outcomes,[7] making it important to fully explore differential diagnoses. Symptom overlap exists between PCBD and major depression, including feelings of sadness, decreased functional status, and suicide risk.[28] With the complex needs of those experiencing grief and bereavement, as well as the risk of medical complications

that can arise from PCBD, forming a network of resources among palliative care, primary care, and mental health providers is increasingly important.[65] Palliative APRNs should conceive of themselves as one part of a supportive team for bereaved persons.

There are several screening instruments to help identify individuals who need a higher level of bereavement services or a mental health referral. The Indicators of Bereavement Adaptation–Cruse Scotland (IBACS) measures severity of grief symptoms and risk of developing complications and has good evidence as a first-step in assessment of grief.[66] The most current version of a commonly used tool, the Inventory of Complicated Grief, now referred to as the PG-13, measures symptoms along four domains: separation, cognitive/emotional, social impairment, and duration.[67] The PG-13 also has a pre-loss version to use with patients prior to an expected death.[68] The Texas Revised Inventory of Grief is another screening tool commonly used in bereavement research.[69] There is empirical support for the use of grief screening tools, with one study suggesting that the use of a screening tool 6 months following the death of a loved one will predict two-thirds of cases of PCBD at 1 year.[70]

STRATEGIES FOR MANAGEMENT

Strategies for management by the palliative APRN include interdisciplinary death preparation, bereavement support, and, when necessary, referral to mental health services. When death is expected, the interdisciplinary team can provide support to patients and families by providing adequate and realistic information on illness progression, supporting families in their caregiving and self-help strategies, validating grief feelings, helping families to anticipate the impending loss, and helping families to reframe and reformulate roles and relationships with the dying patient.[59] Decreasing caregiver stress, use of advance directives, and focusing on the quality of a loved one's death improve the bereavement outcomes of caregivers.[71,72]

Involvement by hospice may also reduce the caregiver's risk for complications of grief, so, when possible and appropriate, palliative APRN's should facilitate the transition to hospice care at the end of life, bearing in mind the importance of follow-up care by the palliative APRN to promote continuity of care.[46,73] Hospices are required by Medicare to provide bereavement services to family members for at least 1 year after the patient dies, though these services may be highly underutilized, thus underscoring the importance of continued support and follow-up from the palliative care team even if no formal bereavement services are offered by that team.[74,75] One study identified preference of family caregivers regarding bereavement services, and they included time alone with the deceased, a quiet room to be alone after the death, sympathy cards from hospital staff, memorial services, chaplain support before/during time of death, and educational grief booklet, grief book recommendations, a check-in phone call from hospital staff, individualized counseling, and a relationship-specific support group.[76] This study also indicated the importance of follow-up screenings for the bereaved 6–12 months post-bereavement to identify those in need of formal psychosocial support.[76]

For those at low risk of complications for grief and who are assessed to be experiencing normal or common grief at the time of follow-up, there is little empirical support for the efficacy of professional intervention by medical or mental health providers.[5,77] For individuals at risk for developing complicated grief and mental health comorbidities, professional intervention may help with their maladaptive thoughts and behaviors.[5] Frequently these interventions focus on these maladaptive thoughts and behaviors and use cognitive-behavioral strategies to provide direct relief.[5] Other strategies that are often incorporated into these traditional interventions include exposure therapy, cognitive restructuring, interpretive therapy, and interpersonal therapy.[5,78–80] The format of these mental health therapies may include bereavement support groups, group therapy, individual psychotherapy, or family therapy.[5] Sometimes the decision is made to use medications to help with symptoms of complicated grief; however, this is controversial and not well-studied, though there is some evidence that antidepressant therapy can improve specific symptoms of depression that occur in the context of grief.[5,81] Drawing from theoretical models of grief, some newer models of grief therapy work to help the bereaved complete necessary tasks for integrating a new sense of meaning and purpose after loss.[82,83] Important components of these therapies include helping the bereaved to find a sense of connection and belonging in the world without their loved one, as well as ways to integrate the loss into a coherent personal narrative that has personal meaning.[82,83]

For palliative APRNs, mindfulness of individual risk factors and physical and emotional sequelae provides the foundation for helping bereaved family caregivers achieve optimal recovery after a loss.

SPECIAL CONSIDERATIONS FOR GRIEF IN CHILDREN

The vast majority of children will experience the death of someone close to them (friend or family member) at some point in their childhood, and approximately 1 in 20 children in the United States will experience the death of a parent before the age of 16.[84] Experiencing the loss of someone close to them often has profound and life-long effects on children and may result in both short- and long-term responses.[84] There are differences in the expression and experience of grief between children and adults, and attention to a child's developmental stage is crucial in providing support and guidance to a grieving child.[5] One of the key differences between grief in children and adults is that, in children, the experience and display of intense emotional and behavioral manifestations of grief may not be continuous. This is due, in part, to the fact that children are not as able as adults to fully explore their thoughts and feelings or the long-term consequences of a loss in real time.[5] While it may appear that children grieve for a shorter period of time than adults, in fact their grief usually lasts longer.[85] Grief needs to be revisited by both children and their caregivers throughout their childhood at different developmental and chronological milestones.[5,86] Expressions and explorations of grief and loss can be seen in play, artwork, schoolwork, behavior, or stories. Children may also naturally take "breaks" from their exploration of grief and appear to be immersed in usual play activities; however, this should not be taken as a sign that the child has stopped grieving.[5] Significant life events, such as important "firsts" throughout childhood, graduation from school, marrying, and experiencing the birth of their own children, may require the child to dip back into the work of grieving, though most children will eventually achieve resolution of their grief.[5] Factors including age, previous experiences with death, cause of death, relationship to the deceased, and stability of family life after the loss will all influence the experience, perception, and trajectory of grief for a child.[87]

Taking into account the child's development stage, three major questions should be addressed with children after a loss including, "Did I cause the death to happen?" "Is it going to happen to me?" and "Who is going to take care of me?"[88] In addressing these themes it is important to provide a child with an explanation of the death. Adults should not keep difficult news from children and should encourage questions, addressing them simply, honestly, and directly. Correct language should be used when discussing death with children because euphemisms (e.g., "passed away," "we lost him," "she is in a better place") can be confusing to children and lead to misinterpretations.[5,85] Using books and children's literature is often very helpful in finding ways to explain death to a child in a developmentally appropriate way and to stimulate conversation with the child about the loss.[89] For older children, social support with other children who have experienced loss can be useful in processing and understanding their own loss. Grief Camps and other group programs have been shown to build resilience in coping with loss in children.[90] Children should be included in rituals related to death and loss. As they feel comfortable, they should be invited to participate in the planning of memorial activities and attend funerals and memorial services. Preparation for what the child might experience at these events (e.g., intense emotions of their own, seeing loved ones cry, the presence of a casket) is important to make sure this is helpful and not harmful to the child.[5]

As with adults, taking time before the death to prepare the child in developmentally appropriate ways may be protective against the development of grief complications in children.[91] Offering children realistic information about their ill loved one can help begin the process of explaining and processing a death.[91] Interventions including art and music therapy with a legacy-building focus can help children process their emotions around an impending loss as well as provide them with a tangible remembrance of their loved one.[92–94]

Some children may develop grief complications, though they look different from those seen in adults. Signs of possible maladaptation to grief can include long-term changes in behavior such as "acting out," regressive or risk-taking behavior, loss of interest in engaging in previously enjoyed activities, or difficulty concentrating in school.[84] In these situations, or if a child appears to be at risk for harming themselves or others, expedient referral to mental health resources is appropriate.[84] Appropriate mental health resources for children may include pediatric psychiatry or psychology, bereavement support groups and camps for children, school-based programs and services, or other mental health professionals trained to counsel grieving children who are also experiencing depression, anxiety, or trauma symptoms.[84] It is important to remember that the goal of providing support for grieving children is not to take away the pain and sorrow that they are experiencing—though it can be tempting to try—but to help them integrate the loss and minimize the negative effects of loss on the child's developmental course.[84]

SELF-CARE

As nursing professionals, particularly in the field of palliative care, a substantial part of the work is bearing witness and tending to suffering.[95] Palliative APRNs and other healthcare providers are not immune to strong emotions, including grief after the death of a patient, and there is substantial evidence that they experience clinically significant grief reactions.[38,96–98] Unacknowledged and unprocessed grief in healthcare providers can lead to burnout, which is generally defined as a state of emotional, mental, and physical exhaustion that results from prolonged periods of stress.[99,100] In addition to burnout, healthcare providers who do not care for their own emotional well-being in the context of the stresses of their work often experience compassion fatigue (declining empathy for suffering), moral distress (a general feeling of helplessness in the context of great responsibility), and loss of personal meaning in their work, which makes them less effective at their jobs and more likely to leave the profession.[101–103] It follows, therefore, that an important part of palliative nursing is to engage in self-care around the work of caring for patients in pain and those who may be near the end of life.

There is very little formal training in nursing and medical education around self-care practices.[96,101,104] Several formal programs that focus on mindfulness, storytelling, self-reflection, and other contemplative practices to help healthcare providers process their emotions around death and dying have been shown to improve well-being, empathy, and job satisfaction while reducing anxiety and symptoms of burnout, though healthcare providers generally have to seek out those programs on their own.[104] There is also evidence to support hospital-based practices to promote processing of grief, which can be as simple as a team debrief after a death.[96,97,105] Many healthcare providers report developing their own self-awareness and self-care plans that include such notions as focusing on "living a good life," developing a sense of spirituality, maintaining a healthy lifestyle (healthy diet, exercise, adequate sleep), fostering hobbies and interests outside of the workplace, and prioritizing relationships with family.[104]

Not all deaths will evoke the same amount of grief or emotional response from the healthcare team. Palliative APRNs should pay close attention to personal, situational, and patient factors that may put them at higher risk for increased emotional response to a patient death. Examples of these factors include identification with a patient or family member, a long-standing relationship with a patient, or complicated patient–family dynamics.[38,95,98] Four ways to address complicated feelings about the loss of a patient are (1) name the feeling, (2) accept the normalcy of the feeling, (3) reflect on the emotion, and (4) consult a trusted colleague.[106] Using appropriate personal and team support systems; paying close attention to emotions, particularly in difficult cases; and seeking individual counseling when necessary may help prevent burnout in palliative APRNs.

SUMMARY

The field of palliative care and bereavement research continues to grow. A need exists for evidence-based interventions for the care of bereaved individuals. Wide-reaching educational efforts should focus on dissemination of best practices in bereavement care for clinicians in primary care, palliative care, psychiatry, and oncology. While the evolution of bereavement research continues along with the creation of evidence-based practice guidelines, palliative APRNs should evaluate the needs of each patient and make referrals to appropriate specialists, including mental health practitioners, to fully support patients struggling with the grieving process.

REFERENCES

1. World Health Organization. The top 10 causes of death. December 9, 2020. https://www.who.int/news-room/fact-sheets/detail/the-top-10-causes-of-death

2. Zisook S PR, Iglewicz A. Grief, depression, and the DSM-5. *J Psychother Pract.* 2013;19(5):386–396. doi:10.1097/01.pra.0000435037.91049.2f

3. World Health Organization. Palliative Care. Facts. August 5, 2020. https://www.who.int/news-room/fact-sheets/detail/palliative-care

4. Shear MK. Grief and mourning gone awry: Pathway and course of complicated grief. *Dialogues Clin Neurosci.* 2012;14(2):119–128. doi:10.31887/DCNS.2012.14.2/mshear

5. PDQ Supportive and Palliative Care Editorial Board. Grief, bereavement, and coping with loss (PDQ): Health professional version. In: *PDQ Cancer Information Summaries [Internet].* Bethesda, MD: National Cancer Institute; December 3, 2020. https://www.ncbi.nlm.nih.gov/books/NBK66052/

6. Stroebe M, Hansson RO, Schutt H, et al. *Handbook of Bereavement Research and Practice: Advances in Theory and Intervention.* Washington DC: American Psychological Association; 2008.

7. Lichtenthal W, Prigerson HG, Kissabe DW. Bereavement: A special issue in oncology. In: Holland JC, Breitbart WS, Jacobsen PB, Lederberg MS, Loscalzo MJ, McCorkle R, eds. *Psycho-Oncology.* 2nd ed. New York: Oxford University Press; 2010: 537–543.

8. Casarett D, Kutner JS, Abrahm, J, et al. Life after death: A practical approach to grief and bereavement. *Ann Intern Med.* 2001;134(3):208–215. doi:10.7326/0003-4819-134-3-200102060-00012

9. Knott J, Wild E. Anticipatory grief and reinvestment. In: Rando T, ed. *Loss and Anticipatory Grief.* Lexington, MA: Lexington Books; 1986: 55–60.

10. Johnson J, Lodhi MK, Cheema U, et al. Outcomes for end-of-life patients with anticipatory grieving: Insights from practice with standardized nursing terminologies within an interoperable internet-based electronic health record. *J Hosp Palliat Nurs.* 2017;19(3):223–231. doi:10.1097/NJH.0000000000000333

11. Vergo M, Whyman J, Li Z, et al. Assessing preparatory grief in advanced cancer patients as an independent predictor of distress in an American population. *J Palliat Med.* 2017;20(1):48–52. doi:10.1089/jpm.2016.0136

12. Holm M, Arestedt K, Alvariza A. Associations between predeath and postdeath grief in family caregivers in palliative home care. *J Palliat Med.* 2019;22(12):1530–1535. doi:10.1089/jpm.2019.0026

13. Bonanno G. Loss, trauma, and human resilience: Have we underestimated the human capacity to thrive after extremely aversive events? *Am Psychol.* 2004;59(1):20–28. doi:10.1037/0003-066X.59.1.20

14. American Psychiatric Association. *Diagnostic and Statistical Manual of Mental Disorders.* 4th ed. Washington DC: American Psychiatric Association; 2000.

15. American Psychiatric Association. *Diagnostic and Statistical Manual of Mental Disorders.* 5th ed. Washington DC: American Psychiatric Association; 2013.

16. Pitman A, King MB, Marston L, Osborn DPJ. The association of loneliness after sudden bereavement with risk of suicide attempt: A nationwide survey of bereaved adults. *Social Psychiatry Psychiatr Epidemiol.* 2020;55:1081–1092. doi:10.1007/s00127-020-01921-w

17. Andriessen K, Krysinska K, Hill NTM, et al. Effectiveness of interventions for people bereaved through suicide: A systematic review of controlled studies of grief, psychosocial and suicide-related outcomes. *BMC Psych.* 2019;19(1):49. Published 2019 Jan 30. doi:10.1186/s12888-019-2020-z

18. Fisher J, Zhou J, Zuleta RF, Fullerton CS, Ursano RJ, Cozza SJ. Coping strategies and considering the possibility of death in those bereaved by sudden and violent death: Grief severity, depression, and posttraumatic growth. *Front Psychiatry.* 2020;11:1–10. doi:10.3389/fpsyt.2020.00749

19. Mitchell K, Anderson H. *All Our Losses, All Our Griefs: Resources for Pastoral Care.* Louisville, KY: Westminster John Knox Press; 2010.

20. Supiano K. The role of theory in understanding grief. *Death Studies.* 2019;43(2):75–78. doi:10.1080/07481187.2018.1456678

21. Archer J. Theories of grief: Past, present, and future perspectives. In: Stroebe M, Hansson RO, Schutt H, Stroebe W, eds. *Handbook of Bereavement Research and Practice: Advanced in Theory and Intervention.* Washington DC: American Psychological Association; 2008: 45–65.

22. Freud S. Mourning and melancholia. In: Strachey J, ed. *The Standard Edition of the Complete Works of Sigmund Freud.* Vol. 14. London: Hogarth Press; 1957: 152–170.

23. Bowlby J. The making and breaking of affectional bonds. I. Aetiology and psychopathology in the light of attachment theory. An expanded version of the fiftieth Maudsley lecture, delivered before the Royal College of Psychiatrists, 19 November 1976. *Br J Psych.* 1977;130:201–210. doi:10.1192/bjp.130.3.201

24. Kubler-Ross E. *On Death and Dying.* New York: Macmillan; 1968.

25. Stroebe M, Schut H, Boerner K. Cautioning health-care professionals. *Omega (Westport).* 2017;74(4):455–473. doi:10.1177/0030222817691870

26. Kubler-Ross E, Kessler D. *On Grief and Grieving: Finding the Meaning of Grief Through the Five Stages of Loss.* New York: Scribner; 2005.

27. Jacobs S. *Pathologic Grief: Maladaptation to Loss.* Washington DC: American Psychiatric Press; 1993.

28. Parkes C, Weiss RS. *Recovery from Bereavement.* New York: Basic; 1983.

29. Bowlby J. Processes of mourning. *Int J Psychoanalysis.* 1961;42:317–338. PMID: 13872076

30. Bowlby J. *Attachment and Loss.* Vols. 1–3. New York: Basic; 1969–1980.

31. Parkes C. *Bereavement: Studies of Grief in Adult Life.* 2nd ed. Madison, WI: International Universities Press; 1987.

32. Neimeyer R. *Meaning Reconstruction & the Experience of Loss.* Washington DC: American Psychological Association; 2001.

33. Broden E, Kurtz Uveges M. Applications of grief and bereavement theory for critical care nurses. *AACN Adv Crit Care.* 2018;29(3):354–359. doi:10.4037/aacnacc2018595

34. Bonanno G, Kaltman S. Toward an integrative perspective on bereavement. *Psychol Bull.* 1999;125:760–786. doi:10.1037/0033-2909.125.6.760

35. Stroebe M, Schut H. The dual process model of coping with bereavement: Rationale and description. *Death Stud.* 1999;23:197–224. doi:10.1080/074811899201046

36. Kacel E, Gao X, Prigerson HG. Understanding bereavement: What every oncology practitioner should know. *J Support Oncol.* 2011;9(5):172–180. doi:10.1016/j.suponc.2011.04.007

37. Prigerson HG, Maciejewski PK. Rebuilding a consensus on valid criteria for disordered grief. *JAMA.* 2017;74(5):435–436. doi:10.1001/jamapsychiatry.2017.0293

38. Granek L, Ben-David M, Shapira S, Bar-Sela G, Ariad S. Grief symptoms and difficult patient loss for oncologists in response to patient death. *Psychooncology.* 2017;26(7):960–966. doi:10.1002/pon.4118

39. Bovero A, Tosi C, Botto R, Fonti I, Torta R. Death and dying on the social network: An Italian survey. *J Soc Work End-of-Life Palliat Care.* 2020;16(3):266–285. doi:10.1080/15524256.2020.1800552

40. Willis E, Ferrucci P. Mourning and grief on facebook: An examination of motivations for interacting with the deceased. *Omega.* 2017;76(2):122–138. doi:10.1177/0030222816688284

41. Egnoto MJ, Sirianni JM, Ortega CR, Stefanone M. Death on the digital landscape: A preliminary investigation into the grief process and motivations behind participation in the online memoriam. *Omega.* 2014;69(3):283–304. doi:10.2190/OM.69.3.d

42. Nuttman-Shwartz O, Shorer S, Dekel R. Long-term grief and sharing courses among military widows who remarried. *Psychol Trauma.* 2019;11(8):828–836. doi:10.1037/tra0000439

43. Näppä U, Björkman-Randström K. Experiences of participation in bereavement groups from significant others' perspectives: A qualitative study. *BMC Palliat Care.* 2020;19(1):124. doi:10.1186/s12904-020-00632-y

44. Schwartz LE, Howell KH, Jamison LE. Effect of time since loss on grief, resilience, and depression among bereaved emerging adults. *Death Stud.* 2018;42(9):537–547. doi:10.1080/07481187.2018.1430082

45. Prigerson HG, Jacobs SC. Caring for bereaved patients. *JAMA.* 2001;286(11):1369–1376. doi:10.1001/jama.286.11.1369

46. Aoun SM, Rumbold B, Howting D, Bolleter A, Breen LJ. Bereavement support for family caregivers: The gap between guidelines and practice in palliative care. *Plos One.* 2017;12(10):e0184750. doi:10.1371/journal.pone.0184750

47. Oechsle K, Ullrich A, Marx G, et al. Prevalence and predictors of distress, anxiety, depression, and quality of life in bereaved family caregivers of patients with advanced cancer. *Am J Hosp Palliat Med.* 2020;37(3):201–213. doi:10.1177/1049909119872755

48. Maciejewski PK, Maercker A, Boelen PA, Prigerson HG. "Prolonged grief disorder" and "persistent complex bereavement disorder", but not "complicated grief", are one and the same diagnostic entity: An analysis of data from the Yale bereavement study. *World Psychiatry.* 2016;15(3):266–275. doi:10.1002/wps.20348

49. Maciejewski PK, Prigerson HG. Prolonged, but not complicated, grief is a mental disorder. *Br J Psych.* 2017;211(4):189–191. doi:10.1192/bjp.bp.116.196238

50. Lundorff M, Holmgren H, Zachariae R, Farver-Vestergaard I, O'Connor M. Prevalence of prolonged grief disorder in adult bereavement: A systematic review and meta-analysis. *J Affect Disord.* 2017;212:138–149. doi:10.1016/j.jad.2017.01.030

51. Prigerson HG, Horowitz MJ, Jacobs SC, et al. Prolonged grief disorder: Psychometric validation of criteria proposed for DSM-V and ICD-11. *PLoS Med.* 2009;6(8):e1000121. doi:10.1371/journal.pmed.1000121

52. Mason TM, Tofthagen CS, Buck HG. Complicated grief: Risk factors, protective factors, and interventions. *J Soc Work*

End-of-Life Palliat Care. 2020;16(2):151–174. doi:10.1080/15524256.2020.1745726.

53. Morris S, Fletcher K, Goldstein R. The grief of parents after the death of a young child. *J Clini Psychol Med Settings.* 2019;26(3):321–338. doi:10.1007/s10880-018-9590-7

54. Eckholdt L, Watson L, O'Connor M. Prolonged grief reactions after old age spousal loss and centrality of the loss in post loss identity. *J Affect Disord.* 2018;227:338–344. doi:10.1016/j.jad.2017.11.010

55. Eisma MC, Rosner R, Comtesse H. ICD-11 prolonged grief disorder criteria: Turning challenges into opportunities with multiverse analyses. *Fron Psych.* 2020;11. doi:10.3389/fpsyt.2020.00752

56. Nakajima S. Complicated grief: Recent developments in diagnostic criteria and treatment. *Philos Trans R Soc Lond B Bio Sci.* 2018;373(1754):20170273. doi:10.1098/rstb.2017.0273

57. White P, Ferszt G. Exploration of nurse practitioner practice with clients who are grieving. *J Am Acad Nurs Practi.* 2009;21(4):231–238. doi:10.1111/j.1745-7599.2009.00398.x

58. Smid GE, Groen S, De La Rie SM, Kooper S, Boelen PA. Toward cultural assessment of grief and grief-related psychopathology. *Psych Serv.* 2018;69(10):1050–1052. doi:10.1176/appi.ps.201700422.

59. Coelho A, De Brito M, Barbosa A. Caregiver anticipatory grief. *Curr Opin Support Palliat Care.* 2018;12(1):52–57. doi:10.1097/SPC.0000000000000321

60. Rogalla KB. Anticipatory grief, proactive coping, social support, and growth: Exploring positive experiences of preparing for loss. *Omega.* 2020;81(1):107–129. doi:10.1177/0030222818761461

61. Davis EL, Deane FP, Lyons GCB, Barclay GD. Is higher acceptance associated with less anticipatory grief among patients in palliative care? *J Pain Symptom Manage.* 2017;54(1):120–125. doi:10.1016/j.jpainsymman.2017.03.012.

62. Milberg A, Liljeroos M, Krevers B. Can a single question about family members' sense of security during palliative care predict their well-being during bereavement? A longitudinal study during ongoing care and one year after the patient's death. *BMC Palliat Care.* 2019;18(1):63. Published 2019 Jul 25. doi:10.1186/s12904-019-0446-1

63. Holm M, Alvariza A, Fürst C-J, Öhlen J, Årestedt K. Psychometric evaluation of the anticipatory grief scale in a sample of family caregivers in the context of palliative care. *Health Qual Life Outcomes.* 2019;17(1):42. doi:10.1186/s12955-019-1110-4

64. Friedman MJ. Seeking the best bereavement-related diagnostic criteria. *Am J Psych.* 2016;173(9):864–865. doi:10.1176/appi.ajp.2016.16050580

65. Patel SR, Cole A, Little V, et al. Acceptability, feasibility and outcome of a screening programme for complicated grief in integrated primary and behavioural health care clinics. *Fam Prac.* 2019;36(2):125–131. doi:10.1093/fampra/cmy050

66. Newsom C, Schut H, Stroebe MS, Wilson S, Birrell J. Initial validation of a comprehensive assessment instrument for bereavement-related grief symptoms and risk of complications: The indicator of bereavement adaptation—Cruse Scotland (IBACS). *Plos One.* 2016;11(10):e0164005. Published 2016 Oct 14. doi:10.1371/journal.pone.0164005

67. Prigerson HG, Maciejewski PK, Reynolds CF, et al. Inventory of complicated grief: A scale to measure maladaptive symptoms of loss. *Psychiatry Res.* 1995;59(1–2):65–79. doi:10.1016/0165-1781(95)02757-2

68. Kiely DK, Prigerson H, Mitchell SL. Health care proxy grief symptoms before the death of nursing home residents with advanced dementia. *Am J Geriatr Psychiatry.* 2008;16(8):664–673. doi:10.1097/JGP.0b013e3181784143

69. Faschingbauer T. *Texas Revised Inventory of Grief Manual.* Houston, TX: Honeycomb; 1981.

70. Thomas K, Hudson P, Trauer T, Remedios C, Clarke D. Risk factors for developing prolonged grief during bereavement in family carers of cancer patients in palliative care: A longitudinal study. *J Pain Symptom Manage.* 2014;47(3):531–541. doi:10.1016/j.jpainsymman.2013.05.022.

71. Wilson DM, Cohen J, Eliason C, et al. Is the bereavement grief intensity of survivors linked with their perception of death quality? *Int J Palliat Nurs.* 2019;25(8):398–405. doi:10.12968/ijpn.2019.25.8.398

72. Bandini JI. Beyond the hour of death: Family experiences of grief and bereavement following an end-of-life hospitalization in the intensive care unit. [published online ahead of print, 2020 Aug 4]. *Health (London).* 2020:1363459320946647. doi:10.1177/1363459320946474

73. Silloway CJ, Glover TL, Coleman BJ, Kittelson S. Filling the void: Hospital palliative care and community hospice: A collaborative approach to providing hospital bereavement support. *J Soc Work End-of-Life Palliat Care.* 2018;14(2–3):153–161. doi:10.1080/15524256.2018.1493627

74. Ghesquiere A, Bagaajav A, Metzendorf M, Bookbinder M, Gardner DS. Hospice bereavement service delivery to family members and friends with bereavement-related mental health symptoms. *Am J Hosp Palliat Med.* 2019;36(5):370–378. doi:10.1177/1049909118812025

75. Ghesquiere A, Thomas J, Bruce ML. Utilization of hospice bereavement support by at-risk family members. *Am J Hosp Palliat Med.* 2016;33(2):124–129. doi:10.1177/1049909114555155

76. Banyasz A, Weiskittle R, Lorenz A, Goodman L, Wells-Di Gregorio S. Bereavement service preferences of surviving family members: Variation among next of kin with depression and complicated grief. *J Palliat Med.* 2017;20(10):1091–1097. doi:10.1089/jpm.2016.0235.

77. Bonanno G, Lilienfeld SO. Let's be realistic: When grief counseling is effective and when it's not. *Prof Psychol Res Pr.* 2008;39(3):377–378. doi:10.1037/0735-7028.39.3.377

78. Boelen PA, de Keijser J, van den Hout MA, van den Bout J. Treatment of complicated grief: A comparison between cognitive-behavioral therapy and supportive counseling. *J Consult Clin Psychol.* 2007;75(2):277–284. doi:10.1037/0022-006X.75.2.277

79. Rosner R, Pfoh G, Kotoučová M. Treatment of complicated grief. *Eur J Psychotraumatol.* 2011;2. doi:10.3402/ejpt.v2i0.7995

80. Rosner R, Rimane E, Vogel A, Rau J, Hagl M. Treating prolonged grief disorder with prolonged grief-specific cognitive behavioral therapy: Study protocol for a randomized controlled trial. *Trials.* 2018;19(1):241. doi:10.1186/s13063-018-2618-3

81. Shear M, Reynolds CF, Simon NM, et al. Optimizing treatment of complicated grief: A randomized clinical trial. *JAMA Psychiatry.* 2016;73(7):685–694. doi:10.1001/jamapsychiatry.2016.0892

82. Lichtenthal WG, Catarozoli C, Masterson M, et al. An open trial of meaning-centered grief therapy: Rationale and preliminary evaluation. *Palliat Support Care.* 2019;17(1):2–12. doi:10.1017/S1478951518000925

83. Harrop E, Morgan F, Longo M, et al. The impacts and effectiveness of support for people bereaved through advanced illness: A systematic review and thematic synthesis. *Palliat Med.* 2020;34(7):871–888. doi:10.1177/0269216320920533

84. Schonfeld DJ, Demaria T. Supporting the grieving child and family. *Pediatrics.* 2016;138(3):e20162147. doi:10.1542/peds.2016-2147

85. O'Toole D, Cory J. *Helping Children Grieve and Grow: A Guide for Those Who Care.* Burnsville, NC: Compassion Books; 1998.

86. Blank NM, Werner-Lin A. Growing up with grief: Revisiting the death of a parent over the life course. *Omega (Westport).* 2011;63(3):271–290. doi:10.2190/OM.63.3.e.

87. Stylianou P, Zembylas M. Dealing with the concepts of "grief" and "grieving" in the classroom: Children's perceptions, emotions, and behavior. *Omega.* 2018;77(3):240–266. doi:10.1177/0030222815626717

88. Worden J. *Children and Grief: When a Parent Dies.* New York: Guilford; 1996.

89. Arruda-Colli MNF, Weaver MS, Wiener L. Communication about dying, death, and bereavement: A systematic review of children's literature. *J Palliat Med.* 2017;20(5):548–559. doi:10.1089/jpm.2016.0494

90. Clute MA, Kobayashi R. Are children's grief camps effective? *J Soc Work End-Of-Life Palliat Care.* 2013;9(1):43–57. doi:10.1080/15524256.2013.758927

91. Jenholt Nolbris M, Enskär K, Hellström A-L. Grief related to the experience of being the sibling of a child with cancer. *Cancer Nurs.* 2014;37(5):E1–E7. doi:10.1097/NCC.0b013e3182a3e585

92. Myers-Coffman K, Baker FA, Daly BP, Palisano R, Bradt J. The resilience songwriting program for adolescent bereavement: A mixed methods exploratory study. *J Music Ther.* 2019;56(4):348–380. doi:10.1093/jmt/thz011

93. Hilliard RE. The effects of Orff-based music therapy and social work groups on childhood grief symptoms and behaviors. *J Music Ther.* 2007;44(2):123–138. doi:10.1093/jmt/44.2.123

94. Foster TL, Dietrich MS, Friedman DL, Gordon JE, Gilmer MJ. National survey of children's hospitals on legacy-making activities. *J Palliat Med.* 2012;15(5):573–578. doi:10.1089/jpm.2011.0447

95. Graetz DE. Finding grace in grief. *J Clin Oncol.* 2020;38(6):645–646. doi:10.1200/JCO.19.02123

96. Ffrench-O'Carroll R, Feeley T, Crowe S, Doherty EM. Grief reactions and coping strategies of trainee doctors working in paediatric intensive care. *Br J Anaesth.* 2019;123(1):74–80. doi:10.1016/j.bja.2019.01.034

97. Fallek R, Tattelman E, Browne T, Kaplan R, Selwyn PA. Helping healthcare providers and staff process grief through a hospital based program. *Am J Nursing.* 2019;119(7):24–33. doi:10.1097/01.NAJ.0000569332.42906.e7

98. Nathoo D, Ellis J. Theories of loss and grief experienced by the patient, family, and healthcare professional: A personal account of a critical event. *J Cancer Ed.* 2019;34(4):831–835. doi:10.1007/s13187-018-1462-1

99. Crowe S, Sullivant S, Miller-Smith L, Lantos JD. Grief and burnout in the PICU. *Pediatrics.* 2017;139(5):e20164041. doi:10.1542/peds.2016-4041

100. Harrad R, Sulla F. Factors associated with and impact of burnout in nursing and residential home care workers for the elderly. *Acta Biomed Health Profess.* 2018;89(7):60–69. doi:10.23750/abm.v89i7-S.7830

101. Rushton CH, Sellers DE, Heller KS, Spring B, Dossey BM, Halifax J. Impact of a contemplative end-of-life training program: Being with dying. *Palliat Support Care.* 2009;7(4):405–414. doi:10.1017/S1478951509990411

102. Zhang Y-Y, Han W-L, Qin W, et al. Extent of compassion satisfaction, compassion fatigue and burnout in nursing: A meta-analysis. *J Nurs Manag.* 2018;26(7):810–819. doi:10.1111/jonm.12589

103. Peters E. Compassion fatigue in nursing: A concept analysis. *Nurs Forum.* 2018;53(4):466–480. doi:10.1111/nuf.12274

104. Sanchez-Reilly S, Morrison L, Carey E, et al. Caring for oneself to care for others: Physicians and their self-care. *J Support Oncol.* 2013;11(2):75–81. doi:10.12788/j.suponc.0003

105. Nyatanga B. Challenges of loss and grief in palliative care nursing. *Br J Comm Nurs.* 2016;21(2):106–106. doi:10.12968/bjcn.2016.21.2.106

106. Meier DE, Back AL, Morrison RS. The inner life of physicians and care of the seriously ill. *JAMA* 2001;286(23):3007–3014. doi:10.1001/jama.286.23.3007

SECTION VIII

SYMPTOMS

39.

ANOREXIA AND CACHEXIA

Robert Smeltz and Renata Shabin

KEY POINTS

- Cachexia and anorexia syndrome is present in most advanced chronic and life-limiting illnesses. The palliative advanced practice registered nurse (APRN) should be vigilant in assessing for its presence.

- Assessment of cachexia and anorexia syndrome requires subjective and objective measures and must take into account the multiple dimensions of the individual.

- Treatment of cachexia and anorexia syndrome requires a multimodal approach using pharmacologic and nonpharmacologic interventions, treating both physical and psychosocial symptoms.

CASE STUDY

RV was a 58-year-old woman with recently diagnosed ovarian cancer with peritoneal carcinomatosis. She had initiated first-line chemotherapy but was hospitalized recently for nausea, weight loss, and abdominal fullness. The palliative APRN was asked to evaluate her and assist with symptom management.

A gastrointestinal (GI) examination revealed positive bowel sounds, distended abdomen, and mild abdominal tenderness. Her height was 5-foot-1 inch and weight 105 pounds, with a 10-pound weight loss. She reported intermittent nausea, denied vomiting. Nausea occurred with eating and with the look and smell of food. She reported daily small bowel movements. She endorsed early satiety. Breakfast included a half a cup of yogurt with a small amount of fruit, with effort; she was often unable to finish due to discomfort. She did not use supplemental nutritional shakes due to their sweetness. She endorsed fatigue, which limited her ability to complete activities of daily living (ADLs). She endorsed feelings of depression and sleep disturbances. She denied pain and denied shortness of breath, coughing, and anxiety.

Psychosocial history revealed that she was married with three adult children with whom she had a close relationship. She stated that cooking and baking were one of her joys, but she no longer had the energy to cook a meal and the sight and smell of food turned her stomach. She reported being raised Catholic and was an active member of her church community.

The palliative advanced practice registered nurse (APRN) engaged in a goals-of-care conversation with RV in which eating and family meals were a focus of joy and pleasure for her and her family. RV wanted to focus on treatment to allow her to eat with her family. She wanted to pursue disease-directed therapies, including chemotherapy. She stated that if things got worse, she would not want to be in pain and would not want to be resuscitated or intubated. She appointed her husband as her healthcare agent.

With this information, the palliative APRN prescribed oral metoclopramide 10 mg AC three times a day for nausea, oral ondansetron 4 mg every 8 hours as needed, and oral mirtazapine 15 mg every evening. A bowel regimen of oral senna, 2 tabs every evening at bedtime and polyethylene glycol each day was added. A referral to a nutritionist was initiated. A plan for daily physical activity was also created.

RV returned to clinic 2 weeks later. She stated that her appetite had not increased but she was able to join her family at meals with less nausea. She reported a weight gain of 1 pound and thought it was due to diet recommendations from the nutritionist. She reported making her own nutrition shakes at home. Her sleep had improved, and her bowel movements were regular.

INTRODUCTION

This chapter defines anorexia and cachexia and their interplay as a syndrome, as seen in most advanced stages of disease. The assessment of anorexia and cachexia is fundamental in establishing an effective treatment plan. A first step in treatment of cachexia and anorexia is setting goals and educating patients and families on the limits of reversing anorexia and cachexia in advanced disease. The use of a multimodal approach with pharmacologic and nonpharmacologic measures delivered by an interdisciplinary care team geared toward treating the whole person is the key strategy to addressing cachexia and anorexia syndrome.

Cachexia is defined as a multifactorial syndrome characterized by an ongoing loss of skeletal muscle mass (with or without loss of fat mass) that cannot be fully reversed by conventional nutritional support and leads to progressive functional impairment. The pathophysiology is characterized by a negative protein and energy balance driven by a variable combination of reduced food intake and abnormal metabolism.[1]

Anorexia in cancer and advanced chronic illness is a decrease in nutritional intake, often accompanied by a loss of appetite. Cachexia and anorexia are often seen together, and this is referred to as *cachexia and anorexia syndrome* (CAS). CAS is seen in cancer, heart disease, kidney failure, chronic lung diseases, and HIV/AIDS. Anorexia is seen in 40% and cachexia is seen in 51% of hospitalized patients with cancer.[2] Anorexia is seen in chronic obstructive pulmonary disease (COPD), end-stage renal disease (ESRD), AIDS, and Parkinson's disease in up to 67%, 64%, 82%, and 13% of patients, respectively.[3] Cachexia is seen in 10.5% of patients with congestive heart failure.[4] Anorexia is seen in 16–20% of elderly persons in the community.[5] Anorexia, cachexia, and dementia increase in prevalence with advancing age in older populations; however, there are little data on the prevalence of CAS in patients with dementia.[6] CAS and dehydration appear to play a role in more than one-third of deaths in dementia.[7]

CAS is a difficult symptom to treat and often becomes refractory toward the end of life.[8] Most pharmaceuticals have limits in terms of efficacy and/or side effects. Dietary counseling seems like a logical choice with no adverse effects, but it is not clear that outcomes are improved.[9] This chapter discusses the role of the palliative APRN in treating CAS. The pathophysiology of CAS, identifying underlying causes, and the importance of using a multimodal approach to treatment are outlined. A review of the psychosocial assessment and how CAS affects the patient and family is offered. Finally, strategies the palliative advanced practice registered nurse (APRN) can offer as part of education and support are described.

PALLIATIVE APRN CONSIDERATIONS

The palliative APRN plays an important role in the assessment, diagnosis, and treatment of anorexia and cachexia. This includes coordinating the patient's interdisciplinary care, advocating for the patient, supporting the patient, and educating the patient and family. The palliative APRN can identify the goals of care in terms of how they relate to addressing CAS and can help the family understand what is realistic within the limits of the disease at its current point in the disease trajectory.[10] The palliative APRN is in a unique position to support the patient and family with the psychological impact of CAS while helping to honor the patient's dignity as a person living with CAS.[11] Living with CAS can cause much distress to the patient and family, and the APRN can serve as a clinical support during this time. The palliative APRN can help the family explore pharmacologic and nonpharmacologic treatment measures and identify a regimen that takes into account the patient's goals as well as caregiver burden.

PATHOPHYSIOLOGY

CAS is produced by multiple factors, including decreased appetite, alterations in metabolism, and increased catabolism. The decrease in appetite is likely multifactorial as well, resulting from decreased drive to feed, early satiety, decreased intestinal motility, and nausea. Decreased food intake results in some of the weight loss but does not explain

all of the wasting seen in CAS.[12] There are disturbances in metabolism in CAS resulting in loss of lean body mass and body fat, unlike initial stages of starvation, where initially body fat is lost.[13]

CAS is believed to be caused, in part, by pro-inflammatory cytokines (interleukin [IL]-1, IL-2 and IL-6; interferon-γ; and tumor necrosis factor-alpha [TNF-α]) in patients with cancer. Other peptides and pathways that influence appetite and catabolism could also be affected by cancer.[13]

TNF appears to increase lipolysis and decrease synthesis of proteins. IL-6 is a pro-inflammatory cytokine, but, like TNF and the other cytokines, it is difficult to understand the specific roles in CAS since there is overlap and redundancy. It is likely that the effects of several cytokines cause CAS, and inhibiting one cytokine has little to no effect on CAS.[13]

Glucagon and other hormonal peptides and neuropeptides play a role in CAS. Specifically, glucagon administration has been shown to reduce food intake, and glucagonemia is associated with some cancers. Corticotropin-releasing factor (CRF) is seen in some cancers, and its presence decreases gastric emptying as well as food intake and appetite. There are several other neuropeptides that appear to affect feeding and weight, but their role in CAS and implications in the treatment of CAS are not known.[14]

Cancer cell metabolism may play a role in CAS. The uncontrolled metabolism and growth of cancer cells inhibit delivery of sufficient oxygen, which prevents creation of energy from the Krebs cycle; instead, the Cori cycle is used to create energy. This creates lactic acid, which needs to be processed in the liver, requiring further energy expenditure. This essentially helps to increase the resting energy expenditure.[13]

CAS is seen in several serious illnesses in addition to cancer. The process of aging likely contributes to CAS in the elderly population.[15] Gastric emptying is decreased in older patients. Senses, including smell, taste, and sight, may be altered, which may have an impact on appetite.[16] Pro-inflammatory cytokines appear to play a role in CAS older patients as well.[17] CAS in amyotrophic lateral sclerosis (ALS) and dementia is not well understood. CAS in ALS is at least partially related to increased dysphagia and decreased mobility and nutritional intake secondary to the progression of the disease.[18] CAS in dementia may also be related to alterations in metabolic homeostasis as well as cognitive and functional decline and dysphagia.[6]

CAS is also seen in advanced heart disease. Pro-inflammatory cytokines appear to be involved. Decreased circulation to the intestines can decrease motility and absorption, which can further contribute to anorexia and cachexia, respectively. There is an increase in muscle protein breakdown. Decreased insulin sensitivity could also play a role in CAS in patients with heart disease.[19]

Inflammatory responses appear to play a role in CAS in COPD. The increased work of breathing likely increases energy expenditure, contributing to CAS. Impaired oxidative capacity in COPD appears to alter protein turnover, worsening CAS further.[20]

ASSESSMENT

The goal of assessment is to identify the presence of cachexia, weight loss, and/or anorexia. It is paramount to complete early nutrition screening to identify at-risk patients. The presence of cachexia is identified with weight loss disproportionate to or without anorexia.[1] The assessment of anorexia and cachexia includes the patient's report of appetite, disturbances in taste and smell, early satiety, and nausea. There are screening tools, but most of them are not practical for daily clinical practice, like the Mini-Nutritional Assessment tool.[21]

New tools for nutrition assessment have been developed, such as the Anorexia/Cachexia Scale (A/CS-12) for use in an outpatient setting for lung cancer patients; this tool was effective at increasing the referral of at-risk patients to nutrition consultations.[22] The cancer patient's food intake should be assessed at the start of treatment and routinely during active cancer treatment.[23]

For all patients with CAS, the number of meals the patient eats per day and the size or the percentage of the meals eaten should be recorded. A variety of tools can be used. The patient can keep a food diary or use applications on computers or handheld devices for tracking food consumption, or healthcare providers can do a calorie count. Tools such as the Patient Generated Subjective Global Assessment (PG-SGA), the Nutritional Risk Screening (NRS), and the Malnutrition Screening Tool (MST) are most frequently referenced. The PG-SGA requires specially trained staff, the NRS considers patients weight loss and food intake, and the MST applies to outpatient oncology patients based on weight and appetite loss. The MST is a quick tool that consists of two questions regarding appetite and weight loss, and the PG-SGA is practical for outpatient oncology patients.[24]

Other causes of reduced food intake should be assessed. These include pain, stomatitis, constipation, dyspnea, depression and anxiety, fatigue, dry mouth, and poor dietary habits.[25] More information on the assessment and treatment of these symptoms can be found throughout this textbook.

The patient's weight should be monitored. Fluid retention should be considered when evaluating weight changes. Body mass index (BMI) is associated with the patient's weight and height. Muscle loss is associated with decreased functional status. Muscle loss, an important end point for assessing cachexia interventions, can be determined through muscle strength and muscle mass. Muscle strength can be assessed using handgrip strength (handgrip dynamometry) and upper extremity and lower extremity strength testing. Muscle mass, a component of lean body mass, is assessed through the mid-upper arm muscle area.[26,27]

Laboratory tests and imaging can be used to measure nutritional status, inflammation, and body composition. Prealbumin is one of the better measures for assessing malnutrition. A low prealbumin level indicates low protein stores, indicative of chronic anorexia. C-reactive protein (CRP) measures systemic inflammation which can be seen in cachexia[1] but cachexia can be present without an increase in C-reactive protein (CRP).[25] Cross-sectional imaging (computed tomography [CT] or magnetic resonance imaging [MRI]), dual energy x-ray imaging (DEXA), anthropometry (mid-arm muscle area), and bioimpedance analysis are tests that can measure muscle mass. One study compared these techniques but found the diagnosis of cachexia was limited.[26]

The palliative APRN must assess the patient's functional status. This can be accomplished through patient report on activities or provider assessment using the Karnofsky scale, the Palliative Performance Scale, or similar measures.[24] In addition, the psychosocial effects of anorexia and cachexia should be assessed. Lack of food intake may alter energy levels and subsequently affect mood.

CACHEXIA AND ANOREXIA MANAGEMENT

Identifying the goals of care and how they relate to management of CAS is important. The palliative APRN can initiate a goals-of-care discussion so that they can inform the patient and family of what is realistic and within the limits of the disease. The patient and family may want to treat CAS to increase body mass, weight, and functional status or to improve appetite for the sake of the pleasure of eating, or they may be simply looking for a way to help the patient. An understanding of the natural progression of disease and the pharmacologic and nonpharmacologic measures (Table 39.1) used to treat CAS will help the patient and family to clarify and meet their goals.

PHARMACOLOGIC MANAGEMENT

Megestrol acetate (MA) is a synthetic progestin used as an antineoplastic agent and to stimulate appetite.[28] MA increases weight by a small amount, but with an increase in adverse events across a variety of serious illnesses when compared to placebo; however, there is no defined optimal dose to maximize weight gain and minimize adverse events.[29] Earlier studies have shown similar results, with an increase in thromboembolic events and mortality.[30] Currently, MA is the most studied and effective pharmaceutical for increasing weight in CAS, but patients should be aware of the side effects and limits of the drug before they start taking it.[29] The typical dosage of MA is 800 mg once a day, or 625 mg with the concentrated formulation.[28] However, there is not enough evidence to support the most effective dosage of MA.[29] MA reaches peak plasma concentrations in 1–5 hours. It is metabolized by the liver and excreted by the kidneys and in the feces.[28]

The American Geriatric Society recommends avoiding MA in older adults.[31] The current evidence for MA in the elderly is mixed, showing some benefit in some and no benefit in other studies.[32] Currently, there is insufficient evidence to recommend megestrol for CAS in heart failure.[33]

Dronabinol and other cannabinoids have been used to improve appetite in CAS resulting from multiple etiologies. Dronabinol, a synthetic cannabinoid, has been approved to

Table 39.1 CACHEXIA AND ANOREXIA SYNDROME (CAS) MANAGEMENT

	INTERVENTION	IMPLEMENTATION	COMMENTS
Pharmacologic	Megestrol	800 mg PO qd	Shown to improve appetite and weight. Increased risk of blood clots and increased mortality. Patients should be aware of this potential adverse effect before implementing.
	Dronabinol	Starting dose is 2.5 mg PO bid (qd in older adult).	Treats anorexia in HIV/AIDS, treats therapy-related nausea in cancer patients
	Glucocorticoids	Starting dose: dexamethasone 4 mg PO qd	Use of this regimen is limited due to side effects. Used often to treat anorexia and cachexia near the end-of-life.
Nonpharmacologic	Dietary counseling	Refer to dietitian in complex cases. Provide instruction to reduce size of meals but increase frequency.	No evidence that this will result in sustained weight gain or improved quality of life in advanced cancer patients. Patients with COPD did benefit from nutritional counseling in terms of increased oral intake, weight gain, and increased strength.
	Oral care	Oral hygiene can prevent oral infection. Keeping the mouth moist can improve mastication and prevent infection.	Low-risk and low-cost interventions

treat anorexia related to HIV/AIDS.[34] There is no evidence to support the use of dronabinol and cannabinoids in CAS related to cancer,[35] but dronabinol is approved to treat cancer treatment–related nausea that is refractory to first-line antiemetics.[34] Research for a similar medication, nabilone, supports its effectiveness in lung cancer; however, more and larger studies are needed before it can be recommended in treating cancer-related CAS.[36] Nabilone is currently only recommended as a cancer treatment–related antiemetic when first-line therapies have failed, with no indication for use in any disease-related CAS.[37]

The starting dose for dronabinol is 2.5 mg before lunch and supper; however, 2.5 mg once daily should be considered for geriatric patients and in patients who experience side effects with more frequent daily dosing. The maximum dosage is 20 mg per day in divided doses.[34] The most common side effects involve the central nervous system and include feeling high, somnolence, and confusion. The initial half-life is 4 hours, but the terminal elimination half-life is 25–36 hours. Steady-state plasma levels are reached in 2 weeks.[34]

Glucocorticoids have shown some efficacy in improving appetite and weight gain, but no better than MA and with a worse toxicity profile.[38] The toxicity may be limited if the drug is given for short periods of time; however, the beneficial effects wear off after the steroids are stopped.[38] The efficacy of glucocorticoids on appetite could depend on patients' baseline status, showing improvement in appetite in patients with higher functional status and without drowsiness.[39]

Mirtazapine is known to produce increased appetite in 17% and weight gain in 12% of patients as a side effect.[40] Although it is has been studied, there is currently insufficient evidence to support the clinical use of mirtazapine in treating CAS related to cancer[41] or in the elderly.[32] Nonsteroidal anti-inflammatory drugs (NSAIDs) have been studied for their effectiveness in managing CAS. The drugs studied include celecoxib, ibuprofen, and indomethacin. Currently, there is insufficient evidence to recommend their use in clinical practice.[42]

Thalidomide is thought to work by anti-inflammatory mechanisms, blocking cytokines or cytokine production and thereby treating the underlying causes of cachexia. Insufficient evidence exists to support the use of thalidomide, and its use is not recommended due to toxicities in the absence of efficacy.[43]

The fatty acids, linoleic acid and icosatetraenoic acid, have been studied to determine their efficacy. It is thought they can reduce the inflammatory factors involved in CAS. Linoleic acid may increase self-report of appetite and daily caloric intake in patients with COPD associated anorexia; however, no change in weight was seen.[44] There currently is insufficient evidence to support the efficacy of eicosapentaenoic acid (EPA), an omega-3 fatty acid, but early studies show promise.[45] Further research will need to be done to determine if fatty acids are effective.

Ghrelin, a peripheral hormone that is secreted from the stomach, is being studied as a treatment for CAS. The release of ghrelin stimulates the release of growth hormone and stimulates orexigenic neurons in the hypothalamus, which is known to increase appetite. Ghrelin has been shown to increase appetite in healthy subjects.[46] Ghrelin has been shown to increase food intake, but its effect on other outcomes is unclear. Given insufficient evidence on efficacy and safety, ghrelin is not recommended for use in treating anorexia and cachexia in patients with serious illness.[47]

L-Carnitine given with celecoxib was compared with L-carnitine with celecoxib and MA. Both treatments were effective in increasing lean body mass and increasing physical daily activity. However, it was not compared to placebo, and the number of people finishing the study was fewer than 60.[48] Another study looked at five types of treatment, with more than 300 patients enrolled. The only group that showed a statistically significant increase in lean body mass was the one taking a combined medication regimen including L-carnitine, MA, EPA, and thalidomide.[49] Despite the limitations of these studies, they suggest that multiple-drug regimens should be looked at more closely, but cannot yet be recommended for clinical practice.

NONPHARMACOLOGIC MANAGEMENT

The palliative APRN is in a unique position to help patients with CAS. Aside from the emotional support provided, APRNs can assess the patient's symptom burden that could be contributing to CAS and prescribe a nonpharmacologic approach that includes engagement of an interdisciplinary team including pharmacists, dieticians, and physical therapists.[50]

Dietary counseling can play an important role in patients with anorexia and cachexia. Dietary counseling includes education on modifying familiar or favorite foods to match patients' changing tastes and needs, adding nutritional supplements, and decreasing the size and increasing the frequency of meals.[51] Standard nutrition supplements alone may not be able to reverse the effects of CAS.[52] There is some evidence to support dietary counseling in patients with COPD. With therapy mainly in the form of nutritional supplements, patients with COPD experienced increased caloric intake, increased weight, and increased grip strength.[53]

Current evidence does not clearly support increased survival, significant weight gain, or improved quality of life with dietary counseling in cancer patients; however, since the risks are low, patients and families may value this kind of support. Dietary counseling should start early with additional nutritional support alongside palliative care.[52]

Providing good oral care to reduce the risk of mucositis and oral mucosal infections can prevent some causes of decreased oral intake.[54] This includes good oral hygiene and a multimodal approach to oral care. Patients at risk (those with reduced immunity, receiving radiation therapy, or receiving chemotherapy) or with mucositis should use a mouth rinse, like bicarbonate solution or a bland mouth wash, regularly.[54] Using sucralfate-based saliva substitutes can provide needed moisture to the mouth to aid with mastication and prevent dryness. Using an antifungal or antibiotic agent in the presence of oral infection should be considered.[54]

Exercise has shown some benefit in improving symptoms related to CAS. One randomized controlled trial found that exercise tracked on an electronic tracker, ActivPal, led to increased compliance.[55] Exercise can be beneficial in a multimodal approach because it can help regulate hormones and improve strength and quality of life.[51] A recent Cochrane review found insufficient evidence demonstrating the effectiveness of exercise on cancer cachexia patients, but there is little harm in incorporating this approach.[56] More evidence is needed to make recommendations on the types and quantity of exercise that work best, but it is likely this could be tailored to the patient. It is important for patients to avoid exercise that causes pain or is too strenuous; safety is always the first consideration.

It has also been determined that patients and families may benefit from psychosocial support while living with CAS and undergoing rigorous cancer treatment. Poor body image can play a significant role in emotional well-being.[51] Assessment of quality of life and mood should be part of standard treatment; one study demonstrated that living with cachexia led to worse qualify of life scores than in non-cachectic patients.[57]

MEDICALLY ADMINISTERED NUTRITION AND HYDRATION

Decisions regarding medically administered nutrition and hydration are challenging. Enteral nutrition is utilized when the cancer patient is unable to have adequate oral intake but has a functioning gastrointestinal (GI) tract.[58] Parenteral feeding can be considered in cancer patients if the patient does not have a functioning GI tract, has active cancer treatment options, and has a prognosis of at least 3 months.[58] Parenteral feeding is often used temporarily prior to treating the gut dysfunction. If prognosis is uncertain, or there is hope of reversing an acute condition, a time-limited trial of medically administered nutrition can occur with clearly outlined treatment goals.[59]

The decision to proceed with enteral feedings and tube placement is multifactorial. Patients with advanced cancer and a poor prognosis likely will not see benefit from enteral or parenteral nutrition and are apt to have more complications.[8] The American Society of Parenteral and Enteral Nutrition (ASPEN) does not recommend medically administered nutritional support to be used for most patients undergoing chemotherapy or radiation, especially in end-stage cancer patients.[9]

In patients with advanced dementia, medically administered nutrition does not improve survival, increase mobility, reverse malnutrition, or prevent aspiration pneumonia and is therefore not recommended.[6] Medically administered enteral feeding is often used in severe dysphagia associated with stroke, when the patient's oral intake is expected to remain impaired for at least 30 days and realistic goals of care are established.[60] Also, patients with head and neck cancers who have lost the ability to swallow as a result of the disease or treatment and are experiencing malnutrition can benefit from enteral feeding through a percutaneous endoscopic gastrostomy (PEG) tube.[61] (See Chapter 56.)

MULTIMODAL APPROACH

CAS is a multifactorial syndrome with multiple components contributing to the symptoms, so it is reasonable to suspect that several modes of treatment, including nutritional, pharmacologic, nonpharmacologic, and exercise measures, will be needed to address the CAS.[56] There are no definitive studies that would allow recommendations to be made for specific treatment regimens (including an exercise program); however, available evidence suggests a trend showing that a multimodal approach could help.[55]

Identifying the patient's goals of care related to treating CAS is an initial step in using a multimodal approach. This will help tailor the interventions and will determine if using a pharmaceutical like MA is prudent. The goals will also inform the instructions provided during nutritional counseling. If patients want to maintain weight during disease-directed therapies, they should eat small meals several times a day, paying attention to the nutritional content of the food. However, if goals are geared toward comfort, instructing patients and families to focus on comfort feeding is important.[62]

PSYCHOSOCIAL SUPPORT

CAS not only affects the body but also has psychosocial implications for patients and families.[63] This is because food is the essence of life. It not only sustains life, but it also plays a central role in most cultures, traditions, and celebrations. Moreover, preparing food is one way we show love and take care of the ones we love. Therefore, food symbolizes life, love, and nurturing. The perception of patients who cannot or do not want to eat can be seen as rejecting that love. The inability to eat over time is a visible reminder of the imminence of death.

The psychosocial dimensions of anorexia and cachexia also result in social isolation. Patients may avoid social situations to avert the rituals of eating if it caused physical distress such as nausea or anxiety around eating. The patient may try to please family and friends and attempt to eat and families may pressure or contently remind the patient to eat, but this can strain relationships.[64] Family members often experience a sense of rejection, guilt, or helplessness when the patient refuses offers of food.[65]

Patients with CAS and their family members may express concern about the patient's decreased appetite, changing appearance, prognosis, and changes in social interactions.[64] Addressing these concerns is important to patients and families,[64] but healthcare professionals may not have the knowledge or training to do so.[63] APRNs specializing in palliative care need to develop expertise in addressing the physical and psychosocial sequelae of CAS.

The palliative APRN can arrange a family meeting to discuss the role of food in the patient's care. This will create an opportunity for the patient and family to discuss their views about eating food in light of the patient's condition and disease. The APRN can establish goals of care as they relate to nutritional intake. This becomes a good time to educate both the patient and family on the impact that progressive illnesses have on appetite and weight loss.

END-OF-LIFE CONSIDERATIONS

During the final days to hours of life, it is not uncommon for patients to eat and drink little to nothing. The family may make requests at this time to address the patient's poor nutritional intake or weight loss. This often includes requests for medically administered nutrition and hydration. It is likely the family is seeking a way to provide care to their loved one. Finding meaningful ways for family members to provide care introduces hope that may not have been realized.

Providing the family with education regarding the risks and limited benefits of medically administered nutrition may be helpful.[66] Some studies demonstrated increased symptoms due to increased fluid burden and no improvement in quality of life, while others stated that hydration is a human right and that it will alleviate thirst.[66] Overall, the use of medically administered nutrition is not recommended at end of life due to increased risks of adverse effects and little to no benefit.[8,67] The body increasingly becomes unable to properly process food due to an underlying inflammatory response and catabolic state. Providing medically administered nutrition is unable to reverse these processes.[8] The APRN can identify the values, preferences, and beliefs influencing these decisions in honest goals-of-care conversations.[8,59] The patients previously stated wishes regarding nutrition and hydration at end of life must be reviewed. If there is a disagreement between family wishes and previously documented goals, hospital policies may need to be referenced.[59]

When goals of care are directed toward treating symptoms and promoting comfort, it is helpful to provide foods in small portions that are easy for the patient to consume and tolerate. Easing diet restrictions and allowing diet modifications can greatly increase food enjoyment at end of life.[62] Any food provided should be the right consistency, texture, and amount.[62] Sometimes a taste is all that is needed; this is referred as to *pleasure feeding* or *eating*. Safety always needs to be considered, along with goals and comfort; patients should not be force fed or made to feel judged regarding their lack of desire to eat.[8]

It is important for families to see the hope they provide to their loved ones by their presence and commitment to care. Having some useful routines of care that family members can provide at the end of life goes a long way in comforting both the patient and the family. The family can utilize aromatherapy, massage, music therapy, and other more advanced options depending on the care site to aid in comforting and nurturing their loved one at the end of life.[68]

SUMMARY

CAS comprises a complex set of symptoms that are difficult to manage; best outcomes can be achieved with early identification and intervention. The cause of CAS can be related to treatment, but, as the end of life nears, it is almost always a manifestation of the progression of disease. Since reversal of this progression is often not possible, alleviating or slowing CAS is difficult, if not impossible. Identifying goals of care for nutrition and weight loss is important. Educating family members and primary care providers about CAS as part of the natural progression of disease is necessary. The palliative APRN can utilize screening tools early to identify nutritional deficiencies and help the patient and family identify a multidisciplinary regimen (pharmacologic and nonpharmacologic) that will maximize the patient's comfort and help slow the development of CAS.[69] Though a palliative care focus cannot eliminate CAS, the palliative APRN can help improve some of the symptoms and can align care with the patient's values to optimize quality of life.[69]

REFERENCES

1. Fearon K, Strasser F, Anker SD, et al. Definition and classification of cancer cachexia: An international consensus. *Lancet Oncol.* 2011;12(5):489–495. doi:10.1016/S1470-2045(10)70218-7

2. Vagnildhaug OM, Balstad TR, Almberg SS, et al. A cross-sectional study examining the prevalence of cachexia and areas of unmet need in patients with cancer. *Support Care Cancer.* 2018;26(6):1871–1880. doi:10.1007/s00520-017-4022-z

3. von Haehling S, Anker MS, Anker SD. Prevalence and clinical impact of cachexia in chronic illness in Europe, USA, and japan: Facts and numbers update 2016. *J Cachexia Sarcopenia Muscle.* 2016;7(5):507–509. doi:10.1002/jcsm.12167

4. Christensen HM, Kistorp C, Schou M, et al. Prevalence of cachexia in chronic heart failure and characteristics of body composition and metabolic status. *Endocrine.* 2013;43(3):626–634. doi:10.1007/s12020-012-9836-3

5. Giezenaar C, Chapman I, Luscombe-Marsh N, Feinle-Bisset C, Horowitz M, Soenen S. Ageing is associated with decreases in appetite and energy intake: A meta-analysis in healthy adults. *Nutrients.* 2016;8(1):28. doi:10.3390/nu8010028. PMID: 26751475; PMCID: PMC4728642.

6. Minaglia C, Giannotti C, Boccardi V, et al. Cachexia and advanced dementia. *J Cachexia Sarcopenia Muscle.* 2019;10(2):263–277. doi:10.1002/jcsm.12380

7. Koopmans RT, van der Sterren KJ, van der Steen JT. The "natural" endpoint of dementia: Death from cachexia or dehydration following palliative care? *Inter J Geri Psych.* 2007;22(4):350–355. doi:10.1002/gps.1680

8. Hui D, Dev R, Bruera E. The last days of life: Symptom burden and impact on nutrition and hydration in cancer patients. *Curr Opin Support Palliat Care.* 2015;9(4):346–354. doi:10.1097/SPC.0000000000000171

9. Childs DS, Jatoi A. A hunger for hunger: A review of palliative therapies for cancer-associated anorexia. *Ann Palliat Med.* 2019;8(1):50–58. doi:10.21037/apm.2018.05.08

10. Hagmann C, Cramer A, Kestenbaum A, et al. Evidence-based palliative care approaches to non-pain physical symptom management in cancer patients. *Semin Oncol Nurs.* 2018;34(3):227–240. doi:10.1016/j.soncn.2018.06.004

11. McClement S. Cancer cachexia and its impact on patient dignity: What nurses need to know. *Asia Pac J Oncol Nurs.* 2016;3(3):218–219. doi:10.4103/2347-5625.189808

12. Esposito A, Criscitiello C, Gelao L, et al. Mechanisms of anorexia-cachexia syndrome and rational for treatment with selective ghrelin receptor agonist. *Cancer Treat Rev.* 2015;41(9):793–797. doi:10.1016/j.ctrv.2015.09.002

13. Zhu R, Liu Z, Jiao R, et al. Updates on the pathogenesis of advanced lung cancer-induced cachexia. *Thorac Cancer.* 2019;10(1):8–16. doi:10.1111/1759-7714.12910

14. Patra SK, Arora S. Integrative role of neuropeptides and cytokines in cancer anorexia-cachexia syndrome. *Clin Chim Acta.* 2012;413(13–14):1025–1034. doi:10.1016/j.cca.2011.12.008

15. Laviano A, Koverech A, Seelaender M. Assessing pathophysiology of cancer anorexia. *Curr Opin Clin Nutr Metab Care.* 2017;20(5):340–345. doi:10.1097/MCO.0000000000000394

16. Jadczak AD, Visvanathan R. Anorexia of aging: An updated short review. *J Nutr Health Aging.* 2019;23(3):306–309. doi:10.1007/s12603-019-1159-0

17. Sanford AM. Anorexia of aging and its role for frailty. *Curr Opin Clin Nutr Metab Care.* 2017;20(1):54–60. doi:10.1097/MCO.0000000000000336

18. Korner S, Hendricks M, Kollewe K, et al. Weight loss, dysphagia and supplement intake in patients with amyotrophic lateral sclerosis (ALS): Impact on quality of life and therapeutic options. *BioMed Central Neurol.* 2013;13(84):1–9. http://www.biomedcentral.com/1471-2377/13/84. doi:10.1186/1471-2377-13-84

19. Saitoh M, Ishida J, Doehner W, et al. Sarcopenia, cachexia, and muscle performance in heart failure: Review update 2016. *Int J Cardiol.* 2017;238:5–11. doi:10.1016/j.ijcard.2017.03.155

20. Ceelen JJ, Langen RC, Schols AM. Systemic inflammation in chronic obstructive pulmonary disease and lung cancer: Common driver of pulmonary cachexia? *Curr Opin Support Palliat Care.* 2014;8(4):339–345. doi:10.1097/SPC.0000000000000088

21. Miller J, Wells L, Nwulu U, Currow D, Johnson MJ, Skipworth RJE. Validated screening tools for the assessment of cachexia, sarcopenia, and malnutrition: A systematic review. *Am J Clin Nutr.* 2018;108(6):1196–1208. doi:10.1093/ajcn/nqy244

22. Berry DL, Blonquist T, Nayak M, et al. Cancer anorexia and cachexia. *Clin J Oncol Nurs.* 2017;22(1):63–68. doi:10.1188/18.CJON.63-68

23. Hendifar AE, Petzel MQB, Zimmers TA, et al. Pancreas cancer-associated weight loss. *Oncologist.* 2019;24(5):691–701. doi:10.1634/theoncologist.2018-0266

24. Castillo-Martinez L, Castro-Eguiluz D, Copca-Mendoza ET, et al. Nutritional assessment tools for the identification of malnutrition and nutritional risk associated with cancer treatment. *Rev Invest Clin.* 2018;70(3):121–125. doi:10.24875/RIC.18002524

25. Arends J, Baracos V, Bertz H, et al. ESPEN expert group recommendations for action against cancer-related malnutrition. *Clinical Nutrition.* 2017;36(5):1187–1196. doi:10.1016/j.clnu.2017.06.017

26. Blauwhoff-Buskermolen S, Langius JAE, Becker A, Verheul HMW, de van der Schueren MAE. The influence of different muscle mass measurements on the diagnosis of cancer cachexia. *J Cachexia Sarcopenia Muscle.* 2017;8(4):615–622. doi:10.1002/jcsm.12200

27. Crawford J. What are the criteria for response to cachexia treatment? *Ann Palliat Med.* 2019;8(1):43–49. doi:10.21037/apm.2018.12.08

28. StatREf. *Gastrointestinal. Antiemetics.* Megestrol Acetate. In: Snow E, ed. AHFS Drug Information. Bethesda, MD: American Society of Health-System Pharmacists; 2021;68:32. http://online.statref.com/document/67KgWosfBzI0s2HFIzAUAj!!

29. Ruiz-Garcia V, Lopez-Briz E, Carbonell-Sanchis R, Bort-Marti S, Gonzalvez-Perales JL. Megestrol acetate for cachexia-anorexia syndrome. A systematic review. *J Cachexia Sarcopenia Muscle.* 2018;9(3):444–452. doi:10.1002/jcsm.12292

30. Ruiz Garcia V, Lopez-Briz E, Carbonell Sanchis R, Gonzalvez Perales JL, Bort-Marti S. Megestrol acetate for treatment of anorexia-cachexia syndrome. *Cochrane Database Sys Rev.* 2013;3:CD004310. doi:10.1002/14651858.CD004310.pub3

31. American Geriatrics Society Beers Criteria Update Expert Panel. American Geriatrics Society 2019 updated AGS Beers criteria(r) for potentially inappropriate medication use in older adults. *J Am Geriatr Soc.* 2019;67(4):674–694. doi:10.1111/jgs.15767

32. Fox C, Treadway AK, Blaszczyk AT, Sleeper R. Megestrol acetate and mirtazapine for treatment of weight loss. *Pharmacotherapy.* 2009 Apr;29(4):383–397. doi:10.1592/phco.29.4.383

33. Kalantar-Zadeh K, Anker SD, Horwich TB, Fonarow GC. Nutritional and anti-inflammatory interventions in chronic heart failure. *Am J Cardiol.* 2008;101(11A):89E–103E. doi:10.1016/j.amjcard.2008.03.007

34. StatREf. *Hormones and Synthetic Substitutes.* Dronabinol. In: Snow E, ed. AHFS Drug Information. Bethesda, MD: American Society of Health-System Pharmacists; 2021. 56:22.92. http://online.statref.com/document/o-RIoPCARPzi6gwmQK_gmt!!

35. Cannabis in Cachexia Study Group, Strasser F, Luftner D, et al. Comparison of orally administered cannabis extract and delta-9-tetrahydrocannabinol in treating patients with cancer-related anorexia-cachexia syndrome: A multicenter, Phase III, randomized,

double-blind, placebo-controlled clinical trial from the cannabis-in-cachexia-study-group. *J Clin Oncol.* 2006;24(21):3394–3400. doi:10.1200/JCO.2005.05.1847

36. Turcott JG, Del Rocio Guillen Nunez M, Flores-Estrada D, et al. The effect of nabilone on appetite, nutritional status, and quality of life in lung cancer patients: A randomized, double-blind clinical trial. *Support Care Cancer.* 2018;26(9):3029–3038. doi:10.1007/s00520-018-4154-9

37. StatREf. *Gastrointestinal. Antiemetics.* Nabilone. In: Snow E, ed. AHFS Drug Information. Bethesda, MD: American Society of Health-System Pharmacists; 2021. 56:22.92. http://online.statref.com/document/yRM6KDBFkQIURBR-3hO_0j!!

38. Loprinzi CL, Kugler JW, Sloan JA, et al. Randomized comparison of megestrol acetate versus dexamethasone versus fluoxymesterone for the treatment of cancer anorexia/cachexia. *J Clin Oncol.* 1999;17(10):3299–3306. doi:10.1200/JCO.1999.17.10.3299

39. Matsuo N, Morita T, Matsuda Y, et al. Predictors of responses to corticosteroids for anorexia in advanced cancer patients: A multicenter prospective observational study. *Support Care Cancer.* 2017;25(1):41–50. doi:10.1007/s00520-016-3383-z

40. Remeron (mirtazapine) tablets, for oral use. Whitehouse Station, NJ: Merck & Co.; Revised June 2021. https://www.merck.com/product/USA/pi_circulars/r/remeron/remeron_tablets_pi.pdf

41. Economos G, Lovell N, Johnston A, Higginson IJ. What is the evidence for mirtazapine in treating cancer-related symptomatology? A systematic review. *Support Care Cancer.* 2020;28(4):1597–1606. doi:10.1007/s00520-019-05229-7

42. Reid J, Hughes CM, Murray LJ, Parsons C, Cantwell MM. Non-steroidal anti-inflammatory drugs for the treatment of cancer cachexia: A systematic review. *Palliat Med.* 2013;27(4):295–303. doi:10.1177/0269216312441382

43. Reid J, Mills M, Cantwell M, Cardwell CR, Murray LJ, Donnelly M. Thalidomide for managing cancer cachexia. *Cochrane Database Syst Rev.* 2012;4:CD008664. doi:10.1002/14651858.CD008664.pub2

44. Ghobadi H, Matin S, Nemati A, Naghizadeh-Baghi A. The effect of conjugated linoleic acid supplementation on the nutritional status of COPD patients. *Int J Chron Obstruct Pulmon Dis.* 2016;11:2711–2720. doi:10.2147/COPD.S111629

45. Dewey A, Baughan C, Dean T, Higgins B, Johnson I. Eicosapentaenoic acid (EPA, an omega-3 fatty acid from fish oils) for the treatment of cancer cachexia. *Cochrane Database Syst Rev.* 2007(1):CD004597. doi:10.1002/14651858.CD004597.pub2

46. Ashby D, Choi P, Bloom S. Gut hormones and the treatment of disease cachexia. *Proc Nutr Soc.* 2008;67(3):263–269. doi:10.1017/S0029665108007143

47. Khatib MN, Shankar AH, Kirubakaran R, et al. Ghrelin for the management of cachexia associated with cancer. *Cochrane Database Syst Rev.* 2018;2:CD012229. doi:10.1002/14651858.CD012229.pub2

48. Madeddu C, Dessi M, Panzone F, et al. Randomized phase III clinical trial of a combined treatment with carnitine + celecoxib + megestrol acetate for patients with cancer-related anorexia/cachexia syndrome. *Clin Nutr.* 2012;31(2):176–182. doi:10.1016/j.clnu.2011.10.005

49. Mantovani G, Maccio A, Madeddu C, et al. Randomized phase III clinical trial of five different arms of treatment in 332 patients with cancer cachexia. *Oncologist.* 2010;15(2):200–211. doi:10.1634/theoncologist.2009-0153

50. Bruggeman AR, Kamal AH, LeBlanc TW, Ma JD, Baracos VE, Roeland EJ. Cancer cachexia: Beyond weight loss. *J Oncol Pract.* 2016;12(11):1163–1171. doi:10.1200/JOP.2016.016832

51. Del Fabbro E. Combination therapy in cachexia. *Ann Palliat Med.* 2019;8(1):59–66. doi:10.21037/apm.2018.08.05

52. Laviano A, Di Lazzaro Giraldi G, Koverech A. Does nutrition support have a role in managing cancer cachexia? *Curr Opin Support Palliat Care.* 2016;10(4):288–292. doi:10.1097/SPC.0000000000000242

53. Collins PF, Stratton RJ, Elia M. Nutritional support in chronic obstructive pulmonary disease: A systematic review and meta-analysis. *Am J Clin Nutr.* 2012;95(6):1385–1395. doi:10.3945/ajcn.111.023499

54. Hong CHL, Gueiros LA, Fulton JS, et al. Systematic review of basic oral care for the management of oral mucositis in cancer patients and clinical practice guidelines. *Support Care Cancer.* 2019;27(10):3949–3967. doi:10.1007/s00520-019-04848-4

55. Solheim TS, Laird BJA, Balstad TR, et al. A randomized phase II feasibility trial of a multimodal intervention for the management of cachexia in lung and pancreatic cancer. *J Cachexia Sarcopenia Muscle.* 2017;8(5):778–788. doi:10.1002/jcsm.12201

56. Grande AJ, Silva V, Maddocks M. Exercise for cancer cachexia in adults: Executive summary of a Cochrane collaboration systematic review. *J Cachexia Sarcopenia Muscle.* 2015;6(3):208–211. doi:10.1002/jcsm.12055

57. Schwarz S, Prokopchuk O, Esefeld K, et al. The clinical picture of cachexia: A mosaic of different parameters (experience of 503 patients). *BMC Cancer.* 2017;17(1):130. doi:10.1186/s12885-017-3116-9

58. Cotogni P. Enteral versus parenteral nutrition in cancer patients: Evidences and controversies. *Ann Palliat Med.* 2016;5(1):42–49. doi:10.3978/j.issn.2224-5820.2016.01.05

59. Hospice and Palliative Nurses Association. *HPNA Position Statement: Medically Administered Nutrition and Hydration.* Pittsburgh, PA: Hospice and Palliative Nurses Association; 2020. https://advancingexpertcare.org/position-statements.

60. Galovic M, Stauber AJ, Leisi N, et al. Development and validation of a prognostic model of swallowing recovery and enteral tube feeding after ischemic stroke. *JAMA Neurol.* 2019;76(5):561–570. doi:10.1001/jamaneurol.2018.4858

61. Lang K, Elshafie RA, Akbaba S, et al. Percutaneous endoscopic gastrostomy tube placement in patients with head and neck cancer treated with radiotherapy. *Cancer Manage Res.* 2020;12:127–136. doi:10.2147/CMAR.S218432

62. Orrevall Y. Nutritional support at the end of life. *Nutrition.* 2015;31(4):615–616. doi:10.1016/j.nut.2014.12.004

63. Amano K, Baracos VE, Hopkinson JB. Integration of palliative, supportive, and nutritional care to alleviate eating-related distress among advanced cancer patients with cachexia and their family members. *Crit Rev Oncol Hematol.* 2019;143:117–123. doi:10.1016/j.critrevonc.2019.08.006

64. Hopkinson JB. Food connections: A qualitative exploratory study of weight- and eating-related distress in families affected by advanced cancer. *Eur J Oncol Nurs.* 2016;20:87–96. doi:10.1016/j.ejon.2015.06.002

65. Reid J, McKenna H, Fitzsimons D, McCance T. Fighting over food: Patient and family understanding of cancer cachexia. *Oncol Nurs Forum.* 2009;36(4):439–445. doi:10.1188/09.ONF.439-445

66. Lembeck ME, Pameijer CR, Westcott AM. The role of intravenous fluids and enteral or parenteral nutrition in patients with life-limiting illness. *Med Clin North Am.* 2016;100(5):1131–1141. doi:10.1016/j.mcna.2016.04.019

67. Blinderman CD, Billings JA. Comfort care for patients dying in the hospital. *N Engl J Med.* 2015;373(26):2549–2561. doi:10.1056/NEJMra1411746

68. Coelho A, Parola V, Cardoso D, Bravo ME, Apostolo J. Use of non-pharmacological interventions for comforting patients in palliative care: A scoping review. *JBI Database System Rev Implement Rep.* 2017;15(7):1867–1904. doi:10.11124/JBISRIR-2016-003204

69. Day T. Managing the nutritional needs of palliative care patients. *Br J Nursing.* 2017;26(21):1151–1159. doi:10.12968/bjon.2017.26.21.1151

40.

BOWEL SYMPTOMS

Kimberly Chow and Lauren Koranteng

KEY POINTS

- Constipation, diarrhea, and malignant bowel obstruction are highly prevalent and distressful symptoms in advanced illness.

- The palliative advanced practice registered nurse (APRN) plays a vital role in assessing, treating, educating, and supporting patients and families with a high symptom burden from bowel dysfunction throughout the disease trajectory.

- Bowel symptoms do not occur in isolation from other symptoms, and proper management requires a global understanding of the patient's experience.

CASE STUDY: CONSTIPATION

AJ was a 40-year-old woman diagnosed with myelodysplastic syndrome 3 years prior. She declined initial curative treatment with standard hypomethylating agent and allogeneic stem cell transplantation. She had a past medical history significant for anal warts, for which she underwent a rectal dilatation with a post-procedure course complicated by pyoderma gangrenosum.

AJ maintained close follow-up with her oncologist for more than 2 years, requiring red blood cell transfusions approximately twice per month. When her disease progressed to acute myeloid leukemia (AML), she agreed to stem cell transplantation. Unfortunately, she relapsed 3 months later, which was indicative of an overall poor prognosis. Despite multiple lines of disease-directed therapies, her AML continued to progress with extensive bone marrow involvement causing severe hip pain. A palliative advanced practice registered nurse (APRN) was consulted to assist with pain management and psychosocial support.

Upon initial consultation, AJ reported not only bone pain, but severe rectal pain with bowel movements that was even more distressing. She expressed frustration that her care providers and family did not focus as much on these symptoms despite her struggles to use the bathroom every morning. The palliative APRN sensitively performed a comprehensive assessment of her bowel history, beginning with the diagnosis of pyoderma gangrenosum and her worsening symptoms over the course of AML therapy. AJ's bowel patterns fluctuated between diarrhea and constipation. Most recently, she reported sensations of incomplete stool evacuation that required at least three consecutive trips to the bathroom to feel fully relieved. By the third attempt, her pain would escalate to 8 out of 10

on the numeric rating scale due to repeated irritation. AJ took only a stool softener out of fear that laxatives would result in diarrhea, which exacerbated rectal inflammation. She became tearful, expressing awareness of her limited life expectancy and inability to participate in anything that she enjoyed due to pain and bowel anxiety. She was unwilling to take opioids due to risk of exacerbating her constipation. In addition to her post-transplant medications, AJ was taking prednisone for the past year for possible graft-versus-host-disease. Her physical exam was significant for erythema and superficial skin tears around the anus. Digital rectal exam was not performed due to pancytopenia and her immunocompromised state. Her abdominal examination was unremarkable.

The palliative APRN worked with AJ to develop a detailed plan of care that addressed both her bowel patterns and pain. A low-dose stimulant laxative was added to the stool softener with a plan to gradually titrate to achieve the goal of more efficient bowel movements in fewer attempts. In collaboration with the transplant team, her steroids were tapered to allow for better tissue healing. AJ's bowels started to normalize within a few days, and she was willing to initiate opioids for pain relief. Unfortunately, she developed opioid-induced constipation despite ongoing titration of laxatives. She was unwilling to add stronger osmotic laxatives due to past experiences with severe diarrhea but was amenable to a trial of low-dose naloxegol that specifically targeted opioid-induced constipation. With this bowel regimen, AJ's bowels and pain remained well controlled as she considered her limited options for further disease-directed therapies. She requested that her palliative APRN participate in ongoing goals-of-care discussions involving her family and primary oncology team because she felt that management of her symptoms in order to actively and comfortably participate in her life was her main priority.

INTRODUCTION

This chapter discusses three common bowel symptoms that are highly prevalent and distressful for palliative care patients: constipation, diarrhea, and obstruction. These symptoms rarely occur in isolation from other clinical manifestations of disease and can affect a person's quality of life and eligibility for treatment; they may even be life-threatening. The palliative advanced practice registered nurse (APRN) must approach care with a global understanding of the patient's individual needs, primary illness, disease-related complications, and past and current treatments. Assessment and management are always provided with respect for the patient's culture, privacy, and goals of care.

CONSTIPATION

Constipation remains a largely subjective symptom that is often quantified by individuals based on what they perceive to be their normal bowel function.[1] Four suggested domains for clinical diagnosis are (1) life-long history of constipation using the Rome Criteria; (2) clinical changes causing or exacerbating constipation; (3) subjective symptoms, including bloating or incomplete defecation; and (4) objective changes, such as frequency and consistency of stools.[2] Constipation is a highly distressing symptom for patients, families, and providers and can lead to a multitude of physical signs and symptoms, including anorexia, nausea, vomiting, abdominal pain, distention, and obstruction.[3–5] In addition to the physical distress, patients also feel the psychological and social effects such as irritability, loss of independence, embarrassment, and social isolation from not wanting to be far from a bathroom.[4]

The American Gastroenterology Association defines constipation as "difficult or infrequent passage of stool, at times associated with straining or a feeling of incomplete defecation."[6] The identification and management of constipation in palliative care have historically been complicated by the lack of a universal definition as well as by disparities between patient and provider opinions on the extent and frequency of the symptom.[5,7]

INCIDENCE

Constipation is one of the most frequently encountered and bothersome symptoms in patients with serious chronic illness.[8] Approximately one-third of older adults experience some degree of constipation.[4] Specific to the palliative care population, estimated prevalence across recent studies remains highly variable and ranges from 7% to 90%.[1,8] Constipation is one of the most common nonmotor symptoms that occur in patients with Parkinson's disease and can affect between 50% and 80% of the population.[9] For those on opioid therapy, an estimated 72–87% of patients will report constipation at some point during treatment.[8] Despite its high prevalence in acute and chronic illness, constipation often remains underrecognized, underreported, and undertreated by providers at every level, with the consequence of unnecessary distress, anxiety, and even hospital admissions.[2,10,11]

PATHOPHYSIOLOGY

Potential causes of constipation may be related to structure, disease, or personal factors and are grouped into primary or secondary causes.[12] Primary (e.g., idiopathic or functional) constipation occurs without an identifiable underlying cause.[13] Gastrointestinal motility is often intact, with reports of difficulty evacuating, hard stools, or dysfunction of the

---

***Box 40.1* SECONDARY CAUSES OF CONSTIPATION**

Medications (e.g., opioids, anticholinergics)
Personal factors (e.g., time, privacy, diet, activity, fluid intake)
Endocrine/Metabolic disorders (e.g., diabetes, hypercalcemia, hypothyroidism)
Cancer-related (e.g., tumor obstruction, spinal cord compression, electrolyte imbalances, cerebral tumors)
Neurologic disease (e.g., cerebrovascular disease, Parkinson's disease)
Psychologic disorders (e.g., anxiety, depression, somatization)

From Farmer et al.[12]; Hagman et al.[16]; Huang[17]; Kittelson et al.[18]; Prichard, Bharucha[19]; and Young.[20]

---

pelvic floor muscles or anal sphincter.[5,12–14] Opioid induced constipation (OIC) is mostly associated with delayed colonic transit due to the binding of opioid agonists to mu-opioid receptors located in the enteric nervous system.[10,15]

Secondary causes of constipation (Box 40.1) are the result of medications, personal factors, or disorders that may be structural, metabolic, or neurologic in nature. In advanced illness, constipation is often multifactorial from decreased activity, anorexia, polypharmacy, older age, side effects of disease and treatment, and psychological effects of disease.[12,16–20] Current recommendations support treating the multiple contributing factors rather than single risk factors, and the palliative APRN should be aware of the common etiologies.

ASSESSMENT

A subjective assessment requires a thorough history of current and past bowel patterns. The palliative APRN should document stool volume, frequency, and appearance, along with the presence of accompanying symptoms, such as flatus, nausea, vomiting, and anorexia.[1,3]

The palliative APRN may want to consider the elements of the *Constipation Assessment Scale* (CAS), a quick, reliable, and validated tool commonly used in palliative care.[8] It assesses for eight symptoms that measure the severity of constipation: (1) abdominal distention or bloating, (2) change in amount of gas passed rectally, (3) less frequent bowel movements, (4) oozing liquid stool, (5) rectal fullness or pressure, (6) rectal pain with bowel movements, (7) smaller stool size, and (8) urge, but inability to pass stool.[21,22] Medication reconciliation can help the APRN to identify common medications (Table 40.1) that may contribute to constipation.[22,23]

It is important to note that several studies emphasize the disconnect between provider assessment and the patient and family experience with constipation.[4,7,11] One exploratory, qualitative study on the experience of constipation assessment and management by palliative care specialists revealed a heavy focus on physical assessment with very little attention paid to the psychological and social impacts of impaired bowel patterns.[4] Patients and families expressed frustration that the

Table 40.1 DRUGS/DRUG CLASSES ASSOCIATED WITH CONSTIPATION

DRUGS/DRUG CLASS	EXAMPLES
Antacids	Calcium carbonate
Anticonvulsants	
Antidepressants	Amitriptyline, doxepin
Antihistamines	Diphenhydramine
Antiparkinsonian agents	Benztropine, bromocriptine
Barium sulfate	
Calcium channel antagonists	Verapamil
Cholestyramine	
Clonidine	
Diuretics	Furosemide, hydrochlorothiazide
Nonsteroidal anti-inflammatory agents	Ibuprofen, naproxen
Opioids	Morphine, hydromorphone
Serotonin receptor antagonists	Ondansetron, granisetron
Phenothiazines	Promethazine
Polystyrene sodium sulfonate	
Vinca alkaloids	Vincristine

From Mooney et al.[22]; Richter.[23]

primary approach was often focused on reactive medication management, rather than lifestyle factors, nonpharmacologic options, and preventive measures. Subjective assessments must include the anxiety, fear, embarrassment, caregiver distress, and social isolation often associated with constipation. Patients and families should be asked about the lifestyle and dietary changes they have implemented and their personal preferences and goals for symptom management to ensure a unified team approach to care. In fact, a growing body of literature is supporting the use of patient reported outcomes (PROs) to incorporate the patient's and family's voice into the regular assessment of palliative care symptoms.[4,24]

When conducting a physical exam, the palliative APRN should always be mindful of privacy and cultural sensitivity. Such an assessment may need to be done with another person present for a sense of safety and comfort. Assessment includes looking for oral lesions and thrush, which can affect diet and nutrition. The abdomen should be assessed for bowel sounds, distention, tenderness, and organomegaly. Fecal masses may be palpable on rectal exam. Box 40.2 lists the differential diagnoses to consider when patients present with constipation. Unless the patient is immunocompromised, rectal exams help rule out fecal impaction, impaired sphincter tone, anal fissures, tumor, and/or hemorrhoids.[14,22,25]

Box 40.2 DIFFERENTIAL DIAGNOSIS OF CONSTIPATION

Psychologic disorders (e.g., anxiety, depression)
Irritable bowel syndrome
Colonic obstruction (e.g., malignant, nonmalignant)
Surgical adhesions
Electrolyte Imbalance
Ileus
Spinal cord compression

From Sharma, Rao[14]; Mooney et al.[22]; Prichard, Bharucha.[25]

Further workup of constipation should be dictated by life expectancy and may include complete blood count, comprehensive metabolic panel, thyroid levels, and abdominal radiograph.[22,23] For palliative care patients, extensive imaging and bloodwork may be costly and provide little benefit.[26] Results may lead to unintentional findings that can complicate the clinical picture and delay care transitions. Thus, any workup should match the patient's goals of care.

MANAGEMENT

PHARMACOLOGIC MANAGEMENT

Optimal pharmacologic management of constipation involves a combination of effective and appropriate prophylactic and treatment doses. Table 40.2 offers prophylactic options to consider.[27,28] Because there is a lack of rigorous data to strongly support the use of one laxative over another, the choice of agents should be influenced by factors such as cost, patient preference, availability, and side effects.[28]

Developing an individualized bowel regimen requires careful thought and monitoring by the palliative APRN as

Table 40.2 OPTIONS FOR PROPHYLACTIC MANAGEMENT OF CONSTIPATION

Start with a basic regimen based on the patient status and preference and titrate to effect.

Patients on opioid therapy should be on constipation prophylaxis unless contraindicated.

Option 1	Senna 17.2 mg at bedtime or 17.2 mg oral (PO) twice daily if taking opioids. Consider stool softener (Docusate 100 mg PO twice daily) if indicated
Option 2	Polyethylene glycol 17g PO once daily
Option 3	Lactulose 30 mL PO once or twice daily
Option 4	Bisacodyl 1 tablet PO once daily

From National Comprehensive Cancer Network[27]; Candy et al.[28]

even the most benign-appearing laxatives carry risks if not prescribed properly. For example, caution should be taken with over-the-counter laxatives, suppositories, and enemas as they may be contraindicated or duplicates of an already prescribed regimen.[22] Before initiating stimulant laxatives, palliative APRNs should assess for partial or complete bowel obstruction because prescribing medications to increase intestinal motility could be life-threatening.[29–31]

Palliative APRNs should also be mindful of minimizing pill burden for patients and especially those with advanced illness. One prospective randomized controlled trial demonstrated that docusate plus sennosides was no more efficacious than sennosides alone in managing constipation in hospice patients.[32] Table 40.3 contains the various classes of laxatives and bowel preparations, initial and maximum daily doses, and special considerations for the palliative APRN.[21,22,33–38]

Table 40.3 MEDICATIONS FOR CONSTIPATION

GENERIC NAME (*BRAND NAME*)	INITIAL DOSE	COMMENTS
Bulk-Forming Agents: Absorb liquid in the gastrointestinal tract and increase the bulk consistency of stool. *Not recommended if unable to tolerate large volume of liquids.*		
Psyllium (*Metamucil*)	2.5 g PO 1–3 times daily	Drink with 8 ounces of liquid Separate dose by at least 2 h from other medications Onset of action: 12–72 h
Methylcellulose (*Citrucel*)	2 g 1–3 times daily as needed MDD: 6 g	Caution in dehydrated patients Onset of action: 24–48 h
Stimulant Laxatives: Stimulate myenteric plexus and initiate peristaltic activity and inhibit water absorption		
Senna (*Senokot*)	17.2 mg PO at bedtime MDD: 68.8 mg	Previously used in combination with docusate May cause cramping Onset of action: 6–12 h
Bisacodyl (*Dulcolax*)	5 mg PO *or* 1 suppository *or* enema (10 mg) PR once daily MDD: 15 mg PO	May cause cramping Onset of action: 6–8 h (oral); 0.25–1 h after rectal administration
Castor Oil (*Emulsoil*)	15–60 mL PO once daily as needed MDD: 60 mL	May cause cramping Onset of action: 2–6 h
Surfactant/Detergent Laxatives: Lower surface tension of stool to allow mixing of aqueous and fatty substances; alter intestinal mucosal permeability		
Docusate salts (*Colace*)	50–300 mg PO in single or divided doses MDD: 240 mg PO for docusate calcium; 360 mg PO for docusate sodium	Onset of action: 24–72 h Recent study suggests no significant benefit of docusate with sennosides versus sennosides alone; should consider use on an individual basis.
Osmotic Laxatives: Cause fluid retention, distending the colon to increase peristalsis		
Lactulose (*Kristalose Chronulac, Constulose, Enulose*)	15–30 mL once daily MDD: variable	Mix with beverage to improve flavor Costly May cause flatulence and cramping Onset of action: 24–48 h
Sorbitol (*Arlex*)	30–45 mL (27–40 g) PO once daily MDD: 45 mL PO; 120 mL PR	Less expensive than lactulose May cause abdominal pain, cramping and diarrhea Onset of action: 0.25–1 h
Magnesium citrate (*Citroma*)	150–300 mL PO as a single or divided dose MDD: 300 mL PO as a laxative	Chill to improve taste May cause cramping Onset of action: 3–6 h
Magnesium hydroxide (*Milk of Magnesia*)	15–60 mL PO daily, preferably at bedtime MDD: 60 mL	May dilute with water prior to administration Onset of action: 0.5–8 h
Magnesium sulfate (*Epsom Salt*)	10–30 g PO as single or divided doses MDD: N/A	Dissolve in a full glass of water prior to intake May use lemon juice for taste Onset of action: 3–6 h
Polyethylene glycol (*Miralax*)	17 g daily MDD: 34 g PO daily	Mix with 8 ounces of water, juice, coffee, or tea Onset of action: 24–96 h

Table 40.3 CONTINUED

GENERIC NAME (*BRAND NAME*)	INITIAL DOSE	COMMENTS
Lubricant Laxatives: Penetrate and soften stool and interferes with reabsorption of water in the colon		
Mineral oil (*Fleet Mineral Oil*)	45 mL PR as single dose MDD: 45 mL	Avoid oral formulation due to risk of lipid pneumonitis if aspirated Adverse effects: mild abdominal pain, fecal urgency, cramps Onset of action: within 0.25 h
Other Agents		
Linaclotide (*Linzess*)	145 μg PO once daily MDD: 290 μg	Take on empty stomach at least 0.5 h before the first meal of the day May cause diarrhea
Lubiprostone (*Amitiza*)	24 μg PO twice daily MDD: 48 μg	May experience nausea, diarrhea, headache, abdominal pain, distension, flatulence Take with food and water
Methylnaltrexone (*Relistor*)	Administered SC based on weight: ≤38 kg: 0.15 mg/kg/day; 38 to <62 kg: 8 mg/day; 62–114 kg: 12 mg/day	For opioid-induced constipation; high cost of administration Onset of action: 0.5–1 h
Naloxegol (*Movantik*)	25 mg PO once daily	For opioid-induced constipation Time to peak <2 h Reduce dose to 12.5 mg if unable to tolerate recommended dose

MDD, Maximum daily dose.

From Sharma, Rao[21]; Mooney et al.[22]; Sykes[33]; Wald[34]; Viscusi et al.[35]; Jamal et al.[36]; Fukudo et al.[37]; Naloxegol.[38]

NONPHARMACOLOGIC INTERVENTIONS

A nonpharmacologic approach is a key part of the care plan and considers personal factors to promote optimal bowel function. Examples include routine upright positioning, increasing activity, and an effective combination of fiber and fluid intake when appropriate. Toileting should allow privacy and ample time. Unless completion of assessment is urgent, the palliative APRN should not interrupt the patient's toileting to complete assessment.[4,5,12,28] Smaller studies have suggested the potential benefits of gentle abdominal massage and acupressure by trained professionals as a nonpharmacologic approach to constipation.[39,40]

MANAGEMENT INTERVENTIONAL TECHNIQUES

Evidence supports the use of digital rectal examination (DRE) in order to exclude fecal impaction if a patient has not had a bowel movement in more than 3 days or if they report feelings of incomplete evacuation.[8,11] Disimpaction can cause severe pain, so proper premedication should be provided. Additionally, any rectal interventions should be used with caution in immunocompromised patients.[22]

PATIENT AND FAMILY EDUCATION

Participating in his or her own plan of care can be extremely helpful to ensure compliance. This approach empowers the patient to detect changes and communicate them to the care team. Education on the nonpharmacologic interventions mentioned here should be reviewed, and caregivers should also be educated about the physical, psychological, and social impact that constipation can have on the patient. Patients and caregivers should understand proper bowel prophylaxis and signs of constipation to report. They can benefit from being aware of and participating in self-care activities, increasing physical activity, and keeping food diaries.

DIARRHEA

Diarrhea has commonly been classified as an increase in stool frequency and liquidity; for the majority of the general population, it is self-limited and does not require medical attention.[41] The objective definition is the passage of three or more unformed stools within a 24-hour period.[34] Acute diarrhea occurs within 24–48 hours of exposure to the offending agent or event and usually subsides within 1–2 weeks.[22] Most cases have a short duration and are infectious in nature. For chronic diarrhea, onset may not occur immediately and can persist for more than 30 days.[35] The goal of management is to determine and treat the underlying etiology while simultaneously providing supportive care.

Subjectively, patients may describe any change in stool frequency, volume, or consistency as diarrhea; this should be clarified.[42] When bowel movements are intense and variable, patients may have discomfort, anxiety, and experience social isolation. Uncontrolled, persistent diarrhea can cause increased weakness, malnutrition, dehydration, and electrolyte imbalances that may be debilitating and even life-threatening.[41] In patients continuing to receive active treatment, severity of symptoms may result in dose reduction or even discontinuation of disease-targeted therapies. The palliative APRN should be mindful of treatments that commonly cause diarrhea in order to provide prompt evaluation and intervention.

INCIDENCE

The incidence of diarrhea in the palliative care population varies by disease and treatment modalities. In HIV-positive patients, diarrhea has been reported in 28–60% of the population treated with combination antiretroviral therapy.[43] In older, frail adults, approximately 10–60% of patients receiving enteral feedings will suffer from diarrhea.[44] While significantly less prevalent than constipation in the palliative care population, diarrhea is a highly distressing symptom, with both physical and psychosocial effects.

Diarrhea occurs frequently throughout the cancer treatment trajectory and has been seen across all treatment approaches, including systemic therapies, radiotherapy, surgery, and even from the primary malignancy itself. Malignancies of the gastrointestinal system, such as pancreatic and colorectal cancers, have the highest frequency of tumor-associated diarrhea, and diarrhea is seen in approximately 20% of these cases.[41] The incidence and severity of chemotherapy-induced diarrhea vary based on the agent and dose, with rates as high as 50–96% with certain regimens.[41,45] Radiation-induced diarrhea has been mostly associated with treatment that involves the lower gastrointestinal tract, with incidence of diarrhea of any level reported in up to 70% of patients and more moderate to severe cases seen in 20–40% of this population.[22,41,46,47]

PATHOPHYSIOLOGY

The pathophysiology of diarrhea is described by the specific cause or causes of increased stool water content and output. Potential causes are listed in Table 40.4 and include increased fluid secretion, decreased fluid absorption, or bowel hypermotility.[22,48,49]

Table 40.4 PATHOPHYSIOLOGY OF DIARRHEA

TYPE	CAUSES
Increased fluid secretion- (Most difficult to control and often not preventable)	Inflammation Hormones Enterotoxins Chemotherapy, radiotherapy
Decreased fluid absorption	Medications (i.e., antibiotics) Hyperosmolar preparations/enteral feedings Laxative overuse Dietary: high sorbitol diet, lactose intolerance Fistulas
Bowel hypermotility	Gastrointestinal malignancies Adhesions, fistulas Biliary/pancreatic or bowel obstructions Chemotherapy

From Mooney et al.[22]; McQuade et al.[48]; and Sauk, Richter.[49]

ASSESSMENT

A careful history and assessment are crucial. The palliative APRN should assess the frequency, appearance, and number of stools and the temporal correlation with medications, treatment, or meals. Secondary effects of diarrhea, such as fatigue, weakness, abdominal pain or cramping, dehydration, dizziness, weight loss, and skin breakdown, should also be identified. Constipation with a sudden onset of diarrhea is suspicious for fecal impaction or obstruction with overflow diarrhea.[16,22] Medications should be reviewed for offending agents, such as laxatives, antibiotics, and chemotherapeutic agents.[42]

Specific signs of dehydration that palliative APRNs should be assessing in patients with moderate to severe diarrhea include dry oral mucosa, skin appearance, and changes in mental status. The physical assessment includes looking for oral candidiasis, hyperactive or hypoactive bowel sounds, abdominal distention, and tenderness. A rectal examination is performed if there is concern for fecal impaction.[16]

Additional testing may include stool specimen examination for pus, blood, fat, ova, or parasites as appropriate. Cultures and sensitivity testing can rule out opportunistic infections, such as *Clostridium difficile* or other gastrointestinal infections that should be on the APRN's differential diagnosis (Box 40.3).[22,49,50] For high-volume output, stool specimens should be collected before suppressing output, and patients should be evaluated for electrolyte imbalance. Severe diarrhea with rapid dehydration can lead to acute renal injury and, in extreme cases, shock. If obstruction is suspected, an abdominal radiograph may be indicated.[16,42] While symptoms of diarrhea may be quite distressing for patients, palliative APRNs must take time to thoroughly assess their patients in order to implement safe prescribing techniques and identify clinical scenarios that may warrant further evaluation, including hospitalization.[27,41,49]

MANAGEMENT

Management first considers treatment of the underlying cause. If this does not lead to resolution of diarrhea, symptom management to thicken stool and slow peristalsis may be necessary. Adequate hydration should be ensured, and modification of medications or dietary factors should be considered.[35]

PHARMACOLOGIC MANAGEMENT

Identifying the cause of diarrhea guides pharmacotherapy. Treatment for specific causes of diarrhea may include pancreatic enzymes for steatorrhea or pancreatic insufficiency, cholestyramine for excess fecal bile acids or radiation-associated diarrhea, histamine antagonists for carcinoid syndrome, antibiotics, and mesalazine for ulcerative colitis.[18] Various nonspecific medications (Table 40.5) can be used for the general treatment of diarrhea and unless contraindicated, may help control the extent of symptoms.[21,51,52]

NONPHARMACOLOGIC INTERVENTIONS

Nonpharmacologic interventions begin with dietary modifications, including a focus on oral rehydration, as tolerated. Bowel rest or consuming clear liquids and simple carbohydrates can often give the gastrointestinal tract a much-needed rest. Proactive management should be provided for patients undergoing treatments highly associated with diarrhea.

Keeping a food log to help determine any food sensitivities is encouraged. Common products that are irritating to normal bowel function are dairy products, caffeine, and high-fiber, spicy, and high-fat foods.[16,22]

MANAGEMENT INTERVENTIONAL TECHNIQUES

For patients with limited mobility, fecal incontinence and persistent diarrhea in the acute care setting may warrant consideration of rectal catheter placement to divert stool away from both impaired and healthy skin. Patients on anticoagulation and antiplatelet therapy have an increased risk of gastrointestinal hemorrhage with rectal tubes and should be monitored closely.[22] The palliative APRN should advocate for appropriate treatments that are in line with the patient's goals of care and improve quality of life as defined by the patient.

PATIENT AND FAMILY EDUCATION

Persistent diarrhea can be quite debilitating and distressing for patients and their families. Implementing changes in the home environment may help the patient feel more secure and comfortable. The goal is to minimize or prevent accidents by attempting to plan and time activities based on predictable bowel patterns. Access to the bathroom should be unobstructed, and the availability of a commode may be helpful to reduce the risk of injury. Beds can be protected with padding, which may be more dignified for the patient compared to wearing diapers. Meticulous skin and perineal care are essential and should be emphasized to patients and caregivers. Application of skin ointment may help with irritation, and odor management with aromatherapy may be soothing for the patient.

BOWEL OBSTRUCTION

INCIDENCE AND DEFINITION

A malignant bowel obstruction (MBO) is defined as an obstruction beyond the ligament of Treitz that is related to an intra-abdominal primary cancer with incurable disease or from a non–intra-abdominal primary cancer with clear intraperitoneal disease.[53,54] MBO occurs in approximately 5–51% of women with ovarian cancer and 10–28% of patients with advanced gastrointestinal cancers.[55] Depending on the type of malignancy, median survival after onset varies between 30 and 90 days; awareness of median survival can aid in prognosticating and decision-making.[47–49]

PATHOPHYSIOLOGY

MBO can occur at single or multiple levels and can be classified as mechanical or functional, partial or complete.[48]

Table 40.5 PHARMACOLOGICAL MANAGEMENT OF DIARRHEA

GENERIC NAME (*BRAND NAME*)	INITIAL DOSE	COMMENTS
Bulk-forming agents: Absorb liquid in the gastrointestinal tract and increase the bulk consistency of stool		
Methylcellulose (*Citrucel*)	2 g 1–3 times daily as needed MDD: 6 g	Take with water to reduce risk of choking Caution in dehydrated patients Onset of action: 24–48 h
Cholestyramine (*Questran*)	2-4 g 2–4 times daily MDD: 24 g	Bile acid-binding resin For chologenic diarrhea
Opioid agents: If cause of diarrhea is unknown and low suspicion for infection		
Codeine	10–60 mg PO 2–4 times daily MDD: Variable	Avoid use in diarrhea caused by poison or bacteria
Diphenoxylate/ Atropine (*Lomotil*)	5 mg/0.05 mg (2 tablets) PO, then 1 tablet (2.5mg/0.025 mg) after each loose stool MDD: 20 mg	Avoid use in diarrhea caused by poison or bacteria Onset of action: 0.75–1 h
Loperamide (*Imodium*)	4 mg PO initially, followed by 2 mg after each unformed stool. MDD: 16 mg	Avoid use in diarrhea caused by poison or bacteria
Opium tincture	50 mg/5 mL solution Take 0.6 mL PO 4 times a day MDD: 6 mL	25 times stronger than paregoric or camphorated tincture of opium Range: 0.3–1 mL per dose Monitor stools Do not abruptly discontinue after prolonged use
Camphorated tincture of opium (*Paregoric*)	2 mg/5 mL solution. Take 5–10 mL PO 1–4 times daily MDD: N/A	Monitor stools Do not abruptly discontinue after prolonged use
Adsorbents: Naturally occurring minerals that have adsorptive capacities		
Kaolin-pectin mixture	15–30 mL PO after each loose BM MDD: 120 mL per 12 h	May decrease the absorption of drugs that chelate with aluminum Onset of action: 24–48 h
Polycarbophil (*Fiber-lax*)	1,000 mg PO 1–4 times daily MDD: 6,000 mg PO	Some products may contain calcium Onset of action: 12–72 h
Salicylates: May have antisecretory, antimicrobial, and anti-inflammatory effects		
Bismuth subsalicylate (*Pepto-Bismol*)	524 mg PO every 30–60 minutes, as needed. MDD: 4.2 g	For nonspecific acute diarrhea Avoid if salicylate hypersensitivity FDA approved for proctitis and ulcerative colitis May discolor stool
Somatostatin Analogues: Inhibit diarrhea caused by hormone-secreting tumors of the pancreas and GI tract		
Octreotide (*Sandostatin*)	300–600 μg/day SC in 2–4 divided doses	May cause diarrhea, abdominal pain, nausea, and drowsiness High cost of administration
Other agents		
Ranitidine (*Zantac*)	150 mg twice daily MDD: 300 mg	May be given with pancrelipase Reduces gastric acidity
Pancrelipase (*Creon*)	Dose varies by brand	Individualize dose; may be given with ranitidine or other H2 blocker
Vancomycin	125 mg daily for 10 days	Diarrhea due to *Clostridium difficile*
Metronidazole (*Flagyl*)	400 mg 3 times daily for 10–14 days	Diarrhea due to *Clostridium difficile*
Cyproheptadine (*Periactin*)	4 mg 3 times daily	Carcinoid syndrome diarrhea

MDD, Maximum daily dose.

From Sharma, Rao[21]; Bharucha et al.[51]; and Lamberts, Hofland.[52]

It can affect bowel function significantly and is considered an oncologic emergency due to the risk of perforation, sepsis, or necrosis.

Intra-abdominal tumors may be intraluminal or intramural. They can impair bowel function by occluding the lumen, causing intussusception or impairing peristalsis. Malignant adhesions can create multiple points of obstruction as they kink the bowel from an extramural site.[46,48] Duodenal obstruction is most related to cholangiocarcinoma and pancreatic malignancies, while distal obstruction is largely associated with primary colon and ovarian carcinomas.[48] In rare cases, obstruction is treatment-related from nonmalignant adhesions following surgery or radiation.

ASSESSMENT

A combination of subjective and objective findings often aids in diagnosing the presence and level of obstruction. The palliative APRN should understand the different characteristics of the location of the bowel obstruction. Duodenal obstruction presents with severe vomiting and emesis often containing undigested food. Pain or distention will often not be noted on examination. Obstructions of the small and large intestine both present with hyperactive bowel sounds with borborygmi. Nausea and vomiting will be more severe with obstruction higher along the gastrointestinal tract, whereas obstructions of the large intestine will produce delayed emesis with abdominal distention and colicky pain.[22,53,55] As part of the initial subjective assessment, palliative APRNs should assess the primary goals of patients with MBO receiving palliative care, and their family, which often includes time at home, avoidance of surgery, and minimizing symptom sequelae.[55]

Radiologic imaging should be employed only if suspected findings can be treated. There tends to be an overreliance on abdominal x-rays, which are more cost-effective but less accurate than contrast radiographs. Computed tomography (CT) scan is the gold standard for diagnosis, with an accuracy of 94% in identifying the etiology of obstruction, and can help the clinician rule out other diagnoses such as ileus, pseudo-obstruction, Ogilvie syndrome, or intrabdominal sepsis.[22,56]

MANAGEMENT

Symptoms associated with MBO have historically been difficult to manage, as nausea, vomiting, colic, and abdominal pains can be quite persistent and bothersome. A number of medical and surgical interventions exist, but the best treatment remains undetermined and should always be based on the patient's goals of care, symptom burden, and prognosis.[22,54,57–59]

PHARMACOLOGIC MANAGEMENT

The goal of pharmacologic management in obstruction is to provide symptomatic relief while minimizing the adverse effects of medications. Individualized treatment approaches may include analgesics, antisecretory drugs, glucocorticoids, and antiemetics. These pharmacologic management options are listed in Table 40.6 and may be the sole treatment or used for symptom relief while anticipating surgical interventions.[54,60,61] For persistent pain, opioid analgesics are recommended but may exacerbate colicky pain. Anticholinergic agents may offer additional pain relief in these scenarios.[54] Given the challenges with oral medications, parenteral, sublingual, and transdermal routes should be considered. The palliative APRN should also keep in mind that while combination regimens can improve quality of life, they often require inpatient admissions due to cost and lack of availability in the community. Treatment approach remains guided by the patient's larger goals of care and unique needs.

NONPHARMACOLOGIC INTERVENTIONS

During the workup and evaluation of potential treatment options, patients should avoid oral intake of food and fluids that may worsen symptoms and increase the risk of perforation with complete obstruction. The palliative APRN may prefer a period of bowel rest to avoid unnecessary surgical interventions. Thirst and the desire for oral intake may be highly distressing, and support as well as meticulous mouth care should be provided.[59]

MANAGEMENT INTERVENTIONAL TECHNIQUES

Multiple factors are associated with the selection of intervention, and several options exist. Initial management often consists of fluid resuscitation, electrolyte repletion, and placement of a nasogastric tube for decompression. Care should be taken when rehydrating patients as excess fluid may worsen bowel edema.[54] Surgical intervention in advanced cancer is controversial and is determined by performance status, extent of disease, level of obstruction(s), presence of ascites, and goals of care.[53,56,59,62] Patients with progressive cancer despite tumor-directed therapy pose the greatest risk for surgeons and often the risk of surgery outweighs any potential benefit, which may be difficult for patients and families to understand and accept.[54,59,63]

Endoscopic procedures, such as gastric or colonic stenting, present a less invasive option and have been associated with quicker recovery in patients with a single focus of obstruction or locally advanced disease.[64–66] Stenting is contraindicated in patients with already established perforation or for rectal tumors as symptoms of tenesmus and incontinence may worsen. Risks include stent migration and perforation.[66–68]

Management in patients with a poor prognosis, overt ascites, and carcinomatosis with multiple levels of obstruction is primarily supportive; placement of a venting gastrostomy tube can help to relieve symptoms. This may or may not allow the patient to tolerate some oral intake for pleasure and decreases pressure in the abdomen.[66,69,70] Nasogastric tubes are often used as a temporary bridge to surgery and can be quite

Table 40.6 PHARMACOLOGICAL MANAGEMENT OF OBSTRUCTION

GENERIC NAME (*BRAND NAME*)	INITIAL DOSE	COMMENTS
Chlorpromazine (*Thorazine*)	10–25 mg q4–6h as needed MDD: 1,000 mg	To control nausea and vomiting Sedating Monitor for extrapyramidal symptoms (EPS) Onset of action: 0.5-1 h
Haloperidol (*Haldol*)	0.5–1 mg q12h *or* q4–6h as needed MDD: 100 mg PO	To control nausea and vomiting Monitor for EPS Onset of action: 0.5–1 h
Metoclopramide (*Reglan*)	10 mg q6–8h MDD: 60 mg PO; single dose not to exceed 20 mg	Prokinetic; avoid in definitive or complete obstruction May cause sedation, fatigue, and restlessness Onset of action: 0.5–1 h
Prochlorperazine (*Compazine*)	10 mg PO q4–6h as needed *or* 25 mg PR q6–12h as needed MDD: 50 mg/day PR; 40 mg/day PO or IM	EPS especially at high doses Onset of action: 0.5–1 h
Hyoscyamine (*Levsin*)	0.25–0.5 mg IV *or* SQ q6h as needed *or* 0.125–0.25 mg PO or SL q4h as needed MDD: 1.5 mg	May cause blurred vision, confusion, constipation, dizziness, drowsiness, ileus, mydriasis, nausea/vomiting, nervousness, palpitations, sinus tachycardia, urinary retention/hesitancy, weakness Onset of action: IV: 2–3 minutes; PO: 20–30 minutes
Octreotide (*Sandostatin*)	50–100 µg IV/ SQ q8h MDD: Variable	High cost of administration May cause diarrhea, abdominal pain, flatulence, nausea, constipation Onset of action: 0.5 h
Scopolamine Transdermal Patch Scopolamine Hydrobromide (*Transderm Scop*)	1.5 mg transdermal q72h; 0.3–0.6 mg IV *or* SQ q4h as needed MDD: 2.4 mg IV 1 transdermal patch q72h	May cause drowsiness, or somnolence Onset of action: Transdermal, 4 h; IV, 15–20 minutes
Dexamethasone (*Decadron*)	4 mg 1–2 times daily MDD: Variable	Long-term use not recommended

MDD, Maximum daily dose.

From Hsu et al.[54]; Obita et al.[60]; Star, Boland.[61]

uncomfortable. These tubes provide short-term symptomatic relief in patients who do not qualify for a gastrostomy tube due to severe ascites or tumor infiltration of the stomach.[54,58,63]

PATIENT AND FAMILY EDUCATION

Patients and caregivers should be taught about the signs and symptoms of obstruction early in the disease course, especially in gastrointestinal and gynecologic malignancies, where obstruction is highly prevalent.[58] Patients may feel that lack of bowel movements is expected in the setting of decreased food and fluid intake and may go weeks without reporting early or late signs of obstruction. MBO is often indicative of the late stages of disease, and access to psychoeducation and support for both patients and caregivers cannot be emphasized enough.

SUMMARY

Bowel symptoms do not occur in isolation and are often accompanied by decreased appetite, fatigue, and general malaise. Patients may experience loss of dignity that can lead to social isolation if not addressed. Adequate support and education can empower patients to play an active role in their disease process and can help build trust between the patient, the family, and the palliative APRN. The palliative APRN must understand conditions, medications, and situations that induce bowel symptoms in order to provide appropriate care throughout the disease trajectory. Crafting an individualized plan of care tailored to specific patient needs is an essential piece of quality care and promotes quality of life.

REFERENCES

1. Erichsén E, Milberg A, Jaarsma T, Friedrichsen M. Constipation in specialized palliative care: Factors related to constipation when applying different definitions. *Support Care Cancer.* 2016;24(2):691–698. doi:10.1007/s00520-015-2831-5
2. Clark K, Currow DC. Constipation in palliative care: What do we use as definitions and outcome measures? *J Pain Symptom Manage.* 2013;45(4):753–762. doi:10.1016/j.jpainsymman.2012.03.016

3. Erichsén E, Milberg A, Jaarsma T, Friedrichsen MJ. Constipation in specialized palliative care: Prevalence, definition, and patient-perceived symptom distress. *J Palliat Med.* 2015;18(7):585–592. doi:10.1089/jpm.2014.0414

4. Hasson F, Muldrew D, Carduff E, et al. "Take more laxatives was their answer to everything": A qualitative exploration of the patient, carer and healthcare professional experience of constipation in specialist palliative care. *Palliat Med.* 2020;34(8):1057–1066. doi:10.1177/0269216319891584

5. Davies A, Leach C, Caponero R, et al. MASCC recommendations on the management of constipation in patients with advanced cancer. *Support Care Cancer.* 2020;28(1):23–33. doi:10.1007/s00520-019-05016-4

6. Bharucha AE, Dorn SD, Lembo A, Pressman A. American Gastroenterological Association medical position statement on constipation. *Gastroenterology (New York, NY 1943).* 2013;144(1):211–217. doi:10.1053/j.gastro.2012.10.029

7. Muldrew DHL, Hasson F, Carduff E, et al. Assessment and management of constipation for patients receiving palliative care in specialist palliative care settings: A systematic review of the literature. *Palliat Med.* 2018;32(5):930–938. doi:10.1177/0269216317752515

8. Zhe H. The assessment and management of constipation among patients with advanced cancer in a palliative care ward in china: A best practice implementation project. *JBI Database System Rev Implement Rep.* 2016;14(5):295–309. doi:10.11124/JBISRIR-2016-002631

9. Andrée-Anne P, Benoit A, Mélissa C, Nicolas M, Thérèse Di P, Denis S. Gastrointestinal dysfunctions in Parkinson's disease: Symptoms and treatments. *Parkinson's Dis.* 2016;2016:6762528–6762523. doi:10.1155/2016/6762528

10. Rossi M, Casale G, Baiali D, et al. Opioid-induced bowel dysfunction: Suggestions from a multidisciplinary expert board. *Support Care Cancer.* 2019;27(11):4083–4090. doi:10.1007/s00520-019-04688-2

11. McIlfatrick S, Muldrew DHL, Beck E, et al. Examining constipation assessment and management of patients with advanced cancer receiving specialist palliative care: A multi-site retrospective case note review of clinical practice. *BMC Palliat Care.* 2019;18(1):57. doi:10.1186/s12904-019-0436-3

12. Farmer AD, Holt CB, Downes TJ, Ruggeri E, Del Vecchio S, De Giorgio R. Pathophysiology, diagnosis, and management of opioid-induced constipation. *Lancet Gastroenterol Hepatol.* 2018;3(3):203–212.

13. Black CJ, Ford AC. Chronic idiopathic constipation in adults: Epidemiology, pathophysiology, diagnosis and clinical management. *Med J Aust.* 2018;209(2):86–91. doi:10.5694/mja18.00241

14. Sharma A, Rao S. Constipation: Pathophysiology and current therapeutic approaches. *Handb Exp Pharmacol.* 2017;239:59–74. doi:10.1007/164_2016_111

15. Chey WD, Webster L, Sostek M, Lappalainen J, Barker PN, Tack J. Naloxegol for opioid-induced constipation in patients with non-cancer pain. *N Engl J Med.* 2014;370(25):2387–2396. doi:10.1056/NEJMoa1310246

16. Hagmann C, Cramer A, Kestenbaum A, et al. Evidence-based palliative care approaches to non-pain physical symptom management in cancer patients. *Semin Oncol Nurs.* 2018;34(3):227–240. doi:10.1016/j.soncn.2018.06.004

17. Huang Z. The assessment and management of constipation among patients with advanced cancer in a palliative care ward in china: A best practice implementation project. *JBI Database System Rev Implement Rep.* 2016;14(5):295–309. doi:10.11124/JBISRIR-2016-002631

18. Kittelson SM, Elie M-C, Pennypacker L. Palliative care symptom management. *Crit Care Nurs Clin North Am.* 2015;27(3):315–339. doi:10.1016/j.cnc.2015.05.010

19. Prichard D, Bharucha A. Management of opioid-induced constipation for people in palliative care. *Int J Palliat Nurs.* 2015;21(6):272–280. doi:10.12968/ijpn.2015.21.6.272

20. Young J. An evidence review on managing constipation in palliative care. *Nursing Times.* 2019;115(5):28–32.

21. Sharma A, Rao S. Constipation: Pathophysiology and current therapeutic approaches. *Gastrointest Pharmacol.* 2016;239:59–74. doi:10.1007/164_2016_111

22. Mooney SN, Patel P, Buga S. Bowel management: Constipation, obstruction, diarrhea, and ascites. In: Ferrell BR, Paice J, eds. *Oxford Textbook of Palliative Nursing.* 5th ed. New York: Oxford University Press; 2019: 217–236.

23. Richter J. Approach to the patient with constipation. In: Goroll AH, Mully AG, eds. *Primary Care Medicine.* 7th ed. Philadelphia: Wolters Kulwer Health; 2014: 529–534.

24. Shu-Yu T, Chung-Yin L, Chien-Yi W, et al. Symptom severity of patients with advanced cancer in palliative care unit: Longitudinal assessments of symptoms improvement. *BMC Palliat Care.* 2016;15:1–7. doi:10.1186/s12904-016-0105-8

25. Prichard DO, Bharucha AE. Recent advances in understanding and managing chronic constipation. *F1000 Res.* 2018;7-F1000 Faculty Rev-1640. Published 2018 Oct 15. doi:10.12688/f1000research.15900.1

26. Clark K, Lam LT, Talley NJ, et al. Assessing the presence and severity of constipation with plain radiographs in constipated palliative care patients. *J Palliat Med.* 2016;19(6):617–621. doi:10.1089/jpm.2015.0451

27. National Comprehensive Cancer Network. NCCN clinical practice guidelines in oncology: Palliative care. Version 1. 2020. https://www.nccn.org/professionals/physician_gls/pdf/palliative.pdf

28. Candy B, Jones L, Goodman ML, et al. Laxatives for the management of constipation in people receiving palliative care. *Cochrane Database Syst Rev.* 2015(5):CD003448. Published 2015 May 13. doi:10.1002/14651858.CD003448.pub4

29. Fernandes AW, Kern DM, Datto C, Chen Y-W, McLeskey C, Tunceli O. Increased burden of healthcare utilization and cost associated with opioid-related constipation among patients with non-cancer pain. *Am Health Drug Benefits.* 2016;9(3):160–170.

30. Wittbrodt ET, Gan TJ, Datto C, McLeskey C, Sinha M. Resource use and costs associated with opioid-induced constipation following total hip or total knee replacement surgery. *J Pain Res.* 2018;11:1017–1025. doi:10.2147/JPR.S160045

31. Søndergaard J, Christensen HN, Ibsen R, Jarbøl DE, Kjellberg J. Healthcare resource use and costs of opioid-induced constipation among non-cancer and cancer patients on opioid therapy: A nationwide register-based cohort study in Denmark. *Scand J Pain.* 2017;15(1):83–90. doi:10.1016/j.sjpain.2017.01.006

32. Sharma A, Rao S. Constipation: Pathophysiology and current therapeutic approaches. *Handb Exp Pharmacol.* 2017;239:59–74. doi:10.1007/164_2016_111

33. Sykes NP. Constipation and diarrhea. In: Cherny N, Fallon M, Kaasa S, Portenoy RK, Currow DC, eds. *Oxford Textbook of Palliative Medicine.* 5th ed. New York: Oxford University Press; 2015: 675–685.

34. Wald A. JAMA patient page. Treating constipation with medications. *JAMA.* 2016;315(12):1299–1299. doi:10.1001/jama.2015.17993

35. Viscusi ER, Barrett AC, Paterson C, Forbes WP. Efficacy and safety of methylnaltrexone for opioid-induced constipation in patients with chronic noncancer pain: A placebo crossover analysis. *Reg Anesthesia Pain Med.* 2016;41(1):93–98 doi:10.1097/AAP.0000000000000341

36. Jamal MM, Adams AB, Jansen J-P, Webster LR. A randomized, placebo-controlled trial of lubiprostone for opioid-induced constipation in chronic noncancer pain. *Am J Gastroenterol.* 2015;110(5):725–732. doi:10.1038/ajg.2015.106

37. Fukudo S, Hongo M, Kaneko H, Takano M, Ueno R. Lubiprostone increases spontaneous bowel movement frequency and quality of life in patients with chronic idiopathic constipation. *Clin Tastroenterol Hepatol.* 2015;13(2):294–301.e295. doi:10.1016/j.cgh.2014.08.026

38. Naloxegol (Movantik) for opioid-induced constipation. *JAMA.* 2016;315(2):194–195. doi:10.1001/jama.2015.17459

39. Dadura E, Stępień P, Iwańska D, Wójcik A. Effects of abdominal massage on constipation in palliative care patients: A pilot study. *Adv Rehabil.* 2017;31(4):19–34.

40. Wang P-M, Hsu C-W, Liu C-T, Lai T-Y, Tzeng F-L, Huang C-F. Effect of acupressure on constipation in patients with advanced cancer. *Support Care Cancer*. 2019;27(9):3473–3478. doi:10.1007/s00520-019-4655-1

41. Bossi P, Antonuzzo A, Cherny NI, et al. Diarrhoea in adult cancer patients: ESMO clinical practice guidelines. *Ann Oncol*. 2018;29(Suppl 4):iv126–iv142. doi:10.1093/annonc/mdy145

42. Camilleri M, Sellin JH, Barrett KE. Pathophysiology, evaluation, and management of chronic watery diarrhea. *Gastroenterology*. 2017;152(3):515–532.e512. doi:10.1053/j.gastro.2016.10.014

43. Logan C, Beadsworth MB, Beeching NJ. HIV and diarrhoea: What is new? *Curr Opin Infect Dis*. 2016;29(5):486–494. doi:10.1097/QCO.0000000000000305

44. Musa MK, Saga S, Blekken LE, Harris R, Goodman C, Norton C. The prevalence, incidence, and correlates of fecal incontinence among older people residing in care homes: A systematic review. *J Am Med Dir Assoc*. 2019;20(8):956–962.e958. doi:10.1016/j.jamda.2019.03.033

45. Lui M, Gallo-Hershberg D, DeAngelis C. Development and validation of a patient-reported questionnaire assessing systemic therapy induced diarrhea in oncology patients. *Health Qual Life Outcomes*. 2017;15(1):249. doi:10.1186/s12955-017-0794-6

46. Jensen NBK, Pötter R, Kirchheiner K, et al. Bowel morbidity following radiochemotherapy and image-guided adaptive brachytherapy for cervical cancer: Physician- and patient reported outcome from the embrace study. *Radiother Oncol*. 2018;127(3):431–439. doi:10.1016/j.radonc.2018.05.016

47. Klopp AH, Yeung AR, Deshmukh S, et al. Patient-reported toxicity during pelvic intensity-modulated radiation therapy: NRG oncology-RTOG 1203. *J Clin Oncol*. 2018;36(24):2538–2544. doi:10.1200/JCO.2017.77.4273

48. McQuade RM, Stojanovska V, Abalo R, Bornstein JC, Nurgali K. Chemotherapy-induced constipation and diarrhea: Pathophysiology, current and emerging treatments. *Front Pharmacol*. 2016;7:414. doi:10.3389/fphar.2016.00414

49. Sauk J, Richter J. Evaluation and management of diarrhea. In: Goroll AH, Mully AG, eds. *Primary Care Medicine*. 7th ed. Philadelphia: Wolters Kulwer Health; 2014: 517–529.

50. Jump RLP, Crnich CJ, Mody L, Bradley SF, Nicolle LE, Yoshikawa TT. Infectious diseases in older adults of long-term care facilities: Update on approach to diagnosis and management. *J Am Geriatr Soc*. 2018;66(4):789–803. doi:10.1111/jgs.15248

51. Bharucha AE, Wouters MM, Tack J. Existing and emerging therapies for managing constipation and diarrhea. *Curr Opin Pharmacol*. 2017;37:158–166.

52. Lamberts SWJ, Hofland LJ. Octreotide, 40 years later. *Eur J Endocrinol*. 2019;181(5):R173–R183. doi:10.1016/j.coph.2017.10.015

53. Krouse RS. Malignant bowel obstruction. *J Surg Oncol*. 2019;120(1):74–77.

54. Hsu K, Prommer E, Murphy MC, Lankarani-Fard A. Pharmacologic management of malignant bowel obstruction: When surgery is not an option. *J Hosp Med*. 2019;14(6):367–373. doi:10.12788/jhm.3187

55. Roses RE, Folkert IW, Krouse RS. Malignant bowel obstruction: Reappraising the value of surgery. *Surg Oncol Clin N Am*. 2018;27(4):705–715. doi:10.1016/j.soc.2018.05.010

56. Santangelo M, Grifasi C, Criscitiello C, et al. Bowel obstruction and peritoneal carcinomatosis in the elderly. A systematic review. *Aging Clin Exp Res*. 2017;29:73–78. doi:10.1007/s40520-016-0656-9

57. Berger J, Lester P, Rodrigues L. Medical therapy of malignant bowel obstruction with octreotide, dexamethasone, and metoclopramide. *Am J Hosp Palliat Care*. 2016;33(4):407–410. doi:10.1177/1049909115569047

58. Daniele A, Ferrero A, Fuso L, et al. Palliative care in patients with ovarian cancer and bowel obstruction. *Support Care Cancer*. 2015;23(11):3157–3163. doi:10.1007/s00520-015-2694-9

59. Lee YC, Jivraj N, Wang L, et al. Optimizing the care of malignant bowel obstruction in patients with advanced gynecologic cancer. *J Oncol Pract*. 2019;15(12):e1066–e1075. doi:10.1200/JOP.18.00793

60. Obita GP, Boland EG, Currow DC, Johnson MJ, Boland JW. Somatostatin analogues compared with placebo and other pharmacologic agents in the management of symptoms of inoperable malignant bowel obstruction: A systematic review. *J Pain Symptom Manage*. 2016;52(6):901–919.e901. doi:10.1016/j.jpainsymman.2016.05.032

61. Star A, Boland JW. Updates in palliative care: Recent advancements in the pharmacological management of symptoms. *Clin Med*. 2018;18(1):11–16. doi:10.7861/clinmedicine.18-1-11

62. Mudumbi SK, Leonard EV, Swetz KM. Challenges and successes in non-operative management of high-grade malignant bowel obstruction. *Ann Palliat Med*. 2017;6(Suppl 1):S95–s98. doi:10.21037/apm.2017.03.07

63. Lilley EJ, Scott JW, Goldberg JE, et al. Survival, healthcare utilization, and end-of-life care among older adults with malignancy-associated bowel obstruction: Comparative study of surgery, venting gastrostomy, or medical management. *Ann Surg*. 2018;267(4):692–699. doi:10.1097/SLA.0000000000002164

64. Gleditsch D, Søreide O, Nesbakken A, Søreide OK. Managing malignant colorectal obstruction with self-expanding stents. A closer look at bowel perforations and failed procedures. *J Gastrointest Surg*. 2016;20(9):1643–1649. doi:10.1007/s11605-016-3186-z

65. Gunnells D, Whitlow C. Malignant bowel obstructions. *Semin Colon Rectal Surg*. 2019;30(3):1-6. https://doi.org/10.1016/j.scrs.2019.100684

66. Horesh N, Dux JY, Nadler M, et al. Stenting in malignant colonic obstruction: Is it a real therapeutic option? *Int J Colorectal Dis*. 2016;31(1):131–135. doi:10.1007/s00384-015-2375-7

67. Hori Y, Naitoh I, Hayashi K, et al. Predictors of stent dysfunction after self-expandable metal stent placement for malignant gastric outlet obstruction: Tumor ingrowth in uncovered stents and migration of covered stents. *Surg Endosc*. 2017;31(10):4165–4173. doi:10.1007/s00464-017-5471-7

68. Imai M, Kamimura K, Takahashi Y, et al. The factors influencing long-term outcomes of stenting for malignant colorectal obstruction in elderly group in community medicine. *Int J Colorectal Dis*. 2018;33(2):189–197. doi:10.1007/s00384-017-2946-x

69. Halpern AL, McCarter MD. Palliative management of gastric and esophageal cancer. *Surg Clin North Am*. 2019;99(3):555–569. doi:10.1016/j.suc.2019.02.007

70. Romeo M, de Los LGM, Cuadra Urteaga JL, et al. Outcome prognostic factors in inoperable malignant bowel obstruction. *Support Care Cancer*. 2016;24(11):4577–4586. doi:10.1007/s00520-016-3299-7

41.

FATIGUE

Shila Pandey

CASE STUDY

Carmen was a 78-year-old African American woman with newly diagnosed acute myeloid leukemia (AML) who presented to the cancer center for treatment options. Her past medical history included Paget's disease in the left breast (status post lumpectomy and radiation 9 years prior), obstructive sleep apnea, gastroesophageal reflux disease, peptic ulcer, refractory lymphedema, hyperlipidemia, depression, and claustrophobia. She had an episode of chest and back pain approximately 2 months ago with a negative cardiac workup. Computed tomography (CT) and magnetic resonance imaging (MRI) showed multiple lytic lesions involving the ribs, T11 vertebral body with a pathologic fracture, and a thyroid nodule measuring 1.7 cm. Abdominal ultrasound showed mild hepatomegaly with a dominant 5.7 × 5.6 cm cyst at the junction of the left and right hepatic lobes. Carmen was admitted for leukocytosis and expedited treatment. Initial presentation showed labs with a blast population of 12% with a white blood count of 21.7. Her hospital course was significant for a bone marrow aspirate and biopsy that confirmed AML, and she was initiated on azacitidine and venetoclax. She received transfusions for anemia and thrombocytopenia.

Review of systems was negative except for diarrhea from the leukemia treatments and fatigue. Physical exam confirmed hyperactive bowel sounds and dry mucous membranes. Several lab values were abnormal, including a hemoglobin of 7.0 g/dL. Carmen had received multiple transfusions, and the plan was to continue with treatment for leukemia. It was deemed that Carmen was not a candidate for future hematopoietic cell transplantation. After a chest wall nerve block, her pain was well controlled, but she rated her fatigue at 10/10. Eastern Cooperative Oncology Group (ECOG) performance status was 2. Additional

medications included hydroxyurea, antidepressant, β-blocker, antiviral, pregabalin, and several vitamins.

Carmen was retired from a government research coordinator position, which remained a source of pride. Carmen was married for more than 50 years before becoming a widow 5 years prior. She had three adult children, aged 50, 48, and 45, each with whom Carmen had distinctive relationships. The family dynamics had changed after the death of her husband. Her eldest daughter, Gina, an internal medicine physician, was most involved her in care. Carmen's children and friends stopped by throughout the week to visit or bring a meal. Her hobbies included reading, drawing, and painting.

Carmen stated that she had very poor quality of life. She reported crying frequently, having little energy to do much of anything around the house or go out with friends, and a diminished appetite. In addition, she admitted to feeling complacent, more anxious, and rather negative. Carmen noted she "just couldn't seem to get moving" and she had "never been this tired in my life." She loved visits and spending time with her children and friends. However, she was relieved when they left so she could lie down and take a nap.

Carmen was referred to palliative care. Prior to the meeting, Carmen's case was reviewed with the palliative care team. At the appointment, the palliative advanced practice registered nurse (APRN) reviewed the purpose of the meeting with Carmen and her daughter Gina. During the consultation, Carmen explained her understanding about the AML. Gina also shared her views of what her mother had been going through. Carmen and her daughter expressed understanding about the ultimate outcome of her disease and that treatment would not provide a cure. She knew she needed to complete an advance directive, but stated, "I can't bring myself to think about it yet." She said, "I'm just so very tired." Gina stated that she was at a loss as to how to help her.

The palliative APRN explained to Carmen and Gina that fatigue is a common symptom of both treatment and cancer. A consult with physical therapy (PT) and occupational therapy (OT) was recommended so that Carmen could learn how to maximize her activity through exercises and other techniques. Meetings with social work and chaplaincy were suggested to work on reframing her disease and creating her legacy. Carmen also agreed to meet with the nutritionist about her decreased appetite and with integrative medicine for massage and other integrative therapies. Carmen was started on methylphenidate 5 mg PO twice daily at 8 AM and 1 PM after she expressed inability to engage in exercise due to fatigue. Her oncologist agreed to a 2-week trial of the drug, which did help her increase physical activity and improved fatigue scores and so it was continued upon discharge.

Over the next 3 months, Carmen saw some improvement in her fatigue levels. Her energy never returned to baseline; she was unable to complete any books or artwork. However, she was able to carry on with most of her activities of daily living. Carmen stated that the appointments with physical and occupational therapy were most helpful, teaching her strategies to walk and conserve energy. The social worker discussed with her ways to reframe her outlook on life in coping with fatigue as well as the disease overall. She was also able to teach her three children ways to support Carmen both emotionally and around the house, in addition to taking care of themselves. Gina found social work and chaplaincy especially helpful in dealing with the role changes.

As expected, Carmen became more ill and was no longer able to continue disease-targeted therapies or the oral methylphenidate. When Carmen was ready, the APRN set up a home hospice visit. Carmen died a peaceful death 3 weeks later on hospice. Gina and her siblings expressed deep gratitude for all that was done for their mother. They were thankful that she did not suffer at the end of her life.

INTRODUCTION

Fatigue is a common symptom experienced by patients with serious conditions and illnesses. For patients receiving palliative care, the prevalence of fatigue ranges from 48% to 78%.[1] The number of people living with three or more chronic diseases is expected to rise from 30.8 million in 2015 to 83.4 million in 2030.[4] In addition, the population continues to age, with the number of people aged 65 or older reaching 23.5% by 2060.[5] In older adults with chronic illnesses the prevalence of fatigue ranges from 40% to 74%.[6] People living with multiple comorbidities tend to have a higher symptom burden, unaddressed symptoms, poor quality of life (QoL), and unmet palliative care needs.[7] These burdens on the population, including economic, are expected to rise by 2030.[8] It is essential that palliative advanced practice registered nurses (APRNs) understand how to manage fatigue in individuals throughout the life span and across illnesses.

See and colleagues[9] conducted a cross-sectional study to investigate symptom burden of patients admitted to a palliative care unit. They found patients with both malignant and nonmalignant illnesses were more likely to have fatigue, pain, and psychological or spiritual symptoms. As people transition to the end of life, symptom burden usually worsens.[10] Fatigue is one of the most reported, severe symptom experienced by patients with cancer due to the disease and its treatment.[11] Its prevalence in patients with advanced-stage cancer ranges from 62% during treatment to 51% during treatment.[12] Adolescents and young adults with cancer have a higher prevalence of severe fatigue when compared with population-based controls.[13] Fatigue is also prevalent in cancer survivors and may be associated with disability.[14] In fact, many breast cancer survivors experience fatigue that may last from months to years.[15]

For patients with heart failure (HF) and cardiovascular disease, shortness of breath and fatigue are the two most commonly reported symptoms, with fatigue as one of the first symptoms of HF.[16,17] In 2019, fatigue was reported as one of the most common symptoms for patients with chronic obstructive pulmonary disease (COPD), with its prevalence at 77% and its severity significantly affecting QoL, causing functional impairment and frequently associated with pain and dyspnea.[18] For patients with chronic kidney disease (CKD), fatigue is the most common symptom irrespective of hemodialysis status.[19] Patients with neurological and autoimmune disorders, such as multiple sclerosis (MS), systemic lupus erythematosus (SLE), diabetes, Sjögren's syndrome, amyotrophic lateral sclerosis, and Parkinson's disease also experience fatigue as one of the most prevalent and debilitating symptoms.[20,21,22,23] After a stroke, fatigue is a common consequence, with the prevalence of post-stroke fatigue reported as high as 85%.[24]

Other chronic conditions such as chronic liver disease, inflammatory bowel disease, chronic graft versus host disease (GvHD), and endometriosis also have a high burden of fatigue.[25,26,27,28] People living with human immunodeficiency virus (HIV) are at elevated risk of fatigue given the hematologic and metabolic changes that result from HIV infection, affecting nearly 90% of this population.[29,30] Fatigue is a symptom that may overlap with many psychiatric illnesses. In major depressive disorder, fatigue is more common in women than men and reported in 95% of patients.[31]

DEFINITIONS OF FATIGUE

Fatigue is a symptom of overwhelming tiredness or malaise associated with many diseases and disorders; in some cases no specific causes can be found.[32] Definitions of fatigue are varied given the complexity of this symptom.[33] Clinical fatigue has been defined by three major features: (1) generalized weakness, resulting in limitations in some activities; (2) easy fatigability and reduced capacity to maintain performance; and (3) mental fatigue resulting in impaired concentration, loss of memory, and emotional lability.[34] The National Comprehensive Cancer Network (NCCN) defines cancer-related fatigue (CRF) as "a distressing, persistent, subjective sense of physical, emotional, and/or cognitive tiredness or exhaustion related to cancer or cancer treatment that is not proportional to recent activity and interferes with usual functioning."[35] Fatigue in advanced illnesses other than cancer is often called *nonmalignant fatigue*.[36] Chronic fatigue syndrome (CFS) or myalgic encephalomyelitis (ME) is characterized by profound fatigue, reduction in ability to perform usual activities, unrefreshing sleep, postexertional malaise, and cognitive dysfunction for more than 6 months.[37] CFS is usually a diagnosis of exclusion and an extreme version of fatigue in the palliative care population and may not be associated with an underlying serious illness. For these reasons and others, CFS is beyond the scope of this chapter. While there is no one agreed-upon definition of fatigue, a common theme is that fatigue affects the patient's physical function, cognition, emotions, and daily activities and is beyond the norm.

PATHOPHYSIOLOGY OF FATIGUE

There are several descriptions in the literature on the pathophysiology of fatigue, with most of the research coming from CRF. The pathophysiology of fatigue is multifactorial and involves a complex interaction of cognitive, emotional, psychosocial, and somatic factors, resulting in highly variable clinical expressions.[38] Matura and colleagues[39] conducted a systematic review of 26 studies to describe the biological mechanisms of fatigue in cancer and chronic illnesses. They synthesized the current state of the literature describing inflammation and alterations in the hypothalamic–pituitary–adrenal (HPA) axis and the autonomic nervous system as possible mechanisms of fatigue in patients with cancer, HF, MS, COPD, CKD, and rheumatoid arthritis (RA). Additional causes of CRF include metabolic or neuroendocrine dysfunction and genetic influence.[40]

Fatigue can also be described as peripheral or central.[37,41–43] Peripheral mechanisms include hypotheses about adenosine triphosphate (ATP) and muscle contractility properties.[37] *Peripheral fatigue* refers to muscle fatigability caused by disorders of muscle and the neuromuscular junction, such as myasthenia gravis and McArdle's disease. Chronic conditions such as cancer damage the sarcoplasmic reticulum and dysregulation of ATP can lead to lower protein synthesis or metabolite production, which causes increased intracellular calcium levels as well as impaired mitochondrial mechanisms for regeneration of skeletal muscle. Hence, this can compromise the individual's ability to perform physical tasks.[37]

Central fatigue is a result of either failed transmission of motor impulses or an inability to perform voluntary activities.[37,41,43] Central mechanisms include hypotheses about cytokines, HPA axis, circadian rhythm, serotonin, and vagal afferent nerve dysfunction. These biological processes affect the body physically and cognitively, thus impairing concentration and energy.[37] Cytokine dysregulation causes a pro-inflammatory state characterized by elevated levels of circulating cytokines, such as c-reactive protein (CRP), interleukin-6 (IL-6), interferons (IFNs), and tumor necrosis factors (TNFs) and is a main driver of fatigue in cancer and chronic illnesses including irritable bowel syndrome (IBS) and Parkinson's disease.[36,41] Central fatigue mechanisms for fatigue are key to presentations of fatigue in autoimmune diseases, such as SLE, MS, type 1 diabetes, celiac disease, CFS, and RA.[42] Autonomic nervous system impairments are pathologic to fatigue in MS and Parkinson's' disease and can present as orthostatic intolerance.[43,44] Interestingly, the severity of central fatigue does not always correlate with the severity of the underlying disease. For example, a patient with MS may experience fatigue in one limb caused by a sustained motor task. Magnetic resonance imaging (MRI) is the primary procedure used to rule out other factors, along with a neuropsychological assessment if cognitive impairment is suspected.

Box 41.1 CONTRIBUTING FACTORS TO FATIGUE[30,37,38]

- Inflammation/cytokines
- Metabolic and neuroendocrine alterations
- Autonomic dysfunction
- Dysregulation of the hypothalamic–pituitary–adrenal (HPA) axis
- Genetic influences
- Adenosine triphosphate (ATP) dysregulation
- Deconditioning
- Dehydration
- Chemotherapy/radiation
- Polypharmacy
- Comorbidities of major organs
- Mental health disorders
- Paraneoplastic syndromes

Conditions that cause fatigue often have both central and peripheral mechanisms at work to cause this symptom.

Muscular, cardiac, and pulmonary deconditioning increases the risk for chronic fatigue. Prolonged hospitalization, treatment-related adverse events, or critical illness can decrease exercise tolerance which further exacerbate fatigue. Highlighted in Box 41.1 are multiple other conditions that contribute to fatigue. Iron deficiency anemia and aplastic anemias are known to manifest fatigue and other symptoms due to low hemoglobin.[45,46] Chronic infections lead to an inflammatory state which can persist after resolution of an infection.[47] Cancer-directed treatments such as chemotherapy and radiation are also offending causes of fatigue.[48] Predisposing risk factors such as history of depression or anxiety, sleep disturbance, pain severity, or lower levels of physical activity may increase risk of fatigue in those with cancer and chronic illnesses.[49,50]

IMPACT OF FATIGUE ON QUALITY OF LIFE

Fatigue affects not only a patient's physical well-being but also psychological, social, and spiritual well-being.[51–54,56,59,60–65] Studies exploring CRF have shown a decrease in functional status, interference with activities of daily living, and limits on quality of life, especially in the elderly. CRF can negatively affect health-related QoL at the time of diagnosis and may last for years in adults and adolescents, including those in remission.[51] Higher severity of fatigue often leads to worse reports of QoL.[52] QoL may remain poor despite stage of cancer or presence of metastasis.[53] Cancers where fatigue occurs in symptom clusters, such as with lung cancer, have strong negative associations with QoL.[54] Akin and colleagues[55] conducted a descriptive-correlational study to investigate the relationship among fatigue, self-efficacy, and QoL in cancer patients who were receiving chemotherapy. They observed significant correlations between fatigue and QoL, with worse fatigue causing lower ratings of QoL. For cancer patients and survivors, long-term fatigue is associated with an increase in depression, sleep disturbance, and neuropathy.[56] Severity of fatigue and its effect on QoL and mental function can play a role in predicting when someone with cancer will return to work.[57] Noncancer patients report fatigue as one of the worst symptoms they experience and describe it as a feeling of tiredness, having little energy, and as a main barrier to functioning.[58,59]

Fatigue experienced by people living with chronic illnesses such as COPD is also negatively associated with QoL.[58,60] Negative impacts of fatigue include alterations in daily life functioning leading to high mental burden, challenged coping, loss of joy in life, and, in some cases, loss of the will to live.[60] For patients with MS, fatigue and depression are closely associated with QoL.[61] However, physical fatigue may have the strongest influence on overall QoL, emotional well-being, role limitations, social function, and other measures of health-related QoL in patients with MS.[62] For older adults, fatigue related to chronic illness is associated with poor physical performance and negative outcomes such as hospitalizations, increased health care utilization, disability, and mortality.[63] Fatigue in neurological diseases not only decreases QoL and functioning but also can be a reason for earlier retirement.[22] Fatigue can also be demoralizing because it robs patients of who they were, leading to grief over loss of roles and responsibilities.[59,64]

Overall, fatigue can negatively impact one's sense of self, cognitive performance, physical function, family care, and social interaction.[65] Figure 41.1 summarizes areas of QoL

affected by fatigue. The burden of fatigue extends into the area of spirituality. Hirsh and Siros[66] examined the association between hope and fatigue across three chronic illnesses (arthritis, IBD, and fibromyalgia) and found that those with greater hope reported less stress and consequent fatigue. However, this may be less true for CRF.[67,68] Cancer patients and non-cancer patients alike experience the profound effects of fatigue. Due to medical advances, people are living longer with these serious illnesses; hence, palliative APRNs should continue to assess QoL.

ASSESSMENT OF FATIGUE

Like pain, fatigue is a subjective experience, requiring dependence on self-report to assess its presence and severity. The assessment of fatigue can be complex given its varied etiology and definitions. Although objective testing may assist with the management of fatigue, patient-reported outcomes remain the gold standard for fatigue assessment.[69] Screening for fatigue in seriously ill patients should be part of a comprehensive assessment by the palliative APRN. It is recommended that patients with cancer and survivors be screened for fatigue at the initial visit, at appropriate intervals during and following treatment, and as clinically indicated.[35,70] This approach can be taken with other serious illnesses including HF and COPD. A common and easy to use assessment is measurement of fatigue by a single-item number scale, using a 0 as "no fatigue" and 10 as "severe fatigue." Similarly, a single-item scale such as the Visual Analogue Scale for Fatigue (VAS-F), which uses a 10 cm, 0–100 mm horizontal line is useful for quick screening.[71]

In addition to the patient's self-report of fatigue, palliative APRNs should use a holistic, patient-centered approach to obtain information to assist in management of this symptom. Fatigue assessment tools may be unidimensional or multidimensional. Unidimensional assessment tools measure the physical impact of fatigue, whereas multidimensional tools assess the physical, mental, and emotional dimensions of fatigue.[1] Multidimensional tools are much longer than unidimensional ones and may be more time-consuming. Shorter form versions have been created for some such as the Multidimensional Fatigue Symptom Inventory-Short Form (MFSI-SF) to address this problem.[72] Other tools, such as the Edmonton Symptom Assessment System (ESAS)[73,74] and the Symptom Distress Scale[75] are single- and multiple-item measures with fatigue items embedded in other scales and are often used in palliative care settings. Palliative APRNs must select the assessment tool that is most appropriate for their patient population.

Multidimensional tools are often used in palliative care since fatigue usually affects other aspects of well-being that cannot be measured in single-item or unidimensional tools. Table 41.1 provides unidimensional (Brief Fatigue Inventory [BFI],[76] Functional Assessment of Chronic Illness Therapy-Fatigue [FACIT-F],[77] Fatigue Severity Scale [FSS],[78] Profile of Mood States Fatigue subscale [POMS-F][79]) and multidimensional tools (Multidimensional Fatigue Inventory [MFI],[80]

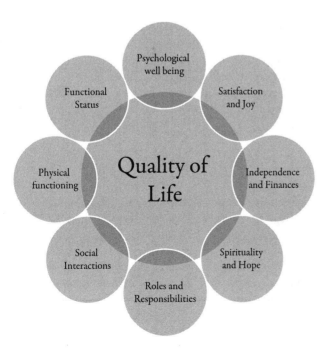

Figure 41.1 Areas of quality of life affected by fatigue.[51,55,60,66]
Unger et al., 2016,[37]; O'Higgins at al., 2018,[38]; Matura et al., 2018,[39]

Table 41.1 FATIGUE ASSESSMENT TOOLS

UNIDIMENSIONAL FATIGUE ASSESSMENT TOOLS		MULTIDIMENSIONAL FATIGUE ASSESSMENT TOOLS	
INSTRUMENT	DESCRIPTION	INSTRUMENT	DESCRIPTION
Brief Fatigue Inventory (BFI)	9 items Measures intensity or severity (present, usual, worst fatigue during past 24 hours) 0–10 scale (0 = no fatigue, 10 = fatigue as bad as one can imagine) Average of 9 items provides a global fatigue severity score (1–3 mild, 4–6 moderate, 7–10 severe)	Multidimensional Fatigue Inventory (MFI)	20 items Likert scale ranging from 1 to 7 Evaluates five dimensions of fatigue: general fatigue, physical fatigue, reduced motivation, reduced activity, and mental fatigue Validated in cancer and chronic fatigue syndrome
Functional Assessment of Chronic Illness Therapy-Fatigue (FACIT-F)	13 items Measures self-reported level of fatigue and its impact during activities of daily living over the past week Likert scale ranging from 0 to 4 0 = "not at all" and 4 = "very much" Score ranges from 0 to 52 with a score <30 indicating severe fatigue	Fatigue Symptom Inventory (FSI)	14 items Evaluates multiple aspects of fatigue Primarily validated in cancer 11-point Likert scale (0–10) 0 = "not at all fatigued" and 10 = "as fatigued as I could be" Global score obtained from all items
Fatigue Severity Scale (FSS)	9 items Designed to differentiate fatigue from clinical depression 1–7, total score divided by 9; 1 indicates "strongly disagree" and 7 indicates "strongly agree." The minimum score = 9 and maximum score possible = 63	Fatigue Questionnaire (FQ)	11 items Assesses mental fatigue and physical fatigue Likert-type scale ranging from 0 ("less than usual") to 3 ("much more than usual") Higher scores indicate more fatigue
Profile of Mood States Fatigue subscale (POMS-F)	7 items Used in cancer and non-cancer population Five-point scale ranging from "not at all" to "extremely"	Fatigue Assessment Scale (FAS)	10 items Likert-type scale ranging from 1 ("never") to 5 ("always") Total scores can range from 10 (lowest level of fatigue) to 50 (highest level fatigue)

References: Chen et al., 2016[76]; Montan et al., 2018[77]; Ozyemisci-Taskiran et al., 2019[78]; Minton, Stone, 2019[79]; Hinz et al., 2020[80]; Hann et al., 1998[81]; Chilcot et al., 2016[82].

Fatigue Symptom Inventory [FSI],[81] Fatigue Questionnaire [FQ],[82] Fatigue Assessment Scale [FAS][83]) that have been developed. Both types of screening tools for fatigue have been studied for validity and reliability.[84] For example, the Fatigue Assessment Scale (FAS) displayed good internal consistency and test-retest reliability to assess fatigue in patients with SLE.[20]

Once screening for fatigue is completed, a focused evaluation will be needed based on the severity of the fatigue. For moderate to severe fatigue, a more detailed history and physical exam is warranted.[35,70] Assessment of fatigue should include a detailed health history of its onset, duration, severity, aggravating and alleviating factors, effect on function, and associated psychosocial effects. A comprehensive review of systems and physical exam should be conducted. A detailed physical exam including a cognitive, neurological, and musculoskeletal evaluation may help to rule out other confounding factors of fatigue. Comorbidities that may cause fatigue include hypo- or hyperthyroidism, HF, infections, COPD, sleep apnea, anemia, autoimmune disorders, IBS, and cancer.[85] A review of medications and potential side effects, nutritional status, and stage of illness

may help identify potentially reversible causes of fatigue.[75] Ordering laboratory tests to detect for anemias, electrolyte abnormalities, or other diagnostics should depend on the goals of care. Furthermore, assessment of functional status can help explain symptom severity and prognosis in palliative care patients.[86] Table 41.2 summarizes key components to consider when assessing fatigue.

Effective fatigue assessment and management can be hindered due to patient, professional, and system barriers. A survey of palliative care providers, mostly nurses, found a lack of confidence in assessing fatigue and completing an individualized management plan.[87] A total of 77.2% of participants did not find fatigue an easy symptom to manage, and fewer than half felt confident assessing and managing it. Although patients may report fatigue as a common symptom, they may not seek help for the symptom.[88] Patients may believe fatigue is to be expected with their illness or age and be hesitant to report the symptom or accept help. These patient and provider factors add to the challenges in treating this common but complicated symptom. Fatigue may be associated with disease progression, and the fear associated with this may be a barrier to patients reporting fatigue to their providers. In

Table 41.2 COMPREHENSIVE ASSESSMENT OF FATIGUE

PHYSICAL EXAM	LABORATORY	CONCERNING COMORBIDITIES	DIAGNOSTICS
Functional status • Karnofsky performance status (KPS) • European Cooperative Oncology Group (ECOG) criteria General appearance • Weight, BMI, vital signs Systems: • Skin, hair, nails: Alopecia, rashes, growths, pallor • Head and neck: Thyroid exam, oral cavity • Cardiac: Heart sounds, edema • Lungs: Respiratory rate and effort, lung sounds • Gastrointestinal: Jaundice, organomegaly, tenderness • Renal: Change in urine color or output • Musculoskeletal: Muscle atrophy, joint appearance, range of motion • Neurological: Mental status, sedation, motor and sensory function • Psychological: Orientation, alertness, affect	Complete blood count (includes white blood cells, hemoglobin, hematocrit, platelet counts) Basic metabolic profile (includes creatinine, blood urine nitrogen, electrolytes) Hepatic profile (includes alkaline phosphate, transaminases) Albumin Total protein Thyroid stimulating hormone Urinalysis Vitamin B_{12}, thiamine, folate, vitamin D levels Basic natriuretic peptide	Malignancy Hypo or hyperthyroid HF Infection COPD, CHF, HIV, CVA Sleep apnea Anemias Autoimmune disorders Irritable bowel syndrome Poor nutritional status Chronic liver disease Parkinson's Disease Renal disease or injury Depression, anxiety	Chest X-ray Electrocardiogram Echocardiogram Computerized tomography scan (CT) Magnetic resonance imaging (MRI) Positron emission tomography (PET)

CHF, congestive heart failure; COPD, chronic obstructive pulmonary disease; CVA, cerebrovascular accident; HF, heart failure.

References: National Comprehensive Cancer Network (NCCN), 2021[35], Nadler, 2016[85]; Hernández-Quiles, et al., 2017[86].

addition, patients get fatigued with questionnaires and assessment forms during their interactions with healthcare systems. System barriers still exist despite repeated recommendations from healthcare societies. These barriers include lack of supportive care referrals, lack of healthcare reimbursement that affects the availability of medications and prescription practices, lack of consistent assessment and documentation between clinical settings, and lack of time to obtain a consult order for supportive services.[70]

MANAGEMENT OF FATIGUE

In the palliative care setting, effective fatigue management requires addressing symptoms that contribute to fatigue and preventing secondary fatigue by maintaining a balance between restorative rest and restorative activity.[89] The primary goal of managing fatigue is to treat any underlying contributory factors (e.g., pain, anemia, medication side effects, emotional distress) that are reversible with pharmacologic and/or nonpharmacologic interventions. When that is not possible, mitigating the effects of fatigue through palliation to maximize energy levels becomes the goal. Often a combination of both pharmacological and nonpharmacologic approaches is needed.[90]

PHARMACOLOGIC MANAGEMENT

For patients whose fatigue is a major hindrance on function and quality of life, there are limited nonspecific pharmacologic options for the management of fatigue. The evidence for the use of psychostimulants, corticosteroids, antidepressants,

and supplements continues to evolve. Table 41.3 summarizes options for pharmacologic management of fatigue.

Psychostimulants

Psychostimulants have been used to help patients with fatigue. Psychostimulants act to increase cortical function by interacting with neurotransmitters and receptors in the brain. These drugs include methylphenidate, modafinil, or dexamphetamine. Different types of psychostimulants work differently in the brain to produce short-term increased energy levels and psychomotor activity.[65] Medications like methylphenidate affect the brain in several areas, whereas modafinil, another type of stimulant, specifically affects the excitatory histamine projections to the hypothalamus, promoting wakefulness.[91] The NCCN[35] reports "some evidence" for using medications for fatigue, but randomized controlled trials (RCTs) have also shown a significant placebo effect. In light of these findings, the NCCN recommends the use of psychostimulants, specifically methylphenidate, for cancer patients undergoing active treatment after other causes of fatigue have been excluded.

In 2015, Mücke and colleagues[92] performed a review of pharmacologic treatments for nonspecific fatigue in patients with advanced cancer and other advanced chronic diseases receiving palliative care. After screening more than 1,645 publications, data from 45 studies, 18 drugs, and 4,696 patients were analyzed. Studies used in the meta-analysis were those that investigated medications (amantadine, pemoline, and modafinil) for patients with MS-related fatigue and for those with advanced cancer and fatigue (methylphenidate and modafinil). Even though methylphenidate for patients with cancer or HIV and amantadine for MS patients showed

Table 41.3 PHARMACOLOGIC INTERVENTIONS FOR FATIGUE

INTERVENTION	CONSIDERATIONS	EXAMPLES WITH COMMON STARTING DOSAGES	AVERAGE COST FOR 1-MONTH SUPPLY
Psychostimulants	Methylphenidate may be used for fatigue associated with cancer and other serious illnesses in carefully selected patients Modafinil can be used in patients with Parkinson disease, obstructive sleep apnea, and HIV but is not recommended for chronic renal failure (CRF) Amantadine is primarily used in multiple sclerosis-related fatigue Caution with use in elderly, severe hypertension, untreated hyperthyroidism or glaucoma, and uncontrolled cardiac arrhythmia	Methylphenidate 5 mg PO every morning or bid (8 AM and 1 PM) Modafinil 50 mg PO every morning Armodafinil 100 mg PO bid Dextroamphetamine 10 mg PO every morning	$$ $$$ $$$ $$$
Corticosteroids	Consider a time-limited course Reserve long-term use for end of life or terminally ill Monitor for multisystem side effects including hyperglycemia	Dexamethasone 4 mg PO daily every morning Betamethasone 4 mg PO daily every morning Methylprednisone 32 mg PO daily Prednisone 7.5 mg PO daily	$$ $$ $$ $
Antidepressants	Insufficient evidence on the use of selective serotonin reuptake inhibitors (SSRIs) for fatigue in cancer and multiple sclerosis Assess for other symptoms and depression Consider long half-life and side-effect profile of drugs before use	Bupropion 150 mg PO daily	$$
Supplements	Insufficient evidence for the use of L-carnitine Ginseng may have therapeutic effects for CRF More research is needed for the use of vitamin D or zinc supplementation	L-Carnitine 500-1,000 mg PO daily Ginseng 800 mg PO daily Coenzyme Q10 500 mg PO daily Zinc 8 mg PO daily Vitamin D 15 µg to 1,200 µg PO daily based on vitamin D levels	$ $ $ $

References: National Comprehensive Cancer Network (NCCN), 2021[35]; National Institute of Health (NCI), 2021[65]; Mücke et al., 2015[92]; Fabi et al., 2020[93]; Miller, Soundy, 2017[98].

superior effect, the authors concluded that no specific medication could be recommended for treating fatigue in patients receiving palliative care. Given this evidence, organizations such as the European Society for Medical Oncology (ESMO) are not able to reach a consensus on the use of psychostimulants.[93] Other reviews have also found mixed results on the efficacy of methylphenidate[94,95] and modafinil[96] for CRF and for MS-related fatigue.[97] Use of modafinil for MS fatigue is cautioned until larger clinical studies are conducted.[98]

Dose of stimulant and length of therapy may be important factors to its utility.[92,99] A prospective, controlled, double-blind, placebo-controlled study found that when methylphenidate was used as needed there was a significant decrease in fatigue after 2 hours (P = 0.004) and 5 hours (P = 0.001), respectively, in patients with advanced cancer.[100] Methylphenidate can be combined with other interventions such as erythropoiesis-stimulating agents or complementary alternative medicine.[101,102,103] The use of erythropoietin is associated with risks and should be carefully considered. At the end of life, there may be little benefit of psychostimulants.[104] Palliative APRNs should be aware of the contraindications for psychostimulant use. These include comorbid advanced arteriosclerosis, cardiac arrhythmias, severe hypertension, untreated hyperthyroidism, or glaucoma.

Corticosteroids

Corticosteroids are used to treat various clinical conditions and have multiple effects on the body.[105] They are used in endocrine disorders, pulmonary conditions, autoimmune disease, infection, and musculoskeletal conditions, and in the form of injections for pain relief. Glucocorticoids such as dexamethasone decrease fatigue by decreasing the inflammatory response and HPA axis function, which are associated with fatigue. The NCCN[35] recommends limiting the use of corticosteroids to the terminally ill, patients with fatigue and concomitant anorexia, and patients with pain related to brain or bone metastasis. Similarly, the ESMO[93] clinical practice guidelines recommend the short-term use of dexamethasone or methylprednisolone for the control of CRF in metastatic cancer patients. Dexamethasone appears to be the most studied glucocorticoid for management of fatigue.

Results of a 2015 Cochrane review[92] revealed a lack of research studies investigating the use of corticosteroids for fatigue, even though this is a common clinical practice. A review by Begley and colleagues[106] also reported varied results of corticosteroids on CRF and recommended more rigorous research. Similarly, Tomlinson and colleagues[101] conducted a meta-analysis and found corticosteroids were not associated with improvement in fatigue in patients with cancer or recipients of hematopoietic stem cell transplantation. Dexamethasone is often used to treat more than one symptom, such as nausea, pain, and fatigue. Yennurajalingam and colleagues[107] performed a secondary analysis of a previously conducted RCT to examine the effects of dexamethasone on symptom clusters in patients with advanced cancer. They found a found significant improvement in the fatigue/anorexia-cachexia/depression cluster scores compared with placebo at day 8 and day 15 of treatment. A retrospective review on the effect of prophylactic use of an oral dexamethasone on fatigue during regorafenib treatment in patients with metastatic colorectal cancer found the incidence of fatigue was significantly lower with dexamethasone than without dexamethasone (P = .022).[108] Steroids may be most helpful for patients with fatigue who are in the terminal phases of serious illness. A retrospective review examined the use of 4 mg per day of betamethasone in 87 hospitalized cancer patients at the end of life.[109] Betamethasone was effective in 42 out of 87 patients, suggesting steroids can have a sufficient effect on CRF for at least 2 weeks in terminally ill patients.

It is well-known that long-term use of steroids is associated with negative side effects, so future studies are warranted, keeping in mind the risk–benefit ratio. Some serious illnesses may require the long-term use of steroids. In such conditions, careful monitoring for adverse effects, particularly those affecting quality of life is essential.[110] Multiple systems can be affected, leading to a wide range of side effects including osteoporosis, myopathy, hyperglycemia, peptic ulcer formation and gastrointestinal bleeding, hypertension, delayed wound healing, mood changes, psychosis, predisposition to infection, oral thrush, and others.[111] For the cancer patient, the palliative APRN should collaborate or consult with the primary oncologist before initialing therapy since corticosteroids may impact the effectiveness of immune-based systemic cancer treatments such as immunotherapy.[112] Palliative APRNs should consider prognosis before initiating long-term use of corticosteroids for management of fatigue. Regular monitoring for clinical response is needed, and one may discontinue or taper the steroid if there is no clinical benefit.

Antidepressants

Fatigue and depression are highly comorbid in people living with serious illnesses. Individuals with either fatigue or depression have an approximately twofold increased risk for comorbid presentation of both traits compared to the general population.[113] Given some similarities in presentation, it may be challenging to differentiate the two diagnoses. Antidepressants have also been used to mitigate fatigue.

Generally, antidepressants affect the serotonin or norepinephrine system or both. Those affecting the serotonin system (selective serotonin reuptake inhibitors [SSRIs]) include fluoxetine, paroxetine, escitalopram, and sertraline. Agents affecting the norepinephrine system include bupropion and mirtazapine. Agents like venlafaxine and duloxetine affect both systems.[114] The SSRIs have been shown to improve depression and anxiety in cancer patients, but studies have failed to reveal improvement in fatigue.[92,115,116] A 2015 Cochrane review on the pharmacologic agents for fatigue in palliative care patients could not find therapeutic effects of paroxetine or fluoxetine for this symptom in COPD, cancer, and other chronic illnesses.[92] Similarly, a review conducted by Miller and Soundy[98] could not find enough data to evaluate the use of antidepressants for MS-related fatigue. Hence, the NCCN and ESMO do not recommend the use of antidepressants for the control of CRF.[35,93]

Bupropion, a norepinephrine/dopamine-reuptake inhibitor antidepressant, has been shown to be more effective for patients with CFS, but there are mixed reviews as to its efficacy in patients with CRF.[35,116] Ashrafi and colleagues[117] conducted a randomized, double-blind, placebo-controlled trial on the effects of bupropion on patients with cancer fatigue. The primary endpoint was change in average daily fatigue from baseline to week 4 using the FACIT-F questionnaire. Cancer patients who received 150 mg bupropion daily had a significant improvement in fatigue and QoL compared to the placebo group (P = 0.000). Similar results were observed by Salehifar and colleagues[118] in a double-blind randomized placebo-controlled clinical trial conducted on bupropion versus placebo in 30 patients with cancer and fatigue. Results showed a significant difference by the end of week 6 (P = 0.006) in the intervention group. Despite the lack of evidence for antidepressants in the management of fatigue alone, these medications may be beneficial for patients with fatigue and depression.

Palliative APRNs should consider the risks and benefits of using antidepressants in the seriously ill. These medications may take 4–6 weeks to take effect. Selection of antidepressants should be based on side-effect profile and patient characteristics. The effectiveness of antidepressants can be evaluated by assessing the degree of symptom reduction and the occurrence of any adverse effects.[119] One must also consider the cost of these medications. Generic and brand names of antidepressants may be expensive or unaffordable for some. In addition, availability of insurance coverage and out-of-pocket costs should be assessed before starting therapy. Patients may fear stigma with antidepressant use, for which the APRN can provide education and counseling.

Supplements

Other supplements have been the subject of evaluation for fatigue, with mixed results. Vitamins have not proven to be effective at reducing CRF.[65] L-Carnitine is thought to be helpful in treating CRF due to its ability to decrease pro-inflammatory cytokines. This nutrient can be depleted from chemotherapeutics. However, studies have not been able to support its effects.[92] Marx and colleagues[120] conducted a meta-analysis to evaluate the effectiveness of L-carnitine supplementation for CRF. The review of 12 studies showed no significant difference in fatigue with carnitine use (P = 0.45). Similarly, two separate reviews of carnitine for MS fatigue found insignificant results and insufficient data to support its use in this population.[98,121] Another systematic review of commonly used supplements, guarana, acetyl-L-carnitine, and co-enzyme Q10, could not confirm any statistical benefit for fatigue in patients with breast cancer.[122]

Ginseng has also been evaluated for treating fatigue. In 2017, Yennurajalingam and colleagues[123] conducted a prospective, open-label study with 30 patients with CRF. Participants received high-dose *Panax* ginseng at 800 mg orally daily for 29 days. The primary endpoint was change in fatigue scores using the FACIT-F. Results showed a significant reduction in mean FACIT-F scores at baseline, day 15, and day 29 with use of *Panax* ginseng (P <0.001). These promising results were replicated in a systematic review conducted by Arring and colleagues[124] of 10 studies on the use of ginseng as a treatment for fatigue in serious illness. They reported significant results and a modest effect of 800–2,000 mg of American and Asian ginseng on fatigue with no reported adverse effects in any of the studies.

Supplementation with other vitamins has also been studied for management of fatigue. Coenzyme Q10 is one of the most popular dietary and nutritional supplement on the market.[125] Sanoobar and colleagues[126] conducted a randomized, double-blinded, placebo-controlled trial to determine the effect of 500 mg per day of coenzyme Q10 supplement versus placebo for 12 weeks on fatigue in 45 patients with MS. Results showed a significant decrease in fatigue for the intervention group (P = 0.001). A prospective, randomized, double-blinded, placebo-controlled study conducted in Portugal found zinc supplementation prevented fatigue and maintained quality of life of patients with colorectal cancer on chemotherapy.[127] Research on vitamin D supplementation for patients with cancer is still evolving. Low vitamin D levels may be associated with higher levels of self-assessed fatigue in men but not women.[128] Supplements are often combined for management of fatigue. However, these studies have limited generalizability, with mixed results.[129,130] The ESMO and NCCN guidelines do not recommend the use of CoQ10, guarana extract, American ginseng, L-carnitine, or other supplements for CRF.[35,93] Patients who are interested in the use of supplements for fatigue should be properly counseled, and potential side effects with disease-targeted treatments should be reviewed.

NONPHARMACOLOGIC INTERVENTIONS

All patients should receive general education on treatment-related fatigue due to chemotherapy and radiation therapy (Table 41.4). General nonpharmacologic strategies include balancing rest and activity, conserving energy, preventing weight loss, optimizing nutrition, and using distraction (e.g.,

Table 41.4 NONPHARMACOLOGIC INTERVENTIONS FOR FATIGUE

INTERVENTION	CONSIDERATIONS	EXAMPLES
Physical activity	Assess functional status, risk of bleeding, orthostatic blood pressure Caution with bone metastasis, fractures, or anemia Consult rehabilitation specialists for patients who are severely deconditioned Therapies should be tailored to patient needs and abilities Review costs and insurance coverage with patient and family and seek discounts with insurance if present.	Walking, biking, aerobics, resistance exercises, swimming Tai Chi High-intensity interval training Yoga Physical therapy Occupational therapy Gym memberships, community health centers, YMCA
Integrative therapies	Review risk of bleeding, history of bleeding disorders prior to engaging in acupuncture Adverse effects of acupuncture may include needling pain, hematoma, bleeding, orthostasis, or more serious conditions such as vasovagal reactions Risks of massage may include infection, bruising, risk of fracture, reactions to lotions, or dislodging thromboses	Acupuncture Acupressure Reflexology Reiki Massage
Psychosocial therapies	Consider home-based sessions using telehealth to increase compliance to therapy These therapies may be delivered with other nonpharmacological or pharmacologic interventions Use interpreters or culturally appropriate modifications for non–English-speaking patients	Cognitive behavioral therapy Behavioral therapies Relaxation techniques Mindfulness based stress reduction Music therapy Art therapy Hypnosis Biofeedback Patient education and counseling

References: National Comprehensive Cancer Network (NCCN), 2021[35]; National Institute of Health (NCI), 2021[65]; Mücke et al., 2015[92]; Fabi et al., 2020[93]; Hilfiker et al., 2018[133].

listening to music, taking short naps, reading).[35,65,93,98,131] Teaching patients how to monitor their fatigue by using a diary increases awareness of when levels vary and allows them to plan their day accordingly.[132] The NCCN guidelines organize nonpharmacologic interventions into three groups: physical activity (e.g., exercise, yoga), integrative therapies (e.g., massage, acupuncture), and psychosocial intervention (e.g., cognitive-behavioral therapy [CBT]).[35] Although important to a comprehensive fatigue management plan, access to nonpharmacologic therapies may be limited in accessibility, availability, and affordability. A limited number of cancer centers have coexisting integrative medicine centers. In addition, not all insurance companies may provide coverage or reimbursement for integrative or complementary therapies. However, APRNs can partner with patients and families to find community programs or community health centers such as the Young Men's Christian Association (YMCA). APRNs may also need to collaborate with insurers to appeal for coverage of these services.

Physical Activity

Research studies have shown exercise to be the most effective intervention for managing fatigue.[56,88,133,134,135] If the patient's functional status permits, there are several activities, such as walking, biking, aerobics, and swimming, that may prove beneficial. Empirical evidence for exercise guidelines is lacking.[93] In 2017, Mustain and colleagues[90] conducted a meta-analysis of 113 unique studies to compare pharmaceutical, psychological, and exercise treatments for CRF. Although all intervention types showed significant moderate improvements in CRF, studies that intervened with exercise demonstrated the largest overall improvement (P < .001). The role of exercise in CRF has been studied in specific tumor populations as well. Zhou and colleagues[136] conducted an RCT on the effects of Tai Chi after chemoradiotherapy in patients with in nasopharyngeal carcinoma. Results showed Tai Chi reduced fatigue scores on multiple subscales of fatigue (P < 0.01 for general, physical, and emotional fatigue). Several studies, including meta-analyses, have shown exercise reduces CRF significantly in men with prostate cancer.[137,138,139]

Hilkiker and colleagues[133] conducted a systematic review and meta-analysis of 245 studies on the effects of exercise for CRF during and after treatment. During cancer treatment, aerobic and resistance training (alone or combined), and yoga had moderate to large effect sizes compared with usual care. After cancer treatment, yoga showed a large effect size for the reduction of CRF, while combined aerobic and resistance training, Tai-Chi, and aerobic or resistance training alone showed moderate effect sizes. Exercise as an effective intervention for fatigue in breast cancer patients and survivors has been well-studied.[140,141,142] Juvet and colleagues[134] conducted a meta-analysis on the effects of exercise during and after treatment on physical functioning and fatigue in breast cancer patients. Of the 25 RCTs in the review, 17 addressed the efficacy of exercise on fatigue.

Results showed exercise reduced fatigue during (standard mean difference [SMD] = −0.19, 95% confidence interval [CI] = −0.31, −0.07) and after chemotherapy or radiotherapy (SMD = −0.52, 95% CI = −0.96, −0.09). A reduction of fatigue was observed at 6 months of follow-up, and greater effects were seen after cancer-directed treatment. Patients with advanced cancer can benefit from exercise as well. An RCT conducted on patients with advanced cancer receiving palliative care and physical therapy for 2 weeks found a significant reduction in fatigue scores.[143] The intervention consisted of 30-minute active exercises, myofascial release, and proprioception neuromuscular facilitation for 2 weeks.

Effects of exercise have also been studied in CFS. Galeoto and colleagues[144] conducted a systematic review, and results showed rehabilitation programs that promote physiotherapy techniques such as exercise, mobilization, and body awareness are the most effective in reducing medium- and long-term fatigue severity in CFS patients. A 2019 Cochrane review of eight RCTs concluded that exercise therapy reduces fatigue in CFS; however, long-term effects are unclear.[145] For patients with MS, an individualized and supervised exercise program with aerobic training, resistance training, flexibility, and balance exercises is part of a multimodal approach to improve function and QoL.[146] Exercise has been shown to be effective in improving MS-related fatigue and other dimensions of well-being in several RCTs.[147,148,149,150] Other chronic illnesses including CKD, COPD, and SLE may benefit from exercise programs to address bothersome fatigue.[151-154] All programs should be tailored to the patient's needs and adjusted as the functional status changes. Caution should be taken with exercise interventions when patients have bone metastases, thrombocytopenia, anemia, fever or active infection, or any limitations secondary to other illnesses.[35] Physical therapy consultations should be made when patients have comorbidities (e.g., heart disease, COPD), recent major surgery, functional or anatomical deficits, or substantial deconditioning.[35]

Physical therapists (PTs) offer methods to manage fatigue with instruction to patients on proper body mechanics, paced breathing, and activity modification to decrease physical exertion.[155] Occupational therapists (OTs) assess and analyze patients' functional problems. In the case of CRF, OTs can teach patients practical interventions, such as energy conservation and lifestyle management.[152,153] The most common interventions provided by OTs include mobility, self-care skills, upper extremity strength and function, educational needs, home management skills, and need for assistive devices.[154] PTs and OTs can adapt activities according to the effects of fatigue on patients' functional abilities and ensure that proper equipment is accessible so patients can maintain as much independence as possible. This, in turn, empowers patients to continue making their own healthcare decisions and, at the same time, preserves their dignity.[154,155] Palliative APRNs are in a key role to assess the severity of fatigue and offer recommendations and referrals to appropriate exercise therapies.

Integrative Therapies

Acupuncture and Acupressure

Integrative therapies, such as acupuncture and massage therapy can be effective in managing a wide range of symptoms in patients with cancer.[155] The NCCN recommends acupuncture for those who have completed treatment and recommends massage therapy for patients with fatigue who have completed cancer treatment or are on active treatment.[35] The Pan-Canadian Practice Guidelines[156] and the ESMO guidelines[93] both could not reach a consensus on the use of acupuncture for CRF. However, the American Society for Clinical Oncology (ASCO) and Society for Integrative Oncology recommend acupuncture for patents who have completed cancer therapy.[157,158] These therapies along with reflexology and Reiki are often used in hospice and palliative care to provide comfort.[159] Evidence from systematic reviews shows promising results using acupuncture in conjunction with patient education to reduce CRF and improve quality of life.[160,161] Zhang and colleagues[161] conducted a meta-analysis of 116 RCTs with 1,346 participants to evaluate the effect of acupuncture on CRF. Results showed acupuncture delivered in 20- to 30-minute sessions 1–3 times a week for 2–6 weeks had a significant reduction on fatigue (P < 0.01). Participants included those who were receiving cancer-directed treatments and those where not. Seven studies in this review reported the occurrence of adverse events. The effects of acupuncture on fatigue were found to depend on the number of sessions, not the duration, frequency, or length of sessions.

Cheng and colleagues[162] conducted a randomized, double-blind, placebo-controlled pilot trial to evaluate the clinical effect of acupuncture on CRF in lung cancer patients. Twenty-eight patients with CRF were randomly assigned to active acupuncture or placebo. The intervention group received acupuncture twice per week for 4 weeks followed by 2 weeks of monitoring. The primary outcome was fatigue scores on the Brief Fatigue Inventory. Results showed a significant reduction in fatigue scores at 2 weeks in the 14 participants who received active acupuncture compared with those receiving the placebo (P < 0.01). At week 6, symptoms improved further (P < 0.001). There were no significant differences in the incidence of adverse events in either group (P > 0.05). Integrative therapies can be used in non-CRF. In patients with CKD, acupuncture can improve symptoms fatigue, pain, and other symptoms.[163] It is thought acupuncture affects the regulation of sympathetic nerves and the activation of bioactive chemicals to provide this benefit. However, a Cochrane review on acupuncture for symptoms of CKD suggests that further evidence is needed to make clear recommendations for this population.[164] Integrative therapies such as acupuncture are frequently used in patients with MS for relief of fatigue and other symptoms.[165]

Acupressure has been studied to be effective in the relief of CRF as well.[166,167,168] Zick and colleagues[169] conducted a Phase 3 randomized, single-blind, clinical trial on the effects of acupressure for fatigue in 424 breast cancer survivors. The intervention group received 6 weeks of daily self-administered relaxing acupressure or stimulating acupressure. The primary outcome was change in the Brief Fatigue Inventory score from baseline to weeks 6 and 10. At week 6, significant results were seen in the number of participants who achieved normal fatigue levels with relaxing acupressure and stimulating acupressure (P < 0.001). Significant results were also seen at week 10 (P < 0.002). Acupressure is often delivered with or without essential oils.[144] Patients who are interested in acupuncture should be screened for thrombocytopenia or bleeding disorders to avoid adverse events.

Massage

Massage, Reiki, and therapeutic touch are common non-pharmacological interventions used to provide comfort to patients in palliative care settings.[170] Similar to acupuncture, massage studies have shown clinical significance in improving fatigue, but larger-scale trials are needed to substantiate its efficacy[171,172] Kinkead and colleagues[173] conducted an early-phase, randomized, single-masked, 6-week investigation on 66 women who were Stage 0–III breast cancer survivors who had received surgery plus radiation and/or chemotherapy with CRF. They compared weekly Swedish massage therapy, light touch, and waitlist control. The primary outcome was scores on the Multidimensional Fatigue Inventory. Results showed a statistically significant 6-week reduction in total fatigue scores within the Swedish massage therapy and light touch groups (P < 0.0001) and a significant increase in fatigue scores within the wait list control group.

A more recent open-label, parallel-group, quasi-randomized controlled pilot study with 46 cancer patients receiving chemotherapy found aromatherapy massage reduced CRF.[174] Primary endpoints included fatigue scores on the Piper Fatigue Scale. Patients in the intervention group received 40-minute hand and foot massage three times per week for 6 weeks during home visits. The control group received standard medical care. Median fatigue scores did not change during weeks 2–6. However, at week 8, the fatigue scores were significantly lower in the intervention group (P < 0.005). Similar results were replicated in a RCT studying effects of foot massage to control CRF in patients with colorectal cancer who were receiving chemotherapy.[175] Results showed significant reduction in fatigue levels in those who received reflexology or classical massage compared to controls in the third (P = 0.030), fourth (P < 0.001), and fifth weeks (P = 0.036) of therapy. More research is needed on the effects of massage for fatigue related to MS.[176] Massage as an intervention can be delivered in hospitals, clinics, or in patient's homes. Massage therapy should be provided by certified practitioners who can tailor therapies to the patient's medical condition. Caution should be taken for patients with fractures, deep vein thrombosis, open skin wounds, or bleeding disorders.

Psychosocial Therapies

Psychosocial therapies are aimed at helping patients cope with their fatigue. These therapies teach patients how their thoughts can influence feelings and behaviors. Cognitive-behavioral therapy (CBT) has been shown to be effective for both non-cancer and cancer patients.[177,178,179,180,181] Use of psychosocial interventions in palliative care has been widely studied.[182] The NCCN, ESMO, and Pan-Canadian Practice Guidelines recommend the use of psychosocial interventions such as CBT, mindfulness-based stress reduction, psycho-education therapies, educational therapies, and supportive expressive therapies.[35,93,158] Poort and colleagues[183] conducted a reviewed of 14 RCTs on psychosocial interventions for fatigue during cancer treatment. Some studies showed psychosocial interventions such as CBT, support group therapies, and energy conservation approaches improved physical functioning directly after the intervention and may improve fatigue at first follow-up. However, this 2017 Cochrane review could not provide clear evidence to support or not support the use of psychosocial interventions for reducing fatigue in this population.

In an RCT, Mendoza and colleagues[184] studied fatigue in cancer and cancer survivors to determine the effects of waking hypnosis with CBT compared to education control. Forty-four participants completed questionnaires before and after the intervention. The instruments included Patient-Reported Outcomes Measurement Information System (PROMIS), Medical Outcomes Survey Sleep Problem Index, the Patient Health Questionnaire Depression Scale (PHQ-8), Pain Catastrophizing Scale (PCS), and the Cancer Treatment Distress Scale. The intervention group received the combined hypnosis and CBT intervention. Results showed significantly greater improvements in sleep problems, fatigue, and average pain intensity ($P < .001$) with the intervention group compared to the control. Secondary outcomes also resulted in significant differences for depression, cancer distress, pain interference, and pain catastrophizing. Effect sizes for all measures were larger following the waking hypnosis with CBT intervention. At follow-up at 3 months, treatment gains remained for all symptoms ($P \leq .001$). Overall results conclude that CBT as an evidenced-based intervention provides extended benefits in helping to control fatigue and other symptoms.

For MS fatigue, CBT provides short-term relief.[185] Use of combined approaches with CBT and therapies known to improve fatigue is recommended in patients with MS.[43,186] More research is needed to evaluate longer term effects of CBT on MS-related fatigue. Mindfulness-based interventions can be effective in reducing fatigue in patients with advanced COPD[187] and chronic HF.[188] These psychosocial interventions can be delivered at place of residence or with the use of telehealth to increase adherence to therapy.[189,190,191] Palliative APRNs should provide appropriate referrals to interdisciplinary specialists who can provide these psychosocial interventions, including nurses and social workers, and provide education to all patients suffering fatigue.

SUMMARY

Fatigue is an almost universal symptom for people with serious illness receiving palliative care. This symptom clearly affects function and quality of life, often occurring with other bothersome symptoms. Palliative APRNs are in a key position to assess for fatigue and provide evidence-based pharmacologic and nonpharmacologic interventions. Careful consideration of disease trajectory, prognosis, and goals of care will guide treatment strategies. A patient-centered approach in management of fatigue, including education of the patient and family unit, is essential to alleviate the burdens of fatigue. Fatigue affects physical, psychosocial, emotional, and other aspect of well-being. The palliative APRN can partner with the interdisciplinary team to identify, assess, and manage fatigue holistically throughout the disease trajectory.

REFERENCES

1. Yennurajalingam, S., Bruera, E. Fatigue and asthenia. In: Cherny N, Fallon M, Kaasa S, Portenoy R, Currow D, eds. *Oxford Textbook of Palliative Medicine*. Oxford: Oxford University Press; 2015: 409–420.
2. Hospice and Palliative Nurses Association. HPNA position statement: Value of the advanced practice registered nurse in palliative care. 2015. https://advancingexpertcare.org/position-statements.%20Accessed%20September%2023
3. Dahlin C, Coyne P. The palliative APRN leader. *Ann Palliat Med*. 2019;8(Suppl 1):S30–S38. doi:10.21037/apm.2018.06.03
4. Partnership to Fight Chronic Disease. What is the impact of chronic disease on America? 2015. Available at https://www.fightchronicdisease.org/sites/default/files/pfcd_blocks/PFCD_US.FactSheet_FINAL1%20%282%29.pdf
5. United States Census Bureau. Older people projected to outnumber children for first time in US history. Press Release. March 13, 2018. Revised Sept 6 2018 and Oct 8, 2019. https://www.census.gov/newsroom/press-releases/2018/cb18-41-population-projections.html.
6. Torossian M, Jacelon CS. Chronic illness and fatigue in older individuals: A systematic review [published online ahead of print, 2020 Jul 11]. *Rehabil Nurs*. 2020;10.1097/RNJ.0000000000000278. doi:10.1097/RNJ.0000000000000278
7. Reinke LF, Vig EK, Tartaglione EV, Rise P, Au DH. Symptom burden and palliative care needs among high-risk veterans with multimorbidity. *J Pain Symptom Manage*. 2019;57(5):880–889. doi:10.1016/j.jpainsymman.2019.02.011
8. Waters H, Graf M. The cost of chronic disease in the U.S. Milken Institute. August 2018. Santa Monica: Milkin Institute. https://milkeninstitute.org/sites/default/files/reports-pdf/ChronicDiseases-HighRes-FINAL_2.pdf.
9. See D, Le B, Gorelik A, Eastman P. Symptom burden in malignant and non-malignant disease on admission to a palliative care unit [published online ahead of print, 2019 Feb 4]. *BMJ Support Palliat Care*. 2019;bmjspcare-2018–001560. doi:10.1136/bmjspcare-2018-001560
10. Kobewka D, Ronksley P, McIsaac D, Mulpuru S, Forster A. Prevalence of symptoms at the end of life in an acute care hospital: A retrospective cohort study. *CMAJ Open*. 2017;5(1):E222–E228. doi:10.9778/cmajo.20160123
11. Roila F, Fumi G, Ruggeri B, et al. Prevalence, characteristics, and treatment of fatigue in oncological cancer patients in Italy: A cross-sectional study of the Italian Network for Supportive Care

in Cancer (NICSO). *Support Care Cancer.* 2019;27(3):1041–1047. doi:10.1007/s00520-018-4393-9

12. Al Maqbali M, Al Sinani M, Al Naamani Z, Al Badi K, Tanash MI. Prevalence of fatigue in patients with cancer: A systematic review and meta-analysis [published online ahead of print, 2020 Aug 5]. *J Pain Symptom Manage.* 2020;S0885-3924(20):30649–7. doi:10.1016/j.jpainsymman.2020.07.037

13. Poort H, Kaal S, Knoop H, et al. Prevalence and impact of severe fatigue in adolescent and young adult cancer patients in comparison with population-based controls. *Support Care Cancer.* 2017;25(9):2911–2918. doi:10.1007/s00520-017-3746-0

14. Jones J, Olson K, Catton P, et al. Cancer-related fatigue and associated disability in post-treatment cancer survivors. *J Cancer Surviv.* 2016;10(1):51–61. doi:10.1007/s11764-015-0450-2

15. Schmidt ME, Chang-Claude J, Seibold P, et al. Determinants of long-term fatigue in breast cancer survivors: Results of a prospective patient cohort study. *Psychooncology.* 2015; 24(1): 40–46.

16. Johnston S, Eckhardt AL. Fatigue and acute coronary syndrome: A systematic review of contributing factors. *Heart Lung.* 2018;47(3):192–204. doi:10.1016/j.hrtlng.2018.03.005

17. Walthall H, Boulton M, Floegel T, Jenkinson C. Patients experience of fatigue in advanced heart failure. *Contemp Nurse.* 2019; 55(1):71–82. doi:10.1080/10376178.2019.1604147

18. Goërtz YMJ, Spruit MA, Van't Hul AJ, et al. Fatigue is highly prevalent in patients with COPD and correlates poorly with the degree of airflow limitation. *Ther Adv Respir Dis.* 2019;13:1753466619878128. doi:10.1177/1753466619878128

19. Wan Zukiman WZH, Yaakup H, Zakaria NF, Shah SAB. Symptom prevalence and the negative emotional states in end-stage renal disease patients with or without renal replacement therapy: A cross-sectional analysis. *J Palliat Med.* 2017;20(10):1127–1134. doi:10.1089/jpm.2016.0450

20. Horisberger A, Courvoisier D, Ribi C. The Fatigue Assessment Scale as a simple and reliable tool in systemic lupus erythematosus: A cross-sectional study. *Arthritis Res Ther.* 2019;21(1):80. doi:10.1186/s13075-019-1864-4

21. Siciliano M, Trojano L, Santangelo G, De Micco R, Tedeschi G, Tessitore A. Fatigue in Parkinson's disease: A systematic review and meta-analysis. *Movement Disorders.* 2018;33(11):1712–1723. doi:10.1002/mds.27461

22. Penner IK, Paul F. Fatigue as a symptom or comorbidity of neurological diseases. *Nat Rev Neurol.* 2017;13(11):662–675. doi:10.1038/nrneurol.2017.117

23. Kostić VS, Tomić A, Ječmenica-Lukić M. The pathophysiology of fatigue in Parkinson's disease and its pragmatic management. *Mov Disord Clin Pract.* 2016;3(4):323–330. doi:10.1002/mdc3.12341

24. Cumming TB, Packer M, Kramer SF, English C. The prevalence of fatigue after stroke: A systematic review and meta-analysis. *Int J Stroke.* 2016;11(9):968–977. doi:10.1177/1747493016669861

25. Gerber LH, Weinstein AA, Mehta R, Younossi ZM. Importance of fatigue and its measurement in chronic liver disease. *World J Gastroenterol.* 2019;25(28):3669–3683. doi:10.3748/wjg.v25.i28.3669

26. Grimstad T, Norheim KB. Fatigue in inflammatory bowel disease. Article in Norwegian. *Tidsskr Nor Laegeforen.* 2016 Nov 8;136(20):1721–1724. doi:10.4045/tidsskr.16.0134. PMID: 27830906

27. Ramin-Wright A, Schwartz ASK, Geraedts K, et al. Fatigue: A symptom in endometriosis. *Hum Reprod.* 2018;33(8):1459–1465. doi:10.1093/humrep/dey115

28. Im A, Mitchell SA, Steinberg SM, et al. Prevalence and determinants of fatigue in patients with moderate to severe chronic GvHD. *Bone Marrow Transplant.* 2016;51(5):705–712. doi:10.1038/bmt.2015.320

29. Barroso J, Leserman J, Harmon JL, Hammill B, Pence BW. Fatigue in HIV-infected people: A three-year observational study. *J Pain Symptom Manage.* 2015;50(1):69–79. doi:10.1016/j.jpainsymman.2015.02.006

30. Perazzo, Joseph, PhD, RN, Webel, Allison, et al. Fatigue symptom management in people living with human immunodeficiency virus. *J Hosp Palliat Nurs.* 2017;19(2):122–127. doi:10.1097/NJH.0000000000000329

31. Ghanean H, Ceniti AK, Kennedy SH. Fatigue in patients with major depressive disorder: Prevalence, burden and pharmacological approaches to management. *CNS Drugs.* 2018;32(1):65–74. doi:10.1007/s40263-018-0490-z

32. Hamdy RC MD, Doman MR MD, Doman KH. Fatigue. In: Auday BC, Buratovich MA, Marrocco GF, Moglia P, ed. *Magill's Medical Guide.* 8th ed. Amenia, NY: Salem Press, 2018: 900–901.

33. Aaronson LS, Teel CS, Cassmeyer V, et al. Defining and measuring fatigue. *J Nurs Scholarsh.* 2007;31(1):45–50. doi:10.1111/j.1547-5069.1999.tb00420.x

34. Yennurajalingam S, Bruera E. Palliative management of fatigue at the close of life: "It feels like my body is just worn out." *JAMA.* 2007;297(3):295–304. doi:10.1001/jama.297.3.295

35. National Comprehensive Cancer Network. NCCN guidelines version 2.2020 Cancer-related fatigue. 2021. Available at https://www.nccn.org/professionals/physician_gls/pdf/fatigue.pdf

36. Koesel N, Synyder R. Fatigue. In: Dahlin C, Morienes Tycon L, Root M, eds. *Core Curriculum for the Hospice and Palliative Advanced Practice Registered Nurse.* 3rd ed. Pittsburgh, PA: Hospice and Palliative Nurses Association; 2020: 603–612.

37. Unger ER, Lin JS, Brimmer DJ, et al. CDC grand rounds: Chronic fatigue syndrome: Advancing research and clinical education. *MMWR Morb Mortal Wkly Rep.* 2016;65(50–51):1434–1438. doi:10.15585/mmwr.mm655051a4

38. O'Higgins CM, Brady B, O'Connor B, Walsh D, Reilly RB. The pathophysiology of cancer-related fatigue: Current controversies. *Support Care Cancer.* 2018;26(10):3353–3364. doi:10.1007/s00520-018-4318-7

39. Matura LA, Malone S, Jaime-Lara R, Riegel B. A systematic review of biological mechanisms of fatigue in chronic illness. *Biol Res Nurs.* 2018;20(4):410–421. doi:10.1177/1099800418764326

40. Saligan LN, Olson K, Filler K, et al. The biology of cancer-related fatigue: A review of the literature [published correction appears in Support Care Cancer. 2015 Sep;23(9):2853. *Support Care Cancer.* 2015;23(8):2461–2478. doi:10.1007/s00520-015-2763-0

41. Borren NZ, van der Woude CJ, Ananthakrishnan AN. Fatigue in IBD: Epidemiology, pathophysiology and management. *Nat Rev Gastroenterol Hepatol.* 2019;16(4):247–259. doi:10.1038/s41575-018-0091-9

42. Zielinski MR, Systrom DM, Rose NR. Fatigue, sleep, and autoimmune and related disorders. *Front Immunol.* 2019;10:1827. doi:10.3389/fimmu.2019.01827

43. Rottoli M, La Gioia S, Frigeni B, Barcella V. Pathophysiology, assessment and management of multiple sclerosis fatigue: An update. *Expert Rev Neurother.* 2017;17(4):373–379. doi:10.1080/14737175.2017.1247695

44. Chou KL, Gilman S, Bohnen NI. Association between autonomic dysfunction and fatigue in Parkinson disease. *J Neurol Sci.* 2017;377:190–192. doi:10.1016/j.jns.2017.04.023

45. Escalante CP, Chisolm S, Song J, et al. Fatigue, symptom burden, and health-related quality of life in patients with myelodysplastic syndrome, aplastic anemia, and paroxysmal nocturnal hemoglobinuria. *Cancer Med.* 2019;8(2):543–553. doi:10.1002/cam4.1953

46. Prochaska MT, Newcomb R, Block G, Park B, Meltzer DO. Association between anemia and fatigue in hospitalized patients: Does the measure of anemia matter?. *J Hosp Med.* 2017;12(11):898–904. doi:10.12788/jhm.2832

47. Blomberg J, Gottfries CG, Elfaitouri A, Rizwan M, Rosén A. Infection elicited autoimmunity and myalgic encephalomyelitis/chronic fatigue syndrome: An explanatory model. *Front Immunol.* 2018;9:229. doi:10.3389/fimmu.2018.00229

48. Reinertsen KV, Engebraaten O, Loge JH, et al. Fatigue during and after breast cancer therapy: A prospective study. *J*

Pain Symptom Manage. 2017;53(3):551–560. doi:10.1016/j.jpainsymman.2016.09.011

49. Bower JE. The role of neuro-immune interactions in cancer-related fatigue: Biobehavioral risk factors and mechanisms. *Cancer.* 2019;125(3):353–364. doi:10.1002/cncr.31790

50. Natelson BH, Lin JS, Lange G, Khan S, Stegner A, Unger ER. The effect of comorbid medical and psychiatric diagnoses on chronic fatigue syndrome. *Ann Med.* 2019;51(7–8):371–378. doi:10.1080/07853890.2019.1683601

51. Scott K, Posmontier B. Exercise interventions to reduce cancer-related fatigue and improve health-related quality of life in cancer patients. *Holist Nurs Pract.* 2017;31(2):66–79. doi:10.1097/HNP.0000000000000194

52. Nunes MDR, Jacob E, Bomfim EO, et al. Fatigue and health related quality of life in children and adolescents with cancer. *Eur J Oncol Nurs.* 2017;29:39–46. doi:10.1016/j.ejon.2017.05.001

53. Rodríguez Antolín A, Martínez-Piñeiro L, Jiménez Romero ME, et al. Prevalence of fatigue and impact on quality of life in castration resistant prostate cancer patients: The VITAL study. *BMC Urol.* 2019;19(1):92. doi:10.1186/s12894-019-0527-8

54. Morrison EJ, Novotny PJ, Sloan JA, et al. Emotional problems, quality of life, and symptom burden in patients with lung cancer. *Clin Lung Cancer.* 2017;18(5):497–503. doi:10.1016/j.cllc.2017.02.008

55. Akin S, Kas Guner C. Investigation of the relationship among fatigue, self-efficacy and quality of life during chemotherapy in patients with breast, lung or gastrointestinal cancer. *Eur J Cancer Care.* 2019;28(1):e12898. doi:10.1111/ecc.12898

56. Joly F, Ahmed-Lecheheb D, Kalbacher E, et al. Long-term fatigue and quality of life among epithelial ovarian cancer survivors: A GINECO case/control VIVROVAIRE I study. *Ann Oncol.* 2019;30(5):845–852. doi:10.1093/annonc/mdz074

57. Porro B, Michel A, Zinzindohoué C, et al. Quality of life, fatigue and changes therein as predictors of return to work during breast cancer treatment. *Scand J Caring Sci.* 2019;33(2):467–477. doi:10.1111/scs.12646

58. Lim KE, Kim SR, Kim HK, Kim SR. Symptom clusters and quality of life in subjects with COPD. *Respir Care.* 2017;62(9):1203–1211. doi:10.4187/respcare.05374

59. Hoffmann S, Ramm J, Grittner U, Kohler S, Siedler J, Meisel A. Fatigue in myasthenia gravis: Risk factors and impact on quality of life. *Brain Behav.* 2016;6(10):e00538. doi:10.1002/brb3.538

60. Kouijzer M, Brusse-Keizer M, Bode C. COPD-related fatigue: Impact on daily life and treatment opportunities from the patient's perspective. *Respir Med.* 2018;141:47–51. doi:10.1016/j.rmed.2018.06.011

61. Schmidt S, Jöstingmeyer P. Depression, fatigue and disability are independently associated with quality of life in patients with multiple sclerosis: Results of a cross-sectional study. *Mult Scler Relat Disord.* 2019;35:262–269. doi:10.1016/j.msard.2019.07.029

62. Biernacki T, Sandi D, Kincses ZT, et al. Contributing factors to health-related quality of life in multiple sclerosis. *Brain Behav.* 2019;9(12):e01466. doi:10.1002/brb3.1466

63. Zengarini E, Ruggiero C, Pérez-Zepeda MU, et al. Fatigue: Relevance and implications in the aging population. *Exp Gerontol.* 2015;70:78–83. doi:10.1016/j.exger.2015.07.011

64. Cajanding RJ. Causes, assessment and management of fatigue in critically ill patients. *Br J Nurs.* 2017;26(21):1176–1181. doi:10.12968/bjon.2017.26.21.1176

65. National Institute of Health. National Cancer Institute. Fatigue (PDQ°). January 28, 2021. http://cancer.gov/cancertopics/pdq/supportivecare/fatigue/HealthProfessional.

66. Hirsch JK, Sirois FM. Hope and fatigue in chronic illness: The role of perceived stress. *J Health Psychol.* 2016;21(4):451–456. doi:10.1177/1359105314527142

67. Davis MP, Lagman R, Parala A, et al. Hope, symptoms, and palliative care. *Am J Hosp Palliat Care.* 2017;34(3):223–232. doi:10.1177/1049909115627772

68. Steffen LE, Cheavens JS, Vowles KE, et al. Hope-related goal cognitions and daily experiences of fatigue, pain, and functional concern among lung cancer patients. *Support Care Cancer.* 2020;28(2):827–835. doi:10.1007/s00520-019-04878-y

69. Schvartsman G, Park M, Liu DD, Yennu S, Bruera E, Hui D. Could objective tests be used to measure fatigue in patients with advanced cancer?. *J Pain Symptom Manage.* 2017;54(2):237–244. doi:10.1016/j.jpainsymman.2016.12.341

70. Partridge AH, Jacobsen PB, Andersen BL. Challenges to standardizing the care for adult cancer survivors: Highlighting ASCO's fatigue and anxiety and depression guidelines. *Am Soc Clin Oncol Educ Book.* 2015;188–194. doi:10.14694/EdBook_AM.2015.35.188

71. Tseng BY, Gajewski BJ, Kluding PM. Reliability, responsiveness, and validity of the visual analog fatigue scale to measure exertion fatigue in people with chronic stroke: A preliminary study. *Stroke Res Treat.* 2010;2010:412964. doi:10.4061/2010/412964

72. Donovan KA, Stein KD, Lee M, Leach CR, Ilozumba O, Jacobsen PB. Systematic review of the multidimensional fatigue symptom inventory-short form. *Support Care Cancer.* 2015;23(1):191–212. doi:10.1007/s00520-014-2389-7

73. Chow S, Wan BA, Pidduck W, et al. Symptoms predictive of overall quality of life using the Edmonton Symptom Assessment Scale in breast cancer patients receiving radiotherapy. *Clin Breast Cancer.* 2019;19(6):405–410. doi:10.1016/j.clbc.2019.05.007

74. Graham J, Gingerich J, Lambert P, Alamri A, Czaykowski P. Baseline Edmonton Symptom Assessment System and survival in metastatic renal cell carcinoma. *Curr Oncol.* 2018;25(4):e319-e323. doi:10.3747/co.25.3935

75. Stapleton SJ, Holden J, Epstein J, Wilkie DJ. A Systematic review of the Symptom Distress Scale in advanced cancer studies. *Cancer Nurs.* 2016;39(4):E9-E23. doi:10.1097/NCC.0000000000000292

76. Chen YW, Coxson HO, Reid WD. Reliability and validity of the Brief Fatigue Inventory and Dyspnea Inventory in people with chronic obstructive pulmonary disease. *J Pain Symptom Manage.* 2016;52(2):298–304. doi:10.1016/j.jpainsymman.2016.02.018

77. Montan I, Löwe B, Cella D, Mehnert A, Hinz A. General population norms for the Functional Assessment of Chronic Illness Therapy (FACIT)-Fatigue scale. *Value Health.* 2018;21(11):1313–1321. doi:10.1016/j.jval.2018.03.013

78. Ozyemisci-Taskiran O, Batur EB, Yuksel S, Cengiz M, Karatas GK. Validity and reliability of fatigue severity scale in stroke. *Top Stroke Rehabil.* 2019;26(2):122–127. doi:10.1080/10749357.2018.1550957

79. Minton O, Stone P. A systematic review of the scales used for the measurement of cancer-related fatigue (CRF). *Ann Oncol.* 2009;20(1):17–25. doi:10.1093/annonc/mdn537

80. Hinz A, Benzing C, Brähler E, et al. Psychometric properties of the Multidimensional Fatigue Inventory (MFI-20), derived from seven samples. *J Pain Symptom Manage.* 2020;59(3):717–723. doi:10.1016/j.jpainsymman.2019.12.005

81. Hann DM, Jacobsen PB, Azzarello LM, et al. Measurement of fatigue in cancer patients: Development and validation of the Fatigue Symptom Inventory. *Qual Life Res.* 1998;7(4):301–310. doi:10.1023/a:1024929829627

82. Chilcot J, Norton S, Kelly ME, Moss-Morris R. The Chalder Fatigue Questionnaire is a valid and reliable measure of perceived fatigue severity in multiple sclerosis. *Mult Scler.* 2016;22(5):677–684. doi:10.1177/1352458515598019

83. Hendriks C, Drent M, Elfferich M, De Vries J. The Fatigue Assessment Scale: Quality and availability in sarcoidosis and other diseases. *Curr Opin Pulm Med.* 2018;24(5):495–503. doi:10.1097/MCP.0000000000000496

84. Al Maqbali M, Hughes C, Gracey J, Rankin J, Dunwoody L, Hacker E. Quality assessment criteria: Psychometric properties of measurement tools for cancer related fatigue. *Acta Oncol.* 2019;58(9):1286–1297. doi:10.1080/0284186X.2019.1622773

85. Nadler PL, Gonzales R. Common symptoms. In: Papadakis MA, McPhee SJ, eds. *Current Medical Diagnosis & Treatment.* 55th ed. New York: McGraw-Hill Education; 2016: 37–38.

86. Hernández-Quiles C, Bernabeu-Wittel M, Pérez-Belmonte LM, et al. Concordance of Barthel Index, ECOG-PS, and Palliative Performance Scale in the assessment of functional status in patients with advanced medical diseases. *BMJ Support Palliat Care*. 2017;7(3):300–307. doi:10.1136/bmjspcare-2015-001073

87. Ingham G, Urban K. How confident are we at assessing and managing fatigue in palliative care patients? A multicentre survey exploring the current attitudes of palliative care professionals. *Palliat Med Rep*. 2020;1:1, 58–65, doi:10.1089/pmr.2020.0005

88. Wang N, Yang Z, Miao J, et al. Clinical management of cancer-related fatigue in hospitalized adult patients: A best practice implementation project. *JBI Database System Rev Implement Rep*. 2018;16(10):2038–2049. doi:10.11124/JBISRIR-2017-003769

89. O'Neil-Page E, Dean GE, Anderson PR. Fatigue. In: Ferrell BR, Paice JA, eds. *Oxford Textbook of Palliative Nursing*. 5th ed. New York: Oxford University Press, 2019: 132–139.

90. Mustian KM, Alfano CM, Heckler C, et al. Comparison of pharmaceutical, psychological, and exercise treatments for cancer-related fatigue: A meta-analysis. *JAMA Oncol*. 2017;3(7):961–968. doi:10.1001/jamaoncol.2016.6914

91. Murillo-Rodríguez E, Barciela Veras A, Barbosa Rocha N, Budde H, Machado S. An overview of the clinical uses, pharmacology, and safety of modafinil. *ACS Chem Neurosci*. 2018;9(2):151–158. doi:10.1021/acschemneuro.7b00374

92. Mücke M; Mochamat, Cuhls H, et al. Pharmacological treatments for fatigue associated with palliative care. *Cochrane Database Syst Rev*. 2015;2015(5):CD006788. doi:10.1002/14651858.CD006788.pub3

93. Fabi A, Bhargava R, Fatigoni S, et al. Cancer-related fatigue: ESMO Clinical Practice Guidelines for diagnosis and treatment. *Annals of Oncology*. 2020;31(6):713–723. doi:10.1016/j.annonc.2020.02.016

94. Andrew BN, Guan NC, Jaafar NRN. The use of methylphenidate for physical and psychological symptoms in cancer patients: A review. *Curr Drug Targets*. 2018;19(8):877–887. doi:10.2174/1389450118666170317162603

95. Hagmann C, Cramer A, Kestenbaum A, et al. Evidence-based palliative care approaches to non-pain physical symptom management in cancer patients. *Semin Oncol Nurs*. 2018;34(3):227–240. doi:10.1016/j.soncn.2018.06.004

96. Qu D, Zhang Z, Yu X, Zhao J, Qiu F, Huang J. Psychotropic drugs for the management of cancer-related fatigue: A systematic review and meta-analysis. *Eur J Cancer Care (Engl)*. 2016;25(6):970–979. doi:10.1111/ecc.12397

97. Cameron MH, McMillan G. Methylphenidate is likely less effective than placebo for improving imbalance, walking, and fatigue in people with multiple sclerosis. *Mult Scler*. 2017;23(13):1799–1801. doi:10.1177/1352458517692421

98. Miller P, Soundy A. The pharmacological and non-pharmacological interventions for the management of fatigue related multiple sclerosis. *J Neurol Sci*. 2017;381:41–54. doi:10.1016/j.jns.2017.08.012

99. Rojí R, Centeno C. The use of methylphenidate to relieve fatigue. *Curr Opin Support Palliat Care*. 2017;11(4):299–305. doi:10.1097/SPC.0000000000000296

100. Pedersen L, Lund L, Petersen MA, Sjogren P, Groenvold M. Methylphenidate as needed for fatigue in patients with advanced cancer: A prospective, double-blind, and placebo-controlled study [published online ahead of print, 2020 May 26]. *J Pain Symptom Manage*. 2020;S0885-3924(20)30427-9

101. Tomlinson D, Robinson PD, Oberoi S, et al. Pharmacologic interventions for fatigue in cancer and transplantation: A meta-analysis. *Curr Oncol*. 2018;25(2):e152-e167. doi:10.3747/co.25.3883

102. Mohandas H, Jaganathan SK, Mani MP, Ayyar M, Rohini Thevi GV. Cancer-related fatigue treatment: An overview. *J Cancer Res Ther*. 2017;13(6):916–929. doi:10.4103/jcrt.JCRT_50_17

103. Pearson EJM, Morris ME, di Stefano M, McKinstry CE. Interventions for cancer-related fatigue: A scoping review. *Eur J Cancer Care (Engl)*. 2018;27(1):10.1111/ecc.12516. doi:10.1111/ecc.12516

104. Mitchell GK, Hardy JR, Nikles CJ, et al. The effect of methylphenidate on fatigue in advanced cancer: An aggregated n-of-1 trial. *J Pain Symptom Manage*. 2015;50(3):289–296. doi:10.1016/j.jpainsymman.2015.03.009

105. Kapugi M, Cunningham K. Corticosteroids. *Orthop Nurs*. 2019;38(5):336–339. doi:10.1097/NOR.0000000000000595

106. Begley S, Rose K, O'Connor M. The use of corticosteroids in reducing cancer-related fatigue: Assessing the evidence for clinical practice. *Int J Palliat Nurs*. 2016 Jan;22(1):5–9. doi:10.12968/ijpn.2016.22.1.5. PMID: 26804950

107. Yennurajalingam S, Williams JL, Chisholm G, Bruera E. Effects of dexamethasone and placebo on symptom clusters in advanced cancer patients: A preliminary report. *Oncologist*. 2016;21(3):384–390. doi:10.1634/theoncologist.2014-0260

108. Fukuoka S, Shitara K, Noguchi M, et al. Prophylactic use of oral dexamethasone to alleviate fatigue during regorafenib treatment for patients with metastatic colorectal cancer. *Clin Colorectal Cancer*. 2017;16(2):e39-e44. doi:10.1016/j.clcc.2016.07.012

109. Kanbayashi Y, Hosokawa T. Predictors of the usefulness of corticosteroids for cancer-related fatigue in end-of-life patients. *Clin Drug Investig*. 37(4):387–392. doi:10.1007/s40261-017-0493-4

110. Jaward LR, O'Neil TA, Marks A, Smith MA. Differences in adverse effect profiles of corticosteroids in palliative care patients. *Am J Hosp Palliat Care*. 2019;36(2):158–168. doi:10.1177/1049909118797283

111. Oray M, Abu Samra K, Ebrahimiadib N, Meese H, Foster CS. Long-term side effects of glucocorticoids. *Expert Opin Drug Saf*. 2016;15(4):457–465. doi:10.1517/14740338.2016.1140741

112. Giles AJ, Hutchinson MND, Sonnemann HM, et al. Dexamethasone-induced immunosuppression: Mechanisms and implications for immunotherapy. *J Immunother Cancer*. 2018;6(1):51. doi:10.1186/s40425-018-0371-5

113. Corfield EC, Martin NG, Nyholt DR. Co-occurrence and symptomatology of fatigue and depression. *Compr Psychiatry*. 2016;71:1–10. doi:10.1016/j.comppsych.2016.08.004

114. Harmer CJ, Duman RS, Cowen PJ. How do antidepressants work? New perspectives for refining future treatment approaches. *Lancet Psychiatry*. 2017;4(5):409–418. doi:10.1016/S2215-0366(17)30015-9

115. Mohandas H, Thevi GVR, Jaganathan SK, Mani MP, Ayyar M. Cancer-related fatigue treatment: An overview. *J Cancer Res Ther*. 2017;13(6):916–929. doi:10.4103/jcrt.JCRT_50_17

116. Zaini S, Guan NC, Sulaiman AH, Zainal NZ, Huri HZ, Shamsudin SH. The use of antidepressants for physical and psychological symptoms in cancer. *Curr Drug Targets*. 2018;19(12):1431–1455. doi:10.2174/1389450119666180226125026

117. Ashrafi F, Mousavi S, Karimi M. Potential role of bupropion sustained release for cancer-related fatigue: A double-blind, placebo-controlled study. *Asian Pac J Cancer Prev*. 2018;19(6):1547–1551. doi:10.22034/APJCP.2018.19.6.1547

118. Salehifar E, Azimi S, Janbabai G, et al. Efficacy and safety of bupropion in cancer-related fatigue, a randomized double blind placebo controlled clinical trial. *BMC Cancer*. 2020;20(1):158. doi:10.1186/s12885-020-6618-9

119. Auday BC PhD. Antidepressants. *Magill's Medical Guide*. In: Auday BC, Buratovich MA, Marrocco GF, Moglia P, ed. *Magill's Medical Guide*. 8th ed. Amenia, NY: Salem Press, 2018:163–164.

120. Marx W, Teleni L, Opie RS, et al. Efficacy and effectiveness of carnitine supplementation for cancer-related fatigue: A systematic literature review and meta-analysis. *Nutrients*. 2017;9(11):1224. doi:10.3390/nu9111224

121. Yang TT, Wang L, Deng XY, Yu G. Pharmacological treatments for fatigue in patients with multiple sclerosis: A systematic review and meta-analysis. *J Neurol Sci*. 2017;380:256–261. doi:10.1016/j.jns.2017.07.042

122. Pereira PTVT, Reis AD, Diniz RR, et al. Dietary supplements and fatigue in patients with breast cancer: A systematic review. *Breast Cancer Res Treat*. 2018;171(3):515–526. doi:10.1007/s10549-018-4857-0

123. Yennurajalingam S, Reddy A, Tannir NM, et al. High-dose Asian ginseng (panax ginseng) for cancer-related fatigue: A preliminary report. *Integr Cancer Ther.* 2015;14(5):419–427. doi:10.1177/1534735415580676

124. Arring NM, Millstine D, Marks LA, Nail LM. Ginseng as a treatment for fatigue: A systematic review. *J Altern Complement Med.* 2018;24(7):624–633. doi:10.1089/acm.2017.0361

125. Raizner AE. Coenzyme Q10. *Methodist Debakey Cardiovasc J.* 2019;15(3):185–191. doi:10.14797/mdcj-15-3-185

126. Sanoobar M, Dehghan P, Khalili M, Azimi A, Seifar F. Coenzyme Q10 as a treatment for fatigue and depression in multiple sclerosis patients: A double blind randomized clinical trial. *Nutr Neurosci.* 2016;19(3):138–141. doi:10.1179/1476830515Y.0000000002

127. Ribeiro SMF, Braga CBM, Peria FM, Martinez EZ, Rocha JJRD, Cunha SFC. Effects of zinc supplementation on fatigue and quality of life in patients with colorectal cancer. *Einstein (Sao Paulo).* 2017;15(1):24–28. doi:10.1590/S1679-45082017AO3830

128. Klasson C, Helde-Frankling M, Sandberg C, Nordström M, Lundh-Hagelin C, Björkhem-Bergman L. Vitamin D and fatigue in palliative cancer: A cross-sectional study of sex difference in baseline data from the Palliative D Cohort. [published online ahead of print, 2020 Sep 16]. *J Palliat Med.* 2020;10.1089/jpm.2020.0283. doi:10.1089/jpm.2020.0283

129. Iwase S, Kawaguchi T, Yotsumoto D, et al. Efficacy and safety of an amino acid jelly containing coenzyme Q10 and L-carnitine in controlling fatigue in breast cancer patients receiving chemotherapy: A multi-institutional, randomized, exploratory trial (JORTC-CAM01). *Support Care Cancer.* 2016;24(2):637–646. doi:10.1007/s00520-015-2824-4

130. Chang YD, Smith J, Portman D, et al. Single institute experience with methylphenidate and american ginseng in cancer-related fatigue. *Am J Hosp Palliat Care.* 2018;35(1):144–150. doi:10.1177/1049909117695733

131. Wendebourg MJ, Heesen C, Finlayson M, Meyer B, Pöttgen J, Köpke S. Patient education for people with multiple sclerosis-associated fatigue: A systematic review. *PLoS One.* 2017;12(3):e0173025. doi:10.1371/journal.pone.0173025

132. Bennett S, Pigott A, Beller EM, Haines T, Meredith P, Delaney C. Educational interventions for the management of cancer-related fatigue in adults. *Cochrane Database Syst Rev.* 2016;11(11):CD008144. doi:10.1002/14651858.CD008144.pub2

133. Hilfiker R, Meichtry A, Eicher M, et al. Exercise and other non-pharmaceutical interventions for cancer-related fatigue in patients during or after cancer treatment: A systematic review incorporating an indirect-comparisons meta-analysis. *Br J Sports Med.* 2018;52(10):651–658. doi:10.1136/bjsports-2016-096422

134. Juvet LK, Thune I, Elvsaas IKØ, et al. The effect of exercise on fatigue and physical functioning in breast cancer patients during and after treatment and at 6 months follow-up: A meta-analysis. *Breast.* 2017;33:166–177. doi:10.1016/j.breast.2017.04.003

135. Scott K, Posmontier B. Exercise interventions to reduce cancer-related fatigue and improve health-related quality of life in cancer patients. *Holist Nurs Pract.* 2017;31(2):66–79. doi:10.1097/HNP.0000000000000194

136. Zhou W, Wan YH, Chen Q, Qiu YR, Luo XM. Effects of tai chi exercise on cancer-related fatigue in patients with nasopharyngeal carcinoma undergoing chemoradiotherapy: A randomized controlled trial. *J Pain Symptom Manage.* 2018;55(3):737–744. doi:10.1016/j.jpainsymman.2017.10.021

137. Bourke L, Smith D, Steed L, et al. Exercise for men with prostate cancer: A systematic review and meta-analysis. *Eur Urol.* 2016;69(4):693–703. doi:10.1016/j.eururo.2015.10.047

138. Yang B, Wang J. Effects of exercise on cancer-related fatigue and quality of life in prostate cancer patients undergoing androgen deprivation therapy: A meta-analysis of randomized clinical trials. *Chin Med Sci J.* 2017;32(1):13–21. doi:10.24920/j1001-9242.2007.002

139. Taaffe DR, Newton RU, Spry N, et al. Effects of different exercise modalities on fatigue in prostate cancer patients undergoing androgen deprivation therapy: A year-long randomised controlled trial. *Eur Urol.* 2017;72(2):293–299. doi:10.1016/j.eururo.2017.02.019

140. Lipsett A, Barrett S, Haruna F, Mustian K, O'Donovan A. The impact of exercise during adjuvant radiotherapy for breast cancer on fatigue and quality of life: A systematic review and meta-analysis. *Breast.* 2017;32:144–155. doi:10.1016/j.breast.2017.02.002

141. Galiano-Castillo N, Cantarero-Villanueva I, Fernández-Lao C, et al. Telehealth system: A randomized controlled trial evaluating the impact of an internet-based exercise intervention on quality of life, pain, muscle strength, and fatigue in breast cancer survivors. *Cancer.* 2016;122(20):3166–3174. doi:10.1002/cncr.30172

142. Kim S, Han J, Lee MY, Jang MK. The experience of cancer-related fatigue, exercise and exercise adherence among women breast cancer survivors: Insights from focus group interviews. *J Clin Nurs.* 2020;29(5-6):758–769. doi:10.1111/jocn.15114

143. Pyszora A, Budzyński J, Wójcik A, Prokop A, Krajnik M. Physiotherapy programme reduces fatigue in patients with advanced cancer receiving palliative care: Randomized controlled trial. *Support Care Cancer.* 2017 Sep;25(9):2899–2908. doi:10.1007/s00520-017-3742-4

144. Galeoto G, Sansoni J, Valenti D, et al. The effect of physiotherapy on fatigue and physical functioning in chronic fatigue syndrome patients: A systematic review. *Clin Ter.* 2018;169(4):e184-e188. doi:10.7417/T.2018.2076

145. Larun L, Brurberg KG, Odgaard-Jensen J, Price JR. Exercise therapy for chronic fatigue syndrome [published online ahead of print, 2019 Oct 2]. *Cochrane Database Syst Rev.* 2019;10(10):CD003200. doi:10.1002/14651858.CD003200.pub8

146. Halabchi F, Alizadeh Z, Sahraian MA, Abolhasani M. Exercise prescription for patients with multiple sclerosis: Potential benefits and practical recommendations. *BMC Neurol.* 2017;17(1):185. doi:10.1186/s12883-017-0960-9

147. Hasanpour Dehkordi A. Influence of yoga and aerobics exercise on fatigue, pain and psychosocial status in patients with multiple sclerosis: A randomized trial. *J Sports Med Phys Fitness.* 2016;56(11):1417–1422.

148. Negaresh R, Motl R, Mokhtarzade M, et al. E Effect of short-term interval exercise training on fatigue, depression, and fitness in normal weight vs. overweight person with multiple sclerosis. *Explore (NY).* 2019;15(2):134–141. doi:10.1016/j.explore.2018.07.007

149. Grubić Kezele T, Babić M, Štimac D. Exploring the feasibility of a mild and short 4-week combined upper limb and breathing exercise program as a possible home base program to decrease fatigue and improve quality of life in ambulatory and non-ambulatory multiple sclerosis individuals. *Neurol Sci.* 2019;40(4):733–741. doi:10.1007/s10072-019-3707-0

150. Razazian N, Yavari Z, Farnia V, et al. Exercising impacts on fatigue, depression, and paresthesia in female patients with multiple sclerosis. *Med Sci Sports Exerc.* 2016;48(5):796–803. doi:10.1249/MSS.0000000000000834

151. Song YY, Hu RJ, Diao YS, Chen L, Jiang XL. Effects of exercise training on restless legs syndrome, depression, sleep quality, and fatigue among hemodialysis patients: A systematic review and meta-analysis. *J Pain Symptom Manage.* 2018;55(4):1184–1195. doi:10.1016/j.jpainsymman.2017.12.472

152. Høgdal N, Eidemak I, Sjøgren P, Larsen H, Sørensen J, Christensen J. Occupational therapy and physiotherapy interventions in palliative care: A cross-sectional study of patient-reported needs [published online ahead of print, 2020 Aug 11]. *BMJ Support Palliat Care.* 2020;bmjspcare-2020-002337. doi:10.1136/bmjspcare-2020-002337

153. Tavemark S, Hermansson LN, Blomberg K. Enabling activity in palliative care: Focus groups among occupational therapists. *BMC Palliat Care.* 2019;18(1):17. doi:10.1186/s12904-019-0394-9

154. Lin D, Borjan M, San Andres SD, Kelly C. The role of PT, OT, and other therapies in palliative care for seriously ill patients. In: Ferrell B, Paice, JA, eds. *Oxford Textbook of Palliative Nursing.* 5th ed. New York: Oxford University Press; 2019:682–689.

155. Lau CH, Wu X, Chung VC, et al. Acupuncture and related therapies for symptom management in palliative cancer care: Systematic review and meta-analysis. *Medicine (Baltimore)*. 2016;95(9):e2901. doi:10.1097/MD.0000000000002901

156. Howell D, Keshavarz H, Braodfield L, et al. A pan-Canadian practice guideline for screening, assessment, and management of cancer-related fatigue in adults. Verson 2- 2015. 2015. https://era.library.ualberta.ca/items/8b8823da-1858-46f1-bb08-8811cd1a5a74

157. Lyman GH, Bohlke K, Cohen L. Integrative therapies during and after breast cancer treatment: ASCO endorsement of the SIO clinical practice guideline summary. *J Oncol Pract*. 2018;14(8):495–499. doi:10.1200/JOP.18.00283

158. Greenlee H, DuPont-Reyes MJ, Balneaves LG, et al. Clinical practice guidelines on the evidence-based use of integrative therapies during and after breast cancer treatment. *CA Cancer J Clin*. 2017;67(3):194–232. doi:10.3322/caac.21397

159. Zeng YS, Wang C, Ward KE, Hume AL. Complementary and alternative medicine in hospice and palliative care: A systematic review. *J Pain Symptom Manage*. 2018;56(5):781-794.e4. doi:10.1016/j.jpainsymman.2018.07.016

160. Wu X, Chung VC, Hui EP, et al. Effectiveness of acupuncture and related therapies for palliative care of cancer: Overview of systematic reviews. *Sci Rep*. 2015;5:16776. doi:10.1038/srep16776

161. Zhang Q, Gong J, Dong H, Xu S, Wang W, Huang G. Acupuncture for chronic fatigue syndrome: A systematic review and meta-analysis. *Acupunct Med*. 2019;37(4):211–222. doi:10.1136/acupmed-2017-011582

162. Cheng CS, Chen LY, Ning ZY, et al. Acupuncture for cancer-related fatigue in lung cancer patients: A randomized, double blind, placebo-controlled pilot trial. *Support Care Cancer*. 2017;25(12):3807–3814. doi:10.1007/s00520-017-3812-7

163. Xiong W, He FF, You RY, et al. Acupuncture application in chronic kidney disease and its potential mechanisms. *Am J Chin Med*. 2018;46(6):1169–1185. doi:10.1142/S0192415X18500611

164. Kim KH, Lee MS, Kim TH, Kang JW, Choi TY, Lee JD. Acupuncture and related interventions for symptoms of chronic kidney disease. *Cochrane Database Syst Rev*. 2016;(6):CD009440. doi:10.1002/14651858.CD009440.pub2

165. Kim S, Chang L, Weinstock-Guttman B, et al. Complementary and alternative medicine usage by multiple sclerosis patients: Results from a prospective clinical study. *J Altern Complement Med*. 2018;24(6):596–602. doi:10.1089/acm.2017.0268

166. Khanghah AG, Rizi MS, Nabi BN, Adib M, Leili EKN. Effects of acupressure on fatigue in patients with cancer who underwent chemotherapy. *J Acupunct Meridian Stud*. 2019;12(4):103–110. doi:10.1016/j.jams.2019.07.003

167. Miller KR, Patel JN, Symanowski JT, Edelen CA, Walsh D. Acupuncture for cancer pain and symptom management in a palliative medicine clinic. *Am J Hosp Palliat Care*. 2019;36(4):326–332. doi:10.1177/1049909118804464

168. Sand-Jecklin K, Reiser V. Use of Seva stress release acupressure to reduce pain, stress, and fatigue in patients hospitalized for cancer treatment. *J Hosp Palliat Nurs*. 2018;20(6):521–528. doi:10.1097/NJH.0000000000000484

169. Zick SM, Sen A, Wyatt GK, Murphy SL, Arnedt JT, Harris RE. Investigation of 2 types of self-administered acupressure for persistent cancer-related fatigue in breast cancer survivors: A randomized clinical trial. *JAMA Oncol*. 2016;2(11):1470–1476. doi:10.1001/jamaoncol.2016.1867

170. Coelho A, Parola V, Cardoso D, Bravo ME, Apóstolo J. Use of non-pharmacological interventions for comforting patients in palliative care: A scoping review. *JBI Database System Rev Implement Rep*. 2017;15(7):1867–1904. doi:10.11124/JBISRIR-2016-003204

171. Shin ES, Seo KH, Lee SH, et al. Massage with or without aromatherapy for symptom relief in people with cancer. *Cochrane Database Syst Rev*. 2016;(6):CD009873. doi:10.1002/14651858.CD009873.pub3

172. Wilson A. Massage with or without aromatherapy for symptom relief in people with cancer. *Res Nurs Health*. 2018;41(6):593–594. doi:10.1002/nur.21916

173. Kinkead B, Schettler PJ, Larson ER, et al. Massage therapy decreases cancer-related fatigue: Results from a randomized early phase trial. *Cancer*. 2018;124(3):546–554. doi:10.1002/cncr.31064

174. Izgu N, Ozdemir L, Bugdayci Basal F. Effect of aromatherapy massage on chemotherapy-induced peripheral neuropathic pain and fatigue in patients receiving oxaliplatin: An open label quasi-randomized controlled pilot study. *Cancer Nurs*. 2019;42(2):139–147. doi:10.1097/NCC.0000000000000577

175. Uysal N, Kutlutürkan S, Uğur I. Effects of foot massage applied in two different methods on symptom control in colorectal cancer patients: Randomised control trial. *Int J Nurs Pract*. 2017;23(3):10.1111/ijn.12532. doi:10.1111/ijn.12532

176. Backus D, Manella C, Bender A, Sweatman M. Impact of massage therapy on fatigue, pain, and spasticity in people with multiple sclerosis: A pilot study. *Int J Ther Massage Bodywork*. 2016;9(4):4–13. doi:10.3822/ijtmb.v9i4.327

177. Wu C, Zheng Y, Duan Y, et al. Nonpharmacological interventions for cancer-related fatigue: A systematic review and Bayesian network meta-analysis. *Worldviews Evid Based Nurs*. 2019;16(2):102–110. doi:10.1111/wvn.12352

178. He J, Hou J, Qi J, Zhang T, Wang Y, Qian M. Mindfulness ased stress reduction interventions for cancer related fatigue: A meta-analysis and systematic review. *Natl Med Assoc*. 2020;112(4):387–394. doi:10.1016/j.jnma.2020.04.006

179. Kwekkeboom K, Zhang Y, Campbell T, et al. Randomized controlled trial of a brief cognitive-behavioral strategies intervention for the pain, fatigue, and sleep disturbance symptom cluster in advanced cancer. *Psychooncology*. 2018;27(12):2761–2769. doi:10.1002/pon.4883

180. Kwekkeboom KL, Bratzke LC. A systematic review of relaxation, meditation, and guided imagery strategies for symptom management in heart failure. *J Cardiovasc Nurs*. 2016;31(5):457–468. doi:10.1097/JCN.0000000000000274

181. Wendebourg MJ, Heesen C, Finlayson M, Meyer B, Pöttgen J, Köpke S. Patient education for people with multiple sclerosis-associated fatigue: A systematic review. *PLoS One*. 2017;12(3):e0173025. doi:10.1371/journal.pone.0173025

182. von Blanckenburg P, Leppin N. Psychological interventions in palliative care. *Curr Opin Psychiatry*. 2018;31(5):389–395. doi:10.1097/YCO.0000000000000441

183. Poort H, Peters M, Bleijenberg G, et al. Psychosocial interventions for fatigue during cancer treatment with palliative intent. *Cochrane Database Syst Rev*. 2017;7(7):CD012030. doi:10.1002/14651858.CD012030.pub2

184. Mendoza ME, Capafons A, Gralow JR, et al. Randomized controlled trial of the Valencia model of waking hypnosis plus CBT for pain, fatigue, and sleep management in patients with cancer and cancer survivors. *Psychooncology*. 2017;26(11):1832–1838. doi:10.1002/pon.4232

185. Chalah MA, Ayache SS. Cognitive behavioral therapies and multiple sclerosis fatigue: A review of literature. *J Clin Neurosci*. 2018;52:1–4. doi:10.1016/j.jocn.2018.03.024

186. Brenner P, Piehl F. Fatigue and depression in multiple sclerosis: Pharmacological and non-pharmacological interventions. *Acta Neurol Scand*. 2016;134 Suppl 200:47–54. doi:10.1111/ane.12648

187. Seyedi Chegeni P, Gholami M, Azargoon A, Hossein Pour AH, Birjandi M, Norollahi H. The effect of progressive muscle relaxation on the management of fatigue and quality of sleep in patients with chronic obstructive pulmonary disease: A randomized controlled clinical trial. *Complement Ther Clin Pract*. 2018;31:64–70. doi:10.1016/j.ctcp.2018.01.010

188. Norman J, Fu M, Ekman I, Björck L, Falk K. Effects of a mindfulness-based intervention on symptoms and signs in chronic heart failure: A feasibility study. *Eur J Cardiovasc Nurs*. 2018;17(1):54–65. doi:10.1177/1474515117715841

189. Zhang Q, Li F, Zhang H, Yu X, Cong Y. Effects of nurse-led home-based exercise and cognitive behavioral therapy on reducing cancer-related fatigue in patients with ovarian cancer during and after chemotherapy: A randomized controlled trial. *Int J Nurs Stud.* 2018;78:52–60. doi:10.1016/j.ijnurstu.2017.08.010

190. Jim HSL, Hyland KA, Nelson AM, et al. Internet-assisted cognitive behavioral intervention for targeted therapy-related fatigue in chronic myeloid leukemia: Results from a pilot randomized trial. *Cancer.* 2020;126(1):174–180. doi:10.1002/cncr.32521

191. Nguyen LT, Alexander K, Yates P. Psychoeducational intervention for symptom management of fatigue, pain, and sleep disturbance cluster among cancer patients: A pilot quasi-experimental study. *J Pain Symptom Manage.* 2018;55(6):1459–1472. doi:10.1016/j.jpainsymman.2018.02.019

42.

NAUSEA AND VOMITING

Katherine E. DeMarco

KEY POINTS

- Nausea and vomiting are different symptom burdens that require the palliative advanced practice registered nurse (APRN) to perform a comprehensive assessment to determine appropriate and personalized interventions for the individual patient.

- When antiemetics are used as part of the management plan, the palliative APRN must consider the etiology of symptoms and use one medication from a pharmacologic class. The simultaneous use of more than one agent from each class is generally avoided to prevent overlapping side effects/toxicities.

- The use of nonpharmacologic interventions as per evidence-based benefits and the patient's condition and values are part of the palliative APRN's approach to the management of nausea and vomiting.

CASE STUDY: NAUSEA AND VOMITING IN CANCER AND PARKINSON'S

Chad was a 75-year-old man with metastatic gastric carcinoma involving his liver and lungs. His past medical history included Parkinson's disease, hypertension (HTN), and gastroesophageal reflux disease (GERD). He reported intermittent nausea and dizziness over the past month and 1–2 episodes of vomiting in the past 3 days. The palliative advanced practice registered nurse (APRN) considered whether his symptoms were due to changes in gastrointestinal (GI) function related to tumor growth in or adjacent to the GI tract (liver metastasis), possible increased intracranial pressure from an undetected central nervous system (CNS) tumor, GERD, constipation, dehydration, reactions to medications, or anxiety.

INTRODUCTION

Both adult and pediatric individuals who have serious or advanced illness can experience nausea and vomiting (N/V). The symptom(s) of N/V affect all the dimensions of quality of life, particularly if the symptoms are protracted.[1,2] Dehydration, electrolyte imbalances, malnutrition, fatigue, and aspiration are common physical sequelae of N/V. Concerns about eating and declining physical function may

lead to feelings of social isolation. The burden of uncontrolled symptoms may lead to feelings of hopelessness and depression. Caregivers may be distressed by their inability to nourish patients. The cost of medications and other direct and indirect care may contribute to distress. If the symptoms are thought to be related to disease-modifying treatments, patients may decide to prematurely stop potentially beneficial therapies. The palliative advanced practice registered nurse (APRN) can positively impact the patient's quality of life and reduce the risk of physical sequelae through a symptom management plan that is based on an understanding of the physiology and pathophysiology of N/V, comprehensive symptom assessment, and formulation of a symptom diagnosis that will direct the use of antiemetic therapies.[1-3] Using national palliative care guidelines, such as the National Consensus Project for Quality Palliative Care *Clinical Practice Guidelines* and the National Comprehensive Cancer Network *Palliative Clinical Practice Guidelines in Oncology* can support the palliative APRN in creating evidence-based and patient-personalized care plans.[4,5]

DEFINITIONS

Although nausea and vomiting are separate symptoms, they are often viewed as a single entity in practice and in the literature. Either may be experienced acutely, chronically, spontaneously, or in response to specific events, such as eating, activity, or medication use. *Nausea* is a subjective unpleasant sensation experienced in the back of the throat and epigastrium and is associated with a perceived need to vomit. Patients may describe queasiness or an upset or unsettled stomach or may use other terms. Nausea may be continuous or intermittent and may have a more negative impact on quality of life than vomiting.[2,6] *Vomiting* is the expulsion of gastric contents through the mouth. It may occur as a single episode or be recurrent. *Retching* or *dry heaves* refers to spasmodic contractions of abdominal muscles and diaphragm that do not result in vomiting.[2,6]

Acute nausea occurs within minutes or hours of a specific event, such as chemotherapy. Temporal co-occurrence of cluster symptoms or delayed N/V occurs at least 24 hours after the stimulus and lasts for 3–7 days.[1] N/V associated with an event may trigger a learned response to similar events in the future, causing anticipatory N/V.[7] Refractory N/V occurs when the symptoms continue to occur even when medications and other interventions are completed.[3] There is no formal definition for chronic nausea. However, in academic research, nausea that last longer than 4 weeks is often considered chronic nausea.[1]

PREVALENCE AND RISK FACTORS

Much of the research and literature on N/V focuses on the experience and management of these symptoms in oncology practice. Up to 80% of adult oncology patients undergoing chemotherapy and/or radiation therapy experience N/V.[7,8] Nausea is more frequently experienced than vomiting. The prevalence rates vary depending on specifics of disease, chemotherapeutic agents used, and anatomic sites of radiation therapy.[7] In oncology patients with advanced disease who are no longer receiving active anti-cancer therapies, the prevalence rate is about 60% for nausea and 30% for vomiting.[7]

N/V is also frequently experienced by patients with other life-limiting or life-threatening illnesses and conditions (Table 42.1). N/V may burden patients with progressive neurological conditions, such as multiple sclerosis and Parkinson's disease.[3,9] As patients near death, the overall prevalence of N/V is 19%, with a range from 8.4% to 70%.[6] A literature review identifies that about 40–70% of individuals experience moderate to severe nausea in the final weeks of life.[10,11] The risk of developing N/V in advanced disease may be higher in patients who are female, are younger, and have a history of low alcohol intake.[7] Other risk factors include treatment with chemotherapy, opioids, antibiotics, and digoxin and the presence of hypercalcemia; fluid and electrolyte imbalances; hepatic, renal, gastrointestinal (GI), and central nervous system (CNS) pathologies; and anxiety.[7,12]

PHYSIOLOGY

The research surrounding chemotherapy-induced N/V (CINV) advanced our understanding of the basic physiology of vomiting. Nausea involves more cerebral involvement and consciousness compared to vomiting,[10] whereas vomiting is a protective reflex designed to rid the body of ingested toxins. Vomiting is controlled in the brainstem by the vomiting center (VC) in the medulla and the chemoreceptor trigger zone (CTZ).[1,10] A number of neurotransmitters and their receptors play an important role in coordination of the reflex. Dopamine/dopamine receptors, γ-aminobutyric acid (GABA), serotonin/5-HT3 receptors, and substance P/neurokinin-1 receptors have the best-described roles.[6,7,10] Cannabinoids and their related receptors, present in the CNS and the GI tract, may also play a role, with synergistic effects on dopamine, serotonin, and neurokinin-1 receptors.[6] Mechanoreceptors in the CNS may also cause N/V symptoms as these receptors are responsive to pressure from stretching and irritation of the meninges.[10]

The vomiting center responds to input from afferent pathways that include the CTZ, the vagus nerve, the cerebral cortex, and the vestibular system. The CTZ is a highly vascular area located in the fourth ventricle of the brain. The lack of a blood–brain barrier at the CTZ allows direct exposure to various drugs, toxins, and metabolites circulating in the blood or cerebrospinal fluid. Dopamine, histamine, serotonin, and substance P are the major neurotransmitters in this pathway.[2,6,7] Studies suggest that there may be synergistic activity between 5-HT3 and neurokinin-1 receptors.[6] In addition, the CTZ responds to signaling from the vagal afferents mediated by the release of serotonin from gastric enterochromaffin cells in response to injury or inflammation of the GI tract, changes in GI motility, and the chemistry of the luminal contents. Oropharyngeal irritants signal the CTZ via the pharyngeal

Table 42.1 PREVALENCE OF NAUSEA AND VOMITING IN NON-ONCOLOGY POPULATION

DISEASE	NAUSEA RATE (%)	VOMITING RATE (%)	NAUSEA AND VOMITING RATE (%)
Liver failure	50		50
Heart failure	50	24	2–48
End-stage renal disease			8–52
HIV/AIDS			41–57
COPD	18	4	4
Motor neuron disease	No data found		
Parkinson's	9.8	4.1	
Dementia			8
Multiple sclerosis	10–40	2	2–78
COVID-19	10–27	8–16	

From Chow et al.[6]; Lee et al.[9]; Higgson et al.[13]; Levinthal et al.[14]; Moens et al.[15]; Elshazli et al.[16]; Dorrell et al.[17]; and Elmunzer et al.[18]

branch of the vagus nerve, with histamine and acetylcholine thought to be the major neurotransmitters. The vagal afferents may also directly stimulate the vomiting center.[10]

The cerebral cortex signals the VC via the midbrain. The primary neurotransmitter may be GABA. Stimuli include anticipation, fear, and memories (e.g., anticipatory vomiting) as well as signals from the senses, such as disturbing sights, smells, or pain. The VC also responds to vestibular input via the inner ear, mediated by histamine and acetylcholine. Motion, certain medications, and changes in intracranial pressure may trigger this pathway. With threshold stimulation of these afferent pathways, the VC triggers the efferent pathways that coordinate the complex sequence of powerful and sustained contractions of the abdominal muscles and diaphragm and relaxation of pyloric and duodenal sphincters that forces expulsion of gastric contents via the mouth.[2,3,12,13]

Physiologic pathways and the central processing of nausea are still poorly understood. At one time, nausea was thought to be caused by subthreshold stimulation of the vomiting pathways, but recent research suggests that the physiology of nausea is different.[14–19] While vomiting is a reflex controlled by lower brain structures, nausea seems to require consciousness and cerebral function.[10] Studies suggest that nausea may be associated with the morphology of the subcortex, along with changes in gastric myoelectrical activity and neuroendocrine responses mediated via the autonomic nervous system and cerebral cortex.[19] The changes in gastric motility are accompanied by a decrease in gastric acid levels and release of cortisol, β-endorphins, epinephrine, and norepinephrine, causing nausea, pallor, cold sweats, tachypnea, tachycardia, and increased salivation.[7,10] The CTZ plays a role in the development of nausea through its effect on GI motility, taste aversion, and food intake.[7]

These different physiological pathways may explain why N/V does not always respond to the same symptom interventions. An example is the continued higher incidence of post-chemotherapy nausea despite the reduced incidence of chemotherapy-induced vomiting with the use of research-based antiemetic guidelines.[20]

ETIOLOGY

Nausea, vomiting, and retching are distinct phenomena that may be experienced acutely, chronically, independently, simultaneously, or sequentially. In palliative care, the etiologies of N/V are often multifactorial and may be related to underlying disease and/or comorbidities, treatment effects, or debility.[1,6,21] Most often, a primary etiology of N/V can be identified and should always be explored.[21]

N/V is often experienced in relation to other symptoms. Clusters of two or more symptoms that consistently occur concurrently may share a common etiology and be synergistic.[22] Studies of N/V in oncology describe clustering of nausea, vomiting, loss of appetite, taste changes, weight loss, and fatigue.[20,22] While not all concurrent symptoms are clusters, the palliative APRN's attention to other symptoms is part of the comprehensive assessment and may suggest etiologies for N/V.

Gastroparesis, occurring in 34–45% of cases, is a common etiology in palliative care that is suggested by intermittent nausea, early satiety, and postprandial bloating relieved by vomiting.[2,21,23] Gastroparesis occurs due to slowed or delayed gastric emptying. Upper GI symptoms such as dyspepsia, N/V, constipation, and gastric outlet obstruction can occur with gastroparesis. Commonly etiologies include a variety of causes, such as diabetic neuropathy, postsurgery of the GI tract, and postinfectious gastroparesis. Lesser common etiologies include stroke, Parkinson's disease, paraneoplastic syndrome, and opioid or anticholinergic medication classes. Since 2000, gastroparesis prevalence has increased in the United States.[24]

Bowel obstruction, occurring in a range of 3% to 30% of cases, may be suggested by the presence of N/V, abdominal pain, altered bowel function, and abdominal distention.[21,25] Bowel obstructions, such as malignant obstructions, occur in 3–15% of individuals with cancer.[25,26] Malignant obstructions can be due to tumor burden or mechanical or functional obstruction, which can occur due to abdominal carcinomatosis, tumor infiltration of the GI musculature, myenteric plexus, or a combination of both. Patients who are diagnosed with ovarian cancer and colon cancer have a higher incidence of bowel obstruction, 20–50% and 10–29%, respectively.[25,26]

Pharyngeal stimulation is suggested by vomiting and gagging associated with cough and difficulty clearing secretions.[21] Persistent nausea unaccompanied by or unrelieved by vomiting may suggest a metabolic and drug-related cause. Opioid use in patients without a previous history of nausea may cause constipation, gastroparesis, and/or stimulation of the CTZ, resulting in a 40% incidence of N/V. Early-morning vomiting associated with headache may suggest increased intracranial pressure. Nausea related to movement may suggest a vestibular component.[21]

Anti-neoplastic interventions are common palliative interventions and are known to have the risk of N/V. It is estimated that 50–80% of patients who receive chemotherapy, immunotherapy, and/or radiation have treatment-induced N/V.[8,27] Chemotherapy, immunotherapy, and radiation therapy can induce N/V acutely and with delayed onset. Radiotherapy-induced N/V (RINV) is identified as an underestimated and underrecognized symptom burden.[28] Anti-neoplastic-induced N/V can impact the patient's ability to continue disease-directed or palliative-focused cancer treatments.

Other etiologies, both acute and chronic, also need to be considered by the APRN in formulating a differential diagnosis and approach to symptom management. In patients with chronic obstructive pulmonary disease (COPD), N/V may be reactions to antibiotics, theophylline, or steroids; steroid-induced GI irritation; gastropathy from circulatory overload; or infection (e.g., thrush, cough and secretions, fatigue, and anxiety). Heart failure may trigger N/V related to cardiac ischemia, digitalis and other medications, congestive gastropathy, impaired renal and/or hepatic function causing hyponatremia, dehydration from diuretics, cough, and anxiety.[2,10,21] Table 42.2 outlines common etiologies of N/V to be considered in formulating a differential diagnosis.

Table 42.2 COMMON ETIOLOGIES OF NAUSEA AND VOMITING

Gastrointestinal	**Drug-induced**
Ascites	Anesthesia
Adhesions	Antibiotics
Biliary obstruction	Anticonvulsants
Cholecystitis	Aspirin and NSAIDs
Constipation	Chemotherapy
Gastric irritation/distention	Digoxin
Gastroparesis	Cannabis/marijuana
Gastric outlet obstruction	Immunotherapy
Gastric reflux	Iron supplements
Hepatitis	Opioids
Hepatic capsular distention	Theophylline
Intestinal obstruction	Buprenorphine/naloxone
Irritable bowel	**Radiation-induced**
Intra-abdominal cancers:	Esophagus
Colon, pancreas, ovarian,	Abdominal
gastric, esophageal	Pelvic
Peritoneal carcinomatosis	Brain
Pancreatitis	
Gastric or duodenal ulcers	
Metabolic	**Increased intracranial**
Fluid and electrolyte imbalances:	**pressure**
Hypercalcemia	Cerebral edema
Hyper-/Hyponatremia	Intracranial tumor
Dehydration	Intracranial bleeding
Adrenocortical insufficiency	Skull metastases
Liver failure	Carcinomatous meningitis
Renal failure	
Diabetic ketoacidosis	
Pregnancy	
Infections	**Psychological**
Candida esophagitis	Fear
Gastroenteritis	Anxiety
Sepsis	
Vestibular	**Pharyngeal**
Motion sickness	Chronic cough
Ménière syndrome	Oropharyngeal secretions
Vestibular problems	

From Dalal[1]; National Consensus Project for Quality Palliative Care[4]; National Comprehensive Cancer Network[5]; Tipton[7];Moorthy, Letizia[10]; Glare et al.[21]; Star, Boland[26]; Horn et al.[29]; and Micromedex.[30]

ASSESSMENT

The palliative APRN's comprehensive symptom assessment includes data from multiple sources, including the patient, family, and caregivers; medical and surgical history; medication history and current utilization of medications, including herbs, vitamins, and cannabis; physical examination and clinical observation; the medical record; and diagnostic tests. The assessment data describe the clinical personhood, the individual's health status, the individual's symptom experience, and other patient-specific factors that will affect the symptom management plan. This includes an understanding of the patient's prognosis, overall goals of care, and specific goals for symptom relief.[10]

A synthesis of the patient-specific data and the palliative APRN's knowledge and understanding of the health problems forms the differential diagnoses and likely cause(s). In conjunction with patient-specific goals, this guides potential further diagnostic testing for therapeutic decision-making and the selection of therapeutic interventions to eliminate or modify the cause of the symptom, if possible, and to alleviate symptom distress related to N/V.

Identifying the presence of the symptom(s) is the first step in assessment. The subjectivity of nausea is expressed by the patient and therefore varies from patient to patient.[1] The patient's report of N/V, either spontaneously or in the clinical interview, is a frequent method of symptom identification. Some patients may be reluctant to report either symptom in the belief that nothing can be done or that symptom management will detract from disease-directed therapies. Palliative APRNs should remain aware that N/V can have associated cluster symptoms and/or multifactorial etiology; symptom assessment is therefore multidimensional.[1] Routine screening for common symptoms using symptom inventory tools, such as the Memorial Symptom Assessment Scale or the Edmonton Symptom Assessment System, is another method of symptom identification.[11,31]

Understanding the patient's experience of N/V begins with the patient's description of the symptom to clarify its nature. The patient's experiential, linguistic, cultural, ethnic, and geographical background may influence the expression and meaning of N/V for the individual. Characteristics of onset, frequency, duration, intensity or severity, and pattern of occurrence; triggering and alleviating factors, such as use of prescription or over-the-counter medications or herbal preparations, exercise or activity, and changes in eating and drinking patterns; and associated symptoms help delineate possible etiologies and therapies. The effects of the N/V on the patient's function, including performance status and quality of life, are essential parts of the assessment. N/V symptoms often change eating patterns and are accompanied by diminished physical functioning and self-care capacity. In turn, social isolation, uncertainty, and concern about how N/V affects the patient's lifestyle, medical therapies, family caregivers, and survival add to symptom distress.[1,10]

If aligned with the patient's personalized medical care plan, clinical evaluation and diagnostics may be beneficial. Analysis of renal, liver, and pancreatic function, along with assessing for metabolic abnormalities (e.g., hyponatremia, hypokalemia, and hypercalcemia) could be necessary. In addition, diagnostics, such as computed tomography (CT) of the brain, abdomen and pelvis, and/or radiographs of the abdomen may assist clinically to connect to the patient's N/V experiences.[1]

In addition to the clinician assessment and history, patient diaries and journals may aid in understanding the patient's perception of and response to N/V.[3] There are also specific assessment tools for evaluating N/V. The *Morrow*

Assessment of Nausea and Vomiting (MANE) and the *Rhodes Index of Nausea and Vomiting* (INVR) enhance the patient's report of the symptom characteristics. Other tools (e.g., the *Functional Living Index-Emesis* and the *Osbana Nausea and Emesis Module*) describe the effect of the symptoms on function and well-being.[6,20] Research investigating novel technology approaches, like machine learning to assess and predict an individual's nausea susceptibility, is being conducted and will likely impact the future of clinical care[19] (Table 42.3).

Table 42.3 ASSESSMENT OF NAUSEA AND VOMITING

General	*Clinical Personhood* Demographics: Age, gender, race, employment, education, place of residence, socioeconomics, health insurance Spiritual: Values/beliefs, faith community, practices, rituals, restrictions Psychosocial: Marital status, sexual preference, culture, coping, social supports, substance use concerns, financial, past experience with health-related issues Current quality-of-life concerns Consider a symptom journal that the patient maintains and shares with palliative APRN	
Health status	Current diagnosis, prognosis, functional status, disease course, and trajectory, including past and current therapies, patient's understanding of disease status, goals of care Medication history; recent history or present anti-neoplastic interventions; current medication list/reconciliation. Herb, substance use; including cannabis and illicit drug history and current use. Assessment for polypharmacy and drug interactions. Past symptom burden history, including history of nausea or vomiting and effective therapies.	
	NAUSEA	**VOMITING**
Symptom experience	Patient description: Nausea, upset stomach, queasiness, sick stomach, other	Description of "throwing up," "upchucking," "barfing"; volume, color, content of emesis
Severity	0 none–10 worst; mild/moderate/severe intensity; episodes per day/week/month; intermittent or constant	Frequency per day/week; volume of emesis, intensity of vomiting
Duration and pattern	Onset; pattern and timing of occurrence	
Modulating factors	What makes your nausea or vomiting better or worse (e.g., time of day, medications, eating, activity, bowel function)?	

Distress/Impact	*Meaning of symptom; interference with function and quality of life:*
	What and how much are you able to eat or drink?
	What concerns you most about the nausea and/or vomiting?
	What worries do you have about what is causing it?
	Do you have an inability to eat or drink? Are you able to eat with family/friends?
	When you do eat, how soon do you become full or satisfied? Is this a change compared to prior?
	What effects does it have on energy and activity?
	Are there family concerns?
	What have been the effects on treatments?
	Have you had concerns about your appetite/weight in the past?
	    Overweight?
	    Underweight?
	    History of anorexia/bulimia?	

Associated symptoms	Fever, cough, oropharyngeal secretions, dizziness, headaches, vision changes, anorexia, dysgeusia, hyperosmia, dysphagia, abdominal pain, bloating, abdominal distention, heartburn, hiccups, constipation, diarrhea, weight changes	
Physical examination	Temperature Weight: If available serial weights, comparison to past weights is helpful Neurological: Level of consciousness; cognition, balance, cranial nerve deficits Oropharynx: Mucositis, secretions, infection, obstruction Blood pressure and pulse: Sitting, lying, standing to assess for postural hypotension from fluid imbalance Abdomen: Distention, bowel sounds, tenderness, masses, ascites Rectal exam: Fecal impaction	

(continued)

Table 42.3 CONTINUED

Diagnostic tests as indicated by: • History and physical findings • patient's health status • goals of care	Laboratory tests for renal and hepatic function, electrolytes, calcium, sodium, potassium Complete blood count Blood or urine cultures if infection is suspected Therapeutic drug level monitoring, if appropriate (digoxin, theophylline, tricyclic antidepressants, etc.) Radiological studies: Computed tomography (CT) or magnetic resonance imaging (MRI) of brain if CNS pathology suspected Chest radiograph if pneumonia suspected Plain film of abdomen to assess for obstruction or constipation CT scan of abdomen to assess for obstruction, ascites, other pathologies Endoscopic evaluation to assess for reflux, esophagitis, obstruction

From Dalal[1]; National Comprehensive Project for Quality Palliative Care[3]; Chow et al.[6]; Tipton[7]; and Moorthy, Letizia.[10]

CASE STUDY: NAUSEA AND VOMITING (CONTINUED)

Chad described persistent, worsening, continuous, moderate-level (5–6/10) nausea in the past 4 weeks. Over the past 3 days, the nausea was accompanied by vomiting of moderate amounts of regurgitated food/liquid or green, sour liquid once or twice each day. Vomiting did not relieve the nausea. He noticed the symptoms were worse when he ate, so he restricted his oral intake, resulting in a 6-pound weight loss in the past month. His bowels were normal for him, having a bowel movement every 2–3 days. He noted some abdominal bloating, which he attributes to gas and "not eating much." He felt abdominal pressure and had an increased abdominal pain, 6/10 at best and 9/10 worst intensity. He periodically modified his normal activities around the house and declined social activities because of worsening tremors and increasing fatigue.

Chad's medications included carbidopa 25 mg/levodopa 100 mg tablet 4 times per day, long-acting morphine tablets 60 mg orally every 12 hours for malignant pain (in the lung and liver), immediate-release morphine 15 mg tablets every 4 hours as needed for moderate to severe pain, senna 2 tablets taken at night, prochlorperazine 10 mg tablet every 6 hours as needed for nausea and/or vomiting, and omeprazole 20 mg tablet daily in the morning. He was opioid-tolerant and had increased the immediate-release morphine due to worsening pain the past 2 weeks. He was in between his chemotherapy cycles at this time.

Chad's assessment and physical exam revealed weight loss; increased upper extremity and hand tremor; abdominal distention, with palpation tenderness to the right upper quadrant of the abdomen; pain at 6/10; and nausea. Restaging scans completed 6 weeks earlier showed stable liver metastasis. His laboratory studies were unremarkable. The symptom diagnosis was N/V likely related to increased morphine use and opioid-induced constipation. There was a concern for worsening performance status as well.

MANAGEMENT STRATEGIES

The goal of antiemetic therapy is to modify or alleviate the patient's experience of N/V by reducing the incidence and severity of both, addressing symptom-related distress, and modifying or eliminating the cause if possible. Broad categories of interventions include patient and family education, psychosocial and spiritual support, behavioral and lifestyle changes, medications, invasive procedures, and etiology-directed therapies. The suspected cause of the N/V, the patient's general condition, comorbidities, current medications, prognosis, goals of care, and the patient's preferences and available resources guide selection of interventions. Table 42.4 summarizes management approaches.

INTERVENTIONS

If the etiology of N/V is diagnosed, it is beneficial to treat the underlying cause(s). The corrective action of the symptom burden treats the patient with enhanced medical optimization.[1] Multimodal management of N/V is often viewed as the mainstay of therapy. When medications are being considered, the personalized medication administration route is a thoughtful patient- and APRN-shared decision. Alternative to the oral route, medication administration that can be considered include sublingual, oral dissolvable tablets, intravenous, subcutaneous, transdermal, suppository, and rectal. The palliative APRN's multimodal and holistic approach encompasses nonpharmacologic and integrative interventions which are safe and personalized to the individual. For all interventions that are considered, the palliative APRN should be mindful to assess accessibility and financial burdens to the patient. Patient and family education centers on causes of N/V for the individual, realistic goals for symptom control, and implementation of the symptom management plan. This may include specific instructions regarding how and when to use medications, other therapies, and self-monitoring journals.[3] Patients and families also receive support and education about how to contact the care team for unexpected or emergent situations.

Nonpharmacologic Interventions

Psychosocial and spiritual support centers on acknowledging the quality of life and functional concerns as well as symptom distress; it that focuses on the meaning and implications of the symptom for the patient. Nursing's presence and understanding the symptom control plan help to decrease the patient's

Table 42.4 APPROACHES TO MANAGING NAUSEA AND VOMITING IN PALLIATIVE CARE

Identification and management of etiology and contributing symptoms

Patient and family education	Likely causes of nausea and vomiting for this patient Functional and exercise goals for symptom management Directions re: specific interventions and self-monitoring, including emergent situations (e.g., symptom journal) Information about how to contact clinical care team
Psychosocial and spiritual support	Acknowledge the psychological, social, cultural, and religious impact of nausea and vomiting as appropriate for patient and family. Refer to social worker, chaplain, or psychiatric support, if needed.
Nutrition counseling	Mouth care[a] Small, frequent meals or snacks[a] Maintain fluid intake but limit fluids with meals[a] Pleasant eating environment[a] Eat bland, cool temperature foods[a] Avoid salty, sweet, spicy foods[a] Use enriched and fortified foods to increased calories and protein. Use of commercial oral liquid nutritional supplements Consultation with qualified nutritionist
Cognitive-behavioral therapies	Includes relaxation, imagery, distraction, self-hypnosis[b]
Integrative therapies	Acupuncture[b] Acupressure[c] Ginger[c] Aromatherapy[c] Music therapy[c] Acupressure bands and relaxation music [c]
Metabolic abnormalities	Correct if possible: hypercalcemia, hypokalemia, hyponatremia.
Medications	Antiemetics see Table 42.5. Medication routes to be evaluated and considered by APRN; risk, burden vs. benefit Constipation management (see Chapter 40, "Bowel Symptoms")
Medically administered hydration and nutrition	May benefit patients with early-stage disease who have temporary limitations in oral intake or those with GI malfunctions but high-performance status. Generally, not tolerated or beneficial in patients who have end-stage disease. Individualized goals of the therapy need to be considered.
Therapeutic Radiation	Radiation therapy for brain metastasis and other CNS conditions
Invasive procedures	For obstructions: Nasogastric tube to suction, surgery, venting gastrostomy tubes, stents

[a] Expert opinion;

[b] Limited data to support use;

[c] Mixed or no data to support use.

From Dalal[1]; Chow et al.[6]; Tipton[7]; Glare et al.[21]; McKenzie et al.[27]; Gyi[32,33]; Peoples et al.[34]; Uster et al.[35]; Zeng et al.[36]; Wei et al.[37]; and Holmer Pettersson, Wengstrom.[38]

and family's sense of loss of control and uncertainty. Involving social workers, a chaplain, and/or psychiatric support may also be helpful. Expert opinion and some research have shown that cognitive therapy is a psychological modality that eases the burdens of N/V.[1] However, due to Grade B research, best practice recommendations include using clinical judgment when referring a patient to cognitive therapy or relaxation therapy.[32] Psychotherapy or counseling may be particularly helpful if medically administered nutrition and hydration, as well as invasive procedures to bypass obstructions, are being considered. Behavioral interventions, such as relaxation, progressive muscle relaxation, and guided imagery, reduce the incidence and intensity of anticipatory chemotherapy-related N/V.[32] These techniques can be taught to patients and may increase their sense of control and decrease distress.[6,7,21]

Lifestyle changes center on self-care activities dealing with physical activity and oral intake. One study reveals that when nutrition and physical exercise are completed systematically, individuals experience a decrease in N/V intensity.[36] Expert opinion suggests that oral care; recommendations on the amount, types, and frequency of intake; and maintaining an environment free of emetogenic sights, sounds, and smells are key points.[6]

The use of integrative therapies has grown, although few studies have been done in palliative care populations.[34] In general, integrative interventions may also help with anxiety and overall stress reduction. Most of these therapies are relatively nontoxic and can be suggested based on N/V evidence in other populations. However most are not covered by insurance. Some studies have highlighted music therapy to ease distress related to N/V. A systematic review and meta-analysis revealed that music interventions can ease anticipatory N/V, chemotherapy-induced vomiting, and other N/V burdens, but these data were mixed and limited.[36,37]

Some studies demonstrate a reduction in the incidence of postoperative and acute CINV through acupuncture.[1,38] Acupressure reduced acute chemotherapy-induced nausea. The use of acupressure wristbands produced mixed results.[36] Specifically, acupuncture, electroacupuncture, acupoint stimulation, acupressure, and transcutaneous electrical nerve stimulation were determined to all ease postoperative N/V.[39] Both acupressure and acupuncture could be considered within a multimodal care plan.

Interest in the spice ginger as an antiemetic exerting weak inhibition on 5-HT3 receptors led to studies and reviews of its use in motion sickness and pregnancy- and chemotherapy-related nausea. Formulations and doses varied, as did reported side effects of heartburn, diarrhea, and bruising. The mixed study results demonstrate no clear evidence of efficacy.[6,29] It is recommended that the APRN considers ginger as part of a multimodal approach with standard antiemetic medications.[33]

If N/V is moderate to severe, recurrent, or prolonged, as with recurrent or persistent GI obstructions, the use of medically administered nutrition and hydration, electrolyte balance, or enteral or parenteral nutrition may be considered. For patients in advanced or terminal stages of disease, the use of these therapies beyond the acute phase of management is a highly individual decision based on goals of care, prognosis, and the perceived benefits, burdens, and outcomes of the interventions.[40]

Pharmacologic Interventions

There are eight classes of drugs used in antiemetic therapy: dopamine receptor antagonists, including prokinetics and neuroleptics (antipsychotics), corticosteroids, serotonin receptor antagonists, NK1 receptor antagonists, cannabinoids, anticholinergics, antihistamines, and benzodiazepines (Table 42.5). There are potentially other medications not used as commonly which may be worth consideration when nausea or vomiting proves intractable (e.g., hydroxyzine). Drug selection may be guided by either a mechanistic or etiological approach or by an empiric approach. The mechanistic approach is evidence-based, utilizing an understanding of the neurotransmitters and neuroreceptors involved in the different emetic pathways and the use of drugs to block their activation/effect.[1] The empiric approach leaves antiemetic selection to the preference of the clinician. Due to limited randomized trials and low-quality studies, there is no clear evidence that one approach or antiemetic class is more effective in palliative care, particularly where the etiology of N/V may be unknown or multifactorial, and only limited studies on antiemetic efficacy in this population exist.[41] Understanding the action and

side effects of the different antiemetics may guide medication selection.[1,10,21] Regardless of the approach, if initial therapies are unsuccessful, adding or rotating to a different class of antiemetics may be beneficial. In the situation of intractable or refractory N/V, combination therapies may be considered.[21]

Dopamine receptor antagonist (D_2) antiemetics are active at the CTZ and in the gut.[42] Commonly used drugs in this class are metoclopramide and neuroleptics such as prochlorperazine, chlorpromazine, haloperidol, and olanzapine. Metoclopramide is the drug of choice for patients who have advanced cancer and a patent GI tract.[5,43] Except for haloperidol, most drugs in the class also block other receptors in the emetic pathway.[21] Haloperidol is commonly prescribed for N/V and is administered via the oral, intravenous, or subcutaneous route. It should be noted that haloperidol is not absorbed through the transdermal route, relegating transdermal gel preparations such as lorazepam, diphenhydramine, and haloperidol (known as ABH Gel) ineffective and dangerous for older adults since these medications all cause significant extrapyramidal effects.[42,44] Dopamine receptor antagonist agents may be most useful for N/V related to chemical or metabolic causes.

Extrapyramidal side effects that range from mild to moderate akathisia (subjective sense of restlessness to motor restlessness), parkinsonian-like changes (masked facies, resting tremor, cogwheel rigidity, shuffling gait, bradykinesia), dystonia (involuntary contraction of major muscles [e.g., torticollis, oculogyric crisis]), and tardive dyskinesia (characterized by lip smacking, rhythmic tongue and/or body movements, grimacing) may be associated with dopamine receptor antagonist use. Management of extrapyramidal symptoms includes discontinuing the drug or reducing the dose. Co-administering a benzodiazepine, a β-blocker, or an anticholinergic may temporarily reduce akathisia and dystonia.[45]

Olanzapine, a second-generation atypical antipsychotic, targets HT3 and histamine receptor sites. Due to the common side effect of drowsiness, olanzapine is recommended as a short-term course for N/V.[46] It is recommended to consider olanzapine when the etiology of nausea is unknown, or when refractory or chronic nausea occurs, or EPS symptoms are present.[8,10] More research is needed to identify its benefit and risk profile when treating anti-neoplastic-induced N/V.[46]

Selective 5-HT3 (serotonin receptor subtype) receptor antagonists (e.g., ondansetron and granisetron) work on receptors in the GI tract, the CTZ, and the VC. In the palliative oncology setting, 5-HT3 receptor antagonists are considered primary intervention for N/V caused by chemotherapy and radiation therapy that affects the digestive system organs.[28,47] Granisetron extended-release can be beneficial with treating delayed-onset CINV.[48] The antiemetic class of 5-HT3 receptor antagonists can also be beneficial for treating postoperative N/V, gastroparesis, and N/V related to bowel obstruction, where chemical and mechanical intestinal stimulation causes release of serotonin from enterochromaffin cells.[9,23,48] They should also be considered if dopamine antagonist agents are ineffective or not tolerated. Constipation and QT prolongation are potential side

Table 42.5 COMMONLY USED ANTIEMETICS

DRUG	SUGGESTED DOSES AND ROUTE	PRIMARY NEURORECEPTOR AFFINITY	COMMON USE	SIDE EFFECTS/ COMMENTS
DOPAMINE RECEPTOR ANTAGONISTS				
Prokinetic agent (Metoclopramide)	Oral, ODT, IV: 10–20 mg, q6–12h	Moderate D_2 (primarily in GI tract) Low 5-HT3 (only at high doses)	Gastroparesis Ileus or partial bowel obstruction	EPS; esophageal spasm; colic in GI tract obstruction; prolonged half-life in renal failure. QT prolongation. Do not use in complete bowel obstruction. Do not co-administer tricyclic antidepressant as it reverses the prokinetic effect.
Butyrophenone (Haloperidol)	Oral: 0.5–5 mg q8–12h IV: 0.5–1 mg q6–8h Caution with subcutaneous route due to risk of haloperidol crystals Not absorbed via transdermal route	High D_2	Chemical and/or metabolic nausea Bowel obstruction	Less sedating than phenothiazines. May cause QT prolongation, EPS, or neuroleptic malignant syndrome. Dose reduction may be needed in hepatic insufficiency. Safe in renal failure.
Phenothiazine (Prochlorperazine)	Oral: 5–10 mg q6–8h PR: 25 mg q12h IV: 10 mg q6h Max dose: 40 mg/24 h	Moderate D_2 Low H_1	Chemical and/or metabolic nausea	EPS; headache; dry mouth; hypotension, drowsiness; QT prolongation Low oral absorption
Chlorpromazine	Oral: 10–25 q6h IV: 12.5–25 mg q6–12h	Moderate D_2 Low H_1	Chemical and/or metabolic nausea	More sedating than prochlorperazine; EPS; QT prolongation
Atypical antipsychotic (Olanzapine)	Oral: 2.5–10 mg q12–24h	D_{1-4}, 5-HT3, H_1	Refractory nausea/ vomiting	Sedation; hyperglycemia; reduced seizure threshold. Associated with weight gain and improved appetite. Lower risk of EPS QT prolongation
CORTICOSTEROID				
Dexamethasone	Oral: 2–4 mg q6–24h IV: 2–4 mg q6–24h	Possibly reduces release of serotonin or activation of corticosteroid receptors in the CNS	Cerebral edema Intracranial tumors Chemotherapy-induced nausea Bowel obstruction	Insomnia; anxiety; euphoria; perirectal burning with IV administration; GI upset; metabolic effects: glycemic changes; infection risk Abrupt discontinuation can cause rebound N/V
Methylprednisolone	See dosing per immunotherapy guidelines.	Anti-inflammatory glucocorticoid used in replacement therapy of adrenocortical deficiencies	Recommended for use of immunotherapy induced N/V and other immunotherapy side effects	Hypertension; body fluid retention; HF; euphoria. Metabolic effects: glycemic control, infection risk. Do not abruptly discontinue; can cause rebound N/V.

(continued)

Table 42.5 CONTINUED

DRUG	SUGGESTED DOSES AND ROUTE	PRIMARY NEURORECEPTOR AFFINITY	COMMON USE	SIDE EFFECTS/ COMMENTS
SEROTONIN ANTAGONISTS				
Ondansetron	Oral/ODT/IV: 4-8 mg q8–12h	High 5-HT3 Both peripherally and centrally	Chemotherapy-induced nausea; delayed-onset of chemotherapy induced N/V Abdominal radiation therapy Postop GI irritants	Constipation Headache Diarrhea Mild sedation QT prolongation
Granisetron	Oral/IV: 1 mg q12h or 2 mg q24h Transdermal patch: 3.1 mg/24 h (lasts 7 days)			
NK1 RECEPTOR ANTAGONISTS				
Aprepitant	125 mg PO chemo day 1, 80 mg PO on chemotherapy day 2 and day 3; give 1 hour prior to chemotherapy Oral capsule, oral suspension, and IV formulations are available. See NCCN guidelines. Dose and frequency of medication are dependent upon risk category of emetogenic chemotherapy and chemotherapy schedule.	P/neurokinin 1 (NK1) receptor antagonist with high selectivity and affinity	Chemotherapy-induced nausea and vomiting, for highly emetogenic and moderately emetogenic chemotherapy Postoperative nausea and vomiting	Hypotension; constipation; diarrhea, asthenia; abdominal pain.
Fosaprepitant	150 mg IV, given with dexamethasone 12 mg orally 30 minutes prior to chemotherapy day 1 and concurrent 5-HT3 receptor antagonist. See NCCN guidelines. Dose and frequency of medication are dependent upon risk category of emetogenic chemotherapy and chemotherapy schedule.	Pro-drug of aprepitant, which is a selective, high-affinity antagonist of human substance P/ neurokinin 1 (NK-1) receptors	Chemotherapy-induced nausea and vomiting, for highly emetogenic and moderately emetogenic chemotherapy	Diarrhea; fatigue; neutropenia; infusion reaction; Stevens-Johnson syndrome.
Rolapitant	180 mg PO within 2 hours of chemotherapy, day 1 and every 2 weeks. Concurrent use of dexamethasone and 5-HT3 receptor antagonist. See NCCN guidelines. Oral capsule and IV formulations are available. Dose and frequency of medication are dependent upon risk category of emetogenic chemotherapy and chemotherapy schedule.	Selective and competitive P/ neurokinin 1 (NK1) receptor antagonist with antiemetic activity. Crosses the blood–brain barrier and occupies brain NK1 receptors	Chemotherapy-induced nausea and vomiting, In combination with other antiemetic agents; including highly emetogenic chemotherapy	Decrease in appetite; neutropenia; dizziness; hiccoughs.
Netupitant/ Palonosetron	300 mg/0.5 mg PO 1 hour prior to chemotherapy on day 1; administration of dexamethasone day 1–4 of chemotherapy. See NCCN guidelines. Dose and frequency of medication are dependent upon risk category of emetogenic chemotherapy and chemotherapy schedule.	P/neurokinin 1 (NK1) receptor antagonist, and palonosetron, a selective serotonin-3 (5-HT3) receptor antagonist	Chemotherapy-induced nausea and vomiting, Acute and delayed	Headache; fatigue; erythema; constipation; indigestions; asthenia; serotonin syndrome.

Table 42.5 CONTINUED

DRUG	SUGGESTED DOSES AND ROUTE	PRIMARY NEURORECEPTOR AFFINITY	COMMON USE	SIDE EFFECTS/ COMMENTS
Fosnetupitant/ Palonosetron	235 mg/0.25 mg IV over 30 minutes, starting 30 minutes prior to chemotherapy. administration of dexamethasone day 1–4 of chemotherapy. See NCCN Guidelines. Dose and frequency of medication are dependent upon risk category of emetogenic chemotherapy and chemotherapy schedule. Decadron also given prior to chemotherapy.	Active metabolite of Fosenetupitant is a selective substance P/neurokinin 1 receptor antagonist. Palonosetron is a 5-HT3 receptor antagonist	Chemotherapy-induced nausea and vomiting, Acute and delayed, associated with highly emetogenic chemotherapy	Headache; fatigue; asthenia; constipation; indigestion; erythema; hypersensitivity reaction; serotonin syndrome.
CANNABINOIDS				
Dronabinol	2–10 mg q8–12h Contains sesame oil	CB_1	Second-line antiemetic	Sedation; dizziness; disorientation; concentration difficulties; euphoria; dysphoria; hypotension; dry mouth; tachycardia.
Nabilone	1–2 mg q8–12h (max dose 6 mg/day)	CB_1	Second-line antiemetic	
ANTICHOLINERGICS				
Hyoscyamine	Oral/IV: 0.125–0.25 mg q4h as needed up to 1.5 mg/day	mAChR (in the vomiting center and peripherally)	Intestinal obstruction Peritoneal irritation, Increased intracranial pressure Excess secretions Motion sickness	Dry mouth; ileus; urinary retention; blurred vision; agitation.
Scopolamine	Transdermal: 1.5 mg q72h (lasts 72 h)			Onset of effect is up to 24 h. Crosses the blood-brain barrier: common side effects are confusion and sedation.
ANTIHISTAMINES				
Promethazine	Oral, PR, or IV: 12.5–25 mg q6–8h (max dose 100 mg/day)	High H_1 Low D_2 Low mAChR	Motion sickness Increased intracranial pressure	Drowsiness Sedation Dry mouth Constipation Dizziness Confusion Blurred vision
Cyclizine	Oral: 25–50 mg q6–8h (max dose 200 mg/day)	H_1		
Diphenhydramine	Oral/IV: 12.5–50 mg q6–8h			
BENZODIAZEPINE				
Lorazepam	Oral/IV: 0.5–1 mg q6–24h	GABA	Anxiety Not FDA approved as antiemetic	Sedation; amnesia; delirium. Depression. Reduce dose in renal or hepatic insufficiency. Not FDA approved as an antinausea or antiemetic.
OTHER				
Octreotide (somatostatin analogue)	SC: 100–150 mg q8h IV continuous infusion: 0.2–0.9 mg/day IM depot: 20–30 mg q3–4 weeks	Somatostatin receptors in brain, pituitary, GI tract	Bowel obstruction. Reduces peristalsis and intestinal secretions	Pain at injection site; worsening GI symptoms. Reduce dose in renal or hepatic insufficiency.
Mirtazapine (antidepressant)	Oral: 7.5–30 mg at bedtime	$5-HT_3$, H_1, mAChR	Gastroparesis	Increased appetite; weight gain, somnolence.

ODT, oral disintegrating tablet; D_2, dopamine; H_1, histamine; 5-HT3, serotonin; CB_1, cannabinoid; mAChR, muscarinic acetylcholine receptors; EPS, extrapyramidal side effects.

From Dalal[1]; Chow et al.[6]; Tipton[7]; Moorthy, Letizia[10]; Wood et al.[20]; Glare et al.[21]; Star, Boland[26]; Miromedex[30]; Walsh et al.[41]; Fletcher et al.[44]; and Gabrail et al.[48]

effects.[7,20,47,48] Insurance coverage may be a factor in access to these medications.[7,47]

Antihistamines block H_1 receptor activity at the CTZ and the VC. They are primarily used to manage N/V caused by vestibular stimulation (e.g., motion sickness, raised intracranial pressure). Promethazine, cyclizine, meclizine, and diphenhydramine are commonly used agents. Sedation and anticholinergic side effects may limit use, particularly the potential for falls and delirium in older adults.[7,21]

Anticholinergic agents are primarily used as antiemetics in combination with other antiemetics for control of N/V associated with dizziness and movement and bowel obstruction.[4,32] They block muscarinic acetylcholine receptors (mAChR) in vestibular nuclei and the autonomic nervous system, resulting in decreased peristaltic tone and movement and reduced intestinal secretions.[4,35] Hyoscyamine and scopolamine are commonly used drugs in this class.

Corticosteroids are often used in antiemetic regimens for CINV, RINV, symptom management in bowel obstruction, and in treatment of raised intracranial pressure. The antiemetic mechanism of these agents is not known. Theorized actions include anti-inflammatory and antisecretory activity and altered permeability of the blood–brain barrier with reduced effect of potential chemical and metabolic stimuli. Dexamethasone with ondansetron, a 5-HT3 receptor antagonists, has been shown to treat RINV.[27] Concerns about gastric irritation, glycemic control, infection risk, proximal muscle weakness with long-term use, and dysphoria and/or delirium may limit their use.[20]

Cannabinoids' activity at the CB_1 receptors in the central and peripheral nervous systems is thought to be the basis of their antiemetic effect. Dronabinol and nabilone are approved by the US Food and Drug Administration (FDA) for use in CINV.[35,36] Cannabinoids are not recommended as first- or second-line antiemetic interventions.[49–51] The effectiveness of other cannabinoid formulations, such as medicinal or recreational state programs, are not established. Cannabis remains a schedule 1 substance despite legalization for medical and recreational purposes in some states. When considering medicinal cannabis, the palliative APRN should implement shared decision-making with the patient. It is recommended to consider financial burdens, state legislation, and patient preferences.[50] Reports of cannabinoid hyperemesis syndrome (CHS) with chronic cannabis use raise the need for further study of this antiemetic class.[52]

Neurokinin-1 receptor antagonists are FDA approved for use in acute and delayed CINV and in the postoperative setting. Drugs in this class are aprepitant, fosaprepitant, and netupitant. Neurokinin-1 receptor antagonists are recommended in conjunction with other antiemetics. Combination therapy is recommended to treat moderate to high-risk emetic anti-neoplastic-associated interventions.[53] A combination of NK1 receptor agonists, such as aprepitant, and a 5-HT3 receptor agonist, such as granisetron, has been shown to relieve chemotherapy- and radiation associated N/V.[27,28] Other multi-class emetic medications, such as netupitant and palonosetron (NEPA), have also been found to ease CINV. Research is still being conducted to evaluate the routine clinical use of NEPA.[54]

Benzodiazepines act on GABA in the cerebral cortex. They are effective in managing anxiety associated with N/V but do not have antiemetic activity.[12,35] Side effects of sedation and amnesia may limit use. Mirtazapine, a tetracyclic antidepressant, has activity as a 5-HT3, H_1, and muscarinic receptor antagonist. Reports of its antiemetic effect in diabetic gastroparesis and idiopathic nausea are indicative of a prokinetic effect that needs further study in the palliative care population.[21]

CASE STUDY: NAUSEA AND VOMITING (CONTINUED)

Initial interventions for Chad's presumed opioid-induced constipation focused on his bowel regimen: senna 2 tablets twice a day and lactulose 30 mg solution 1–3 times a day, with a goal of a bowel movement at least every other day. Due to the increasing duration and intensity of the N/V, his antiemetic was changed. Prochlorperazine was discontinued and replaced by mirtazapine 7.5 mg tablet at night, for its pro-kinetic effect, which enhanced the bowel regimen. This antiemetic rotation was aimed to benefit Chad's performance status because the prochlorperazine could have been interacting with his Parkinson's disease medications, carbidopa/levodopa.

MANAGEMENT OF GASTROPARESIS-INDUCED N/V

Concurrent treatment for the primary etiology of gastroparesis and gastroparesis-induced N/V is recommended. Evidence has found that transdermal granisetron eases N/V and other associated symptoms such as postprandial fullness, upper abdominal pain, early satiety, and loss of appetite.[23] Motility agents such as metoclopramide or mirtazapine can be considered. Specifically, the pro-motility effect of metoclopramide on the upper GI tract and its activity at the CTZ make it a useful first-line antiemetic.[55] However, it should be avoided in patients with complete bowel obstruction.[21]

MANAGEMENT OF OPIOID-INDUCED N/V

There is limited evidence to guide management of opioid-induced N/V.[56,57] These symptom burdens may result from gastroparesis, constipation, CTZ stimulation, and/or vestibular stimulation. Some experts observe that opioid-induced N/V may be time limited, with symptoms easing within 5–7 days of starting the opioid.[41] In the acute setting, concurrent or preemptive use of metoclopramide to ease morphine-induced N/V was not recommended. With use of metoclopramide, there was an increase in dizziness without reducing morphine-induced N/V.[58] A preliminary study retrospectively identified that administering naldemedine tosylate, a peripheral acting nonselective opioid receptor antagonist, could have secondary benefits and help ease early-onset opioid-induced N/V.[59] Given limited evidence, managing associated symptoms, such as constipation and anticipatory N/V, by preemptively treating the symptoms can still be considered. Although there are no specific recommendations in the literature, opioid rotation also seems reasonable.[41,57] Higher quality research is needed to guide management of opioid-induced N/V.

MANAGEMENT OF CHEMOTHERAPY-INDUCED NAUSEA AND VOMITING

Chemotherapy-induced N/V (CINV) is a common adverse and stressful side effect that individuals experience. Both acute- and delayed-onset N/V are associated with antineoplastic treatments. The American Society of Clinical Oncology (ASCO) and National Comprehensive Cancer Network (NCCN) are the clinical organizational leaders that provide best practice and expert opinion and compile evidence-based antiemetic guidelines.[22,60] Updated research and clinical guidelines support using a multiple classes of antiemetic medications to prevent and ease CINV. Considering the high emetic risk, a combination of an NK-1 receptor antagonist and a 5-HT3 receptor antagonist, along with dexamethasone and olanzapine were found to prevent, treat, and overall ease CINV.[8] Cannabinoids have insufficient evidence and are therefore not recommended to treat CINV.[49] Some findings have reported undermanagement of CINV events.[61] It is best practice for the palliative APRN to develop an antiemetic care plan that is personalized to the patient and aligned with the known emetic risk profile of the chemotherapy being administered.[8]

MANAGEMENT OF CANNABINOID HYPEREMESIS SYNDROME

CHS has become more common as medicinal and recreational laws have increasingly been passed by state legislatures. A systematic review of literature identifies that management of CHS can be difficult. The palliative APRN should provide CHS education about the etiology and treatment of CHS. Recommendations to treat CHS include the individual decreasing or eliminating the use of cannabinoids and consideration for the use lorazepam as an anticipatory antiemetic or haloperidol or topical capsaicin to relieve vomiting.[52] In general, the prevalence of cannabis use is likely to increase so additional high-quality research is needed to establish evidence-based guidelines.

MANAGEMENT OF BOWEL OBSTRUCTION

Bowel obstruction requires immediate intervention. Decisions about surgical, interventional, and/or medical management are based on the etiology of the obstruction and the patient's condition and goals of care. Symptom management in bowel obstructions focuses on relief of pain, N/V, and abdominal distension. Surgical interventions for bowel obstructions are intended on removing or minimizing the tumor burden. Postsurgical morbidity, mortality, and reobstruction are all common risks and burdens.[26] If the bowel obstruction is deemed to be inoperable, the palliative APRN should review illness severity, trajectory, prognosis, and other recommended interventions with the patient.[25]

If surgical options are not appropriate, the use of venting gastrostomy tubes or stents may offer symptom relief. If the patient has a high-performance status, life expectancy greater than 30 days, and an obstruction at the gastric outlet, proximal small bowel, or colon, then insertion of self-expanding metal stents placed via endoscopy or interventional radiology may be considered. Although often successful in relieving symptoms, stents may cause perforation and bleeding; if the stent migrates, reobstruction may occur.[26,62] Prolonged nasogastric intubation is possible to relieve distension and vomiting but is limited by discomfort from nasal and pharyngeal irritation and/or infections, difficulty clearing oral secretions, and aspiration pneumonias. An alternative is a venting gastrostomy tube (g-tube) that is placed surgically or percutaneously during an endoscopic procedure to allow drainage of gastric contents. With a venting g-tube in place, limited oral intake may be tolerated, which can be psychosocially satisfying for both the patient and family. Large-volume ascites, carcinomatosis, and tumor infiltration of the stomach may preclude g-tube placement. Complications include pain at the insertion site, leakage of gastric fluid with resulting skin irritation, and the need for periodic replacement if used in long-term therapy[62,63] (see Chapter 40, "Bowel Symptoms," for further information).

Chad resumed palliative chemotherapy to treat the tumor. He continued his optimized bowel regimen and opioid pain management plan, as well as oral mirtazapine and depot octreotide to minimize recurrent symptoms.

SUMMARY

N/V is highly distressing that many palliative care patients experience as a result of disease or therapies, even those that are palliative- or symptom-focused. The palliative APRN provides expert, compassionate clinical care while contributing to the expanding evidence base for managing these symptoms in palliative care. Successful management of these complex symptoms requires that the APRN conducts an ongoing comprehensive assessment to describe the patient's experience and associated factors, formulate a symptom diagnosis based on an understanding of likely etiologies, and use appropriate nonpharmacologic and pharmacologic management strategies based on best evidence, expert opinion, and patient acceptability.

REFERENCES

1. Dalal S. Chronic nausea and vomiting. In: Yennurajalingam S, Bruera E, eds. *Oxford American Handbook Hospice and Palliative Medicine and Supportive Care*, 2nd ed. New York: Oxford University Press, 2016: 125–136.
2. Leach C. Nausea and vomiting in palliative care. *Clin Med (Lond)*. 2019;19(4):299–301. doi:10.7861/clinmedicine.19-4-299
3. National Comprehensive Cancer Network. NCCN guidelines for patients. Nausea and Vomiting. Supportive care book series. 2016. https://www.NCCN.org/patients/guidelines/content/PDF/nausea-patient.pdf
4. National Consensus Project for Quality Palliative Care. Clinical Practice Guidelines for Quality Palliative Care, 4th ed. Richmond, VA: National Coalition for Hospice and Palliative Care. 2018. https://www.nationalcoalitionhpc.org/ncp/.
5. National Comprehensive Cancer Network. Palliative care guidelines. Version 2.2021. Available at https://jnccn.org/view/journals/jnccn/19/7/article-p780.xml
6. Chow K, Cogan D, Mun S. Nausea and vomiting. In: Ferrell BR, Paice J. *Oxford Textbook of Palliative Nursing*. 5th ed. New York: Oxford University Press, 2019. https://oxfordmedicine.com/view/10.1093/med/9780190862374.001.0001/med-9780190862374-chapter-12#med-9780190862374-chapter-12-bibItem-772
7. Tipton J. Nausea and vomiting. In: Yarbro CH, Wujcik D, Gobel BH, eds. *Cancer Symptom Management*. Burlington, MA: Jones and Bartlett; 2014: 213–233.
8. Whitehorn A. 2. Evidence summary. Chemotherapy induced nausea and vomiting: Antiemetics. The Joanna Briggs Institute EBP Database, https://www.library.ucdavis.edu/database/joanna-briggs-institute-jbi-evidence-based-practice-database/.2019; JBI22776.
9. Lee MA, Prentice WM, Hildreth AJ, Walker RW. Measuring symptom load in idiopathic Parkinson's disease. *Parkinsonism Related Dis*. 2007;13(5):284–289. doi: 10.1016/j.parkreldis.2006.11.009
10. Moorthy GS, Letizia M. The management of nausea at the end of life. *J Hosp Palliat Nurs*. 2018;20(5):442–449. doi:10.1097/NJH.0000000000000453
11. Henson LA, Maddocks M, Evans C, Davidson M, Hicks S, Higginson IJ. Palliative care and the management of common distressing symptoms in advanced cancer: Pain, breathlessness, nausea and vomiting, and fatigue. *J Clin Oncol*. 2020;38(9):905–914. doi:10.1200/JCO.19.00470
12. Postoperative nausea and vomiting: Drug therapy. Micromedex Solutions. Greenwood Village, CO: Truven Health Analytics. http://micromedex.com/. Last updated July 2021. https://www.micromedexsolutions.com/micromedex2/librarian/CS/DFF13C/ND_PR/evidencexpert/ND_P/evidencexpert/DUPLICATIONSHIELDSYNC/3746CD/ND_PG/evidencexpert/ND_B/evidencexpert/ND_AppProduct/evidencexpert/ND_T/evidencexpert/PFActionId/evidencexpert.IntermediateToDocumentLink?docId=9269&contentSetId=50&title=Postoperative+Nausea+and+Vomiting+-+Drug+Therapy&servicesTitle=Postoperative+Nausea+and+Vomiting+-+Drug+Therapy
13. Higginson IJ, Hart S, Silber E, Burman R, Edmonds P. Symptom prevalence and severity in people severely affected by multiple sclerosis. *J Palliat Care*. 2006;22(3):158–165.
14. Levinthal DJ, Rahman A, Nusrat S, O'Leary M, Heyman R, Bielefeldt K. Adding to the burden: Gastrointestinal symptoms and syndromes in multiple sclerosis. *Mult Scler Int*. 2013;2013:319201. doi:10.1155/2013/319201
15. Moens K, Higginson IJ, Harding R; Euro Impact. Are there differences in the prevalence of palliative care-related problems in people living with advanced cancer and eight non-cancer conditions? A systematic review. *J Pain Symptom Manage*. 2014;48(4):660–677. doi:10.1016/j.jpainsymman.2013.11.009
16. Elshazli RM, Kline A, Elgaml A, et al. Gastroenterology manifestations and COVID-19 outcomes: A meta-analysis of 25,252 cohorts among the first and second waves. *J Med Virol*. 2021;93(5):2740–2768. doi:10.1002/jmv.26836
17. Dorrell RD, Dougherty MK, Barash EL, Lichtig AE, Clayton SB, Jensen ET. Gastrointestinal and hepatic manifestations of covid-19: A systematic review and meta-analysis [published online ahead of print, 2020 Nov 21]. *JGH Open*. 2020;5(1):107–115. doi:10.1002/jgh3.12456
18. Elmunzer BJ, Spitzer RL, Foster LD, et al. Digestive manifestations in patients hospitalized with coronavirus disease 2019. *Clin Gastroenterol Hepatol*. 2021;19(7):1355–1365.e4. doi:10.1016/j.cgh.2020.09.041
19. Ruffle JK, Patel A, Giampietro V, et al. Functional brain networks and neuroanatomy underpinning nausea severity can predict nausea susceptibility using machine learning. *J Physiol*. 2019;597(6):1517–1529. doi:10.1113/JP277474
20. Wood JM, Chapman K, Eilers J. Tools for assessing nausea, vomiting, and retching. *Cancer Nurs*. 2011;34(1):E14–E24. doi:10.1097/ncc.0b013e3181e2cd79
21. Glare P, Miller J, Nikolova T, Tickoo R. Treating nausea and vomiting in palliative care: A review. *Clin Interv Aging*. 2011;6:243–259. doi:10.2147/CIA.S13109
22. National Comprehensive Cancer Network. Antiemesis. 2021, version 1. https://www.nccn.org/professionals/physician_gls/pdf/antiemesis.pdf
23. Midani D, Parkman HP. Granisetron transdermal system for treatment of symptoms of gastroparesis: A prescription registry study. *J Neurogastroenterol Motil*. 2016;22(4):650–655. doi:10.5056/jnm15203
24. Bharucha AE. Epidemiology and natural history of gastroparesis. *Gastroenterol Clin North Am*. 2015;44(1):9–19. doi:10.1016/j.gtc.2014.11.002
25. Boland JW, Boland EG. Constipation and malignant bowel obstruction in palliative care. *Medicine*. 2019; 48(1), 18–22. https://www.sciencedirect.com/science/article/abs/pII/S1357303919302488.
26. Star A, Boland JW. Updates in palliative care: Recent advancements in the pharmacological management of symptoms. *Clin Med (Lond)*. 2018;18(1):11–16. doi:10.7861/clinmedicine.18-1-11
27. McKenzie E, Chan D, Parsafar S, et al. Evolution of antiemetic studies for radiation-induced nausea and vomiting within an outpatient palliative radiotherapy clinic. *Support Care Cancer*. 2019;27(9):3245–3252. doi:10.1007/s00520-019-04870-6

28. Chiu N, Chiu L, Popovic M, et al. Latest advances in the management of radiation-induced pain flare, nausea and vomiting. *Ann Palliat Med*. 2016;5(1):50–57. doi:10.3978/j.issn.2224-5820.2015.08.01

29. Horn CC, Wallisch WJ, Homanics GE, Williams JP. Pathophysiological and neurochemical mechanisms of postoperative nausea and vomiting. *Eur J Pharmacol*. 2014;722:55–66. doi:10.1016/j.ejphar.2013.10.037

30. Micromedex. Nausea and vomiting. 2021. https://www.micromedexsolutions.com/

31. Watanabe SM, Nekolaichuk C, Beaumont C, Johnson L, Myers J, Strasser F. A multicenter study comparing two numerical versions of the Edmonton symptom assessment system in palliative care patients. *J Pain Symptom Manage*. 2011;41(2):456–468. doi:10.1016/j.jpainsymman.2010.04.020

32. Gyi AA. 1. Evidence summary. Chemotherapy induced nausea and vomiting: Cognitive behavior distraction therapy and deep relaxation therapy. The Joanna Briggs Institute EBP Database, https://www.library.ucdavis.edu/database/joanna-briggs-institute-jbi-evidence-based-practice-database/. 2018; JBI20527.

33. Gyi AA. 2. Evidence summary. Chemotherapy-induced nausea and vomiting: Ginger. The Joanna Briggs Institute EBP Database. https://www.library.ucdavis.edu/database/joanna-briggs-institute-jbi-evidence-based-practice-database/. 2018; JBI967.

34. Peoples AR, Culakova E, Heckler CE, et al. Positive effects of acupressure bands combined with relaxation music/instructions on patients most at risk for chemotherapy-induced nausea. *Support Care Cancer*. 2019;27(12):4597–4605. doi:10.1007/s00520-019-04736-x

35. Uster A, Ruehlin M, Mey S, et al. Effects of nutrition and physical exercise intervention in palliative cancer patients: A randomized controlled trial. *Clin Nutr*. 2018;37(4):1202–1209. doi:10.1016/j.clnu.2017.05.027

36. Zeng YS, Wang C, Ward KE, Hume AL. Complementary and alternative medicine in hospice and palliative care: A systematic review. *J Pain Symptom Manage*. 2018;56(5):781–794.e4. doi:10.1016/j.jpainsymman.2018.07.016

37. Wei TT, Tian X, Zhang FY, Qiang WM, Bai AL. Music interventions for chemotherapy-induced nausea and vomiting: A systematic review and meta-analysis. *Support Care Cancer*. 2020;28(9):4031–4041. doi:10.1007/s00520-020-05409-w

38. Holmér Pettersson P, Wengström Y. Acupuncture prior to surgery to minimise postoperative nausea and vomiting: A systematic review. *J Clin Nurs*. 2012;21(13–14):1799–1805. doi:10.1111/j.1365-2702.2012.04114.x

39. Elvir-Lazo OL, White PF, Yumul R, Cruz Eng H. Management strategies for the treatment and prevention of postoperative/postdischarge nausea and vomiting: An updated review. *F1000Res*. 2020;9:F1000 Faculty Rev-983. doi:10.12688/f1000research.21832.1

40. Hospice and Palliative Nursing Association. *HPNA position statement: Medically administered hydration and nutrition*. Pittsburgh, PA: HPNA. 2020. https://advancingexpertcare.org/position-statements/

41. Walsh D, Davis M, Ripamonti C, Bruera E, Davies A, Molassiotis A. 2016 updated MASCC/ESMO consensus recommendations: Management of nausea and vomiting in advanced cancer. *Support Care Cancer*. 2017;25(1):333–340. doi:10.1007/s00520-016-3371-3

42. Murray-Brown F, Dorman S. Haloperidol for the treatment of nausea and vomiting in palliative care patients. *Cochrane Database Syst Rev*. 2015;2015(11):CD006271. doi:10.1002/14651858.CD006271.pub3

43. Prommer E. Role of haloperidol in palliative medicine: An update. *Am J Hosp Palliat Care*. 2012;29(4):295–301. doi:10.1177/1049909111423094

44. Fletcher DS, Coyne PJ, Dodson PW, Parker GG, Wan W, Smith TJ. A randomized trial of the effectiveness of topical "ABH gel" (Ativan(*), Benadryl(*), Haldol(*)) vs. placebo in cancer patients with nausea. *J Pain Symptom Manage*. 2014;48(5):797–803. doi:10.1016/j.jpainsymman.2014.02.010

45. Marder S, Stroup TS. In: Stein M eds. Schizophrenia in adults: Maintenance therapy and Side effect management. UpToDate. Waltham, MA: Uptodate. April 22, 2021 https://www.uptodate.com/contents/schizophrenia-in-adults-maintenance-therapy-and-side-effect-management

46. Whitehorn A. Evidence summary. Chemotherapy induced nausea and vomiting: Olanzapine. The Joanna Briggs Institute EBP Database. https://www.library.ucdavis.edu/database/joanna-briggs-institute-jbi-evidence-based-practice-database/. 2019; JBI22824.

47. Whitehorn A. 3. Evidence summary. Chemotherapy induced nausea and vomiting: 5-HT3 receptor antagonists. The Joanna Briggs Institute EBP Database. https://www.library.ucdavis.edu/database/joanna-briggs-institute-jbi-evidence-based-practice-database/. 2019; JBI22775

48. Gabrail N, Yanagihara R, Spaczyński M, et al. Pharmacokinetics, safety, and efficacy of apf530 (extended-release granisetron) in patients receiving moderately or highly emetogenic chemotherapy: Results of two phase II trials. *Cancer Manag Res*. 2015;7:83–92. doi:10.2147/CMAR.S72626

49. Howard P, Twycross R, Shuster J, Mihalyo M, Wilcock A. Cannabinoids. *J Pain Symptom Manage*. 2013;46(1):142–149. doi:10.1016/j.jpainsymman.2013.05.002

50. Whitehorn A. 1. Evidence summary. Chemotherapy induced nausea and vomiting: Cannabinoids. The Joanna Briggs Institute EBP Database. https://www.library.ucdavis.edu/database/joanna-briggs-institute-jbi-evidence-based-practice-database/. 2019; JBI22822

51. Chow R, Valdez C, Chow N, et al. Oral cannabinoid for the prophylaxis of chemotherapy-induced nausea and vomiting-a systematic review and meta-analysis. *Support Care Cancer*. 2020;28(5):2095–2103. doi:10.1007/s00520-019-05280-4

52. Richards JR, Gordon BK, Danielson AR, Moulin AK. Pharmacologic treatment of cannabinoid hyperemesis syndrome: A systematic review. *Pharmacotherapy*. 2017;37(6):725–734. doi:10.1002/phar.1931

53. Whitehorn A. 5. Evidence summary. Chemotherapy induced nausea and vomiting: Nk-1 receptor antagonists. The Joanna Briggs Institute EBP Database. https://www.library.ucdavis.edu/database/joanna-briggs-institute-jbi-evidence-based-practice-database/. 2019; JBI22823

54. Whitehorn A. 4. Evidence summary. Chemotherapy induced nausea and vomiting: Netupitant plus palonosetron (NEPA). The Joanna Briggs Institute EBP Database. https://www.library.ucdavis.edu/database/joanna-briggs-institute-jbi-evidence-based-practice-database/. 2019; JBI22837

55. Cherwin CH. Gastrointestinal symptom representation in cancer symptom clusters: A synthesis of the literature. *Oncol Nurs Forum*. 2012;39(2):157–165. doi:10.1188/12.ONF.157-165

56. Moola S. Evidence summary. Intravenous morphine (nausea and vomiting): Prophylactic metoclopramide. The Joanna Briggs Institute EBP Database. https://www.library.ucdavis.edu/database/joanna-briggs-institute-jbi-evidence-based-practice-database/. 2019; JBI5505

57. Sande TA, Laird BJA, Fallon MT. The management of opioid-induced nausea and vomiting in patients with cancer: A systematic review. *J Palliat Med*. 2019;22(1):90–97. doi:10.1089/jpm.2018.0260

58. Rowland K, Fuehrer J, Motov SM. American Academy of Emergency Medicine (AAEM): Clinical practice statement: Should antiemetics be given prophylactically with intravenous opioids while treating acute pain in the emergency department? Reviewed and Updated June 7, 2019. https://www.aaem.org/UserFiles/file/PostCPCAntiemetic.pdf

59. Sato J, Tanaka R, Ishikawa H, Suzuki T, Shino M. A preliminary study of the effect of naldemedine tosylate on opioid-induced nausea and vomiting. *Support Care Cancer*. 2020;28(3):1083–1088. doi:10.1007/s00520-019-04884-0

60. Henson LA, Maddocks M, Evans C, Davidson M, Hicks S, Higginson IJ. Palliative care and the management of common

distressing symptoms in advanced cancer: Pain, breathlessness, nausea and vomiting, and fatigue. *J Clin Oncol.* 2020;38(9):905–914. doi:10.1200/JCO.19.00470

61. Mahendraratnam N, Farley JF, Basch E, Proctor A, Wheeler SB, Dusetzina SB. Characterizing and assessing antiemetic underuse in patients initiating highly emetogenic chemotherapy. *Support Care Cancer.* 2019;27(12):4525–4534. doi:10.1007/s00520-019-04730-3

62. Frago R, Ramirez E, Millan M, Kreisler E, del Valle E, Biondo S. Current management of acute malignant large bowel obstruction: A systematic review. *Am J Surg.* 2014;207(1):127–138. doi:10.1016/j.amjsurg.2013.07.027

63. Ripamonti CI, Easson AM, Gerdes H. Bowel obstruction. In: Cherny NI, Fallon MT, Kassa S, Portemoy RK, Currow DC, eds. *Textbook of Palliative Medicine.* 5th ed. New York: Oxford University Press; 2015: 919–929.

43.

PAIN

Judith A. Paice

KEY POINTS

- Expert assessment skills, including highly developed history-taking and physical examination skills, are essential to effective pain management in palliative care

- Palliative advanced practice registered nurses (APRNs) with comprehensive knowledge of pain management options can prescribe appropriate therapies, educate patients and families regarding safe and effective medication use, and consult colleagues who might provide other essential interventions, such as physical or occupational therapy, interventional techniques, cognitive-behavioral strategies and integrative therapies.

- Safe prescribing practices are vital for patients, families, and society at large.

CASE STUDY

Mr. J was a 66-year-old African-American man with metastatic non-small-cell lung cancer for whom a full pain assessment was conducted. He recently developed right hip pain and was found to have a pathologic fracture of the right femur, which was treated with open reduction and internal fixation and x-ray therapy (XRT) 3 months prior. This pain had resolved, but he then presented with low back pain and right rib pain these were consistent with sites of metastatic disease on his positron emission tomography (PET) scan. The back pain was distributed over the low lumbar area, described as aching without radiculopathy. The intensity was 2 at rest but 8 when standing for more than a few minutes. The rib pain was also aching and throbbing and was worse when lying on that side or taking a deep inspiration. He had been given hydrocodone/acetaminophen with little relief, although he took less than the prescribed dose. He denied adverse effects. Further investigation revealed no personal history of substance misuse, but his son had died from a heroin overdose. He was extremely worried about becoming addicted and anxious regarding constipation. Review of the prescription drug monitoring program revealed only a few refills of small amounts of hydrocodone, all prescribed by his oncologist. Urine toxicology was negative except for opioids.

Extensive education provided by the palliative advanced practice registered nurse (APRN) reassured Mr. J about safe medication use and storage. Constipation prevention and management were discussed and a bowel program was initiated. The hydrocodone/acetaminophen was changed to oxycodone to reduce potential toxicities associated with excess acetaminophen. After consistent use of oxycodone, a fentanyl patch was added to provide a baseline level of relief. Radiotherapy was consulted for palliation of bone metastases. A home palliative nurse was consulted to ensure his environment was safe, provide ongoing assessment of pain, and reinforce teaching. Transition to hospice occurred when disease progressed, and he died peacefully.

INTRODUCTION

Pain is greatly feared by those experiencing a life-threatening illness. In most cases, patients and their loved ones can be reassured that this symptom can be relieved, but in some cases pain can be extremely challenging to control. This is in part because the subjectivity of the pain experience, along with the absence of specific laboratory or imaging markers, complicates assessment and management. The biopsychosocial model of pain provides a framework that can guide palliative APRNs in understanding the many variables that contribute to the experience of pain (Figure 43.1).[1,2] Biological, psychological, social, and spiritual factors should be considered part of a complete assessment and serve as a guide for development of a comprehensive plan of care.

The palliative advanced practice registered nurse (APRN) is in a unique position to provide this "whole-person" care. Blending knowledge of the common pain syndromes seen in life-threatening illness, sophisticated assessment skills, and awareness of interventions used to relieve pain while employing stellar education and communication strategies, the APRN can provide safe and effective pain relief for the majority of palliative care patients with pain.

GOALS OF PAIN MANAGEMENT

The goals of comprehensive and effective pain management include prevention of pain, relief of pain, improved function and quality of life, safety, and the prevention of adverse societal effects (such as diversion). In a perfect world, all pain would be prevented. Yet acute pain serves as an important warning sign. Therefore, although preventing acute pain is neither reasonable nor desired in all circumstances, there are situations in palliative care where the APRN can work to

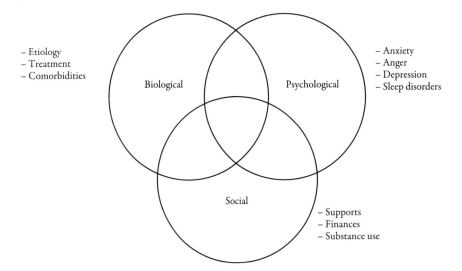

Figure 43.1 The biopsychosocial model of pain.
From Sutton LM, Porter LS, Keefe FJ. Cancer pain at the end of life: A biopsychosocial perspective. *Pain*. 2002;99(1–2):5–10[1]; and Syrjala KL, Jensen MP, Mendoza ME, Yi JC, Fisher HM, Keefe FJ. Psychological and behavioral approaches to cancer pain management. *J Clin Oncol*. 2014;32(16):1703–1711.[2]

develop strategies to prevent pain. Procedural pain, such as that experienced with bone marrow aspiration or other interventions, can be reduced or prevented with adequate local and/or systemic analgesics, education, and preparation. There is ample evidence that unrelieved postoperative pain correlates with chronic pain syndromes, such as post-mastectomy pain.[3] Thus, prevention of acute pain may preclude or limit persistent pain syndromes.

When pain cannot be prevented, relief is imperative. This requires a balance among analgesia, increased function, and safety, and these goals are based on the state of the patient's illness. For the actively dying, the scale may tip toward analgesia, with less emphasis on function. For the patient who is a long-term survivor, the goal of enhanced function supersedes complete pain control.[4] Regardless of the patient's overall stage of disease, safety needs are paramount. Adverse effects must be prevented, minimized, or controlled. Medications must be used by the patient, and only the patient, in a manner that will limit untoward events. This includes preventing access to controlled substances by family, friends, caregivers, or others for inappropriate use (sharing with others or selling the medications).[5,6]

PAIN SYNDROMES IN PALLIATIVE CARE

An awareness of common pain syndromes seen in life-threatening illness assists the APRN in identifying the etiology and guides treatment.[7,8] Differentiating acute from chronic syndromes will help determine the course and treatment options. Specific pain syndromes common in those with cancer have been identified, but unfortunately the types of pain associated with other life-threatening illnesses have not been fully categorized (Table 43.1).[9–11] Understanding the

Table 43.1 SELECTED CANCER PAIN SYNDROMES

Tumor-Related Pain Syndromes
- Bone metastases
- Hepatic capsule distention due to metastases
- Plexus involvement by tumor

Treatment-Related Pain Syndromes

Surgical Pain Syndromes
- Post-amputation phantom pain
- Post-thoracotomy pain
- Post-mastectomy pain

Chemotherapy-Related Pain Syndromes
- Chemotherapy-induced peripheral neuropathy
- Osteonecrosis from corticosteroids

Radiation-Related Pain Syndromes
- Chest pain/tightness
- Cystitis
- Enteritis
- Fistula formation
- Myelopathy
- Osteoporosis
- Osteoradionecrosis
- Pelvic fractures
- Peripheral nerve entrapment
- Plexopathies
- Proctitis
- Secondary malignancies

Stem Cell Transplant-Mediated Chronic Graft-versus-Host Disease
- Scleroderma-like skin changes
- Eye pain and dryness
- Oral pain and reduced jaw motion
- Dysuria
- Dyspareunia, vaginal pain
- Paresthesias
- Arthralgias, myalgias

Hormonal Therapy-Related Pain Syndromes
- Osteoporotic compression fractures
- Arthralgias

Pain Unrelated to Tumor or Treatment
- Comorbid conditions, such as diabetic neuropathy, arthritis

From Paice[4]; Paice et al.[6,11]

etiology may lead to treatment options beyond analgesic therapies, such as radiotherapy for new bone metastases or surgery to repair joints affected by avascular necrosis (discussed later in this chapter).

Another strategy for grouping pain syndromes is by their quality: somatic, neuropathic, visceral, or mixed.[8] Understanding the quality of the patient's pain informs the analgesic regimen. One paradigm is as follows:

- *Somatic pain*: Usually managed by non-opioids and opioids

- Neuropathic pain: Treated with adjuvant analgesics and opioids (little or no response to non-opioids)

- Visceral pain: May be controlled by opioids and, in some cases, corticosteroids or other adjuvant analgesics

PAIN ASSESSMENT

The APRN is uniquely trained to obtain a comprehensive pain assessment in palliative care. This includes a thorough history, a careful physical examination, and, in some cases, interpretation of laboratory values or imaging results.[12–14] The history can be guided by the biopsychosocial model, considering all components of the pain experience. Box 43.1 provides a sample template for a comprehensive pain assessment.

While conducting a thorough history, it is useful to consider those patients at risk for inadequate assessment and management of pain (Box 43.2).[15–17] The use of tools designed for special populations can improve the accuracy of assessment findings. Table 43.2 provides a list of instruments designed to assess pain in adult populations at risk for inadequate assessment.[18]

The physical examination begins when first meeting the patient. Observing the patient's gait while they approach the examination room or evaluating posture while sitting or lying in bed provides essential information. Pay special attention to nonverbal cues of pain. This is followed by close inspection of painful sites, evaluating areas of trauma, skin breakdown, changes in bony or joint structures, and trophic changes, such as reduced hair growth or thickened nails. Palpate areas for tenderness or masses (including signs of obstipation). Perform range of motion in affected extremities to determine if there are contractures or disorders of the joint that elicit pain. Auscultation can reveal crackles, rhonchi, or decreased breath sounds that may signal painful respiratory complications (such as pneumonia) or hyperactive bowel sounds, suggesting bowel obstruction. Percussion can assist in revealing fluid accumulation in ascites. A careful neurological evaluation can identify allodynia, dermatomal distribution of pain, and other sensorimotor changes.

Coupled with a thorough physical examination, radiographic studies and laboratory evaluation may be useful in identifying the etiology of pain. However, these tools may not be readily accessible in all settings, they may place the patient at risk for discomfort (e.g., lying on a hard table

---

Box 43.1 TEMPLATE FOR COMPREHENSIVE PAIN HISTORY DOCUMENTATION

Chief Report

Mr. J is a 56-year-old African-American male diagnosed with metastatic non-small-cell lung cancer (NSCLC) after experiencing a chronic cough that did not resolve with antibiotic therapy; we were asked to see him by Dr. Washington for concerns related to back pain. Briefly, he was diagnosed with NSCLC 8 months ago and underwent 4 courses of chemotherapy (carboplatin and pemetrexed). He recently developed right hip pain and was found to have a pathologic fracture of the right femur that was treated with open reduction and internal fixation and x-ray therapy (XRT) 3 months ago. He now presents with low back pain and right rib pain which are consistent with sites of metastatic disease on recent positron emission tomography (PET) scan.

Pain History

Location(s), referral, radiating pattern
Duration
Intensity (last 24 hours, at rest, with movement)
Quality
Timing
Aggravating/alleviating factors
Other symptoms associated with pain
Functional changes/interference with daily activities

Current Therapies

- Medications duration, response
- Radiation therapy
- Other nerve blocks, kyphoplasty/vertebroplasty, physical therapy (PT)/occupational therapy (OT), acupuncture, etc.

Prior Treatment, Response, Adverse Effects, Reason for Discontinuing

- Medications dose, duration, adverse effects
- Radiation therapy (sites)
- Other nerve blocks, kyphoplasty/vertebroplasty, PT/OT, acupuncture, etc.

Past Medical History

The PMH includes *relevant* serious illness, chronic diseases, surgical procedures, and injuries the patient has experienced.

Social History

Marital status/partnered
Children/grandchildren
Type of home (access), who lives in home, who provides support
Work history, education

Substance Use History

Smoking
Alcohol consumption (ETOH)
Cannabis medical card, adult use
Recreational drug use
Family history of addictive disease
Physical, emotional or sexual abuse, especially as preteen or teenager; post traumatic stress disorder (PTSD)

Medication History

Current medications, including prescription and nonprescription medications, name and dosage for each.

Review of Systems

Perform a review of symptoms (ROS) that may occur along with pain. May use Edmonton Symptom Assessment Scale (ESAS) or other symptom assessment tool in place of ROS. The following is the ROS for Mr. J.
GENERAL: Endorses fatigue, sleep
HEENT: Xerostomia, denies dysphagia
CV: Denies chest pain
RESP: Denies SOB, cough
GI: Last BM x days ago, consistency x, appetite [poor/good], nausea and vomiting
GU: Denies urgency, frequency, incontinence, or dysuria
MS: Denies tripping or falls
NEURO: Denies neuropathy
SKIN: Denies rash or open wounds
PSYCH: Endorses feeling sad/depressed, finds strength through [name the focus, strategy, or intervention]

Performance Status

May use ECOG, Karnofsky, Palliative Performance, Scale or other tool. This helps determine function and prognosis and track change over time.

Physical Exam

List the physical assessment findings that are "remarkable" or contribute to understanding the pain experience and/or etiology.

Patient Goals

What the patient hopes to achieve if pain is relieved (e.g., return to work, play with grandchildren, go to church).

Impression/Recommendations

1.

2.

3.

Box 43.2 GROUPS AT RISK FOR INADEQUATE ASSESSMENT AND UNDERTREATMENT OF PAIN

- Infants and children
- Elderly
- Cognitively impaired
- Nonverbal individuals
- People with mental health disorders
- Minorities
- Non–English-speaking individuals
- Long-term survivors
- Socioeconomically disadvantaged
- Uninsured
- Those with current or past substance use disorders

From Stein et al.[15]; Gunnardottir et al.[16]; and Kwon.[17]

during a lengthy scan), and they may increase the financial burden to patients and families. These diagnostic tools should not be employed if they are not going to alter the course of therapy.

Table 43.2 ASSESSMENT TOOLS FOR SPECIAL ADULT POPULATIONS

TOOL	INTENDED POPULATION
Assessment of Discomfort in Dementia (ADD)	Dementia
Behavioral Pain Scale (BPS)	Intensive care, unresponsive adults
Checklist of Nonverbal Pain Indicators (CNPI)	Dementia
Critical Care Pain Observation Tool (CPOT)	Intensive care, unresponsive adults
Doloplus 2	Dementia, palliative care
Nursing Assistant-Administered Instrument to Assess Pain in Demented Individuals (NOPPAIN)	Dementia
Pain Assessment Scale for Seniors with Limited Ability to Communicate (PACSLAC)	Dementia
Pain Assessment in Advanced Dementia (PAINAD)	Dementia

From Herr et al.[18]; and Booker, Herr.[19]

PHARMACOLOGIC MANAGEMENT OF PAIN

There are three broad categories of medications used to relieve pain: non-opioids, opioids, and adjuvant analgesics. In most cases, a strong analgesic regimen employs multimodal therapies, including more than one pharmacologic agent along with nonpharmacologic strategies. The palliative APRN with prescribing privileges must adhere to safe prescribing principles as well as bearing in mind financial and regulatory concerns.

NON-OPIOIDS

Acetaminophen (also called paracetamol) is analgesic and antipyretic and is found in a variety of combination prescription and over-the-counter compounds. These may include admixtures with opioids (e.g., acetaminophen with codeine, hydrocodone, or oxycodone), or over-the-counter cold, sinus, or sleep remedies (e.g., acetaminophen with diphenhydramine). Hepatic toxicity can result from excessive use, and a firm limit on daily consumption has not been established.[20,21] Some sources recommend no more than 2,000 mg per day, while others suggest up to 3,000 mg may be safe. This needs to be tailored to the patient. Altered hepatic function, excessive alcohol intake, and other comorbid factors may place some patients at elevated risk, and these individuals should be advised to avoid acetaminophen. Renal toxicity is another potential adverse effect of this agent. Acetaminophen is available in oral formulations (including liquids), suppositories, and an injectable formulation which has been used to treat pain and fever.[22] The adult dosage (adults weighing >50 kg) is 1 g given intravenously every 6 hours with a maximum of 4 g per day; patients with renal or hepatic disease should be given a decreased dose or should avoid this drug. The price may preclude use in many palliative care settings.

Nonsteroidal anti-inflammatory drugs (NSAIDs) are analgesic, antipyretic, and anti-inflammatory. They are generally useful for nociceptive or musculoskeletal pain syndromes.[22–24] Adverse effects include gastrointestinal bleeding (which can be prevented with the addition of a prostaglandin analog or a proton pump inhibitor), renal dysfunction, platelet aggregation abnormalities (generally reversible when stopping the drug, except for aspirin, which has an irreversible effect on platelets), and cardiovascular events, such as myocardial infarction and stroke in those at risk.[25–27] Most NSAIDs are available in oral formulations, some in liquids or suppositories. Ketorolac is available for parenteral use and is highly potent; however, prolonged use is contraindicated due to an elevated risk of adverse effects. Topical formulations, including gels, patches, and creams, of several NSAIDs are now available over the counter or with a prescription. These formulations are generally considered to be safe with little systemic absorption.[28]

OPIOIDS

Opioids are useful in treating nociceptive and neuropathic pain, although higher doses are generally required to relieve nerve pain.[29,30] A wide array of opioids is available, allowing rotation when one opioid is ineffective or produces uncontrolled adverse effects. Immediate-release agents provide faster onset to provide rescue when breakthrough pain occurs, and controlled-release products allow more constant control of pain. Various routes of administration allow personalized care when oral delivery is not feasible. Table 43.3 lists opioids available in the United States.[8,29,31] Prevention and management of adverse events is crucial, as is education of patients, family members, and caregivers regarding safe use of these agents.[32]

There are significant differences between opioids. Codeine is a prodrug and must be metabolized to morphine by the action of the CYP2D6 enzyme.[33,34] Inadequate analgesia can result in patients who are poor metabolizers, while increased toxicity and overdose have been reported in individuals (or a breastfeeding baby) who are ultra-rapid metabolizers of this enzyme.[35,36] Tramadol is a weak opioid agonist and a serotonin-norepinephrine reuptake inhibitor. Due to this dual action, it has a ceiling of 300 mg per day, and naloxone will not completely reverse overdose.[37] Tramadol should be avoided in patients with seizure risk or suicidal ideation. Dizziness is the most common adverse effect. Tapentadol is also an opioid agonist and norepinephrine reuptake inhibitor, with little action on serotonin reuptake.[38] Caution is warranted when adding antidepressants that act on the serotonin system to either tramadol or tapentadol to prevent serotonin syndrome. As with tramadol, naloxone will not completely reverse the effects of overdose with tapentadol.

Methadone can be a highly effective analgesic: it may prevent or limit hyperalgesia, it appears to be useful for neuropathic pain, it can be crushed and used via enteral tubes while retaining its long-acting property, and it is inexpensive.[39,40] Several challenges complicate the use of methadone, and several guidelines recommend a palliative care consultation when considering its use. As a result, palliative APRNs must be highly skilled in the use of this opioid. Specific issues in methadone use include the long and variable half-life, which complicates dose escalation and conversions; the prolonged QTc that can result; lack of clarity on equianalgesic ratios; and many drug–drug interactions.[40–42] Box 43.3 provides guidelines for use of this drug.[29,42] Table 43.4 lists potential drug–drug interactions with methadone involving medications commonly employed in palliative care.[39,41,43] Box 43.4 lists chemotherapeutic agents that can result in prolonged QTc when given in combination with methadone.[44]

When analgesia is incomplete despite appropriate titration of the opioid, or when adverse effects persist despite aggressive management, opioid rotation is warranted.[13,41–48] Box 43.5 provides general guidelines for opioid rotation. An excellent handbook is available to guide the APRN who is new to equianalgesic dosing: *Demystifying Opioid Conversion Calculations: A Guide for Effective Dosing.*[31] Although online calculators are available, the palliative APRN must thoroughly understand the calculations to provide safe dosing and to teach other colleagues how to use them appropriately.

Table 43.3 OPIOID ANALGESICS: AVAILABLE FORMULATIONS AND EQUIANALGESIC GUIDELINES

OPIOID EQUIANALGESIC TABLE

| DRUG | DOSAGE FORM/STRENGTHS | APPROXIMATE EQUIVALENCE | |
		IV/SQ	ORAL
Buprenorphine	**Transdermal** Butrans 5, 7.5, 10, 15, 20 μg/h	0.3–0.4 mg	See package insert
	Buccal Strip: Belbuca™ 75,150, 300, 450, 600, 750, 900 μg q12–24h		
	Injection 0.3 mg/mL		
	Medication-assisted therapy (MAT), for treatment of opioid use disorder; not typically used for pain control; requires specialized waiver (see https://www.samhsa.gov/medication-assisted-treatment) • Buprenorphine/naloxone sublingual strips or tablets		
Codeine	**Rarely recommended:** A pro-drug dependent on CYP2D6; significant percentage of people are poor metabolizers and cannot obtain relief		200 mg
Fentanyl Parenteral		100 μg	
Fentanyl Transdermal Long-acting; Not for opioid-naïve patients	**Fentanyl Transdermal** Duragesic® and generic 12, 25, 37.5, 50, 62.5, 75, 87.5, 100 μg/h • Not for postop/acute pain • 12–24h for full onset • 12–24h to leave system		100 μg patch q2–3 days ≈ 200 mg oral morphine q24 h
Fentanyl Transmucosal Immediate-Release Fentanyl (TIRF) Not for opioid-naïve patients	**Buccal Oral Lozenge** Actiq® and generic 200, 400, 600, 800, 1200, 1600 μg **Buccal Oral Tablet** Fentora® 100, 200, 400, 600, 800 μg **Sublingual Tablet** Abstral® Fentanyl SL 100, 200, 400, 800 μg **Sublingual Spray** Subsys® 100, 200, 400, 600, 800 μg spray **Nasal Spray** Lazanda® 100, 300, 400 μg **Requires TIRF-REMS compliance** https://www.tirfremsaccess.com/TirfUI/rems/home.action	–	See package inserts
Hydrocodone	**Hydrocodone/Acetaminophen Tablets:** Vicodin® 5/300 mg; Vicodin® ES 7.5/300 mg, Lorcet® or Vicodin® HP 10 mg/300 mg Lortab® 2.5/500 mg, 5/500 mg 7.5/500 mg, 10/500 mg Norco® 5/325 mg, 7.5/325 mg, 10/325 mg **Liquid:** Hycet® 7.5/325/15 mL **Hydrocodone/Ibuprofen Tablets:** Vicoprofen® and generic 7.5/200 mg **Extended-Release:** Hysingla® ER (q 24h) -20, 30, 40, 60, 80, 100, 120 mg Zohydro® ER (q 12h) 10, 15, 30, 40, 50 mg	–	20–30 mg
Hydromorphone	**Tablets** Hydromorphone (Dilaudid® and generic) 2, 4, 8 mg **Liquid:** Hydromorphone (Dilaudid®) 1 mg/mL **Injection:** 1, 2, 4 mg/mL and Dilaudid® HP 10 mg/mL **Suppository:** Hydromorphone 3 mg Extended-Release (Exalgo®) 8, 12, 16, 32 mg q24 h	1.5 mg	7.5 mg

Table 43.3 CONTINUED

OPIOID EQUIANALGESIC TABLE

| DRUG | DOSAGE FORM/STRENGTHS | APPROXIMATE EQUIVALENCE | |
		IV/SQ	ORAL
Methadone	Equivalency ratios for methadone are complex because of its long half-life, potency, and individual variations in pharmacokinetics.	–	Consult with Pain/Palliative Care Specialist
Morphine	**Immediate-Release Tablets** Morphine Sulfate Immediate-Release 15, 30 mg	10 mg	30 mg
	Liquid: Morphine Sulfate Immediate-Release Solution 2 mg/mL, 4 mg/mL, 20 mg/mL		
	Extended or Sustained Release Tablet or Capsules: Generic 10,15, 20, 30, 45,50, 60, 75, 80, 90, 100, 120, 200 mg q12 h MS Contin® 15, 30, 60, 100, 200 mg q8h or q12h Kadian® 10, 20, 30, 40, 50, 60, 70, 80, 100, 200 mg q12–24h		
	Injection: 2, 4, 5, 8, 10 mg/mL **Suppository:** Rectal morphine sulfate (RMS) 5, 10, 20, 30 mg		
Oxycodone	**Immediate-Release Tablets:** Oxycodone IR 5, 10, 15, 20, 30 mg Oxaydo 5, 7.5 mg Roxicodone® 15, 30 mg	–	20 mg
	Oxycodone/Acetaminophen Tablets: Endocet® 5/325, 7.5/325, 10/325 mg Percocet® and generics 2.5/325, 5/325, 7.5/325, 10/325 mg Primlev™ 2.5/300, 5/300, 7.5/300, 10/300 mg		
	Extended- or Sustained-Release Tablets: Oxycodone ER 10, 20, 40, 80 mg q12h OxyContin® 10, 15, 20, 30, 40, 60, 80 mg Xtampza® ER ***– 9, 13.5, 18, 27, 36 mg q12h		
	Liquid: Oxycodone 5 mg/5 mL, 20 mg/mL		
Oxymorphone	**Tablets** Opana® 5, 10 mg, Generⁱc IR 5, 10 mg Generic ER 7.5, 10, 15, 20, 30, 40 mg q12h	1 mg	10 mg
	Injection: 1 mg/mL		
Tapentadol (opioid and norepinephrine reuptake inhibitor)	**Tapentadol Tablets** Nucynta® 50, 75, 100 mg	–	150 mg
	Extended-Release Nucynta®ER– 50, 100, 150, 200, 250 mg q12h		
Tramadol (opioid and SNRI reuptake inhibitor)	**Tramadol Tablets** Generic 50, 100 mg Generic– 37.5/325 mg acetaminophen	–	300 mg
	Extended-Release: ConZip and generic 100, 200, 300 mg q24h		
	Liquid Qdolo™ 5 mg/mL		

From Swarm et al.[8]; Caraceni et al.[29]; Bennett et al.[32] Reprinted with permission from ELNEC.

ADJUVANT ANALGESICS

Adjuvant analgesics include agents that have other purposes but have been found to be analgesic, primarily in the management of neuropathic pain. Table 43.5 includes common agents, starting doses, and potential adverse effects.[8,13,41,49,50] Because these agents act via different mechanisms, patients with complex pain may require multimodal therapy that includes one agent from each drug class. There are few studies exploring the efficacy of these drugs in the palliative care setting, and results often conflict with observations from clinical practice.

Corticosteroids are important adjuvant analgesics for the relief of neuropathic pain as well as some visceral pain syndromes that involve inflammation around masses (e.g., ovarian or gastrointestinal malignancies).[51,52] These agents can be highly effective in reducing the tumor burden of lymphoma, which can open airway or gastrointestinal obstructions from this malignancy.

Table 43.4 SELECTED METHADONE DRUG–DRUG INTERACTIONS

INDUCERS (DECREASE METHADONE LEVELS)	INHIBITORS (INCREASE METHADONE LEVELS)
• Abacavir	• Cimetidine
• Amprenavir	• Ciprofloxacin
• Barbiturates	• Diazepam
• Carbamazepine	• Diltiazem
• Cocaine	• Disulfiram
• Dexamethasone	• Fluconazole
• Efavirenz	• Grapefruit
• Heroin	• Haloperidol
• Lopinavir + Ritonavir	• Ketoconazole
• Nelfinavir	• Macrolides (erythromycin, clarithromycin)
• Nevirapine	• Metronidazole
• Phenytoin	• Omeprazole
• Rifampin	• Sorafenib
• Spironolactone	• Selective serotonin reuptake inhibitors (SSRIs; fluoxetine, paroxetine, nefazodone, sertraline)
• St. John's wort	

From Edmonds et al.[44]; McPherson et al.[45]; World Health Organization.[46]

Added benefits of corticosteroids include improved appetite for approximately 2 weeks, and activation, which can relieve fatigue and possibly depression.[51] Systematic reviews find the evidence for analgesia associated with corticosteroids to be generally weak despite anecdotal clinical experiences suggesting these agents can provide efficacy in some settings.[52,53] Study design issues, including inclusion criteria, limit the extrapolation of these findings to most people with cancer pain. Important drug–drug interactions with dexamethasone are listed in Box 43.6.

Lidocaine and other local anesthetics have been limited by the lack of an oral formulation. Topical solutions and patches may relieve more superficial pain syndromes. Spinal delivery, either alone or in combination with opioids and other agents, can be useful, but administration requires specialists to insert catheters and potentially complicated and/or expensive delivery systems (e.g., catheter care, external or implanted pumps). Infusions of parenteral lidocaine, particularly in the face of intractable neuropathic pain, may be effective.[54,55]

Table 43.5 ADJUVANT ANALGESICS

DRUG CLASS	USUAL ADULT DAILY STARTING DOSE	ROUTES OF ADMINISTRATION	ADVERSE EFFECTS
Antidepressants	Nortriptyline 10–25 mg qhs	PO	Anticholinergic effects
	Venlafaxine 37.5 mg bid	PO	Nausea, dizziness
	Duloxetine 30 mg qd		Nausea
Antiepilepsy drugs	Gabapentin 100 mg tid	PO	Dizziness
	Pregabalin 50 mg tid	PO	Dizziness
	Clonazepam 0.5–1 mg qhs, bid, or tid	PO	Sedation
Corticosteroids	Dexamethasone 2–20 mg qd	PO/IV/SQ	"Steroid psychosis" Dyspepsia
Lidocaine	Lidocaine patch 5% qd (also 4% patch over the counter along with creams/gels) Lidocaine infusion	Topical IV/SQ	Rare skin erythema Perioral numbness, cardiac changes
N-Methyl-D-aspartic acid antagonists	Ketamine (see following text section on ketamine for dosing)	PO/IV	Hallucinations

From Swarm et al.[8]; Fallon et al.[13]

Ketamine is an N-methyl-D-aspartic acid antagonist that is thought to be useful in relieving neuropathic pain, in reducing opioid doses when high doses appear ineffective, or in the management of opioid-induced hyperalgesia.[56,57] Yet clinical trials have not supported the benefits of ketamine for pain control in palliative care. In a controlled trial of ketamine versus placebo in neuropathic cancer pain, ketamine was equivalent to placebo.[58] Case reports suggest this agent may be useful for refractory depression at the end of life.[59] Box 43.7 provides a sample protocol for use in palliative care. Palliative APRNs with prescribing privileges should check state and institutional rules regarding their ability to prescribe this medication. Additional well-controlled studies are needed to evaluate the role of ketamine for those with central sensitization who might be experiencing neurotoxicity and hyperalgesia to opioids at the end of life, as well as the efficacy in treating severe depression and suicidal ideation in those with serious illness.

Box 43.6 DRUG–DRUG INTERACTIONS INVOLVING DEXAMETHASONE: POTENTIAL TO DECREASE BLOOD LEVELS OF TARGETED THERAPIES

Erlotinib
Gefitinib
Ibrutinib
Lapatinib
Pazopanib
Ruxolitinib
Sorafenib
Sunitinib
Temsirolimus

The role of cannabinoids in relieving pain is often questioned, and palliative APRNs will be asked by professionals, patients, and the public about the use of these compounds.[60,61] Research is limited, in part because of inadequate funding and lack of availability of an approved study drug.[62] Possible harms include hyperemesis syndrome (seen more often with inhaled cannabis) and psychiatric or cardiovascular effects (seen more frequently with edible cannabinoids).[63] As the APRN reviews current literature, it is helpful to understand the different formulations of cannabinoids. This is particularly important as more states approve either medical or adult use (formerly called recreational use) of cannabinoids.[64] Box 43.8 clarifies the variety of formulations of cannabinoids.[65,66]

NONPHARMACOLOGIC INTERVENTIONS FOR PAIN

The biopsychosocial model clarifies the need for both pharmacologic and nonpharmacologic techniques to relieve pain. The findings from the complete pain history and physical examination help the palliative APRN in designing a treatment plan that incorporates appropriate interventions. Many of these interventions require the expertise of specialists and other team members, including radiologists, surgeons, psychologists, physical therapists, chaplains, social workers, and many others. Close communication with these consultants and team members will ensure continuity of care and will increase the chances of meeting the patient's goals for pain relief. Education is an essential component of all successful pain relief regimens.[67] Table 43.6 lists selected nonpharmacologic interventions.[2,68–70] Challenges to the incorporation of these interventions into the treatment plan include lack of reimbursement, limited access to practitioners with expertise in these interventions, and reluctance on the part of some patients and family members to accept these techniques.[71]

Purpose

This is an adjunct medication often considered for pain refractory to opioids or intractable side effects from opioids, particularly if the pain is neuropathic in nature or if a high degree of morphine tolerance is suspected.

Definition

Ketamine is an N-methyl-D-aspartate receptor (NMDA) agent that may be opioid-sparing.

Protocol

ORAL DOSING

- The typical starting dose is 10–15 mg PO every 6 hours. Reversal of morphine tolerance may occur at low doses such as this, while management of neuropathic pain is likely to require higher doses.

- There is no commercially available oral product. The injectable product may be diluted from its standard concentration of 50 mg/mL or 100 mg/mL with cherry syrup or cola to mask the bitter taste when given orally.

- Consider decreasing long-acting opioid by 25–50%.

- Dosing may be increased *daily* by 10 mg every 6 hours until pain is relieved or side effects occur. Do not increase doses more frequently than every 24 hours.

- Major side effects include dizziness, a dreamlike feeling, and auditory or visual hallucinations. If intolerable side effects occur, ketamine should be decreased to the previous dose or discontinued. Resolution may not occur for 24 hours.

- Oral doses as high as 1,000 mg per day have been reported in the neuropathic pain literature, with average oral doses of 200 mg per day in divided doses required for pain relief.

IV DOSING

- Ketamine may be given intravenously or subcutaneously if the oral route is not available.

- Some facilities allow a ketamine challenge. A trial of 10 mg IV can be considered, which may be repeated in 15–30 minutes.

- The starting infusion dose of 0.2 mg/kg/h can be increased by 0.1 mg/kg/h q6h, with upward titrations to 0.5 mg/kg/h or 800 mg in 24 h.

- Consider decreasing long-acting opioid dose by 25–50%.

- The injectable solution is irritating and the subcutaneous needle may need to be changed daily.

- For side effects of hallucinations or a dreamlike state, benzodiazepines can be given prophylactically or Haldol can be given when the effects occur.

Box 43.8 FORMULATIONS OF CANNABINOIDS

Endocannabinoids

- Endogenous neurotransmitters arachidonic acid derivatives (e.g., anandamide)

Phytocannabinoids (Also Called Botanical Cannabis)

- Compounds found in *Cannabis sativa* plant (e.g., THC, CBD, many others)

- Primarily smoked, vaporized, ingested or applied topically

Synthetic Cannabinoids

- Laboratory-produced congeners of THC, CBD

- Dronabinol (Marinol) tablet, approved in United States for chemotherapy-induced nausea and vomiting and AIDS-associated anorexia

- Nabilone (Cesamet) approved in United States for chemotherapy- induced nausea and vomiting that has not responded to traditional treatments

- Nabiximols oral spray indicated for neuropathic pain, spasticity (not yet approved in United States)

- Cannabidiol (Epidiolex) a oral solution approved in United States for drug-resistant seizures

From Volkow et al.[65]; Devinsky et al.[66]

Table 43.6 BIOPSYCHOSOCIAL MODEL: NONPHARMACOLOGIC INTERVENTIONS

BIOLOGICAL	PSYCHOLOGICAL/ SOCIAL/SPIRITUAL
Disease-modifying therapies • Chemotherapy, immunotherapy • Radiation therapy	Cognitive-behavioral therapies
Kyphoplasty/vertebroplasty	Mindfulness/Meditation
Nerve blocks	Guided imagery
Ablative procedures	Hypnosis
Physical/occupational and other rehabilitation therapies	Biofeedback
Exercise	Prayer
Heat/cold/bracing/orthotics	Music
Massage	Art therapy
Acupuncture and other integrative procedures	Support groups

From Syrjala et al.[2]; Swarm et al.[8]; Kwekkeboom, Bratzke[68]; Sadeghi-Naini et al.[72]; Cheville et al.[73,74]; Dikmen, Terzioglu[75]; Zollfrank et al.[76]; Kang, Formenti[77]; Mark et al[78]; and Park et al.[79]

Pain management in palliative care will include the use of drugs with a high potential for abuse. To provide safe and effective pain control, palliative APRNs must work to prevent misuse and diversion.

SAFE STORAGE

Education of patients and their family members regarding safe storage and disposal is essential. Studies suggest that patients, including oncology and palliative care patients, are not employing these practices.[80,81] Medications should be kept locked, not stored in the medicine cabinet or out on the kitchen counter. Medications should never be shared and should be used only for pain relief. Many find that these medications enhance sleep, improve mood, and relieve anxiety, particularly during initial exposure, in part due to the sedating effect. But tolerance quickly develops to the soporific or sedative effect, and patients will find the need to escalate doses to obtain the original response. Dose escalation can lead to serious complications, including oversedation or other toxicities as the dose is increased. Compounding this is the stigma held by many about taking psychotropic medications, which are more appropriate in managing anxiety, depression, sleep issues, or other mood disorders.[82]

SAFE DISPOSAL

Safe disposal of medications prevents access by others (e.g., children, pets, individuals with intent to use the drugs recreationally or sell these agents) and limits impact on the environment.[81] Municipalities are detecting medications in the water supply, in part as a result of drugs being flushed into the sanitary system. The Environmental Protection Agency advises against flushing medications (https://www.epa.gov/hwgenerators/collecting-and-disposing-unwanted-medicines), preferring incineration.

The Drug Enforcement Agency (DEA) offers a twice-yearly National Prescription Drug Take-Back Program and allows collection receptacles in places such as law enforcement stations, hospitals, and pharmacies, the locations for which can be found at DEA website (https://apps2.deadiversion.usdoj.gov/pubdispsearch/spring/main?execution=e1s1).

The Food and Drug Administration (FDA) recommends that if a take-back program is not available, medications (except for opioids) should be mixed with moistened kitty litter or used coffee grounds, placed in a sealed plastic bag, and thrown away in the trash. Empty pill bottles or other packaging should be blacked out so that the drug or individual cannot be identified. However, the FDA still requires that if a take-back program is not available, opioids must be flushed down the sink or toilet due to safety concerns (https://www.fda.gov/drugs/safe-disposal-medicines/disposal-unused-medicines-what-you-should-know#Flushing_list).

Because there is no absolute predictor for who might misuse medications, chronic pain management experts recommend the use of "universal precautions." Although studies are ongoing regarding their efficacy, particularly in palliative care, many prescribers are adopting all or some of these recommendations.[83–86] Box 43.9 outlines key aspects of universal precautions.[87] Numerous tools are available to screen for misuse or high-risk behaviors (e.g., CAGE, Current Opioid Misuse Measure [COMM], Opioid Risk Tool [ORT]). Few have been validated in a palliative care population.

Random urine drug testing through toxicology screening can help determine if patients are taking illicit drugs or not taking the drugs prescribed.[88,89] However, caution is advised in the interpretation of these results; false negatives and positives abound (see Table 43.7). For example, a patient receiving transdermal fentanyl will have a test result that is negative for opioids. The palliative APRN obtaining random urine toxicology must seek expert advice regarding interpretation of the results before making decisions regarding whether a patient should no longer be prescribed an opioid.

Statewide prescription drug monitoring programs (PDMPs) are now available in 49 states (Missouri has a modified program). Although the information provided by each state varies, most allow prescribers to view the controlled substances that have been prescribed for a particular patient, the date and number of tablets/patches dispensed, the method of payment (insurance vs. self-pay), the pharmacy where the drug was dispensed, and the name of the prescriber.[90] Many state PDMPs can access data from other states. Although sometimes viewed as a method to "catch" offenders, more often these programs help identify the medications taken by patients who do not bring in their medications or do not know the name of the drug (e.g., the "blue pill"). Several states and institutions have mandated review of the PDMP prior to prescribing a controlled substance. The palliative APRN must be aware of the associated regulations to appropriately and safely prescribe.

Box 43.9 UNIVERSAL PRECAUTIONS

Assess

- Pain and function

- Risk for addiction/diversion

Opioid management agreements or "contracts" have limited evidence in palliative care.

Adherence Monitoring

- Urine drug testing

- Pill counts

- Prescription drug monitoring programs

From Arthur, Bruera.[87]

Table 43.7 URINE DRUG TESTING

TEST	TYPE OF TEST	GENERAL PURPOSE	INTERPRETATION ISSUES: EXAMPLES

Brief Screen	Immunoassay
	More rapid results usually within hours
	Less expensive
		Detects the presence of drugs: amphetamines, barbiturates, benzodiazepines, cocaine, opiates, phencyclidine, δ-9-tetrahydrocannabinol (THC)	False negatives:
			    Cannot detect synthetic opioids such as oxycodone
			    May not detect ketamine, clonidine, non-benzodiazepine hypnotics (e.g., zolpidem)
			False positives:
			    Selective serotonin reuptake inhibitor (SSRI) intake positive benzodiazepine
			    Ephedrine positive amphetamines
			    Nonsteroidal anti-inflammatory drugs (NSAIDs) positive barbiturates

Confirmation	Liquid or gas chromatography/mass spectrometry May take days for results More expensive; not all insurance covers	Can identify specific opioids and other controlled substances along with their metabolites	Timing of collection may alter results: A delay from ingestion to sampling may produce negative results for hydrocodone and positive results for hydromorphone (a metabolite of hydrocodone) Consider the metabolites of each opioid during interpretation

Table 43.8 CONTROLLED SUBSTANCES SCHEDULES

SCHEDULE	EXAMPLES SELECTED	APRN ABILITY TO PRESCRIBE
Schedule I	Heroin Lysergic acid diethylamide (LSD) Marijuana (cannabis)	No currently accepted medical use in the United States; available only for research purposes
Schedule II/IIN (2/2N)	Schedule II Amphetamine Cocaine Codeine Fentanyl Hydrocodone Hydromorphone Methadone Meperidine Methamphetamine Methylphenidate Morphine Opium Oxycodone Pentobarbital	**Allowed by national DEA registration.** **Each state has its own statutes as to whether APRN can prescribe.** **Transmucosal immediate-release fentanyl products (TIRF REMS) require REMS (https://www.tirfremsaccess.com/TirfUI/rems/home.action)**
Schedule III/IIIN (3/3N)	Buprenorphine Codeine/acetaminophen Ketamine Testosterone	**Allowed by national DEA registration.** **Each state has its own statutes as to whether APRN can prescribe.** **Buprenorphine requires medication-assisted therapy (MAT) for treatment of opioid use disorder; requires specialized waiver (see https://www.samhsa.gov/medication-assisted-treatment)**
Schedule IV	Tramadol Alprazolam Clonazepam Diazepam Lorazepam Midazolam	**Allowed by national DEA registration.** **Each state has its own statutes as to whether APRN can prescribe.**
Schedule V	Cough preparations containing not more than 200 mg of codeine per 100 mL or per 100 grams	**Allowed by national DEA registration.** **Each state has its own statutes as to whether APRN can prescribe.**

Adapted from http://www.deadiversion.usdoj.gov/schedules/#define

Another component of safe prescribing is the provision of naloxone, an opioid antagonist, in the event of an accidental overdose by the patient or loved ones (e.g., a grandchild finding and eating a tablet, thinking it is candy).[91] Naloxone is available as a nasal formulation, an auto-injector, or in vials for intravenous administration. Long used by first responders to treat opioid overdose, nasal naloxone is now available as a generic formulation, by prescription, although many national retail pharmacies will provide it without a prescription. Additionally, although initially costing patients approximately $150, most insurance companies now cover this charge. To save costs, some settings have used improvised atomizers to deliver naloxone; however, there is concern this does not deliver a full dose of the medication and must be avoided. Patients and family members require education about the symptoms of an opioid overdose, including inability to wake the person verbally or by shaking them, very slow or shallow breathing, and fingernails or lips turning blue. In addition to explaining how to use the nasal naloxone, they should be informed to call 911 after administering naloxone as the duration of effect is from 30 to 90 minutes, much shorter than most opioids. Although co-prescribing with opioids is recommended, it is unclear how often this medication is currently provided to those receiving palliative care in the home. For more information about delivery systems, patient teaching and access, see https://www.drugabuse.gov/drug-topics/opioids/opioid-overdose-reversal-naloxone-narcan-evzio.

Palliative APRNs must also be aware of the DEA schedule system so they can comply with prescribing regulations in their own state and institution. Table 43.8 lists substances that may be used in palliative care for pain and symptom control. Lack of awareness of any changes to an agents schedule can result in delays in patients obtaining needed medications. For more information, see https://www.dea.gov/drug-scheduling.

Risk evaluation and mitigation strategies (REMS) have been instituted to advance safe prescribing of a variety of substances. Two of these strategies involve opioids and have implications for APRNs who might prescribe these agents. Use of the strategy for transmucosal immediate-release fentanyl products (TIRF REMS) (https://www.tirfremsaccess.com/TirfUI/rems/home.action) is required for prescribers of these products. An online educational module and exam can be completed for provider enrollment in this program. When these medications are prescribed for an individual patient, he or she signs an online agreement affirming that he or she understands appropriate use of these products. The strategy for extended-release and long-acting opioid analgesics is highly recommended to improve the knowledge of both providers and patients (http://www.er-la-opioidrems.com/IwgUI/rems/home.action).

Despite all of these measures and safeguards, there may be times when patients exhibit what seems to be aberrant drug-taking behavior. The palliative APRN must assess further requests for early or frequent refills. Box 43.10 describes the differential diagnosis for these requests so that the underlying problem can be appropriately addressed[92,93] (see Chapter 47, "Patients with Substance Use Disorder and Dual Diagnoses").

Box 43.10 DIFFERENTIAL DIAGNOSIS OF ABERRANT DRUG-TAKING BEHAVIOR

Addiction (Substance Use Disorder)

PSEUDO-ADDICTION (INADEQUATE ANALGESIA)

- Amount of drug ordered too low dose, number of tablets
- Partial fill provided by pharmacy
- Insurance limits, prior authorization

OTHER PSYCHIATRIC DISORDERS

- Chemical coping
- Mood disorders (anxiety, depression)
- Encephalopathy
- Borderline personality disorder

INABILITY TO FOLLOW A TREATMENT PLAN

- Low literacy
- Use of pain medication to treat other symptoms (sleep, anxiety, depression)
- Misunderstanding regarding "prn" or as needed dosing
- Fear of pain returning

CRIMINAL INTENT

From Yennurajalingam et al.[92]; and Arthur, Hui.[93]

SUMMARY

Effective pain management in palliative care requires knowledge of common pain etiologies, as well as skill in conducting a thorough assessment. The palliative APRN who is devising a treatment plan must consider the available pharmacologic and nonpharmacologic therapies, using the biopsychosocial model as a guide. Consulting with other team members is imperative to provide optimal control including pain services for interventions such as a neurolytic block, radiation oncology for radiation, and surgery for kyphoplasty or vertebroplasty. Safety is crucial: the palliative APRN must use tools such as prescription drug monitoring programs and urine toxicology. Education of patients and families regarding appropriate use, storage, and disposal of pain medications is essential.

REFERENCES

1. Sutton LM, Porter LS, Keefe FJ. Cancer pain at the end of life: A biopsychosocial perspective. *Pain*. 2002;99(1–2):5–10. doi:10.1016/s0304-3959(02)00236-1

2. Syrjala KL, Jensen MP, Mendoza ME, Yi JC, Fisher HM, Keefe FJ. Psychological and behavioral approaches to cancer pain management. *J Clin Oncol.* 2014;32(16):1703–1711. doi:10.1200/JCO.2013.54.4825

3. Schreiber KL, Martel MO, Shnol H, et al. Persistent pain in postmastectomy patients: Comparison of psychophysical, medical, surgical, and psychosocial characteristics between patients with and without pain. *Pain.* 2013;154(5):660–668. doi:10.1016/j.pain.2012.11.015

4. Paice JA. Pain in cancer survivors: How to manage. *Curr Treat Options Oncol.* 2019;20(6):48. doi:10.1007/s11864-019-0647-0

5. Peck KR, Harman JL, Anghelescu DL. Family and peer-group substance abuse as a risk-factor for opioid misuse behaviors for a young adult with cancer-related pain-a case study. *J Adolesc Young Adult Oncol.* 2018;7(1):137–140. doi:10.1089/jayao.2017.0055

6. Paice JA, Portenoy R, Lacchetti C, et al. Management of chronic pain in survivors of adult cancers: American Society of Clinical Oncology clinical practice guideline. *J Clin Oncol.* 2016;34(27):3325–3345. doi:10.1200/JCO.2016.68.5206

7. van den Beuken-van Everdingen MH, Hochstenbach LM, Joosten EA, Tjan-Heijnen VC, Janssen DJ. Update on prevalence of pain in patients with cancer: Systematic review and meta-analysis. *J Pain Symptom Manage.* 2016;51(6):1070–1090 e1079. doi:10.1016/j.jpainsymman.2015.12.340

8. Swarm RA, Paice JA, Anghelescu DL, et al. Adult cancer pain, version 3.2019, NCCN clinical practice guidelines in oncology. *J Natl Compr Canc Netw.* 2019;17(8):977–1007. doi:10.6004/jnccn.2019.0038

9. Ma JD, El-Jawahri AR, LeBlanc TW, Roeland EJ. Pain syndromes and management in adult hematopoietic stem cell transplantation. *Hematol Oncol Clin North Am.* 2018;32(3):551–567. doi:10.1016/j.hoc.2018.01.012

10. Kane CM, Hoskin P, Bennett MI. Cancer induced bone pain. *BMJ.* 2015;350:h315. doi:10.1136/bmj.h315

11. Paice JA, Mulvey M, Bennett M, et al. AAPT diagnostic criteria for chronic cancer pain conditions. *J Pain.* 2017;18(3):233–246. doi:10.1016/j.jpain.2016.10.020

12. Fink RM, Gallagher E. Cancer pain assessment and measurement. *Semin Oncol Nurs.* 2019;35(3):229–234. doi:10.1016/j.soncn.2019.04.003

13. Fallon M, Giusti R, Aielli F, et al. Management of cancer pain in adult patients: ESMO clinical practice guidelines. *Ann Oncol.* 2018;29 Suppl 4:iv166–iv191. doi:10.1093/annonc/mdy152

14. Bennett MI, Eisenberg E, Ahmedzai SH, et al. Standards for the management of cancer-related pain across Europe: A position paper from the EFIC task force on cancer pain. *Eur J Pain.* 2019;23(4):660–668. doi:10.1002/ejp.1346

15. Stein KD, Alcaraz KI, Kamson C, Fallon EA, Smith TG. Sociodemographic inequalities in barriers to cancer pain management: A report from the American Cancer Society's Study of Cancer Survivors-II (SCS-II). *Psychooncology.* 2016;25(10):1212–1221. doi:10.1002/pon.4218

16. Gunnarsdottir S, Sigurdardottir V, Kloke M, et al. A multicenter study of attitudinal barriers to cancer pain management. *Support Care Cancer.* 2017;25(11):3595–3602. doi:10.1007/s00520-017-3791-8

17. Kwon JH. Overcoming barriers in cancer pain management. *J Clin Oncol.* 2014;32(16):1727–1733. doi:10.1200/JCO.2013.52.4827

18. Herr K, Coyne PJ, Ely E, Gelinas C, Manworren RCB. ASPMN 2019 position statement: Pain assessment in the patient unable to self-report. *Pain Manag Nurs.* 2019;20(5):402–403. doi:10.1016/j.pmn.2019.07.005

19. Booker SQ, Herr KA. Assessment and measurement of pain in adults in later life. *Clin Geriatr Med.* 2016;32(4):677–692. doi:10.1016/j.cger.2016.06.012

20. Saccomano SJ. Acute acetaminophen toxicity in adults. *Nurse Pract.* 2019;44(11):42–47. 10.1097/01.NPR.0000586020.15798.c6

21. Wiffen PJ, Derry S, Moore RA, et al. Oral paracetamol (acetaminophen) for cancer pain. *Cochrane Database Syst Rev.* 2017;7:CD012637. doi:10.1002/14651858.CD012637.pub2

22. Vardy J, Agar M. Nonopioid drugs in the treatment of cancer pain. *J Clin Oncol.* 2014;32(16):1677–1690. doi:10.1200/JCO.2013.52.8356

23. Magee DJ, Jhanji S, Poulogiannis G, Farquhar-Smith P, Brown MRD. Nonsteroidal anti-inflammatory drugs and pain in cancer patients: A systematic review and reappraisal of the evidence. *Br J Anaesth.* 2019;123(2):e412–e423. doi:10.1016/j.bja.2019.02.028

24. Strawson J. Nonsteroidal anti-inflammatory drugs and cancer pain. *Curr Opin Support Palliat Care.* 2018;12(2):102–107. doi:10.1097/SPC.0000000000000332

25. Bjarnason I, Scarpignato C, Holmgren E, Olszewski M, Rainsford KD, Lanas A. Mechanisms of damage to the gastrointestinal tract from nonsteroidal anti-inflammatory drugs. *Gastroenterology.* 2018;154(3):500–514. doi:10.1053/j.gastro.2017.10.049

26. McGettigan P, Henry D. Cardiovascular risk with non-steroidal anti-inflammatory drugs: Systematic review of population-based controlled observational studies. *PLoS Med.* 2011;8(9):e1001098. doi:10.1371/journal.pmed.1001098

27. Olsen AS, McGettigan P, Gerds TA, et al. Risk of gastrointestinal bleeding associated with oral anticoagulation and non-steroidal anti-inflammatory drugs in patients with atrial fibrillation: A nationwide study. *Eur Heart J Cardiovasc Pharmacother.* 2020;6(5):292–300. doi:10.1093/ehjcvp/pvz069

28. Honvo G, Leclercq V, Geerinck A, et al. Safety of topical non-steroidal anti-inflammatory drugs in osteoarthritis: Outcomes of a systematic review and meta-analysis. *Drugs Aging.* 2019;36(Suppl 1):45–64. doi:10.1007/s40266-019-00661-0

29. Caraceni A, Hanks G, Kaasa S, et al. Use of opioid analgesics in the treatment of cancer pain: Evidence-based recommendations from the EAPC. *Lancet Oncol.* 2012;13(2):e58–68. doi:10.1016/S1470-2045(12)70040-2

30. Wiffen PJ, Wee B, Derry S, Bell RF, Moore RA. Opioids for cancer pain: An overview of Cochrane reviews. *Cochrane Database Syst Rev.* 2017;7:CD012592. doi:10.1002/14651858.CD012592.pub2

31. McPherson ML. *Demystifying Opioid Conversion Calculations: A Guide for Effective Dosing.* 2nd ed. Bethesda, MD: American Society of Health-System Pharmacists; 2018.

32. Bennett M, Paice JA, Wallace M. Pain and opioids in cancer care: Benefits, risks, and alternatives. *Am Soc Clin Oncol Educ Book.* 2017;37:705–713. doi:10.1200/EDBK_180469

33. Straube C, Derry S, Jackson KC, et al. Codeine, alone and with paracetamol (acetaminophen), for cancer pain. *Cochrane Database Syst Rev.* 2014(9):CD006601. doi:10.1002/14651858.CD006601.pub4

34. Linares OA, Fudin J, Schiesser WE, Daly Linares AL, Boston RC. CYP2D6 phenotype-specific codeine population pharmacokinetics. *J Pain Palliat Care Pharmacother.* 2015;29(1):4–15. doi:10.3109/15360288.2014.997854

35. Bateman DN, Eddleston M, Sandilands E. Codeine and breastfeeding. *Lancet.* 2008;372(9639):625; author reply 626. doi:10.1016/S0140-6736(08)61266-0

36. Madadi P, Koren G, Cairns J, et al. Safety of codeine during breastfeeding: Fatal morphine poisoning in the breastfed neonate of a mother prescribed codeine. *Can Fam Physician.* 2007;53(1):33–35. PMID: 17872605

37. Wiffen PJ, Derry S, Moore RA. Tramadol with or without paracetamol (acetaminophen) for cancer pain. *Cochrane Database Syst Rev.* 2017;5:CD012508. doi:10.1002/14651858.CD012508.pub2

38. Vadivelu N, Chang D, Helander EM, et al. Ketorolac, oxymorphone, tapentadol, and tramadol: A comprehensive review. *Anesthesiol Clin.* 2017;35(2):e1–e20. doi:10.1016/j.anclin.2017.01.001

39. Kreutzwiser D, Tawfic QA. Methadone for pain management: A pharmacotherapeutic review. *CNS Drugs.* 2020;34(8):827–839. doi:10.1007/s40263-020-00743-3

40. Nicholson AB, Watson GR, Derry S, Wiffen PJ. Methadone for cancer pain. *Cochrane Database Syst Rev.* 2017;2:CD003971. doi:10.1002/14651858.CD003971.pub4

41. McPherson ML, Walker KA, Davis MP, et al. Safe and appropriate use of methadone in hospice and palliative care: Expert consensus white paper. *J Pain Symptom Manage.* 2019;57(3):635–645 e634. doi:10.1016/j.jpainsymman.2018.12.001

42. Chou R, Cruciani RA, Fiellin DA, et al. Methadone safety: A clinical practice guideline from the American Pain Society and College on Problems of Drug Dependence, in collaboration with the Heart Rhythm Society. *J Pain.* 2014;15(4):321–337. doi:10.1016/j.jpain.2014.01.494

43. Hanna V, Senderovich H. Methadone in pain management: A systematic review. *J Pain.* 2020;22(3). doi:10.1016/j.jpain.2020.04.004

44. Edmonds KP, Saunders IM, Willeford A, Ajayi TA, Atayee RS. Emerging challenges to the safe and effective use of methadone for cancer-related pain in paediatric and adult patient populations. *Drugs.* 2020;80(2):115–130. doi:10.1007/s40265-019-01234-6

45. McPherson ML, Costantino RC, McPherson AL. Methadone: Maximizing safety and efficacy for pain control in patients with cancer. *Hematol Oncol Clin North Am.* 2018;32(3):405–415. doi:10.1016/j.hoc.2018.01.004

46. World Health Organization. *WHO Guidelines for the Pharmacological and Radiotherapeutic Management of Cancer Pain in Adults and Adolescents.* Geneva: World Health Organization; 2018. https://www.who.int/publications/i/item/who-guidelines-for-the-pharmacological-and-radiotherapeutic-management-of-cancer-pain-in-adults-and-adolescents

47. Reddy A, Yennurajalingam S, Reddy S, et al. The opioid rotation ratio from transdermal fentanyl to "strong" opioids in patients with cancer pain. *J Pain Symptom Manage.* 2016;51(6):1040–1045. doi:https://doi.org/10.1016/j.jpainsymman.2015.12.312

48. Tan C, Wong JF, Yee CM, Hum A. Methadone rotation for cancer pain: An observational study. *BMJ Support Palliat Care.* 2020; Apr 22;bmjspcare-2019-002175. doi:10.1136/bmjspcare-2019-002175

49. Yennurajalingam S, Williams JL, Chisholm G, Bruera E. Effects of dexamethasone and placebo on symptom clusters in advanced cancer patients: A preliminary report. *Oncologist.* 2016;21(3):384–390. doi:10.1634/theoncologist.2014-0260

50. Chow E, Meyer RM, Ding K, et al. Dexamethasone in the prophylaxis of radiation-induced pain flare after palliative radiotherapy for bone metastases: A double-blind, randomised placebo-controlled, phase 3 trial. *Lancet Oncol.* 2015;16(15):1413–1472. doi:10.1016/S1470-2045(15)00199-0

51. Paulsen O, Aass N, Kaasa S, Dale O. Do corticosteroids provide analgesic effects in cancer patients? A systematic literature review. *J Pain Symptom Manage.* 2013;41(1):96–105. doi:10.1016/j.jpainsymman.2012.06.019

52. Haywood A, Good P, Khan S, et al. Corticosteroids for the management of cancer-related pain in adults. *Cochrane Database Syst Rev.* 2015;(4):CD010756. doi:10.1002/14651858.CD010756.pub2

53. Lim FMY, Bobrowski A, Agarwal A, Silva MF. Use of corticosteroids for pain control in cancer patients with bone metastases: A comprehensive literature review. *Curr Opin Support Palliat Care.* 2017;11(2):78–87. doi:10.1097/SPC.0000000000000263

54. Seah DSE, Herschtal A, Tran H, Thakerar A, Fullerton S. Subcutaneous lidocaine infusion for pain in patients with cancer. *J Palliat Med.* 2017;20(6):667–671. doi:10.1089/jpm.2016.0298

55. Lee JT, Sanderson CR, Xuan W, Agar M. Lidocaine for cancer pain in adults: A systematic review and meta-analysis. *J Palliat Med.* 2019;22(3):326–334. doi:10.1089/jpm.2018.0257

56. Jonkman K, van de Donk T, Dahan A. Ketamine for cancer pain: What is the evidence? *Curr Opin Support Palliat Care.* 2017;11(2):88–92. doi:10.1097/SPC.0000000000000262

57. Bell RF, Eccleston C, Kalso EA. Ketamine as an adjuvant to opioids for cancer pain. *Cochrane Database Syst Rev.* 2017;6:CD003351. doi:10.1002/14651858.CD003351.pub3

58. Fallon MT, Wilcock A, Kelly CA, et al. Oral ketamine vs placebo in patients with cancer-related neuropathic pain: A randomized clinical trial. *JAMA Oncol.* 2018;4(6):870–872. doi:10.1001/jamaoncol.2018.0131

59. Rodriguez-Mayoral O, Perez-Esparza R, Dominguez-Ocadio G, Allende-Perez S. Ketamine as augmentation for the treatment of major depression and suicidal risk in advanced cancer: Case report. *Palliat Support Care.* 2020;18(1):110–112. doi:10.1017/S1478951519000580

60. Briscoe J, Kamal AH, Casarett DJ. Top ten tips palliative care clinicians should know about medical cannabis. *J Palliat Med.* 2019;22(3):319–325. https://doi.org/10.1089/jpm.2018.0641

61. Boland EG, Bennett MI, Allgar V, Boland JW. Cannabinoids for adult cancer-related pain: Systematic review and meta-analysis. *BMJ Support Palliat Care.* 2020;10(1):14–24. doi:10.1136/bmjspcare-2019-002032

62. Savage SR, Romero-Sandoval A, Schatman M, et al. Cannabis in pain treatment: Clinical and research considerations. *J Pain.* 2016;17(6):654–668. doi:10.1016/j.jpain.2016.02.007

63. Monte AA, Shelton SK, Mills E, et al. Acute illness associated with cannabis use, by route of exposure: An observational study. *Ann Intern Med.* 2019;170(8):531–537. doi:10.7326/M18-2809

64. Byars T, Theisen E, Bolton DL. Using cannabis to treat cancer-related pain. *Semin Oncol Nurs.* 2019;35(3):300–309. doi:10.1016/j.soncn.2019.04.012

65. Volkow ND, Compton WM, Weiss SR. Adverse health effects of marijuana use. *N Engl J Med.* 2014;370(23):2219–2227. doi:10.1056/NEJMra1402309

66. Devinsky O, Cross JH, Wright S. Trial of cannabidiol for drug-resistant seizures in the Dravet syndrome. *N Engl J Med.* 2017;377(7):699–700. doi:10.1056/NEJMc1708349

67. Oldenmenger WH, Geerling JI, Mostovaya I, et al. A systematic review of the effectiveness of patient-based educational interventions to improve cancer-related pain. *Cancer Treat Rev.* 2017;63:96–103. doi:10.1016/j.ctrv.2017.12.005

68. Kwekkeboom KL, Bratzke LC. A systematic review of relaxation, meditation, and guided imagery strategies for symptom management in heart failure. *J Cardiovasc Nurs.* 2016;31(5):457–468. doi:10.1097/JCN.0000000000000274

69. Lee SH, Kim JY, Yeo S, Kim SH, Lim S. Meta-analysis of massage therapy on cancer pain. *Integr Cancer Ther.* 2015;14(4):297–304. doi:10.1177/1534735415572885

70. Paley CA, Johnson MI, Tashani OA, Bagnall AM. Acupuncture for cancer pain in adults. *Cochrane Database Syst Rev.* 2015(10):CD007753. doi:10.1002/14651858.CD007753.pub3

71. Janke EA, Cheatle M, Keefe FJ, Dhingra L, Society of Behavioral Medicine Health Policy C. Society of Behavioral Medicine (SBM) position statement: Improving access to psychosocial care for individuals with persistent pain: Supporting the national pain strategy's call for interdisciplinary pain care. *Transl Behav Med.* 2018;8(2):305–308. doi:10.1093/tbm/ibx043

72. Sadeghi-Naini M, Aarabi S, Shokraneh F, Janani L, Vaccaro AR, Rahimi-Movaghar V. Vertebroplasty and kyphoplasty for metastatic spinal lesions: A systematic review. *Clin Spine Surg.* 2018 Jun;31(5):203–210. doi:10.1097/BSD.0000000000000601

73. Cheville AL, Moynihan T, Herrin J, Loprinzi C, Kroenke K. Effect of collaborative telerehabilitation on functional impairment and pain among patients with advanced-stage cancer: A randomized clinical trial. *JAMA Oncol.* 2019;5(5):644–652. doi:10.1001/jamaoncol.2019.0011

74. Cheville AL, Smith SR, Basford JR. Rehabilitation medicine approaches to pain management. *Hematol Oncol Clin North Am.* 2018;32(3):469–482. doi:10.1016/j.hoc.2018.02.001

75. Dikmen HA, Terzioglu F. Effects of reflexology and progressive muscle relaxation on pain, fatigue, and quality of life during chemotherapy in gynecologic cancer patients. *Pain Manag Nurs.* 2019;20(1):47–53. doi:10.1016/j.pmn.2018.03.001

76. Zollfrank AA, Trevino KM, Cadge W, et al. Teaching health care providers to provide spiritual care: A pilot study. *J Palliat Med.* 2015;18(5):408–414. doi:10.1089/jpm.2014.0306

77. Kang J, Formenti SC. Metastatic osseous pain control: Radiation therapy. *Semin Intervent Radiol.* 2017;34(4):322–327. doi:10.1055/s-0037-1608703

78. Mark D, Gilbo P, Meshrekey R, Ghaly M. Local radiation therapy for palliation in patients with multiple myeloma of the spine. *Front Oncol.* 2019;9:601. doi:10.3389/fonc.2019.00601

79. Park KR, Lee CG, Tseng YD, et al. Palliative radiation therapy in the last 30 days of life: A systematic review. *Radiother Oncol.* 2017;125(2):193–199. doi:10.1016/j.radonc.2017.09.016

80. Silvestre J, Reddy A, de la Cruz M, et al. Frequency of unsafe storage, use, and disposal practices of opioids among cancer patients presenting to the emergency department. *Palliat Support Care.* 2017;15(6):638–643. doi:10.1017/S1478951516000158

81. de la Cruz M, Reddy A, Balankari V, et al. The impact of an educational program on patient practices for safe use, storage, and disposal of opioids at a comprehensive cancer center. *Oncologist.* 2017;22(1):115–121. doi:10.1634/theoncologist.2016-0266

82. Volkow ND, McLellan TA. Curtailing diversion and abuse of opioid analgesics without jeopardizing pain treatment. *JAMA.* 2011;305(13):1346–1347. doi:10.1001/jama.2011.369

83. Merlin JS, Patel K, Thompson N, et al. Managing chronic pain in cancer survivors prescribed long-term opioid therapy: A national survey of ambulatory palliative care providers. *J Pain Symptom Manage.* 2019;57(1):20–27. doi:10.1016/j.jpainsymman.2018.10.493

84. Paice JA. Navigating cancer pain management in the midst of the opioid epidemic. *Oncology (Williston Park).* 2018;32(8):386–390, 403. PMID: 30153316

85. Paice JA. Cancer pain management and the opioid crisis in America: How to preserve hard-earned gains in improving the quality of cancer pain management. *Cancer.* 2018 Jun 15;124(12):2491–2497. doi:10.1002/cncr.31303

86. Paice JA. Under pressure: The tension between access and abuse of opioids in cancer pain management. *J Oncol Pract.* 2017;13(9):595–596. doi:10.1200/JOP.2017.026120

87. Arthur J, Bruera E. Balancing opioid analgesia with the risk of nonmedical opioid use in patients with cancer. *Nat Rev Clin Oncol.* 2019;16(4):213–226. doi:10.1038/s41571-018-0143-7

88. Arthur J, Lu Z, Nguyen K, et al. Random vs targeted urine drug testing among patients undergoing long-term opioid treatment for cancer pain. *JAMA Oncol.* 2020;6(4):580–581. doi:10.1001/jamaoncol.2019.6756

89. Arthur JA, Edwards T, Lu Z, et al. Frequency, predictors, and outcomes of urine drug testing among patients with advanced cancer on chronic opioid therapy at an outpatient supportive care clinic. *Cancer.* 2016;122(23):3732–3739. doi:10.1002/cncr.30240

90. Ali MM, Dowd WN, Classen T, Mutter R, Novak SP. Prescription drug monitoring programs, nonmedical use of prescription drugs, and heroin use: Evidence from the national survey of drug use and health. *Addict Behav.* 2017;69:65–77. doi:10.1016/j.addbeh.2017.01.011

91. Mitchell MT. Dancing with deterrents: Understanding the role of abuse-deterrent opioid formulations and naloxone in managing cancer pain. *Oncologist.* 2019;24(12):1505–1509. doi:10.1634/theoncologist.2019-0340

92. Yennurajalingam S, Edwards T, Arthur JA, et al. Predicting the risk for aberrant opioid use behavior in patients receiving outpatient supportive care consultation at a comprehensive cancer center. *Cancer.* 2018;124(19):3942–3949. doi:10.1002/cncr.31670

93. Arthur J, Hui D. Safe opioid use: Management of opioid-related adverse effects and aberrant behaviors. *Hematol Oncol Clin North Am.* 2018;32(3):387–403. doi:10.1016/j.hoc.2018.01.003

44.

RESPIRATORY SYMPTOMS

Ember S. Moore and Kathleen Broglio

KEY POINTS

- Dyspnea and cough are symptoms that affect individuals with advanced diseases and may worsens toward the end of life.

- The advanced practice registered nurse (APRN) should assess dyspnea and cough using a biopsychosocial approach, with the understanding that these symptoms affect the entire person.

- The APRN should actively seek opportunities to participate in research to extend the current body of evidence related to dyspnea and cough.

CASE STUDY: SHORTNESS OF BREATH

Carey was a 64-year-old woman with past medical history of chronic obstructive pulmonary disease (COPD), hypertension (HTN), and severe osteoarthritis woman who quit smoking 15 years ago. Three months ago, after a 30-pound unexplained weight loss, she was diagnosed with adenocarcinoma of the lung with metastases to the liver. She initiated chemotherapy and was referred to palliative care for assistance in management of her dyspnea and cough. The palliative advanced practice registered nurse (APRN) performed an assessment to elicit information about her respiratory status. Prior to her diagnosis, she was able to walk around her neighborhood with her dog, about one-half mile without having to stop to rest. Carey reported she was unable to ambulate 50 feet without becoming short of breath. Additionally, her chronic cough has worsened over the week, and it exacerbated the pain in her right upper quadrant of the abdomen. Carey reported taking ipratropium bromide/albuterol inhaler as well as guaifenesin as needed, which did not help her shortness of breath or cough. She wondered if having oxygen at home will help her feel better.

INTRODUCTION

Dyspnea and cough are two common symptoms that often contribute to decreased quality of life (QoL) and can be exceptionally distressing symptoms near end of life for individuals and their caregivers. Each can be associated with several underlying acute and chronic disease states or develop as symptoms of a new disease process or acute complication of treatment, such as a malignant pleural effusion or chemotherapy induced pneumonitis. Although very common

in palliative care, dyspnea and cough have relatively limited research dedicated to understanding the effects of these symptoms on the total person. This may be due to the difficulty of appreciating and measuring the different severity of symptoms. As an example, a person may say "I can't catch my breath" or "I'm suffocating!" but has oxygen saturations within normal limits and no observed work of breathing.[1]

Dyspnea and cough may exacerbate or influence each other as well as symptoms such as anxiety, pain, and depression.[2] These relationships highlight the need to better understand and address the complexity of interactions between physiologic, psychologic, environmental, and interpersonal factors that affect the quality of life—and the quality of death.[3,4] (In lieu of robust research and treatment guidelines in palliative care, much of the evidence is extrapolated from research of these symptoms in the general population as well as specific populations such as those with chronic obstructive pulmonary disease [COPD] or congestive heart failure [CHF]).

Although individuals often present with both symptoms, dyspnea and cough are two distinct symptoms, each with complex pathophysiology. Advanced practice registered nurses (APRNs) must accurately assess the situation, treat the underlying cause when possible, and manage dyspnea and cough much like managing "total pain"[5] to enhance the person's QoL and alleviate suffering.

DYSPNEA

DEFINITION

Dyspnea is a medical term for a symptom or sign usually associated with an underlying condition. It has been defined by the American Thoracic Society as "a subjective experience of breathing discomfort that consists of qualitatively distinct sensations that vary in intensity."[6 (pp. 436–437)] The group adds that the "experience of dyspnea derives from interactions of physiological, psychological, social, and environmental factors and may induce secondary physiological and behavioral responses."[6 (pp. 436–437)] Bausewein et al. (2018) differentiate the medical term "dyspnea" from the common term "breathlessness," "a unique and subjective experience to the individual reflecting the patient's perspective based on the daily experience."[7 (p. 48)] *Breathlessness* can better encompass the many dimensions of a person's experience of dyspnea, and breathlessness may persist as a chronic symptom despite optimal treatment of underlying conditions.[7]

Dyspnea is a symptom that often arises from physiologic impairment from a disease process or subsequent therapies, and it may be independent of physiologic signs of respiratory compromise, such as tachypnea. The person experiences physical sensations that are commonly described as "suffocating," "can't get enough air," or being "out of breath"[8] that can be rated in degree of unpleasantness as well as the reaction to these sensations.[9] The reactions, an affective response of the central nervous system, are associated strongly with other symptoms such as depression, fear, and anxiety.[10]

Neuroimaging study results demonstrate the relationship between the affective response and reported symptom severity. Additionally, these neuroimaging studies have shown the effect that opioids have in altering the affective response.[1,8,10,11] This new information may increase the understanding of why some individuals who experience dyspnea over time, such as those with COPD, may have different experiences of dyspnea during different time periods of disease course.

A person with COPD may have chronic experiences of activity intolerance or exacerbations of dyspnea. These experiences may be due to increased anxiety and fear related to a learned affective response compared to those with cancer, where dyspnea tends to occur toward end of life and is more limited to episodic events.[12,13] Individuals with COPD tend to rate their symptoms of dyspnea worse than those with cancer or CHF. This may be due to anticipatory responses learned over time mediated by the amygdala and hippocampus.[1,10,14] Understanding this relationship can help target treatments and future study to better palliate all aspects of dyspnea.

Descriptive qualities of dyspnea have been separated into three categories (air hunger, work, and tightness); each may arise from different pathophysiologic processes such as COPD, CHF, advanced cancer, lung fibrosis, and neuromuscular disease and may indicate the need for different management approaches.[4] Acute dyspnea and chronic breathlessness can also be differentiated. Although acute dyspnea can be considered a palliative care emergency, it is important to differentiate it from the chronic experience that many individuals with serious illness experience.[15] Chronic breathlessness may be viewed as a syndrome that is associated with anxiety, depression, and declining activity tolerance. It has been "defined as "breathlessness that persists despite optimal treatment of the underlying pathophysiology and that results in disability."[16 (p. 1)]

PREVALENCE

Dyspnea may be experienced by up to 2.9% of the general population.[15,17] The majority of people living with COPD experience some dyspnea, and 80% frequently experience moderate to severe dyspnea.[18,19] Dyspnea is also experienced by 51% of individuals with lung cancer[12,20] and up to 52% of those with dementia at the end of life.[12,21] Activity-related breathlessness is twice as high in woman compared to men and is likely explained by the general gender difference in absolute lung volume.[19,22]

Although the recorded prevalence in these special populations is relatively high, the percentage of seriously ill individuals experiencing dyspnea may be underappreciated secondary to challenges in measuring dyspnea and consistently documenting it as a symptom.[9] Underappreciated symptoms may be most significant in populations that have historically experienced significant dyspnea burden such people with COPD, CHF, advanced local or metastatic cancer, idiopathic lung disease, pulmonary hypertension, and motor neuron disease/amyotrophic lateral sclerosis. Individuals may not be aware that there may be better treatment for this pervasive symptom.[7,23] The individual may experience frustration, vulnerability, and shame related to dyspnea and may not appreciate that symptoms of anxiety, insomnia, and depression may be rooted in their experience of dyspnea. Therefore, the palliative APRN should be keenly aware that individuals may underreport the impact or the decreased QoL related to dyspnea.[20,24]

The quality and intensity of dyspnea may vary across disease states.[25] In a qualitative study of individuals with cancer, COPD, CHF, and motor neuron disease, there were individual variations in the experience of dyspnea.[26] Those with COPD had higher levels of breathlessness over time, whereas those with lung cancer experienced worsening dyspnea toward the end of life.[25] In a consecutive cohort hospice study, dyspnea was worse in those with non-cancer diagnoses but increased significantly for individuals with cancer in the last 8–10 days of life.[12,27] Among individuals with advanced cancer, those with metastases to lung, liver, and lymph nodes were strongly predisposed to more severe dyspnea,[28] pointing to the need for the palliative APRN to personalize treatment.

ETIOLOGIES

The APRN must understand the multifactorial etiologies of dyspnea to design the best treatment plan. Pulmonary causes of dyspnea can be from malignant or nonmalignant sources, whereas cardiac causes of dyspnea are generally related to nonmalignant pathology. Dyspnea may occur related to increased respiratory effort in obstructive processes, increases in ventilatory requirements, restrictive processes, ventilatory mismatch, fatigue, or musculoskeletal weakness.[11,29] Systemic causes of dyspnea may be secondary to advancing disease as well as the side effects of treatments. Psychological states including mood and expectation influence the experience of and can also provoke dyspnea[11] (see Table 44.1).

PATHOPHYSIOLOGY AND MECHANISMS

The sequences of pathophysiological mechanisms that result in the symptom of dyspnea are not completely understood. Studies to date have led to the development of several constructs of physiologic mechanisms and affective states that interact in the whole person.[11,29,30] A person with COPD may have dyspnea at rest and severe exertional dyspnea and anxiety and related depression due to decreased functional ability, while a person with CHF may have severe exertional dyspnea with disease exacerbation with mild anxiety and no depression (see Box 44.1).

Table 44.1 POTENTIAL CAUSES OF DYSPNEA IN ADVANCED DISEASE

PULMONARY	CARDIAC	SYSTEMIC	TREATMENT-RELATED	PSYCHOLOGICAL
Airway obstructions	CHF	Cachexia	Surgical	Anxiety
Carcinomatosis	Ischemia	Steroid myopathy	Lobectomy	Panic
Chest wall infiltrations	Pericardial	Hepatomegaly	Pneumonectomy	
COPD	effusion	Ascites	Chemotherapy	
Interstitial lung disease	Pulmonary	Anemia	Pulmonary or cardiac toxicity	
Effusions	hypertension	Metabolic abnormalities	Radiation side effects	
Embolism		Obesity	Pneumonitis	
Pneumonia		Hyperventilation	Fibrosis	
Pneumothorax		Neuromuscular	Pericarditis	
Superior vena cava		abnormalities		
obstruction				
Tumor				

This is only a partial list of more common causes.

Adapted from Chan et al.[30]

It is generally accepted that the experience of dyspnea emanates from changes in activity in central and peripheral chemoreceptors, imbalance in feedback between efferent and afferent signals from sensory receptors in the body to the brain's respiratory processing centers (thought to be in the medulla and cortex), and the effects of increased activation of affective

response to these changes in the limbic and paralimbic brain areas. This results in a sensation of "unpleasantness."[29]

Independent of changes in respiratory activity, levels of hypoxia, and hypercarbia have been shown to generate equivalent levels of air hunger in humans and can induce a sense of "unpleasantness" or "air hunger."[31] Changes in mechanoreceptor and ergoreceptor activity in the lung, chest wall, upper airway, and facial receptors can also contribute to dyspnea by relaying feedback to the somatosensory cortex.[29,32,33] It is hypothesized that these neuromechanical changes drive many responses, such as changes in breath rate and depth and affective response. Affective responses may lead to modification of overall activity.

Over time, limitation of physical activity to avoid these triggers leads to muscle deconditioning that has at least two further effects that contribute to dyspnea in chronic conditions.[29] First, it can contribute to overall muscle deconditioning, including that of the diaphragm, which can affect the ability to respond with optimal lung volumes for inspiration. This may cause changes to mechanoreceptor stimulation and decrease overall spirometry. Second, increased anaerobic muscle metabolism may result from global deconditioning. This may cause increased systemic acidosis with muscle activity that may increase chemoreceptor stimulation, thus further driving the cycle of dyspnea.[29,31] Dyspnea can arise from a sense of increased work of breathing in those with fatigue, weakened respiratory muscles, or obstructive diseases. Neuromechanical dissociation, a mismatch between incoming information from the respiratory system and outgoing commands from the brain center, can also cause dyspnea.[29,34]

Results of neural imaging studies have demonstrated that the limbic and paralimbic areas of the brain are active when a person experiences dyspnea and are known to be active in people experiencing fear and reaction to learned responses.[11,29] In imaging studies of opioids used for activity-induced dyspnea, brain activity in the limbic and paralimbic areas was interrupted.[1,35] This finding offers one explanation of the affective mechanisms and experience of dyspnea. Further investigation may lead to a better understanding of the central processes involved in the perception of and response to

Box 44.1 POTENTIAL MECHANISMS FOR DYSPNEA

Decreased lung volume

Gender difference: Women have smaller spirometric lung volume

Central chemoreceptor changes

Acidosis
Hypoxia
Hypercapnia

Mechanoreceptor and ergoreceptor stimulation

Lung, chest wall, upper airway, facial area

Respiratory and general muscle effort

Fatigue/obstructive processes
Generalized deconditioning

Neuromechanical disassociation

Mismatch between respiratory and brain command center increasing neural inspiratory drive (IND) stimulating medulla and cortex areas of the brain

Affective and learned response

Psychologic response to IND stimulation with activity: mortal distress, fear, anxiety driving decrease in physical activity and subsequent deconditioning

From Marlow et al.[11]; McKenzie et al.[29]; Moosavi et al.[31]; Kako et al.[32]; Swan et al.[33]; and Nishino.[34]

breathlessness, which are not fully explained by currently accepted mechanisms.[11]

CLINICAL ASSESSMENT

The palliative APRN should ensure that a routine assessment of dyspnea is incorporated fully into practice in a similar routine to that of pain.[7] Many people with serious illness may not appear in distress yet experience acute or chronic dyspnea. They and their caregivers may not volunteer to report symptoms of chronic breathlessness, and, without routine assessment, symptom distress may be underappreciated and undertreated.[36] McCaffery's (1968) original description of the subjectivity of "pain as being what the person says it is when experienced"[37 (p.95)] implies the complexity of the pain experience and the need first to assess symptoms in a similarly robust manner based on the implications of that experience. Similarly, the subjectivity of dyspnea needs to be recognized as a combined mind and body phenomenon.[36]

The palliative APRN's clinical assessment of dyspnea initially focuses on eliciting the underlying pathology, either from previous consultations or by appropriate assessment and diagnostic workup. A biopsychosocial assessment is imperative because the individual's experience and interpretation of dyspnea and preferences for treatment may vary and change with disease progression.[7,9,26]

Experts recommend dyspnea assessment and tracking over time.[6,36] The APRN can adapt the PQRST mnemonic for pain assessment to guide dyspnea assessment.[38]

- Provoking/palliating factors
- Quality/characteristics
- Relationship to other symptoms, such as fatigue, anxiety, and depression
- Severity, using a unidimensional scale
- Timing (constant or intermittent)

In individuals with cancer, the APRN should assess not only the effects of tumor burden, but also the post-treatment effects of radiation, chemotherapy, and immunotherapies that may contribute to dyspnea. In individuals with cardiac, pulmonary, or motor neuron diseases, the palliative APRN should inquire about the appropriate use of disease-modifying therapies that affect the respiratory system. Lifestyle factors should be explored because exposure to environmental toxins like tobacco smoke may contribute to dyspnea.

Multiple dyspnea assessment tools have been developed, yet many are unidimensional or disease-specific or do not address dyspnea's affective component or dyspnea in advanced disease.[36] The American Thoracic Society and the American College of Chest Physicians have not endorsed the use of any specific scale.[6] The modified Borg Scale,[39] visual analogue scale (VAS),[40] and numeric rating scale (NRS)[41] are unidimensional scales that measure dyspnea severity but do not elicit affective components of dyspnea. Although they are simple, these tools have been validated and are indicated in initial and follow-up assessments as part of a short dyspnea assessment. For assessment of individuals who have cognitive challenges, the categorical verbal descriptor scale (VDS) using "none," "mild," "moderate," and "severe" has shown good correlation with the VAS and NRS scales and may be ideal for continued assessment in certain individuals.[23] Individual self-assessment tools in those with advanced disease such as the Memorial Symptom Assessment Scale (MSAS)[42] and the Edmonton Symptom Assessment System (ESAS),[43] measure the severity of multiple symptoms. Psychometrically valid tools, such as the Dynspnoea-12, tested in those with CHF, COPD, and interstitial lung disease (ILD),[44] and the Cancer Dyspnea Scale (CDS), tested in those with cancer,[45] address both the physical and affective components of dyspnea. For individuals who cannot self-report, the Respiratory Distress Observation Scale (RDOS) is a validated, simple-to-use tool that may help the clinician to evaluate the trend and response to treatment.[46,47] However, this seems to be used mostly in the intensive care unit and at end of life. Caregivers' reports, through use of unidimensional scales such as NRS or VDS, may be useful if the individual cannot report the severity of dyspnea. It is important for the APRN to use the above-mentioned tools when appropriate and reassess at regular intervals.[36,48]

The clinical interview and the use of psychometrically validated tools for dyspnea assessment should be coupled with physical examination and diagnostic testing as appropriate. In considering the choice of diagnostic testing for evaluating dyspnea, the palliative APRN should understand potential causes for dyspnea related to the disease state. Further diagnostic testing should be coupled with consideration of the goals of care and the effects of additional information on the management of disease or symptom (see Box 44.2).

MANAGEMENT

The palliative APRN must ensure optimal management of both the disease and the dyspnea. Disease-specific therapies should be optimized to decrease dyspnea when the benefit outweighs the risk and if consistent with goals of care. Toward the end of life, dyspnea management may preclude the treatment of the underlying pathology.[4]

Although there has been progress in understanding the mechanisms of dyspnea, the treatment of dyspnea has not progressed significantly. Despite the lack of high-quality studies and gaps in evidence for recommended therapies, the palliative APRN can manage dyspnea and improve QoL.[3,4,49] Regardless of the state of disease, the APRN should utilize pharmacologic, nonpharmacologic, and psychoeducational strategies as well as breathlessness services, if available, to decrease symptom distress.[3,7,49,50]

Dyspnea management in the palliative care population may vary considerably related to the underlying diseases, phase of advanced disease, and individual treatment preferences related to goals of care. The palliative APRN role is vital to assess and acknowledge a distressing symptom that may be underreported in a person who has lived with serious illness prior to palliative care involvement. The APRN discusses goals of care to frame management recommendations. In this population, the palliative APRN utilizes therapies that may not be used in the general population to best control symptoms as end of life approaches (see Table 44.2 and Table 44.3).

Pharmacologic Management

Opioids

Dyspnea has been compared to pain in terms of the need to address it as a basic human right for treatment—the evidence is there for opioid therapy—and to deny it is to deny a human right.[51] Opioids are the first-line pharmacologic treatment for dyspnea. Low-dose opioids may reduce dyspnea by decreasing the respiratory drive without inducing respiratory depression even in individuals who are opioid-naïve.[4,35,49] It is thought that the positive effect on the "unpleasantness" of dyspnea from low-dose opiates is due to the suppression of respiratory system signaling in the brainstem as well as higher brain centers. This is thought to interrupt the affective response and may be of most importance when considering opioid's therapeutic use.[1,10] There is strong evidence for the treatment effect of opioids on COPD; even a single dose of morphine may improve exertional dyspnea ratings.[52] Consensus on optimal dose, route, and how opioids may relieve dyspnea in some populations, such as CHF and ILD, remains less defined.[35]

Morphine, the most widely studied opioid, has been shown to be effective for dyspnea.[35,53–55] In a systematic review and meta-analysis of 26 randomized controlled trials (RCTs) ($n = 526$), dyspnea improved with opioid therapy compared to placebo.[56] Recent evaluation of that meta-analysis noted selection bias and recommended reassessment and a revised recommendation of a moderate level of evidence for the use of opioids to relieve dyspnea.[57] A few small studies have demonstrated the efficacy and safety of buccal fentanyl compared to immediate-release morphine for rapid relief of episodic dyspnea in cancer.[58,59]

In a multisite RCT of patients with chronic dyspnea, 54% of participants had COPD and were treated with extended release once-daily morphine (10–30 mg), which remained

Table 44.2 SELECTED PHARMACOLOGIC TREATMENT OPTIONS FOR DYSPNEA IN SERIOUS ILLNESS

MEDICATION	COMMENT
Opioids (IV, SC, PO)	May be considered first-line treatment for dyspnea related to cancer, COPD May consider in CHF Optimal dosing not determined; start low dose and may titrate more rapidly for severe dyspnea Adult starting morphine doses range from 2.5 mg to 5 mg orally (or IV/SQ equivalent) q4h as needed Other opioids may also be effective if morphine is contraindicated Consider low dose, extended release opioid if tolerating immediate release opioids
Benzodiazepines (IV, PO)	Not a first-line recommendation Consider as second or third line or combination with opioids for refractory dyspnea at end of life. Potentially useful for refractory dyspnea and dyspnea-associated anxiety
Furosemide	Nebulized furosemide cannot be recommended due to equivocal evidence May be useful in COPD
Corticosteroids (IV, PO, INH)	May be beneficial and well-tolerated in cancer associated dyspnea May reduce airway inflammation and edema leading to dyspnea.
Oxygen	Beneficial in hypoxemia Beneficial in ILD to support activity related hypoxemia Questionable benefit in absence of hypoxemia, trial is warranted
Noninvasive ventilation (NIV)	Long term use effective in dyspnea associated with neuromuscular or restrictive thoracic diseases Benefits not clear long-term in stable COPD Benefits shown when combined with opioid therapy in hypercarbic COPD For patients foregoing intubation yet with hope for more time, may be beneficial in combination with opioid therapy for short-term survival
High-flow nasal therapy	May provide benefit to reduce work of breathing and respiratory rate May improve exercise tolerance especially with combined opioid therapy

CHF, congestive heart failure; COPD, chronic obstructive pulmonary disease; ILD, interstitial lung disease.

From Ambrosino, Fracchia[3]; Pisani et al.[4]; Johnson, Currow[35]; Strieder et al.[49]; Simon et al.[60]; Ekstrom et al.[61]; Faverio et al.[62]; Rochwerg et al.[63]; and Koyauchi et al.[64]

effective over time.[53] There is a call to consider oral extended-release low dose (10–30 mg per day) opioids for the treatment of dyspnea standard in care as the risks are relatively low and side effects such as constipation, nausea, and vomiting can be controlled.[35,65]

The potential for improvement in health-related QoL should be of high value in palliative care.[1,11] Common barriers in prescribing opioids for dyspnea have been their association with respiratory depression or lack of provider experience in prescribing opioids for the treatment of dyspnea.[50] Results from studies of individuals with COPD,[66] cancer,[67] or CHF[68] evaluating the use of opioids for dyspnea failed to demonstrate a relationship between opioids and respiratory compromise.

Limited studies have been conducted to confirm the opioid dose needed to manage dyspnea. This is partially due to the inherent difficulty of conducting RCTs in vulnerable populations and the heterogeneity of the populations with dyspnea. The proposed starting dose of morphine for opioid-naïve individuals with acute dyspnea in the acute care setting is 1–2 mg intravenous (IV) every 15 minutes with titration until dyspnea improves.[4] In those who can take oral medications, the recommended dose is 2.5–5 mg oral morphine (or morphine equivalent) every 4 hours as needed.[69] In individuals who can take medications orally with chronic breathlessness, experts recommend starting with 10 mg of extended-release oral morphine daily, with titration to control symptoms to 30 mg daily,[35] combined with 2 mg immediate-release oral morphine every 4 hours as needed for dyspnea.

Based on the variation of proposed doses, APRNs should use the same approach as when treating pain: "start low and go slow." There is an exception when managing dyspnea toward the end of life in an acute care setting, where opioids may be given IV and the dose rapidly titrated. The palliative APRN should anticipate and prevent opioid-related side effects such as nausea, vomiting, and constipation, and the dose may need to be adjusted for those who are older and frail with multiple comorbidities and as disease progresses.[55] Although there are limited studies on the use of other opioids for dyspnea, the APRN can use opioids other than morphine for those with renal dysfunction due to accumulation of morphine metabolites M-3-glucuronide and M-6-gluconoride, which may add to the adverse effects of opioids.[58]

Nebulized opioids may be attractive to individuals who may not want to take oral medications, yet the evidence of the effects of nebulized opiates are equivocal due in part to the low-quality evidence to date.[4,56] Therefore, the use of nebulized opioids should be evaluated on a case-by-case basis[70,71] but may be considered if oral or parenteral opioids fail to provide benefit.

Benzodiazepines

Benzodiazepines have been used for dyspnea and may treat the affective response to dyspnea. In a systematic review (eight studies in advanced cancer and COPD) benzodiazepines were not of significant benefit regardless of type, dose, or route.[60] Anxiolytics (including benzodiazepines) have not been recommended by the American and Canadian thoracic societies for dyspnea in individuals with COPD.[6,72] However, benzodiazepines have been shown to be effective in some small studies.[73–75]

Although quality studies are needed to further evaluate their potential efficacy, benzodiazepines may be used for dyspnea refractory to opioids or other nonpharmacologic

Table 44.3 NONPHARMACOLOGIC AND
INTERVENTIONAL THERAPIES FOR DYSPNEA IN
SERIOUS ILLNESS

INTERVENTIONAL

Tunneled catheter	May provide almost immediate relief of dyspnea in malignant and non-malignant pleural effusions
	More consistent success compared with pleurodesis
	Infection rate similar to pleurodesis
Pleurodesis	May decrease dyspnea due to pleural effusions
	High failure rate
	Tunneled catheter has better success rate
Bronchial stenting	First line for to re-establish airway patency in obstructions and relief of dyspnea if aligned with individual's goals

NONPHARMACOLOGIC

Rehabilitation	Breath training
	COPD and HF may have benefit
	Low risk, low cost
	Pulmonary rehabilitation
	Usually combination of physical and respiratory therapy over several weeks;
	Strong evidence for improvement in chronic dyspnea, health related quality of life in COPD,
	Some evidence in cancer and ILD
	Not possible in severe dyspnea and at end of life
Psychoeducational	Counseling, education, relaxation, Internet-based self-management
	May increase self-efficacy
	May be included in holistic breathlessness services
	May have positive effect on affective component of dyspnea
Fans	May be beneficial
	Low-risk and low-cost treatment
Acupuncture	May be beneficial, some inconsistent evidence

COPD, chronic obstructive pulmonary disease; HF, heart failure; ILD, interstitial lung disease.

From Brighton et al.[2]; Ambrosino, Fracchia[3]; Pisani et al.[4], Bausewein et al.[7]; Kako et al.[32]; Strieder et al.[49]; Vitacca et al.[76]; Frost et al.[77]; Bausewein et al.[78]; Bittencourt et al.[79]; and Gysels et al.[80]

measures, especially in those who have anxiety.[60] Midazolam is recommended in the symptomatic hospitalized patient at end of life due rapid onset of action, short half-life, and ease in IV titration to desired effect.[81] In non-acute situations, it is reasonable to consider low-dose oral lorazepam due to the relatively short half-life and availability in liquid form. Dosing can start at 0.5 mg orally or sublingually every 4 hours. Individuals with significant anxiety, who may not be approaching the end of life, may also benefit from treatment of anxiety with agents such as selective serotonin reuptake inhibitors.[4]

Furosemide

In individuals with dyspnea secondary to lung congestion, as in CHF, or in those who have had lymph destruction from therapy such as radiation, IV furosemide and diuretics may be helpful in treatment. In a review of nebulized medications for dyspnea, furosemide showed potential benefit in those with dyspnea related to COPD.[4] Yet, in a recent double-blind randomized crossover trial, no relief of exercise-induced dyspnea was noted in healthy men using nebulized furosemide.[82] In a systematic review of the use of furosemide for dyspnea in cancer, only two small RCTs were identified, and nebulized furosemide was not beneficial for dyspnea.[83] Given the paucity of studies, the use of nebulized furosemide should be reserved for those who do not respond to first-line therapies.[3,4]

Corticosteroids

Although corticosteroids are often used in palliative care for many symptoms, there is conflicting evidence on their efficacy in treating dyspnea.[3,4] However, in RCTs, dexamethasone was well-tolerated and reduced severe dyspnea symptoms in individuals with cancer.[84,85] Due to limited evidence, steroid use for dyspnea may be considered in disease processes involving inflammation and in those with malignancy.[4,84]

Oxygen

Standard Supplemental Oxygen Therapy. Oxygen is generally the first treatment clinicians consider when someone is dyspneic. The use of oxygen is warranted if dyspnea is related to a physiologic event limiting the delivery of necessary oxygen to the body, such as for those with COPD[3,4,49,61] and fibrotic lung diseases.[62] However, in advanced disease, the oxygen saturation and carbon dioxide status may not correlate with the perception of dyspnea. Abernethy and colleagues (2010) compared the effects of oxygen versus room air delivered by nasal cannula in those with advanced disease in a multisite RCT and found that the subjective feeling of dyspnea was relieved in those who were treated with air by nasal cannula at the same rates as those treated with oxygen therapy, thus questioning the need for oxygen therapy and calling for ongoing evaluation of alternative strategies.[86] Ekström and colleagues (2016) concluded that there is modest evidence that dyspnea with activity was improved with the use of oxygen therapy in those with COPD who were mildly hypoxemic or not hypoxemic and would not have qualified for home oxygen therapy.[61]

Oxygen use in ILD is standard practice although there is little evidence of improvement of dyspnea. However, oxygen may improve health-related QoL and exercise tolerance in this population.[62,87] There have not been any high-quality studies assessing the efficacy of oxygen use in those with CHF, yet for those with comorbid obstructive sleep apnea, nocturnal oxygen may improve QoL.[88–90]

Despite wide use of oxygen for those with dyspnea in many advanced disease states, most results from systematic reviews do not support its long-term use in individuals without hypoxemia.[61,88,91] The palliative APRN's best approach may be a time-limited trial of oxygen therapy to evaluate the response in dyspneic individuals with advanced disease who are not hypoxemic or only mildly hypoxemic.

Noninvasive ventilation. Noninvasive ventilation (NIV) delivers assisted airway pressure through the upper airways by a face mask or pronged nasal mask. NIV is able to provide this oxygen support without the use of oropharyngeal or tracheostomy tubes. NIV has commonly been used to provide continuous positive airway pressure (CPAP), and/or for those who need lower expiratory airway pressure for better tolerance, bilevel positive airway pressure (BiPAP). This ventilation is provided in and out of the hospital setting for treatment of obstructive sleep apnea and illness states with hypoxemia. NIV has been established in international guidelines as treatment for respiratory distress and dyspnea in acute COPD exacerbation, acute pulmonary edema, chest trauma, and postoperative weaning or post-extubation respiratory distress.[61,63,88,91] NIV combined with exercise training and pulmonary rehabilitation has been shown to improve dyspnea and health-related QoL measures in those with heart failure.[81] Vitacca and colleagues (2018) found that in individuals with COPD and restrictive thoracic diseases, NIV improved exercise endurance but not dyspnea symptoms.[76]

In a systematic review of NIV in palliative care, there is strong support for its use in treating dyspnea in many illnesses including acute exacerbations of COPD and end-stage neuromuscular diseases yet equivocal and limited evidence on the effects on NIV on dyspnea at end of life. The widespread use of NIV at end of life may be more related to specific goals of care such as treating dyspnea and achieving short-term survival goals while avoiding oral intubation at end of life.[92] The treatment of dyspnea related to motor neuron diseases poses additional challenges. Individuals must make decisions related to the use of both noninvasive and invasive ventilation not only to manage dyspnea but also to prolong life. Based on lack of evidence on the treatment of dyspnea in a wide variety of advanced disease and end of life, the American Thoracic Society was unable to provide a firm recommendation for the use of NIV as a palliative care tool yet was able to note the possibility of use as a therapy for certain disease states.[6]

High-Flow Nasal Therapy. Compared to traditional nasal cannula oxygen delivery that is usually limited to 15 liters of oxygen flow, high-flow nasal therapy (HFNT) is a type of NIV delivered through nonocclusive nasal cannulation that allows for delivery of warmed and humidified gas flow up to 100% the fraction of inspired oxygen (FiO_2). Up to 60 liters of oxygen per minute can be delivered while also providing some positive end expiratory pressure (PEEP) and providing washout of carbon dioxide in physiologic dead space. The warmed and humidified therapy may contribute to individual's increased ability to mobilize secretions. The physical apparatus allows for the individual to better communicate and tolerate oral intake compared with NIV that uses face masks. HFNT has not been provided out of the hospital setting, mostly due to high oxygen use demands that usually are not able to be delivered in most home settings as most home oxygen concentrators deliver only up to 10 liters per minute.

In recent decades, HFNT has been shown to provide a number of beneficial effects such as decreased work of breathing and reduced respiratory rate.[92] It has been used for prevention and treatment of acute respiratory failure in individuals with CHF and pneumonia.[3,4,93] HFNT improves respiratory distress by decreasing respiratory rate and work of breathing in CHF,[94] cystic fibrosis,[95] and ILD,[62,64] and by counterbalancing auto-PEEP in those with COPD.[96]

Although the study of HFNT in all illnesses has not consistently demonstrated decreased dyspnea, it has been shown to decrease work of breathing by reducing the respiratory rate in many disease states.[62,96] For individuals seeking to avoid intubation at the end of life who also want symptoms of respiratory distress managed and short-term life prolongation,[62,93-95] HFNT may be well-tolerated.[62,93-95] HFNT will likely be more widely used in palliative care as technology changes, which may enable its use in the home care setting. Until that time, palliative APRNs should discuss the goal of the HFNT, especially if lung disease will not enable the individual to transition to oxygen therapy that is available at home or in a skilled or assisted living facility. A potential scenario may be that HFNT would be utilized to allow family or friends to visit the individual prior to discontinuation to allow natural death.

Pisani and colleagues (2018) highlight the need for the palliative APRN to address symptom management in the context of individual goals of care to guide decision-making when considering oxygen therapy, HFNT, and NIV.[4] NIV may be indicated in individuals who do not want intubation but are seeking symptom relief mainly from dyspnea. If that individual will not be able to live without continued ventilatory support, yet wishes to maintain cognition and prolong life, NIV in combination with pharmacologic agents may support these combined goals as the individual approaches the end of life.[4] In acute situations and near end of life, the individual may wish to utilize these therapies in the short term to achieve certain goals, such as seeing family members prior to their death.

Interventional Therapy

The palliative APRN may consider referrals for interventional therapies to reduce dyspnea if consistent with the individual's goals of care. Disease-modifying therapies that may reduce dyspnea, such as chemotherapy and radiation therapy, should be explored as first-line treatments for obstructions secondary to tumor burden.[97] Mechanical or chemical pleurodesis may reduce dyspnea secondary to pleural effusions. For those with more advanced disease, the placement of a tunneled catheter for management of pleural effusions has been shown to be the most effective option.[77,98] For those with malignant airway obstruction, interventional bronchoscopy as well as or instead of stenting may provide benefit.[99] However, the increased risk of infection secondary to stenting should be balanced against the possible benefit of decreased feelings of dyspnea.

Nonpharmacologic Management

Treatment for dyspnea is best managed using an individualized multimodal approach. When considering the inclusion of pharmacologic and nonpharmacologic treatments, it is important to consider the individual's beliefs, the perceived relevance, insurance coverage, short-term benefits, convenience in administration, and caregiver involvement, as well as the stage and trajectory of the disease.[99,100]

Therapies

A Cochrane review assessed various therapies used for breathlessness. There was high-level evidence for the use of neuromuscular electrical stimulation (NMES) applied to quadriceps for dyspnea improvement over several weeks in individuals with COPD. Chest wall vibration also improved dyspnea in individuals with COPD and in one study for those with neuromuscular disease. In malignant and nonmalignant disease states, walking aids and breath training had a moderate level of evidence to support their use, and acupuncture showed improvement in dyspnea symptoms with low quality of evidence.[78] There is a paucity of studies of these therapies on those with ILD and therefore these therapies can only be recommended with weak evidence.[62]

Pulmonary Rehabilitation

There is strong evidence for the use of pulmonary rehabilitation (PR) to improve QoL and dyspnea in individuals with COPD,[101–103] CHF,[104,105] and ILD.[106] These programs may be safe for individuals who are not in acute respiratory distress or failure and may be combined with other therapies such as NIV or a combination of breath training with aerobic training to have maximal benefit.[76,79] In a prospective RCT of individuals with CHF, inspiratory muscle training (IMT) with computer-assisted measurement and guidance was added to standard PR aerobic training. Both groups in PR showed improvement in exercise tolerance and dyspnea, yet individuals who had IMT with standard PR showed significantly higher improvement in exercise tolerance and dyspnea symptom reduction at peak exercise.[104] It is important to recognize that improvement in exercise tolerance, dyspnea symptoms, and QoL may be gradual as many of these programs take place over many weeks or months. The study of PR in individuals with cancer is sparse, yet there are many areas of potential for the possibility of improving QoL, exercise tolerance, and perhaps dyspnea with PR, thus much more research is needed to answer these questions.[107]

Psychoeducational Interventions

The authors of a systematic review on noninvasive interventions for lung cancer concluded that nursing intervention programs may improve dyspnea.[108] Counseling, education, exercise, and relaxation techniques to manage breathlessness have been beneficial in individuals with various serious illnesses and most effective when combined with PR to extend the effectiveness of training.[2] In a RCT of an internet-based self-management support program compared to face-to-face care and general health education for individuals with COPD, dyspnea was not reduced, but there was satisfaction with participation in the program and increased self-efficacy.[109] Cognitive-behavioral interventions have been shown to have a positive effect on anxiety and depression.

Doyle and colleagues (2017) demonstrated that the addition of volunteer-based neutral befriending conversations in addition to standard cognitive training demonstrated improved and longer-lasting reduction of anxiety in those with COPD versus cognitive training alone.[110] A common theme in these programs is the inclusion of education, social support, and empowerment of individuals who may be isolated by their illness, which may increase self-efficacy and improve self-management of dyspnea.[2]

Breathlessness Intervention Services

In those with serious illness, the effects of breathlessness on a person's life may compromise their dignity or feelings of self-respect or worth. Targeting holistic treatment to illness-related concerns can benefit the individual's breathlessness symptoms and dignity.[2,26,109,111] A newer concept in the treatment of dyspnea, *holistic breathlessness services*, may increase understanding and self-efficacy, decrease feelings of isolation and distress, and optimize person-centered care. This comprehensive approach to treating dyspnea includes combining palliative care specialists and respiratory physiotherapists as holistic breathlessness services who work together to manage dyspnea and reduce distress in individuals with advanced disease.[80]

An RCT (2014) of individuals with refractory breathlessness and breathlessness at rest were treated with usual care or seen by a holistic breathlessness service for 6 weeks. The service combined palliative, respiratory, occupational, and physical therapy. Those who participated with holistic services had about 16% improvement in rating mastery of breathlessness over those in standard care group. Although findings were not significant, anxiety rating were more improved in the intervention group.[112] Ultimately, optimizing person-centered care has the potential to treat and maintain dignity for individuals with breathlessness and serious illness.[80,112] Although these services may not be available to the palliative APRN working in rural settings, working to collaborate and include respiratory physiotherapists in the assessment and management of dyspnea may improve outcomes.

Fans

The use of fans has been advocated for the relief of dyspnea because airflow has been shown to relieve dyspnea.[33] It has been hypothesized that cool air on the nasoreceptors decreases the subjective feeling of dyspnea. In a randomized controlled crossover trial evaluating the use of a handheld fan on the leg and face, results showed a positive effect on dyspnea with the use of the fan on the face.[113] Results from a meta-analysis demonstrated that fan therapy was effective in treating dyspnea in individuals with terminal cancer.[32] Due to its low risk and cost, a trial of a fan is warranted, except for those with facial pain secondary to trigeminal neuralgia or a neuropathic process that may be aggravated by the air on the face. At the time of this writing, with the prevalence COVID-19, an airborne virus, the use of fans may not be appropriate due to the risk of infection spread. These are a cost-effective intervention for patients in residential, home settings, in hospice programs, and who live in less resourced areas.

Acupuncture

Acupuncture has been shown to be beneficial for dyspnea symptoms in people with advanced disease, yet many studies have been small and heterogeneous or lacked a control group.[114] Results from a recent RCT in individuals with lung cancer undergoing chemotherapy demonstrated significant improvement in dyspnea symptoms in the acupressure group.[115] If available without undue burden to the individual, acupuncture may be a consideration as part of a multimodal therapeutic approach.

Management at the End of Life

Dyspnea may worsen in both pulmonary and nonpulmonary disease states toward the end of life. The palliative APRN should optimize pharmacologic management at this time to relieve suffering. In the acute care setting, the use of an opioid infusion may treat both dyspnea and pain and may be rapidly titrated. Benzodiazepines in combination with opioids may improve moderate to severe dyspnea when opioids alone have failed.[3,4] Although there may be concern that opioids and benzodiazepines may hasten death, the principle of the double effect justifies their use to relieve dyspnea at the end of life.[67] In home care settings, use of sublingual or rectal routes of opioids and benzodiazepines may alleviate dyspnea at end of life. For a select few who experience intractable dyspnea, the use of palliative sedation may be a consideration if dyspnea cannot be controlled with opioids and benzodiazepines (see Chapter 57, "Palliative Sedation").

At the time of this writing, there is a worldwide pandemic secondary to severe acute respiratory syndrome coronavirus 2 (SARS-VoV-2 or COVID-19). Due to the acute and potentially chronic injury to the pulmonary system, the individual may experience resulting chronic dyspnea. Depending on the individual's physiologic status, underlying comorbidities, and goals of care, treatment focus may preclude the ability to reverse the disease trajectory. In these cases, the focus will shift to the management of dyspnea to relieve suffering, and methods utilized in other disease states would also be used in this setting.

CASE STUDY: SHORTNESS OF BREATH (CONTINUED)

Carey was able to attend her son's wedding. She took an average of morphine 4 mg about 8 times a day for her dyspnea and was transitioned to extended-release morphine 15 mg two times daily with 4 mg morphine available every 2 hours as needed. After 2 months, she returned to the clinic in a wheelchair with a 15-pound weigh loss, and worsened and more painful cough. She felt that the morphine wasn't helping her dyspnea as it had in the past. Her lung sounds were very diminished throughout the right lung fields, and she described extremely thick yellow sputum with

her cough. On chest radiograph she had a large right pleural effusion and a small left pleural effusion.

After discussion about her goals in care, she shared that she was hoping that she and her family could have hospice support to help her remain at home with her family as much as possible and enjoy time outside during the warm weather. With those goals in mind she agreed to referral to interventional radiology for palliative pleural drainage catheter placement with the hope of managing the pleural effusion at home.

COUGH

Acute and chronic cough secondary to multiple etiologies, including premorbid conditions, medical therapies, and advanced diseases, can be a debilitating symptom. Individuals seek medical attention for cough due to concerns about serious illness, sleep disturbances, difficulties with tasks such as speaking on the phone, urinary incontinence, and the impact on family, friends, and co-workers who may be disturbed by the cough.[116] Cough as a primary symptom can also create and exacerbate other symptoms and is often part of a symptom cluster that includes pain, dyspnea, and lack of appetite.[117] The additive effect of multiple distressing symptoms can impact the individual's QoL, thus highlighting the need for the palliative APRN to possess the skills to manage multiple related symptoms in the individual with serious illness.

Cough due to viral infections of the respiratory system is one of the leading causes of visits to medical providers.[118] The prevalence of chronic cough, which is defined as cough that persists for longer than 8 weeks, is estimated to be 10% worldwide, with higher prevalence in Oceania, Europe, and America.[119] Internationally, cough is more predominant in women; two-thirds of the individuals seeking medical care for chronic cough were women in their 60s.[116]

Although cough is a major symptom seen in those with serious illness, there is a dearth of high-quality studies conducted in the palliative care population.[117,120] The mainstay of cough management in palliative care is extrapolated from the guidelines for the management of cough in the general population.[116,118,121–123]

CASE STUDY: SHORTNESS OF BREATH (CONTINUED)

Carey was assessed by the hospice nurse. Her dyspnea was better controlled with the pleural catheter placement; however, it was more difficult to clear her thick secretions. She reported the constant presence of cough since her teenage years.

PHYSIOLOGY

Cough is a complex protective neuronal reflex that protects the lungs from chemical and thermal irritants, clears secretions, prevents aspiration, but also spreads infectious disease. The complex physiology, which is still not completely understood, is outlined briefly here. Cough receptors (nerve endings of sensory vagal nerves) innervate the pharynx, trachea, carina, and bronchi. Mechanical and chemical stimuli and inflammatory mediators (tachykinins, bradykinin, and prostaglandins) activate the cough receptors located in the epithelium of larynx, trachea, and bronchi. These receptors detect the stimuli and transmit the signal to the cerebral cough center via the myelinated A-delta (fast-adapting and slow-adapting mechanoreceptors) and the nonmyelinated C-fibers.

Cough is then generated by motor neuron reflexes under the influence of the neurons in the medulla oblongata. The influence of the brain on cough is seen with cough suppression, idiopathic or refractory cough, and the absence of cough during anesthesia. The cough reflex can also be activated via extrapulmonary sources such as rhinosinusitis, even though vagal nerves are not located in the nose or sinuses. The current thought is that, in these cases, trigeminal nerve fibers are involved in the activation and relief of cough.

The cough reflex can be modulated by blocking multiple transient receptor potential (TRP) ion channels, N-methyl-D-aspartate (NMDA) and γ-aminobutyric acid (GABA), which provides opportunities for treatment strategies. To add to the complexity of cough pathophysiology, hypersensitivity of the cough reflex may occur through peripheral sensitization and central neuronal changes, thus leading to chronic idiopathic or refractory cough.[118,124] Chronic refractory, idiopathic cough, more commonly referred to as *cough hypersensitivity syndrome* (CHS), has been likened to neuropathic pain, which often has central neuronal changes.[125] With this emerging understanding related to the physiology of cough, the possibilities of treatment can be expanded to include agents that are utilized in the treatment of neuropathic pain.

It is helpful to think of the cough event in three separate phases: (1) the inspiratory phase to produce enough volume for the cough; (2) the compression phase, where the larynx closes and the chest wall, diaphragm, and abdominal wall muscles contract, thus increasing intrathoracic pressure; and (3) the expiratory phase, during which the glottis opens, and there occurs an expiration of air that may dislodge mucous or foreign materials.[126]

COMMON ETIOLOGIES

Cough has been classified based on its duration into three phases: acute 1–3 weeks, subacute 3–8 weeks, and chronic cough greater than 8 weeks. Recurrent acute cough is that which recurs several times yearly and lasts up to 3 weeks[118] (see Table 44.4).

Acute Cough

Acute cough is most commonly associated with viral infections of the respiratory tract and generally resolves within a

Table 44.4 ETIOLOGIES OF COUGH IN THE GENERAL POPULATION

Acute (1–3 weeks)	Viral infections Asthma Inhalation intoxication Pulmonary embolism Pneumothorax Acute congestive heart failure
Subacute (3–8 weeks)	Viral infection Postviral rhinosinusitis Pneumonia Pleuritis
Chronic (>8 weeks)	Upper airway cough syndrome (UACS) Cough variant asthma Nonasthmatic eosinophilic bronchitis GERD Chronic bronchitis secondary to COPD ACE inhibitors Obstructive sleep apnea Chronic idiopathic cough or UCC/CHS

COPD, chronic obstructive pulmonary disease; CHS, cough hypersensitivity syndrome; UCC, unexplained chronic cough.

From Morice et al.[116]; Kardos et al.[118]; Lai et al.[121]; Gibson et al.[123]; Spanevello et al.[127]; and Song, Morice.[128]

few weeks without specific treatment. The various causes of acute cough include not only viral infections, but also asthma and inhalation intoxication such as from smoke, as well as acute lung pathologies, such as pulmonary embolism, pneumothorax, or acute CHF exacerbation.[118]

Subacute Cough

Similar to acute cough, the most common reason for subacute cough that persists from 3 to 8 weeks is a viral infection. The cough may also be a result of postviral rhinosinusitis due to bronchial hyperreactivity or may be secondary to lung pathology such as pneumonia and pleuritis.[118]

Chronic Cough

Cough lasting more than 8 weeks, labeled chronic cough, has many potential causes. Airway diseases responsible for chronic cough include chronic upper airway diseases; chronic bronchitis secondary to COPD; cough variant asthma, including nonasthmatic eosinophilic bronchitis; obstructive sleep apnea; lung cancer; cystic fibrosis; and environmental irritants (smoke); as well as systemic disease with lung involvement or rare diseases of the tracheobronchial system. Extrapulmonary diseases that can cause chronic cough are gastroesophageal reflux disease (GERD), angiotensin-converting enzyme (ACE) inhibitors, and cardiac diseases that produce lung congestion and endocarditis. Chronic idiopathic cough, also termed *unexplained chronic cough* (UCC), is also a consideration if diagnostic workup is negative for the just listed pathologies.[118,123,127] Emerging evidence suggests that chronic cough even in some of the above-mentioned disease states may be due to CHS.[116,127,128]

BRIEF OVERVIEW FREQUENT CAUSES OF COUGH

Upper Airway Cough Syndrome

Upper airway cough syndrome (UACS), which has also been referred to as *postnasal drip syndrome*, *rhinitis*, or *rhinosinusitis* has been assumed to be one of the most common cause of chronic cough. With the evolution in the understanding of chronic cough, some question whether the cough that has been attributed to UACS may actually be cough secondary to CHS.[116]

Cough Variant Asthma/Nonasthmatic Eosinophilic Bronchitis

Asthma is characterized by chronic or recurrent respiratory symptoms associated with airway inflammation and variable airflow obstruction. Most individuals experience wheeze, dyspnea, and cough. Some individuals with asthma who have cough-predominant symptoms without signs of bronchial obstruction can be classified as having cough-variant asthma.[116,118] A third disorder classified under asthma that causes a chronic cough, not secondary to bronchoconstriction or hyperresponsiveness is nonasthmatic eosinophilic bronchitis.[116]

COPD

Cough is a common symptom for those with COPD who have chronic bronchitis. Variations of cough in COPD types may not be fully understood and appreciated. Cough secondary to bronchitis is generally defined as cough that has occurred for at least 3 months a year for 2 years and is not attributable to other causes. Madison and Irwin (2020) have raised concerns that other potential causes of chronic cough in those with COPD such as UACS, GERD, and asthma may be overlooked and thus further diagnostics and treatments could be missed.[129]

GERD

Chronic cough secondary to GERD has been one of the most frequently cited.[127] At present, GERD is viewed as one of the possible triggers for chronic cough due to hypersensitivity of the cough reflex.[118] There is also controversy about the role of reflux in chronic cough and the possibility that esophagopharyngeal reflux may be the actual problem.[116]

ACE Inhibitors

Cough associated with ACE inhibitors, which is a class effect, was first reported with the medication captopril in 1985.[130] The incidence of cough secondary to ACE inhibitors varies from 3.9% to 35%. Approximately 20% of individuals discontinue ACE inhibitors due to cough. The cough tends to be dry, is not dose-related, and time to onset varies; it can occur within hours or months after starting treatment and can persist for months after discontinuation of treatment.[131]

UCC and CHS

Chronic idiopathic or refractory cough, also termed UCC, was a category utilized to define chronic cough that did not seem to be associated with the conditions known to cause cough.[123] A relatively new paradigm, CHS, has been proposed to describe unexplained cough that may arise from increased sensitivity to chemical, thermal, mechanical, or emotional triggers. CHS is thought to arise from dysregulation of the neural pathways that regulate the cough reflex and neural alterations that regulate cough processing. Clinical measurement tools are lacking and antitussives may not be effective, whereas agents that work centrally, such as gabapentinoids and opioids, may be helpful.[127,128]

ETIOLOGIES OF COUGH IN INDIVIDUALS WITH SERIOUS ILLNESS

In the palliative care population, cough may be a common symptom seen in those individuals with ineffective swallowing, malignancies (most commonly lung and surrounding structures), and infections in those with diseases such as COPD and cystic fibrosis. Common causes of cough such as UACS, viral infections, and GERD can also occur in those with serious illness and may not be related to the life-limiting illness.[132] Consideration for aspiration as a causative factor of cough should be considered in those with dementia,[133,134] neuromuscular diseases,[135] and Parkinson's disease[136] as there may be decreased cough sensitivity which results in aspiration.[133–136]

In individuals with cancer, cough is most commonly associated with primary cancers arising from the airways, lungs, pleura, and other mediastinal structures as well as primary tumors metastasizing to the mediastinum.[117,137] Indirect causes include pulmonary embolism, atelectasis, pleural effusion, pericardial effusion, and infections such as pneumonia or empyema.[132] Radiation therapy has also been known to cause fibrosis of the lung, which can cause chronic cough.[117]

Targeted agents such as immunotherapies utilized in advanced lung cancer are known to cause pneumonitis, in which cough and dyspnea are the predominant symptoms. At the time of this writing, COVID-19 infection is a worldwide pandemic. Lung involvement, with bilateral pneumonia has been reported in up to 80% of symptomatic individuals. Given similar symptomatology (dyspnea and cough), it may be challenging to initially determine the causative factor[138] (see Table 44.5).

ASSESSMENT

The palliative APRN's comprehensive assessment will help guide symptom management. In an individual with serious illness and cough, the APRN may already have some ideas about the causative factor of the cough based on the underlying disease. However, determining the etiology of cough in an individual with serious illness can be challenging. Multiple etiologies need to be considered given the likelihood of chronic

Table 44.5 ETIOLOGIES COUGH IN INDIVIDUALS WITH SERIOUS ILLNESS

Pulmonary	COPD
	Cystic fibrosis
	Interstitial lung disease
Neurologic	Amyotrophic lateral sclerosis
	Cerebrovascular disease
	Dementia
	Multiple sclerosis
Cardiac	CHF
Systemic	HIV
	Tuberculosis
Cancer	**Direct Causes**
	Tumor/tumor microemboli
	Pulmonary parenchymal involvement
	Lymphangitic carcinomatosis
	Intrinsic or extrinsic airway obstruction
	Pleural effusion
	Indirect Causes
	Chemotherapy, targeted therapy
	Radiation therapy
	GERD infection
	Paraneoplastic syndrome
	Pulmonary embolus
	Smoking

This list is not exhaustive. Consider etiologies of cough in general population in addition to those listed.

CHF, congestive heart failure; COPD, chronic obstructive pulmonary disease; GERD, gastroesophageal reflux disease.

From Molassiotis et al.[117]; Spanevello et al.[127]; von Gunten, Buckholz[132]; and Harle et al.[137]

Table 44.6 COUGH ASSESSMENT

Clinical interview	Onset, duration, severity, productive/non-productive, exacerbating/alleviating factors
	Use of disease-modifying therapies that could induce/control cough
	Lifestyle factors: Smoke exposure, environmental triggers
Assessment tools	The Leicester Cough (LCQ) Questionnaire
	Cough-Specific Quality-of-Life Questionnaire (CQLQ)
	Visual analogue scale (VAS)
Physical examination (tailored to potential cause of cough)	General: Observation type/frequency of cough
	Ears, nose, and throat: Signs of rhinitis/pharyngitis, swallow and gag reflex
	Pulmonary: Respiratory rate and quality, lung sounds, sputum production
	Cardiac: Heart sounds, jugular venous pressure, edema
Diagnostic testing (if indicated to assess for etiology)	**Asthma**
	Spirometry, methacholine challenge, induced sputum
	GERD
	24-hour pH testing, esophageal manometry
	UACS
	Sinus radiography or computed tomography, laryngoscopy, videofluoroscopic swallow evaluation; nasopharyngoscopy
	Cardiopulmonary
	Chest radiograph, computed tomograph (CT) scan of the chest/neck, bronchoscopy, echocardiogram
	Esophageal
	Modified barium swallow, endoscopy

GERD, gastroesophageal reflux disease; UACS, Upper airway cough syndrome.

From Morice et al.[116]; Kardos et al.[118]; Lai et al.[121]; Spanevello et al.[127]

---

comorbidities. The APRN should differentiate between acute versus subacute versus chronic cough, infectious versus noninfectious cough, life-threatening versus non–life-threatening causes, and cancerous versus noncancerous or chronic conditions.

By conducting a comprehensive assessment, the palliative APRN may be able to differentiate between the acute or new pathology and comorbid conditions contributing to cough (see Table 44.6). Assessment of cough begins with a thorough review of the individual's medical history, review of systems, and current medications. The APRN should inquire about environmental factors such as current and past occupation, tobacco or cannabis use, exposure to secondhand smoke or other irritants or allergens known to cause cough. A review of medications will help determine if the individual is taking medications that may cause cough (i.e., ACE inhibitors) and which medications have been ineffective in controlling cough.

The APRN should conduct a thorough individual evaluation of the cough, including the intensity and quality of the cough (wet, dry, productive), its temporal onset (acute, subacute, chronic), frequency, precipitating, aggravating and alleviating factors, accompanying symptoms, and the resulting emotional stress. Assessment should include inquiry into potential red flags (fever, weight loss, vocal changes) that may

indicate a new concerning pathology or infection. Changes in environmental triggers should also be assessed as a potential cough trigger.[125,139]

For those with acute cough, the APRN should first consider the most common causes of cough, such as rhinoviruses, especially in those reporting nasal congestion and rhinitis or postnasal drip. Assessment for GERD should be considered when there are reports of acid regurgitation or retrosternal pain. Acute respiratory infections should be considered if the individual reports cough with purulent sputum production.[121,123]

The palliative APRN should focus questions related to the organ system that is most likely associated with the cough. For example, in individuals with COPD, the APRN should inquire about the presence of fever/chills, productive or nonproductive sputum, hemoptysis, and increased dyspnea. The APRN should ask individuals with CHF about weight gain, increased edema, orthopnea, activity intolerance, and increased use/need for oxygen.[121,125] The APRN should consider the use of cough assessment tools such as the Leicester Cough (LCQ) Questionnaire[140] and the Cough-Specific Quality-of-Life Questionnaire (CQLQ),[141] which are valid and reliable for use in adults. Although widely used, the Visual Analogue Scale (VAS) has insufficient data to support its use.[116,142]

In individuals with chronic cough, the APRN should consider if there may be more than one etiology of the cough, especially in individuals with multiple comorbidities. To consider appropriate management, the APRN may need to consider if the source of cough in an individual with lung cancer is secondary to the tumor, the treatment, or a comorbidity such as COPD or GERD.

When conducting the physical examination, the palliative APRN should take into consideration the individual's medical history and the clinical interview. Consideration should be given to several different organ systems that may be the etiology of the cough; this includes examination of the ears, nose, throat, heart, and lungs.[121] The APRN may also assess the individual's swallowing and gag reflex to assess for possible presence of aspiration that could be contributing to the cough. However, in the frail individual, such as the person with dementia, the cough reflex may be impaired or even absent and thus contribute to the development of repeated aspiration pneumonia.[133]

DIAGNOSTIC EVALUATION

With the information obtained from the interview and physical examination, the APRN can determine what type of diagnostic evaluation may be necessary. In the population without life-limiting illnesses, workup of some of the most common causes of cough include the following:

- Asthma: Spirometry, methacholine challenge (a drug used to induce bronchoconstriction that can be measured by spirometry), and induced sputum test

- GERD: Twenty-four-hour ambulatory pH monitoring, and esophageal manometry

- UACS: Plain sinus radiography and CT of the sinuses[118,125]

Normal chest radiography usually excludes bronchiectasis, persistent pneumonia, sarcoidosis, and tuberculosis.[125] If aspiration is suspected, a clinical assessment and tests such as the modified barium swallow can determine the degree of dysphagia.[143]

In those with serious illnesses, such as cancer or advancing COPD, the APRN should consider whether more comprehensive diagnostic tests such as CT scans are warranted. If the APRN is in a consultative role, involvement of the primary specialists (oncologists, pulmonologists, cardiologists) may help tailor the type of evaluation needed and avoid the possibility of duplicate diagnostic evaluations.

CASE STUDY: SHORTNESS OF BREATH (CONTINUED)

Although Carey had previously declined medications for cough, she was interested in a retrial of guaifenesin 600 mg extended-release every 12 hours to help thin her pulmonary secretions. She occasionally utilized 4 mg of oral morphine about 2–3 times daily for severe cough with dyspnea, but she preferred to avoid sedating medications. Carey also utilized relaxation techniques that not only helped her cough but also her dyspnea.

Four weeks after placement of a pleural catheter and hospice admission, Carey developed a fever and worsening dyspnea after her grandson who lived out of state visited her. He later tested positive for COVID-19. Carey's cough and dyspnea worsened, and she developed a fever. She did not want to seek any further medical workup. Carey was able to stay at home with the priority of comfort over alertness at the end of her life. Her oral morphine dose was titrated up and lorazepam was utilized to manage her dyspnea and cough. She died peacefully with her family around her.

MANAGEMENT

Palliative APRNs play an instrumental role in the care of individuals with life-limiting illnesses. Management of cough in this population may vary considerably from that of the general population. In the general population, managing cough is directed at treating reversible causes. Although the diagnostic workup and treatment may include some modalities seen in the general population, those same methods may not be feasible for individuals with advanced disease if they are approaching the end of life.

Pharmacologic Therapies

The goal of cough management is to treat the underlying cause and either help promote cough (expectorants) or suppress cough (antitussives). For acute cough related to the common cold, individuals often use antihistamines, decongestants, nonsteroidal anti-inflammatories, and over-the-counter cough suppressives. However, due to the paucity of high-quality studies, there are no specific recommendations.[144] For those with subacute cough (3–8 weeks), individuals often use over-the-counter antitussives and inhaled corticosteroids. However, results of studies do not support the use of any pharmacologic agents for subacute cough not related to COPD or asthma.[145]

Targeted therapy should be considered in individuals with chronic cough related to conditions that affect the general population, such as UACS, asthma, GERD, and chronic bronchitis, with the primary aim being the treatment of the underlying cause of the cough. For these conditions medications such as expectorants and inhaled corticosteroids (UACS), antacids (GERD), inhaled/oral corticosteroids (asthma/bronchitis), and bronchodilators (bronchitis) may be the mainstay of treatment for cough.[116,118,143] With the recent evolution in the understanding of UCC and CHS, treatment may include neuromodulatory agents utilized to treat neuropathic pain such as gabapentinoids and tricyclic antidepressants.[123] Medications are in development that target the cough reflex pathway, which may change treatment options for those with UCC.[128,146]

It is important to recognize that, for many individuals receiving palliative care, cough may be related to a comorbid condition that is not the life-limiting illness. The palliative APRN may have the opportunity to provide guidance for treatment of the cough to the clinician managing these comorbid conditions. In individuals receiving palliative care, there is a lower threshold for empiric treatment to manage the distressing symptom of cough especially if the overall care is directed toward alleviating distressing symptoms. A pragmatic approach has been proposed that includes stepwise treatment, much in the same way as pain is treated based on severity.[147] In the case of worsening cough and advancing disease, opioids may be the medication class of choice if the cough is severe and not responsive to other measures.[116] A brief description of pharmacologic agents will help the palliative APRN determine the best treatment in those with serious illness (see Table 44.7).

Expectorants

Expectorants decrease the viscosity of mucus, allowing for improved expulsion. This can be helpful for the individual with excessive or thick mucus production. Guaifenesin, the only expectorant available in the United States, is utilized in many over-the-counter products for cough and cold. However, it can also be utilized in conditions where mucus hypersecretion and cough are present, such as in chronic bronchitis. It is relatively safe, well-tolerated, and is available in both immediate-release and extended-release formulations.[148] Simple nebulized saline solution and substances that lessen irritation, such as thyme cough syrup, can also be effective. Other medications, such as acetylcysteine and ambroxol hydrochloride, are also utilized but may not be available in the United States.[121,149] Caution should be exercised when prescribing expectorants in individuals with neuromuscular diseases, such as amyotrophic lateral sclerosis, due to impaired cough.[149]

Opioids

When the cough's etiology has been determined and effectively treated, the goal may be to suppress the cough with antitussives. Cough suppressants are classified as central and peripheral antitussive drugs. Peripheral agents act on receptors in the cough reflex arch, whereas central agents act on the cough center in the medulla oblongata.[121] Therefore, centrally acting medications may produce side effects like sedation.[149] Among centrally acting medications, opioids, such as codeine and morphine, bind to the μ-opioid receptor and suppress the cough center.[121,150]

Even though codeine has long been promoted as an antitussive, its efficacy has not been demonstrated in clinical trials.[149] Codeine exerts its effect by converting codeine to morphine through cytochrome P450 2D6 activity. Some

Table 44.7 SELECTED PHARMACOLOGIC TREATMENTS OF COUGH IN PALLIATIVE CARE

MEDICATION	SUGGESTED DOSES (IF APPLICABLE)
Guaifenesin (expectorant)	200–400 mg PO q4h 600–1,200 mg ER PO bid
Opioids/Opioid derivatives (cough not responsive to reversal of pathology)	
Morphine	5 mg PO/SL q2–4h PRN
Hydrocodone	5 mg PO q4h PRN
Dextromethorphan (opioid derivative)	15–30 mg PO q4h PRN
Anesthetics (chronic refractory cough)	
Lidocaine (fentanyl and opioid associated cough)	3–5 mL of 4% nebulized bid-tid or 0.5–1.5 mg/kg IV once
Benzonatate	100–200 mg PO tid
Neuromodulatory agents (used in UCC/CHS)	
Gabapentin	300–2,700 mg PO tid
Pregabalin	75–150 mg PO bid
Baclofen	30–60 mg PO tid
Amitriptyline	10–100 mg PO daily
Miscellaneous medications (refer to dosing guidelines)	
Inhaled, nasal or oral corticosteroids (cough secondary to cough variant asthma, eosinophilic bronchitis, lung cancer) Glycopyrrolate (anticholinergic utilized at end of life to decrease secretions) Ketamine, propofol, dexmedetomidine, pheniramine maleate, lidocaine (opioid-induced cough)	

List is not all-inclusive.

From Morice et al.[116]; Molassiotis et al.[117]; Harle et al.[147]; Bausewein, Simon[149]; Morice, Kardos[151]; Lim et al.[152]; and Bishop-Freeman et al.[153]

individuals may be rapid metabolizers and others slow metabolizers; therefore it is difficult to predict its action. In those who are rapid metabolizers, there is a risk of oversedation and respiratory depression. Thus, while it had been an antitussive of choice in children, the risks outweigh the benefits and it should be avoided.[151] Moreover, in many places it is being eliminated from formularies since there are better medications to use.

In palliative care, morphine is the preferred opioid because it also can treat distressing symptoms, such as dyspnea, which can often co-occur with cough. In an earlier randomized, double-blind, placebo-controlled trial ($n = 27$), daily cough score was reduced by 40% with 5–10 mg of daily morphine.[154] In a recent small double blind, placebo-controlled crossover study ($n = 22$) of those with chronic cough treated with morphine, 78% of individuals had decreased cough frequency with low-dose morphine.[155]

The use of nebulized medications to treat symptoms has been an interest in palliative care. However, the evidence for use of nebulized morphine for cough is limited to case reports,[156] thus it should not be considered unless no other options are available to treat the cough. Hydrocodone is another opioid commonly prescribed for cough. Some hydrocodone products also contain the anticholinergic homatropine (1.5 mg/5 mL hydrocodone) to reduce deliberate overdose.[157] In a small ($n = 20$) Phase 2 study of hydrocodone in individuals with lung neoplasms, 19 individuals experienced at least 50% improvement in cough with a median dose of hydrocodone 10 mg daily.[158] Although widely used, there have not been more robust studies about the efficacy of hydrocodone. Because it is an opioid, it may provide benefit for those unable to utilize morphine. Dextromethorphan is an opioid derivative and NMDA receptor antagonist with antitussive efficacy and low toxicity that could be considered for cough suppression.[120,147]

Corticosteroids

Corticosteroids are utilized in individuals with serious illness to treat multiple distressing symptoms such as pain, nausea, lack of appetite, and fatigue. Generally, their use is limited by the long-term side-effect profile. Although there is not supporting evidence, inhaled corticosteroids are often utilized in acute or subacute cough.[145] Inhaled or nasal corticosteroids may be effective in chronic cough for those individuals who have cough variant asthma and eosinophilic bronchitis.[116,118,127,159] Even though there is a paucity of studies, in those with cough related to lung cancer, a trial of corticosteroids is warranted, if not contraindicated by other health conditions or chemotherapy regimens.

Anesthetics

The most commonly used peripherally active antitussives are inhaled local anesthetics, such as bupivacaine 0.25% or lidocaine 2%.[117] There is evidence for the use of nebulized lidocaine for cough that has not responded to other antitussives.[117,149,160] Although there have been concerns for safety, reports from case series on the use of inhaled lidocaine for intractable cough did not reveal serious adverse effects.[159,161] While there is evidence supporting the use of lidocaine for intractable cough, there is a dearth of quality studies.[160] Intravenous lidocaine may be effective in preventing opioid-induced cough,[162] particularly fentanyl-associated cough.[153] IV lidocaine could be helpful for individuals requiring opioids such as fentanyl in settings such as the intensive care unit. Benzonatate, a peripherally acting oral local anesthetic, may be helpful for cough unresponsive to other antitussives.[117,147] Individuals with pulmonary disease may utilize this medication on a chronic basis. Caution needs to be exercised due to the possibility of toxicity if taken at higher than prescribed doses because it can cause seizures and cardiac collapse.[163]

Neuromodulatory Agents

CHS is believed to contribute to chronic refractory cough (also known as UCC) that is not relieved by treatment of the underlying pathology or through antitussives. This cough is thought to have a neuropathic component, thus current treatments have focused on agents that treat neuropathic pain, with the most widely studied being the gabapentinoids.[164–166] Amitriptyline, a tricyclic antidepressant also utilized for neuropathic pain, has been evaluated for chronic cough.[164]

In a study comparing gabapentin and amitriptyline over 6 months, both had short-term efficacy. Individuals in both arms dropped out due to lack of efficacy, but there was a higher discontinuation rate among those in the amitriptyline arm.[164] An RCT compared gabapentin and baclofen for refractory cough secondary to GERD. More than 50% of individuals showed improvement, but gabapentin was better tolerated.[166] As the understanding of chronic refractory cough evolves, treatment modalities may be developed that more effectively treat cough. Studies of medications that exert their effect on the different areas of cough reflex neural pathways are in progress.[128]

Miscellaneous

Other miscellaneous agents utilized for opioid-induced cough include dexmedetomidine,[161,167] propofol, or ketamine.[161] In one study, the antihistamine pheniramine maleate was more effective than lidocaine for the reduction of fentanyl-induced cough.[168] Anticholinergics, such as glycopyrrolate, may be helpful during the dying phase as decreasing secretions may also decrease cough.[132] Given that these agents are utilized for other purposes, they may provide a secondary benefit in palliating cough.

Nonpharmacologic Interventions

Nonpharmacologic techniques for cough management may help the individual strengthen their cough (cough augmentation) for airway clearance or control their cough (cough suppression).[169] These techniques have not been widely studied in the palliative care population. However, the palliative APRN managing symptoms for individuals with chronic progressive diseases such as amyotrophic lateral sclerosis may find benefit from cough augmentation strategies. Individuals with advancing diseases with chronic cough may also benefit from nonpharmacologic techniques of cough suppression or augmentation (see Box 44.3).

Complementary and Alternative Therapies

Individuals may utilize home remedies and preparations to control cough or improve expectoration. Eucalyptus and myrtol have been used in preparations as expectorants.[121] Traditional Chinese Medicine formulas are included in the Chinese Thoracic Society's guidelines for treatment of cough (2018). These formulas have also been utilized to treat cough, even in the cases of cough unexplained by any pathology.[121] Individuals may utilize honey to reduce cough. Studies evaluating honey for acute cough secondary to cold have been conducted in the pediatric population. Honey was not more effective than dextromethorphan, but may be more effective than diphenhydramine or no treatment. Zinc was found to reduce cold symptoms that include cough if administered within 24 hours of onset of symptoms.[144] These treatments, although marketed as natural, may have unwanted side effects or interactions with the individual's medical treatment. Thus, the palliative APRN should always inquire about the use of complementary or alternative therapies.

Cough Suppression Nonpharmacologic Therapies

Most studies on cough suppression therapies have been conducted on individuals with chronic cough without life-limiting illnesses. However, in a multicenter randomized controlled study aimed at testing the feasibility of a nonpharmacologic intervention for the management of a respiratory distress symptom cluster (breathlessness, cough, fatigue), individuals participated in a respiratory distress symptom intervention that included controlled breathing techniques, cough easing techniques, acupressure, an information packet, and psychoeducation. This type of study intervention was deemed feasible and acceptable by the participants, but a fully powered trial is necessary for definitive conclusions.[172]

Nonpharmacologic therapies for cough suppression have often been delivered by speech and language therapists or physiotherapists. Cough suppression therapies utilized in key studies can be grouped into four categories: (1) patient education, (2) cough control/suppression techniques, (3) vocal/laryngeal hygiene and hydration, and (4) psychoeducational counseling. These nonpharmacologic interventions have been shown to improve QoL and in some cases decrease cough frequency and severity.[169,170]

Cough Control/Suppression Techniques

Cough control techniques may be most effective for those individuals with UCC or CHS not adequately controlled through treatment of the underlying pathology or use of pharmacotherapeutic agents. Expert guidelines recommend a trial of cough suppression nonpharmacologic therapy.[116,123] Simple measures that the individual can utilize include sipping water, chewing gum, and sucking nonmedicated sweets. Speech and language therapists or physiotherapists teach breathing techniques or respiratory training exercises in addition to counseling and education. Therapeutic techniques varies between therapists, thus it has been a challenge to measure efficacy.[170]

The efficacy of speech and language therapy for UCC was evaluated in a recent Cochrane Review (2019), where only two studies met the criteria for evaluation. Findings were significant for decreased cough frequency and improved health-related QoL, but these improvements were not sustained over time.[171] In a small ($n = 40$) RCT of individuals with chronic cough, the combination of speech pathology treatment with the neuromodulatory agent pregabalin was superior to speech pathology alone in reported improved QoL and reduced cough symptoms.[173] Although clinicians in another center increased referrals to speech and language therapy for those with chronic cough, they were not able to evaluate the efficacy of the addition of this therapy.[174] High-quality research is needed to determine those aspects of speech and language therapy that provide benefit and how to sustain benefits over time.[170,171]

Education/Psychoeducational Counseling

An integral component of cough management is education about the anatomy of cough reflex, identification of cough triggers, and the benefits of nonpharmacologic interventions. Psychoeducational counseling can motivate individuals to participate in treatments such as breathing exercises and cough suppression measures and to manage the stress and anxiety that can trigger cough. Through education and counseling, individuals can gain an understanding of cough physiology and acquire skills in ways to avoid cough triggers to control cough.[169,170]

Vocal/Laryngeal Hygiene and Hydration

Laryngeal irritation due to throat dryness is a cough trigger. Vocal/laryngeal hydration measures include adequate water intake, reduction of caffeine and alcohol, nasal breathing, and nasal douching.[169,170] These therapies rely on individual motivation and involvement for success, thus the need for continued education and reinforcement.

Cough Augmentation

Techniques for cough augmentation can be utilized to prevent aspiration through enhancing effective airway clearance. Individuals with cerebrovascular accidents, Parkinson's disease, multiple sclerosis, neuromuscular diseases, and spinal cord injury, as well as those who are intubated and mechanically ventilated, may have decreased respiratory strength or endurance and may benefit from therapies to decrease the risk of aspiration.[169]

Hyperinflation and Compression

Mechanical or manual hyperinflation (positive pressure mechanical ventilation or non-resuscitation bag) delivered by therapists may increase the inspiratory peak cough flow (PCF) to a level necessary for airway clearance. Hyperinflation may be more effective than unassisted cough for individuals with neuromuscular diseases or spinal cord injury. Thoracic, abdominal, or thoracoabdominal compression are cough augmentation techniques that can help those with expiratory muscle weakness and may be useful in the aforementioned populations.[169]

Mechanical Insufflation-Exsufflation Therapy

This therapy involves a series of maneuvers: positive airway pressure (insufflation) followed by a pause, followed by applying negative airway pressure (exsufflation). It has been utilized in those with neuromuscular disease to augment cough and has been evaluated as a means for augmenting cough when weaning individuals from mechanical ventilation.[175,176] Although widely used and recommended for those with neuromuscular disease, the actual efficacy is unknown due to the paucity of high-quality studies.[175] There is low-quality evidence for cough augmentation through the use of mechanical insufflation-exsufflation as a measure to improve successful extubation from mechanical ventilation. Yet, due to limited studies, actual harms could not be determined.[176] These techniques may be important for further study, especially given the prolonged time on ventilatory support that may be experienced due to the respiratory effects of COVID-19.

Abdominal Electrical Stimulation, Abdominal Binding, Oscillation Techniques

For those with amyotrophic lateral sclerosis and spinal cord injury, abdominal electrical stimulation has been utilized to improve cough in the expulsive phase. Abdominal binding has also been utilized for cough augmentation in those with spinal cord injury, but efficacy is uncertain.[169] In those with bronchiectasis, the use of airway clearance techniques (high-frequency oscillation techniques or airway oscillatory devices) may improve sputum expectoration and QoL.[177]

Respiratory Muscle Training

Individuals can participate in respiratory muscle training to improve muscle strength in the inspiratory and expiratory phase and endurance for cough augmentation.[169] Individuals with Parkinson's disease showed significant improvement with the use of expiratory muscle strength training.[178] A Cochrane review of respiratory training evaluated individuals with multiple sclerosis. There was low-quality evidence that the training improves predicted inspiratory muscle strength. However, conclusions about cough efficacy and QoL were not included in the study results, thus it is unclear if this therapy would be of benefit to this population.[179] In those with acute stroke, the use of respiratory muscle training was no more effective than no intervention. In this RCT, cough improved even without training.[180]

Most of these therapies have not been supported by high-quality studies and may not be appropriate as disease progresses and the individual experiences functional decline. Additionally, these therapies may not be available for those who live in rural areas or those without robust multidisciplinary services. The APRN must weigh the potential benefit versus burden and overall goals of care before recommending these therapies.

Interventional Techniques

Cough may be relieved if the underlying pathology is treated (as outlined earlier in the interventional treatment of dyspnea). In those with lung cancer, for example, disease-modifying treatments such as chemotherapy, immunotherapy, or radiation may decrease tumor burden and thus relieve cough. Where available, if the individual has cough secondary to tumor burden not relieved by disease-modifying treatment, endobronchial brachytherapy may be a treatment option.[117,181] For those with pleural effusions, thoracentesis may relieve the cough. The decision to undergo interventions to address underlying pathology depends on the individual's goals of care and the benefit versus burden of the proposed intervention. The palliative APRN can be instrumental in assisting the individual in decision-making, especially as disease progresses.

PATIENT AND FAMILY EDUCATION

APRNs are in an optimal position to provide essential components of care that include information and education. Individuals and families should understand the potential causes of dyspnea and cough and treatments that may address the underlying pathology and those that will provide symptom relief. Discussions should include information about multimodal treatment, including pharmacologic and non-pharmacologic modalities for dyspnea and cough.[109,149,169,170] Identification and education about simple, low-cost, and low-risk interventions such as breathing techniques and the use of fans may establish trust and build confidence in individual self-management of dyspnea.[32,112] Reinforcement of the practice of cough suppression techniques and vocal/laryngeal hydration therapies may help the individual better manage cough.[169,170] Depending on the disease trajectory and goals of care, education about smoking cessation may be appropriate since smoking cessation may help with both dyspnea and cough. There is a strong evidence base for the use of individual counseling by trained smoking cessation specialists.[182] Thus, if the palliative APRN does not feel skilled in smoking cessation counseling, the individual can be referred to these specialists if available. If specialized counseling is not available, there are online resources available to assist the individual in smoking cessation.[183]

Individual and caregiver involvement is key to providing personalized treatment.[7,149] Caregivers may experience psychological distress secondary to increased caregiving.[184] They may feel isolated, especially when there are longer trajectories of illness, and they may benefit from social work involvement and referral to community support agencies.[7] Given the multidimensional nature of dyspnea and cough, a multi-modal plan that is individual and family-centered is essential to ensure appropriate effective management.[7,170,185]

SUMMARY

The effective treatment of dyspnea and cough, which may co-occur, involves the optimal treatment of the underlying pathology (when appropriate) and the associated affective response and distress related to the symptoms. During the clinical assessment, the palliative APRN should assess the characteristics of dyspnea and cough and their impact on the individual's life. The palliative APRN should recognize that many individuals may experience multiple distressing symptoms unrelated to cough or dyspnea, as well as symptoms associated with dyspnea or cough such as pain, incontinence, depression, anxiety, anorexia, and fatigue. The APRN should evaluate and manage co-occurring symptoms or those that are secondary to dyspnea or cough. Pharmacologic and nonpharmacologic approaches can decrease dyspnea and cough and their impact on the individual's QoL. Further research is necessary to optimize the most effective treatments for dyspnea and cough. Palliative APRNs have a essential role to play in contributing to the further development of this evidence base.

REFERENCES

1. Hayen A, Wanigasekera V, Faull OK, et al. Opioid suppression of conditioned anticipatory brain responses to breathlessness. *Neuroimage.* 2017;150(Apr):383–394. doi:10.1016/j.neuroimage.2017.01.005
2. Brighton LJ, Miller S, Farquhar M, et al. Holistic services for people with advanced disease and chronic breathlessness: A systematic review and meta-analysis. *Thorax.* 2018;74(3):270–281. doi:10.1136/thoraxjnl-2018-211589
3. Ambrosino N, Fracchia C. Strategies to relieve dyspnoea in patients with advanced chronic respiratory diseases. A narrative review. *Pulmonology.* 2019;25(5):289–298. doi:10.1016/j.pulmoe.2019.04.002
4. Pisani L, Hill NS, Pacilli AMG, Polastri M, Nava S. Management of dyspnea in the terminally ill. *Chest.* 2018;154(4):925–934. doi:10.1016/j.chest.2018.04.003
5. Saunders C. A personal therapeutic journey. *Br Med J.* 1996;313(7072):1599–1601. doi:10.1136/bmj.313.7072.1599
6. Parshall MB, Schwartzstein RM, Adams L, et al. An official American Thoracic Society statement: Update on the mechanisms, assessment, and management of dyspnea. *Am J Respir Crit Care Med.* 2012;185(4):435–452. doi:10.1164/rccm.201111-2042ST
7. Bausewein C, Schunk M, Schumacher P, Dittmer J, Bolzani A, Booth S. Breathlessness services as a new model of support for patients with respiratory disease. *Chron Respir Dis.* 2018;15(1):48–59. doi:10.1177/1479972317721557
8. Booth S, Chin C, Spathis A. The brain and breathlessness: Understanding and disseminating a palliative care approach. *Palliat Med.* 2015;29(5):396–398. doi:10.1177/0269216315579836
9. Chowienczyk S, Javadzadeh S, Booth S, Farquhar M. Association of descriptors of breathlessness with diagnosis and self-reported severity of breathlessness in patients with advanced chronic obstructive pulmonary disease or cancer. *J Pain Symptom Manage.* 2016;52(2):259–264. doi:10.1016/j.jpainsymman.2016.01.014
10. Herigstad M, Hayen A, Evans E, et al. Dyspnea-related cues engage the prefrontal cortex: Evidence from functional brain imaging in COPD. *Chest.* 2015;148(4):953–961. doi:10.1378/chest.15-0416
11. Marlow LL, Faull OK, Finnegan SL, Pattinson KTS. Breathlessness and the brain: The role of expectation. *Curr Opin Support Palliat Care.* 2019;13(3):200–210. doi:10.1097/SPC.0000000000000441
12. Guirimand F, Sahut d'Izarn M, Laporte L, Francillard M, Richard J-F, Aegerter P. Sequential occurrence of dyspnea at the end of life in palliative care, according to the underlying cancer. *Cancer Med.* 2015;4(4):532–539. doi:10.1002/cam4.419
13. McKenzie E, Hwang MK, Chan S, et al. Predictors of dyspnea in patients with advanced cancer. *Ann Palliat Med.* 2018;7(4):427–436. doi:10.21037/apm.2018.06.09
14. Pattinson K. Functional brain imaging in respiratory medicine. *Thorax.* 2015;70(6):598–600. doi:10.1136/thoraxjnl-2014-206688
15. Currow DC, Plummer JL, Crockett A, Abernethy AP. A community population survey of prevalence and severity of dyspnea in adults. *J Pain Symptom Manage.* 2009;38(4):533–545. doi:10.1016/j.jpainsymman.2009.01.006
16. Johnson MJ, Yorke J, Hansen-Flaschen J, et al. Towards an expert consensus to delineate a clinical syndrome of chronic breathlessness. *Eur Respir J.* 2017;49(5):1602277 doi:10.1183/13993003.02277-2016
17. von Winckelmann K, Renier W, Thompson M, Buntinx F. The frequency and outcome of acute dyspnoea in primary care: An observational study. *Eur J Gen Pract.* 2016;22(4):240–246. doi:10.1080/13814788.2016.1213809
18. Carette H, Zysman M, Morelot-Panzini C, et al. Prevalence and management of chronic breathlessness in COPD in a tertiary care center. *BMC Pulm Med.* 2019;19(1):1–7. doi:10.1186/s12890-019-0851-5
19. Müllerová H, Lu C, Li H, Tabberer M. Prevalence and burden of breathlessness in patients with chronic obstructive pulmonary disease managed in primary care. *PLoS One.* 2014;9(1):70–80. doi:10.1371/journal.pone.0085540
20. Sung JH, Brown MC, Perez-Cosio A, et al. Acceptability and accuracy of patient-reported outcome measures (proms) for surveillance of breathlessness in routine lung cancer care: A mixed-method study. *Lung Cancer.* 2020;147:1–11. doi:10.1016/j.lungcan.2020.06.028. Epub 2020 Jun 24. PMID: 32634651.
21. Hendriks SA, Smalbrugge M, Galindo-Garre F, Hertogh CMPM, van der Steen JT. From admission to death: Prevalence and course of pain, agitation, and shortness of breath, and treatment of these symptoms in nursing home residents with dementia. *J Am Med Dir Assoc.* 2015;16(6):475–481. doi:10.1016/j.jamda.2014.12.016
22. Ekström M, Schiöler L, Grønseth R, et al. Absolute values of lung function explain the sex difference in breathlessness in the general population. *Eur Respir J.* 2017;49(5):1–9. doi:10.1183/13993003.02047-2016
23. Wysham NG, Miriovsky BJ, Currow DC, et al. Practical dyspnea assessment: Relationship between the 0-10 numerical rating scale and the four-level categorical verbal descriptor scale of dyspnea intensity. *J Pain Symptom Manage.* 2015;50(4):480–487. doi:10.1016/j.jpainsymman.2015.04.015
24. Kochovska S, Chang S, Morgan DD, et al. Activities forgone because of chronic breathlessness: A cross-sectional population prevalence study. *Palliat Med Rep.* 2020;1:166–170. doi:10.1089/pmr.2020.0083
25. Hutchinson A, Barclay-Klingle N, Galvin K, Johnson MJ. Living with breathlessness: A systematic literature review and qualitative synthesis. *Eur Respir J.* 2018;51(2):1701477. doi:10.1183/13993003.01477-2017
26. Gysels MH, Higginson IJ. The lived experience of breathlessness and its implications for care: A qualitative comparison in cancer, COPD, heart failure and MND. *BMC Palliat Care.* 2011;10:q15 doi:10.1186/1472-684X-10-15
27. Currow DC, Smith J, Davidson PM, Newton PJ, Agar MR, Abernethy AP. Do the trajectories of dyspnea differ in prevalence and intensity by diagnosis at the end of life? A consecutive cohort study. *J Pain Symptom Manage.* 2010;39(4):680–690. doi:10.1016/j.jpainsymman.2009.09.017

28. McKenzie E, Zhang L, Chan S, et al. Symptom correlates of dyspnea in advanced cancer patients using the Edmonton symptom assessment system. *Support Care Cancer.* 2020;28(1):87–98. doi:10.1007/s00520-019-04787-0

29. O'Donnell DE, James MD, Milne KM, Neder JA. The pathophysiology of dyspnea and exercise intolerance in chronic obstructive pulmonary disease. *Clin Chest Med.* 2019;40(2):343–366. doi:10.1016/j.ccm.2019.02.007

30. Chan K, Tse DMW, Sham MMK, Thorsen AB. Palliative medicine in malignant respiratory diseases. In: Hanks G, Fallon M, Cherny NI, Christakis NA, Portenoy RK, Kaasa S, eds. *Oxford Textbook of Palliative Medicine.* 4th ed. New York: Oxford University Press; 2010:1107–1144.

31. Moosavi SH, Golestanian E, Binks AP, Lansing RW, Banzett RB. Hypoxic and hypercapnic drives to breathe generate equivalent levels of air hunger in humans. *J Appl Physiol.* 2003;94:141–154. doi:10.1152/japplphysiol

32. Kako J, Kobayashi M, Oosono Y, Kajiwara K, Miyashita M. Immediate effect of fan therapy in terminal cancer with dyspnea at rest: A meta-analysis. *Am J Hosp Palliat Med.* 2020;37(4):294–299. doi:10.1177/1049909119873626

33. Swan F, Newey A, Bland M, et al. Airflow relieves chronic breathlessness in people with advanced disease: An exploratory systematic review and meta-analyses. *Palliat Med.* 2019;33(6):618–633. doi:10.1177/0269216319835393

34. Nishino T. Dyspnoea: Underlying mechanisms and treatment. *Br J Anaesth.* 2011;106(4):463–474. doi:10.1093/bja/aer040

35. Johnson M, Currow D. Opioids for breathlessness: A narrative review. *BMJ Support Palliat Care.* 2020;10(3):287–295. doi:10.1136/bmjspcare-2020-002314

36. Elliott-Button HL, Johnson MJ, Nwulu U, Clark J. Identification and assessment of breathlessness in clinical practice: A systematic review and narrative synthesis. *J Pain Symptom Manage.* 2020;59(3):724–733.e19. doi:10.1016/j.jpainsymman.2019.10.014

37. McCaffery M. *Nursing Practice Theories Related to Cognition, Bodily Pain, and Man-Environment Interactions.* Los Angeles: University of California at Los Angeles Press; 1968: 95.

38. Twycross RG. The assessment of pain in advanced cancer. *J Med Ethics.* 1978;4(3):112–116. doi:10.1136/jme.4.3.112

39. Borg G. Perceived exertion as an indicator of somatic stress. *Scand J Rehabil Med.* 1970;2(2):92–98.

40. Gift A. Validation of a vertical visual analogue scale as a measure of clinical dyspnea. *Rehabil Nurs.* 1989;14(6):323–325.

41. Gift, AG; Narsavage G. Validity of the numeric rating scale as a measure of dyspnea. *Am J Crit care.* 1998;7(3):200–204. doi:10.1002/j.2048-7940.1989.tb01129.x

42. Portenoy, RK; Thaler, HT; Kornblith AB, et al. The memorial symptom assessment scale: An instrument for the evaluation of symptom prevalence, characteristics and distress. *Eur J Cancer.* 1994;30A(9):1326–1336. doi:10.1016/0959-8049(94)90182-1

43. Bruera E, Kuehn N, Miller MJ, Selmser P, Macmillan K. The Edmonton Symptom Assessment System (ESAS): A simple method for the assessment of palliative care patients. *J Palliat Care.* 1991;7(2):6–9.

44. Yorke J, Moosavi SH, Shuldham C, Jones PW. Quantification of dyspnea using descriptors: Development and initial testing of the dyspnoea-12. *Thorax2.* 2010;65(1):21–26. doi:10.1136/thx.2009.11852

45. Tanaka K, Akechi T, Okuyama T, Nishiwaki Y Uchitomi Y. Development and validation of the cancer dyspnoea scale: A multidimensional, brief, self-rating scale. *Br J Cancer.* 2000;82(4):800–805. doi:10.1054/bjoc.1999.1002

46. Campbell ML, Kero KK, Templin TN. Mild, moderate, and severe intensity cut-points for the respiratory distress observation scale. *Heart Lung.* 2017;46(1):14–17. doi:10.1016/j.hrtlng.2016.06.008

47. Persichini R, Gay F, Schmidt M, et al. Diagnostic accuracy of respiratory distress observation scales as surrogates of dyspnea self-report in intensive care unit patients. *Anesthesiology.* 2015;123(4):830–837. doi:10.1097/ALN.0000000000000805

48. Stevens JP, Dechen T, Schwartzstein R, et al. Prevalence of dyspnea among hospitalized patients at the time of admission. *J Pain Symptom Manage.* 2018;56(1):15–22.e2. doi:10.1016/j.jpainsymman.2018.02.013

49. Strieder M, Pecherstorfer M, Kreye G. Symptomatic treatment of dyspnea in advanced cancer patients: A narrative review of the current literature. *Wien Med Wochenschr.* 2018;168(13–14):333–343. doi:10.1007/s10354-017-0600-4

50. Smallwood N, Currow D, Booth S, Spathis A, Irving L, Philip J. Differing approaches to managing the chronic breathlessness syndrome in advanced COPD: A multi-national survey of specialists. *COPD.* 2018;15(3):294–302. doi:10.1080/15412555.2018.1502264

51. Currow DC, Abernethy AP, Ko DN. The active identification and management of chronic refractory breathlessness is a human right. *Thorax.* 2014;69(4):393–394. doi:10.1136/thoraxjnl-2013-204701

52. Abdallah SJ, Wilkinson-Maitland C, Saad N, et al. Effect of morphine on breathlessness and exercise endurance in advanced COPD: A randomised crossover trial. *Eur Respir J.* 2017;50(4):1701235. doi:10.1183/13993003.01235-2017

53. Currow D, Louw S, McCloud P, et al. Regular, sustained-release morphine for chronic breathlessness: A multicentre, double-blind, randomised, placebo-controlled trial. *Thorax.* 2020;75(1):50–56. doi:10.1136/thoraxjnl-2019-213681

54. Ferreira DH, Ekström M, Sajkov D, Vandersman Z, Eckert DJ, Currow DC. Extended-release morphine for chronic breathlessness in pulmonary arterial hypertension: A randomized, double-blind, placebo-controlled, crossover study. *J Pain Symptom Manage.* 2018;56(4):483–492. doi:10.1016/j.jpainsymman.2018.07.010

55. Johnson M, Cockayne S, Currow D, et al. Oral modified release morphine for breathlessness in chronic heart failure: A randomized placebo- controlled trial. *ESC Heart Fail.* 2019;6:1149–1160. doi:10.1002/ehf2.12498

56. Barnes H, McDonald J, Smallwood N, Manser R. Opioids for the palliation of refractory breathlessness in adults with advanced disease and terminal illness. *Cochrane Database Syst Rev.* 2016;3(3):CD011008. Published 2016 Mar 31. doi:10.1002/14651858.CD011008.pub2

57. Ekström M, Bajwah S, Bland JM, Currow DC, Hussain J, Johnson MJ. One evidence base; three stories: Do opioids relieve chronic breathlessness? *Thorax.* 2018;73(1):88–90. doi:10.1136/thoraxjnl-2016-209868

58. Simon ST, Köskeroglu P, Gaertner J, Voltz R. Fentanyl for the relief of refractory breathlessness: A systematic review. *J Palliat Med.* 2013;46(6):874–886. doi:10.1016/j.jpainsymman.2013.02.019

59. Simon ST, Kloke M, Alt-Epping B, et al. Effendys: Fentanyl buccal tablet for the relief of episodic breathlessness in patients with advanced cancer: A multicenter, open-label, randomized, morphine-controlled, crossover, Phase II trial. *J Pain Symptom Manage.* 2016;52(5):617–625. doi:10.1016/j.jpainsymman.2016.05.023

60. Simon ST, Higginson IJ, Booth S, Harding R, Weingärtner V, Bausewein C. Benzodiazepines for the relief of breathlessness in advanced malignant and non-malignant diseases in adults. *Cochrane Database Syst Rev.* 2016;10(10):CD007354. doi:10.1002/14651858.CD007354.pub3

61. Ekström M, Ahmadi Z, Bornefalk-Hermansson A, Abernethy A, Currow D. Oxygen for breathlessness in patients with chronic obstructive pulmonary disease who do not qualify for home oxygen therapy. *Cochrane Database Syst Rev.* 2016;11(11):CD006429 doi:10.1002/14651858.CD006429.pub3

62. Faverio P, De Giacomi F, Bonaiti G, et al. Management of chronic respiratory failure in interstitial lung diseases: Overview and clinical insights. *Int J Med Sci.* 2019;16(7):967–980. doi:10.7150/ijms.32752

63. Rochwerg B, Brochard L, Elliott MW, et al. Official ERS/ATS clinical practice guidelines: Noninvasive ventilation for acute respiratory failure. *Eur Respir J.* 2017;50(2):1602426. doi:10.1183/13993003.02426-2016

64. Koyauchi T, Hasegawa H, Kanata K, et al. Efficacy and tolerability of high-flow nasal cannula oxygen therapy for hypoxemic

respiratory failure in patients with interstitial lung disease with do-not-intubate orders: A retrospective single-center study. *Respiration.* 2018;96(4):323–329. doi:10.1159/000489890

65. Verberkt CA, van den Beuken-van Everdingen MHJ, Schols JMGA, et al. Respiratory adverse effects of opioids for breathlessness: A systematic review and meta-analysis. *Eur Respir J.* 2017;50(5):1701153. doi:10.1183/13993003.01153-2017

66. Ekström MP, Bornefalk-Hermansson A, Abernethy AP, Currow DC. Safety of benzodiazepines and opioids in very severe respiratory disease: National prospective study. *BMJ* 2014;348:g445. Published 2014 Jan 30. doi:10.1136/bmjg445

67. Currow DC, McDonald C, Oaten S, et al. Once-daily opioids for chronic dyspnea: A dose increment and pharmacolvigilance study. *J Pain Symptom Manage.* 2011;42(3):388–399. doi:10.1016/j.jpainsymman.2010.11.021

68. Tanaka M, Maeba H, Senoo T, et al. Efficacy of oxycodone for dyspnea in end-stage heart failure with renal insufficiency. *Intern Med.* 2018;57(1):53–57. doi:10.2169/internalmedicine.9216-17

69. Crombeen AM, Lilly EJ. Management of dyspnea in palliative care. *Curr Oncol.* 2020;27(3):142–145. doi:10.3747/co.27.6413

70. Afolabi TM, Nahata MC, Pai V. Nebulized opioids for the palliation of dyspnea in terminally ill patients. *Am J Health Syst Pharm.* 2017;74(14):1053–1061. doi:10.2146/ajhp150893

71. Boyden JY, Connor SR, Otolorin L, et al. Nebulized medications for the treatment of dyspnea: A literature review. *J Aerosol Med Pulm Drug Deliv.* 2015;28(1):1–19. doi:10.1089/jamp.2014.1136

72. Marciniuk DD, Goodridge D, Hernandez P, et al. Managing dyspnea in patients with advanced chronic obstructive pulmonary disease: A Canadian Thoracic Society clinical practice guideline. *Can Respir J.* 2011;18(2):69–78. doi:10.1155/2011/745047

73. Clemens KE, Klaschik E. Dyspnoea associated with anxiety—symptomatic therapy with opioids in combination with lorazepam and its effect on ventilation in palliative care patients. *Support Care Cancer.* 2011;19:2027–2033. doi:10.1007/s00520-010-1058-8

74. Navigante AH, Castro MA, Cerchietti LCC. Morphine versus midazolam as upfront therapy to control dyspnea perception in cancer patients while its underlying cause is sought or treated. *J Pain Symptom Manage.* 2010;39(5):820–830. doi:10.1016/j.jpainsymman.2009.10.003

75. Navigante AH, Cerchietti LCA, Castro MA, Lutteral MA, Cabalar ME. Midazolam as adjunct therapy to morphine in the alleviation of severe dyspnea perception in patients with advanced cancer. *J Pain Symptom Manage.* 2006;31(1):38–47. doi:10.1016/j.jpainsymman.2005.06.009

76. Vitacca M, Kaymaz D, Lanini B, et al. Non-invasive ventilation during cycle exercise training in patients with chronic respiratory failure on long-term ventilatory support: A randomized controlled trial. *Respirology.* 2018;23(2):182–189. doi:10.1111/resp.13181

77. Frost N, Ruwwe-Glösenkamp C, Raspe M, et al. Indwelling pleural catheters for non-malignant pleural effusions: Report on a single centre's 10 years of experience. *BMJ Open Respir Res.* 2020;7(1):1–5. doi:10.1136/bmjresp-2019-000501

78. Bausewein C, Booth S, Gysels M, Higginson IJ. Non-pharmacological interventions for breathlessness in advanced stages of malignant and non-malignant diseases. *Cochrane Database Syst Rev.* 2008;(2):CD005623. Published 2008 Apr 16. doi:10.1002/14651858.CD005623.pub2

79. Bittencourt HS, Cruz CG, David BC, et al. Addition of non-invasive ventilatory support to combined aerobic and resistance training improves dyspnea and quality of life in heart failure patients: A randomized controlled trial. *Clin Rehabil.* 2017;31(11):1508–1515. doi:10.1177/0269215517704269

80. Gysels M, Reilly CC, Jolley CJ, et al. Dignity through integrated symptom management: Lessons from the breathlessness support service. *J Pain Symptom Manage.* 2016;52(4):515–524. doi:10.1016/j.jpainsymman.2016.04.010

81. Prommer E. Midazolam: An essential palliative care drug. *Palliat Care Soc Pract.* 2020;14:1–12. doi:10.1177/2632352419895527

82. Waskiw-Ford M, Wu A, Mainra A, et al. Effect of inhaled nebulized furosemide (40 and 120 mg) on breathlessness during exercise in the presence of external thoracic restriction in healthy men. *Front Physiol.* 2018;9:86. doi:10.3389/fphys.2018.00086

83. Jeba J, George R, Pease N. Nebulised furosemide in the palliation of dyspnoea in cancer: A systematic review. *BMJ Support Palliat Care.* 2014;4(2):132–139. doi:10.1136/bmjspcare-2013-000492

84. Hui D, Kilgore K, Frisbee-Hume S, et al. Dexamethasone for dyspnea in cancer patients: A pilot double-blind, randomized, controlled trial. *J Pain Symptom Manage.* 2016;52(1):8–16.e1. doi:10.1016/j.jpainsymman.2015.10.023

85. Yennurajalingam S, Frisbee-Hume S, Palmer JL, et al. Reduction of cancer-related fatigue with dexamethasone: A double-blind, randomized, placebo-controlled trial in patients with advanced cancer. *J Clin Oncol.* 2013;31(25):3076–3082. doi:10.1200/JCO.2012.44.4661

86. Abernethy AP, McDonald CF, Frith PA, et al. Effect of palliative oxygen versus room air in relief of breathlessness in patients with refractory dyspnoea: A double-blind, randomised controlled trial. *Lancet.* 2010;376(9743):784–793. doi:10.1016/S0140-6736(10)61115-4

87. Visca D, Mori L, Tsipouri V, et al. Effect of ambulatory oxygen on quality of life for patients with fibrotic lung disease (AMBOX): A prospective, open-label, mixed-method, crossover randomised controlled trial. *Lancet Respir Med.* 2018;6(10):759–770. doi:10.1016/S2213-2600(18)30289-3

88. Asano R, Mathai SC, Macdonald PS, et al. Oxygen use in chronic heart failure to relieve breathlessness: A systematic review. *Heart Fail Rev.* 2020;25(2):195–205. doi:10.1007/s10741-019-09814-0

89. Johnson MJ, Clark AL. The mechanisms of breathlessness in heart failure as the basis of therapy. *Curr Opin Support Palliat Care.* 2016;10(1):32–35. doi:10.1097/SPC.0000000000000181

90. Nakao YM, Ueshima K, Yasuno S, Sasayama S. Effects of nocturnal oxygen therapy in patients with chronic heart failure and central sleep apnea: CHF-HOT study. *Heart Vessels.* 2016;31(2):165–172. doi:10.1007/s00380-014-0592-6

91. Bell EC, Cox NS, Goh N, et al. Oxygen therapy for interstitial lung disease: A systematic review. *Eur Respir Rev.* 2017;26(143):1–7. doi:10.1183/16000617.0080-2016

92. Diaz De Teran T, Barbagelata E, Cilloniz C, et al. Non-invasive ventilation in palliative care: A systematic review. *Minerva Med.* 2019;110(6):555–563. doi:10.23736/S0026-4806.19.06273-6

93. Stefan MS, Priya A, Pekow PS, et al. The comparative effectiveness of noninvasive and invasive ventilation in patients with pneumonia. *J Crit Care.* 2018;43:190–196. doi:10.1016/j.jcrc.2017.05.023

94. Roca O, Pérez-Terán P, Masclans JR, et al. Patients with New York Heart Association class III heart failure may benefit with high flow nasal cannula supportive therapy: High flow nasal cannula in heart failure. *J Crit Care.* 2013;28(5):741–746. doi:10.1016/j.jcrc.2013.02.007

95. Sklar MC, Dres M, Rittayamai N, et al. High-flow nasal oxygen versus noninvasive ventilation in adult patients with cystic fibrosis: A randomized crossover physiological study. *Ann Intensive Care.* 2018;8(1):1–9. doi:10.1186/s13613-018-0432-4

96. Spoletini G, Alotaibi M, Blasi F, Hill NS. Heated humidified high-flow nasal oxygen in adults: Mechanisms of action and clinical implications. *Chest.* 2015;148(1):253–261. doi:10.1378/chest.14-2871

97. Narang M, Mohindra P, Mishra M, Regine W, Kwok Y. Radiation oncology emergencies. *Hematol Oncol Clin North Am.* 2020;34(1):279–292. doi:10.1016/j.hoc.2019.09.004

98. Fysh ETH, Waterer GW, Kendall PA, et al. Indwelling pleural catheters reduce inpatient days over pleurodesis for malignant pleural effusion. *Chest.* 2012;142(2):394–400. doi:10.1378/chest.11-2657

99. Akram MJ, Khalid U, Bakar MA, Ashraf MB, Butt FM, Khan F. Indications and clinical outcomes of fully covered self-expandable metallic tracheobronchial stents in patients with malignant airway diseases. *Expert Rev Respir Med.* 2020;14(11):1173–1181. doi:10.1080/17476348.2020.1796642

100. Grosu HB, Eapen GA, Morice RC, et al. Stents are associated with increased risk of respiratory infections in patients undergoing airway interventions for malignant airways disease. *Chest.* 2013;144(2):441–449. doi:10.1378/chest.12-1721

101. Polkey MI, Qiu ZH, Zhou L, et al. Tai chi and pulmonary rehabilitation compared for treatment-naive patients with COPD: A randomized controlled trial. *Chest.* 2018;153(5):1116–1124. doi:10.1016/j.chest.2018.01.053

102. McCarthy B, Casey D, Devane D, Murphy K, Murphy E, Lacasse Y. Pulmonary rehabilitation for chronic obstructive pulmonary disease. *Cochrane Database Syst Rev.* 2015;CD003793. Published 2015 Feb 23. doi:10.1002/14651858.CD003793.pub3

103. Gloeckl R, Andrianopoulos V, Stegemann A, et al. High-pressure non-invasive ventilation during exercise in COPD patients with chronic hypercapnic respiratory failure: A randomized, controlled, cross-over trial. *Respirology.* 2019;24(3):254–261. doi:10.1111/resp.13399

104. Adamopoulos S, Schmid JP, Dendale P, et al. Combined aerobic/inspiratory muscle training vs. Aerobic training in patients with chronic heart failure: The vent-heft trial: A European prospective multicentre randomized trial. *Eur J Heart Fail.* 2014;16(5):574–582. doi:10.1002/ejhf.70

105. Wu J, Kuang L, Fu L. Effects of inspiratory muscle training in chronic heart failure patients: A systematic review and meta-analysis. *Congenit Heart Dis.* 2018;13(2):194–202. doi:10.1111/chd.12586

106. Tonelli R, Cocconcelli E, Lanini B, et al. Effectiveness of pulmonary rehabilitation in patients with interstitial lung disease of different etiology: A multicenter prospective study. *BMC Pulm Med.* 2017;17(1):1–9. doi:10.1186/s12890-017-0476-5

107. Cavalheri V, Granger CL. Exercise training as part of lung cancer therapy. *Respirology.* 2020;25(Suppl 2):80–87. doi:10.1111/resp.13869

108. Rueda JR, Solà, Pascual A, Casacuberta MS. Non-invasive interventions for improving well-being and quality of life in patients with lung cancer. *Cochrane Database Syst Rev.* 2011:CD004282. Published 2011 Sep 7. doi:10.1002/14651858.CD004282.pub3.

109. Steindal SA, Torheim H, Oksholm T, et al. Effectiveness of nursing interventions for breathlessness in people with chronic obstructive pulmonary disease: A systematic review and meta-analysis. *J Adv Nurs.* 2019;75(5):927–945. doi:10.1111/Jan.13902

110. Doyle C, Bhar S, Fearn M, et al. The impact of telephone-delivered cognitive behaviour therapy and befriending on mood disorders in people with chronic obstructive pulmonary disease: A randomized controlled trial. *Br J Health Psychol.* 2017;22(3):542–556. doi:10.1111/bjhp.12245

111. Nguyen HQ, Donesky D, Reinke LF, et al. Internet-based dyspnea self-management support for patients with chronic obstructive pulmonary disease. *J Pain Symptom Manage.* 2013;46(1):43–55. doi:10.1016/j.jpainsymman.2012.06.015

112. Higginson IJ, Bausewein C, Reilly CC, et al. An integrated palliative and respiratory care service for patients with advanced disease and refractory breathlessness: A randomised controlled trial. *Lancet Respir Med.* 2014;2(12):979–987. doi:10.1016/S2213-2600(14)70226-7

113. Kako J, Morita T, Yamaguchi T, et al. Fan therapy is effective in relieving dyspnea in patients with terminally ill cancer: A parallel-arm, randomized controlled trial. *J Pain Symptom Manage.* 2018;56(4):493–500. doi:10.1016/j.jpainsymman.2018.07.001

114. von Trott P, Oei SL, Ramsenthaler C. Acupuncture for breathlessness in advanced diseases: A systematic review and meta-analysis. *J Pain Symptom Manage.* 2020;59(2):327–338.e3. doi:10.1016/j.jpainsymman.2019.09.007

115. Doğan N, Taşcı S. The effects of acupressure on quality of life and dyspnea in lung cancer: A randomized, controlled trial. *Altern Ther Health Med.* 2020;26(1):49–56.

116. Morice AH, Millqvist E, Bieksiene K, et al. ERS guidelines on the diagnosis and treatment of chronic cough in adults and children. *Eur Respir J.* 2020;55(1):1–20. doi:10.1183/13993003.01136-2019

117. Molassiotis A, Smith JA, Mazzone P, et al. Symptomatic treatment of cough among adult patients with lung cancer: Chest guideline and expert panel report. *Chest.* 2017;151(4):861–874. doi:10.1016/j.chest.2016.12.028

118. Kardos P, Dinh QT, Fuchs KH, et al. German respiratory society guidelines for diagnosis and treatment of adults suffering from acute, subacute and chronic cough. *Respir Med.* 2020;170:105939. doi:10.1016/j.rmed.2020.105939

119. Song WJ, Chang YS, Faruqi S, et al. The global epidemiology of chronic cough in adults: A systematic review and meta-analysis. *Eur Respir J.* 2015;45(5):1479–1481. doi:10.1183/09031936.00218714

120. Wee B, Browning J, Adams A, et al. Management of chronic cough in patients receiving palliative care: Review of evidence and recommendations by a task group of the Association for Palliative Medicine of Great Britain and Ireland. *Palliat Med.* 2012;26(6):780–787. doi:10.1177/0269216311423793

121. Lai K, Shen H, Zhou X, et al. Clinical practice guidelines for diagnosis and management of cough: Chinese Thoracic Society (CTS) asthma consortium. *J Thorac Dis.* 2018;10(11):6314–6351. doi:10.21037/jtd.2018.09.153

122. Rhee CK, Jung JY, Lee SW, et al. The Korean cough guideline: Recommendation and summary statement. *Tuberc Respir Dis (Seoul).* 2016;79(1):14–21. doi:10.4046/trd.2016.79.1.14

123. Gibson P, Wang G, McGarvey L, Vertigan AE, Altman KW, Birring SS. Treatment of unexplained chronic cough: Chest guideline and expert panel report. *Chest.* 2016;149(1):27–44. doi:10.1378/chest.15-1496. Epub 2016 Jan 6. PMID: 26426314; PMCID: PMC5831652.

124. Canning BJ, Chang AB, Bolser DC, Smith JA, Mazzone SB, McGarvey L. Anatomy and neurophysiology of cough: Chest guideline and expert panel report. *Chest.* 2014;146(6):1633–1648. doi:10.1378/chest.14-1481

125. Achilleos A. Evidence-based evaluation and management of chronic cough. *Med Clin North Am.* 2016;100(5):1033–1045. doi:10.1016/j.mcna.2016.04.008

126. Polverino M, Polverino F, Fasolino M, Andò F, Alfieri A, De Blasio F. Anatomy and neuro-pathophysiology of the cough reflex arc. *Multidiscip Respir Med.* 2012;7(1):5. doi:10.1186/2049-6958-7-5

127. Spanevello A, Beghé B, Visca D, Fabbri LM, Papi A. Chronic cough in adults. *Eur J Intern Med.* 2020;78:8–16 doi:10.1016/j.ejim.2020.03.018

128. Song WJ, Morice AH. Cough hypersensitivity syndrome: A few more steps forward. *Allergy, Asthma Immunol Res.* 2017;9(5):394–402. doi:10.4168/aair.2017.9.5.394

129. Madison JM, Irwin RS. Chronic cough and COPD. *Chest.* 2020;157(6):1399–1400. doi:10.1016/j.chest.2020.02.012

130. Sesoko S, Kaneko Y. Cough associated with the use of captopril. *Arch Intern Med.* 1985;145(8):1524. doi:10.1001/archinte.1985.00360080206033

131. Yılmaz İ. Angiotensin-converting enzyme inhibitors induce cough. *Turkish Thorac J.* 2019;20(1):36–42. doi:10.5152/TurkThoracJ.2018.18014

132. von Gunten C, Buckholz G. In: Bruera, E. ed. Palliative care: Overview of cough, stridor, and hemoptysis. UpToDate. Waltham, MA: Uptodate. Updated July 2, 2021. https://www.uptodate.com/contents/palliative-care-overview-of-cough-stridor-and-hemoptysis

133. Ebihara S, Sekiya H, Miyagi M, Ebihara T, Okazaki T. Dysphagia, dystussia, and aspiration pneumonia in elderly people. *J Thoracic Dis.* 2016;8(9):632–639. doi:10.21037/jtd.2016.02.60

134. Ebihara T, Gui P, Ooyama C, Kozaki K, Ebihara S. Cough reflex sensitivity and urge-to-cough deterioration in dementia with Lewy bodies. *ERJ Open Res.* 2020;6(1):00108–02019. doi:10.1183/23120541.00108-2019

135. Benditt JO, Boitano LJ. Pulmonary issues in patients with chronic neuromuscular disease. *Am J Respir Crit Care Med.* 2013;187(10):1046–1055. doi:10.1164/rccm.201210-1804CI

136. Troche MS, Brandimore AE, Okun MS, Davenport PW, Hegland KW. Decreased cough sensitivity and aspiration in Parkinson disease. *Chest.* 2014;146(5):1294–1299. doi:10.1378/chest.14-0066

137. Harle A, Molassiotis A, Buffin O, et al. A cross sectional study to determine the prevalence of cough and its impact in patients with lung cancer: A patient unmet need. *BMC Cancer.* 2020;20(1):1–8. doi:10.1186/s12885-019-6451-1

138. Rossi E, Schinzari G, Tortora G. Pneumonitis from immune checkpoint inhibitors and covid-19: Current concern in cancer treatment. *J Immunother Cancer.* 2020;8(2):8–10. doi:10.1136/jitc-2020-000952

139. Michaudet C, Malaty J. Chronic cough: Evaluation and management. *Am Fam Physician.* 2017;96(9):575–580. doi:10.1111/j.1745-7599.2002.tb00123.x

140. Birring SS, Prudon B, Carr AJ, Singh SJ, Morgan L, Pavord ID. Development of a symptom specific health status measure for patients with chronic cough: Leicester Cough Questionnaire (LCQ). *Thorax.* 2003;58(4):339–343. doi:10.1136/thorax.58.4.339

141. French CT, Irwin RS, Fletcher KE, Adams TM. Evaluation of a cough-specific quality-of-life questionnaire. *Chest.* 2002;121(4):1123–1131. doi:10.1378/chest.121.4.1123

142. Schmit KM, Coeytaux RR, Goode AP, et al. Evaluating cough assessment tools: A systematic review. *Chest.* 2013;144(6):1819–1826. doi:10.1378/chest.13-0310

143. Jalil AAA, Katzka DA, Castell DO. Approach to the patient with dysphagia. *Am J Med.* 2015;128(10):1138.e17–23. doi:10.1016/j.amjmed.2015.04.026

144. Malesker MA, Callahan-Lyon P, Ireland B, Irwin RS, Chest Expert Cough Panel. Pharmacologic and nonpharmacologic treatment for acute cough associated with the common cold: Chest Expert Panel report. *Chest.* 2017;152(5):1021–1037. doi:10.1016/j.chest.2017.08.009

145. Speich B, Thomer A, Aghlmandi S, Ewald H, Zeller A, Hemkens LG. Treatments for subacute cough in primary care: Systematic review and meta-analyses of randomised clinical trials. *Br J Gen Pract.* 2018;68(675):e694–e702. doi:10.3399/bjgp18X698885

146. Song WJ, Chung KF. Pharmacotherapeutic options for chronic refractory cough. *Expert Opin Pharmacother.* 2020;21(11):1345–1358. doi:10.1080/14656566.2020.1751816

147. Harle ASM, Blackhall FH, Smith JA, Molassiotis A. Understanding cough and its management in lung cancer. *Curr Opin Support Palliat Care.* 2012;6(2):153–162. doi:10.1097/SPC.0b013e328352b6a5

148. Albrecht HH, Dicpinigaitis PV, Guenin EP. Role of guaifenesin in the management of chronic bronchitis and upper respiratory tract infections. *Multidiscip Respir Med.* 2017;12(1):1–11. doi:10.1186/s40248-017-0113-4

149. Bausewein C, Simon ST. Shortness of breath and cough in patients in palliative care. *Dtsch Arztebl Int.* 2013;110(33–34):563–572. doi:10.3238/arztebl.2013.0563

150. Morice AH, Shanks G. Pharmacology of cough in palliative care. *Curr Opin Support Palliat Care.* 2017;11(3):147–151. doi:10.1097/SPC.0000000000000279

151. Morice A, Kardos P. Comprehensive evidence-based review on European antitussives. *BMJ Open Respir Res.* 2016;3(1):1–8. doi:10.1136/bmjresp-2016-000137

152. Lim KG, Rank MA, Hahn PY, Keogh KA, Morgenthaler TI, Olson EJ. Long-term safety of nebulized lidocaine for adults with difficult-to-control chronic cough: A case series. *Chest.* 2013;143(4):1060–1065. doi:10.1378/chest.12-1533

153. Tan W, Li S, Liu X, et al. Prophylactic intravenous lidocaine at different doses for fentanyl-induced cough (FIC): A meta-analysis. *Sci Rep.* 2018;8(1):1–8. doi:10.1038/s41598-018-27457-3

154. Morice AH, Menon MS, Mulrennan SA, et al. Opiate therapy in chronic cough. *Am J Respir Crit Care Med.* 2007;175(4):312–315. doi:10.1164/rccm.200607-892OC

155. Al-Sheklly B, Mitchell J, Issa B, et al. S35 randomised control trial quantifying the efficacy of low dose morphine in a responder group of patients with refractory chronic cough. *Thorax.* 2017; 72:A24.2–A25. doi:10.1136/thoraxjnl-2017-210983.41

156. An HJ, Kim I-K, Lee JE, Kang Y-J, Kim CH, Kim H-K. Nebulized morphine for intractable cough in advanced cancer: Two case reports. *J Palliat Med.* 2015;18(3):278–281. doi:10.1089/jpm.2014.0126

157. Food and Drug Administration. Hycodan. Prescribing information. Revised June 2018. Available at https://www.accessdata.fda.gov/drugsatfda_docs/label/2018/005213s039lbl.pdf

158. Homsi J, Walsh D, Nelson KA, et al. A phase II study of hydrocodone for cough in advanced cancer. *Am J Hosp Palliat Care.* 2002;19(1):49–56. doi:10.1177/104990910201900110

159. Lee SE, Lee JH, Kim HJ, et al. Inhaled corticosteroids and placebo treatment effects in adult patients with cough: A systematic review and meta-analysis. *Allergy, Asthma Immunol Res.* 2019;11(6):856–870. doi:10.4168/aair.2019.11.6.856

160. Truesdale K, Jurdi A. Nebulized lidocaine in the treatment of intractable cough. *Am J Hosp Palliat Care.* 2013;30(6):587–589. doi:10.1177/1049909112458577

161. Slaton RM, Thomas RH, Mbathi JW. Evidence for therapeutic uses of nebulized lidocaine in the treatment of intractable cough and asthma. *Ann Pharmacother.* 2013;47(4):578–585. doi:10.1345/aph.1R573

162. Shuying L, Ping L, Juan N, Dong L. Different interventions in preventing opioid-induced cough: A meta-analysis. *J Clin Anesth.* 2016;34:440–447. doi:10.1016/j.jclinane.2016.05.034

163. Bishop-Freeman SC, Shonsey EM, Friederich LW, Beuhler MC, Winecker RE. Benzonatate toxicity: Nothing to cough at. *J Anal Toxicol.* 2017;41(5):461–463. doi:10.1093/jat/bkx021

164. Bowen AJ, Nowacki AS, Contrera K, et al. Short- and long-term effects of neuromodulators for unexplained chronic cough. *Otolaryngol—Head Neck Surg.* 2018;159(3):508–515. doi:10.1177/0194599818768517

165. Shi G, Shen Q, Zhang C, Ma J, Mohammed A, Zhao H. Efficacy and safety of gabapentin in the treatment of chronic cough: A systematic review. *Tuberc Respir Dis (Seoul).* 2018;81(3):167–174. doi:10.4046/trd.2017.0089

166. Dong R, Xu X, Yu L, et al. Randomised clinical trial: Gabapentin vs baclofen in the treatment of suspected refractory gastro-oesophageal reflux-induced chronic cough. *Aliment Pharmacol Ther.* 2019;49(6):714–722. doi:10.1111/apt.15169

167. Wu H, Hu W, Tan G. Efficacy and safety of prophylactic intravenous dexmedetomidine on opioid-induced cough: A systematic review and meta-analysis. *Int J Clin Exp Med.* 2016;9(5):7655–7667

168. Arslan Z, Çalık ES, Kaplan B, Ahiskalioglu EO. The effect of pheniramine on fentanyl-induced cough: A randomized, double blinded, placebo controlled clinical study. *Brazilian J Anesthesiol.* 2016;66(4):383–387. doi:10.1016/j.bjane.2014.11.018

169. Spinou A. Non-pharmacological techniques for the extremes of the cough spectrum. *Respir Physiol Neurobiol.* 2018;257:5–11. doi:10.1016/j.resp.2018.03.006

170. Chamberlain Mitchell SAF, Ellis J, Ludlow S, Pandyan A, Birring SS. Non-pharmacological interventions for chronic cough: The past, present and future. *Pulm Pharmacol Ther.* 2019;56(Jun):29–38. doi:10.1016/j.pupt.2019.02.006

171. Slinger C, Mehdi SB, Milan SJ, et al. Speech and language therapy for management of chronic cough. *Cochrane Database Syst Rev.* 2019;7(7):CD013067. Published 2019 Jul 23. doi:10.1002/14651858.CD013067.pub2

172. Yorke J, Lloyd-Williams M, Smith J, et al. Management of the respiratory distress symptom cluster in lung cancer: A randomised controlled feasibility trial. *Support Care Cancer.* 2015;23(11):3373–3384. doi:10.1007/s00520-015-2810-x

173. Vertigan AE, Kapela SL, Ryan NM, Birring SS, McElduff P, Gibson PG. Pregabalin and speech pathology combination therapy for refractory chronic cough: A randomized controlled trial. *Chest.* 2016;149(3):639–648. doi:10.1378/chest.15-1271

174. Al-Sheklly B, Satia I, Badri H, et al. Chronic cough: Are we integrating non-pharmacological therapies into treatment plans? *Eur Respir J.* 2017;50(Suppl 61):PA717. doi:10.1183/1393003.congress-2017.PA717

175. Auger C, Hernando V, Galmiche H. Use of mechanical insufflation-exsufflation devices for airway clearance in subjects with neuromuscular disease. *Respir Care.* 2017;62(2):236–245. doi:10.4187/respcare.04877

176. Rose L, Adhikari NK, Leasa D, Fergusson DA, McKim D. Cough augmentation techniques for extubation or weaning critically ill patients from mechanical ventilation. *Cochrane Database Syst Rev.* 2017;1(1):CD011833. Published 2017 Jan 11. doi:10.1002/14651858.CD011833.pub2

177. Lee AL, Burge AT, Holland AE. Airway clearance techniques for bronchiectasis. *Cochrane Database Syst Rev.* 2015;Nov(11):CD008351. Published 2015 Nov 23. doi:10.1002/14651858.CD008351.pub3

178. Troche MS, Rosenbek JC, Okun MS, Sapienza CM. Detraining outcomes with expiratory muscle strength training in Parkinson disease. *J Rehabil Res Dev.* 2014;51(2):305–310. doi:10.1682/JRRD.2013.05.0101

179. Rietberg MB, Veerbeek JM, Gosselink R, Kwakkel G, van Wegen EE. Respiratory muscle training for multiple sclerosis. *Cochrane Database Syst Rev.* 2017;12(12):CD009424. Published 2017 Dec 21. doi:10.1002/14651858.CD009424.pub2

180. Kulnik ST, Birring SS, Moxham J, Rafferty GF, Kalra L. Does respiratory muscle training improve cough flow in acute stroke? Pilot randomized controlled trial. *Stroke.* 2015;46(2):447–453. doi:10.1161/STROKEAHA.114.007110

181. Molassiotis A, Bailey C, Caress A, Tan J-Y. Interventions for cough in cancer. *Cochrane Database Syst Rev.* 2015;5(5):CD007881. doi:10.1002/14651858.CD007881.pub3

182. Lancaster T, Stead LF. Individual behavioural counselling for smoking cessation. *Cochrane Database Syst Rev.* 2017;3(3):CD001292. doi:10.1002/14651858.CD001292.pub3

183. Centers for Disease Control and Prevention. Tips from former smokers. How to Quit Smoking. Last reviewed: June 21, 2021 Available at https://www.cdc.gov/tobacco/campaign/tips/quit-smoking/index.html?s_cid=OSH_tips_GL0004&utm_source=google&utm_medium=cpc&utm_campaign=Quit+2020%3BS%3BWL%3BBR%3BIMM%3BDTC%3BCO&utm_content=Quit+Smoking+-+General_P&utm_term=quit+smoking&gclid=Cj0KCQjwxNT8BRD

184. Ellis J, Wagland R, Tishelman C, et al. Considerations in developing and delivering a nonpharmacological intervention for symptom management in lung cancer: The views of patients and informal caregivers. *J Pain Symptom Manage.* 2012;44(6):831–842. doi:10.1016/j.jpainsymman.2011.12.274

185. Malik FA, Gysels M, Higginson IJ. Living with breathlessness: A survey of caregivers of breathless patients with lung cancer or heart failure. *Palliat Med.* 2013;27(7):647–656. doi:10.1177/0269216313488812

45.

COGNITIVE IMPAIRMENT

Abraham A. Brody and Donna E. McCabe

KEY POINTS

- The palliative advanced practice registered nurse (APRN) must understand the multiple forms of cognitive impairment in order to optimize treatment of each specific form.

- The palliative APRN should perform a thorough assessment of unmet needs and use nonpharmacologic interventions as the first line of therapy for treating behavioral and psychological symptoms of dementia (BPSD) or developmental disability (DD) because pharmacologic interventions have limited efficacy.

- The APRN's prime focus of treatment should be maintaining physical activity and preventing functional decline.

- Advance care planning should occur early in the disease process, when the person living with dementia (PLWD) still has the ability to participate.

CASE STUDY

Diane was a 78-year-old African American woman admitted to the hospital following left-sided hemiparesis. Her history included hypertension, hyperlipidemia, two past minor strokes, bilateral knee osteoarthritis, and cognitive impairment, with a St. Louis University Mental Status Exam (SLUMS) score of 24/30 (1 year ago). Her medications included clopidogrel, atorvastatin, lisinopril, HCTZ, and amlodipine. According to her daughter Lisa, her primary caregiver, prior to this most recent stroke, Diane had been experiencing slow, progressive loss of short-term memory and physical function. She also became more socially isolated and spent much of the day inside with the shades drawn, and she had stopped smiling or eating as much. Lisa spent approximately 20 hours per week caring for her mother, who lived in their home. Lisa had two small children and a husband who was often out of town for work. Regarding care planning, Lisa stated that her mom had previously stated that when it is her time to go, she didn't want "extra measures," but wanted to be left comfortable and wanted to die at home. The advanced practice registered nurse (APRN) queried further and found that Diane would not want medically administered nutrition or hydration if she wasn't able to eat; however, if she had a simple infection, she wanted it treated.

On assessment, Diane was alert and oriented to person and place only and had a new SLUMS score of 14/30, as well as a positive screen for depression. Diane had 2/5 strength of her left leg and arm, and required a max 1 person assist to transfer. She became physically and verbally aggressive with any attempt to begin physical activity or when passive range-of-motion (ROM) exercises of the lower extremities were performed. Lisa appeared very stressed and scored a 20/26 on the Modified Caregiver Strain Index (MCSI). The computed tomography (CT) scan revealed a new focal hyperattenuation in the primary motor cortex on the right side of the brain (new stroke) and several old deep lesions, 10 mm in diameter, in the lacunar area of the brain consistent with prior CT (old lacunar infarcts). There was also overall moderate brain atrophy (consistent with Alzheimer's disease).

Based on this clinical picture, the APRN diagnosed Diane with mixed dementia and depression. After a discussion with Lisa, the APRN performed an assessment of unmet needs and found that Diane was depressed, had pain, and this had limited her physical exercise and caused aggressive behaviors when moved. The APRN initiated acetaminophen 1,000 mg three times daily for osteoarthritic knee pain. After the first dose of acetaminophen, she reassessed and found Diane was no longer physically or verbally aggressive with ROM exercises or transfer. She also found that Diane loved swing music, so started on a daily regimen of 1 hour of music as a therapy with active engagement (reminiscing and dancing) and started her on citalopram 5 mg daily PO for 1 week, then increased to 10 mg. The APRN ordered physical therapy (PT) and occupational therapy (OT) for post-stroke rehab. The APRN completed a physician order for life-sustaining treatment (POLST) for do-not-attempt-resuscitation (DNAR), limited interventions, and no medically administered nutrition and hydration, but antibiotics for infection. Diane was discharged home with home PT, OT, safety evaluation, and short-term home health aide services to assist the Lisa during the transition period. A follow-up appointment was made for 1 week, at which time there was a discussion of whether to start Diane on an acetylcholinesterase inhibitor and an N-methyl-D-aspartate (NMDA) receptor antagonist (memantine) as well as her long-term plan of care and trajectory. While Diane was not eligible for hospice, further palliative follow-up was recommended for symptomatic care. The APRN discussed the importance of self-care with Lisa. The social worker consulted with Lisa to continue psychoeducation on disease progression and to monitor and treat caregiver strain. Lisa was also referred to the local Alzheimer's Association chapter for caregiver training and support groups.

INTRODUCTION

Cognitive impairment, in its many forms, is a devastating illness that has significant effects on the individual with the impairment and his or her family and caregivers. The most common form of cognitive impairment is dementia, mainly Alzheimer's disease (AD), with an estimated 5.8 million people living with AD in 2019 in the United States.[1] As the population rises over the next 35 years, this number will increase to 13.8 million. Dementia is a heterogeneous illness; there are more than 25 known etiologies, the most common forms being Alzheimer's dementia (approximately 60% of cases), followed by vascular dementia, Lewy body dementia, and frontotemporal dementia (FTD). The remaining etiologies combined represent less than 1% of cases of dementia. Palliative advanced practice registered nurses (APRNs) will be caring for many people living with dementia (PLWD).

Regardless of the etiology, the cognitive symptoms and progression of dementia can alter how the person is perceived by others and endanger their personhood. The language used by clinicians can affect how a person is seem by others. The term "person living with dementia" reinforces personhood and is the preferred term, rather than "dementia patient." Similarly, while we will refer to behavioral and psychological symptoms of dementia (BPSD) herein from a clinical perspective, with the PLWD or family, these issues should be addressed under the rubric of "unmet needs" rather than BPSD or neuropsychiatric symptoms, to reduce stigma.

In addition to dementia, there are many other etiologies of cognitive impairment, the most common of which include Down syndrome, delirium, paraneoplastic syndrome, and neoplastic and benign tumors. While many of the principles provided will relate to forms of cognitive impairment other than dementia, particularly advance care planning and goals-of-care conversations, identification and management of symptoms, and caregiving, this chapter will primarily frame the conversation in terms of care for PLWD. This includes cognitive decline, as in persons with developmental disability (DD), particularly Down syndrome, because these individuals are highly likely to develop dementia in older age. Moreover, it is important to recognize that many individuals with serious illness will have a different primary serious illness, but their care will be complicated due to cognitive impairment. Therefore, this chapter is important even for those who primarily see cancer, heart failure, or renal populations, where the disease is often concomitant.

CLINICAL BACKGROUND AND DIFFERENTIAL DIAGNOSIS IN DEMENTIAS

Dementia is highly underdiagnosed. It estimated that approximately half of those with dementia and their caregivers are not aware of their diagnosis. Also, people with a known dementia are often diagnosed with just "dementia," not a specific form of the disease. The different types of dementia have different presentations, prognosis, disease progression, and, in some cases, appropriate therapies. The most common causes of dementia and cognitive impairment to be included in the differential are listed in Table 45.1. While the final diagnosis should be made by a trained geriatrician, neurologist, neuropsychologist, geriatric nurse practitioner, or interprofessional team at an Alzheimer's Disease Center, these resources are not always accessible. Often the primary care provider or inpatient care team may not have made the diagnosis, completed an assessment for the etiology of dementia, or even identified the symptoms of cognitive impairment. It therefore may become part of the palliative care team members' work to make the diagnosis and develop a working diagnosis of the etiology. In certain cases the palliative APRN may also need to ensure that a reversible cause of dementia has not been overlooked.

The assessment should begin by evaluating the person's level of cognitive function using an appropriate screening instrument. There are several valid and appropriate tests available. The Mini-Cog, a brief assessment for cognitive impairment that takes about 2 minutes to complete, can be a starting point[2] for cognitive assessment. It consists of a three-item registration, a clock drawing test, and a three-item recall. The Montreal Cognitive Assessment (MOCA) and the St. Louis University Mental Status Exam (SLUMS), which have good reliability and validity, are easy and quick to administer and are not biased toward education and socioeconomic status, as is the more traditionally used Mini Mental Status Exam (MMSE) (Table 45.2). As of September 2019, the MOCA requires training and certification for the user, making the SLUMS the most accessible test for evaluation if needed after the Mini-Cog.[3] An additional benefit of the MOCA and SLUMS tests are that they are sensitive for mild cognitive impairment.

While screening tools estimate the severity of dementia along a continuum from mild to severe, several rating scales exist to provide more accurate staging. The gold standard tool for staging, the Clinical Dementia Rating (CDR) scale, assesses domains of home life, community life, and personal care in addition to memory, orientation, and problem-solving.[4] The Quick Dementia Rating Scale (QDRS) is another valid and reliable tool, which, as the name suggests, is brief and takes less time than the CDR, approximately 3–5 minutes.[5] The cutoff scores for these tools are summarized in Table 45.2.

The palliative APRN should obtain a history. The PLWD or DD should participate to the degree they are able, along with the key informant for the PLWD. The history should include the length and progression of the cognitive impairment as well as the symptoms and their duration and severity. Information on the degree to which function has been impaired related to the cognitive impairment should be ascertained. This information will help determine the type of dementia and can also distinguish if the PLWD has delirium or depression superimposed on dementia. The syndromes of dementia, delirium, and depression, known as the "3Ds," can often coexist.

If the PLWD has sudden onset or clear and sudden worsening of an existing cognitive deficit over a short period, delirium should be strongly considered because dementia has a slower and more progressive course. One common cause of delirium is medication, so the person's medication list should

Table 45.1 DIFFERENTIAL DIAGNOSIS OF DEMENTIA

POTENTIALLY REVERSIBLE CAUSES OF DEMENTIA	COMMON DEMENTIAS	UNCOMMON DEMENTIAS
Depression	Alzheimer's disease	Alcoholic dementia
Infection	Vascular dementia	Huntington's disease
Anemia	Mixed dementia	Progressive supranuclear palsy
Hypothyroidism	Dementia with Lewy bodies	Multiple system atrophy
Syphilis	Parkinson's dementia	Corticobasal degeneration
B_{12} deficiency	Frontotemporal dementia	Hydrocephalus
Folate deficiency		AIDS dementia
Drugs (anticholinergic activity)		HSV encephalopathy
Tumors		Traumatic brain injury
Sensory issues (hearing/vision loss)		Prion diseases
Electrolyte disturbances, dehydration		Paraneoplastic syndrome
Increased intracranial pressure		Multiple sclerosis
Other metabolic disorders (hypo-/hyperglycemia, storage disorders)		Drug-induced
		Progressive multifocal leukoencephalopathy
		Subacute sclerosing panencephalitis
		Whipple's disease

be reviewed to rule out the etiology of cognition-reducing medications (e.g., anticholinergics, antipsychotics, opioids, antiepileptics, sedatives, anxiolytics). Other common causes of delirium in the seriously ill are infection (urinary tract infection and pneumonia in particular), recent surgery with or without anesthesia, dehydration, electrolyte imbalances, and encephalopathies caused by renal or liver failure or viral infections such as herpesvirus, which occur particularly in those who are immunocompromised.

Depression can be a symptom of, a prodrome to, or coexist with dementia. Major depressive disorder can mimic cognitive impairment and can lead to worsened cognitive function. Screening instruments such as the Geriatric Depression Scale 15 or PHQ-9 can be used in persons without cognitive impairment as well as in those with mild to moderate dementia. Persons who screen positive should then receive further evaluation for depressive disorders. Table 45.3 highlights major differences in the presentation of persons with major depression

Table 45.2 DEMENTIA SCREENING INSTRUMENT CUTOFF SCORES

	SLUMS	MOCA	MMSE	CDR	QDRS
Normal	27–30[a] 25–30[b]	27–30	28–30	0	0–1
Mild cognitive impairment	21–26[a] 20–24[b]		25–27	0.5–4.0 (questionable to very mild)	2–5
Mild dementia	15–19	18–26	19–24	4.5–9	6–12
Moderate dementia	11–14	10–17	10–18	9.5–15.5	13–20
Severe dementia	>11	>10	>10	16–18	20–30

[a]High school education.

[b]Less than high school education.

From Galvin.[5]

Table 45.3 PRESENTATION OF DEPRESSION VERSUS DEMENTIA

MAJOR DEPRESSION	DEMENTIA
Acute	Progressive
Oriented	Impaired orientation
Gives up easily	Tries hard even if incorrect
Fewer symptoms at night	Sundowning
Self-referred	Others refer
Diminished concentration ability	Short-term memory deficit
Normal language	Impaired language capabilities
Draws attention to memory problems	Minimized memory problems
Severely depressed	Minor or no depression
Blunted or flat affect	Full range of emotions
Apathy or anhedonia over weeks	Apathy or anhedonia gradual over time
Common suicidal thoughts	Rare suicidal thoughts
Guilt is common	Guilt is uncommon
Sudden sleep pattern/ability changes	Gradual sleep disturbance development
Major weight changes	Gradual weight loss over time

versus dementia. Depression also carries a strong risk for developing Alzheimer's dementia, and up to half of older adults with dementia have concomitant depression and dementia depending on the setting.[6] Thus, the two are not mutually exclusive and often need to be treated simultaneously.

Once a longer-standing cognitive impairment has been established based on the scores from screening instruments and informant and patient interviews, lab tests are performed to rule out potentially reversible causes of dementia (if they have not already been performed). Labs should include B_{12} and folate (deficiency), TSH (hypothyroidism), a complete blood count (severe anemia), and an RPR (syphilis) and HIV test can be considered based on the person's history. Assuming these tests are negative, the next step is to consider imaging based on symptom presentation. A head computed tomography (CT) scan without contrast can rule out tumors and hydrocephalus and examine whether any brain atrophy, white matter changes, or strokes have occurred.

A specialty positron emission tomography (PET) imaging technique using tracers such as florbetapir F-18 (Amyvid) has been approved by the US Food and Drug Administration (FDA); it shows the presence of amyloid plaques, a major cause of AD. However, the test is nondefinitive and does not add to certainty in diagnosis in most cases. Therefore, it should be ordered only by a dementia expert in certain highly specific circumstances where there is atypical presentation.[7] There are also now biomarkers of Alzheimer's dementia that can be used for preclinical symptom diagnosis through serum analysis. At this point, despite recent advances, these biomarkers, including amyloid-β accumulation levels, should only be used for research purposes.[8]

Once the appropriate tests are performed to rule out non-dementia causes of impairment and combined with the symptomatic presentation, a clinical diagnosis can be made. Table 45.4 summarizes the presenting symptoms of the five most common forms of dementia. Each is discussed in greater detail herein.

Table 45.4 DIFFERENTIATION OF MAJOR CAUSES OF DEMENTIA

ALZHEIMER'S	VASCULAR	MIXED	LEWY BODY	FRONTOTEMPORAL
Short-term memory loss	Impaired executive function	Includes symptoms of both Alzheimer's and vascular	Fluctuating cognition	Disinhibition
Forgetfulness	Motor deficits		Recurrent visual hallucinations	Expressive or receptive aphasia
Difficulty learning new tasks	Difficulty retrieving memories		Parkinsonian movement	Stubbornness
Poor attention	Aphasia		Rapid eye movement (REM) sleep disorder	Selfishness
Difficulty finding words	Inefficiency of thought		Sensitivity to neuroleptics	Facial recognition difficulty
Difficulty with complex tasks	Poor problem solving		Autonomic dysfunction	Emotional distance
Poor recognition			Systematic delusions	Apathy
			Repeated falls	

ALZHEIMER'S DISEASE

AD is characterized by a progressive loss of memory, beginning with short-term memory loss and leading to long-term memory loss, including the loss of decades of life memories. In addition to memory loss, there is at minimum an alteration in one other cognitive domain such as executive function or language that interferes with daily functioning. As AD progresses, the loss of activities of daily living (ADLs) and instrumental ADLs (IADLs) progresses, and eventually loss of speech and coordinated muscle movements, such as swallowing, occurs. The average life span following diagnosis is 8 years, and people usually spend the last 40% of that time in the moderate to severe stage.[1] Between 60% and 80% of all dementias diagnosed are of the Alzheimer's type, though up to 40% of people may have mixed etiology with vascular dementia (see the section on mixed dementia).[9] The disease is caused by a number of changes in the brain, including formation of amyloid plaques and tau tangles, leading to the damage and destruction of neurons, causing the brain to atrophy. While most individuals diagnosed with AD are older than 65, early-onset AD is thought to progress more quickly.[10]

Prior to the onset of AD, the individual can often develop mild cognitive impairment in the form of some memory problems and perhaps some movement difficulties and changes in smell. Not all people will advance from mild cognitive impairment to AD. Mild cognitive impairment is defined as short-term memory deficit and is largely stable over time; it does not affect functional status.

AD is generally divided into mild, moderate, and severe categories, and people will progress over time (https://www.alz.org/alzheimers-dementia/stages). In mild AD, the person will start to lose short-term memory, which can lead them to become confused in complex situations, such as with driving. They may become lost, have difficulty managing their financial affairs, ask repetitive questions, forget to turn off the stove after starting to cook a meal, and start to show some alteration in personality, particularly due to the frustration of declining memory. Many PLWD attempt to hide these deficits, and therefore it is often a family member or friend who will make sure that the deficits are brought to the attention of a medical provider. The mild Alzheimer's stage is where these deficits become clear enough for family to recognize and is therefore where the majority of cases are diagnosed. The median time spent in the mild stage is 3.6–5 years, with those older at the shorter end of the spectrum and younger at the longer end.[10]

The moderate or middle-stage of AD can last for many years. In this stage, PLWD begin losing the ability to learn new tasks or pieces of information, may no longer recognize family and friends, begin to have difficulty performing complex ADLs such as dressing, and start to have significant impairment in executive function. Assessment of function and interventions to simplify tasks are useful at this stage. PLWD will start to lose more long-term memory, such as where they went to school, what year they are living in, and the fact that they have grandchildren or that their adult children are married. They cannot compare situations and therefore cannot make decisions about most future care (e.g., advance directives). They can no longer live safely and independently in the community and therefore require help with ADLs and IADLs. Many PLWD may develop significant behavioral problems at this stage, although they are generally manageable with appropriate interventions (see later sections). The behavioral and mood problems include agitation, depression, and aggression. Some individuals may develop delusions or hallucinations, though these are more common in Lewy body dementia. Caregiver strain can also become prominent at this stage.

Severe AD is characterized by complete loss of ability to communicate needs and dependence in all ADLs. PLWD in this stage may be able to string together a few words, but the words are not generally meaningful, and they will eventually lose speech altogether. In this stage, the PLWD can also often also develop difficulty with swallowing because they can no longer coordinate movement. Aspiration pneumonias may become frequent and are often a cause of death. People generally enter the severe stage 6 years from diagnosis, depending on the study cited, and the stage generally lasts 1–2 years.[11] The median survival time is approximately 8 years from diagnosis, although the older the person was at diagnosis, the shorter the life span. Men are likely to die sooner than women. Race and ethnicity have been also been found to influence survival time due to multiple factors including differences in medical comorbidities as well as social support after diagnosis.[12]

VASCULAR DEMENTIA

Vascular dementia is caused by ischemic or hemorrhagic damage to the brain, primarily through stroke. It is the second most common form of dementia after AD, accounting for approximately 10–15% of all dementias[13] (excluding mixed dementia). Risk factors for dementia are cerebrovascular in nature (Box 45.1).[14] Unlike in AD, progression is variable and highly dependent upon cardiovascular status and risk for future stroke. Therefore, mortality is also highly variable and difficult to determine, although in general the survival is shorter than in Alzheimer's dementia.

Symptoms of vascular dementia are highly variable and may be sudden or gradual depending on the size and location of the stroke. Early symptoms include impaired executive function, ineffective memory, perseveration, changes in personality, poor verbal fluency, sleep disturbances, and cortical symptoms such as visual disturbances and difficulty doing mathematical calculations. A stepped progression is common as the symptoms worsen with new infarcts that may or may not be recognized.

Some strokes are major and easily perceived, leading to a clear functional loss. Others may be smaller and occur over time, leading to declines in cognitive capacity. One typical form of small stroke is a *lacunar infarct*. Multiple small lacunar infarcts are a common, slow, insidious form of vascular dementia that is often missed until later stages if cognitive screening is not performed frequently.

MIXED DEMENTIA

Mixed dementia occurs when the person develops both AD and vascular dementia. Symptoms from both diseases will be present, as discussed earlier. In addition, individuals with mixed dementia experience depressed mood, motor and sensory changes, and gait abnormalities with higher frequency than those with either AD or vascular dementia separately.[15] The prevalence of mixed dementia is about 22%[16]; many cases that are diagnosed as AD turn out to be mixed dementia as determined at autopsy or through symptomatic and radiographic findings. The median survival time of mixed dementia has been estimated at 4.5 years in older populations, with slightly longer survival in younger populations.[17]

LEWY BODY DEMENTIA

Lewy body dementia is an overarching term for two separate diseases, dementia with Lewy bodies and Parkinson's dementia. The primary distinction between the two is whether the cognitive symptoms occur at the same time as movement symptoms (dementia with Lewy bodies) or the movement symptoms are followed at least 2 years later by cognitive symptoms (Parkinson's dementia). Lewy body dementia is caused by the formation in the brain of *Lewy bodies*, which

are abnormal clumps of α-synuclein, a protein. It is unclear what causes these bodies to develop, though in most cases it is thought to be genetic–environment interaction. In Parkinson's dementia, Lewy bodies form as well, but the primary pathophysiology is the degeneration of dopaminergic neurons in the substantia nigra.

The movement disorder features of both include resting tremor, shuffling gait, rigidity, and eventually akinesia, which includes both hypokinesia (decreased frequency or absence of movement) and bradykinesia (slowed movement). Behavioral and psychological symptoms include sleep disturbance, including rapid eye movement (REM) sleep disorder, fluctuation in alertness and attention, recurrent visual hallucinations, visual-spatial problems, and depression. People living with Lewy body dementia have sensitivity to antipsychotic medications, so the correct diagnosis must be made before prescribing an antipsychotic for dementia symptoms. Approximately 4.6% of dementia cases are diagnosed as Lewy body dementia,[18] and the average survival time from diagnosis is approximately 4.4 years.[19]

FRONTOTEMPORAL DEMENTIA

FTD is an umbrella term used to describe a group of dementias caused by progressive neuronal degeneration in the frontal and/or temporal lobes of the brain. It generally occurs in individuals younger than 65 (median in studies is 52 to 60).[20] Survival is highly variable and depends on the subtype of disease, ranging from 3 years in motor neuron disease variants to 12 years in semantic dementia and 9 years in behavioral variant and progressive nonfluent aphasia. People with genetic risk factors make up about 30–50% of cases, although clinicians do not generally test for these markers, and the remainder of cases occur for unknown reasons, although head trauma and thyroid disease are thought to be potential risk factors. Overall, approximately 2.7% and 10.2% of cases of dementia are from FTD in older and younger adults, respectively.[21]

BEHAVIORAL VARIANT

The behavioral variant of FTD, formerly known as *Pick's disease*, is the most common form. Individuals generally present with personality changes and impaired social behaviors. These symptoms vary and can include disinhibition, including inappropriate touching or sexual behavior; impulsiveness; loss of empathy or sympathy; overeating; compulsive behaviors; apathy; and loss of executive function. The nature of these symptoms in the behavioral variant of FTD can be misidentified as a psychiatric disorder, delaying the correct diagnosis. As the disease progresses, symptoms will start to worsen, and people will also begin to have more memory problems and issues with planning and attention in the moderate stage. In the severe stage, people will express severe memory loss and language difficulty, and behavioral symptoms will continue to decline.

SEMANTIC DEMENTIA

People with left-sided semantic dementia commonly present with word-finding difficulties; a "pencil" might be a "writing thing" and an "orange" might be "that fruit." In right-sided semantic dementia, people tend to present with decreased awareness of other people's emotions. In both cases, memory remains more or less intact. The disease progresses to the moderate phase, generally about 2–3 years after diagnosis. At this time, people with left- and right-sided disease begin to show a more merged symptom presentation, including trouble with comprehending statements and recognizing faces, and some of the behavioral and psychological symptoms common to the behavioral variant of FTD. As individuals move into the severe stage of the disease, their BPSD worsen and they lose the ability to communicate.

PROGRESSIVE NONFLUENT APHASIA

Unlike those with semantic dementia, people with progressive nonfluent aphasia retain the ability to understand language and know the words they want to say; the first signs of disease relate to their ability to actually produce the speech they wish. This expressive aphasia will continue to worsen over time, and, within 3–4 years, they will enter the moderate stage, where they will only be able to use short phrases to express their needs. They can still, however, read and write well in most cases, so a dry-erase board or paper and notebook can help with communication in this stage. Approximately 5–7 years from diagnosis, people will become completely unable to speak and will start to develop the behavioral and psychological symptoms common to the behavioral variant of FTD.

MOTOR NEURON DISEASE

Motor neuron disease is the most severe form of FTD and causes a precipitous decline. Symptoms are similar to those of the behavioral variant, but people also exhibit muscle weakness, stiffness and atrophy, and loss of coordination and fine motor movement as motor neurons slowly disintegrate, similar to that seen in amyotrophic lateral sclerosis. Eventually the individual will present with dysphagia and dysarthria and are at high risk for developing aspiration pneumonia.

DOWN SYNDROME

Down syndrome, also known as trisomy 21, is generally diagnosed very early in life or during pregnancy through chromosomal or blood testing. The disease is caused by the abnormal development of a third full or partial chromosome 21 during early development. Individuals have a distinct appearance, which includes some but not always all of the following: upward-slanting eyes, flattened facial features, short hands and fingers, protruding tongue, and short stature. Severity is highly variable: some individuals exhibit mild cognitive deficits and others have severe cognitive difficulty, up to the levels seen in advanced dementias.

Life expectancy in Down syndrome is currently 60 years of age; it has increased dramatically over the past 50 years.[22] While a certain segment of the population will die in childhood, those individuals who live to adulthood generally develop the same health issues as the general public, though in a more rapid fashion. More than 70% of individuals with Down syndrome over the age of 35 may develop Alzheimer's dementia superimposed on Down syndrome.[23] Persons living with Down syndrome generally start to develop functional, cognitive, and health declines around the age of 40. The greatest causes of death in this population include congenital heart defect, dementia-related causes (e.g., aspiration pneumonia, falls), and cancers.[24] Persons living with Down syndrome toward the end of life often present with issues similar to PLWD; specifically issues related to functional decline such as dysphagia, pressure ulcers, and agitation, particularly around baths and personal care. Persons living with Down syndrome are often shuttled between group care homes and nursing homes as they enter the last several years of their lives, and multiple studies have found that the greater the number of transfers, the higher the risk of deterioration; transfers should therefore be limited as much as possible.[25]

ADVANCE CARE PLANNING

Advance care planning (ACP) in those with cognitive impairment can be a difficult process. Ideally, individuals will have discussed their wishes with their family/proxy before diagnosis or at least during the early phase of their disease. However, this is often not the case. Studies have shown that those with mild and even early moderate disease may be able to select a healthcare proxy or surrogate decision-maker[26] and take part in some healthcare decision-making.[27] Depending on the level of cognitive impairment, the level of decision-making permissible may be more or less complex, and a capacity assessment is essential in this process. It is important during this capacity assessment to see if the individual can consistently verbalize their wishes, reasoning, and ability to understand both the short- and long-term risks and benefits of decisions they would be making. Therefore, many decisions are discussed with the healthcare proxy or surrogate decision-maker. However, to the extent possible, the individual should be consulted and input taken in forming a decision.

The most important items to focus on in ACP for those with cognitive impairment include the aggressiveness and amount of care versus quality of life (hospitalization, resuscitation status, intubation, antibiotics, feeding tube placement) and the preferred setting of care based on available caregiving and financial status (home, group home, continuing care community, assisted living, nursing home). In states where orders for out-of-hospital life-sustaining treatments (physician/provider order for life-sustaining treatment [POLST] or medical orders for life-sustaining treatment [MOLST]) are accepted, these documents should be used to help provide clear, across-setting orders for the individual's wishes (for more information, see Chapter 32, "Advance Care Planning").

MANAGEMENT OF DECLINE AND SYMPTOMS

There are many challenges in caring for individuals with cognitive impairment related to both cognitive and functional decline and BPSD. These challenges often go hand in hand and require a comprehensive management approach that focuses on the unmet needs of individuals. In this section we first present cognitive and functional decline, and then focus on a philosophy of assessing unmet needs to treat BPSD. BPSD domains can be found in Table 45.5. As a first step toward addressing BPSD, unmet needs should first be assessed and addressed. One useful approach for assessing these unmet needs utilizes the PIECES pneumonic, which stands for Physical, Intellectual, Emotional, Capabilities, Environmental, and Social causes. Information on this approach can be found at http://pieceslearning.com/. Should these approaches not address the underlying BPSD, recommended nonpharmacologic (preferred) and pharmacologic (secondary) treatments can be found in Table 45.6 by domain.

COGNITIVE DECLINE

There are currently no pharmacologic or nonpharmacologic agents to reverse cognitive decline in dementia. Two classes of drugs are approved for slowing the progress of Alzheimer's dementia and Lewy body dementia: acetylcholinesterase inhibitors and NMDA receptor agonists. The former include donepezil (Aricept), galantamine (Razadyne), and rivastigmine (Exelon) and are indicated in mild and moderate dementia. These drugs have been shown to slightly decrease the rate of progression of the disease both cognitively and functionally and are more effective in Lewy body dementia than in AD. While these drugs do have some efficacy, they can also have significant side effects that are worse than the slight benefit of the medication. The most prominent side effect is gastrointestinal disturbance and upset, particularly diarrhea; this can lead to reduced oral intake and fluid/electrolyte imbalances. When starting this class of medication, the benefits and risks should be weighed and discussed with the individual and proxy. These drugs are not miracle cures, so it is important to set expectations appropriately. After initiation, if side effects are significant and do not dissipate, then a discussion needs to occur. Once this class of medication is stopped, the person will lose whatever effect the medication had and will not return to that level if it is restarted.

The second class of drugs, NMDA receptor agonists, consists of only one medication, memantine (Namenda). Memantine is indicated for use in moderate or severe AD; there is limited evidence for use in other forms of dementia. Studies have shown that combining memantine with an acetylcholinesterase inhibitor when the individual reaches the moderate stage of AD has a synergistic effect in slowing the disease greater than one or the other alone; however, the effect size is small at best.[28] The drug has limited side effects, so the cost versus small benefit should be discussed and weighed with the PLWD or family.

A third drug, aducanumab (Aduhelm) was recently approved by the Food and Drug Administration for use in individuals with mild cognitive impairment and early stage Alzheimer's disease. However, this was with considerable

Table 45.5 DOMAINS OF BEHAVIORAL AND PSYCHOLOGICAL SYMPTOMS OF DEMENTIA (BPSD)

DOMAIN	BEHAVIORS	NEUROPSYCHIATRIC INVENTORY-QUESTIONNAIRE (NPI-Q) CATEGORIES
Psychosis	Delusions and hallucinations	Delusions Hallucinations
Psychomotor agitation	Pacing, wandering, repetitive movements, physical aggression, dressing/undressing	Agitation/Aggression Disinhibition Motor disturbance Anxiety
Aggression	Yelling, calling out, repetitive speech, and verbal aggression	Agitation/Aggression Irritability/Lability
Depression	Depressed mood, other symptoms can vary Depression can also lead to other BPSD	Elation/Euphoria Apathy/Indifference Depression Disinhibition
Apathy	Social isolation, withdrawal	Nighttime behaviors Appetite/Eating
Sleep disturbances	Sundowning, diurnal sleep, rapid eye movement (REM) sleep disorder	Nighttime behaviors

From Corey-Bloom et al.[15], Custodio et al.[16]

Table 45.6 TREATMENTS FOR BEHAVIORAL AND PSYCHOLOGICAL SYMPTOMS OF DEMENTIA (BPSD)

BPSD DOMAIN	NONPHARMACOLOGICAL INTERVENTIONS	MEDICATION CLASS TO CONSIDER
Psychosis	Reduce environmental stimuli Address sensory impairments Do not dismiss concerns, assure person's safety	Only indication for antipsychotic[a,b]
Psychomotor agitation	Redirect and distraction Reduce environmental stimuli	Cholinesterase inhibitors, Memantine
Aggression	Acknowledge person's feelings Don't argue or react defensively Redirection and distraction	Cholinesterase inhibitors Memantine SSRI Trazadone (evening use only)[a]
Depression	Exercise Music as therapy Reminiscence therapy	SSRI (citalopram, sertraline, escitalopram)
Apathy	Socialization Actively involving the person in an activity	Cholinesterase inhibitors Methylphenidate[a,c] SSRIs
Sleep disturbances	Exercise Limit napping Good sleep hygiene	Melatonin Trazadone

[a] Off label use.

[b] Black box warning for increased risk of death, cardiovascular accident, myocardial infarction; requires informed consent prior to prescribing.

[c] Contraindicated in those with concurrent cardiovascular disease; do not use in cases where other BPSD domains other than depression are present.

SSRI, selective serotonin reuptake inhibitor.

From Corey-Bloom et al.[15], Custodio et al.[16]

---

controversy due to its lack of efficacy, being approved based on a surrogate endpoint with no proof of clinical improvement and with substantial side effects that can require intensive monitoring.

There is limited evidence about medication use once a person reaches end-stage dementia (e.g., needs help with all ADLs except walking, limited speech capability). Studies have shown that, in severe dementia, there is potentially some improvement in quality of life and reduction in depression symptoms, but these are not at the end stage, and similarly little evidence is available regarding what to do when a person has entered hospice care. Therefore, a conversation should occur with family about the goals of care and potential benefits and burdens of continuing the medication.

An additional method for reducing cognitive decline in PLWD is to ensure that cardiovascular disease, atrial fibrillation, and diabetes management are maintained in place, including both pharmacologic interventions *and* physical activity.[29,30] There are strong links between these conditions and cognitive decline, likely due to the effects of the illness on brain health, and they may even be one of the causes of the individual's dementia, depending on the type and etiology. While maintaining these in place, it is important for palliative care clinicians to consider how to best support the person and family in self-management.[31,32]

FUNCTIONAL DECLINE

As people decline over the course of disease, more and more issues will arise related to physical function. This decline can lead to aggression and agitation on the part of the person and to caregiver stress, burden, and burnout, among other issues. The goal is therefore to maintain function or find "work-arounds" for function for as long as possible. Physical and occupational therapists can be highly effective partners in this.[33,34] They can suggest home modifications and assistive devices, help train caregivers in how to perform transfers or exercises with the PLWD, or help by providing direct therapy to assist with function or strength. Especially with the removal of restrictions on physical and occupation therapy services to persons with no potential for improvement, there are greater opportunities to use these skilled rehabilitation therapists in these areas.

DYSPHAGIA

One of the most common functional problems facing PLWD as they reach the severe stage of dementia is dysphagia. This is a normal part of the disease process. PLWD often lose their ability to coordinate swallowing movements as well as their ability to feed themselves, leading to a high risk for developing aspiration pneumonias. This often brings up discussions of whether tube feeding would be appropriate. Multiple studies have shown that tube feeding does not prevent aspiration and is no better than spoon feeding, and the potential benefits are far outweighed by the burdens.[35] It is therefore important to educate PLWD and family about these benefits and burdens. The earlier in the disease process this can be discussed the better, allowing time for multiple conversations.

An additional issue, particularly in hospices, is voluntarily cessation of eating and drinking by the PLWD or for the family to stop assisting the person to eat and drink. Morally, ethically, and legally, if a person has made a clear statement or advance directive stating the wish to not be hand-fed or hydrated or receive medically administered nutrition and hydration, then we must respect these wishes.[36] However, if the person has not voiced the wishes directly and clearly (and ideally in writing), this is more of a legal, moral, and ethical gray area, with cultural and religious elements. Therefore, referrals should be placed for legal and ethical consultation, because laws vary state by state in this regard. Eventually the person who stops eating and drinking voluntarily will die rather comfortably, within an average of 8–10 days, from dehydration.

UNMET NEEDS

Many, though not all, BPSD can be addressed through recognizing the unmet needs of the PWLD or DD such as Down syndrome. One rememberable program for assessing for unmet needs is through using the PIECES Learning and Development Model (accessible at https://pieceslearning.com/), which is an evidence-based model. The pneumonic stands for Physical, Intellectual, Emotional health, Supportive strategies to maximize Capabilities, social and physical Environment, and Social self, and it serves as a comprehensive assessment for identifying underlying unmet needs. Some of these unmet needs may require pharmacologic or medical intervention, such as physical elements which can include pain, delirium due to an underlying acute illness, or constipation. Others fall more into psychosocial aspects, such as communication issues (intellectual), depression (emotional), loss of function (capabilities), noise or light (environmental), or isolation (social) that more often than not are sensitive to nonpharmacologic interventions.

BEHAVIORAL AND PSYCHOLOGICAL SYMPTOMS

PLWD and those with DD may present with a variety of behavioral and psychological symptoms related to their condition. Even though Down syndrome and DDs are separate illness from dementia (though often these individuals can develop dementia later in life), for the purposes of simplicity we will refer to behavioral symptoms as BPSD herein, and treatments

(unless otherwise noted) are applicable to both groups. There are six primary clusters of symptoms, and 13 symptoms within that we tend to focus on. When beginning to assess for symptoms, one way to do so in a holistic but straightforward fashion is to use the Neuropsychiatric Inventory–Questionnaire (NPI-Q).[37] The NPI-Q is performed with a caregiver and assesses for the presence and severity of the 13 BPSD and how distressing they are to the caregiver. This can be used to prioritize which symptom (or two) to tackle first and can be used to monitor progress in both treating the BPSD and managing caregiver distress. It takes about 10 minutes to complete and can be performed prior to your visit. Completing the NPI-Q, along with utilizing PIECES, are keys to achieving effective BPSD management. Next we discuss the six clusters and effective nonpharmacologic and pharmacologic treatments specific to each.

AGGRESSION

Physical and verbal aggression are highly prevalent in PLWD and DD. This aggression may be caused by any number of issues, usually unmet needs, so assessment using PIECES is necessary to treat the baseline problem. The most prevalent causes include bathing and personal care (see later discussion), unidentified or undertreated pain or depression, and a poor relationship between the care recipient and the caregiver.[34] Other potential causes include sensory perception issues (hearing, vision), delirium, medication side effects, and environmental factors (noise, temperature). To reduce aggression, the root cause needs to be identified and treated. Antipsychotics, which are frequently prescribed, are not appropriate and do not work for aggressive behaviors; they only sedate the individual, leading to sleep–wake cycle disturbances which can increase caregiver stress and increase patient morbidity and mortality. Similarly, mood stabilizers such as divalproex sodium have not been found effective. Caregivers need to stay calm because any show of strong emotion (e.g., yelling, threatening movements) will only make the aggression worse. Redirection can be a useful method when aggression is not related to an immediately identifiable and treatable cause. Music therapy, physical activity, and aromatherapy are additional nonpharmacologic modalities. From a pharmacologic perspective the only medication that *has* been found to be effective are the selective serotonin reuptake inhibitors (SSRIs). In older adults, the preferred SSRI include citalopram, escitalopram, and sertraline.

BATHING AND PERSONAL CARE

One of the most difficult areas that PLWD and their caregivers struggle with is bathing and personal care. The loss of dignity that occurs when the PLWD can no longer care for him- or herself after a long life of independence, coupled with cognitive impairment, often leads to verbal or physical aggression. To prevent or reduce aggression, a highly person-centered approach needs to be taken.[31] Effective, personally tailored interventions may include the following:

- Assessing the person prior to the care for pain and current physical and mental state and altering the routine or stopping the care until these can be better managed

- Addressing the environment such as reducing noise, introducing soothing music

- Adhering to routine, including stopping and interacting with the person prior to initiating personal care, covering private parts to the extent possible, ensuring as much privacy as possible

- Ensuring that the caregiver has developed a relationship with the PLWD and clearly shares step by step what he or she is going to do before doing it. For instance, "Now I'm going to pull your arm through your shirt. Now I am going to lift it over your head. Now I am going to wash you."

- If performing a bed bath, ensure that the PLWD is only exposed in the area being cleaned, which can both reduce discomfort from being cold or from feeling overexposed.

- Ensuring appropriate water temperature (e.g., warm but not scalding)

- When resistance is encountered, try again a few minutes later (or in the case of a bath a few hours later), provide reasons for the personal care or bath (e.g., "You've been working hard, wouldn't it feel good to freshen up?"), and/or changing the type of bath (e.g., bath, using a shower chair, bed bath with warm wet towels).

PSYCHOMOTOR AGITATION

Psychomotor agitation includes hyperactive behaviors such as repetitive actions, pacing, restlessness, and dressing and undressing. This form of agitation is common in Lewy body dementia and can also result from the overuse of antipsychotics. Removing these medications may stop these behaviors. Other options include physical therapy to help PLWD or those with DD focus on completing specific tasks rather than aimless hyperactivity. Increasing stimulation and companionship may also help reduce this symptom.

PSYCHOSIS

The psychosis cluster includes hallucinations, delusions, and misidentification of people and objects. From a person- and family-centered perspective, the term "psychosis" should not be used, only the individual symptom experienced, as the term "psychosis" can have negative connotations that will cause unease. This cluster of symptoms is the only time when it may be beneficial to use antipsychotics. If the hallucination, delusion, or misidentification is not distressing or causing harm to the PLWD or caregiver, pharmacologic treatment should *not* be prescribed, as the risks outweigh any benefits. If, however, the PLWD is experiencing multiple distressing visual or auditory hallucinations, delusions, or misidentifications, antipsychotic use can be considered. It is important to "start low and

go slow." Moreover, different antipsychotics have different properties (e.g., quetiapine is sedating whereas olanzapine is activating), so the medication must be given at the appropriate time of day, and an activated PLWD should not be given an activating antipsychotic (or vice versa). For persons with Lewy body dementia or Parkinson's dementia, the only viable medications are quetiapine and clozapine, though the latter requires frequent blood testing for agranulocytosis. While pimavanserin was approved specifically for this population by the FDA in 2016, it is not currently recommended as a first-line therapy for those with Lewy body or Parkinson's dementia due to sparse evidence.[38]

Whenever considering prescribing an antipsychotic, whether typical or atypical, the PLWD, where appropriate, and proxy need to be informed of the black-box warning and the risks for increased heart attack or stroke and must clearly consent to the medication. PLWD or those with DD are also at a higher risk for falls when taking these medications, and certain medications have other significant side effects. For instance, olanzapine causes disturbances in blood sugar in individuals with diabetes. Therefore, the palliative APRN must be knowledgeable about the specific medication prior to prescribing. The conversation, including all side effects, needs to be documented in the chart.

APATHY

Apathy, including social isolation, withdrawal, and lack of interest, is common in PLWD. Nonpharmacologic measures to engage the PLWD or those with DD are important: music therapy, multisensory behavioral interventions, physical activity, dancing, singing, and talking have been found to be effective.[39] Pharmacologically, acetylcholinesterase inhibitors have shown to be mildly beneficial in some studies but not others, but the side effects likely outweigh the benefits, and other classes, such as stimulants and neuroleptics, have not shown any efficacy.[40]

DEPRESSION

Depression can be identified using the Geriatric Depression Scale in mild to moderate dementia[41] and the Cornell Scale for Depression in Dementia,[42] an informant-based interview, can be used for individuals living with moderate to severe dementia. Treating depression in PLWD can often lead to significant decreases in other BPSDs, so the person should be assessed for depression early on. Treatment for depression should focus on nonpharmacologic measures (e.g., music, reminiscence, and physical activity).[39] Pharmacologic interventions have not shown efficacy in improving depression using depression scales in this population[43]; however, as discussed earlier, they lead to significant improvement in agitative behaviors and thus may not be the best measure to use. If the APRN chooses to use a pharmacologic treatment to augment nonpharmacologic treatments, then citalopram, sertraline, or escitalopram, which present fewer issues in the geriatric population, are preferred.

SLEEP DISTURBANCE

Sleep disturbances occur in approximately 38% of the dementia population and can have significant consequences, including significantly increasing caregiver stress.[44] One of the most common disturbances is alteration of the diurnal sleep pattern. PLWD are often sleepy and take long naps during the day, becoming restless in the early evening. This early evening agitation is often called *sundowning*. The most important way to avoid or decrease these sleep-pattern changes is to prevent the PLWD from taking long naps throughout the day. This requires the person to be engaged and not socially isolated. The physical environment should be kept bright, if possible with natural light or specialized lights that mimic daylight. Only one nap of no more than 1.5 hours should be permitted. Sleep medications in this population can cause significant side effects and can lead to falls. Stimulants during the day (pharmacologic or nonpharmacologic, such as caffeine) can cause agitation and should therefore be avoided as much as possible. Melatonin has shown limited efficacy in this population, although no substantial side effects occurred in doses of 1–3 mg. Alcohol should also be avoided. Finally, regular physical activity can help to maintain the proper sleep–wake cycle.

A second type of sleep disturbance is *REM sleep disorder*, which is more prevalent in Lewy body dementia than in other forms. In REM sleep disorder, individuals act out their dreams in ways such as walking, talking, screaming, or displaying physical aggression. Clonazepam is the suggested treatment in individuals who have REM sleep disorder, but it is not recommended in PLWD due to the risk for rebound agitation. Melatonin has shown some efficacy in treating this disorder, and acetylcholinesterase inhibitors such as donepezil have shown some efficacy, though the evidence is limited.[45]

PAIN

While pain in and of itself is not associated with cognitive impairment, identifying and managing pain in this population can be difficult. PLWD and those with DD still experience pain, though they often cannot communicate that they do. In general, older adults may not identify pain by using the word "pain," instead describing it in terms of soreness, achiness, "the arthritis," or having difficulty with "that" (e.g., using their hands, walking).[46,47] While the rating scale of choice (faces, numeric, or verbal descriptor) can all be used in individuals with mild and early moderate dementia, PLWD should be assessed at times other than when they are resting because they may forget that they had pain with movement. The assessment should be done immediately after the PLWD completes a movement, or even during the movement. The palliative APRN should observe for pain behaviors such as bracing, verbalizations, and facial expressions indicating pain and should examine the person's problem list for potential painful conditions (e.g., osteoarthritis, compression fractures, neuropathies). In individuals with moderate and severe dementia, a pain assessment instrument specifically for use in this population should be used (e.g., the PAINAD) in addition to the person's subjective report and reporting from the primary caregiver.[45]

Once identified, treatment of pain in this population generally follows the same recommendations as for other populations—with some differences. Mild pain should be treated using nonpharmacologic interventions. Medications should be given on a scheduled basis rather than as needed because the PLWD may not request or will forget to request pain medicine. For mild to moderate pain, acetaminophen is the first-line treatment, not exceeding 3 g per day. If pain is not controlled with acetaminophen, nonsteroidal anti-inflammatory drugs (NSAIDs) are generally the next step for short-term treatment, potentially a COX-2 inhibitor for longer term treatment. Most pain in older adults comes from osteoarthritis and lower back pain, and opioids have not been shown to be effective in this group and thus should not be prescribed.[48] For other forms of pain, such as from fractures, pressure injuries, or cancer, opioids may be a more evidence-based approach.

SPIRITUAL SUPPORT

Spiritual support can improve the quality of life for both the PLWD or those with DD and their caregivers. Higher religiosity has been found to slow cognitive and behavioral decline in dementia. Spiritual support can give meaning to the caregiver's experiences, reducing stress[49] and improving his or her overall mental health.[50] Therefore PLWD or those with DD and their caregivers should be encouraged to use spiritual support, whether in the community, an assisted living facility, nursing home, or hospital setting. The palliative APRN should facilitate such services as appropriate and possible.

WORKING WITH CAREGIVERS

Caregivers for PLWD and those with DD have a high risk of burden, stress, and burnout. Caregivers, especially spouses, may become ill themselves, even necessitating hospital admission. If the caregiver's needs are not met, the PLWD is significantly more likely to be placed in a nursing home or other long-term care facility rather than remaining at home. Paid caregivers, if they become burned-out and leave, cause further trauma to the PLWD and family because they have to develop a new therapeutic relationship, which can cause further decline. PLWD are also at higher risk to be victims of elder abuse, possibly perpetrated by caregivers. Assessing caregiver stress can reduce the possibility for abuse or maltreatment. The palliative APRN should also routinely screen for abuse among PLWD or those with DD.[51]

Providing support for the caregiver is just as important as support for the PLWD or those DD. This can take many forms, such as training sessions from the local Alzheimer's Association (applicable regardless of type of dementia), adult day health programs for the care recipient to give the caregiver some personal time, or respite care in a facility. The most important part of helping the caregiver is to manage BPSD, as outlined earlier, and to manage the caregiver's expectations. When working with the caregiver to manage BPSD it is important to understand what are the most concerning BPSD and what potential evidence-based nonpharmacologic and pharmacologic treatments they would be willing to implement, and then to implement changes in a way that does not overwhelm them. Generally, start with one symptom and 1–2 changes to make and monitor from there.

Caregivers should be monitored for burden, stress, and burnout. The NPI-Q, mentioned earlier, measures both severity of BPSD and distress to caregivers and can be used as a proxy. The Modified Caregiver Strain Index is also a quick and easy tool to use with the caregiver to measure their strain. Some additional instruments include the Pines Burnout Inventory[52] and the Zarit Burden Inventory.[53] When the caregiver's stress starts to rise, it is important to identify the source, correct it, and, if necessary, provide some form of respite.

HOSPICE CARE

While PLWD should begin to receive palliative care early in the disease trajectory, they are not eligible for hospice care until they have very severe dementia. Depending on the region, PLWD must meet the FAST 7C level of debility, which means they cannot speak more than six distinct intelligible words and they have functional dependence with the exception of ambulation, or FAST 7A plus debility in 50% of ADLs. Of note, the FAST scale should only be used in AD and not in other forms of dementia or DD. Instead, the Palliative Performance Scale is another way to determine eligibility, for those individuals who score at or below a 40. PLWD frequently also must have a secondary condition, which could include a recent history of multiple Stage 3 or 4 pressure ulcers, aspiration pneumonia, septicemia, pyelonephritis, recurrent fever, or inability to maintain sufficient intake of food and fluids (as defined by loss of 10% weight in a 6-month period or an albumin level of <2.5 g/dL). It is important to understand the hospice's understanding of what their Medicare Administrative Contractor requires as eligibility.

Once a PLWD is deemed eligible and admitted to hospice, the palliative care team must closely scrutinize standing orders prior to signing the order set. For instance, the emergency kit often provided to PLWD in homes usually includes lorazepam or another short-acting benzodiazepine. Because benzodiazepines can cause rebound confusion and delirium in older adults, particularly those with cognitive impairment, including this in the kit should be discouraged. Haloperidol, prochlorperazine, and promethazine are often included in these kits; these medications should not be permitted in cases where the person has Lewy body dementia or Parkinson's dementia because they have dopaminergic blocking activity and may worsen symptoms.

Once admitted to hospice, it is important to continue following the PLWD because many (though not all) hospice clinicians have limited knowledge of dementia care. They may need help with recognizing and developing a plan of care for treating pain, BPSD, or other symptoms. Given that PLWD tend to have longer stays in hospice than persons with cancer and experience significant functional disability associated with end-stage dementia, special attention needs to be paid to skin integrity. When working with hospices, it is often important to request occupational and physical therapy consultation to help train the caregiver to prevent contractures and prolong function (specifically ambulation) as long as possible and to evaluate for home safety. These therapists can also train the caregiver in how to perform transfers when the PLWD cannot ambulate even with assistance, thus preventing caregiver injury. OTs are experts at providing "workarounds" for functional and cognitive limitations, and PTs can be of great help in teaching caregivers about exercises they can use to help the PLWD maintain strength as long as possible and prevent contractures once the PLWD has lost too much strength to bear weight. These services are included within the hospice benefit but are often not provided unless directly requested. Finally, some PLWD are live-discharged from hospice due to a "stabilization" of their condition. It is important to closely follow the transition away from hospice as it can be an incredibly stressful time for the caregiver due to loss of the substantial services provided by hospice.

ROLE OF THE APRN

The palliative APRN has a wide role in managing cognitively impaired individuals. While a specific diagnosis should probably not be made without consulting a neurologist, geriatrician, AD center, or geriatric APRN, most treatment falls well within the scope of practice and range of knowledge of the palliative APRN. This includes managing nonpharmacologic and pharmacologic interventions for BPSD; advance care planning; referral to physical or occupational therapy for exercise regimens and physical function; assessing and managing caregiver stress, burden, and burnout; and directing care or attending on hospice care.

SUMMARY

Most forms of dementia are irreversible and progressive. While those with DD are not necessarily progressive, they are at higher risk for dementia and early death. The most significant problems related to this group of diseases are the presentation and worsening of BPSD over time, progressive decline in functional status, and progressive increase in caregiver burden, stress, and burnout, leading to placement in a nursing home or other institutional setting. Therefore, the palliative APRN must (1) create a clear plan of care early in the disease, if possible with the PLWD and proxy present; (2) provide clear expectations to the caregiver about the PLWD's course; (3) implement nonpharmacologic and pharmacologic interventions to manage functional decline and BPSD; and (4) train caregivers to provide appropriate care. These steps can help the PLWD or those with DD and their caregivers deal with this devastating group of diseases to the greatest extent possible.

REFERENCES

1. 2021 Alzheimer's disease facts and figures. *Alzheimers Dement.* 2021;17(3):327–406. doi:10.1002/alz.12328
2. Borson S, Scanlan J, Brush M, Vitaliano P, Dokmak A. The Mini-Cog: A cognitive "vital signs" measure for dementia screening in multi-lingual elderly. *Int J Geriatr Psychiatry.* 2000;15(11):1021–1027. doi:10.1002/1099-1166(200011)15:11<1021::aid-gps234>3.0.co;2-6
3. Borson S, Sehgal M, Chodosh J. Monetizing the MOCA: What now? *J Am Geriatr Soc.* 2019;67(11):2229–2231. doi:10.1111/jgs.16158
4. Morris JC. Clinical dementia rating: A reliable and valid diagnostic and staging measure for dementia of the Alzheimer type. *Int Psychogeriatr.* 1997;9 Suppl 1:173–176; discussion 177–178. doi:10.1017/s1041610297004870
5. Galvin JE. The Quick Dementia Rating System (QDRS): A rapid dementia staging tool. *Alzheimers Dement (Amst).* 01 2015;1(2):249–259. doi:10.1016/j.dadm.2015.03.003
6. Leyhe T, Reynolds CF, 3rd, Melcher T, et al. A common challenge in older adults: Classification, overlap, and therapy of depression and dementia. *Alzheimers Dement.* Jan 2017;13(1):59–71. doi:10.1016/j.jalz.2016.08.007
7. Johnson KA, Minoshima S, Bohnen NI, et al. Appropriate use criteria for amyloid pet: A report of the amyloid imaging task force, the society of nuclear medicine and molecular imaging, and the Alzheimer's association. *Alzheimers Dement.* 2013;9(1):e-1–16. doi:10.1016/j.jalz.2013.01.002
8. Khoury R, Ghossoub E. Diagnostic biomarkers of Alzheimer's disease: A state-of-the-art review. *Biomarkers Neuropsychiatry.* 2019;1:100005. doi:Https://doi.org/10.1016/j.bionps.2019.100005
9. Vermunt L, Sikkes SAM, van den Hout A, et al. Duration of preclinical, prodromal, and dementia stages of Alzheimer's disease in relation to age, sex, and apoe genotype. *Alzheimers Dement.* 2019;15(7):888–898. doi:10.1016/j.jalz.2019.04.001
10. Sinforiani E, Bernini S, Picascia M. Disease progression in relation to age at onset in a population with Alzheimer's dementia. *Aging Clin Exp Res.* 2019;31(5):723–725. doi:10.1007/s40520-018-1027-5
11. Brookmeyer R, Johnson E, Ziegler-Graham K, Arrighi HM. Forecasting the global burden of Alzheimer's disease. *Alzheimers Dement.* 2007;3(3):186–191. doi:10.1016/j.jalz.2007.04.381
12. Mayeda ER, Glymour MM, Quesenberry CP, Johnson JK, Perez-Stable EJ, Whitmer RA. Survival after dementia diagnosis in five racial/ethnic groups. *Alzheimers Dement.* 2017;13(7):761–769. doi:10.1016/j.jalz.2016.12.008
13. Wolters FJ, Ikram MA. Epidemiology of vascular dementia. *Arterioscler Thromb Vasc Biol.* 2019;39(8):1542–1549. doi:10.1161/ATVBAHA.119.311908
14. Tariq S, Barber PA. Dementia risk and prevention by targeting modifiable vascular risk factors. *J. Neurochem.* 2018;144(5):565–581. doi:10.1111/jnc.14132
15. Corey-Bloom J, Galasko D, Hofstetter CR, Jackson JE, Thal LJ. Clinical features distinguishing large cohorts with possible ad, probable ad, and mixed dementia. *J Am Geriatr Soc.* 1993;41(1):31–37.
16. Custodio N, Montesinos R, Lira D, Herrera-Perez E, Bardales Y, Valeriano-Lorenzo L. Mixed dementia: A review of the evidence. *Dement Neuropsychol.* 2017;11(4):364–370. doi:10.1590/1980-57642016dn11-040005
17. Strand BH, Knapskog AB, Persson K, et al. Survival and years of life lost in various aetiologies of dementia, mild cognitive impairment (MCI) and subjective cognitive decline (SCD) in Norway. *PLoS One.* 2018;13(9):e0204436. doi:10.1371/journal.pone.0204436
18. Kane JPM, Surendranathan A, Bentley A, et al. Clinical prevalence of Lewy body dementia. *Alzheimers Res Ther.* 15 2018;10(1):19. doi:10.1186/s13195-018-0350-6
19. McKeith IG, Boeve BF, Dickson DW, et al. Diagnosis and management of dementia with Lewy bodies: Fourth consensus report of the DLB consortium. *Neurology.* 2017;89(1):88–100. doi:10.1212/WNL.0000000000004058
20. Onyike CU, Diehl-Schmid J. The epidemiology of frontotemporal dementia. *Intl Rev Psychiatry.* 2013;25(2):130–137. doi:10.3109/09540261.2013.776523
21. Hogan DB, Jette N, Fiest KM, et al. The prevalence and incidence of frontotemporal dementia: A systematic review. *Can J Neurol Sci.* 2016;43 Suppl 1:S96–S109. doi:10.1017/cjn.2016.25
22. Motegi N, Morisaki N, Suto M, Tamai H, Mori R, Nakayama T. Secular trends in longevity among people with Down syndrome in japan, 1995–2016. *Pediatr Int.* 2020;63(1):94–101. doi:10.1111/ped.14354
23. Hithersay R, Startin CM, Hamburg S, et al. Association of dementia with mortality among adults with Down syndrome older than 35 years. *JAMA Neurol.* 2019;76(2):152–160. doi:10.1001/jamaneurol.2018.3616
24. Landes SD, Stevens JD, Turk MA. Cause of death in adults with Down syndrome in the us. *Disabil Health J.* 2020;13(4):100947. doi:10.1016/j.dhjo.2020.100947
25. Fredericksen J, Fabbre V. Down syndrome and Alzheimer's disease: Issues and implications for social work practice. *J Gerontol Soc Work.* 2018;61(1):4–10. doi:10.1080/01634372.2017.1393480
26. Mezey M, Teresi J, Ramsey G, Mitty E, Bobrowitz T. Decision-making capacity to execute a health care proxy: Development and testing of guidelines. *J Am Geriatr Soc.* 2000;48(2):179–187. doi:10.1111/j.1532-5415.2000.tb03909.x
27. Bosisio F, Barazzetti G. Advanced care planning: Promoting autonomy in caring for people with dementia. *Am J Bioeth.* 2020;20(8):93–95. doi:10.1080/15265161.2020.1781958
28. Dou KX, Tan MS, Tan CC, et al. Comparative safety and effectiveness of cholinesterase inhibitors and memantine for Alzheimer's disease: A network meta-analysis of 41 randomized controlled trials. *Alzheimers Res Ther.* 2018;10(1):126. doi:10.1186/s13195-018-0457-9
29. Stefanidis KB, Askew CD, Greaves K, Summers MJ. The effect of non-stroke cardiovascular disease states on risk for cognitive decline and dementia: A systematic and meta-analytic review. *Neuropsychol Rev.* 2018;28(1):1–15. doi:10.1007/s11065-017-9359-z
30. Laver K, Dyer S, Whitehead C, Clemson L, Crotty M. Interventions to delay functional decline in people with dementia: A systematic review of systematic reviews. *BMJ Open.* 2016;6(4):e010767. doi:10.1136/bmjopen-2015-010767
31. Grey M, Schulman-Green D, Knafl K, Reynolds NR. A revised self- and family management framework. *Nurs Outlook.* 2015;63(2):162–170. doi:10.1016/j.outlook.2014.10.003
32. Ibrahim JE, Anderson LJ, MacPhail A, Lovell JJ, Davis MC, Winbolt M. Chronic disease self-management support for persons with dementia, in a clinical setting. *J Multidiscip Healthc.* 2017;10:49–58. doi:10.2147/JMDH.S121626
33. Laver K, Cumming R, Dyer S, et al. Evidence-based occupational therapy for people with dementia and their families: What clinical practice guidelines tell us and implications for practice. *Aust Occup Ther J.* 2017;64(1):3–10. doi:10.1111/1440-1630.12309
34. El-Bizri I, Catic AG. Management of physical function in older adults with dementia. In: Catic AG, ed. *Dementia and Chronic Disease: Management of Comorbid Medical Conditions.* Cham: Springer; 2020: 11–21.
35. American Geriatrics Society. American Geriatrics Society feeding tubes in advanced dementia position statement. *J Am Geriatr Soc.* 2014;62(8):1590–1593. doi:10.1111/jgs.12924
36. Christenson J. An ethical discussion on voluntarily stopping eating and drinking by proxy decision maker or by advance directive. *J Hosp Palliat Nurs.* 2019;21(3):188–192. doi:10.1097/NJH.0000000000000557
37. Kaufer DI, Cummings JL, Ketchel P, et al. Validation of the NPI-Q, a brief clinical form of the neuropsychiatric inventory. *J Neuropsychiatry Clin Neurosci.* 2000;12(2):233–239. doi:10.1176/jnp.12.2.233

38. Tampi RR, Tampi DJ, Young JJ, Balachandran S, Hoq RA, Manikkara G. Evidence for using pimavanserin for the treatment of Parkinson's disease psychosis. *World J Psychiatry.* 2019;9(3):47–54. doi:10.5498/wjp.v9.i3.47

39. Theleritis C, Siarkos K, Politis AA, Katirtzoglou E, Politis A. A systematic review of non-pharmacological treatments for apathy in dementia. *Int J Geriatr Psychiatry.* 2018;33(2):e177–e192. doi:10.1002/gps.4783

40. Harrison F, Aerts L, Brodaty H. Apathy in dementia: Systematic review of recent evidence on pharmacological treatments. *Curr Psychiatry Rep.* 2016;18(11):103. doi:10.1007/s11920-016-0737-7

41. Lach HW, Chang YP, Edwards D. Can older adults with dementia accurately report depression using brief forms? Reliability and validity of the geriatric depression scale. *J Gerontol Nurs.* 2010;36(5):30–37. doi:10.3928/00989134-20100303-01

42. Alexopoulos GS, Abrams RC, Young RC, Shamoian CA. Cornell scale for depression in dementia. *Biol Psychiatry.* 1988;23(3):271–284. doi:10.1016/0006-3223(88)90038-8

43. Dudas R, Malouf R, McCleery J, Dening T. Antidepressants for treating depression in dementia. *Cochrane Database Syst Rev.* 2018;8:CD003944. doi:10.1002/14651858.CD003944.pub2

44. Webster L, Costafreda Gonzalez S, Stringer A, et al. Measuring the prevalence of sleep disturbances in people with dementia living in care homes: A systematic review and meta-analysis. *Sleep.* 2020;43(4):zsz251. doi:10.1093/sleep/zsz251

45. Muntean, ML., Sixel-Döring, F. & Trenkwalder, C. REM sleep behavior disorder in Parkinson's disease. *J Neural Transm* 121 (Suppl 1), 41–47 (2014). doi:10.1007/s00702-014-1192-4

46. Horgas AL. Pain assessment in older adults. *Nurs Clin North Am.* 2017;52(3):375–385. doi:10.1016/j.cnur.2017.04.006

47. Warden V, Hurley AC, Volicer L. Development and psychometric evaluation of the Pain Assessment in Advanced Dementia (PAINAD) scale. *J Am Med Dir Assoc.* 2003;4(1):9–15. doi:10.1097/01.JAM.0000043422.31640.F7

48. Krebs EE, Gravely A, Nugent S, et al. Effect of opioid vs nonopioid medications on pain-related function in patients with chronic back pain or hip or knee osteoarthritis pain: The space randomized clinical trial. *JAMA.* 2018;319(9):872–882. doi:10.1001/jama.2018.0899

49. Coin A, Perissinotto E, Najjar M, et al. Does religiosity protect against cognitive and behavioral decline in Alzheimer's dementia? *Curr Alzheimer Res.* 2010;7(5):445–452. doi:10.2174/156720510791383886

50. Marquez-Gonzalez M, Lopez J, Romero-Moreno R, Losada A. Anger, spiritual meaning and support from the religious community in dementia caregiving. *J Religion Health.* 2012;51(1):179–186. doi:10.1007/s10943-010-9362-7

51. Unson C, Flynn D, Glendon MA, Haymes E, Sancho D. Dementia and caregiver stress: An application of the reconceptualized uncertainty in illness theory. *Iss Ment Health Nurs.* 2015;36(6):439–446. doi:10.3109/01612840.2014.993052

52. Malakh-Pines A, Aronson E, Kafry D. *Burnout: From Tedium to Personal Growth.* New York: Free Press; 1981.

53. Bedard M, Molloy DW, Squire L, Dubois S, Lever JA, O'Donnell M. The Zarit Burden Interview: A new short version and screening version. *Gerontologist.* 2001;41(5):652–657. doi:10.1093/geront/41.5.652

46.

SERIOUS MENTAL ILLNESS

Kristyn Pellecchia and Ryan Murphy

KEY POINTS

- The palliative advanced practice registered nurse (APRN) should have baseline knowledge of psychiatry in the palliative care context and of how serious mental illness (SMI) can intersect with other life-limiting illnesses.

- The palliative APRN can identify barriers and use a trauma-informed care approach to work alongside a patient population that is often stigmatized.

- The palliative APRN benefits from understanding primary pharmacologic management of SMI diagnoses and how to utilize interdisciplinary resources to facilitate best outcomes.

CASE STUDY 1: THE PATIENT WITH SERIOUS MENTAL ILLNESS

AM was a 44-year-old woman with medical history that included hypertension, Stage IV chronic kidney disease, Stage IV anal carcinoma with metastases to liver and lung, and an unclear, under-treated serious mental illness (SMI). She was referred to palliative care for pain management during an acute admission. Nursing reported that AM was actively using heroin immediately prior to admission and often had difficulty engaging with the nurses or following treatment plans. The palliative APRN agreed to follow AM in the outpatient clinic and slowly built rapport. While trying to create a comprehensive treatment plan for AM, the palliative advanced practice registered nurse (APRN) made referrals to oncology, psychiatry, primary care, and physical therapy. At the next visit, AM reported not following-up with any of the referrals, noting she would not be able to follow a schedule with all of those providers, so she wanted to focus on just oncology and palliative care.

The palliative APRN recognized that even though physical symptoms were controlled quickly, AM benefited from weekly or biweekly visits for psychosocial support. After trust was established, AM shared her history of long-standing physical and emotional abuse, illicit drug use, and multiple admissions to psychiatric facilities for paranoia and hallucinations that started in her teenage years. Antipsychotic medications were offered and AM adamantly refused, citing a history of adverse effects from the medications. The palliative APRN attempted to adapt practice to meet the needs of AM, not necessarily to focus on perfect health outcomes, in line with the harm reduction model. Though AM had a mistrust of the medical field, after about a year she

allowed the palliative APRN to assist with an inpatient medical admission when her cancer had progressed. Workup revealed that she had multiple-level bowel obstructions secondary to tumor burden, and no surgical intervention was offered. AM was transitioned to inpatient hospice due to symptom burden, and she died comfortably in a safe space.

INTRODUCTION

There are many challenges to treating individuals with concurrent mental illness and life-threatening illness. This patient population presents with a unique set of needs that often go unmet.[1] As seen in Case Study 1, patients with serious mental illnesses (SMI) often have a difficult time navigating the healthcare system. These individuals are labeled as "difficult patients" because symptoms of their illness may lead to frequently missed appointments, declined therapies and interventions, and poor or irregular adherence to treatment regimens.[2]

Patients with SMI may have difficulty understanding their illness trajectory, the risks and benefits of treatment, and the necessary goals of care pertaining to the treatment plan, reflecting changes in capacity for medical decision-making. These situations can further be complicated when individuals are actively using illicit substances or have a history of illicit substance use to treat pain or symptom burdens. Substance use disorder (SUD), discussed in a separate chapter, is common in populations with SMI,[3] with about half of patients with SMI having a comorbid SUD.[4] The symptom burden of SMI is high and is the source of multiple areas of suffering; these patients will present with poor relationships and lack of social structure, poverty, homelessness, history of incarceration, and inability to care for themselves.

The palliative APRN is in a unique position to support this patient population; SMI is a chronic, often life-limiting illness that is inherently accompanied by significant psychosocial and spiritual distress. Care of this population necessitates meticulous assessment, collaboration, and communication. It also requires a holistic approach to recognize the complexity of patient needs, something that can be best met through interdisciplinary work and truly patient-centered care to optimize health outcomes.

To start, it is important to understand what constitutes SMI. Mental illness is highly prevalent, with nearly one in five individuals in the United States living with some sort of qualifying condition.[4] In 2017, it was estimated that 4.5% of all US adults carried an SMI diagnosis: approximately 11.2 million people. Mental illnesses can have a varying effect on all aspects of daily life, with SMI resulting in "serious functional impairment, which substantially interferes with or limits one or more major life activities."[4] Classically, SMIs include schizophrenia, schizoaffective disorder, severe bipolar disorder, and severe major depression. However, other mental disorders such as severe personality disorders and eating disorders may also be included if the functional impairment is serious enough.

This patient population warrants a more compassionate approach to care due not only to high symptom burden, but also to expected decrease in life span. While the average life span in the United States is nearly 79 years, in contrast, a person with SMI has a shortened life expectancy less by a range of 15–25 years.[1] This mortality gap is theorized to be 25% due to suicide, homicide, and accidental deaths and 75% due to poor physical health.[5] The *standardized mortality ratio* describes the observed number of deaths within a study population compared to the standard population[6]; a ratio greater than 1.0 means there are excess deaths in the study population. That said, people with SMI have an increased mortality ratios for cancer (2.4), cardiovascular disease (3.6), and chronic obstructive pulmonary disease (9.9).[1] Poor physical health may be due to medication side effects, reduced access to medical care, and/or higher rates of substance abuse (including tobacco).[3]

Palliative APRNs can draw from cornerstone philosophies within the specialty to impact the care of these individuals. Historically, palliative care has aimed to alleviate suffering in a more comprehensive way than other areas of medicine. A pioneer in the field of end of life care, Dame Cicely Saunders made a point to educate on the concept of "total pain": the idea that suffering is the summation of someone's physical, psychological, social, spiritual, and emotional struggles,[7] with the emphasis that, "mental distress may be perhaps the most intractable pain of all."[8] The idea of total pain becomes particularly important when working with palliative care patients with SMI who regularly present with complex trauma and burden profiles. Case Study 1 depicts a woman who experienced significant, life-long, multidimensional suffering. Like other SMI patients, AM often had high burden from both her mental and physical diseases due to fear of seeking medical assistance, lack of social network, poor emotional coping skills, and inability to self-advocate for assistance that could result in relief of suffering. Only addressing one aspect of pain would leave that patient at risk for experiencing retraumatization, lack of opportunity for closure in her personal relationships, and/or death with uncontrolled symptom burden.

Palliative care principles, consisting of effective communication, holistic assessment of symptom burden, evaluation of decision-making capacity, advance care planning alongside decision-makers, and interdisciplinary care (including psychiatric care when possible) should be applied to these patients.[3] The Palliative APRN in Case 1 used the therapeutic approach of careful and compassionate rapport-building to establish a trusting relationship that likely allowed AM to accept palliation of her symptoms and a peaceful end of life. This chapter also aims to introduce trauma-informed care and harm reduction, principles that are helpful when trying to create a

trusting relationship like the one in the case study. Palliative APRNs can be the leaders in reframing care to focus on all aspects of suffering for patients with SMI by using the inherent philosophy of care that nurses employ in relationship-building and holistic care along with the framework of total pain as advocated by Saunders.

In fact, psychiatry and palliative care have long shared similar ideals in treatment planning that is focused on detailed assessment based on the biopsychosocial model, successful communication, rapport-building, symptom management, family-centered care, and interdisciplinary management.[9] SMIs, such as schizophrenia and bipolar disorder, for example, are not curable disorders and thus the approach is focused on relief of symptoms and improved quality of life, clearly in line with palliative care.[9] Psychiatry and palliative care both focus on relationships with the patient and family and understand the therapeutic benefit of being with suffering that cannot be cured. Hence, palliative psychiatry is an "emerging subspecialty discipline at the intersection of palliative medicine and psychiatry"[10] that clearly adds value to the core palliative team. Since many psychiatric disorders are chronic and have high rates of relapse, palliative psychiatry aims to address symptom burden and optimize quality of life in these patients. The palliative psychiatrist and the palliative psychiatric APRN work collaboratively with palliative care teams and provide expertise in the following areas:

- Complex treatment planning (i.e., psychopharmacological and nonpharmacological interventions as well as psychotherapies)

- Diagnostic challenges in the assessment of psychiatric symptoms in a terminally ill patient

- Clarification of ethical issues (e.g., decisional capacity assessment)

- Advice and support to the palliative care team

- Assistance in identifying risk for complex grief and in bereavement care

Just as in primary palliative care, palliative psychiatry recognizes that best health outcomes may be met by focusing on the debility of the symptoms rather than the disease itself. While this chapter is focused on assisting palliative APRNs, it is important to recognize the growing need to incorporate palliative psychiatric providers into the team.

GENERAL APPROACH TO WORKING WITH SMI PATIENTS

To successfully engage with this patient population, the palliative APRN can understand the barriers to care, pull from both trauma-informed care and harm reduction practices, become self-aware of personal biases, and utilize interdisciplinary teams when available. In Case Study 1, AM did not disclose a history of psychiatric hospitalizations to the palliative APRN for months. She reported that she felt a significant shift in how healthcare providers interacted with her after learning about a psychiatric diagnosis. Healthcare providers may be less comfortable with the management of these patients due to lack of knowledge of SMI disease trajectories or treatment plans. Moreover, in palliative care settings, clinicians may be confused about *when and if* patients are able to engage in their own advance care planning based on their current capacity, as discussed later in this chapter. These patients are clinically complex on many levels, with a wide variety of barriers in the way of successful outcomes.

In the face of these barriers, a different approach may be useful to create therapeutic relationships with this patient population. *Trauma-informed care* is an approach that assumes that most, if not all, individuals have experienced some level of trauma in their pasts.[11] As such, an individual's view of self, others, and systems are influenced by that trauma. Proponents of this care assert that the trauma-informed lens should be uniformly integrated in all patient assessments. When implemented systemically, this concept has the ability to shift the mindset of the clinician from "what is wrong with this person?" to "what has happened to this person?"[12] Trauma-informed care consists of five key principles: safety, choice, collaboration, trustworthiness, and empowerment, further explored in Table 46.1.

While trauma-informed care can be used to benefit all patients, there is a clear application within those of the SMI patient population who have life-limiting illness. Whether trauma is formally a part of their SMI diagnosis, such as posttraumatic stress disorder (PTSD), or other health conditions have created more implicit traumas over time, this lens helps the provider recognize that behavior may be a symptom of trauma. Due to the fact that the patient accessing palliative care has a life-limiting (thus implicitly traumatic) illness, the incidence of posttraumatic stress symptoms is high in the terminally ill population. The palliative APRN can use the trauma-informed principles to create a meaningful, therapeutic relationship with these at-risk individuals.

Another useful clinical lesson can be derived from the world of addiction medicine. Harm reduction is similar to trauma-informed care in its aim to make care patient-centered, formally allowing for the patient to partner in the creation of expectations and desired health outcomes.[13] Harm reduction also does not penalize the patient if health outcomes are not met or even if the patient engages in behaviors that negatively affect well-being.[14] For example, partnering with a patient to reduce the amount and frequency of methamphetamine use, if not altogether stopping use, is considered harm reduction. Again, this type of care comes with core principles, seen in Table 46.2, which can be applied to patients within this population.[15]

This framework can be useful for the palliative APRN when initiating care of individuals with SMI. This philosophy supports the idea that all patients are the true experts of their experience. While the healthcare provider provides guidance based on evidence based practice, to date, the patient has survived and navigated their illnesses without the help of the healthcare provider. When approaching the care of patients with SMI and life-threatening illness, harm reduction principles create an environment of honesty, realistic expectations, and true partnership.

When working alongside these patients, it is also important for the clinician to be aware of implicit and personal biases. It is clear that mental illness is stigmatized in our society,[16] and, even with the best intentions, those stigmas can lead to implicit or explicit biases.[17] The palliative APRN can reflect on their experiences of working with patients who have concurrent SMI to try to identify which patients or encounters have made them uncomfortable. Is the APRN able to recognize moments of transference or countertransference when in a difficult situation? Being self-aware of biases and even one's own personal traumas is an important factor in creating a collaborative, successful partnership with SMI patients.

Assessment of patients with SMI is the same as with all other palliative care patients and should be holistic, systematic, and compassionate. A psychiatric history, including past treatments, hospitalizations, symptoms of mania and psychosis, and suicide attempts should be obtained at the start of treatment. Assessing the support system of the patient and finding collateral information from past psychiatric providers, past psychiatric hospitalizations, outpatient mental health centers, and case managers will also contribute to the assessment. Patients with SMI often receive care within silos,[18] contributing to care disparities at end of life. These patients find themselves with medical illnesses that psychiatric providers are uncomfortable managing as well as with psychiatric illnesses that palliative providers have less experience in treating. Good palliative care means breaking down these silos and working together with psychiatric providers who may have been the biggest source of support for these patients. The patient's psychiatric provider can assist the palliative APRN in better understanding their SMI diagnosis, treatment plan,

Table 46.1 TRAUMA-INFORMED CARE PRINCIPLES

PRINCIPLE	DEFINITION	IN PRACTICE
Safety	Ensuring physical and emotional safety	Clinical areas are welcoming and privacy is respected
Choice	Establishing individual patient choice and control	Individuals are given clear messages about their rights and responsibilities to help design their care plans
Collaboration	Making decisions with the individual, sharing power	Individuals are provided a significant role in planning and evaluating healthcare services
Trustworthiness	Providing clarity, consistency, and interpersonal boundaries	Respectful and professional boundaries are maintained during clinical encounters
Empowerment	Prioritizing empowerment and skill building	Affirmation and validation are provided at every clinical encounter

From University at Buffalo.[12]

Table 46.2 HARM REDUCTION PRINCIPLES

PRINCIPLE	DEFINITION	APPROACHES
1. Humanism	Providers value, care for, respect, and dignify patients as individuals. Recognize that individuals with serious mental illness (SMI) may choose a different path. It is important to recognize that people do things for a reason; harmful health behaviors provide some benefit to the individual, and those benefits must be assessed and acknowledged to understand the balance between harms and benefits. Understanding why individuals make decisions is empowering for providers.	Moral judgments made against individuals do not produce positive health outcomes. Compassion at end of life is imperative. Grudges based on past behavior are not held against individuals. A respectful death is a right for everyone. Palliative care services are user-friendly and responsive to patients' needs. The palliative APRN accepts patients' choices.
2. Pragmatism	No individual will ever achieve perfect health behaviors. The palliative APRN must be accepting of the individual with SMI. Health behaviors and the ability to change them are influenced by social and community norms; behaviors do not occur within a vacuum.	A range of palliative, supportive approaches is provided. The palliative APRN provides care messages about actual harms to individuals as opposed to moral or societal standards.
	The palliative APRN must understand the social determinants of health (SDOH) of the individual with SMI.	
3. Individualism	Every person presents with his or her own needs and strengths. The palliative APRN seeks to find those in the individual with SMI. People present with spectrums of harm and receptivity and therefore require a spectrum of intervention options.	The palliative APRN assesses strengths and needs for each individual, and no assumptions are made based on harmful health behaviors. The palliative APRN does not have one universal application of protocol or messaging for individuals with SMI. Instead, the APRN tailors messages and interventions for each individual and maximizes treatment options.
	The palliative APRN facilitates collaborative care for the individual with SMI.	
4. Autonomy	Although the palliative APRN offers suggestions and education regarding individuals' medications and treatment options, individuals ultimately make their own choices about medications, treatment, and health behaviors to the best of their abilities, beliefs, and priorities.	The palliative APRN–patient partnerships is important, and is exemplified by patient-driven care, shared decision-making, and reciprocal learning. Care negotiations are based on the current state of the individual.
5. Incrementalism	The palliative APRN understands that any positive change is a step toward improved health, and positive change can take years. The palliative APRN understands and plan for backward movements or return of unhealthy behaviors.	The palliative APRN can help individuals celebrate any positive movement. It is important to recognize that, at times, all people experience plateaus or negative trajectories. The palliative APRN provides valuable positive reinforcement.
6. Accountability without termination	Individuals are responsible for their choices and health behaviors. Individuals are not "fired" for not achieving goals. Individuals have the right to make harmful health decisions, and palliative APRNs can still help them to understand that the consequences are their own.	While helping individuals to understand the impact of their choices and behaviors is valuable, backward movement is not penalized. The palliative APRN works in collaboration with and the support of a team to discuss an individual's care.

From Hawk et al.[15]

and disease trajectory and provide assistance in assessing decisional capacity in patients with psychotic disorders.

In addition to working with the psychiatric provider, the palliative APRN works with the other members of the interdisciplinary team to provide good care. Social workers can assist with completing an in-depth biopsychosocial and spiritual evaluation that may highlight areas of distress, particularly if that patient now has a terminal diagnosis and is approaching end of life. A pharmacist may be needed to confirm the safety of medication regimens for both SMI and palliative needs (e.g., in identifying medication interactions that may be significant with psychotropics). The palliative APRN can promote the patient's wellness by being the leader in communication between all of the involved caregivers.

The next section reviews major psychotic disorders and bipolar disorders to assist the palliative APRN in being be more attuned to the symptoms and burdens of these patient populations. In addition, PTSD will be discussed because it has particular relevance and high prevalence in the palliative care population. The authors encourage readers to consult with psychiatry resources for more in-depth information and to consult with psychiatric colleagues if available and whenever possible.

PSYCHOTIC DISORDERS, MOOD DISORDERS, POSTTRAUMATIC STRESS DISORDER

PSYCHOSIS

First, it is important to understand the phenomenon of psychosis. This symptom, characterized by hallucinations and/or delusions, can be seen in patients with varying psychiatric disorders, which are categorized as primary and secondary psychotic disorders. Schizophrenia, schizoaffective disorder, and delusional disorder are the main primary psychotic disorders of which psychosis is the cardinal symptom. Affective disorders, such as bipolar and major depression, as well as anxiety disorders, such as obsessive compulsive disorder (OCD) and PTSD, may also present with psychosis when severe.

Secondary psychotic disorders are those in which psychosis is prominent and there is evidence that it is the direct pathophysiological consequence of a medical condition or a substance or medication. Secondary psychotic disorders may be seen in Alzheimer's dementia, Parkinson's disease, diffuse Lewy body disease, frontotemporal lobar degeneration, cerebrovascular disease (including cerebrovascular accident [CVA] and brain tumor), Huntington's disease, prion disease, traumatic brain injury, and HIV, among others (Box 46.1).[19] *It is important to remember that patients with severe and persistent mental illness may also develop secondary psychotic disorders, when new or different psychotic symptoms arise. Proper assessment diagnosis, and treatment are essential.*

SCHIZOPHRENIA SPECTRUM AND OTHER PSYCHOTIC DISORDERS

Schizophrenia, schizoaffective disorder, and delusional disorder fall under the umbrella of the schizophrenia spectrum and other psychotic disorders (as described in the *Diagnostic and Statistical Manual of Mental Disorders* [DSM-5]).[21] These disorders are diagnosed after all other potential reasons for the psychosis are ruled out (e.g., neurocognitive disorders, substance use, delirium). Schizophrenia is a heterogenous syndrome with a cluster of symptoms that are significant enough to cause an impairment in occupational or social functioning. The primary symptoms of schizophrenia are two or more of the following: delusions, hallucinations, disorganized speech/thought, grossly disorganized or catatonic behavior, and/or negative symptoms. Cognitive impairment is often seen

---

Box 46.1 PSYCHIATRIC SYMPTOMS DEFINITIONS

Hallucinations are defined as sensory perceptions without the presence of an external stimulus and may be visual, tactile, auditory, gustatory, or olfactory. Hallucinations may or may not cause distress to the patient, and the patient may or may not have insight into the fact that the hallucination is not based in reality. In schizophrenia and other primary psychotic disorders, hallucinations are primarily auditory, followed by visual, and are often negative in nature, speaking in a derogatory manner to or about the patient. Visual hallucinations in schizophrenia are usually surrealistic, featuring "denatured people, parts of bodies, unidentifiable things and superimposed things."[20] Hallucinations occurring in delirium are usually distressing to the patient and are most often visual hallucinations of different animals or shapes. In PTSD, patients may experience visual and auditory hallucinations consistent with the theme of the trauma or of a depressive nature, and paranoid delusions as well. Hallucinations experienced in Alzheimer's dementia, Lewy body disease, and other organic brain syndromes are predominantly visual and may or may not be distressing. In Parkinson's disease, visual hallucinations predominate and are often not disturbing to the patient. In affective disorders, hallucinations are often auditory and congruent with their mood, whether elevated (i.e., in mania) or depressed. Not all hallucinations are considered pathological; for example, hearing one's voice called or a comforting voice in times of distress, seeing a deceased loved one, or the lights and visions seen or voices heard during profound religious experiences are considered within the range of normal.[20] Often, when a person is close to death, comforting visions will appear and reassure them.

Delusions are fixed, false beliefs, and their content may reflect a variety of themes (e.g., persecutory, referential, grandiose, erotomanic, somatic, religious, or nihilistic).[21] The most common delusions are persecutory and are often referred to as *paranoia*; these are seen frequently in schizophrenia spectrum disorders as well as neurocognitive disorders. Delusions seen in schizophrenia spectrum disorders are often bizarre while those in neurocognitive disorders are less so and reflect more ordinary life experiences. A common delusion in Alzheimer's disease, for example, is that people are stealing from the patient, reflecting the fact that they do not remember what happened to an item. Another non-bizarre and common delusion is that one is being spied on or that someone is poisoning the patient's food. A bizarre delusion example would be that aliens have implanted devices into one's brain and record everything one does to report back to the mother ship. Other bizarre delusions include thought withdrawal or insertion, where the patient believes that their thoughts are being controlled by an outside force. Delusions, like hallucinations, may also be more or less disturbing to the patient, a fact that should be understood when considering potential treatments.

Thought disorders (i.e., disorganized thinking) are prevalent in schizophrenia and schizoaffective disorders and are often identified through the patient's speech.[21] When one is talking with a person with a thought disorder, the observer will feel as if the patient is not making any sense or that they are very difficult to follow. The patient may switch from one topic to another quickly, with little association between thoughts (*derailment* or *loose associations*) or thoughts may be *tangential*, with vaguely related ideas connecting them. Thoughts (and hence speech) may also be completely incoherent, which is described as "word salad." Disorganized or abnormal motor behavior exists along a spectrum "from childlike 'silliness' to unpredictable agitation" as well as catatonia (i.e., marked decrease in reactivity to the environment).[21] Negative symptoms include diminished emotional expression and *avolition*. Patients with these symptoms will not express emotion; their voice sounds flat and monotone, and their facial expression is blunted. Avolition includes diminished desire to participate in work, social activities or hobbies, or even self-care. Other negative symptoms include diminished speech, lack of ability to experience pleasure, and lack of interest in social activities.

From American Psychiatric Association.[21]

in schizophrenia and leads to functional impairment, but does not de facto imply lack of capacity for medical decision-making. It is distinguished from schizoaffective disorder or major depressive disorder with psychosis by the lack of significant mood disturbances.

Lifetime prevalence of schizophrenia is about 0.3–0.7%, and most patients are chronically ill, require daily living supports, and they experience exacerbations and remissions of active symptoms. Schizophrenia generally develops in the late teenage to early adulthood years, but onset, particularly in women, may occur during middle age as well. Over the life course of a patient with schizophrenia, generally the psychotic symptoms diminish while the cognitive symptoms remain stable.

Schizophrenia is one of the top 10 most common disorders in the world, and the long-term disability burden is by far the highest among all mental illnesses. Drug and alcohol use are more prevalent in patients with schizophrenia than in the general population, and the prevalence of comorbid substance use disorder is approximately 42%.[22] Methamphetamine and cannabis in particular can initiate psychosis in patients who are susceptible to schizophrenia, which has a strong hereditary component, and these substances can contribute to worsened disease trajectory and quality of life.

Due to their symptomatology and resulting functional impairments as well as the stigma against them, patients with SMI, and in particular schizophrenia, avoid healthcare and experience many healthcare disparities leading to lower quality and quantity of life.[23] These vulnerable patients have a higher rate of hospital mortality, fewer advance care plans, higher use of long-term institutional care, and are less likely to receive opioids and significantly less likely to access palliative care.[1,3] They have lower rates of specialist use, worse survival after a cancer diagnosis, and more unnecessary aggressive and invasive interventions.[1,3] In addition, these patients at end of life present with complex ethical situations related to decisional capacity and autonomy (in the form of refusing care and involuntary treatment) as well as stigma, necessitating strong interdisciplinary teamwork with psychiatry, outpatient care, social work, and clinical ethicists. Of note and discussed later, most patients with SMI, when not in the throes of an acute exacerbation and who are stabilized on medication, have decisional capacity.

Schizoaffective disorder is a psychotic disorder similar to schizophrenia in that the patient has primary symptoms of schizophrenia as well as major mood episodes (manic or depressive). The psychosis occurs outside of the mood disorders, as opposed to a patient with bipolar or major depression who may become psychotic only during the mood episodes. Negative symptoms may be less severe than seen in schizophrenia. Schizoaffective disorder is less common than schizophrenia, with a prevalence rate of 0.3%.

Delusional disorder is a psychotic disorder in which a patient presents with delusions but not usually with hallucinations. Functioning is not usually as impaired as in schizophrenia and schizoaffective disorder outside of the impact of the delusion. This type of psychotic illness can be difficult to identify as their behavior appears normal when their delusional ideas are being discussed or acted on. However, these patients can become hostile, litigious, and aggressive if their delusions are challenged. This can be particularly difficult when addressing delusions that are persecutory, erotomanic, or rooted in jealousy.

In Case Study 1, the palliative APRN surmised that AM had previously been diagnosed with a schizophrenia spectrum disorder. AM presented to the office disheveled, physically agitated, and reported her needs in a way that was very difficult to follow. AM was not forthcoming about psychiatric history and unwilling to engage with psychiatry referral, making multidisciplinary care challenging. The palliative APRN had to take time to interpret her speech and try to elicit more direct responses with motivational interviewing, despite AM's clear thought disorder. This became easier over time as rapport was built. Even though communication was challenging due to AM's untreated psychosis, it was determined that she had decisional capacity related to her medical decision-making as she clearly articulated the risks and benefits of both adhering and not adhering to proposed treatments. Through careful exploration of her wishes, the APRN learned that the patient's goals included being pain free and living as long as possible, even though the patient did not always agree with oncology or primary medical treatment plans. Despite her fear of medical facilities, through use of trauma-informed care, a trusting relationship was eventually created. AM felt comfortable coming into the hospital when she felt she was acutely decompensating, eventually dying on inpatient hospice service.

CASE STUDY 2: THE PATIENT WITH BIPOLAR DISORDER

EM was a 32-year-old woman with medical history including hypertension, asthma, lupus, rheumatoid arthritis, fibromyalgia, seizure disorder, anxiety, and depression. She was referred to palliative care for pain/symptom management and psychosocial support. EM had frequent acute medical events leading to admission, including asthma exacerbations requiring intubation and lupus flares with pain crisis. She shared with the palliative service that she had little social support in the community and often felt she did not have the necessary resources to care for her three young daughters.

During an assessment with the palliative licensed social worker (LCSW), EM confided that she had been previously hospitalized for a suicide attempt. She was starting to feel that she would be "better off if I never woke up again," but never had any regular relationship with a psychiatrist. She described a history of shift in mood to feeling very irritable and anxious, accompanied with a very high energy level, only sleeping 3 hours per night and spending money on unnecessary items, leaving her without enough funds for rent and food. During these episodes EM experienced asthma crises and pain crises which would often correspond with more despondent and suicidal moods.

The palliative APRN successfully linked EM to a psychiatric provider who diagnosed these as manic episodes from bipolar disorder; he suggested the mood stabilizer and antiepileptic agent valproic acid (Depakote), which significantly reduced her manic episodes, regulated her sleep, and reduced her anxiety. EM experienced significantly less frequent asthma exacerbations and eventually was able to start on duloxetine for her pain associated with fibromyalgia and depression. Once her mental illness was under more control, the palliative care team was able to address her deeper relational wounds with her family caused by many years of untreated mania.

BIPOLAR DISORDER

Bipolar disorders are considered the "bridge" between psychotic disorders and depressive disorders. [21] Distinctions are made between bipolar I and bipolar II disorders (with bipolar II displaying less severe functional impairments during hypomania and lack of psychosis); however, both cause serious functional impairment over the course of a lifetime. The defining feature of bipolar disorders is the presence of at least one manic/hypomanic episode as well as at least one depressive episode in their lifetime. Some patients have more manic and hypomanic episodes than depressive, while others have more depressive, and still others have mixed episodes or rapidly cycle between mania and depression. *Mania* is an altered mood state that is distinct from the patient's normal or depressed moods and is abnormal and persistently elevated, expansive (i.e., very enthusiastic, grandiose, extremely friendly), or irritable accompanied by high energy. Patients who are manic will engage in multiple projects (i.e., increase in goal-directed activity), particularly in areas that they are not knowledgeable about, and they may engage in these projects at all hours. During this time the patient will also experience symptoms of inflated self-esteem or grandiosity, decreased need for sleep (i.e., only needing 3 hours of sleep as opposed to their normal 8 hours), increased or pressured speech, mood lability, flight of ideas or thoughts, distractibility (i.e., inattention), psychomotor agitation, and/or excessive involvement in activities that have a high potential for painful consequences.[21] A person who is manic may be loud, difficult to interrupt, highly distractible, unable to focus, forceful or pressured in their speech, and may become psychotic as well. The high impulsivity and extremely poor judgment during manic episodes may increase the risk of danger to self and others.

Rapid cycling is a high-risk situation, defined as four or more mood episodes in a year. Patients with rapid cycling have a poorer long-term prognosis, more suicide attempts, and poorer response to pharmacotherapy.[24] Rapid cycling is seen more often in patients with a history of childhood trauma.[25] Antidepressant therapy in the absence of a mood stabilizer may also induce rapid cycling, which underlies the importance of proper assessment and history-taking in any patient with a history of depression. When a patient with bipolar disorder has episodes with mixed features, this indicates that the mood state has both manic and depressive features, and it is a sign of more severe illness and poorer treatment response.[26, 27] Mixed states are extremely uncomfortable and distressing for patients and are associated with higher rates of comorbidity, psychosis, suicide, and substance abuse.[27] Recognizing that a patient has bipolar disorder (i.e., has a history of mania or hypomania) is a key task in the assessment of the patient with SMI for both safety and well-being and should trigger referral or consult with a psychiatric provider.

In Case Study 2, EM's manic episodes were clearly defined by irritable mood and a reduced need for sleep, accompanied by increased energy and impulsive buying which caused her to not be able to provide for the basic needs of her family. This elevated activity level with little rest often led to exacerbations in her asthma, sometimes requiring acute admission. Once admitted, EM rarely could follow nursing care or directions from medical providers. This discord led to her being loud and sometimes agitated. In addition, her pain crises often corresponded with depressed mood. The palliative APRN successfully identified the need for psychiatric evaluation, which led to proper diagnosis and stabilization through appropriate pharmacology interventions. After the SMI was addressed, continued support allowed for decreased psychosocial distress with ongoing counseling to promote successful personal relationships.

CASE STUDY 3: THE PATIENT WITH POSTTRAUMATIC STRESS DISORDER

JH was a 37-year-old man with medical history of posttraumatic stress disorder (PTSD) and active IV drug use leading to endocarditis following bioprosthetic valve replacements, septic pulmonary embolism, splenic abscess, and osteomyelitis. He was referred to palliative care for pain management, support, and goals of care during an acute admission for severe sepsis with multifocal infection. In conjunction with the pain and addiction medicine service, JH was placed on methadone for both opioid use disorder and pain management.

The palliative APRN and LCSW utilized motivational interviewing to get to know JH on a deeper level. He revealed that he was previously in the Navy and had been involved in the 9/11 terrorism attack response. JH shared that these experiences resulted in physical, emotional, and psychological traumas that manifested in severe physical pain. This pain is what led JH to seek analgesia through illicit drug use, specifically heroin. JH had multiple admissions for sepsis, with frequent signing out against medical advice (AMA), although after methadone induction JH was able to remain admitted until discharge.

JH remained homeless and experienced difficulty in initiating follow-up with the methadone clinic due to severe mistrust of medical providers, hypervigilance related to his PTSD, and deep spiritual pain in the context of drug use. However, the palliative APRN and team continued to work diligently with JH, even though he experienced multiple relapses. The team celebrated his successes when he was able to stay off heroin, referred him to a clean needle program, and provided a nonjudgmental and caring safe place for the patient to receive care for his many wounds. Treatment consisted of adjuvant pain medications, methadone treatment for pain and opioid use disorder, sertraline for his PTSD symptoms, and social work assistance in finding safe shelter, food, clothing, and a shower. Over time JH was able to sustain longer and longer periods of time off heroin, experienced fewer hospitalizations, and was able to reestablish contact with a long-lost daughter. He retained capacity for decision-making and refused the recommendation of amputation. He eventually died comfortably in the hospital after admission related to his osteomyelitis.

POSTTRAUMATIC STRESS DISORDER

While PTSD may not always be considered a SMI, the incidence increases from 8% in the general population to 35% in cancer patients, making it a significant mental illness in the palliative care context. Furthermore, significantly ill or terminal individuals are at risk of experiencing significant PTSD symptoms at high rates, though they may not meet all DSM-5 criteria for formal diagnosis (68% in a study of breast cancer patients, 64% in ICU patients with various life-threatening conditions, and up to 88% in a study of terminal cancer patients).[28] Patients with a history of trauma, particularly in childhood, have worse health outcomes, including chronic health conditions, depression, and substance abuse.[29]

PTSD develops as a reaction to actual or threatened death, serious injury, or sexual violence that is experienced directly to self, is witnessed, or that has occurred to a loved one. It may also be experienced as secondary trauma by medical professionals and first responders who bear witness to their patients' traumas. Symptoms include intrusive reexperiencing of the trauma (e.g., nightmares, flashbacks), hyperarousal and increased reactivity (e.g., hyperstartle, hypervigilance), and avoidance of reminders of the event(s), as well as negative alterations in cognition and mood. These patients often have dysfunctional coping mechanisms, irritable and depressed mood, difficulty trusting authority, and withdrawal from social support, all leading to challenges with relationships, adherence to treatment, and maintaining work, and spiritual distress. Substance use and mood disorders are frequently comorbid, pain sensation is altered, somatization may occur, and sleep is frequently problematic as well.[30]

In Case Study 3, JH reported to the team that after being a 9/11 first responder, his untreated emotional pain led to physical pain. Eventually the pain was so intense JH sought out analgesia through illicit drug use. He noted that after injecting heroin and fentanyl, his body and mind both "felt quiet for the first time" since being in the service. He also deeply distrusted medical providers (a symptom of PTSD) which caused him to leave the hospital before treatment was complete and experience recurring infection.

Patients who have a history of PTSD are at increased risk for a return of symptoms at end of life, even if their disorder has been previously under control, because they now are facing impending death. In addition, in a study by Bickel et al., Veterans Administration patients who suffer from PTSD have increased symptom burden at end of life, and PTSD may be a risk factor for terminal delirium and increased antipsychotic usage in the last week of life.[30] (see Chapter 23 "Care of the Veteran With Palliative Care Needs," for information on PTSD in the Veteran.)

Whether the trauma that has caused PTSD is more recent or in the distant past, patients with active PTSD symptoms are at risk for a less than desirable dying experience due to several factors. Communication may be worsened due to the coping factor of avoidance of reminders of death. Anger, irritability, and mistrust are common symptoms of PTSD that may lead to breakdown of important discussions with providers regarding end-of-life decision-making, and they also may cause poorer family and social relationships and support. Life review has been shown to increase quality of life and depression and anxiety scores, and it leads to a greater sense of meaning at end of life; however, due to avoidance symptoms seen in PTSD, patients may not engage in life review and, if they do, may experience retraumatization and increased symptoms.[28]

NONPHARMACOLOGICAL AND PHARMACOLOGICAL APPROACHES TO SERIOUS MENTAL ILLNESS

Treatment of psychosis in palliative care includes pharmacological and nonpharmacological approaches and is based on the etiology, assessment of the risks and benefits of treatment and nontreatment, reversibility of the condition, and concomitant symptoms, along with the consideration and discussion of goals of care for the patient. Improved level of functioning, including the ability to resolve relationship issues and perform other end-of-life tasks, should be considered.

NONPHARMACOLOGICAL APPROACHES

Patients with serious mental illness and psychotic disorders in particular have many factors that contribute to a poor quality of life. A palliative approach to this patient population aims at enhancing their quality of life not only through medication but also through many nonpharmacological approaches. A qualitative study by Sweers et al. (2013) showed that patients with schizophrenia—no different from most individuals—desire warm, trusting, and skilled companionship at end of life; absence of pain and physical deterioration; respect for and promotion of their autonomy; social support and to not die alone[31]; and attendance to spiritual concerns (i.e., finding meaning in suffering, illness, and death). As a provider, cultivating a compassionate presence for patients with SMI will go a long way in developing the trust and rapport necessary to providing beneficial palliative care.

Meeting basic needs such as housing, relationship/social, food, hygiene, and recreation and entertainment are tantamount to living a higher quality of life but are often unmet in the SMI population. Needless to say, these basic needs should be thoroughly addressed by the palliative care team. Research in patients with SMI has shown that cognitive-behavioral therapy (CBT) can also be potentially beneficial in addressing needs, if appropriate to the patient's medical condition.[32] Mobilizing social support for help in decision-making may also contribute to improved quality of life and avoidance of aggressive interventions at end of life.

For patients with PTSD, traditional pharmacotherapy and psychotherapy approaches may not be helpful and may worsen symptoms in patients with a life-limiting illness, particularly if the primary trauma is disease-related. Standard psychotherapeutic approaches often cause worsened symptoms before improvement, and this process may be too time-intensive and will also not be effective as long as the primary trauma continues. Standard pharmacological treatment (i.e., selective serotonin reuptake inhibitors [SSRIs] sertraline and paroxetine) also may take too long to reach their therapeutic potential, similar to treatment for depression at end of life. Benzodiazepines are contraindicated in PTSD and are too often used inappropriately for treatment of PTSD-related anxiety, frequently causing worsened symptoms, presumably due to disinhibition. General approaches to patients with PTSD include cultivating compassionate presence, allowing the patient to feel in control of decisions and situation, validation of their experience, avoidance of triggers such as loud noises and restraints, and a focus on strengths and resilience.[33] In addition, psychoeducation about PTSD and when symptoms are likely to be exacerbated should occur with families and patients, which will help the patient mentally prepare and improve trust between provider and patient.

Other approaches to treatment of PTSD at end of life have been developed including modified CBT, modified eye movement desensitization reprocessing (EMDR), a stepwise psychosocial model guided by palliative care social workers, and life review techniques (including meaning-centered psychotherapy and *dignity therapy*, a short course of psychotherapy that focuses on highlighting meaning and purpose when someone is at end of life[34]), as well as spiritually oriented psychotherapeutic techniques to address areas of spiritual pain frequently seen in patients with PTSD.[33] Complementary and alternative medicine (CAM) techniques may be helpful for patients with PTSD but caution is necessary to avoid triggering traumatic memories (e.g., massage in patients with sexual trauma).[33]

The palliative APRN should adhere to principles of trauma-informed care in the approach to patients with a history of trauma. It is not recommended to probe into the trauma history as this may cause a resurgence of symptoms. However, if a patient discloses trauma, the APRN should respond with gentle and compassionate acknowledgment of the suffering and difficulty the patient has experienced. Recognize symptoms of trauma and refer the patient accordingly to social work, psychology, and/or psychiatry. If the patient has a 3-month or longer life expectancy, consider an SSRI such as sertraline or paroxetine. Trauma-informed care is congruent with a palliative approach in its focus on partnering with the patient to empower them to make informed choices and participate in their own care, as well as in its focus on interdisciplinary collaboration. Taking steps to ensure the patient's physical and emotional safety is key, as well as developing good rapport as a trustworthy provider who informs the patient of the details of what proposed treatments entail, what are expected outcomes, and potential risks, as well as identifying who will be involved in providing care (Box 46.2).

Box 46.2 APPROACH TO PATIENT WITH TRAUMA HISTORY

1. Respond gently and acknowledge suffering.

2. Recognize symptoms of trauma.

3. Make appropriate referrals.

4. If life expectancy >3 months, consider starting an SSRI.

5. Focus on partnering with patient and give control to patient as much as possible.

6. Ensure emotional as well as physical safety.

Racine, Killam, Madigan[11], University at Buffalo. Buffalo Center for Social Research.[12]

PHARMACOLOGICAL TREATMENT

For patients with psychotic disorders, first- and second-generation antipsychotics are utilized in addition to treatment of any underlying organic disorder that may be causing psychosis. Antipsychotics, reviewed in Table 46.3, are also used in treatment-refractory depressive disorders or depression with psychosis, as well as in patients with severe OCD. Antipsychotics are also appropriate for patients with bipolar illness because they have mood stabilizing properties and particularly in patients who are psychotic while manic. As the stress of medical illness may worsen psychotic symptoms in patients, it is important to be cautious about de-prescribing antipsychotics in patients who are not imminently dying.[3] Care should be taken regarding antipsychotic dosages in psychotic disorders because these are usually much higher than when used for treatment of delirium and nausea. Likewise, it is recommended to utilize psychiatric provider consultation if needing to stop antipsychotic therapy for any medical contingency. Antipsychotic therapy may also improve the psychotic patient's ability to participate in decision-making, which is not an insignificant consideration.

Patients with bipolar illness require a mood stabilizer such as lithium or valproic acid to control symptoms of decreased need for sleep, severe irritability and/or grandiosity, mood lability, and impulsivity seen in mania and hypomania in particular. Lithium is also protective against suicide. In addition to lithium and valproic acid, other first-line mood stabilizers include carbamazepine and lamotrigine. The palliative APRN is reminded to consult prescribing guides for mood stabilizers and seek psychiatric consultation for more detailed pharmacologic information. Antipsychotics are second-line, but are often prescribed as well for psychosis associated with bipolar and/or mood stabilization. Avoid antidepressant use that is unopposed by a mood stabilizer as it may trigger manic episodes and rapid cycling.

ANTIPSYCHOTIC CAUTIONS

Use of antipsychotics in elderly patients with dementia increases risk of stroke and all-cause mortality by about two

Table 46.3 FIRST- AND SECOND-GENERATION ANTIPSYCHOTICS

NEUROTRANSMITTER	FIRST-GENERATION "TYPICAL" ANTIPSYCHOTICS (FGAS) D_2 ANTAGONISTS	SECOND-GENERATION "ATYPICAL" ANTIPSYCHOTICS (SGAS) $D_2/5$-HT_{2A} ANTAGONISTS (*WITH 4 NOTABLE EXCEPTIONS)
Side effects	Higher risk of EPS (dyskinesia, parkinsonism, akathisia, dystonia), tardive dyskinesia QTc prolongation Hyperprolactinemia Falls Sedation Anticholinergic effects Lowered seizure threshold Cholestatic jaundice Sexual dysfunction *Rare but potentially fatal:* Agranulocytosis, neuroleptic malignant syndrome (NMS), sudden death	More variation in neurotransmitter action than in FGAs, thus more variation in side effect profiles, Lower risk of EPS QTc prolongation Hyperprolactinemia Falls Sedation Higher risk of metabolic syndrome, hyperlipidemia, diabetes mellitus, weight gain Sexual dysfunction *Rare but potentially fatal:* NMS, sudden death, agranulocytosis, DRESS, myocarditis, cardiomyopathy
	Black box risk in patients with dementia: 1.6 to 1.7-fold increased risk of mortality when used to treat behavioral symptoms of dementia	
Examples	*High potency:* Fluphenazine, haloperidol, loxapine, perphenazine, pimozide, thiothixene, and trifluoperazine *Low potency:* Chlorpromazine, thioridazine	Olanzapine, risperidone, quetiapine, clozapine, ziprasidone, brexipiprazole *exceptions: Pimavanserin (no D_2 affinity) Aripiprazole and brexipiprazole (D_2 receptor partial agonists) Cariprazine (D_3-preferring D_3/D_2 receptor partial agonist)
Dosages	*High potency:* 1–10 mg of a high potency antipsychotic medication (higher risk of EPS) *Low potency:* 100-800 mg of a low potency antipsychotic medication (higher risk of sedation, orthostatic hypotension, dry mouth, constipation)	Variable
Efficacy	No notable differences in efficacy between FGAs and SGAs Chosen for individual efficacy (history of good effect) and side-effect profile	

Drug reaction with eosinophilia and systemic symptoms (DRESS), extrapyramidal symptoms (EPS).

From: Shalev Fields, Shapiro[1], Shalev, Brewster, Levenson[3] Trachsel et al.[9], Fairman, Irwin[10] Shalev, Brewster, Arbuckle, Levenson.[37]

---

times, and this is considered to be a black-box risk of all antipsychotics. Antipsychotics should be used with great caution in patients with dementia after clear and documented risk-benefit discussions with the surrogate decision-maker.

Antipsychotics increase the risk of seizures by lowering the seizure threshold: typically, the more sedating the antipsychotic and the higher the dose, the higher the risk. Additionally, antipsychotics cause and worsen parkinsonism of any etiology. Pimavanserin is the only antipsychotic approved by the US Food and Drug Administration (FDA) for treating psychosis in Parkinson's disease, and it does not carry the same risk as most other antipsychotics in worsening parkinsonism because it does not have any affinity for dopamine receptors.[35] In addition, clozapine and low-dose quetiapine have a lower risk of worsening movement symptoms and may be considered in treating problematic psychosis in Parkinson's disease and atypical parkinsonian disorders along with dopamine agonist tapering.

Antipsychotics are metabolized through P450 pathways and thus serious interactions may occur from induction or inhibition of hepatic metabolism (e.g., antiemetics, methadone, or certain antibiotics and antivirals). Hence, it is important to consult pharmacists and also perform drug–drug interaction checks before prescribing these agents. In addition, antipsychotics pose a risk of dose-dependent QT prolongation and resulting torsade de pointes. Additive effects of antipsychotics with other medications may also occur, such as increased sedation, hypotension, and QT prolongation. Antipsychotics may also reduce the effect of antiparkinsonian medications.[36] As with all treatments, a proper risk-benefit analysis and discussion should occur before using these medications.

OTHER ISSUES WITH SMI PATIENTS

DECISIONAL CAPACITY AND ADVANCE CARE PLANNING

Assessment of capacity to make medical decisions in patients with schizophrenia spectrum disorders can be challenging due to questions regarding capacity, refusal of care, and presence or history of suicidal behavior. Thus, issues related to determining capacity may present a barrier to advance care planning and complex decision-making in these patients. Research shows that many patients with schizophrenia spectrum disorders that are in remission *can* participate in end-of-life decision-making and have the same concerns as nonpsychiatric patients in regards to fear of physical pain, fear of dying alone, and hope for self-determination.[37] It is important to note that legal guardians may not always be able to make decisions related to healthcare, and these patients may not have the social support or skills to engage and enlist healthcare proxies in advance care planning. While barriers exist to determining decision-making capacity, advance care planning is vital to the provision of good palliative care and should include psychiatric as well as medical contingencies. Consultation and collaboration with psychiatry will help in determining the level of decision-making capacity the patient has, treatment of psychiatric symptoms to improve capacity, identification of potential healthcare surrogates, and engagement of the patient in complex medical and psychiatric decision-making.[37] In addition, training caregivers and surrogate decision-makers in end-of-life communication and legal issues may improve palliative care for these patients.

PAIN PERCEPTION

Patients with schizophrenia have difficulty with identifying and reporting pain,[3] which may contribute to reports that these patients have lower utilization of opioids. Utilizing caregivers who have a good relationship and are familiar with the patient, building trust and rapport, and using the Pain Assessment in Advanced Dementia Scale (PAINAD) may be helpful, even though the PAINAD scale has not yet been validated in this patient population.[3]

RISK OF VIOLENCE

While some patients with schizophrenia may exhibit hostility, most schizophrenic patients are not aggressive and are more likely to be victimized than to commit a violent act. Nonetheless, aggressive behavior has been diagnostically linked to schizophrenia, mania, alcohol abuse, organic brain syndrome (i.e., delirium and dementia), seizure disorder, and personality disorders,[38] with an increased risk of aggression in an acute psychiatric setting seen in younger males, and with nonadherence to treatment, substance abuse, impulsivity, and a history of violence.[38] The higher the degree of impulsivity combined with observed dysphoric and irritable affective state, the higher the risk of aggression, which is seen in patients with schizophrenia and bipolar disorder, as well as

dementia, implying that aggression is related to a complex serotonergic dysfunction.[39] The palliative APRN should identify and screen for factors that increase risk of violence and enlist psychiatric provider assistance in further assessment and proper management. Signs of increasing impulsivity, dysphoric and/or irritable mood, substance use, history of violence, and untreated paranoia and command hallucinations, no matter the etiology, should be given serious attention and warrant further assessment and mitigation of risk.

SUICIDE

Increased risk for suicide is associated with previous attempts and recent psychiatric hospitalization along with history of multiple hospitalizations; comorbid psychiatric, somatic, and substance use disorders; rapid cycling or predominantly depressive states; current mixed or depressed state; and longer duration of untreated illness.[40] Sociodemographic risk factors include being divorced, living in social isolation, being an unmarried parent, having occupational problems, age (<35 or >75 years), and having acute stressors. Impulsive and depressive personality traits and family history of suicide also indicate higher risk.

Suicide risk is high in patients with schizophrenia and schizoaffective disorder, with about 5–6% of patients with these disorders dying of suicide; 10–50% will at some point attempt suicide.[41] Command hallucinations increase suicide risk, as do comorbid substance use, depressive symptoms, feelings of hopelessness, being unemployed, and after a psychotic episode or hospital discharge.[21] Risk of suicide is higher in newly diagnosed patients with schizophrenia.[41]

Important in the care of the patient with bipolar illness is that the combination of impulsivity, poor judgment, psychosis, and/or irritability increases the danger for violence, which is particularly high in this patient population. In fact, the lifetime risk of suicide is 20–30 times higher than that of the general population, and 15–20% of bipolar patients die of suicide.[42] One-third to one-half of all bipolar patients attempt suicide at least once in their lifetime.[42] Referral to a psychiatric provider is preferred in patients with untreated bipolar disorder, and, if not possible, curbside consult may be fruitful.

EM, the patient in Case Study 2, alternated between depression with passive suicidal thoughts and mania, with her poor treatment adherence and associated asthma exacerbations leading to hospitalization. When working with SMI patients in a palliative care setting, a thorough suicide risk assessment along with assessment of their current mental state at every visit, along with timely referrals to psychiatric care, is very important in caring for this population.

SUMMARY

Working with the SMI patient population in a palliative care setting presents unique challenges. SMI causes substantial interference with everyday life, thereby increasing the potential domains of suffering.[4] The SMI patient population is at risk for increased symptom burden, worse health outcomes, and early mortality,[5] not only due to higher incidence of suicide and accidents, but also to lifestyle risk factors such as cigarette smoking; physical illnesses such as cardiovascular, respiratory, and metabolic disease; and worse access to care when compared to patients without SMI. This becomes particularly important and challenging when these individuals experience a life-limiting or terminal condition in addition to their mental health disorder. The care of these patients can be greatly positively impacted by the involvement of a palliative APRN.

Palliative care and psychiatry hold similar values, noting that treatment should include detailed biopsychosocial and spiritual assessment, successful communication, symptom management, family-centered care, and interdisciplinary management.[43] Regardless of the SMI diagnosis, or if the patient has experience psychosis or mania, the palliative APRN can use the notion of "total pain" to recognize that suffering is multidimensional and may need special care in the context of a life-threatening or terminal diagnosis. Concepts such as trauma-informed care and harm reduction can be used to create successful, therapeutic, and lasting relationships with this patient population. This patient-centered care can also help to recognize the individual's health-related goals rather than the goals of the healthcare system. It is important for the palliative APRN to have a baseline knowledge of each of the SMI diagnoses in order to best collaborate with the patient's mental health provider. The palliative APRN should initiate communication when talking to psychiatry and other medical specialties to ensure the best possible health outcomes for this patient population, and the palliative APRN may be positioned to advocate for palliative psychiatry to be integrated into the primary palliative care team for improved patient and team care.

REFERENCES

1. Shalev D, Fields L, Shapiro PA. End-of-life care in individuals with serious mental illness. *Psychosomatics.* 2020;61(5):428–435. doi:10.1016/j.psym.2020.06.003
2. Donald EE, Stajduhar KI. A scoping review of palliative care for persons with severe persistent mental illness. *Palliat Support Care.* 2019;17(4):479–487. doi:10.1017/S1478951519000087
3. Shalev D, Brewster KK, Levenson JA. End-of-life care for patients with schizophrenia #332. *J Palliat Med.* 2017;20(7):787–788. doi:10.1089/jpm.2017.0164
4. National Institute of Mental Health. Mental illness. From 2019 National Survey of Drug Use and Health (NSDUH) Releases. Available at https://www.nimh.nih.gov/health/statistics/mental-illness.shtml#:~:text=Serious mental illness (SMI) is,or more major life activities.
5. Fiorillo A, Luciano M, Pompili M, Sartorius N. Editorial: Reducing the mortality gap in people with severe mental disorders: The role of lifestyle psychosocial interventions. *Front Psychiatry.* 2019;10:434. doi:10.3389/fpsyt.2019.00434
6. Lomholt LH, Andersen DV, Sejrsgaard-Jacobsen C, et al. Mortality rate trends in patients diagnosed with schizophrenia or bipolar disorder: A nationwide study with 20 years of follow-up. *Int J Bipolar Disord.* 2019;7(1):4–11. doi:10.1186/s40345-018-0140-x
7. Saunders C. *The Management of Terminal Malignant Disease.* Baltimore, MD: E. Arnold; 1984.
8. Saunders C. The treatment of intractable pain in terminal cancer. *Dublin J Med Sci.* 1905;119(4):294–297. doi:10.1007/BF02971564
9. Trachsel M, Irwin SA, Biller-Andorno N, Hoff P, Riese F. Palliative psychiatry for severe persistent mental illness as a new approach to psychiatry? Definition, scope, benefits, and risks. *BMC Psychiatry.* 2016;16(1):1–6. doi:10.1186/s12888-016-0970-y
10. Fairman N, Irwin SA. Palliative care psychiatry: Update on an emerging dimension of psychiatric practice. *Curr Psychiatry Curr Psychiatry Rep.* 2013;15(7):374. doi:10.1007/s11920-013-0374-3
11. Racine N, Killam T, Madigan S. Trauma-informed care as a universal precaution, beyond the adverse childhood experiences questionnaire. *JAMA Pediatr.* 2020;174(1):5–6.
12. University at Buffalo. Buffalo Center for Social Research. What is trauma informed care? The Institute on Trauma and Trauma-Informed Care. What is Trauma-Informed Care? Buffalo, NY: University of Buffalo. 2015. http://socialwork.buffalo.edu/social-research/institutes-centers/institute-on-trauma-and-trauma-informed-care/what-is-trauma-informed-care.html
13. Marlatt GA. Harm reduction: Come as you are. *Addict Behav.* 1996;21(6):779–788. doi:10.1016/0306-4603(96)00042-1
14. McNeil R, Guirguis-Younger M, Dilley LB, Aubry TD, Turnbull J, Hwang SW. Harm reduction services as a point-of-entry to and source of end-of-life care and support for homeless and marginally housed persons who use alcohol and/or illicit drugs: A qualitative analysis. *BMC Public Health.* 2012;12:312. Published 2012 May 17. doi:10.1186/1471-2458-12-312
15. Hawk M, Coulter RWS, Egan JE, et al. Harm reduction principles for healthcare settings. *Harm Reduct J.* 2017;14(1):70. doi:10.1186/s12954-017-0196-4
16. Bloomer MJ, O'Brien AP. Palliative care for the person with a serious mental illness: The need for a partnership approach to care in Australia. *Prog Palliat Care.* 2013;21(1):27–31. doi:10.1179/1743291X12Y.0000000033
17. Snowden LR. Bias in mental health assessment and intervention: Theory and evidence. *Am J Public Health.* 2003;93(2):239–243. doi:10.2105/AJPH.93.2.239
18. Horvitz-Lennon M, Kilbourne AM, Pincus HA. From silos to bridges: Meeting the general health care needs of adults with severe mental illnesses. *Health Aff.* 2006;25(3):659–669. doi:10.1377/hlthaff.25.3.659
19. Arciniegas DB. Psychosis. *Contin Lifelong Learn Neurol.* 2015;21(3):715–736. doi:10.1212/01.CON.0000466662.89908.e7
20. Chaudhury S. Hallucinations: Clinical aspects and management. *Ind Psychiatry J.* 2010;19(1):5. doi:10.4103/0972-6748.77625
21. American Psychiatric Association. *Diagnostic and Statistical Manual of Mental Disorders.* 5th ed. Arlington, VA: American Psychiatric Association; 2013.
22. Hunt GE, Large MM, Cleary M, Man H, Lai X, Saunders JB. Prevalence of comorbid substance use in schizophrenia spectrum disorders in community and clinical settings, 1990-2017: Systematic review and meta-analysis. *Drug Alcohol Depend.* 2018;191:234–258. doi:10.1016/j.drugalcdep.2018.07.011
23. Sweers K, Dierckx de Casterlé B, Detraux J, De Hert M. End-of-life (care) perspectives and expectations of patients with schizophrenia. *Arch Psychiatr Nurs.* 2013;27(5):246–252. doi:10.1016/j.apnu.2013.05.003
24. Gigante AD, Barenboim IY, Dias R da S, et al. Psychiatric and clinical correlates of rapid cycling bipolar disorder: A cross-sectional study. *Rev Bras Psiquiatr.* 2016;38(4):270–274. doi:10.1590/1516-4446-2015-1789
25. Aas M, Henry C, Bellivier F, et al. Affective lability mediates the association between childhood trauma and suicide attempts, mixed episodes and co-morbid anxiety disorders in bipolar disorders. *Psychol Med.* 2017;47(5):902–912. doi:10.1017/S0033291716003081
26. Muneer A. Mixed states in bipolar disorder: Etiology, pathogenesis and treatment. *Chonnam Med J.* 2017;53(1):1. doi:10.4068/cmj.2017.53.1.1

27. Solé E, Garriga M, Valentí M, Vieta E. Mixed features in bipolar disorder. *CNS Spectr.* 2017;22(2):134–140. doi:10.1017/S1092852916000869

28. Feldman DB. Stepwise psychosocial palliative care: A new approach to the treatment of posttraumatic stress disorder at the end of life. *J Soc Work End-of-Life Palliat Care.* 2017;13(2–3):113–133. doi:10.1080/15524256.2017.1346543

29. Shonkoff JP, Garner AS, Siegel BS, et al. The lifelong effects of early childhood adversity and toxic stress. *Pediatrics.* 2012;129(1):e232–e246. doi:10.1542/peds.2011-2663

30. Bickel KE, Kennedy R, Levy C, Burgio KL, Bailey FA. The relationship of post-traumatic stress disorder to end-of-life care received by dying veterans: A secondary data analysis. *J Gen Intern Med.* 2020;35(2):505–513. doi:10.1007/s11606-019-05538-x

31. Sweers K, Dierckx de Casterlé B, Detraux J, De Hert M. End-of-life (care) perspectives and expectations of patients with schizophrenia. *Arch Psychiatr Nurs.* 2013;27(5):246–252. doi:10.1016/j.apnu.2013.05.003

32. Jauhar S, Laws KR, Mckenna PJ. CBT for schizophrenia: A critical viewpoint. *Psychol Med.* 2019;49(8):1233-1236. doi:10.1017/S0033291718004166. Epub 2019 Feb 13. PMID: 30757979.

33. Glick DM, Cook JM, Moye J, Kaiser AP. Assessment and treatment considerations for post traumatic stress disorder at end of life. *Am J Hosp Palliat Med.* 2018;35(8):1133–1139. doi:10.1177/1049909118756656

34. Chochinov HM, Hack T, Hassard T, Kristjanson LJ, McClement S, Harlos M. Dignity therapy: A novel psychotherapeutic intervention for patients near the end of life. *J Clin Oncol.* 2005;23(24):5520–5525. doi:10.1200/JCO.2005.08.391

35. Katz M, Goto Y, Kluger BM, et al. Top ten tips palliative care clinicians should know about Parkinson's disease and related disorders. *J Palliat Med.* 2018;21(10):1507–1517. doi:10.1089/jpm.2018.0390

36. Howard P, Twycross R, Shuster J, Mihalyo M, Wilcock A. Therapeutic reviews. *J Pain Symptom Manage.* 2011;41(5):956–965. doi:10.1016/j.jpainsymman.2011.03.002

37. Shalev D, Brewster K, Arbuckle MR, Levenson JA. A staggered edge: End-of-life care in patients with severe mental illness. *Gen Hosp Psychiatry.* 2017;44:1–3. doi:10.1016/j.genhosppsych.2016.10.004

38. Noffsinger SG, Resnick PJ. Violence and mental illness. *Curr Opin Psychiatry.* 1999;12(6):683–687. doi:10.1097/00001504-199911000-00017

39. Krakowski MI, Czobor P. Depression and impulsivity as pathways to violence: Implications for antiaggressive treatment. *Schizophr Bull.* 2014;40(4):886–894. doi:10.1093/schbul/sbt117

40. Dome P, Rihmer Z, Gonda X. Suicide risk in bipolar disorder: A brief review. *Med.* 2019;55(8):403. Published 2019 Jul 24. doi:10.3390/medicina55080403

41. Ventriglio A, Gentile A, Bonfitto I, et al. Suicide in the early stage of schizophrenia. *Front Psychiatry.* 2016;7(Jun):1–9. doi:10.3389/fpsyt.2016.00116

42. Miller JN, Black DW. Bipolar disorder and suicide: A review. *Curr Psychiatry Rep.* 2020;22(2):6. Published 2020 Jan 18. doi:10.1007/s11920-020-1130-0

43. Lindblad A, Helgesson G, Sjöstrand M. Towards a palliative care approach in psychiatry: Do we need a new definition? *J Med Ethics.* 2019;45(1):26–30. doi:10.1136/medethics-2018-104944

47.

PATIENTS WITH SUBSTANCE USE DISORDERS AND DUAL DIAGNOSES

Jeannine M. Brant and Tonya Edwards

KEY POINTS

- Substance use disorders (SUDs) are a growing concern across the United States and pose significant challenges in assessment and management.

- Co-occurring substance use and mental health disorders commonly exist.

- A variety of risk assessment tools exist to help identify and manage patients with SUDs.

- Criteria from the *Diagnostic and Statistical Manual of Mental Disorders* (DSM-5) are used to diagnose SUDs.

- Palliative advanced practice registered nurses (APRNs) who manage patients with SUDS monitor the 5 A's at each visit: analgesic response, activities of daily living, adverse events, affect, and aberrant behaviors.

CASE STUDY: A PATIENT WITH SUBSTANCE USE DISORDER

William was a 43-year-old man who recently reported to the emergency room with abdominal pain. He has a newly diagnosis of metastatic colon cancer and was treatment-naïve. A computed tomography (CT) scan revealed concern for a small bowel obstruction. He admitted to current polysubstance abuse. His CAGE questionnaire was 4/4. He previously completed drug rehabilitation and was no longer in touch with a drug rehabilitation sponsor. He rated his abdominal pain 8/10 and stated he had taken hydrocodone, 2 tabs, twice today with no pain relief. During examination, he was very drowsy, with slurred speech. William was placed on a 24-hour observation for further assessment and monitoring.

The palliative advanced practice registered nurse (APRN) was requested to see the patient for symptom control; the APRN ordered a stat urine drug screen with additional confirmatory screening. Results were positive for cocaine, amphetamines, THC, benzodiazepines, and hydrocodone. After completing a medical history, opioid risk assessment, and psychological assessment, the APRN ordered short-acting morphine for acute pain control. Naloxone was also added to the medication list. William's pain decreased to 3/10 within the hour, and he was discharged the next day with a pain level of 2/10. At discharge, the results of his positive urine drug screen test were discussed with him. Discharge included extensive opioid education, a 1-week supply of short-acting morphine, stool softeners/bowel stimulants, and details on naloxone nasal spray use in case of overdose. A referral was placed for social work to reconnect the patient with drug rehabilitation and to schedule a follow-up outpatient clinic appointment in 1 week.

The palliative APRN saw William for follow-up in the outpatient clinic 1 week later. A pill count was conducted. William reported he ran out of his morphine tablets early, although he appeared comfortable. The palliative APRN suspected a diagnosis of opioid diversion or opioid misuse. The palliative APRN set boundaries and arranged for an intervention that same day with a specialized opioid interdisciplinary team. The purpose of the intervention was to reduce opioid misuse, abuse, diversion, and the frequency of drug-related aberrant behaviors. The patient was placed in the high-risk category, and a care agreement was signed. After evaluation, he was given a 1-week supply of morphine and an appointment to return for a 1-week follow-up.

INTRODUCTION

Substance use disorder (SUD) is defined as substance abuse and/or dependence, ranging from mild to severe, as characterized by 11 diagnostic criteria: hazardous use, interpersonal problems, neglected responsibilities, withdrawal, tolerance, increased use over time, failed attempts to quit, time spent focused using the substance, mental and health problems, abandoned interests, and cravings.[1] *Dual diagnosis* is defined as a co-occurring SUD and diagnosed mental health condition.[2]

Palliative advanced practice registered nurses (APRNs) are on the frontline of managing symptoms in patients with serious illnesses, and inevitably some of these patients will have a SUD, and, often, a diagnosis of a mental disorder coexists. Managing these patients is challenging for palliative APRNs: prescribing opioids can contribute to the problem, yet underprescribing can lead to suboptimal pain management. Fears about loss of licensure can also surface, reinforcing the need for palliative APRNs to have adequate knowledge about caring for this population. This chapter provides an overview of SUD and dual diagnoses and describes implications for the palliative APRN in assessing and providing care for patients with SUD and dual diagnoses.

SUDs are a growing concern in the United States. According to the Substance Abuse and Mental Health Services Administration 2019 survey, 13% of the US population used an illicit drug in the past month, an increase from 9.2% in 2012. Yet the prevalence of those with a diagnosed SUD remained stable between 2015 and 2019. Of those with a SUDs, 71.1% reported an alcohol use disorders in the past year, 40.7% an illicit drug use disorders, and 11.8% a combined alcohol disorder and SUD. Prescription drug use disorders are also a concern; encouragingly, the rate decreased from 0.9% in 2015 to 0.6% in 2019.[3]

Patients with SUDs often have co-occurring mental health issues (i.e., dual diagnosis) which further complicate their care.[2] Approximately 24.5% of adults aged 18 or older had either a mental illness or SUD in 2019. Of those individuals, 16.8% had only a mental illness, 3.9% had only a SUD, and 3.8% had both.[3] Patients with chronic pain are also at a greater risk for SUDs. Two meta-analyses found that nonmedical use of prescription opioids has been found to be as high as 48–60%, whereas five systematic reviews estimated prevalence to range from 0.05% to 81%. The wide variability is due to varying definitions within studies.[4]

While the exact incidence of SUD in palliative care patients is unknown, it is likely close to that of the general population. Some data are available on patients with cancer. One systematic review of 28 studies found opioid use disorders ranging from 2% to 35% and alcohol disorders from 18% to 25.5%.[5] Of 482,688 veterans with a cancer diagnosis, 6.64% were found to have a SUD.[6] Another study found opioid use disorders among patients with gastrointestinal cancers rose substantially between 2005 and 2014, with a compound annual growth rate of approximately 22%.[7] Given this current crisis, palliative APRNs need to better understand SUDs, how to identify them, and how to manage pain and symptoms safely, according to the risk stratification of the specific patient. A tailored approach to care will ensure the best possible outcomes while minimizing abuse, misuse, and diversion.

DEFINITIONS

Many definitions apply to the concepts of addiction and substance abuse. Some definitions, such as *tolerance* and *physical dependence*, can be confusing and are often used erroneously when referring to patients with SUDs. For example, *addiction* involves genetic and biobehavioral influences, whereas *tolerance* and *physical dependence* are strictly physiologic phenomena.[8–10] Table 47.1 defines terms related to this topic.

BARRIERS

Multiple barriers exist in the assessment and management of patients with SUD and/or dual diagnoses. One of the challenges of working with patients with SUDs is the lack of knowledge as well as the lack of standardized practices and guidelines in place for palliative care programs. One qualitative study of healthcare professionals who provided care

for patients during a palliative trajectory perceived that care for patients with SUD is often fragmented, with providers lacking knowledge about how to manage their multiplicity of care needs. Moreover, the study suggested that care was experience-based, rather than practiced with a foundation of evidence.[11] Increased education for both hospice and palliative care providers and better infrastructure for care are essential for quality and patient safety.[12]

Stigma is another barrier associated with SUDs, which is often rooted in shame and guilt. The more stigmatized patients feel, the less likely they are to disclose a SUD. Using judgment-free language, avoiding terms like *drug-seeking* or *junkie*, and categorizing substance abuse as a disorder can encourage a more open therapeutic relationship. One educational training program, Improving Addiction Care Team (IMPACT), focused on improving providers' attitudes, beliefs, and experiences about SUD treatment. The IMPACT team, comprised of a physician, social worker, and two addiction counseling peer partners, provided patient consultation in patients with SUDs and helped to guide hospital-based care. Their role-modeling and SUD therapy-directed interventions resulted in improved perceptions about SUD and better patient engagement and communication.[13] These types of programs are recommended to provide a more humanized approach to the care of patients with SUDs.

PATHOPHYSIOLOGY

SUDs and addiction are complex phenomena that involve an interplay of neurobiological, genetic, and behavioral components. A wide array of neuroadaptive theories apply to the development of these disorders and the permanent brain changes that occur, but, overall, the pathology involves three stages: binge/intoxication, withdrawal/negative affect, and preoccupation/anticipation. Impulsivity is common with use disorders because these are often relied on to relieve tension and anxiety. Impulsivity then leads to compulsivity, which drives the ongoing behavior.[14,15] Dopamine plays a major role in all stages and specifically drives negative reinforcement; that is, drugs are taken to avoid negative emotions rather than to feel good.[16] The individual then becomes preoccupied on obtaining the substance for escape.

Physiologically, neural systems, including dopamine neurons and the mesolimbic system, are sensitized when introduced to a potentially addictive substance. Changes in the glutamatergic connections within various parts of the brain (ventral tegmental area, nucleus accumbens, prefrontal cortex, and amygdala) are thought to contribute to this sensitization. Neurocognitive imbalance between the impulsive amygdala, which signals pleasure, and the prefrontal cortex, which signals future decision-making, is also thought to occur. These brain changes endure even after the individual stops taking the substance, which explains why relapse rates for addiction remain high. Up to 92% of patients relapse within 8 weeks of tapering buprenorphine.[17] Sex-related differences have been recently recognized and indicate that women experience a more rapid escalation to addiction, have

Table 47.1 DEFINITION OF TERMS RELATED TO SUBSTANCE USE DISORDER

TERM	DEFINITION
Aberrant behaviors	Any medication-related behaviors that depart from strict adherence to the prescribed therapeutic plan of care
Addiction	A neurobiological disorder with genetic and environmental influences that results in psychological dependence on the use of substances for their psychic effects; characterized by craving and compulsive use despite harm
Compulsive	An irresistible urge, especially against conscious wishes
Craving	A strong desire to obtain and use a psychoactive substance for its intoxicating effects
Drug misuse	Use of prescription or over-the-counter drugs that does not follow medical indications or prescribed dosing
Drug abuse	Use of a drug for nontherapeutic purposes to obtain psychotropic effects
Diversion	Unlawful channelling of pharmaceuticals from legal sources to the illegal marketplace
Euphoria	A sense of intense happiness and well-being
Illicit drug	A drug that is not legally permitted or authorized
Nonmedical use	Use of a prescription drug without a prescription or in a manner that is not prescribed
Physical dependence	A physiological neuroadaptation characterized by a withdrawal syndrome if the drug is stopped or decreased abruptly or if an antagonist is administered
Pseudotolerance	A need to increase dosage that is due not to tolerance but to other factors, such as disease progression, new disease, increased physical activity, lack of compliance, change in medication, drug interaction, addiction, and deviant behavior
Pseudoaddiction	A pattern of drug-seeking behavior in patients with pain who are receiving inadequate pain management; can be mistaken for addiction
Substance abuse	The use of any substance for nontherapeutic purposes to obtain psychotropic effects
Tampering	Manipulation of a pharmaceutical to change its drug delivery performance
Tolerance	A physiologic response resulting from the regular use of a drug in which an increased dosage is needed to produce the same effect

From Federation of State Medical Boards of the United States[8]; and Smith et al.[10]

---

a more profound withdrawal response, and are more vulnerable to treatment outcomes.[18] Genetic influences are also involved, and more than 1,500 human addiction genes have been identified. The highest heritability has been found to be opioid addiction.[19] Further research is needed to determine which genes play the greatest role and to understand the exact influence the genes have on the development of addiction.

Environmental factors, stress, reward-based learning, and conditioning effects with potential epigenetic effects also contribute to the development of addiction. Stress and traumatic experience early in life that result in externalizing psychopathology has been linked to SUDs and addiction.[20] This also decreases an individual's ability to self-regulate, further complicating the problem.[21] This pattern underlies the stimulus–response habits, aberrant memories, and maladaptive behaviors that characterize addiction (Figure 47.1).[20] Interestingly, the neurobiological and genetic aspects of substance addiction parallel changes observed in behavioral addictions, such as gambling, internet/video game use, and shopping. Figure 47.1 provides the pathophysiologic aspects of addiction.

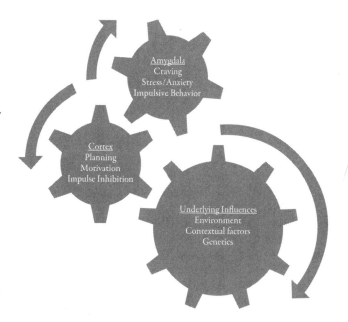

Substance abuse and addiction result from the imbalance between the cortex and the amygdala. Underlying influences can contribute to the phenomena.

Figure 47.1 The pathophysiologic aspects of addiction.

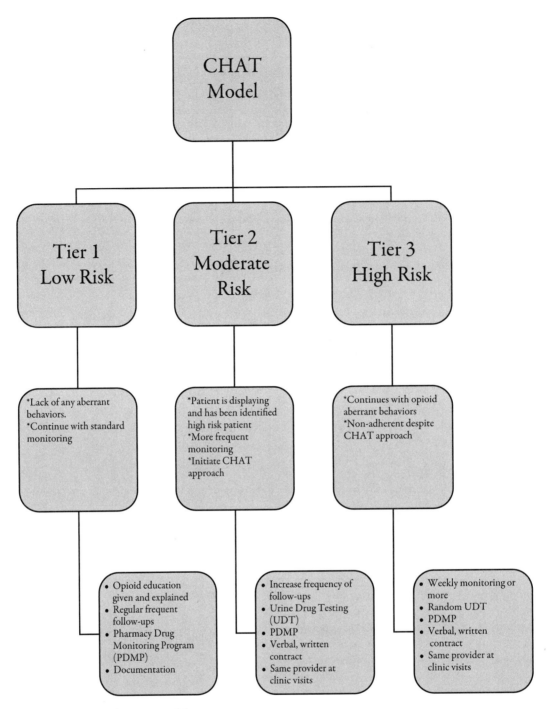

Figure 47.2 The Compassionate High Alert Team model.
From Dalal S, Bruera E.[73], Arthur J, Edwards T, Reddy S, et al.[43]

ASSESSMENT

A detailed patient history, opioid assessment tools, urine drug screens, and the prescription drug monitoring program (PDMP) are effective tools for discovering SUDs.[22] First, the palliative APRN must obtain a baseline history and physical examination, which includes screening all patients for opioid risk prior to starting opioid therapy. Universal precautions should be practiced consistently when assessing, diagnosing, and managing all pain in the palliative care setting (Box 47.1).[23] This methodology, which overall involves preliminary monitoring of all patients to determine their level of risk of substance misuse, any history of non-adherence with opioids, and past substance abuse or family history of abuse.[22,24] If detected, the APRN should implement an effective ongoing opioid monitoring strategic plan that is reassessed at each patient encounter. However, accurate assessment of opioid history and substance abuse is fraught with potential stigma linked to substance abuse and lack of trust, thus necessitating skilled, open interviewing techniques.[25]

Identifying patients at greatest risk for substance abuse is a key component of the assessment. Sociodemographic,

Box 47.1 UNIVERSAL PRECAUTIONS AND ASSESSMENT GUIDE

1. Use therapeutic interview skills:
   - Withhold judgment until ample evidence is available.
   - Spend adequate time with the patient to assess verbal and nonverbal behaviors.
   - Focus on the patient, not specifically on the pain or other symptom.
   - Explore patient fears, expectations of treatment, goals.
   - Use reflective listening—reflect back using a slight modification of what the patient said.
     - Clarify understanding.
     - Encourage the patient to keep talking.
     - Communicate a therapeutic alliance.

2. Perform a thorough physical examination to make a pain diagnosis, including:
   - Pain and symptom assessment
   - Effect of pain on sleep, mood, function, relationships, sex, recreation
   - Medical history
   - Functional assessment: how the pain and symptoms affect function

3. Conduct a psychosocial history and psychological exam, informing the patient that this is a routine part of the assessment which includes:
   - Adverse childhood events and family upbringing
   - History of sexual or physical abuse
   - Family and social support
   - History of depression, anxiety, psychiatric disorders
   - Substance use history
   - Screening for addiction risk in all potential candidates for chronic opioid therapy
   - Access the prescriptive drug monitoring program prior to the visit to determine the patient's use of prior medications, pharmacy use, and areas of concerns
   - Urine drug screening at baseline

4. Determine potential treatment options, discuss benefits and burdens of proposed intervention, and provide informed consent.

5. Complete a treatment agreement.

6. Conduct an opioid trial or controlled substance.

7. Assess the impact of the opioid intervention on pain and function, with regular assessment of the 5 A's of opioid therapy: Analgesic response, Activities of daily living, Adverse events, Affect, and Aberrant behaviors.

8. Regularly review the diagnosis, comorbidities, substance use disorders, and treatment plan.

9. Summarize each visit with the patient, reviewing treatment plan, goals of treatment, and follow-up.

10. Document each visit and ongoing treatment planning.

Data from Kim et al.[35]; Arthur[40]; and Christo et al.[42]

psychological factors, drug-related factors, family history, and genetics have all been linked to addiction risk.[25] The strongest link appears to be the presence of psychosocial, drug-related, and genetic factors combined. Therefore, a social history must include a history of drug abuse and a family history of alcoholism and sexual abuse.[26]

Psychological assessment deserves special recognition as there is a high prevalence of mood disorders accompanying both chronic pain and SUD.[27] Mental health conditions like depression, anxiety, and personality disorders can contribute to and also complicate the presentation of the SUD.[26,27] For example, patients with a SUD are more likely to have increased mental health concerns, including use of higher doses of opioids, higher levels of alcohol use, higher rates of tobacco use, and higher rates in the use of benzodiazepines, and have a higher rate of depression.[26,27] Multiple tools are available to monitor for depression, anxiety, and other mental conditions. Being aware of an underlying mental health disorder can lead to earlier detection of problems. If aberrant behaviors are detected, the palliative APRN should carefully interpret the meaning of the behaviors and their influence on the treatment plan.[28]

RISK ASSESSMENT TOOLS

Opioid risk assessment is an important part of initial and ongoing assessment and surveillance.[29] Several screening tools exist to identify potential problems (Table 47.2). Some of the more common tools include the CAGE, which is widely used to assess for alcoholism, and the Screener and Opioid Assessment for Patients with Pain-Revised (SOAPP-R) and the Opioid Risk Tool (ORT), which screen for opioid abuse.[29] The SOAPP-R has been shown to be a valid tool to screen patients with cancer for substance abuse.[30] The Current Opioid Misuse Measure (COMM), can be used during the monitoring phase. A score of 9 or higher is associated with a higher degree of aberrant behaviors. A systematic review of tools used to monitor ongoing opioid therapy indicated that further testing of these tools is needed because there is limited evidence to support their ability to detect misuse and SUDs in patients taking opioids.[29] While these tools have good internal consistency, they are not "lie detector tests," and the accuracy of the assessment depends on how honestly the individual completes the responses.[29]

Using objective measures to assess the risk for substance use can help to eliminate implicit biases around individuals with SUDs. For example, the palliative APRN may overestimate the risk in an individual who is a heavily tattooed construction worker and underestimate the risk in a well-dressed, high-profile bank manager. Racial biases lead to overestimation of SUD. One study reported that Black patients were more likely to undergo urine drug testing, required to attend more office visits, and received more restrictive opioid prescriptions than White patients.[31] Patients with poorly managed pain can also exhibit addictive behaviors (i.e., pseudoaddiction).

Table 47.2 SUBSTANCE USE DISORDERS RISK SCREENING TOOLS

TOOL	DESCRIPTION	COMMENTS
CAGE (Cut, annoyed, guilty, eye)	4 items	Interview to screen for alcohol use One positive response warrants caution. Two affirmative responses are considered a positive result.
CAGE–AID (Adapted to include drugs)	4 items	Interview to screen for drug and alcohol use Consider modifying yes/no questions to open-ended questions.
COMM (Current Opioid Misuse Measure)	17 items	Self-administered Use during chronic opioid monitoring. Score of 9 or higher suggests aberrancy.
DAST (Drug Abuse Screening Test)	20 items	Self-administered Questions refer to past 12 months.
DSM-V Structured Clinical Interview	Interview	Assessment of the 11 characteristics in the DSM-V criteria Takes 30–60 minutes to complete
ORT (Opioid Risk Tool)	5 items	Self-administered For initial visit for pain treatment Predictive of substance abuse
PDUQ (Prescription Drug Use Questionnaire)	42 items	Interview Score >15 indicates a substance use disorders. Predictive of substance abuse
RAFFT (Relax, alone, friends, family, trouble)	5 items	Self-administered Three affirmative responses are considered a positive result.
SOAPP-R (Screener and Opioid Assessment for Patients with Pain-Revised)	24 items	Self-administered or interview to screen for drug and alcohol use Intended for patients with chronic pain on long-term opioid therapy Score of 7 or higher indicates the person is likely to abuse. Validated in patients with cancer

Data from Yasin et al.[30]; Webster, Dove[32]; and Fishman.[33]

Aberrant behaviors and risk factors for substance abuse are included in Table 47.3. Risk should be evaluated so that strategies can be employed to regain control over the plan.

PRESCRIPTION DRUG MONITORING PROGRAMS

PDMPs, state-based electronic databases that track controlled substances to prevent misuse, abuse, and diversion, provide additional assessment data. Databases contain prescriber-and patient-level data on drugs with high misuse and abuse potential, including opioids and benzodiazepines.[38] They are used to evaluate patient risk by ensuring appropriate prescribing and dispensing of controlled substances. The PDMP should be used in conjunction with other screening tools and ongoing assessment for aberrant behaviors. While not diagnostic, PDMPs are another tool that should be used at baseline and during follow-up to evaluate aberrant behaviors and drug use patterns.

Using individual Drug Enforcement Agency (DEA) numbers, palliative APRNs can register for their state's PDMP and access the database to examine patterns of prescription drug use in patients. Databases will reveal if a patient is using multiple prescribers or multiple pharmacies, which suggests abuse or illegal activities. One study found that using the PDMP for patient assessment resulted in an 8.9% reduction in opioids dispensed.[39] Efforts are under way to link state PDMPs to detect misuse, abuse, or diversion of opioids across state lines.

URINE DRUG TESTING

Urine drug testing is another assessment tool available to monitor for controlled substance misuse, abuse, and diversion.[40] This results in immediate action to increase or modify opioid safety practices. Urine drug testing can be an operative tool for adherence to opioid pain medication treatment. However, urine drug testing is infrequently used, and there is a lack of knowledge and standardized practices that limit its use.[40]

Urine drug testing has two types: screening assays and confirmatory testing.[22] *Screening test assays* detect antibodies or drug metabolites and report only a positive or negative result. Urine *confirmatory tests* specify separated molecules by a chromatograph and are analyzed using a mass spectrometer. Although the confirmatory testing is more expensive, the results reveal specific drug identification.[41] Abnormal urine drug testing can show illicit drug or alcohol abuse or an abstinence of prescribed opioids.[42] However, interpretation can be challenging; therefore, the palliative APRN

BEHAVIORS LESS SUGGESTIVE OF ADDICTION	BEHAVIORS MORE SUGGESTIVE OF ADDICTION	RISK FACTORS FOR ADDICTION
Drug hoarding when symptoms are improved	High opioid dose	White male
Acquiring drugs from multiple medical sources	Selling prescription drugs	Younger age
Aggressive complaining about the need for a higher dose	Forgery of prescriptions	Higher pain intensity and lower pain tolerance
Unapproved use of a medication to treat a symptom (e.g., use of an opioid to treat anxiety)	Concurrent illicit drug use	More pain complaints
Unsanctioned dose escalation (once or twice)	Multiple prescription/medication losses	More pain-related limitations
Reporting psychic effects	Ongoing unsanctioned dose escalations	Depression and psychotropic medications in younger populations
Requesting specific drugs	Stealing or borrowing drugs	Psychological comorbidity: panic, anxiety, depression, agoraphobia, low self-reported health status
Second opinion for pain requested	Obtaining prescription drugs from nonmedical sources	Substance abuse history; positive CAGE-AID results
Smoking cigarettes to relieve pain	Repeated resistance to change—inflexibility	Genetic predisposition
Drinking alcohol to relieve pain	Prostitution for drugs or for money to obtain drugs	Financial distress
Urine toxicology screens positive	Unanticipated positive results in urine toxicology	
Nonadherence to appointments	Frequent pain clinic or emergency department visits	
	Financial distress	

Data from Yennurajalingam et al.[28]; Pinkerton, Hardy[34]; Kim et al.[35]; Childers et al.[36]; and Sehgal et al.[37]

should have essential knowledge of test interpretation grounded in an understanding of drug metabolic pathways. An understanding of the metabolism of opioids to explain the presence pro-drugs and of apparent un-prescribed drugs is essential.

The APRN should routinely request a urine drug testing for low-risk patients, minimally once per year; moderate-risk patients should be tested two times yearly; and high-risk patients should be tested three or more times per year.[40] Often, a urine drug test is collected at baseline, or random testing can be employed within the first 3 months upon initiation of opioid therapy. The purpose for undergoing urine drug testing is based on current guidelines (see Table 47.4).[43]

When ordering urine drug testing, the APRN should communicate the key intention of obtaining the test, which is to safeguard the patient on opioid therapy.[41] If the urine drug test yields abnormal results, the APRN should initiate a nonconfrontational open dialog with the patient. Understanding pro-drugs and metabolites will enable the palliative APRNs to interpret results correctly[40]

(see Chapter 43, "Pain," for information on interpreting results of the urine drug test).

DIAGNOSIS

Diagnosing SUDs can be a long and arduous process. It often cannot occur during the first appointment unless the diagnosis is preestablished and overt. Otherwise, patients can be observed over time, and a diagnosis or dual diagnosis often emerges over time.

SUBSTANCE USE DISORDER

The palliative APRN can use the *Diagnosis Statistical Manual of Mental Disorders* (DSM-5) criteria to diagnose a SUD.[1] The DSM-5 classification includes an amendment for prescription opioid use disorders.[26] Key changes recently occurred with elimination of the words "tolerance"

Table 47.4 PALLIATIVE CARE URINE DRUG TESTING RECOMMENDATIONS

CATEGORY	RECOMMENDATION AND COMMENTS	RATIONALE
1. Who to test	Test all palliative care patients receiving chronic opioid therapy (>3 months).	Removes palliative APRN subjectivity and makes testing consistent with chronic disease management paradigm
2. How to test	Explain the urine drug testing and it purpose to ensure patient understanding.	Removes fear; informs patients that urine drug testing is not punitive but rather part of standard procedures
	Review the urine drug testing parameters may be included in a Controlled Substance Agreement for pain management from palliative care.	Clearly delineates urine drug testing role in therapy
	Conduct comprehensive medication testing, which includes illicit drugs, opioids, and other substances, such as benzodiazepines.	Tests for suspected therapeutic metabolites and other substances
	Develop collaborative relationship with the Clinical Laboratory Improvement Amendments (CLIA)-certified laboratory with knowledge about urine drug testing performing urine drug testing on palliative patients, with results available on same day.	Results can be falsely positive or negative; laboratory proficiency will minimize this variability.
	Use Point-of-care (POC) testing on the initial palliative care consultation visit, but inconsistent results should be verified with urine drug testing.	POC testing is for screening only.
	Ensure accurate sampling and monitoring . . . etc.	Indicates if the sample has been tampered with
3. When to test	Initiate urine drug testing when starting palliative care patient on chronic opioid therapy.	Aids in risk stratification
	Test according to assessment of risk stratification via SOAPP-R/ORT and other factors.	Allows for more frequent screening for high-risk patients
	Develop palliative care program procedure to determine frequency of urine drug testing while maintaining minimum requirements (e.g., having patient flip a coin or roll dice at each visit).	Removes burden from palliative care staff tracking while providing fairness for random testing
4. How to interpret results	Confirm appropriate interpretation from laboratory that performs testing.	Identifies the type of aberrant medication use so that behavior can be specifically addressed
	Classify findings as (1) prescribed drug not detected, (2) illicit drug detected, (3) nonprescribed drug of concern detected.	
	Construct pathways for palliative care patients in constructing a differential diagnosis if (1) drug not detected (e.g., diversion, hoarding, lab error); may need additional testing to determine absence; (2) illicit drug detected (e.g., addiction, seeking additional pain relief, lab error); (3) nonprescribed drug detected (e.g., multiple providers).	Allows the palliative APRN to understand the finding; absence of prescribed drug with presence of illicit drug requires immediate action
5. How to handle test result discrepancies	Verify discrepancies with laboratory.	Lab results should always be verified.
	Schedule an immediate follow-up visit to discuss findings with patient in non-judgmental manner.	The patient may disclose the reason for the discrepancy; promotes therapeutic communication.
	Develop a plan based on the findings.	The plan will vary and depends on the problem detected.

Data from Peppin et al.[44]; and Arthur et al.[45]

and "withdrawal symptoms" for patients who are prescribed opioids by a medical professional.[26] The DSM-5's 11 criteria combine substance abuse and dependence into a single disorder and a stratified graded structure.[1] Criteria include the following:

- Perceptions about use, such as taking more of a substance than intended, desire to cut down or stop using the substance, craving the substance, and being consumed with obtaining the substance

- Functional elements, including inability to manage current roles and responsibilities and forgoing opportunities (e.g., family outings, social relationships)[25]

- Continued use despite harm and endangerment physically, psychologically, and socially[25]

- Development of tolerance and physical withdrawal[26]

Mild SUDS require the presence of two or three symptoms from the list, a moderate SUD includes four or five symptoms, and six or more symptoms indicate a severe SUD. A long-standing criticism of the DSM criteria is that patients with cancer often exhibit some of these symptoms and yet they may not have a SUD. The diagnosis of a SUD is not valid if the opioid is taken as prescribed.

DUAL DIAGNOSIS

A dual diagnosis of a SUD and a psychiatric disorder is well-recognized in the literature, and both genetic and environmental risks are proposed. Of those individuals with a SUD in the United States, approximately 45% have a coexisting psychiatric disorders.[3] One recent study found co-occurring SUDs ranged from 26.4% with alcohol and 10.6% for methamphetamine.[46] Within the palliative care and cancer population, one study found that 12.4% of patients with advanced cervical cancer had a dual diagnosis.[47]

Diagnostic pitfalls exist, and identifying the actual problem may be challenging. For example, the onset of each disorder can be variable. According to one study, two-thirds of patients were diagnosed with late-onset SUD and mood disorders (after age 18). Psychotic disorders, on the other hand, were more prevalent with an early-onset (before age 18) diagnosis. When compared to the late-onset group, the early-onset group had a higher number of psychiatric admissions.[48] The palliative APRN may therefore be the first to detect the dual diagnosis, depending on the patient's situation.

Another complicating factor is that the relationship between mental illness and SUD is bidirectional, indicating that they affect one another and can cloud the assessment. For example, substances can lead to manic activity, but this can also be exhibited in anxiety and attention-deficit hyperactivity disorders (ADHD).[49] Obtaining a detailed history is important to understand how each problem contributes to the current situation. Assessment tools for anxiety, depression,

and addiction are warranted, as are reports from family members and other mental health professionals. If not previously evaluated, the palliative APRN may need to consult psychiatry or clinical psychology to conduct a full evaluation of the patient.[49]

Overall, the interplay between substance use and mental illness is complex, and caution should be taken in making a formal diagnosis of SUD and/or a dual diagnosis. Building a relationship with the patient and assessing and managing the patient over time will ensure a more accurate conclusion.

MANAGEMENT

Managing pain and symptoms and providing overall care in patients with SUDs can be challenging. Many palliative care patients will require chronic opioid therapy or other treatments, such as benzodiazepines, that may pose risks for those with SUDs. Risk of relapse for those in remission is a valid fear, and yet undertreatment of pain and symptoms is also common due to a lack of understanding of the appropriate care of these patients. Balancing comfort with opioids along with the risk of opioid misuse, abuse, and diversion is imperative in this population.[24] For patients with a co-occurring SUD and mental illness (see Chapter 46, "Serious Mental Illness"), pain and symptom management may be even more challenging. Management of the existing depression, anxiety, or mood disorder is foundational to managing the patient's pain.[50,51] Having a well-defined plan in place that focuses on the goals of care and stratifies patients according to addiction risk allows for individualized pain and symptom care while monitoring patients for aberrant behaviors and signs of addiction.[45] This will provide the best care for the patient while at the same time preventing misuse, abuse, and diversion.

RISK STRATIFICATION

Risk stratification is one of the first steps of the management plan. The palliative APRN should make a clinical assessment if aberrant opioid behaviors are discovered based on obtained clinical, history, risk assessment tools, the PDMP, and urine drug testing.[28] The palliative APRN can make an opioid safety plan for prevention of known aberrant opioid behaviors. A strategic opioid therapy plan provides a basis for managing patients with SUDs; it includes ongoing risk assessment and monitoring and deploys a corrective personalized action plan.[43] Stratifying patients according to their risk for a SUD is the first step in the management plan. Prominent risk factors have been recognized and associated with high risk for substance abuse, such as family history of SUD or mental health issues, young male gender, and tobacco or alcohol use.[52] The APRN can observe the patient's behaviors and adherence over time (Table 47.5).

Table 47.5 MANAGEMENT ACCORDING TO RISK

RISK STRATIFICATION	RISK ASSESSMENT TOOLS	OTHER RISK CONSIDERATIONS	MANAGEMENT STRATEGIES
Low	SOAPP-R score <10 ORT score <4	No family history No past/current history of substance use disorders No psychological comorbidity	Annual adherence monitoring Review prescription drug monitoring program (PDM) twice per year Urine drug testing every 1–2 years
Medium	SOAPP-R score 10–21 ORT score 4–7	Family history positive Past history of treated substance use disorders; can be on pharmacotherapy for addiction Psychological comorbidity, past or current <25 years of age	Adherence monitoring every 6 months Review PDM 3 times per year Urine drug testing every 6 months to 1 year
High	SOAPP-R score >21 ORT score <7	Current substance use disorders or addiction Current aberrant behaviors (those more suggestive of addiction) Major psychiatric disorders that is untreated	Weekly to monthly adherence monitoring Management by pain and addiction specialists recommended Review PDM 4 times per year Urine drug testing every 3–6 months Prescribe opioids cautiously; chronic opioid therapy may be prohibitive in terms of risk to the patient.

Data from Dalal, Bruera[22]; Yennurajalingam et al.[28]; Yasin et al.[30]; and Gourlay, Heit.[53]

GOALS OF CARE

Pain and symptom management goals provide a foundation for measuring the success of the plan of care. The 5 A's can be used to measure the success of a management plan: analgesia, activities of daily living, adverse events, aberrant behaviors, and affect[8] (Table 47.6). The palliative APRN should document the 5 A's at each visit to assess the patient's response to the treatment plan. Goals should be clear to the patient when treatment is started. Physiologic and psychosocial functioning should be included in the plan because they reflect an improvement in overall quality of life. Affect is especially important to patients with dual diagnoses.

Both pain and SUDs lead to dysfunction, so management should lead to optimal functioning. This focus on function allows the palliative APRN to individualize care and prescribing options.

MANAGEMENT OF PAIN

The pain management plan should be based on a systematic approach that includes the following:

- Diagnosis of the problem with consideration of potential dual diagnoses

Table 47.6 5 A'S OF OPIOID THERAPY MANAGEMENT

5 A'S	DEFINITION	ASSESSMENT
Analgesia	Level of comfort	Decrease in pain intensity Effectiveness of the intervention on the pain
Activities of daily living	Functional status	Increased physical capabilities Psychologically intact Family/social relationships intact Appropriate medication and healthcare utilization
Adverse events	Side effects related to treatment	Sedation Euphoria Other physical and psychological effects
Aberrant activities	Behaviors that warn of potential substance misuse, abuse, or addiction	Behaviors that suggest concern; see Table 47.3
Affect	Psychological functioning	Improved psychological affect Ability to cope with illness

Data from Hwang et al.[7] and Volkow et al.[21]

- Conservative approaches (e.g., physical therapy, non-opioids, co-analgesics to assist in opioid-sparing)

- Nonpharmacologic modalities

- Therapeutic interventions such as anesthetic blocks

- Chronic opioid therapy and other controlled co-analgesics (e.g., benzodiazepines) only when conservative approaches are not effective.

(See Chapter 43, "Pain," for more information about pain management.)

Often practitioners feel that opioids should be avoided in patients with SUDs; however, current literature suggests that many of these patients can be safely managed using a detailed and vigilant monitoring program.[24,54] Dosing can be challenging in this population, especially in terms of drug tolerance. Patients with active opioid use will be tolerant of opioids and may require higher doses, but aberrant behaviors may preclude the palliative APRN from prescribing opioids for these patients. Contributing to addiction and diversion can result in loss of licensure, so caution is warranted. The most important component is careful surveillance for all patients: some high-risk patients may show substantially improved function using opioids, while some low-risk patients may experience deterioration in function.

Prescribing medications may be complicated. Palliative APRNs may prescribe certain medications for pain management but not for substance abuse, unless they have completed addiction graduate education or specific coursework. APRNs should consider training to prescribe medications as appropriate for SUDs. For example, naltrexone and nalmefene are approved for patients with alcohol use disorders; methadone and buprenorphine can be prescribed for opioid use disorders.[55] Specific barriers exist for palliative APRNs in managing patients with SUDs. State-by-state variation in APRNs' prescribing privileges for opioids reveals restrictions for medication management and buprenorphine prescribing. Palliative APRNs may prescribe buprenorphine after they complete 24 hours of training; are licensed in a state where they can prescribe Schedule III, IV, or V medications; and can demonstrate the ability to treat and manage opioid use disorders.[56] APRNs should refer to state laws regarding license requirements.

Determining the right opioid can be difficult because all opioids can be potentially abused. Oxycodone has been shown to have a higher abuse potential compared to morphine and hydrocodone,[57] and tapentadol has a low abuse potential although risk still exists.[58,59] One exception is buprenorphine, which has been found to have a lower abuse potential. In terms of formulation, long-acting dosing should be optimized while the need for breakthrough doses is minimized. This allows for a therapeutic blood level to control pain while avoiding peaks and troughs and "clock-watching" to take the next dose.[60] Abuse-deterrent opioid formulations are another option. These opioids resist manipulation, such as crushing, dissolving, or extracting; any attempts to do so will inactivate the opioid.[61,62] While this property can be of benefit in

high-risk patients, these drug formulations can be expensive, and more evidence is needed to determine their role in managing high-risk patients taking chronic opioid therapy. Some reports indicate that those on abuse-deterrent opioid formulations may inadvertently be encouraged to use heroin, resulting in more safety concerns.[63]

While methadone cannot be crushed and abused due to its high protein-binding affinity, safety concerns relate to the potential for accumulation, oversedation, and potential death.[64,65] Palliative APRNs can prescribe methadone for pain, but only licensed methadone maintenance clinics can prescribe it for addiction. Buprenorphine, a partial opioid agonist that is used in opioid addiction, may be useful for pain management and has been shown to have the lowest abuse potential.[66] While APRNs can prescribe buprenorphine for pain, restrictions also exist on prescribing this agent for addiction. Buprenorphine has a ceiling dose and therefore should be used only in patients with anticipated lower doses of opioids.[67]

Naloxone co-prescription is an important consideration for APRNs ordering any opioid therapy. This short-acting opioid antagonist has been shown to be especially beneficial in patients with nonmedical opioid use. One study found a 47% reduction in opioid-related emergency department visits per month at 6 months and 63% fewer visits at 1 year for patients who received a naloxone prescription.[68] Naloxone recommendations are included in Box 47.2.

SUBSTANCE USE AGREEMENTS

Substance use agreements, also known as contracts, are an additional optional component of the management plan. Substance use agreements have been shown to improve provider satisfaction, decrease emergency department visits, and improve patient adherence. Substance use agreements are highly controversial, and yet some experts recommend that

---

Box 47.2 NALOXONE CO-PRESCRIPTION RECOMMENDATIONS

These are the Centers for Disease Control and Prevention (CDC)[69] recommendations:

- History of drug overdose

- History of a SUD

- Requiring large opioid doses ≥50 mg morphine equivalents/day

- Concurrent use of benzodiazepines

Other appropriate indications:

- Morphine equivalent doses >100 mg/day[70]

- Patients on methadone[71]

- Pulmonary, renal, or hepatic disease comorbidities[70]

- Recent history of incarceration[68]

they be employed for all patients taking controlled medications or chronic opioid therapy for greater than 3 months, regardless of risk.[24,72] Agreements should spell out the risks and benefits of treatment, provide education about the plan of care, outline the responsibilities of the patient and the palliative APRN, and allow a transparent conversation to occur between the patient and the APRN. Agreements should include the following:

- Designated prescriber
- Designated pharmacy
- Frequency of refills
- Times when refills are prohibited (e.g., after hours, weekends)
- Dosage changes
- Screening and consequences for positive screens (e.g., urine, blood, pill counts)
- Need to secure medications and dispose of them safely if needed
- Supportive therapy requirements (e.g., psychiatry)
- Safe use of medications

CHAT MODEL OF CARE

Applying all assessment components and care concepts to the management plan deserves a calculated and planned approach. To determine the best plan of care, the palliative APRN should be reminded that risk stratification guides the management plan. The higher the risk, the more frequent the monitoring and the more cautious the dosing of opioids should be. The Compassionate High Alert Team (CHAT) model (Figure 47.2) provides a solid framework for a tiered opioid risk stratification and for the appropriate care needed for palliative care patients.[73]

The palliative APRN should engage other team members and encourage them to use the CHAT model for high-risk patients. When diversion is suspected, the palliative APRN and team should follow the 5 S's plan: limiting the opioid supply, selecting a drug with a lower street value, scheduling more frequent visits, scheduling more frequent urine drug testing, and involving a substance abuse specialist. Actual proof of diversion calls for the discontinuation of opioids. APRNs should follow the rules listed in the substance use agreement, which may include discharge from the practice, discontinuance of opioids, transition to non-opioids, and the need to include substance abuse providers. All efforts should be made to maintain the patient within the practice, even though opioids may not be continued. When the palliative APRN decides to discontinue opioids, a plan of tapering medications should be initiated.

If a patient is placed in the high-risk category, the palliative APRN can involve the CHAT specialized interdisciplinary team. The CHAT approach involves an APRN or a physician, a registered nurse, a psychologist or counselor, a pharmacist, a patient advocate, a social worker, and/or security personnel.[22,43] A pre-huddle takes place prior to the patient visit, and the CHAT team meets together with the patient to discuss a strategy and an opioid safety plan.[43] During the collective meeting with the patient, the palliative APRN will address concerning matters related to current opioid use, including expectations, the need to establish trust, goals of safe opioid therapy, and risks and dangers with opioid misuse, abuse, or addiction.[22,43] The APRN will continue to engage in a compassionate, nonjudgmental fashion. A post visit huddle with the team only is the final step of the visit. All disciplines document their roles and the outcomes specific to their specialty to ensure a successful subsequent opioid treatment plan.[43]

SUMMARY

The assessment and management of patients with SUDs and dual diagnoses is complex and calls for advanced skills and a calculated interdisciplinary approach to care. The palliative APRN should understand the challenges inherent in managing patients with SUDs and those with co-occurring mental illness but should still approach patients with compassion and in a nonjudgmental manner. As with William in the chapter's case study, the palliative APRN can often successfully manage SUD and dual diagnoses using appropriate guidelines and an interdisciplinary collaborative approach. While occasionally opioids will need to be discontinued because of diversion or other reasons, palliative APRNs should understand that by using a systematic approach and a chronic disease model, the majority of patients can be well-managed and can achieve both comfort and an improved quality of life.

REFERENCES

1. American Psychiatric Association. Substance use disorders. In: *Diagnostic and Statistical Manual of Mental Disorders*. 5th ed. Arlington, VA: American Psychiatric Association; 2013.
2. Antai-Otong D, Theis K, Patrick DD. Dual diagnosis: Coexisting substance use disorders and psychiatric disorders. *Nurs Clin North Am*. 2016;51(2):237–247. doi:10.1016/j.cnur.2016.01.007
3. Substance Abuse and Mental Health Services Administration. *Results from the 2012 National Survey on Drug Use and Health: Summary of National Findings*. Research Triangle Park, NC: US Department of Health and Human Services; 2012. https://www.samhsa.gov/data/sites/default/files/NSDUHnationalfindingresults2012/NSDUHnationalfindingresults2012/NSDUHresults2012.htm
4. Voon P, Karamouzian M, Kerr T. Chronic pain and opioid misuse: A review of reviews. *Subst Abuse Treat Prev Policy*. 2017;12(1):36–36. doi:10.1186/s13011-017-0120-7
5. Yusufov M, Braun IM, Pirl WF. A systematic review of substance use and substance use disorders in patients with cancer. *Gen Hosp Psychiatry*. 2019;60:128–136. doi:10.1016/j.genhosppsych.2019.04.016
6. Ho P, Rosenheck R. Substance use disorder among current cancer patients: Rates and correlates nationally in the Department of Veterans Affairs. *Psychosomatics*. 2018;59(3):267–276. doi:10.1016/j.psym.2018.01.003

7. Hwang J, Shen JJ, Kim SJ, et al. Opioid use disorders and hospital palliative care among patients with gastrointestinal cancers: Ten-year trend and associated factors in the us from 2005 to 2014. *Medicine.* 2020;99(25):e20723. doi:10.1097/md.0000000000020723

8. Federation of State Medical Boards of the United States. *Model Guidelines for the Use of Opioid Analgesics in the Treatment of Chronic Pain.* Euless, TX: Federation of State Medical Boards; 2013. https://pcssnow.org/wp-content/uploads/2013/10/FSMB-Model-Pain-Policy_July-2013.pdf

9. Sinha R. The clinical neurobiology of drug craving. *Curr Opin Neurobiol.* 2013;23(4):649–654. doi:10.1016/j.conb.2013.05.001

10. Smith SM, Dart RC, Katz NP, et al. Classification and definition of misuse, abuse, and related events in clinical trials: Action systematic review and recommendations. *Pain.* 2013;154(11):2287–2296. doi:10.1016/j.pain.2013.05.053

11. Ebenau A, Dijkstra B, Ter Huurne C, Hasselaar J, Vissers K, Groot M. Palliative care for patients with substance use disorder and multiple problems: A qualitative study on experiences of healthcare professionals, volunteers and experts-by-experience. *BMC Palliat Care.* 2020;19(1):8. Published 2020 Jan 14. doi:10.1186/s12904-019-0502-x

12. Gabbard J, Jordan A, Mitchell J, Corbett M, White P, Childers J. Dying on hospice in the midst of an opioid crisis: What should we do now? *Am J Hosp Palliat Care.* 2019;36(4):273–281. doi:10.1177/1049909118806664

13. Englander H, Collins D, Perry SP, Rabinowitz M, Phoutrides E, Nicolaidis C. "We've learned it's a medical illness, not a moral choice": Qualitative study of the effects of a multicomponent addiction intervention on hospital providers' attitudes and experiences. *J Hospital Medicine.* 2018;13(11):752–758. doi:10.12788/jhm.2993

14. Koob GF, Volkow ND. Neurobiology of addiction: A neurocircuitry analysis. *Lancet Psychiatry.* 2016;3(8):760–773. doi:10.1016/s2215-0366(16)00104-8

15. Kozak K, Lucatch AM, Lowe DJE, Balodis IM, MacKillop J, George TP. The neurobiology of impulsivity and substance use disorders: Implications for treatment. *Ann N Y Acad Sci.* 2019;1451(1):71–91. doi:10.1111/nyas.13977

16. Solinas M, Belujon P, Fernagut PO, Jaber M, Thiriet N. Dopamine and addiction: What have we learned from 40 years of research. *J Neural Transm (Vienna).* 2019;126(4):481–516. doi:10.1007/s00702-018-1957-2

17. Uhl GR, Koob GF, Cable J. The neurobiology of addiction. *Ann N Y Acad Sci.* 2019;1451(1):5–28. doi:10.1111/nyas.13989

18. Becker JB. Sex differences in addiction. *Dialogues Clin Neurosci.* 2016;18(4):395–402. doi:10.31887/DCNS.2016.18.4/jbecker

19. Wang SC, Chen YC, Lee CH, Cheng CM. Opioid addiction, genetic susceptibility, and medical treatments: A review. *Int J Mol Sci.* 2019;20(17). doi:10.3390/ijms20174294

20. Sarvet AL, Hasin D. The natural history of substance use disorders. *Curr Opin Psychiatry.* 2016;29(4):250–257. doi:10.1097/yco.0000000000000257

21. Volkow ND, Michaelides M, Baler R. The neuroscience of drug reward and addiction. *Physiol Rev.* 2019;99(4):2115–2140. doi:10.1152/physrev.00014.2018

22. Dalal S, Bruera E. Pain management for patients with advanced cancer in the opioid epidemic era. *Am Soc Clin Oncology Educ Book.* 2019;39:24–35. doi:10.1200/edbk_100020

23. Arthur J, Hui D. Safe opioid use: Management of opioid-related adverse effects and aberrant behaviors. *Hematol Oncol Clin North Am.* 2018;32(3):387–403. doi:10.1016/j.hoc.2018.01.003

24. Arthur J, Bruera E. Balancing opioid analgesia with the risk of nonmedical opioid use in patients with cancer. *Nat Rev Clin Oncol.* 2019;16(4):213–226. doi:10.1038/s41571-018-0143-7

25. Moussas GI, Papadopoulou AG. Substance abuse and cancer. *Psychiatriki.* 2017;28(3):234–241. doi:10.22365/jpsych.2017.283.234

26. Boscarino JA, Hoffman SN, Han JJ. Opioid-use disorder among patients on long-term opioid therapy: Impact of final DSM-5 diagnostic criteria on prevalence and correlates. *Subst Abuse Rehabil.* 2015;6:83–91. doi:10.2147/SAR.S85667

27. Kaye AD, Jones MR, Kaye AM, et al. Prescription opioid abuse in chronic pain: An updated review of opioid abuse predictors and strategies to curb opioid abuse: Part 1. *Pain Physician.* 2017;20(2s):S93–s109.

28. Yennurajalingam S, Edwards T, Arthur JA, et al. Predicting the risk for aberrant opioid use behavior in patients receiving outpatient supportive care consultation at a comprehensive cancer center. *Cancer.* 2018;124(19):3942–3949. doi:10.1002/cncr.31670

29. Jamison RN, Mao J. Opioid analgesics. *Mayo Clin Proc.* 2015;90(7):957–968. doi:10.1016/j.mayocp.2015.04.010

30. Yasin JT, Leader AE, Petok A, Garber G, Stephens B, Worster B. Validity of the Screener and Opioid Assessment for Patients with Pain-Revised (SOAPP-R) in patients with cancer. *J Opioid Manag.* 2019;15(4):272–274. doi:10.5055/jom.2019.0512

31. Becker WC, Starrels JL, Heo M, Li X, Weiner MG, Turner BJ. Racial differences in primary care opioid risk reduction strategies. *Ann Fam Med.* 2011;9(3):219–225. doi:10.1370/afm.1242

32. Webster LR, Dove B. *Avoiding Opioid Abuse While Managing Pain.* North Branch, MN: Sunrise River Press; 2007.

33. Fishman SM. *Responsible Opioid Prescribing: A Physician's Guide.* 2nd ed. Washington, DC: Waterford Life Sciences; 2014.

34. Pinkerton R, Hardy JR. Opioid addiction and misuse in adult and adolescent patients with cancer. *Intern Med J.* 2017;47(6):632–636. doi:10.1111/imj.13449

35. Kim YJ, Dev R, Reddy A, et al. Association between tobacco use, symptom expression, and alcohol and illicit drug use in advanced cancer patients. *J Pain Symptom Manage.* 2016;51(4):762–768. doi:10.1016/j.jpainsymman.2015.11.012

36. Childers JW, King LA, Arnold RM. Chronic pain and risk factors for opioid misuse in a palliative care clinic. *Am J Hosp Palliat Care.* 2015;32(6):654–659. doi:10.1177/1049909114531445

37. Sehgal N, Manchikanti L, Smith HS. Prescription opioid abuse in chronic pain: A review of opioid abuse predictors and strategies to curb opioid abuse. *Pain Physician.* 2012;15(3 Suppl):ES67–92.

38. Centers for Disease Control and Prevention. Drug overdose. PDMPs: What States Need to Know. Reviewed May 19, 2021. https://www.cdc.gov/drugoverdose/pdmp/states.html

39. Winstanley EL, Zhang Y, Mashni R, et al. Mandatory review of a prescription drug monitoring program and impact on opioid and benzodiazepine dispensing. *Drug Alcohol Depend.* 2018;188:169–174. doi:10.1016/j.drugalcdep.2018.03.036

40. Argoff CE, Alford DP, Fudin J, Adler JA, Bair MJ, Dart RC, . . . Webster LR. Rational urine drug monitoring in patients receiving opioids for chronic pain: Consensus recommendations. *Pain Medicine (Malden, Mass.).* 2018;19(1):97–117. doi:10.1093/pm/pnx285

41. Arthur JA. Urine drug testing in cancer pain management. *Oncologist.* 2019. doi:10.1634/theoncologist.2019-0525

42. Christo PJ, Manchikanti L, Ruan X, et al. Urine drug testing in chronic pain. *Pain Physician.* 2011;14(2):123–143.

43. Arthur J, Edwards T, Reddy S, et al. Outcomes of a specialized interdisciplinary approach for patients with cancer with aberrant opioid-related behavior. *Oncologist.* 2018;23(2):263–270. doi:10.1634/theoncologist.2017-0248

44. Peppin JF, Passik SD, Couto JE, et al. Recommendations for urine drug monitoring as a component of opioid therapy in the treatment of chronic pain. *Pain Med.* 2012;13(7):886–896. doi:10.1111/j.1526-4637.2012.01414.x

45. Arthur JA, Haider A, Edwards T, et al. Aberrant opioid use and urine drug testing in outpatient palliative care. *J Palliat Med.* 2016;19(7):778–782. doi:10.1089/jpm.2015.0335

46. Jones CM, McCance-Katz EF. Co-occurring substance use and mental disorders among adults with opioid use disorder. *Drug Alcohol Depend.* 2019;197:78–82. doi:10.1016/j.drugalcdep.2018.12.030

47. Rubinsak LA, Terplan M, Martin CE, Fields EC, McGuire WP, Temkin SM. Co-occurring substance use disorder: The impact on treatment adherence in women with locally advanced cervical cancer. *Gynecol Oncol Rep.* 2019;28:116–119. doi:10.1016/j.gore.2019.03.016

48. Subodh BN, Sahoo S, Basu D, Mattoo SK. Age of onset of substance use in patients with dual diagnosis and its association with clinical

characteristics, risk behaviors, course, and outcome: A retrospective study. *Indian J Psychiatry.* 2019;61(4):359–368. doi:10.4103/psychiatry.IndianJPsychiatry_454_18

49. Iqbal MN, Levin CJ, Levin FR. Treatment for substance use disorder with co-occurring mental illness. *Focus (Am Psychiatr Publ).* 2019;17(2):88–97. doi:10.1176/appi.focus.20180042

50. Vitali M, Mistretta M, Alessandrini G, et al. Pharmacological treatment for dual diagnosis: A literature update and a proposal of intervention. *Riv Psichiatr.* 2018;53(3):160–169. doi:10.1708/2925.29419

51. Tirado Muñoz J, Farré A, Mestre-Pintó J, Szerman N, Torrens M. Dual diagnosis in depression: Treatment recommendations. *Adicciones.* 2018;30(1):66–76. doi:10.20882/adicciones.868

52. Dev R, Parsons HA, Palla S, Palmer JL, Del Fabbro E, Bruera E. Undocumented alcoholism and its correlation with tobacco and illegal drug use in advanced cancer patients. *Cancer.* 2011;117(19):4551–4556. doi:10.1002/cncr.26082

53. Gourlay DL, Heit HA. Risk management is everyone's business. *Pain Med.* 2007;8(2):125–127. doi:10.1111/j.1526-4637.2006.00294.x

54. Merlin JS, Young SR, Arnold R, et al. Managing opioids, including misuse and addiction, in patients with serious illness in ambulatory palliative care: A qualitative study. *Am J Hosp Palliat Care.* 2020;37(7):507–513. doi:10.1177/1049909119890556

55. Butelman ER, Kreek MJ. Medications for substance use disorders (SUD): Emerging approaches. *Expert Opin Emerg Drugs.* 2017;22(4):301–315. doi:10.1080/14728214.2017.1395855

56. American Society of Addiction Medicine. Buprenorphine waiver management. 2021. Available at https://www.asam.org/advocacy/practice-resources/buprenorphine-waiver-management

57. Wightman R, Perrone J, Portelli I, Nelson L. Likeability and abuse liability of commonly prescribed opioids. *J Medical Toxicol.* 2012;8(4):335–340. doi:10.1007/s13181-012-0263-x

58. Vosburg SK, Beaumont J, Dailey-Govoni ST, Butler SF, Green JL. Evaluation of abuse and route of administration of extended-release tapentadol among treatment-seeking individuals, as captured by the Addiction Severity Index-Multimedia Version (ASI-MV). *Pain Med.* 2020;21(9):1891–1901. doi:10.1093/pm/pnz250

59. Vosburg SK, Severtson SG, Dart RC, et al. Assessment of tapentadol API abuse liability with the researched abuse, diversion and addiction-related surveillance system. *J Pain.* 2018;19(4):439–453. doi:10.1016/j.jpain.2017.11.007

60. Cicero TJ, Ellis MS, Kasper ZA. Relative preferences in the abuse of immediate-release versus extended-release opioids in a sample of treatment-seeking opioid abusers. *Pharmacoepidemiol Drug Saf.* 2017;26(1):56–62. doi:10.1002/pds.4078

61. Pergolizzi JV, Jr., Taylor R, Jr., LeQuang JA, Raffa RB. What's holding back abuse-deterrent opioid formulations? Considering 12 us stakeholders. *Expert Opin Drug Deliv.* 2018;15(6):567–576. doi:10.1080/17425247.2018.1473374

62. Webster LR. Interpreting labels of abuse-deterrent opioid analgesics. *J Opioid Manage.* 2017;13(6):415–423. doi:10.5055/jom.2017.0418

63. Alpert A, Powell D, Pacula RL. Supply-side drug policy in the presence of substitutes: Evidence from the introduction of abuse-deterrent opioids. *American Economic Journal: Economic Policy.* 2018;10(4):1–35. doi:10.1257/pol.20170082

64. Taveros MC, Chuang EJ. Pain management strategies for patients on methadone maintenance therapy: A systematic review of the literature. *BMJ Support Palliat Care.* 2017;7(4):383–389. doi:10.1136/bmjspcare-2016-001126

65. Chou R, Cruciani RA, Fiellin DA, et al. Methadone safety: A clinical practice guideline from the American Pain Society and College on Problems of Drug Dependence, in collaboration with the Heart Rhythm Society. *J Pain.* 2014;15(4):321–337. doi:10.1016/j.jpain.2014.01.494

66. Comer SD, Sullivan MA, Vosburg SK, et al. Abuse liability of intravenous buprenorphine/naloxone and buprenorphine alone in buprenorphine-maintained intravenous heroin abusers. *Addiction (Abingdon, UK).* 2010;105(4):709–718. doi:10.1111/j.1360-0443.2009.02843.x

67. Jones KF. Buprenorphine use in palliative care. *J Hospice Palliat Nurs.* 2019;21(6):540–547. doi:10.1097/njh.0000000000000598

68. Coffin PO, Behar E, Rowe C, et al. Nonrandomized intervention study of naloxone coprescription for primary care patients receiving long-term opioid therapy for pain. *Ann Intern Med.* 2016;165(4):245–252. doi:10.7326/M15-2771

69. Guy GP, Jr., Haegerich TM, Evans ME, Losby JL, Young R, Jones CM. Vital signs: Pharmacy-based naloxone dispensing: United States, 2012–2018. *MMWR Morb Mortal Wkly Rep.* 2019;68(31):679–686. doi:10.15585/mmwr.mm6831e1

70. Bohnert AS, Valenstein M, Bair MJ, et al. Association between opioid prescribing patterns and opioid overdose-related deaths. *JAMA.* 2011;305(13):1315–1321. doi:10.1001/jama.2011.370

71. Walley AY, Doe-Simkins M, Quinn E, Pierce C, Xuan Z, Ozonoff A. Opioid overdose prevention with intranasal naloxone among people who take methadone. *J Subst Abuse Treat.* 2013;44(2):241–247. doi:10.1016/j.jsat.2012.07.004

72. Starrels JL, Becker WC, Alford DP, Kapoor A, Williams AR, Turner BJ. Systematic review: Treatment agreements and urine drug testing to reduce opioid misuse in patients with chronic pain. *Ann Intern Med.* 2010;152(11):712–720. doi:10.7326/0003-4819-152-11-201006010-00004

73. Edwards T, Foster T, Brant JM. Managing cancer pain in patients with opioid and substance use disorders. *Semin Oncol Nurs.* 2019;35(3):279–283. doi:10.1016/j.soncn.2019.04.009

48.

ANXIETY

Kira Stalhandske

KEY POINTS

- Anxiety and existential distress occur across the continuum of chronic and serious illness and impact the patient and family.

- The National Consensus Project for Quality Palliative *Clinical Practice Guidelines* outlines the need for the palliative interdisciplinary team to addresses psychological and psychiatric aspects of care in the context of serious illness.

- Assessment and treatment of anxiety by the palliative advanced practice registered nurse (APRN) is essential and should be individualized to address all aspects of suffering: emotional, social, physical, and spiritual.

CASE STUDY: A PATIENT WITH ANXIETY AND DISTRESS

Mr. C was a 48-year-old married man who worked in academia. His past medical history was significant for asthma, obstructive sleep apnea necessitating continuous positive airway pressure (CPAP) at night, NYHA Class II heart failure, and anxiety. He was referred to palliative care for metastatic pancreatic cancer.

Mr. C had been in his usual state of health until 2 months prior to presentation, which including occasional anxiety due to shortness of breath on exertion due to his asthma and heart failure. when he began developing a sense of unease and increased anxiety, coinciding with being at home during the COVID-19 pandemic. Approximately 6 weeks prior to diagnosis he began experiencing intermittent abdominal pain described as a sharp ache that was in a "V shape extending down to the pelvis" and that radiated to his back. He found leaving his home and being outdoors relieved his anxiety and pain.

Mr. C's symptoms were initially attributed to progressive anxiety in the setting of a global pandemic and being at home in quarantine. His primary care provider prescribed buspirone 15 mg twice daily, clonazepam 0.5–0.75 mg at night as needed for anxiety, and cyclobenzaprine 10 mg at night as needed for pain and anxiety. He took extra-strength acetaminophen with no relief. He had a known intolerance to nonsteroidal anti-inflammatory drugs (NSAIDs).

Mr. C presented to the emergency department with a 1-week history of progressive abdominal pain and 25–30 pounds of unintentional weight loss. Workup revealed a pancreatic mass concerning for malignancy, with multiple hepatic masses and pulmonary nodules consistent with metastatic disease. He was admitted for biopsy of the liver mass, which confirmed metastatic pancreatobiliary adenocarcinoma. Upon admission to the hospital, the clonazepam and cyclobenzaprine were discontinued. He was continued on buspirone 15 mg twice daily and lorazepam 0.5 mg every 6 hours as needed. He was started on hydromorphone 4 mg orally every 4 hours as needed for pain.

At the palliative care consultation, Mr. C's most burdensome symptoms were anxiety, adjustment and coping with new diagnosis of metastatic pancreatic cancer, cancer-related pain, constipation, and intermittent nausea. His regimen was continued. He shared that he felt a sense of "calm" and decreased anxiety with the confirmation of a diagnosis and was motivated to figure out a treatment plan. He explored fears of loss of function and prolonged debility with progressive advanced illness. Mr. C shared that he was most concerned about his spouse and reflected on their relationship and partnership. His spouse was a consistent presence at his bedside during restricted visiting hours because of the pandemic.

The palliative advanced practice registered nurse (APRN) communicated with the various teams about Mr. C's preference for information. Mr. C wanted direct information about his disease and to participate in conversations about his care and any future decisions. The palliative APRN provided anticipatory guidance about his transition home after hospitalization and provided an overview of the role of outpatient palliative care.

Mr. C was discharged after a week-long hospitalization with plans for outpatient follow-up with oncology and palliative care. He had a chest port placed for anticipated chemotherapy. At the follow-up visit, the palliative APRN adjusted his pain medications and he was continued on buspirone.

The following week Mr. C had increased anxiety and saw his primary care provider, at which time he was initiated on citalopram 40 mg daily. The oncologist started him on olanzapine 5 mg at night for reports of worsening nausea. He had improvement with his nausea, insomnia, and anxiety with initiation of olanzapine. After a few days, he reported increased daytime jitteriness, which was attributed to high-dose citalopram. He was in contact with the palliative APRN, and there was discussion about clarifying the prescribing roles for the various providers.

One week later, Mr. C presented to his outpatient oncologist for further management. He was visibly jaundiced and hypotensive and was readmitted for evaluation for possible biliary obstruction or liver failure due to rapid progression of his cancer. After further imaging and evaluation, he was found to have multifocal biliary obstruction due to intrahepatic metastases which were too small for endoscopic intervention. Given rapid progression of his cancer and liver failure, Mr. C and his spouse decided to go home with hospice. Mr. C died at home with his spouse by his side a few days after discharge.

This case study highlights assessment by the palliative APRN to address physical and psychological symptoms associated with Mr. C's advanced cancer. The palliative APRN engaged in rapport-building, reflective listening and feedback, normalization of emotional and psychological reactions of the patient and family to coping with serious illness, anticipatory guidance, and communication and collaboration with healthcare providers across healthcare settings (inpatient providers, outpatient/ambulatory care providers, and community-based hospice). The palliative APRN supported patient and family decision-making over the trajectory of his illness from diagnosis to exploration of cancer-directed treatment to pursuit of hospice care.

INTRODUCTION

Anxiety is present in the everyday lives of humans. Anxiety is unique and specifically identified within the National Consensus Project for Quality Palliative Care's (NCP) *Clinical Practice Guidelines* (NCP) Domain 3: Psychological and Psychiatric Aspects of Care: "The interdisciplinary team assesses and addresses psychological and psychiatric aspects of care based on the best available evidence to maximize patient and family coping and quality of life,"[1] Due to the physical, affective, behavioral, and cognitive responses that anxiety may escalate, it can be clinically implicated in several of the domains of the NCP *Clinical Practice Guidelines*, such as Domain 1: Physical Aspects of Care; Domain 2: Physical Aspects of Care; Domain 4: Social Aspects of Care; and Domain 7: Care of the Patient at the End of Life.

Anxiety is a multidimensional subjective and objective experience with manifestations of physical, affective, behavioral, and cognitive responses.[2] As such, it can be considered both positive and negative. The experience is the physiological reaction that occurs in response to a perceived harmful attack or threat to survival. These include feelings of worry, apprehension, tension, and nervousness that are unpleasant and distressful, but they are a common response for patients and family members when faced with a serious diagnosis.

Anxiety is a natural and expected part of the coping process that helps us adapt to everyday concerns. However, extreme distressful anxiety can impair daily function, causing disability and disruptions in quality of life for patients, family, and caregivers. Specific differentiation between anxiety as a normal response and a specific diagnostic criterion that requires professional intervention and treatment is outlined according to the fifth edition of the *Diagnostic and Statistical Manual of Mental Disorders* (DSM-5-TR).[3] The experience of apparent uncontrollable physical, affective, behavioral, and cognitive symptoms having no specific stimulus warrants consideration of a pathological disorder. Anxiety disorders are categorized according to criteria and range in complexity and severity from panic attacks, acute stress disorder, generalized anxiety disorder, social anxiety disorders, phobias,

Table 48.1 ASSOCIATED CAUSES AND MIMICS OF ANXIETY

Acute emotional disruption	Interpersonal stresses
Anger	Legitimate worries and concerns
Anxiety disorders	Loss of control
Coping style (poor pattern)	Pain
Delirium	Physical symptoms
Fear	Side effects of medications
Financial concerns	Spiritual and existential crisis
Grief and bereavement	Withdrawal states

From National Consensus Project for Quality Palliative Care[1]; Loving, Dahlin[2]; and Borneman, Brown-Saltzman.[7]

obsessive-compulsive disorder, PTSD, anxiety secondary to a medical condition, and substance-induced anxiety disorders.[4]

Common situations, medical conditions, medications, and substances are associated with and can cause nonspecific anxiety symptoms. Existential and psychosocial concerns increase anxiety when a person is faced with mortality; long-term or permanent disability; loss of control; family and financial crisis; loss of meaning, hope, and purpose; and religious or spiritual crisis.[5,6] There is also considerable overlap and confusion among the anxiety, depression, and delirium that commonly arise as part of an illness trajectory and that can either lead, progress to, or continue in a vicious downward cycle when not recognized and treated appropriately (Table 48.1).

Despite the importance of mental health and the increasing prevalence of mental health disorders, US healthcare delivery systems are complex and fragmented, and patients and families are offered little guidance in navigating these systems to manage medical conditions effectively. The result is that anxiety is underestimated, untreated or undertreated, and unrecognized by healthcare professionals. Furthermore, intensified financial stress and social economic burden contribute to anxiety. Given this, anxiety is a contributory factor for caregiver burden, chronic distress, mortality, and comorbidity of the family and caregivers.[7,8] Barriers to appropriate professional intervention are also created by the lack of an integrated palliative care curriculum, inadequate professional resources, personal experiences, limited assessment skills and clinical knowledge, and personal biases associated with the stigma and stereotypes related to diagnosis. This often leads to acceptance of not treating anxiety or its physical, emotional, and psychosocial manifestations.

This chapter presents palliative care from the palliative advanced practice registered nurse (APRN) perspective, focusing on APRN competencies as an effective team member or leader for patient- and family-centered care. Assessment and management of anxiety are based on national quality clinical practice guidelines, evidence-based research, and recommendations by national professional organizations.

DEFINITIONS AND THE DISTRESS CONTINUUM

Any serious illness, such as cancer, is a life-altering experience. In the 1970s, Weissman and Worden identified the first 100 days after the diagnosis of cancer as an "existential plight" in which patients suddenly confront their mortality. This is an extremely fragile period filled with fear and anxiety. Information, communication, and overall psychosocial support are priority needs for the patient's mental well-being.

How anxiety is defined when an individual is diagnosed with a serious illness ranges from normal adjustment issues to syndromes that meet the diagnostic criteria for mental disorders. It occurs on a continuum of increasing levels and severity of psychosocial distress ranging from normal adjustment to adjustment disorders and subthreshold mental disorders to diagnosable mental disorders (Figure 48.1).[9–11] Anxiety can manifest as physical and emotional symptoms, and it impacts individuals; ability to cope with serious illness.[12] As healthcare professionals, palliative APRNs must appreciate a variety of related concepts and the distinctions between normal adjustment issues and mental disorders along the distress continuum to anticipate potential or actual needs, treatments, and interventions (Table 48.2).

Normal adjustment or psychosocial adaptation is not defined as a single event or as occurring in a specific moment in time. Adjustment and adaptation are constant and represent an ongoing process. Coping behaviors are continually integrated as the individual learns to manage life and relationships that incorporate and integrate a serious illness into daily activities. As personal, professional, and family relationships change, the individual is confronted with solving and mastering cancer-related and other illness-related emotion issues, and situations.[13–15]

Psychosocial distress has been defined as an unpleasant experience of an emotional, psychological, social, or spiritual nature that interferes with the ability to cope with treatment. It extends along a continuum, from common normal feelings of vulnerability, sadness, and fears, to problems that are disabling, such as depression, anxiety, panic, and feeling isolated or in a spiritual crisis.[9–15]

Adjustment disorders are a diagnostic category in DSM-5-TR. For some, the psychosocial stressors associated with a cancer diagnosis are identifiable, having a reactive psychopathology less severe than the diagnosable mental disorders that impair social or occupational behavior significantly. The DSM-5-TR anxiety disorders are a group of mental disorders whose common symptoms include excessive, unwarranted, often illogical anxiety, worry, fear, apprehension, and/or dread.[4]

PREVALENCE AND INCIDENCE: ANXIETY, DEPRESSION, MENTAL DISTRESS, AND CHRONIC DISEASE CONNECTION

There is a close relationship between the prevalence of anxiety and depression and the incidence of chronic illness. In 2018, more than half (51.8%) of US adults had at least 1 of 10 the following chronic conditions (arthritis, cancer, chronic obstructive pulmonary disease, coronary heart disease, current asthma, diabetes, hepatitis, hypertension, stroke, and weak or failing kidneys), and 27.2% of US adults had multiple chronic conditions.[16] Anxiety and depression are common in patients with serious or life-limiting illness. Receiving a diagnosis of a serious illness can be traumatic and debilitating. There is an increased incidence of PTSD symptoms for patients with a cancer diagnosis.[17] Progression of disease, increased medical interventions, hospitalizations, and intensive or critical care have been associated with psychological trauma.[18] There is a higher association of severe anxiety and depression symptoms for those with multiple medical conditions and for those with higher physical symptom burden.[16,19–21]

The US Centers for Disease Control and Prevention (CDC) and the National Center for Chronic Disease Prevention and Health Promotion (NCCDPHP), Division of Population Health recognized that chronic diseases can exacerbate symptoms of depression, and depressive disorders can lead to chronic diseases.[22] Anxiety, when unrecognized, unassessed, and undertreated, with other comorbid conditions, potentiates adjustment disorders. The CDC report *Mental Illness Surveillance Among Adults in the United States*, which supplements the CDC's *Morbidity and Mortality Weekly Report* (MMWR), compiled the first national data to measure the prevalence and effect of anxiety and other mental health conditions for adults in the United States. It underscored the correlation between

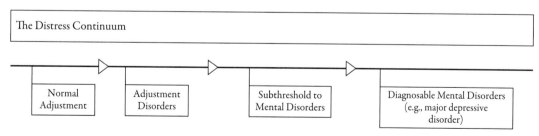

Figure 48.1 The distress continuum.

From PDQ Supportive and Palliative Care Editorial Board. Adjustment to cancer: Anxiety and distress (PDQ®): Health Professional Version. In: *PDQ Cancer Information Summaries*. Bethesda (MD): National Cancer Institute; March 6, 2019.[11]

Table 48.2 SUMMARY OF PSYCHOSOCIAL DISTRESS DEFINITIONS

Normal adjustment	Ongoing life processes and coping responses associated with living with cancer to: • Manage emotional distress • Solve specific cancer-related problems • Gain mastery or control over cancer-related life events
Psychosocial distress	Extends along a continuum ranging from: • Common normal feelings of vulnerability, sadness, and fears to problems that are disabling (i.e., depression, anxiety, panic) • Feeling isolated • Spiritual crisis Unpleasant experience of: • Emotional, psychological, social, or spiritual nature that interferes with the ability to cope with cancer treatment
Adjustment disorders	A diagnostic category of the fifth revised edition of the American Psychiatric Association's *Diagnostic and Statistical Manual of Mental Disorders* (DSM-5-TR): • Reactions to an identifiable psychosocial stressor with a degree of psychopathology • Less severe than diagnosable mental disorders yet in excess of what would be expected • Result in significant impairment in social or occupational functioning (i.e., major depressive disorder, generalized anxiety disorder)
Anxiety disorders	Group of mental disorders whose common symptoms include excessive, unwarranted, often illogical anxiety, worry, fear, apprehension, and/or dread. The DSM-5-TR examples include generalized anxiety disorder, panic disorder, agoraphobia, social anxiety disorder, specific phobia, obsessive-compulsive disorder, and posttraumatic stress disorder.

From PDQ Supportive and Palliative Care Editorial Board.[11]

mental illness and chronic illness.[23] Executive highlights pertaining to chronic disease and anxiety/mental illness are as follows:

- 25% of all US adults have a mental illness, and nearly 50% of US adults will develop at least one mental illness during their lifetime.

- Mental illness is associated with increased occurrence of chronic diseases such as cardiovascular disease, diabetes, obesity, asthma, epilepsy, and cancer.

- Treatment of mental illnesses associated with chronic illness reduces the effects of both and supports better outcomes.

- Chronic diseases can coexist in people who have suffered from depression[23,24] (Table 48.3).

Table 48.3 ANXIETY AND CHRONIC DISEASE PREVALENCE

MEDICAL CONDITIONS	EXAMPLES
Cardiovascular	Angina, congestive heart failure, hypovolemia, mitral valve prolapse, myocardial infarction, paroxysmal atrial tachycardia
Endocrine	Carcinoid syndrome, Cushing's disease, hyperglycemia, hypoglycemia, hyperthyroidism, hypothyroidism, pheochromocytoma
Immune	HIV/AIDS, systemic lupus erythematosus
Metabolic	Anemia, hypercalcemia, hyperkalemia, hypoglycemia, hyponatremia, hyperthermia
Respiratory	Asthma, chronic obstructive pulmonary disease, hypoxia, pneumonia, pulmonary disease, pulmonary edema, pulmonary embolus
Neurological	Akathisia, encephalopathy, brain lesion, seizure disorders, post-concussion syndrome, vertigo, cerebral vascular accident, dementia
Neoplasms	Islet cell adenomas, pheochromocytoma
Cancer	Hormone-producing tumors, pheochromocytoma

From Loving, Dahlin[2]; Noufi et al.[5]; and Borneman, Brown-Saltzman.[7]

ANXIETY AND THE OTHER SIDE OF THE DISTRESS CONTINUUM: ADJUSTMENT, INTEGRATION, AND LIFE TRANSFORMATION

Anxiety, whether positive or negative, occurs throughout life. It is a continual process with many revolving cycles, not a linear progression. When a patient is diagnosed with a serious illness, anxiety is often identified and separated into categories based on different life experiences. Palliative care practice differs because it embraces and incorporates the integrative nature and multidimensional holistic human needs approach to care, which challenges the assumption that anxiety and disease are separate processes. Anxiety needs to be viewed as a multidimensional experience within an integrated whole. Life and serious illness need to be understood as a whole, not as separate entities. The role of the palliative APRN is to understand and address anxiety from an interdisciplinary team perspective and to support adjustment from a medical and holistic perspective.

Cancer and serious illness are experienced within a continuum ranging from positive to negative in terms of adjustment. Positive adjustment is the patient's psychosocial adaptation process or increased ability to cope. Negative adjustment is the patient's inability to cope or the presence of anxiety and mental disorders that may require professional treatment.[24]

Palliative care professionals encourage patients and families to focus on life rather than on the illness. The patient's life and illness are not separate but coexist in a way that can be balanced, meaningful, and purposeful, integrating the illness into a whole that also includes the patient's many roles, responsibilities, personal identity, and life experiences.[25] Integration is not just a matter of incorporating disease management into one's daily activities but rather integrating the disease experience physically, mentally, emotionally, and spiritually.[24]

The clinical courses of cancer are prediagnosis, diagnosis, treatment, post-treatment, remission, reoccurrence/palliative care, and survivorship.[24] Within each clinical course there is an anxiety experience, normal adjustment and support, and an adjustment period.[26] Other diagnoses such as heart conditions, respiratory illnesses, and neurological conditions include diagnoses, treatment, adjustment, progression, with a continuing cycle of treatment, adjustment and progression leading to palliative care. Anxiety and adjustment are natural parts of the illness experience. The clinical courses should not be considered as separate entities but rather as an ongoing experience of anxiety, challenges, and adjustment (Tables 48.4, 48.5, and 48.6). Anxiety adjustment goes beyond the natural state of adaptation, coping, and integration. Adjustment outcomes have been identified in different categories, such as healing, psychosocial and spiritual pain in palliative care, posttraumatic growth, stress-related growth, benefit-finding resilience, subjective well-being, and self-actualization.[27–29]

Life-transforming change can result from the illness experience. Some patients experience a total paradigm shift, where unanticipated discovery of personal abilities and untapped resources helps the patient overcome the challenges of a serious illness diagnosis and life challenges outside of illness. With this shift, the patient's life is taken to a previously unknown level where he or she experiences a more fulfilling, purposeful, and meaningful life, one with greater depth psychosocially and spiritually (Figure 48.2).

Some patients describe a reduction in negative experiences; others identify an increase in positive experiences. These changes can occur in the areas of self-care, relationships, spirituality, being true to oneself, personal strength, and priorities or purpose. The "domains" of this change are pre-diagnosis, diagnosis of a serious illness, adaptive beliefs and attributes, pragmatic actualization, and transformation, extrapolated from research in the cancer experience. Each domain has its own categories and process themes.[25]

A pre-illness, such as pre-cancer, is trauma and healing. The process theme focuses on the pre-illness state and diagnosis as a challenging event. The domain of the illness or cancer has three subcategories: debilitation, challenges to normal life, and coping. The debilitation subcategory focuses on the process themes of symptoms and treatment side effects. The challenges to normal life subcategory focuses on the process themes of uncertainty, heightened awareness, and loss. The major view expressed by patients

Table 48.4 SUMMARY OF ADJUSTMENT STAGES WHEN DIAGNOSED WITH CANCER OR ANOTHER SERIOUS ILLNESS: PRE-DIAGNOSIS AND DIAGNOSIS

PHASE	ANXIETY EXPERIENCE	NORMAL ADJUSTMENT AND SUPPORT	ADJUSTMENT PERIOD
Prediagnosis	Normal levels of anxiety and concern Crisis: Psychological and existential	Support systems, personal, religious, spiritual	1 week
Diagnosis			
Phase 1	Disbelief Denial Shock High level of distress, emotions Inability to remember or understand	Compassionate communication skills to deliver "bad news,"	Variable, 1–2 weeks
Phase 2 Dysphoria	Distress ranges: Illness-death depression, anxiety, insomnia, anorexia Poor concentration: Inability to function in daily roles Hope: Increased with understanding and awareness of treatment	Education and information	Variable, 1–2 weeks
Phase 3 Adaptation	Coping strategies: Problem-focused Emotion-focused Meaning-focused	Personalized coping styles and strategies	Variable, 1–2 weeks

From PDQ Supportive and Palliative Care Editorial Board.[11]

Table 48.5 SUMMARY OF ADJUSTMENT STAGES WHEN DIAGNOSED WITH CANCER OR OTHER
SERIOUS ILLNESSES: TREATMENT, POST-TREATMENT, REMISSION

TREATMENT	POST-TREATMENT	REMISSION
Anxiety experience: Treatment fears and focuses: Side effects Disruptions in daily life Effectiveness Survival	Anxiety experience: Positive anticipation, ambivalence, vulnerability Fear: Lack of physician connection and medical care	Anxiety experience: Normal anxiety regarding recurrence
Normal adjustment and support: Understanding Short-term discomforts outweigh long-term gains	Normal adjustment and support: Balance of positive expectations, reality of fears, apprehensions	Normal adjustment & support: Coping strategies Expression of emotions (i.e., honesty, nonjudgmental acceptance)
Adjustment period: Variable	Adjustment period: Variable	Adjustment period: Variable

From PDQ Supportive and Palliative Care Editorial Board.[11]

in this subcategory is "it's not just about the diagnosis (e.g. heart disease, cancer)." Support comes in the form of education and lowering distress.

The adaptive beliefs and attributes domain has two subcategories: personal life and hope. Personal life focuses on the process themes of maintaining a personal life, tolerance and the expectation that life could be improved, mastery of life skills, and improved situational challenges. The hope category's process themes focus on motivation, protection, and surrounding oneself with people who provide support and offer grounding in personal truth and what is found as meaningful.

The domain of pragmatic actualization entails turning hope into reality. It has two subcategories: exploring and resources. Exploring focuses on the process themes of proactive learning, research, personal decisions and choices, and active experimentation. The resources subcategory focuses on

Table 48.6 SUMMARY OF ADJUSTMENT STAGES WHEN DIAGNOSED WITH CANCER OR ANOTHER SERIOUS ILLNESS: PALLIATIVE CARE AND SURVIVORSHIP

PALLIATIVE CARE	SURVIVORSHIP
Anxiety experience Disbelief, denial, shock, crying, withdrawal, isolation, spiritual/ religious anger Shift: palliative curing to healing	Anxiety experience Greater appreciation, reprioritizing of life values, strengthening of spiritual or religious beliefs
Normal adjustment and support: Palliative care: Hope through what is meaningful	Normal adjustment and support: National organizations (i.e., programs, tools, resources) Physical, emotional well-being support
Adjustment period: Weeks	Adjustment period: Gradual over many years

From PDQ Supportive and Palliative Care Editorial Board.[11]

gathering and giving in a wide range of meaningful relationships, unexpected resources, expanded spirituality, and conservation of resources in times of greater need.

The domain of transformation focuses on a recurrent process theme, "it's not just about the diagnosis," in terms of applying newly discovered personal resources and heightened skills to non-diagnosis issues. Applying these new-found personal resources and abilities ultimately leads to a greater sense of gratitude, life appreciation, and empathy and a higher interest in life-fulfilling pursuits.[25]

SCREENING AND ASSESSMENT

The sequential screening, evaluation, and referral process is undertaken when anxiety or psychosocial issues arise. Formal validated screening assessment tools should be utilized to evaluate the patient's and family's coping.[30–34] For cancer related anxiety, guidelines from the American Society of Clinical Oncology (ASCO) and the National Comprehensive Cancer Network (NCCN) recommend screening for anxiety at time of initial cancer diagnosis and periodically when clinically indicated or at changes in cancer status, treatment plan, or transitions in care.[9,31,35]

Screening tools for other diagnoses that use a brief, self-report questionnaire method can be used in a variety of practice settings for evaluation of anxiety and depression symptoms. The Anxiety Screening Index (ASI) is a 16-item self-report index, with scores rated on a scale of 0 to 4. Higher scores are associated with increasing levels anxiety.[2,34] Initial screening for anxiety and depression may use the Patient Health Questionnaire for Depression and Anxiety (PHQ-4). If the patient screens positive for depression, the PHQ-9 can be used to monitor depression and treatment over time.[2,35] The seven-item GAD-7 questionnaire can be used for screening and monitoring over time.[35] The patient's score establishes the level and severity of distress to guide next steps. If distress is high, a referral for an in-depth psychosocial assessment by an appropriate mental health professional is made.[26]

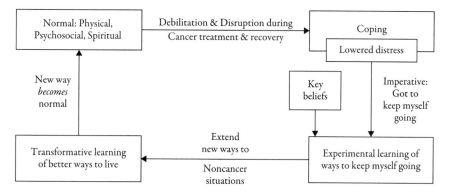

Figure 48.2 Cancer-related life transformation change process.
From Skeath P, Norris S, Katheria V, et al. The nature of life-transforming change among cancer survivors. *Qual Health Res.* 2013;23(9):1155–1167.[25]

The expression of, assessment for, and interventions for anxiety are placed in the cultural and spiritual domains of the NCP *Clinical Practice Guidelines*. Domain 5 addresses spiritual, religious, and existential aspects of palliative care. Domain 6 addresses cultural aspects of care.[1] Inappropriate or incomplete awareness of cultural, religious, and spiritual beliefs or needs can lead to inappropriate and unacceptable plans of care, resulting in unnecessary and undue anxiety and distress.

Comprehensive anxiety assessment includes performing a detailed history, review of systems, physical exam, and diagnostic and laboratory evaluation. A detailed history to identify contributing or predisposing factors to anxiety includes reviewing an individual's medications that mimic anxiety symptoms, substance use history, anxiety-associated medical conditions, and lifestyle contributions. Common cognitive and physical manifestations of anxiety can be detected by a review of systems. Physical examination is appropriate and may reveal symptoms of tachycardia, tachypnea, diaphoresis, skin changes, tongue changes, palpitations, rapid speech, restlessness, and tremors.[2,34] Physiological derangements may be contributing to anxiety symptoms and can be identified by laboratory testing, including complete blood cell counts, metabolic panels, cardiac studies, hormonal studies (e.g., thyroid), infectious workup, and toxicologies. Comprehensive assessment of psychosocial and spiritual assessments of the patient and family, support systems and coping are critical to creating a treatment plan Assessment of patient and family understanding of medical condition, expectations and treatment preferences.

CAREGIVER AND FAMILY-FOCUSED ASSESSMENT

Screening and assessment are not just patient-focused but are also family-focused, based on the standards of the NCP *Clinical Practice Guidelines*.[1] Family members are the most common caregivers, and their needs often go unaddressed. Many are easily overwhelmed physically, mentally, socially, and financially. Caregiver stress and burden can lead to increased health risks in terms of heart disease, hypertension, immune impairment, and cognitive functioning that may meet DSM-V criteria for a psychiatric condition.[36] Caregiver stress can also contribute to decline in the care recipient.[37] When assessing caregivers, the palliative APRN should identify the specific problems, needs, strengths, and resources they have for themselves and those that affect the patient's care.[38] Use of the CARES framework is recommended in oncologic settings for a systematic assessment and approach to support family caregivers and is appropriate to other settings: **C**onsidering caregivers as part of the unit of care, **A**ssessing the caregiver's situation and needs, **R**eferring to appropriate services and resources, **E**ducating about practical aspects of caregiving, and **S**upporting caregivers through bereavement.[39]

Communication with patients and family members and their participation as partners in care are key. By partnering with them, the palliative APRN can identify their needs and set out the next steps. The patient and family are part of the process since assessment is a combination of self-report and evaluation by members of the professional team. This approach to assessing caregivers' needs and strengths can improve the overall health and quality of life for both the patient and caregivers.[40] The five major components of the caregiver experience that provide insight into caregiver stress are caregiver context, primary stressors, secondary stressors, resources, and outcomes.[41]

Caregiver context addresses sociodemographic information, history of illness, and caregiving and living arrangements. *Primary stressors* from the patient experience are symptoms, impairments, activities of daily living, behavioral and cognitive issues, and the caregiver's subjective burden. *Secondary stressors* are tension and conflicts of employment, relationships, and maintaining roles and responsibility. *Resources* are social, financial, emotional, and gains from experience. *Outcomes* are either positive or negative health outcomes related to the caregiver.[8] Assessment of family caregiver distress and identification of bereavement resources, support groups, and counseling should be provided to family caregivers who have high levels of distress and anxiety because they have higher risk for complicated grief, distress, and anxiety following the patient's death.[42]

The National Center on Caregiving (https://www.caregiving.org) offers support and guidance in the development of policy, resources, and programs. It serves as a central resource on caregiving and long-term care issues.[43]

TREATMENT

The palliative care approach to treatment occurs across a continuum, with many different and simultaneous dependent, independent, and collaborative team approaches and interventions. Referral to psychiatric or mental health specialist is appropriate when the patient has preexisting psychiatric pathologies, suicidal ideation, or when anxiety symptoms interfere with the patient's ability to function or are persistent and progressive despite intervention.[35]

PHARMACOLOGIC MANAGEMENT

Common medications and substances that can cause nonspecific anxiety symptoms are listed in Table 48.7. Pharmacologic agents used to manage anxiety are listed in Table 48.8.

When considering treatment, the APRN should evaluate the extent or severity of the patient's anxiety symptoms and their impact on function, quality of life, and prognosis to determine if there is time to benefit from treatment.[12,48–51] For patients with limited prognosis of days or weeks, the use of rapid-acting agents such as benzodiazepines and antipsychotics is preferred.

Table 48.7 ANXIETY-CAUSING MEDICATIONS AND SUBSTANCES

ALCOHOL AND NICOTINE WITHDRAWAL	BRONCHODILATORS AND SYMPATHOMIMETICS
Analgesics	Caffeine (stimulants)
Anticholinergic	Cannabis
Anticonvulsants	Cocaine
Antidepressants	Corticosteroids and anabolic steroids
Antiemetics	Digitalis toxicity
Antihistamines and decongestants	Epinephrine
Antihypertensives	Hallucinogens
Antiparkinsonian drugs	Sedatives (hypnotic withdrawal and paradoxical reaction)
Antipsychotics	
Anesthetics and analgesics	
Benzodiazepines (and their withdrawal)	

From references Loving, Dahlin[2]; Noufi et al.[5]; and Borneman, Brown-Salzman.[7]

Benzodiazepines are commonly used for the relief of acute anxiety and may be used alone or as combination therapy with an antidepressant. They have a rapid onset and can reduce nausea. Common side effects include sedation, memory loss, delirium, confusion, and gait instability. Acute toxicity and overdose can cause respiratory suppression, especially in patients with lung disease, and can cause cognitive impairment.[50] With long-term use of benzodiazepines, there are risks for physical dependency, abuse, and addiction.[12,49] Use of long-acting agents can prevent the loss of efficacy that can occur with shorter-acting agents.[12,49]

Most antidepressants are effective for treating anxiety, although therapeutic effect may take several weeks to months to be reached, and lower doses are tolerated best. Antidepressant selection may depend on prior antidepressant use and potential drug–drug interactions. Many clinicians treating anxiety disorders use serotonergic agents, selective serotonin reuptake inhibitors (SSRIs), or serotonin-norepinephrine reuptake inhibitors (SNRIs) as their first choice due to these agents' reliability and effectiveness for panic, generalized anxiety disorders, PTSD, and obsessive-compulsive disorder. Common side effects are managed with low-dose titration. SSRIs have no adjuvant therapeutic effect on neuropathic pain, unlike SNRIs.[5] Tricyclic antidepressants are effective and inexpensive, and they serve as an adjuvant for neuropathic pain. Tricyclics can promote sleep and appetite but have a high side-effect burden.

Antipsychotics are reliable, but long-term use can produce the side effect of movement disorders. This risk makes them a second-line treatment. They are valuable when a rapid anxiolytic effect is needed and if the patient cannot tolerate benzodiazepines or has respiratory compromise.[52]

Ketamine (S-ketamine), an analgesic used for refractory pain (operative/postsurgical and cancer-related pain), has positive effects on severe psychological distress and has a rapid effect on stress, anxiety, and depression.[53] A single dose of oral ketamine has been demonstrated to provide rapid and sustained relief of anxiety and depression.[44] When used for analgesia, ketamine is commonly administered in a continuous intravenous infusion and now in an approved intranasal preparation for depression. Ketamine can be compounded to be used in various routes of administration, including oral and buccal.

The geriatric population has special considerations, and medication adjustments are required. Treatment of anxiety often reflects the balance between goals and the length of life remaining. This is especially true in geriatric palliative care evaluation and treatment. For patients with less than a few months to live who are minimally ambulatory, the palliative APRN can prescribe benzodiazepines for rapid relief of symptoms or brief treatment. They are considered a second-line drug based on their longer half-life, which causes adverse drug effects. Benzodiazepines overall have a paradoxical effect that may actually cause more anxiety, especially in the elderly, and they are not recommended because they can increase confusion. Typically, tricyclic antidepressants and β-adrenergic agents are not well-tolerated. The most common side effects in the elderly are ataxia, cognitive impairment, and excessive

Table 48.8 COMMON PHARMACOLOGIC TREATMENT OPTIONS FOR ANXIETY

GENERIC NAME	APPROXIMATE ORAL DAILY DOSE AND RANGES (MG)	COMMENT
Benzodiazepines		
Alprazolam	0.25–2 tid–qid	Short-acting
Clonazepam	0.5–2 bid–qid	Long-acting
Diazepam	5–10 bid–qid	Long-acting; rapid onset with single PO dosage
Lorazepam	0.5–2 tid–qid	Short-acting; multiple routes, PO, SL, IV, IM. Preferred for patients with impaired hepatic function, no metabolites.
Midazolam	Infusion dosing sedation: 0.5-1 mg/h, effective dose range 1–20 mg/h.	Use for terminal agitation. Most commonly used medication for palliative sedation. Routes IV or SC.
Azapirones		
Buspirone	5–20 tid	Extended time to peak effect similar to antidepressants Low potential for abuse and toxicity
Antidepressants		
Serotonin reuptake inhibitors		
Citalopram	20–40 daily	Risk for QT interval prolongation. Not recommended for use greater than 40 mg daily.
Fluoxetine	10–80 daily	Longest half-life among serotonin reuptake inhibitors
Paroxetine	10–60 daily	Short half-life, side effects-sedation
Sertraline	50–200 daily	Few drug–drug interactions
Tricyclics		All have moderate risk for QTc prolongation, Dual indication for neuropathic pain
Nortriptyline	10–150 at bedtime	Less anticholinergic side effects
Amitriptyline	10–75 at bedtime	Anticholinergic side effects
Desipramine	12.5–150 daily	Least sedating tricyclic antidepressant
Imipramine	12.5–150 daily	High risk for orthostatic hypotension
Serotonin-norepinephrine reuptake inhibitors		Role for treatment of neuropathic and central pain. Activating effects can help with energy. Consider dosage in the morning to avoid insomnia.
Duloxetine	30–60 daily	Avoid use in hepatic and renal impairment (CrCL <30 mL/min)
Venlafaxine	75–375 daily	Can be utilized in immediate release formulation the setting of renal impairment.
Other Antidepressants		
Mirtazapine	7.5–60 daily	Promotes sleep and appetite at low doses Oral disintegrating tablets available
Bupropion	100 mg immediate release bid, 150 mg extended release bid	Risk of seizures at doses >450 mg/daily
Antipsychotics/Neuroleptics		
Olanzapine	5–15 daily[a]	PO, SL, and IM routes. Oral disintegrating tablets available. Has less extrapyramidal side effects and less demonstrated QTc effects compared to Haloperidol.
Quetiapine	25–200 daily[a]	Preferred for patients with Parkinson's disease
Risperidone	1–3 daily[a]	

Table 48.8 CONTINUED

GENERIC NAME	APPROXIMATE ORAL DAILY DOSE AND RANGES (MG)	COMMENT
Haloperidol	0.5–2 q2–12h	Inexpensive and multiple routes of administration (IV, PO, and IM)
Chlorpromazine	12.5–50 q4–12h	IV, PO and PR. Side effects sedation, extrapyramidal side effects and hypotension. Most common use for palliative sedation with terminal delirium/agitation.
Antihistamines		
Hydroxyzine	25–50 q4–6h	Risk of anticholinergic side effects and delirium
GABAergic		
Gabapentin	600–2,400 mg/day	Use for social and generalized anxiety and panic disorders.
Ketamine		Multiple routes IV, oral, buccal and intranasal. May require compounding. Dosing is variable to use and route. A single oral dose of 0.5 mg/kg has been demonstrated to provide anxiety relief. (Irwin)

ᵃ In divided doses

From Noufi et al.[5]; Irwin, Hirst[35]; Irwin, Iglewicz[44]; Felton et al.[45]; Prommer[46]; and Garakani et al.[47]

sleepiness. Opioids are indicated for treatment of anxiety secondary to dyspnea in terminally ill patients.[54]

NONPHARMACOLOGIC TREATMENT

Dignity therapy (DT) is a brief, individualized psychotherapy to relieve psychological and existential distress in patients with a serious and life-limiting illness, allowing them to reflect on memories and issues important to them and to recall or share with others.[55] The interdisciplinary team should explore opportunities for patients to engage in life review, legacy-making activities, and honoring future moments.

Palliative care includes holistic integrative therapies as well as conventional therapies. Holism and palliative care philosophy are inseparable since they both focus on the total person, with the belief that the mind, body, and spirit are inseparable and interdependent and that health, illness, and dying are manifestations of the life processes of the whole person.[54–59,62] In both holistic and palliative care, the partnership among the patient, family, and provider generates a sense of empowerment and enables healing (if not necessarily a cure) and transcendence. Nonpharmacologic therapies used for anxiety are outlined in Table 48.9.

There are many integrative holistic therapies that can be used to decrease anxiety. They can improve the overall quality of life for patients and families. Maximum benefits with minimal risk can be achieved when complementary/alternative medicine and therapies are integrated with conventional treatments. This can be accomplished through collaborative interdisciplinary team processes as a component of the overall plan of care (Table 48.10).

Table 48.9 NONPHARMACOLOGIC ANXIETY TREATMENT

MIND-BODY THERAPY	POSTURE AND MOBILITY	TOUCH AND BODY WORK ENERGETIC THERAPIES	SENSE THERAPY
Biofeedback	Movement therapy	Massage	Aromatherapy
Psychotherapy	Tai Chi	Reflexology	Music therapy
Guided Imagery	Yoga	Acupressure	Kinesthetics
Hypnosis		Healing touch	
Meditation		Reiki	
Cognitive therapy		Therapeutic touch	
Behavioral therapy		Polarity therapy	
Reminiscence/Life review, Centering			
Creating intention			
Journaling			
Dignity therapy			

From Freeman[56]; Dossey, Keengan[57]; Lindquist et al.[58]; Matzo, Sherman[59]; Fulton et al.[60]; and Satsangi, Brugnoli.[61]

Table 48.10 INTEGRATIVE HOLISTIC TREATMENT OF ANXIETY

NUTRITIONAL THERAPY	EASTERN THERAPIES	INTEGRATIVE HOLISTIC PROVIDERS
Herbology/Herbal Medicine Nutritional supplements	Traditional Chinese Medicine Acupuncture AMMA therapy Shiatsu Jin shin jyutsu	Ayurveda medicine Naturopathic medicine Homeopathic medicine Integrative holistic medicine

From Freeman[56]; Dossey, Keengan[57]; Lindquist et al.[58]; Matzo, Sherman.[59]

SUMMARY

Anxiety contributes to increased suffering and impacts coping and provision of care for the patient and family. Palliative care is a comprehensive, evidence-based specialty provided by a supportive interdisciplinary team that addresses patient- and family-centered needs. Whether the illness is life-threatening, chronic, progressive, advanced, or terminal, the identification and management of anxiety are central to effective treatment. Anxiety is a common response in patients and family members and is manifested in various physical, affective, behavioral, and cognitive responses. Palliative care incorporates anxiety into professional practice standards with the goal of anticipating, identifying, assessing, and addressing it via core and interdisciplinary team approaches.

The interdisciplinary team, through supportive listening and exploration of the patient's history and an understanding of their medical condition, expectations, fears, hopes, and adjustment to illness, can align delivery of care to meet the needs of the patient and family. Social workers assess and address adjustment to illness, coping, support systems, and needs and provide therapeutic grief and bereavement counseling and support of emotional and logistical aspects of care. Chaplains or spiritual care providers explore aspects of faith, existential distress, and coping and may provide prayer, support of faith-based traditions or practices, and connection with community-based spiritual care providers. Child life specialists facilitate developmentally based interventions for coping and communication for children and adolescents.

Palliative APRNs assess diagnose, treat, and evaluate the effectiveness of anxiety management. They provide anticipatory guidance and support to the patient and family and collaborate with other health providers and specialists to ensure the patient and family receive clear, direct, and compassionate information about their medical condition, treatments, and prognosis.

REFERENCES

1. National Consensus Project for Quality Palliative Care. *Clinical Practice Guidelines for Quality Palliative Care.* 4th ed. Richmond, VA: National Coalition for Hospice and Palliative Care; 2018. https://www. nationalcoalitionhpc.org/ncp; 7
2. Loving NG, Dahlin CM. Anxiety, depression and delirium. In: Matzo M, Sherman D, eds. *Palliative Care Nursing: Quality of Care to the End of Life.* 5th ed. New York: Springer; 2018: 545–580.
3. Thalén-Lindström A, Larsson G, Glimelius B, Johansson B. Anxiety and depression in oncology patients: A longitudinal study of a screening, assessment, and psychosocial support intervention. *Acta Oncol.* 2013;52(1):118–127. doi:10.3109/0284186X.2012.707785
4. American Psychiatric Association. *Diagnostic and Statistical Manual of Mental Disorders.* 5th ed. Arlington, VA: American Psychiatric Association; 2013. DSM.psychiatryonline.org.
5. Noufi P, Raza H, Pao M. Depression and anxiety in palliative care. In: Berger A, O'Neill J, eds. *Palliative Care and Supportive Oncology.* 5th ed. Philadelphia, PA: Lippincott Williams & Wilkins; 2021: 990–1041.
6. Salman J, Wolfe E, Patel SK. Anxiety and depression. In: Ferrell BR, Paice JA, eds. *Oxford Textbook of Palliative Nursing.* 5th ed. Oxford: Oxford University Press; 2019: 309–318.
7. Borneman T, Brown-Saltzman K. Meaning in illness. In: Ferrell BR, Paice JA, eds. *Oxford Textbook of Palliative Nursing.* 5th ed. Oxford: Oxford University Press; 2019: 456–466.
8. Witt-Sherman D. Family caregivers. In: Matzo M, Sherman D, eds. *Palliative Care Nursing: Quality Care to the End of Life.* 5th ed. New York: Springer; 2018:165–186.
9. National Comprehensive Cancer Network. NCCN clinical practice guidelines in oncology (NCCN©). *Distress management Ver 2.* 2021. https://www.nccn.org/professionals/physician_gls/pdf/distress.pdf
10. Kostopoulou S, Parpa E, Tsilika E, et al. Advanced cancer patients' perceptions of dignity: The impact of psychologically distressing symptoms and preparatory grief. *J Palliat Care.* 2018;33(2):88–94. doi:10.1177/0825859718759882
11. PDQ Supportive and Palliative Care Editorial Board. Adjustment to cancer: Anxiety and distress (PDQ®): Health Professional Version. June 23, 2021. In: *PDQ Cancer Information Summaries.* Bethesda (MD): National Cancer Institute; Available from: https://www.ncbi.nlm.nih.gov/books/NBK65960/.
12. Salt S, Mulvaney CA, Preston NJ. Drug therapy for symptoms associated with anxiety in adult palliative care patients. *Cochrane Database Syst Rev.* 2017;5(5):CD004596. Published 2017 May 18. doi:10.1002/14651858.CD004596.pub3
13. Bickel KE, Levy C, MacPhee ER, et al. An integrative framework of appraisal and adaptation in serious medical illness. *J Pain Symptom Manage.* 2020;60(3):657–677.e6. doi:10.1016/j.jpainsymman.2020.05.018
14. Teo I, Krishnan A, Lee GL. Psychosocial interventions for advanced cancer patients: A systematic review. *Psychooncology.* 2019;28(7):1394–1407. doi:10.1002/pon.5103
15. Fashoyin-Aje LA, Martinez KA, Dy SM. New patient-centered care standards from the commission on cancer: Opportunities and challenges. *J Support Oncol.* 2012;10(3):107–111. doi:10.1016/j.suponc.2011.12.002
16. Boersma P, Black LI, Ward BW. Prevalence of multiple chronic conditions among us adults, 2018. Prev *Chronic Dis.* 2020;17:E106. doi:10.5888/pcd17.200130
17. Unseld M, Krammer K, Lubowitzki S, et al. Screening for post-traumatic stress disorders in 1017 cancer patients and correlation with anxiety, depression, and distress. *Psychooncology.* 2019;28(12):2382–2388. doi:10.1002/pon.5239
18. Ganzel BL. Trauma-informed hospice and palliative care. *Gerontologist.* 2018;58(3):409–419. doi:10.1093/geront/gnw146
19. Read JR, Sharpe L, Modini M, Dear BF. Multimorbidity and depression: A systematic review and meta-analysis. *J Affect Disord.* 2017;221:36–46. doi:10.1016/j.jad.2017.06.009

20. Niles AN, Dour HJ, Stanton AL, et al. Anxiety and depressive symptoms and medical illness among adults with anxiety disorders. *J Psychosom Res*. 2015;78(2):109–115. doi:10.1016/j.jpsychores.2014.11.018

21. Hofmann S, Hess S, Klein C, Lindena G, Radbruch L, Ostgathe C. Patients in palliative care-development of a predictive model for anxiety using routine data. *PLoS One*. 2017;12(8):e0179415. doi:10.1371/journal.pone.0179415

22. Chapman DP, Perry GS, Strine TW. The vital link between chronic disease and depressive disorders. *Prev Chronic Dis*. 2005;2(1):A14. Epub December 15, 2004.

23. Centers for Disease Control and Prevention. Morbidity and Mortality Weekly Report (MMWR): Mental illness surveillance among adults in the United States. 60(3)Supplements:1–32. http://www.cdc.gov/mmwr/preview/mmwrhtml/su6003a1.htm?s_cid=su6003a1.

24. Whittem R, Dixon J. Chronic illness: The process of integration. *J Clin Nurs*. 2008;17:177–187. doi:10.1111/j.1365-2702.2007.0224

25. Skeath P, Norris S, Katheria V, et al. The nature of life-transforming change among cancer survivors. *Qual Health Res*. 2013;23(9):1155–1167.

26. Holland JC, Wiesel TW. Principles of psycho-oncology. In: Holland JC, Frei E, Bast RC, eds. *Holland-Frei Cancer Medicine*. 9th ed. Hoboken, NJ: Wiley Blackwell; 2017: 531–536.

27. Tartaro J, Roberts J, Nosarti C, et al. Who benefits?: Distress, adjustment and benefit finding among breast cancer survivors. *J Psychosoc Oncol*. 2005;23(2–3):45–64.

28. Johnson J. An overview of psychosocial support services: Resources for healing. *Cancer Nurs*. 2000;23(4):310–3. doi:10.1097/00002820-200008000-00009

29. Lam WWT, Mitchell AJ. Screening and assessment for distress. In: Breibart W, Butow P, Jacobsen P, eds. *Psycho-Oncology*. 4th ed. Oxford: Oxford University Press; 2021: 121–129.

30. Ferrell BR, Twaddle ML, Melnick A, Meier DE. National consensus project clinical practice guidelines for quality palliative care guidelines, 4th edition. *J Palliat Med*. 2018;21(12):1684–1689. doi:10.1089/jpm.2018.0431

31. Ferrell BR, Temel JS, Temin S, et al. Integration of palliative care into standard oncology care: American society of clinical oncology clinical practice guideline update. *J Clin Oncol*. 2017;35(1):96–112. doi:10.1200/JCO.2016.70.1474

32. Osman H, Shrestha S, Temin S, et al. Palliative care in the global setting: ASCO resource-stratified practice guideline. *J Glob Oncol*. 2018;4:1–24. doi:10.1200/JGO.18.00026

33. Smith CB, Phillips T, Smith TJ. Using the new ASCO clinical practice guideline for palliative care concurrent with oncology care using the team approach. *Am Soc Clin Oncol Educ Book*. 2017;37:714–723. doi:10.1200/EDBK_175474

34. Ford JA. The complexity of assessment and treatment for anxiety in patients with a terminal illness. *J Hospice Palliat Nurs*. 2016;18(2):131–138. doi:10.1097/NJH.0000000000000223

35. Irwin SA, Hirst JM. In: Block S, ed. Overview of Anxiety in Palliative Care. UpToDate. Waltham, MA: UptoDate. July 21, 2021. https://www.uptodate.com/contents/overview-of-anxiety-in palliative-care.

36. Family Care Giver Alliance. Caregiver assessment: Principles, guidelines, and strategies for change. Report from a national consensus development conference, 2006. Vol. 1. San Francisco, CA: Family Caregiver Alliance. 2006. http://www.caregiver.org/caregiver/jsp/content/pdfs/v1_consensus.pdf.

37. Moss KO, Kurzawa C, Daly B, Prince-Paul M. Identifying and addressing family caregiver anxiety. *J Hosp Palliat Nurs*. 2019;21(1):14–20. doi:10.1097/NJH.0000000000000489

38. Vanderwerker LC, Laff RE, Kadan-Lotick NS, McColl S, Prigerson HG. Psychiatric disorders and mental health services use among caregivers of advanced cancer patients. *J Clin Oncol*. 2005;23(28):6899–907.

39. Alam S, Hannon B, Zimmermann C. Palliative care for family caregivers. *J Clin Oncol*. 2020;38(9):926–936. doi:10.1200/JCO.19.00018

40. Fineberg L, Houser A. Fact Sheet 258. *Assessing Family Caregiver Needs: Policy and Practice Considerations*. Washington DC: AARP Public Policy Institute. June 2012. https://www.caregiving.org/wp-content/uploads/2010/11/AARP-caregiver-fact-sheet.pdf

41. Kutner KS, Kilbourn KM. Bereavement: Addressing challenges faced by advanced cancer patients and their caregivers, and their physicians. *Prim Care*. 2009;36(4):825–44. doi:10.1016/j.pop.2009.07.004

42. Oechsle K, Ullrich A, Marx G, et al. Prevalence and predictors of distress, anxiety, depression, and quality of life in bereaved family caregivers of patients with advanced cancer. *Am J Hosp Palliat Care*. 2020;37(3):201–213. doi:10.1177/1049909119872755

43. AARP and National Alliance for Caregiving. *Caregiving in the United States* 2020. Washington, DC: AARP; May 14, 2020. https://doi.org/10.26419/ppi.00103.001

44. Irwin SA, Iglewicz A. Oral ketamine for the rapid treatment of depression and anxiety in patients receiving hospice care. *J Palliat Med*. 2010;13(7):903–908. doi:10.1089/jpm.2010.9808

45. Felton M, Weinberg R, Pruskowski J. Olanzapine for nausea, delirium, anxiety, insomnia, and cachexia #315. *J Palliat Med*. 2016;19(11):1224–1225. doi:10.1089/jpm.2016.0220

46. Prommer E. Midazolam: An essential palliative care drug. *Palliat Care Soc Pract*. 2020;14:2632352419895527. Published 2020 Jan 13. doi:10.1177/2632352419895527

47. Garakani A, Murrough JW, Freire RC, et al. Pharmacotherapy of anxiety disorders: Current and emerging treatment options. *Front Psychiatry*. 2020;11:595584. doi:10.3389/fpsyt.2020.595584

48. Johnson RJ 3rd. A research study review of effectiveness of treatments for psychiatric conditions common to end-stage cancer patients: Needs assessment for future research and an impassioned plea. *BMC Psychiatry*. 2018;18(1):85. doi:10.1186/s12888-018-1651-9

49. Guina J, Merrill B. Benzodiazepines I: Upping the care on downers: The evidence of risks, benefits and alternatives. *J Clin Med*. 2018;7(2):17. doi:10.3390/jcm7020017

50. Atkin N, Vickerstaff V, Candy B. "Worried to death": The assessment and management of anxiety in patients with advanced life-limiting disease, a national survey of palliative medicine physicians. *BMC Palliat Care*. 2017;16(1):69. doi:10.1186/s12904-017-0245-5

51. Nutt DJ. Overview of diagnosis and drug treatments of anxiety disorders. *CNS Spectr*. 2005;10(1):46–59. doi:10.1017/s1092852900009901

52. Ravindran LN, Stein MB. The pharmacologic treatment of anxiety disorders: A review of progress. *J Clin Psychiatry*. 2010;71:839–854. doi:10.4088/JCP.10r06218blu

53. Falk E, Schlieper D, van Caster P, et al. A rapid positive influence of s-ketamine on the anxiety of patients in palliative care: A retrospective pilot study. *BMC Palliat Care*. 2020;19(1):1. Published 2020 Jan 3. doi:10.1186/s12904-019-0499-1

54. Morrison RS, Meier D. *Geriatric Palliative Care*. New York: Oxford University Press; 2014; 286–298.

55. Martínez M, Arantzamendi M, Belar A, et al. "Dignity therapy," a promising intervention in palliative care: A comprehensive systematic literature review. *Palliat Med*. 2017;31(6):492–509. doi:10.1177/0269216316665562

56. Freeman L. *Mosby's Complementary and Alternative Medicine: A Research-Based Approach*. 3rd ed. St. Louis, MO: Mosby Elsevier; 2008.

57. Dossey B, Keengan L, eds. *Holistic Nursing, A Handbook for Practice*. 7th ed. Burlington, MA: Jones and Bartlett Learning; 2016.

58. Lindquist R, Tracy MF, Snyder M. *Complementary and Alternative Therapies in Nursing*. 8th ed. New York: Springer; 2018.

59. Matzo M, Sherman D, *Palliative Care Nursing: Quality of Care to the End of Life*. 5th ed. New York: Springer; 2018.

60. Fulton JJ, Newins AR, Porter LS, Ramos K. Psychotherapy targeting depression and anxiety for use in palliative care: A meta-analysis. *J Palliat Med*. 2018;21(7):1024–1037. doi:10.1089/jpm.2017.0576

61. Satsangi AK, Brugnoli MP. Anxiety and psychosomatic symptoms in palliative care: From neuro-psychobiological response to stress, to symptoms' management with clinical hypnosis and meditative states. *Ann Palliat Med*. 2018;7(1):75–111. doi:10.21037/apm.2017.07.01

62. Quinn J. Transpersonal human caring and healing. In: Dossey B, Keengan L, eds. *Holistic Nursing: A Handbook for Practice*. 7th ed. Burlington, MA: Jones & Bartlett; 2016: 101–110.

49.

DELIRIUM

Bonnie D. Evans and Erica J. Hickey

<table>
<tr><td>

KEY POINTS

- Delirium is commonly encountered across palliative care settings and at the end of life and is associated with distressing symptoms and negative outcomes for both patients and family caregivers.

- Awareness of risk factors that can precipitate a delirium by the palliative advanced practice registered nurse (APRN) can help to prevent delirium, as well as target interventions to limit the duration and severity once it has developed.

- Evaluating the potential burden of interventions for delirium versus benefit in palliative care patients, especially at end of life, can be challenging and requires an individualized, family-centered approach and ethical healthcare decision-making.

- Multicomponent, nonpharmacological interventions should be the first approach for the prevention and management of delirium, and the role of pharmacological treatment continues to be evaluated.

- More research is needed to better understand the underlying pathophysiology of delirium and to develop evidence-based interventions for modifiable risk factors, pharmacological management, and effective family caregiver support.

</td></tr>
</table>

CASE STUDY: POLYPHARMACY

Anna was an 89-year-old woman living with her daughter and scheduled to start 6 weeks of radiation therapy (XRT) with weekly chemotherapy for Grade II squamous cell esophageal cancer. Anna had declined to have a stent or feeding tube placed, and her primary care physician (PCP) requested a palliative care consultation prior to beginning treatment. On the initial home visit, the palliative advanced practice registered nurse (APRN) found a frail-appearing woman who was a fair historian and aware of her cancer diagnosis. Anna had completed an advance directive which signified her daughter as the designated surrogate decision-maker or healthcare proxy. However, there had been little discussion around any limitations of treatment, except for feeding tubes. Anna stated that she hoped to live to be 90 and to be kept comfortable. An out-of-hospital order for life-sustaining treatments had not been completed.

Review of systems was positive for fatigue, weight loss, dysphagia, dyspnea on exertion, poor appetite, radicular low back pain, history of falls, and mild memory problems; she reported that she felt "down" but denied suicidality. Her past medical history (PMH) included coronary artery disease (CAD), atrial fibrillation (AF), anticoagulation therapy, systolic heart failure, hyperlipidemia, chronic obstructive pulmonary disease (COPD), chronic kidney disease (CKD) Stage 3, depression, anxiety, insomnia, mild cognitive impairment, spinal stenosis, and hearing impairment.

Anna had a complex medication regimen including digoxin 0.125 mg PO daily, metoprolol 50 mg PO twice daily, furosemide 60 mg PO daily, warfarin 2.5 mg PO daily, gabapentin 300 mg PO twice daily, sertraline 50 mg PO daily, ipratropium bromide/salbutamol inhaler 1 puff 4 times daily, and simvastatin 20 mg PO daily. She had three as-needed medications: ondansetron 8 mg PO every 8 hours as needed for nausea, tramadol 50 mg PO every 6 hours as needed for pain, and diphenhydramine 25 mg PO at bedtime as needed for insomnia.

Anna appeared thin and fatigued with some short-term memory deficits. Her vital signs included a blood pressure 98/66, apical rate 90/min. She had 3+ pitting edema to mid-calf bilaterally; her albumin level was 2.7 g/dL, body mass index was 21, and Eastern Cooperative Oncology Group (ECOG) Performance Status Score was 2.

The palliative APRN was concerned about Anna's high risk for complications during her cancer treatment. She had several predisposing risk factors for developing a delirium: her advanced age and multiple comorbidities, especially esophageal cancer, depression, and mild cognitive impairment. Malnutrition, frailty with a recent fall, and hearing loss also added to her risk. Anna's precipitating risk factors for delirium included polypharmacy, pain, dysphagia, and the potential side effects of her planned radiation and chemotherapy. The care plan developed by the palliative APRN focused on trying to limit complications from treatment, including delirium.

1. *Polypharmacy*: A stepwise approach to tapering and simplifying Anna's medications was discussed with her PCP. Due to hypotension and poor oral intake, her furosemide dose was decreased. The simvastatin was discontinued, and the warfarin would be stopped if she had another fall. The use of diphenhydramine was discontinued since it appeared on the list of medication unsafe for older adults due to its anticholinergic properties. Tramadol was also discontinued since it was contraindicated with sertraline and gabapentin. It was replaced with low-dose oxycodone 2.5 mg PO every 6 hours as needed for pain.

2. *Optimal nutrition*: Speech and language pathology was consulted for swallowing evaluation and safe intake. Nutrition was consulted for optimal foods for calories, protein, and nutritional value.

3. *Family caregiver education*: The palliative APRN reviewed the medication list for safe administration. She also discussed safety precautions in the home, given Anna's increasing weakness and falls; sleep hygiene techniques; pain management strategies; and changes to report in Anna's condition, including mental status.

After 2 weeks of daily XRT and two chemotherapy infusions, Anna was started on a scopolamine patch for copious oral secretions and on a fentanyl patch 12.5 μg/h every 3 days for increasing pain at the radiation site. After another fall, she was evaluated at the emergency department (ED) and treated for dehydration. Her furosemide and warfarin were discontinued. Two days after the ED visit, Anna's daughter called the palliative APRN to report that her mother was sleeping more and seemed confused. Upon arrival, the palliative APRN noted that Anna did not recognize her and was lethargic and dozing unless stimulated. She could not maintain eye contact or follow commands and was oriented to self only. Anna had been not eating, and the palliative APRN noted the new prescriptions for fentanyl and scopolamine.

Based on delirium diagnostic criteria, Anna was exhibiting an acute change from her baseline cognitive status. She was unable to maintain attention, had an altered level of alertness with lethargy, and disturbances in memory and orientation. The daughter had not noticed any hallucinations or agitation. The palliative APRN reviewed her findings with the daughter that were consistent with a hypoactive delirium. As Anna's healthcare proxy, her daughter wanted her transferred to the hospital. The palliative APRN facilitated the hand-off to the ED. Anna's delirium was treated with hydration, antibiotics for a urinary tract infection, and pain management, but it was slow to resolve. Anna again declined the placement of any feeding tubes and did not want to resume her cancer treatment. Hospice was requested, and she returned to her daughter's home where she died a month later.

This case prompted the palliative APRN to research educational materials for family caregivers on delirium and to investigate assessment tools for delirium screening for family caregivers to use in the home care setting, such as the FAM CAM[1] or the Single Question in Delirium (SQiD).[2]

INTRODUCTION

Delirium may develop at any age. The etiology may be due to myriad factors including an acute illness, the adverse effect of a medication, hospitalization, or surgery. Underlying patient vulnerabilities, such as advanced illness and multiple comorbidities, add to this risk.[3] Palliative care is specialized care for patients and families coping with a progressive illness. Therefore, by definition, palliative care patients are at increased risk for the development of a delirium, and this risk increases toward the end of life.[4] The palliative APRN needs education in the assessment, diagnosis, prevention, and management of delirium and its associated symptoms. Family caregivers of patients with delirium also need support and education to better understand it and to participate in nonpharmacological interventions.

DEFINITIONS

Delirium is an acute and complex neurocognitive disorder.[5] There are no definitive laboratory or diagnostic tests for delirium because it is based on clinical presentation.[5] The syndrome of delirium in the American Psychiatric Association's *Diagnostic and Statistical Manual of Mental Disorders* (DSM-5) is defined by five features[6] (see Box 49.1). The disturbances in attention and awareness described are based on an abrupt change from the individual patient's baseline cognitive status. This can be challenging to identify when the patient is not known to the provider, when the symptoms fluctuate, or if symptoms overlap with the features of depression or dementia, all of which can contribute to the underdiagnosis or misdiagnosis of delirium.[4,7] Delirium may be first identified by the family or a consistent family caregiver who recognizes the altered mental status. In evaluating the patient, especially in the acute care setting or during care transitions, the palliative APRN should locate someone familiar with the patient in order to elicit their baseline and establish a timeline for any changes.

The patient with delirium, in addition to being easily distractible, may also exhibit varying levels of awareness of the environment, from hypervigilance to lethargy. Sleep–wake cycle disturbances are common and have been used as a diagnostic criterion.[4] The patient may sleep during the day and become active or agitated at night. The DSM-5 further delineates delirium by the duration of symptoms from acute (lasting hours to days) to persistent (lasting weeks or months).[6] Delirium can also be described as subsyndromal and terminal (see Box 49.2).

Box 49.1 **THE FIVE FEATURES OF DELIRIUM IN THE *DIAGNOSTIC AND STATISTICAL MANUAL OF MENTAL DISORDERS* (DSM-5)**

1. Disturbance in attention and awareness: Reduced ability to direct, focus, sustain, and shift attention along with reduced orientation to the environment.

2. Develops over a short period of time: Usually hours to days, and symptoms tend to fluctuate in severity over the course of the day

3. At least one additional disturbance in cognition: Memory deficit, disorientation, alteration in language, visuospatial or perceptual distortion

4. Changes from baseline of points 1 and 3 that cannot be explained by a preexisting, established, or evolving neurocognitive disorder

5. History and physical and/or diagnostics should provide evidence that the disturbances are the consequence of another medical condition, substance intoxication or withdrawal, exposure to a toxin, or due to multiple etiologies

From American Psychiatric Association.[6]

Patients with delirium can present with four different subtypes of psychomotor activity: hyperactive, hypoactive, mixed, and non-motor subtype[4,6,8,9] (Table 49.1). There is concern that patients with a hypoactive delirium may be less likely to be recognized (e.g., symptoms may be interpreted as a mood disorder or fatigue) and that the poor prognosis noted in some studies may be iatrogenic.[8,10,11] Across all motor subtypes, newly diagnosed delirium in the setting of advanced illness is indicative of a potentially life-threatening clinical situation that needs prompt evaluation and discussions regarding treatment options.[10,12] In the palliative care setting, the underlying etiology of delirium is usually viewed as multifactorial, requiring a comprehensive approach.[4] The role of the family caregiver in the context of delirium can be significant because they offer familiarity and can assist in nonpharmacological management techniques. A family caregiver is defined as the spouse, family member, partner, or friend who is the primary person assisting with care.[13]

PATHOPHYSIOLOGY

Delirium occurs across multiple medical conditions and can be associated with a wide range of signs and symptoms. Moreover, as stated earlier, it is often multifactorial. This contributes to the challenge of clarifying the dysregulation of neuronal activity that occurs, and a variety of theories have been postulated. Based on changes noted in electroencephalography and

Table 49.1 FOUR PSYCHOMOTOR BEHAVIOR
SUBTYPES OF DELIRIUM

Hyperactive	A extremely high level of psychomotor activity, often combined with mood lability, agitation, refusal to cooperate with medical care, perceptual disturbances.
Hypoactive	A abnormally low level of psychomotor activity, often may be accompanied by reduced motor activity, sluggishness, lethargy that can approach stupor, and perceptual disturbances.
Mixed	Includes individuals whose activity level fluctuates between extremely high and abnormally low.
Non-motor	Normal or no motor features.

From Bush et al.[4]; American Psychiatric Association[6]; Evensen et al.[8]; and
Meagher et al.[9]

resting-state functional magnetic resonance imaging in delirium, Shafi et al.[14] propose that delirium is the result of a breakdown in brain connectivity and brain plasticity that can occur when individuals are exposed to a stressor. Potential stressors could include surgery, anesthesia, systemic inflammation, infections, and psychotropic drugs, as well as neurodegenerative disorders such as dementia and comorbid conditions.[14]

A review of the literature by Maldonado[15] identified seven significant theories or mechanisms to explain the underlying pathophysiology of delirium: neuroinflammation, neuronal aging, oxidative stress, neurotransmitter deficiency, neuroendocrine aberrations, diurnal dysregulation, and neuronal network disconnectivity. More than likely, these mechanisms overlap or complement each other. The most common changes in neurotransmitters in delirium include reduced cholinergic activity and/or melatonin availability; an excess of dopamine, norepinephrine, and/or glutamate; and variable changes in serotonin, histamine, and γ-aminobutyric acid.[15] In one study, patients who developed postoperative delirium were positive for a central nervous system biomarker (phosphorylated neurofilament heavy subunit [pNF-H]) that is consistent with dysfunction of the blood–brain barrier.[16] These results lend support to the role of neuroinflammation in the development of delirium in this population.

To date, the dopaminergic–cholinergic imbalance has largely been the focus of the pharmacological approach to the treatment of delirium symptoms.[4] However, the role of antipsychotic medications for delirium symptoms remains unclear.[17] An integrative literature review of neuroimaging evidence of delirium across 11 studies was done by Kalvas and Monroe.[18] Commonly noted structural abnormalities included impaired white matter integrity, brain atrophy, ischemic lesions, edema, and inflammation. These findings were frequently found in the frontal lobe and limbic system, which are areas involved in attention, the stress response, and emotional regulation, thus offering some possible explanation for the symptoms of delirium.

To further the understanding of the neurobiology of the four delirium clinical motor subtypes, FitzGerald[19] conducted a review of the literature that included 61 studies and found evidence of four key characteristics of motor disturbances in delirium. Delirium motor subtypes appear to be connected with levels of arousal/cognitive function, reactions to delirium phenomenology (e.g., delusions or psychosis), disturbances in circadian rhythm, and clinical context (e.g., medications and underlying medical conditions).[19] Longitudinal studies are recommended to further investigate the factors that influence delirium motor subtypes. As additional disturbances in neurotransmission are investigated, new therapeutic options for the prevention and treatment of delirium may evolve, and the palliative APRN needs to stay current on the literature to adapt clinical practice guidelines accordingly.

INCIDENCE AND PREVALENCE

Delirium is commonly found across all palliative care settings and is most prevalent prior to death. A systematic literature review indicated, for patients 65 years of age or older on a general medical unit, a prevalence rate (present on admission) for delirium of 18–35% and an incidence rate (new onset) for delirium of 11–14%.[7] In the intensive care unit, the higher prevalence rate for delirium was 7–50% and the incidence rate was 19–82%. In this same study, up to 40% of nursing home residents presented to the ED with a delirium.[7] Following hip surgery, one study revealed that patients aged 80 years or older were two times more likely to develop a postoperative delirium; if patients had a diagnosis of dementia, they were six times more likely to develop a postoperative delirium.[20] These numbers demonstrate the increased vulnerability to delirium with advanced age and cognitive impairment.

A meta-analysis of 42 studies across palliative care settings revealed prevalence estimates of delirium to be 4–12% in the community on initial assessment, 9–57% in the acute care setting at the time of the first palliative care consultation, and 6.6–73% on admission to an inpatient palliative care unit.[21] Pooling these data revealed that up to one-third of patients had a diagnosis of delirium at the time of admission to an inpatient palliative care unit, and the cumulative incidence rate over the entire admission was 7–45%. Prior to death, the prevalence of delirium was higher at 58–88% in the inpatient palliative care setting and 42–44% in the community.[21] The lower rates of terminal delirium in the community could indicate that the familiar environment of home may be protective against the development of delirium and/or that the caregiver burden of managing associated symptoms and behaviors may prompt admission to an inpatient palliative care or hospice facility.

RISK FACTORS

The development of delirium is complex and multifactorial; key to the prevention and treatment of delirium is an understanding of factors that put individuals at risk.[4,7] Risk factors for delirium have been categorized as either *predisposing*, which implies a nonmodifiable, host-related vulnerability (e.g., age or preexisting medical conditions), or *precipitating*, which implies a potentially modifiable risk and can contribute to the development of delirium (e.g., medications or surgery)[7] (Table 49.2). A conceptual model for delirium by Inouye and Charpentier[22] describes the baseline vulnerability of a patient and precipitating risk factors as highly interrelated and cumulative. Fewer precipitating risk factors may be sufficient to trigger a delirium in patients with a higher number of predisposing risk factors.[22]

There are common predisposing factors for delirium: older age, dementia, functional disability, and a high burden of comorbid conditions, as well as male sex, visual or hearing impairment, history of alcohol abuse, and depression.[7,10] Delirium is more common in combination with dementia, and dementia is more likely to develop after delirium.[7,23] It can be challenging to recognize delirium in older adults with cognitive impairment. In these cases, a distinction must be made between the baseline cognitive disturbance and an acute decline in mental status. Age, as an independent factor, may

Table 49.2 RISK FACTORS FOR THE DEVELOPMENT OF DELIRIUM

PREDISPOSING FACTORS: NONMODIFIABLE	PRECIPITATING FACTORS: POTENTIALLY MODIFIABLE
Age >70 years	Polypharmacy
Male gender	Use of psychoactive (e.g., benzodiazepines and opiates) and anticholinergic medications
Multiple comorbidities	Infection
Dementia/Cognitive impairment	Electrolyte disturbances
Depression	Dehydration
History of transient ischemic attack or stroke	Hypoxia
Brain metastases	Surgical or general anesthesia
Frailty	Organ failure (especially renal)
Functional impairment	Pain
Poor nutritional status	Sleep alterations
Visual or hearing impairment	Restraints
History of alcohol abuse	Change in environment

From Seiler et al.[3]; Bush et al.[4]; Inouye et al.[7]; and Shenvi et al.[24]

relate to functional age and frailty rather than actual chronological age.

Precipitating factors frequently reported for delirium include medications, acute illness, infection, electrolyte imbalances, hypoxia, dehydration, surgery, anesthesia, and high pain levels.[4,10] Medications that can cause or worsen delirium include anticholinergic medications (including tricyclic antidepressants, antihistamines, muscle relaxants, promethazine, typical antipsychotics), sedative hypnotics (benzodiazepines, zolpidem), corticosteroids, high-dose opioids, and polypharmacy of four or more drugs.[24,25]

A nursing assessment tool was developed to improve screening for potentially reversible risk factors for delirium in patients at the end of life, with the acronym CHIMBOP[26,27] (Box 49.3). The risk factors in this assessment tool for delirium are common, although not specific, to patients at the end of life. Pain is included, and inadequate pain management has been associated with an increased risk of delirium.[28] Assessing pain in patients with delirium who are unable to report their pain requires additional expertise and the use of pain assessment tools for the nonverbal and/or cognitively impaired patient.

Environmental risk factors for delirium in hospitalized patients that have been identified are physical restraints, frequent environmental/room changes, absence of clock or watch, lack of reading glasses, disruption of day/night cycles, noise and light disturbances, no visible daylight, isolation room, and no visitors.[29,30] The potential for lack of visitors in health facilities has increased due to policies protecting patients and staff from COVID-19, which, if they continue, could negatively impact patients who are at risk for or are experiencing a delirium.

Over the past decade there has been an increase in delirium research in hospitalized patients, particularly in the critically ill.[31] Delirium risk factors, for example, have been the focus of study in critically ill trauma patients[32] and postoperative head and neck cancer patients.[33] There has, however, been limited data collected regarding delirium risk factors in community-dwelling older adults. One prospective study of older adults living in the community (86.5% in their homes) who presented to the hospital with a delirium found that 80% had either a cognitive (mainly dementia) or other neurological disorder (cerebrovascular disease or Parkinson's disease) and 23% had depression, revealing that neurological deficits were a strong predisposing risk factor for delirium in this community setting.[34] In addition, infections of primarily the lung and urinary tract (49%), adverse effects of drugs (30.8%), dehydration (26%), and electrolyte disturbances (18.7%) were the most frequent precipitating risk factors for delirium in this same study population. The researchers underscore that a significant finding was the relatively higher incidence of infections as a precipitating risk factor for delirium when compared to most inpatient studies. For the palliative APRN working in the community, this study emphasizes careful monitoring of patients with underlying neurological disorders for any change in mental status. Moreover, the correct diagnosis and rapid treatment of community-acquired infections could help to limit further neurological decline, as always based on the goals of care.

A prospective, observational study of delirium risk factors was conducted in 410 hospitalized palliative care patients with a high prevalence of delirium (55.9%). On multivariate regression, the most relevant predisposing risk factors for the development of delirium in these palliative care patients were frailty, impaired hearing and vision, brain neoplasms, and male gender. Frailty was measured across the component of mobility/function and it was associated with a 15-fold increased risk of developing delirium. The most relevant precipitating risk factors for delirium in this population were acute renal failure and pressure ulcers.[3] Given the vulnerability

and medical complexity of palliative care patients and the multifactorial etiology of delirium, it can be challenging to distinguish between predisposing and precipitating risk factors in this population. Accordingly, the palliative APRN's approach to prevention and management should be broad and multifaceted.

Potentially modifiable or precipitating risk factors for delirium can vary by clinical setting, whereas predisposing risk factors are host-related and nonmodifiable.[34] However, the age, gender, or medical conditions most commonly treated in a particular specialty unit or clinic, may be somewhat specific. Accordingly, awareness of the predisposing and precipitating delirium risk factors most relevant to the APRN's clinical setting and patient population is needed to provide optimal care.

OUTCOMES

Although delirium is considered an acute syndrome, evidence suggests that cognitive and functional impairments can persist. Hospitalized patients are most at risk for long-term cognitive and functional decline.[35] Following elective surgery, patients who developed delirium had persistent (for up to 18 months) and clinically meaningful impairment of functional recovery compared to those who did not develop delirium.[36] In another study, critically ill ICU patients diagnosed with a delirium were followed and their cognitive and executive function evaluated at 3 months and 12 months post-discharge. At 3 months, 40% had cognitive scores consistent with moderate traumatic brain injury and 26% had cognitive scores consistent with mild dementia; there was minimal improvement at 12 months (34% and 24%, respectively). The duration of delirium in this study was found to be associated with worse cognitive scores.[37] These study results point to the need for functional and cognitive assessments prior to discharge in patients treated for delirium, given the possibility that they may not have returned to their pre-admission baseline status. It is important to recognize that the cognitive disturbances associated with delirium can affect language, memory, orientation, and the ability to communicate. Patients experiencing delirium are less likely to be able to participate in discussions around symptom management or treatment preferences.[4]

Persons with dementia who develop delirium have even worse outcomes than those with delirium alone. This includes higher rates of rehospitalization, institutionalization, mortality, and subsequent cognitive decline.[38] The interrelationship of dementia and delirium is not fully understood. Delirium may reveal an underlying vulnerability of the brain or unrecognized dementia and/or it may lead to neuronal damage and chronic cognitive impairment/dementia. These are ongoing hypotheses that need further study.[38]

Delirium has also been associated with an increased risk of institutionalization post-discharge. In one meta-analysis, older adults who developed a delirium had higher rates of institutionalization (33.4%) versus controls (10.7%).[39] Similarly, patients who had surgery to repair a hip fracture and developed postoperative delirium (POD), were more likely to be discharged to a nursing home than patients who did not experience POD.[40] Interestingly, in a study of critically ill patients, 80% were found to have subsyndromal delirium (SSD) or cognitive dysfunction that did not meet diagnostic criteria for delirium. The duration of SSD was found to have an independent association with increased odds for being discharged to an institution. Those with SSD for 5 days were 4.2 times more likely to be discharged to an institution than those with SSD for 1.5 days.[41] The prognostic implications of subsyndromal delirium support the need to assess and report all delirium symptoms (even when they do not validate a diagnosis of delirium) with the goals of reducing complications and preventing progression to delirium.

Critically ill patients who developed delirium were compared to those without delirium in one systematic review and delirium was found to be associated with a longer length of stay, longer duration of mechanical ventilation, and a greater than twofold increase in hospital death.[42] In an exploratory analysis of hospitalized older adults followed for 3 years, delirium was strongly associated with mortality, finding that 81% of those who had developed a delirium died within 3 years versus 49% of those without delirium.[43] Similarly, in a retrospective analysis of mortality rates in Medicare beneficiaries who had an emergency room visit and were diagnosed with delirium, there was a fivefold increase in mortality within 30 days of discharge when compared to those without a delirium diagnosis. This increased risk in mortality persisted over the 12 months of the study.[44] These studies illustrate that delirium is a poor prognostic indicator associated with an increased risk of hospital death and that the increased mortality risk can continue post-discharge.

Study results on mortality and delirium vary when factoring in delirium subtypes. One systematic review of ICU patients found a consistent association between mortality and hypoactive delirium.[45] Another study of older adults admitted to a subacute unit with delirium indicated that although hyperactive delirium was the most prevalent motor subtype, only hypoactive delirium was associated with higher mortality.[46] However, Evensen et al. studied geriatric patients for 12 months following a hospitalization for delirium and found significant mortality (43%) but no statistical difference in mortality across the 4 delirium motor subtypes.[8] The exact relationship between delirium and mortality is unclear. Delirium may be a marker for disease severity and not causatively linked to mortality. The significant negative short- and long-term outcomes and complications associated with delirium demand preventive interventions for patients at high risk and timely recognition and treatment for those who develop it.

ASSESSMENT SCALES

There is a wide variety of delirium assessment tools available that vary in the number of items, level of training required, and ease of administration, as well as the optimal setting and patient population for the use of each one. In practice, the palliative APRN should choose the most appropriate tool for the clinical situation and use it consistently and regularly because standardized screening can increase the chance of detection.[47] It is best practice that the team is uses one assessment tool for consistency.

Delirium scales have been developed for different purposes, such as identification of delirium, diagnosis, determining the level of severity, and delineating delirium motor subtypes.[4] Table 49.3 lists details of the delirium assessment scales reviewed in this chapter. Two delirium assessment instruments that are considered the gold standard for delirium screening, alongside the clinical diagnosis using DSM-IV criteria, are the Confusion Assessment Method (CAM)[48] and the Delirium Rating Scale–Revised-98 (DRS-R-98).[49] They both require additional training and expertise.[50] The CAM is a clinical algorithm developed by expert panel consensus in 1990 to allow non-psychiatric clinicians to assess for delirium; it is based on four of the nine features of delirium originally described in the DSM-III–Revised (see Figure 49.1). The CAM assessment, which has been translated into at least 12 languages, shows high sensitivity (94%) and specificity (89%) and is widely used in practice.[7]

THE DRS-R-98 includes inattention and motor subtypes and rates symptom severity over a 24-hour time frame. The DRS-R-98 and the Memorial Delirium Assessment Scale (MDAS)[51] were found by a panel of experts reviewing delirium assessment tools to be the best options for monitoring delirium severity in the context of palliative care.[52] Another study of newly consulted palliative care patients in both inpatient and outpatient settings also found the MDAS to be a valid and reliable tool for delirium screening and severity monitoring in palliative care settings; however, there is still a lack of consensus regarding the optimum cutoff scores for a positive screen.[53,54] Jones et al. also evaluated delirium severity instruments and did a methodological review of 11 tools.[55] Based on the results, six instruments of high quality were selected that best captured delirium symptoms and severity on a continuous and quantitative scale: the CAM–Severity Score (CAM-S),[56] DRS-R-98,[49] MDAS,[51] Confusional State Examination (CSE),[57] Delirium-O-Meter (DOM),[58] and the Delirium Observation Screening Scale (DOS).[59] Accurately identifying and monitoring the severity of delirium can help to target treatment, monitor response to clinical care, and provide meaningful prognostic information.[55]

The Neelon-Champagne Confusion Scale (NEECHAM)[60] and the Nursing Delirium Screening Scale (Nu-Desc)[61,62] are both shorter versions of delirium screening tools designed to be used by nurses during routine clinical practice. The Delirium Motor Subtype Scale (DMSS)[9] was developed to improve the identification and subsequent understanding of the four motor subtypes of delirium: hyperactive, hypoactive, mixed, and nonmotor. Using the DMSS, a study of older adults who developed delirium following hip fracture surgery showed that the majority demonstrated variable motor subtypes over the course of their delirium, supporting the need for frequent assessment.[63]

In a review by delirium research experts on the assessment of delirium in palliative care, the authors concluded that there is no one tool that can capture the complexity of delirium in palliative care patients and that more validation studies are needed for the use of current instruments in palliative care

Table 49.3 SUMMARY OF DELIRIUM ASSESSMENT SCALES

ASSESSMENT TOOL	DESCRIPTION	NUMBER OF ITEMS AND TIME TO COMPLETE	PRIMARY USE COMMENTS
Confusion Assessment Method (CAM)[48] Short Version Long Version	Requires training. Includes brief formal cognitive testing.	4, 3 minutes 10, 5 minutes	Screening scale; widely used in hospitalized older patients[64] Validated for use in palliative care[53,65]
CAM-ICU[66]	Requires training.	8, 2–3 minutes	Screening scale For use with nonverbal or intubated ICU patients
CAM-Severity Score[56] CAM-S Long Version CAM-S Short Version	Requires training. Scores symptoms noted in the CAM, combined with formal cognitive testing.	10, 10–15 mins 4, <5 minutes	Severity scale
FAM-CAM[1]	Requires training. Uses input from family caregivers, in person, by telephone or electronically	11, 5–10 minutes	Screening scale
Delirium Rating Scale Revised-98 (DRS-R-98)[49]	Requires training. Differentiates delirium from dementia, depression and schizophrenia.[53]	16, 20–30 minutes	Diagnosis and severity scale Initial assessment and repeated measurement Use validated in palliative care[52]
Memorial Delirium Assessment Scale (MDAS)[51]	Requires clinician training.	10, >10 minutes	Diagnosis and severity scale Validated for use in palliative care[52–54]
Confusional State Examination (CSE)[57]	Requires training.	22, 30 minutes	Screening and severity scale
Delirium-O-Meter (DOM)[58]	No training, observation scale for nurses at the bedside.	12, 3—5 minutes	Severity scale
Delirium Observation Screening Scale (DOS)[59]	Requires training. Based on observations over an 8-hour nursing shift.	13, 5 minutes	Severity scale; early recognition
Neelon-Champagne Confusion Scale (NEECHAM)[60]	Requires training. Observation scale for nurses at the bedside.	9, 10 minutes	Screening and monitoring scale
Nursing Delirium Screening Scale (Nu-DESC)[61,62]	Requires training. Observation scale for nurses at the bedside.	5, 1–2 minutes	Screening scale
Single Question in Delirium (SQiD)[2]	Requires training. One question for family caregiver on confusion.	1, < 1 minute	Screening scale Use has been supported in oncology patients[53]
Delirium Motor Subtype Scale (DMSS)[9]	Can be used by a variety of clinical staff.	11	Identifies four motor subtypes
DMSS-4[67,68]	Shortened version.	4	Valid and reliable in the ICU setting

across a variety of medical conditions and palliative care settings.[52] The palliative APRN should have a basic understanding of the range of delirium assessment tools available and how to choose the most appropriate tool for the clinical setting and population being targeted. Table 49.4 offers guidance. This is by no means an exhaustive review of available assessment tools for delirium. For more information, the website for the Network for Investigation of Delirium Unifying Scientists

(NIDUS) has a list of Delirium Measurement Resources available at https://deliriumnetwork.org/measurement/.[69]

ASSESSMENT

Delirium is a clinical diagnosis, one that requires the ability to determine the baseline cognitive status of the individual

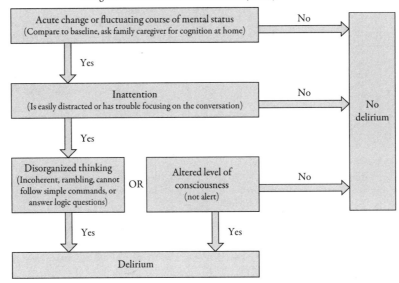

Delirium Diagnostic Criteria
Using the Confusion Assessment Method (CAM)

Acute change or fluctuating course of mental status
(Compare to baseline, ask family caregiver for cognition at home) — No → No delirium

↓ Yes

Inattention
(Is easily distracted or has trouble focusing on the conversation) — No → No delirium

↓ Yes

Disorganized thinking
(Incoherent, rambling, cannot follow simple commands, or answer logic questions)   OR   Altered level of consciousness (not alert) — No → No delirium

↓ Yes   ↓ Yes

Delirium

Figure 49.1 Delirium diagnostic criteria.
From Inouye, van Dyck Alessi et al.[48]

along with a time frame for any acute mental status changes. Input from family caregivers or other informants may be needed for an accurate assessment. Not knowing the baseline cognitive status is reported to be a common reason for most missed diagnoses of delirium.[25] If delirium is suspected, brief cognitive screening tools and bedside observation for key clinical features aid in diagnosis.[25] Examples of brief cognitive screening tools are the Mini-Cog and the Short Portable Mental Status Questionnaire.[70,71] Validated delirium screening tools are numerous and based on standard diagnostic DSM-V criteria.[6] Given the relative subjectivity of delirium observational tools, evidence-based guidelines recommend

Table 49.4 KEY FEATURES AND QUESTIONS TO AID IN THE SELECTION OF A DELIRIUM ASSESSMENT TOOL IN PALLIATIVE CARE

FEATURES	QUESTIONS
Intended use	What is the purpose of use? • Clinical, research, quality assurance What types of tools are available? What is the intended focus of the tool? • Screening, diagnostic, severity, neuropsychological assessment In what types of palliative care settings will the tool be used? • Acute/tertiary palliative care, hospice, outpatients How will the assessments be documented, reported, and used?
Ease of use	Who will administer the tool –ideally and/or practically? • Nurses, physicians, advanced practice providers, other staff What types of additional resources may be needed? What type of additional training is required? Is there a formal training program and/or availability of a training manual? How much time is required to administer the tool? How often will the tool be administered? What is the level of patient, family, and staff burden?
Psychometric properties	*Comprehensiveness* Which domains of delirium should be represented in an ideal tool? Which domains of delirium are represented in the tool? Which domains are not represented? *Reliability and validity* What types of reliability and validity evidence have been gathered in palliative care settings? What is the sensitivity and specificity of the tool in palliative care?

From Leonard et al.[52 (pp. 176–190)]

that clinicians use observational instruments in conjunction with tools that directly assess cognition.[72] Delirium symptoms can fluctuate and therefore patients may need frequent assessments throughout the day to screen for delirium and monitor severity.

History-taking should focus on known predisposing risk factors, especially older age and a previous diagnosis of mild cognitive impairment or dementia. Precipitating risk factors may be noted on initial presentation and may also accrue during an acute illness or hospitalization (e.g., polypharmacy, immobilization, urinary catheter). A careful review of current medications looking for categories of drugs associated with incident delirium and any new medications or recent changes in dosages may reveal additional instigating factors.

A hallmark for the diagnosis of delirium is that it is due to the presence of an underlying medical condition. Common causes of delirium that present to the ED have been identified as infections (estimated at 30–40%), followed by acute neurological disorders (hemorrhage, stroke, intracranial mass), and adverse effects of medications.[24] A detailed physical and neurological exam should incorporate an assessment for dehydration, urinary retention, constipation, infection, or pain. The differential diagnosis for delirium includes distinguishing it from depression, dementia, delirium superimposed on dementia, or psychosis (Table 49.5 summarizes key characteristics of each). Cognitive status at baseline may not be known or symptoms may be atypical or overlapping, and this adds to the challenge of an accurate diagnosis.[73] Of note, acute onset and an altered level of consciousness is most suggestive of a delirium. Dementia has a more gradual and insidious progression of cognitive decline. Neurovegetative symptoms associated with depression could also present similarly to a hypoactive delirium with apathy and lethargy. Standardized depression screening tools are available that are designed to measure depression based on the age of the patient, such as the Geriatric Depression Scale (GDS).[74]

Lab work and diagnostics should be tailored to the patient, but a basic evaluation should include an electrocardiogram, complete blood count, metabolic panel, glucose level, and urinalysis with culture.[24] Additional diagnostics or neuroimaging may be needed if the etiology is unclear or there is a history of falls, worsening neurological findings or focal deficits, or the patient is on anticoagulants.[24,25,75] The extent of any diagnostic testing should be guided by the goals of care and any advance directives, along with the overall assessment of prognosis. The focus of treatment can vary from a full investigation into the underlying etiology with high-risk interventions, to looking for more easily reversible risk factors and/or minimizing the distress of associated symptoms.

Terminal delirium in dying patients denotes a particularly poor prognosis, and the extent of evaluation and treatment can be challenging to determine. The potential for additional time or enhanced ability to communicate with the patient may be extremely valuable to the family, and a timed trial of hydration or antibiotics can sometimes help to determine if the delirium is potentially or even partially reversible. One study of patients with advanced cancer in an inpatient palliative care unit estimated that approximately 50% of delirium

Table 49.5 DISTINGUISHING THE CLINICAL FEATURES OF DELIRIUM, DEMENTIA, DEPRESSION AND PSYCHOSIS

CHARACTERISTIC	DELIRIUM	DEMENTIA	DEPRESSION	PSYCHOSIS
Onset	Abrupt (hours to days)	Insidious	Variable: can be associated with major life changes	Variable
Course	Fluctuates	Progressive	Variable	Chronic with exacerbations
Reversibility	Potentially	Irreversible	Potentially	Potentially
Duration	Hours to months	Months to years	Variable (at least 2 weeks)	Months to years
Level of alertness	Fluctuates	Generally normal	Normal	Normal
Orientation	Fluctuates	Impaired	Selective impairment	Normal
Memory	Impaired	Impaired recent memory worse	Selective impairment	Intact
Attention	Impaired	Normal until end stage	Generally normal	May be impaired
Psychomotor behavior	Variable	Generally normal	Variable (vegetative or agitation)	Variable
Perception/illusions hallucinations, or delusions	Common	Usually absent	Absent except in severe cases	Common
Sleep–wake cycle	Disrupted, cycle may be reversed	Fragmented	Early morning awakening common	Variable

From Shenvi et al.[24]; Weng et al.[76]; Loving and Dahlin[77]; and Milisen et al.[78]

episodes could not be reversed.[79] Impending death and the increased likelihood of irreversible terminal delirium distinguishes the experience of delirium in hospice and palliative care from other settings or contexts.[80]

PREVENTION AND MANAGEMENT

There is limited evidence for both pharmacological and nonpharmacological approaches to the management of delirium symptoms, especially in the palliative care patient population. Clinical guidelines for delirium vary widely in quality and often do not include tools for implementation.[81] Yet, as discussed previously in this chapter, delirium places significant burdens on patients, caregivers, and staff.[82] While the evidence for symptomatic management of delirium is scarce, fortunately the literature on nonpharmacological prevention of delirium is more robust. Primary prevention is almost always preferable to treating a problem once it has occurred, and delirium prevention is paramount. A review of current research also suggests that it is possible to successfully treat reversible causes of delirium in 20–50% of palliative care patients who are not actively dying,[83] making identification and treatment of root causes a priority. Many of the nonpharmacological interventions for prevention also continue to be applicable in delirium management.

Before addressing specific interventions, it is important to note that palliative care patients often have different needs from the general population, especially when approaching end of life, and the specific needs of palliative care patients must shape an APRN's approach to both delirium prevention and management. Above all, the individual patient's values and goals of care as well as prognosis should help to guide any delirium prevention or management interventions.

NONPHARMACOLOGICAL PREVENTION

The standard for delirium prevention is to use a multicomponent, nonpharmacological intervention that targets known delirium risk factors, as exemplified by Inouye et al.'s Hospitalized Elder Life Program (HELP).[84] The HELP program employed an interdisciplinary team and used eight interventions to address delirium risk factors (sleep deprivation, dehydration, immobility, cognitive impairment, and vision or hearing impairment) in hospitalized, older adults. The outcome was a significant reduction in both the total number of risk factors for individual patients, total number of delirium episodes, total number of days with delirium, and new delirium cases.[85] Multicomponent, nonpharmacological prevention interventions have been shown to be highly effective in reducing the incidence of delirium and falls in hospitalized (non-ICU) adults, [86] and there is moderate-quality evidence that multicomponent, nonpharmacological prevention approaches decrease the incidence of delirium by approximately 30% in this same population (although the effect of these interventions on patients with a history of dementia is uncertain).[87] Box 49.4 summarizes current recommendations for multicomponent, nonpharmacological

Box 49.4 ENVIRONMENTAL NONPHARMACOLOGICAL INTERVENTIONS FOR PREVENTION OF DELIRIUM

Levels of light in the patient's room should correspond to the time of day (light during the day, dark at night).

Decrease environmental noise and stimulation during sleep hours and reduce staff/family interruption when possible.

Discourage daytime napping and caffeinated beverages late in the day.

Assist with safe feeding and hydration, if necessary.

Consider implementing a toileting schedule, if necessary.

Whenever possible, provide a healthcare team that knows the patient well and with whom the patient is familiar.

Encourage family and friends to visit and involve them as much as possible in care.

Avoid switching patients between different rooms.

Use a clock, posted schedule, or orientation white board to help remind patients of the date and time.

Make sure patients have access to their glasses, hearing aids, and dentures. Use an interpreter when needed.

Assess for and treat impacted cerumen.

Communicate clearly and consistently and reorient frequently.

Avoid restraints as much as possible to avoid immobility, injury, and discomfort.

Encourage and assist with mobility, up out of bed when possible, and range of motion.

Avoid urinary catheterization if possible.

From Marcantonio[10]; Bush et al.[83]; Inouye et al.[84]; National Institute for Health and Care Excellence[88]; and Hosker, Bennett.[89]

delirium prevention interventions to guide palliative APRN practice.

The relatively straightforward interventions in the HELP protocol (e.g., promote sleep, mobility, and adequate nutrition)[85] are applicable to the practice of palliative APRNs across all healthcare settings and in the hospice and home settings. Palliative APRNs may be in a position to work on quality improvement projects in hospital or long-term care settings and to educate nursing and medical staff to incorporate these interventions into their practice and unit-based procedures. Inpatient or community palliative APRNs should take the opportunity to educate high-risk patients and their family caregivers about how they can maintain relevant preventive measures at home, when applicable. In the inpatient setting, this should also be incorporated into discharge planning and education. The American Geriatrics Society (AGS) has combined the HELP interventions with Geriatrics principles to form the AGS CoCare: HELP program, designed as a comprehensive care model for hospitalized older adults.[90] This can be a helpful tool for palliative APRNs looking to actualize the HELP protocols in their institution. Further information and resources for implementation are available on the website: https://americangeriatrics.org/programs/ags-cocare-helptm

While the majority of research on multicomponent nonpharmacological interventions has not focused on palliative care patients but rather on populations of hospitalized adults and older adults,[85-87] the risks of nonpharmacological interventions for delirium prevention are low, the potential benefits are significant, and the interventions are in line with basic nursing care. They are currently the best tools that palliative APRNs have to prevent delirium, as long as they are tailored to the individual patient.

TREATING REVERSIBLE ETIOLOGIES

In the general population the first step in managing delirium symptoms is to address any modifiable precipitating causes, such as infections, medication adverse effects, or electrolyte imbalances.[88] This can be challenging in palliative care patients with advanced illnesses who often have multiple possible risk factors and potential precipitating factors.[4] In the palliative care setting, addressing reversible etiologies of delirium can still be a critically important step, though as mentioned earlier, clinicians must be sure to take an individualized approach. The palliative APRN is positioned to counsel patients and families about their treatment options and to formulate a plan that is in line with the patient's goals of care. In an article on clinical assessment and management of delirium in palliative care patients, Bush, Tierney, and Lawlor[4] outline an approach to decision-making when considering whether to address reversible causes of delirium for patients at end of life. They suggest a thorough discussion of several topics with patients and/or proxy decision-makers, including "clarification of the known clinical status; the trajectory of the illness and the suspected or known delirium precipitants; the functional status prior to the episode of delirium; the desire for further investigation, based on the patient's prior expressed goals of care; and the risk and burden of further investigation or treatment."[4 (p. 1630)] If there is considerable ambivalence as to whether an intervention should be pursued, especially in patients with advanced disease, it is often helpful to consider a time-limited trial of the intervention and then re-evaluate the plan of care with the patient and family. Box 49.5, adapted from the European Society for Medical Oncology (ESMO) *Clinical Practice Guidelines* for delirium in adult cancer patients,[83] lists examples of interventions that may be helpful in treating the root causes of delirium.

NONPHARMACOLOGICAL MANAGEMENT

The efficacy of nonpharmacological strategies in managing delirium symptoms after their onset has limited evidence-based support. A systematic review by Siddiqi et al.[87] examined 39 delirium prevention studies that focused on hospitalized adults (age 16 and older, non-palliative care–specific; ICU patients were excluded) and found that it is uncertain whether multicomponent, nonpharmacological preventive interventions have any effect on delirium severity or duration. Yet several clinical recommendations and guidelines for delirium management still encourage continuing the use of the interventions in Box 49.4 as part of good nursing care to promote patient safety, sleep, and cognition/orientation.[10,88,89] These recommendations are based on clinical experience, in the

---

Box 49.5 COMMON INTERVENTIONS FOR TREATING REVERSIBLE DELIRIUM ETIOLOGIES

Consider stopping or tapering psychoactive or anticholinergic medications.

For patients on opioid therapy, consider opioid rotation or dose reduction.

Consider steps to improve oral hydration or consider intravenous hydration, if necessary, for dehydration.

Consider electrolyte supplementation for electrolyte imbalance.

Consider antibiotics, antifungals, or antivirals as appropriate for infection.

If known brain metastases or tumors, consider dexamethasone in consultation with oncology and neurology.

If antineoplastic treatments may be contributing to delirium, consider discussion with oncology about alternatives or discontinuation.

Initiate or escalate bowel regimen for constipation.

From Bush et al.[83]

---

context of limited support for other approaches.[10] Additional nonpharmacological interventions for patients with a hyperactive delirium can help to maintain safety (see Box 49.6).

PHARMACOLOGICAL PREVENTION

Current literature does not support the role of pharmacological interventions in delirium prevention. A systematic review by Siddiqi et al.[87] found that the efficacy of using pharmacological approaches to prevent delirium remains uncertain. Of the studies reviewed in this paper, there was no clear evidence for the use of donepezil (a cholinesterase inhibitor), antipsychotics as a general drug class, or melatonin in delirium prevention. This was due to very low-quality evidence, study imprecision/inconsistency, and study heterogeneity, respectively.[87] The ESMO *Clinical Practice Guidelines* for adult patients with cancer also do not recommend pharmacological prevention of delirium in cancer patients due to a lack of available evidence, though they do conclude that de-prescribing medications may be helpful in older patients.[83] At this time

---

Box 49.6 NONPHARMACOLOGIC SAFETY INTERVENTIONS FOR PATIENTS WITH HYPERACTIVE DELIRIUM

Educate nursing staff or caregivers to use de-escalation techniques

Use bed alarms or floor mat alarms to prevent wandering or getting up unassisted

Clear the floor of unnecessary objects (e.g., wastepaper bins, shoes, trash, IV poles)

Remove potentially dangerous objects (e.g., cutlery, sharp objects, scissors, phone cords) from the room

Consider a one-on-one sitter or family member to be with patient at all times

---

nonpharmacological interventions remain the standard of care for delirium prevention.

PHARMACOLOGICAL MANAGEMENT

The evidence is equivocal regarding the efficacy and safety of using medications such as antipsychotics or benzodiazepines for delirium symptoms in both adult palliative care patients and hospitalized adult patients in general. One significant exception is the routine use of benzodiazepines in the treatment of alcohol and benzodiazepine withdrawal and the delirium associated with these conditions.[91,92] Current delirium management guidelines recommend avoiding pharmacological intervention for non–withdrawal-related delirium in mild-moderate cases, and palliative APRNs should avoid using medications to treat delirium unless symptoms become severe and distressing to the patient or the patient is at risk of harming themselves or others.[83,88] Table 49.6 summarizes the recent literature related to pharmacological delirium management. It is important to note that recent systematic reviews differ in their study inclusion and exclusion criteria and hence on the evidence they examine,[93] which may account for their disparate findings.

While clinical guidelines are in agreement that using pharmacological agents to treat severe/distressing delirium may be appropriate, there is no current consensus on which agents to use. Table 49.7 summarizes the National Institute for Health and Care Excellence (NICE) and ESMO guidelines for using medications in severe delirium.[83,88] It is important to note that distressing symptoms do not manifest only in hyperactive delirium. Patients with hypoactive delirium may also experience distress from psychotic symptoms, which may benefit from treatment with antipsychotics.[88] When considering using antipsychotics or benzodiazepines to treat severe delirium, palliative APRNs should evaluate the risks and benefits of the particular medication in light of the individual patient's clinical condition, goals of care, and the potential adverse effects of the drug and take into consideration the policies of the APRN's specific institution. Consultation with a pharmacist may also be helpful. In the palliative care population, the benefits of treating distressing symptoms may outweigh the risks of certain adverse effects, such as prolonged QTC or sedation, especially in patients at the end of life. It is also important to note that the use of antipsychotics or benzodiazepines for delirium is off-label in the United States and not FDA approved.[10] If prescribing antipsychotics or benzodiazepines for severe delirium, consider the following points:

1. Always start with the lowest clinically effective dose and titrate up slowly.[10,83,88]

2. Start with as-needed (prn) administration. If scheduled dosing is required, limit use to the shortest period of time possible.[83]

3. If doses need to be continued after hospital discharge, discharge teaching should include a clear plan as to when and under what conditions the medication will be discontinued.[10]

4. Monitor carefully for adverse effects.

Table 49.8 summarizes common medications used in delirium management, including doses, routes, adverse effects, cost, and other pertinent considerations.

MANAGEMENT OF REFRACTORY TERMINAL DELIRIUM

Symptoms of terminal delirium that are distressing and refractory to nonpharmacological measures, as well as a trial of as-needed or scheduled pharmacological measures as a last resort, are a unique challenge in caring for patients at the end of life. For patients who are actively dying with severe, refractory delirium, historically the next step has been to consider palliative sedation, usually with IV benzodiazepines or other sedative medications. Chapter 57, "Palliative Sedation" provides comprehensive information on the process. However, it is important to note that, as with most aspects of delirium management, the literature on palliative sedation for management of terminal delirium is weak, and the evidence base is evolving. A systematic review by Beller et al.,[94] which looked at 14 different studies, found that delirium was still challenging to manage despite palliative sedation. Beller et al.[94] found "no evidence from randomised controlled trials (RCTs) and limited evidence from observational studies about the efficacy of palliative sedation in terms of a person's quality of life or symptom control, compared with non-sedated people,"[94 (p. 15)] though they cautioned that the studies they had evaluated were of low quality. Nonetheless, for severe, refractory terminal delirium, a trial of palliative sedation may be the only available option and can be considered as a possible approach for these cases.[83,89,93]

THE FAMILY CAREGIVER EXPERIENCE

Delirium is not experienced in isolation: it is an unpredictable and distressing syndrome shared by patients, their family caregivers, and the healthcare professionals involved.[80] Symptoms of delirium can result in different burdens for the patient who is experiencing them versus the family who is witnessing them. A literature review by Partridge et al.[95] (2013) indicated that the distress may be even greater in relatives witnessing the delirium and can have long-term psychological impact. In retrospective, qualitative interviews of elderly patients who had experienced a delirium during a hospitalization, their family caregivers, and nursing staff were analyzed and three common themes of delirium-related burden were revealed.[82] There were shared burdens, albeit from different perspectives, related to the symptoms of delirium (e.g., disorientation, hallucinations), the emotional response to the delirium (e.g., fear, helplessness), and the situational factors (e.g., loss of control, lack of knowledge).

Some specific concerns described by caregivers included not knowing if the symptoms would resolve, the inability to communicate, and changes in the patient's personality.[82] Anxiety

AUTHOR (YEAR)	DESIGN	POPULATION	STUDY DESCRIPTION	FINDINGS AND CONCLUSIONS
Grassi et al.[96] (2015)	Review article	Palliative care patients	Examines the management of delirium in palliative care.	Typical and atypical antipsychotics are equally effective in treating delirium in palliative care. The authors find no basis on which to make recommendations about other classes of drugs.
Kishi et al. [97] (2016)	Meta-analysis	Adults	Examined the use of antipsychotics to treat adults with delirium. The primary outcome measure was the response rate. Secondary outcome measures were time to response, Clinical Global Impression-Severity Scale (CGI-S), severity of delirium, adverse effects, and discontinuation rate.	Antipsychotics showed a greater efficacy than placebo or usual care in terms of response rate, CGI-S scores, time to response, and delirium severity scale scores. There was a higher incidence of sedation and dry mouth with antipsychotics vs. placebo or usual care. There was a lower incidence of extrapyramidal symptoms (EPS) and time to response was shorter with second-generation antipsychotics vs. haloperidol. The authors conclude that second generation antipsychotics are safer and more efficacious at treating delirium than haloperidol, though they suggest the need for further research using larger sample sizes.
Neufeld et al.[98] (2016)	Systematic review and meta-analysis	Adult medical or surgical inpatients	Evaluated the use of antipsychotics for delirium prevention and treatment, examining 19 randomized controlled trials and cohort studies.	The authors found no association between antipsychotic use and change in delirium severity, duration, ICU length of stay (LOS), or hospital LOS. They found no association between antipsychotics and mortality. They reported a high level of study heterogeneity and concluded that there is not sufficient evidence to support the use of antipsychotics for treatment of delirium.
Cerveira et al.[99] (2017)	Systematic review	Elderly patients (>60)	Examines the efficacy of pharmacological and nonpharmacological modalities for treating delirium.	The authors found that olanzapine and haloperidol decreased delirium severity; droperidol decreased hospital LOS and improved the delirium remission rate; and rivastigmine improved cognitive function, decreased caregiver burden, and decreased the duration of delirium. The authors suggest that pharmacological treatments are effective at improving delirium duration and severity in the elderly, though they recognize that overall the studies on this subject are few and the sample sizes are small.
Lawley, Hewison[100] (2017)	Integrative literature review	Adult patients with advanced cancer	Examined the clinical management of delirium in advanced cancer patients.	The author finds limited evidence for the efficacy of the reviewed interventions (opioid rotation, atypical antipsychotics, methylphenidate hydrochloride, celiac plexus block, and exercise therapy), concluding that there is currently no clear evidence to guide practice in delirium management and there is a need for further research.
Burry et al.[101] (2018)	Systematic review	Hospitalized adults	Evaluated the efficacy of antipsychotics vs. non-antipsychotics or placebo on delirium duration, severity and resolution, hospital length of stay, mortality, health-related quality of life, adverse effects, and discharge disposition. Evaluated the efficacy of typical vs. atypical antipsychotics to improve the above outcomes.	The authors did not find evidence for the efficacy of antipsychotics in decreasing delirium severity, altering mortality, or resolving symptoms, though the data were of poor quality. There were no data to assess the efficacy of antipsychotics to change delirium duration, health-related quality of life, hospital LOS, or discharge disposition. There was no difference in the frequency of EPS between antipsychotic and non-antipsychotic drug regimens or typical and atypical antipsychotics.

(continued)

Table 49.6 CONTINUED

AUTHOR (YEAR)	DESIGN	POPULATION	STUDY DESCRIPTION	FINDINGS AND CONCLUSIONS
Bush, et al.[83] (2018)	Literature review for Guidelines	Adult cancer patients	Review of the literature on pharmacological management of delirium to inform clinical guidelines.	Haloperidol and risperidone are not recommended for use in treating symptoms of mild-moderate delirium. Olanzapine, quetiapine, and aripiprazole may be beneficial for managing delirium symptoms. "Methylphenidate may improve cognition in hypoactive delirium in which neither delusions nor perceptual disturbance are present and for which no cause has been identified."[75 (p. iv156)] Benzodiazepines may be helpful to use for sedation and anxiolysis in the treatment of severe, distressing, delirium symptoms. Pharmacological agents should be used only when symptoms have become distressing to the patient or when those symptoms are causing safety concerns. Medications should be used only for short periods of time and at the lowest effective dose.
Wu et al.[102] (2019)	Network meta-analysis	Adults in any setting	Examined the evidence for pharmacological delirium treatment and prevention methods, including only randomized controlled trials.	The authors conclude that haloperidol plus lorazepam may be the best pharmacological treatment for delirium symptoms and that ramelteon may be the best drug to use for delirium prevention. They did not find any increase in all-cause mortality for any of the pharmacological interventions studied.
Finucane et al.[93] (2020)	Systematic review	Terminally ill adult patients	Examined the safety and efficacy of pharmacologic management of delirium symptoms.	The authors found no high-quality evidence that either supports or refutes pharmacological management of delirium symptoms in terminally ill adults. They found possible slight worsening of delirium symptoms with haloperidol or risperidone vs. placebo (low-quality evidence). And they found possible slight increases in EPS with haloperidol and risperidone (moderate- to low-quality evidence).
Hui et al.[103] (2020)	Single center, double-blind, randomized trial	Adult advanced cancer patients with terminal delirium and refractory agitation on a palliative care/ supportive care unit	Examined IV haloperidol dose escalation vs. neuroleptic rotation to chlorpromazine vs. haloperidol + chlorpromazine and the effects of these regimens on Richmond Agitation Sedation Scale (RASS) scores.	RASS score decreased significantly within 30 mins and remained decreased at 24 hours in all three groups. There was no significant difference in RASS scores between the groups. Hypotension was the most common serious side effect, and there were no treatment-related deaths. The authors conclude that while the study was small and limited by design (no placebo group), these three different antipsychotic regimens may decrease agitation in patients with terminal agitated delirium.
Li et al.[104] (2020)	Systematic review	Adult patients in non-ICU healthcare settings	Evaluated the efficacy and safety of benzodiazepines in treating non-withdrawal related delirium.	Two studies (RCTs) were identified that fit selection criteria. The authors found insufficient evidence of benzodiazepine efficacy in treating delirium in non-ICU patients. The current evidence does not support the routine use of benzodiazepines to treat delirium in this patient population.
van der Vorst et al.[105] (2020)	Multicenter, randomized controlled, phase III trial	Adult, hospitalized advanced cancer patients	Examined the efficacy and tolerability of olanzapine vs. haloperidol in treating delirium.	The authors did not find a statistically significant difference in efficacy between haloperidol and olanzapine. While they found less adverse effects with olanzapine vs. haloperidol overall, this difference was not statistically significant.

ORGANIZATION	AUTHOR (YEAR)	GUIDELINE TITLE	FINDINGS/RECOMMENDATIONS
European Society for Medical Oncology (ESMO)	Bush et al. (2018)[83]	Delirium in adult cancer patients: ESMO Clinical Practice Guidelines	Question the use of antipsychotic medications in general for severe delirium • Concerns for potential lack of efficacy • Concern for adverse effects Recommend against using haloperidol or risperidone • Lack of evidence to support the efficacy of these agents in even mild-moderate delirium • Possibility of causing harm Recognize a potential role for olanzapine, quetiapine, and aripiprazole in managing delirium symptoms • Less risk of extrapyramidal symptoms (EPS) • Evidence for efficacy is still insufficient Recognize a possible role for benzodiazepines in acute cases • Anxiolytic and sedating effects may be helpful • Concern for significant adverse effects, including sedation, risk of falls, and risk of contributing to delirium symptoms
National Institute for Health and Care Excellence (NICE)	NICE[88] (last updated March 14, 2019)	Delirium: Prevention diagnosis and management	Recommend consideration of short-term (less than 1 week) haloperidol for patients who have not responded to de-escalation and who: • Have become distressed • Pose a danger to themselves or others Use antipsychotic medications with caution or avoid completely in Parkinson's disease or Lewy body dementia.

Table 49.8 COMMONLY USED MEDICATIONS FOR SYMPTOMATIC TREATMENT OF SEVERE DELIRIUM

MEDICATION CLASS	GENERAL CONSIDERATIONS
Antipsychotics	Consider lowering the initial dose in elderly and frail patients or if administering with a benzodiazepine.[83] Caution if seizure hx. May lower seizure threshold.[106–111] May cause agranulocytosis. If not at end of life and if in line with goals of care, monitor CBC if history of leukopenia or neutropenia, and d/c if ANC <1,000 or if unexplained drop in WBC count.[106–111] Antipsychotics carry a black box warning for increased risk of mortality in elderly dementia patients (cardiovascular and infectious events).[106–111] If possible, avoid antipsychotics in older adults and in older adults with dementia.[112,113] Avoid first-generation antipsychotics, such as haloperidol, in patients with Parkinson's disease and Lewy body dementia due to risk of significant adverse effects, including worsening extrapyramidal symptoms (EPS) and worsening parkinsonian symptoms.[114,115] For a detailed review of the management of delirium in patients with Parkinson's disease, see the article *Management of Delirium in Parkinson's Disease* by Ebersbach et al, 2019.[114] When possible, avoid IM administration in palliative care and especially comfort care patients

DRUG NAME	DOSE/ROUTE*	DRUG-SPECIFIC CONSIDERATIONS	RETAIL COST
Haloperidol (first-generation antipsychotic)	Initial Dose: 0.5–1 mg PO or SubQ STAT or q 1 hr. PRN (0.25–0.5 mg if elderly or frail) For scheduled dosing, give q8–12h Routes: PO, SubQ, IM, IV	Adverse effects include: prolonged QTc and extrapyramidal side effects (EPS)[83,110] Avoid in patients with Parkinson's or Lewy body dementia due to increased risk of EPS [83,114,115] If long-term use, taper gradually to prevent withdrawal. Do not discontinue abruptly.[110] If administering via IV, requires electrocardiogram (ECG) monitoring,[83] if not at end of life.	Low: This is a generic medication and relatively affordable. 0.5 mg tablets are approximately $0.83 /pill.[116]
Chlorpromazine (first-generation antipsychotic)	Initial Dose: 12.5–25 mg PO or rectal STAT For scheduled dosing, give q6–12h. Routes: PO, rectal, deep IM, IV (diluted, slow push or infusion)	Adverse effects include: sedation, prolonged QTc, EPS, orthostatic hypotension, anticholinergic effects, local irritation from IV infusion.[83,107] Avoid in patients with Parkinson's or Lewy body dementia due to increased risk of EPS.[114,115] Use cautiously in hepatic or renal insufficiency.[83]	Moderate: $6.23 per pill (10 mg)[117]

(continued)

Table 49.8 CONTINUED

DRUG NAME	DOSE/ROUTE*	DRUG-SPECIFIC CONSIDERATIONS	RETAIL COST
Risperidone (second-generation antipsychotic)	Initial Dose: 0.5 mg PO (0.25–0.5 mg if elderly or frail) STAT For scheduled dosing, give up to q12h Routes: PO, ODT	Adverse effects include: EPS, hypotension, sedation, insomnia, anxiety.[83,109] May worsen parkinsonian symptoms in patients with Parkinson's disease.[114] Caution if severe hepatic or renal insufficiency (reduce dose).[83]	Low: $0.6/tab (0.5 mg), though prices vary widely according to tablet strength.[118]
Olanzapine (second-generation antipsychotic)	Initial Dose: 2.5–5 mg PO or SubQ STAT (reduce dose if elderly or frail) For scheduled dosing, start with nightly dosing Routes: PO, ODT, or IM	Adverse effects include EPS, sedation, orthostatic hypotension as well as weight gain, hyperglycemia, and hyperlipidemia with long-term use.[83,108] May worsen parkinsonian symptoms in patients with Parkinson's disease.[114] Use caution if concomitant benzodiazepine use due to increased risk of respiratory depression and sedation.[83] Caution if hepatic insufficiency (reduce dose).[83] In patients with Lewy body dementia may still cause high levels of adverse effects.[119]	Moderate: $6.87/pill[120]
Quetiapine (second-generation antipsychotic)	Initial Dose: 25 mg (immediate release) PO STAT (12.5–25 mg if elderly or frail) For scheduled dosing, give q12h. Routes: PO	Adverse effects include: sedation, prolonged QTc, EPS, orthostatic hypotension, anticholinergic effects.[111] Caution if hepatic insufficiency (reduce dose).[83] The most practical choice for delirium in Parkinson's disease (lower risk of worsening symptoms), but efficacy has not been proven.[114] Use with caution, as it may still exacerbate EPS.[111] In patients with Lewy body dementia may still cause high levels of adverse effects.[119]	Moderate: $3.43/pill[121]
Aripiprazole (third-generation antipsychotic)	Initial Dose: 5 mg PO or IM STAT (reduce dose if elderly or frail) For scheduled dosing, give daily. Routes: PO, IM, ODT	Adverse effects include EPS, orthostatic hypotension. Insomnia, dizziness, drowsiness, agitation, headache.[83,106] May worsen parkinsonian symptoms in patients with Parkinson's disease.[114] Use caution in patients with impaired cytochrome P450 2D6 metabolism (reduce dose).[83] May have cytochrome P450 2D6 and 3A4 drug–drug interactions.[83]	High: $9.13–32.23 per pill[122]

MEDICATION CLASS	GENERAL CONSIDERATIONS
Benzodiazepines	First-line treatment for delirium related to alcohol or benzodiazepine withdrawal.[91,92] Consider lower initial dose in elderly and frail patients or if administering with an antipsychotic.[83] Use cautiously in patients with severe liver disease, renal disease, myasthenia gravis, or severe pulmonary insufficiency, unless using for end of life care.[83,123–124] Use caution if concurrent high-dose olanzapine treatment. There are reports of fatalities with concurrent use of these medications.[83] May be considered for patients with Parkinson's disease and Lewy body dementia,[4] taking into account possible adverse effects listed below, though note that no studies have examined their use for managing delirium in this population.[114] When possible, avoid IM administration in palliative care and especially in comfort care patients

Table 49.8 CONTINUED

DRUG NAME	DOSAGE/ROUTE*	DRUG-SPECIFIC CONSIDERATIONS	COST
Lorazepam	Initial Dose: 0.5–1 mg PO, SubQ or IV STAT and q1h PRN (0.25–0.5 mg if elderly or frail) Max Dose: 2 mg Routes: PO, SubQ, IM, IV, sublingual	Adverse effects include: sedation, worsening of delirium symptoms, increased fall risk, paradoxical agitation, and local irritation with SubQ injection.[83,123] Avoid IM/IV use in renal failure and use IM/IV route cautiously in renal impairment (avoid frequent dosing or high doses) due to risk of propylene/polyethylene glycol toxicity.[123] Avoid using in hepatic failure.[123]	Low: $0.80 /pill[125]
Midazolam	Initial Dose: 2.5 mg IV or SubQ STAT and q1h. PRN (0.5–1 mg if elderly or frail) Max Dose: 5 mg maximum cumulative dose Routes: IV, SubQ, IM	Adverse effects include: sedation, worsening of delirium symptoms, increased fall risk, anxiety, insomnia, dizziness, and paradoxical agitation.[83,124] Caution if administering subcutaneously (may cause site irritation).[83]	Low: $10.48/2 vials (1 mL) of 5 mg/mL[126]

*Dosages and routes are adapted from Bush et al. 2017, 2018[4,83], and Marcanonio, 2017[10]

Antipsychotics and benzodiazepines are not approved by the US Food and Drug Administration (FDA) for treatment of delirium symptoms. While the authors have endeavored to include accurate dosing and side effect information, please always consult with a pharmacist, pharmaceutical reference book, or the drug manufacturer data sheet when prescribing. Lists of adverse effects in this table are those of most concern in the palliative care population, but they are not comprehensive.

related to the sense of losing their loved one even before they died has been noted in families of patients with delirium in the palliative care setting.[80] The inability to communicate may lead to frustration and fear in the patient and also heighten distress in the family who worries that they may not be able to resolve issues or say their final good-byes. Terminal delirium with agitation was a significant determinant of family distress identified by bereaved family members of palliative care patients.[127] In addition, family caregivers can have ambivalent feelings regarding the balance of relieving delirium-related suffering with sedation and the desire to maintain consciousness and communicate.[80,127]

A literature review of 15 studies on the role of family caregivers of palliative care patients with delirium identified three themes regarding caregiver participation in the management of delirium: detection/prevention, symptom monitoring, and advocating for the patient[80] (Box 49.7). In general, the family caregivers studied were positive about participating in caring and advocating for patients with delirium at the end of life. Facilitating this participation could be highly valued and meaningful for many caregivers; however, the authors point out that the optimal level of family caregiver participation may vary and requires an individualized approach and more investigation.

Interventions for the family caregivers of patients with delirium fall into two general categories: education and support.[80] Education found to be helpful by caregivers includes information regarding the risk factors, causes, symptoms, expected progression, implications, and treatments for delirium, as well as advice on how to respond to the patient with delirium.[80,128,129] Delirium may linger beyond a hospitalization or develop in the home, therefore, family caregivers in the community could also benefit from education regarding delirium. A review of seven studies on delirium education for family caregivers, revealed four teaching methods: verbal

instruction, informational leaflets, both verbal instruction and leaflets, and training in the use of a delirium assessment tool for caregivers to report delirium symptoms electronically. There were no conclusions regarding an optimal method, and the authors emphasize the need for more evidence-based educational interventions for caregivers.[13]

Caregiver support is described as either support for the caregivers themselves to improve the caregiver experience and well-being or support that enhances the ability of the caregiver to improve patient outcomes (e.g., reduce delirium incidence, severity, or duration).[80] A patient outcome in the context of terminal delirium could also include a peaceful death. Given the high levels of caregiver distress associated with delirium, techniques to improve the caregiver experience can include providing therapeutic presence, discussing coping skills, and investigating ways to maintain the patient–caregiver relationship.[127]

Caregiving from a physical distance is a new phenomenon as the result of the COVID-19 pandemic and may continue into the future. An editorial in the *Journal of the American Geriatrics Society* voiced the concern that restricted visitation, isolation from staff, personal protective equipment, and workload demands all place older hospitalized and nursing home patients at increased risk of delirium and necessitate a redoubling of preventive and management strategies. The editorial recommends that family caregivers be seen as essential healthcare workers and that visitor passes be given to caregivers of COVID-19-negative patients with cognitive impairment or delirium. And it suggested recommendations to allow them to have hospital health screening and education about personal protective equipment to allow their participation, clearly underlying their importance.[130] Assisting family caregivers to connect virtually to receive education about delirium and collaborate on goals of care and treatment may

increasingly need to be offered through a variety of methods,
especially when direct patient contact is restricted.

RESEARCH

The multifactorial etiology of delirium, combined with the
range of comorbidities (vulnerabilities) in patients with
advanced disease, presents a particular challenge to the study of
delirium in palliative care. Despite the relatively high incidence
and prevalence of delirium in this population, the breakdown
in neuronal networks that leads to a disruption in cognition
and attention is not completely understood and may vary with
the different psychomotor subtypes. Hypotheses regarding the
pathophysiology of delirium require further testing, and more
biomarkers need to be identified to advance the science and
improve on the current evidence-based guidelines.

Many of the strategies for the prevention of delirium are
nursing-driven, and palliative APRNs play a significant role
in the development and testing of clinical guidelines, policies, and prevention programs relevant to palliative care and
hospice settings. In the palliative care population, particularly at the end of life, symptom management may be the
focus, and currently there is no one drug approved for the
treatment of delirium. Research is needed on the best pharmacological options based on patient symptoms, along with
pharmacological approaches for severe, refractory terminal
delirium. Multicomponent nonpharmacological approaches
for delirium are recommended; however, identifying the best
combinations for improving patient outcomes needs further
study. Continued research into the optimal interventions
for the support and education of family caregivers is another
important area where palliative APRNs offer significant contributions, especially with the emerging dilemma of physical
distancing and restrictions on visitation.

SUMMARY

Delirium is associated with poor outcomes, is a poor prognostic indicator, and preventing it from developing is the ideal.

However, once it has been diagnosed, each episode is unique
and careful assessment of predisposing and precipitating risk
factors can help to determine the most appropriate interventions. Working collaboratively with the interdisciplinary
team, patients, and family caregivers, is the palliative APRN's
best approach to the treatment of delirium, given its multifactorial nature. The consistent use of validated screening tools to
identify delirium early and monitor treatment is a key component to reducing severity and duration. In the palliative care
population, balancing the burden of even minimally invasive
interventions with the potential for benefit, in the context of
the goals of care, should be incorporated into treatment decisions. Terminal delirium demands additional considerations
when communication can be impaired and opportunities for
closure and good-byes limited, all of which can have a long-
lasting impact on the family.

REFERENCES

1. Steis M, Evans L, Hirschman K, et al. Screening for delirium using
family caregivers: Convergent validity of the family confusion
assessment method and interviewer-rated confusion assessment
method. *J Am Geriatr Soc.* 2012;60(11):2121–2126. doi:10.1111/
j.1532-5415.2012.04200.x
2. Sands MB, Dantoc BP, Hartshorn A, Ryan CJ, Lujic S. Single
Question in Delirium (SQID): Testing its efficacy against psychiatrist interview, the confusion assessment method and the memorial delirium assessment scale. *Palliat Med.* 2010;24(6):561–565.
doi:10.1177/0269216310371556
3. Seiler A, Schubert M, Hertler C, et al. Predisposing and precipitating risk factors for delirium in palliative care patients. *Palliat
Support Care.* 2019:1–10. doi:10.1017/S1478951519000919
4. Bush SH, Tierney S, Lawlor PG. Clinical assessment and
management of delirium in the palliative care setting. *Drugs.*
2017;77(15):1623–1643. doi:10.1007/s40265-017-0804-3
5. Oh ES, Akeju O, Avidan MS, et al. A roadmap to advance delirium
research: Recommendations from the nidus scientific think tank.
Alzheimers Dement. 2020;16(5):726–733. doi:10.1002/alz.12076
6. American Psychiatric Association (APA). Delirium. *Diagnostic
and Statistical Manual of Mental Disorders.* 5th ed. Arlington, VA:
American Psychiatric Association; 2013: 596–602. doi-org.db29.
linccweb.org/10.1176/appi
7. Inouye SK, Westendorp RGJ, Saczynski JS. Delirium in
elderly people. *Lancet.* 2014;383(9920):911–922. doi:10.1016/
s0140-6736(13)60688-1
8. Evensen S, Saltvedt I, Lydersen S, Wyller TB, Taraldsen K, Sletvold
O. Delirium motor subtypes and prognosis in hospitalized geriatric patients: A prospective observational study. *J Psychosom Res.*
2019;122:24–28. doi:10.1016/j.jpsychores.2019.04.020
9. Meagher D, Moran M, Raju B, et al. A new data-based motor
subtype schema for delirium. *J Neuropsychiatry Clin Neurosci.*
2008;20(2):185–193. doi:10.1176/jnp.2008.20.2.185
10. Marcantonio ER. Delirium in hospitalized older adults. *N Engl J
Med.* 2017;377(15):1456–1466. doi:10.1056/NEJMcp1605501
11. Avelino-Silva TJ, Campora F, Curiati JAE, Jacob-Filho W.
Prognostic effects of delirium motor subtypes in hospitalized older
adults: A prospective cohort study. *PLoS One.* 2018;13(1):e0191092.
Published 2018 Jan 30. doi:10. 1371/journal.pone.0191092
12. Agar MR, Quinn SJ, Crawford GB, et al. Predictors of mortality for
delirium in palliative care. *J Palliat Med.* 2016;19(11):1205–1209.
doi:10.1089/jpm.2015.0416
13. Carbone MK, Gugliucci MR. Delirium and the family caregiver:
The need for evidence-based education interventions. *Gerontologist.*
2015;55(3):345–352. doi:10.1093/geront/gnu035.

14. Shafi MM, Santarnecchi E, Fong TG, et al. Advancing the neurophysiological understanding of delirium. *J Am Geriatr Soc.* 2017;65(6):1114–1118. doi:10.1111/jgs.14748

15. Maldonado JR. Neuropathogenesis of delirium: Review of current etiologic theories and common pathways. *Am J Geriatr Psychiatry.* 2013;21(12):1190–1222. doi:10.1016/j.jagp.2013.09.005

16. Mietani K, Sumitani M, Ogata T, et al. Dysfunction of the blood-brain barrier in postoperative delirium patients, referring to the axonal damage biomarker phosphorylated neurofilament heavy subunit. *PLoS One.* 2019;14(10):e0222721. doi:10.1371/journal.pone.0222721

17. Oldham MA, Flanagan NM, Khan A, Boukrina O, Marcantonio ER. Responding to ten common delirium misconceptions with best evidence: An educational review for clinicians. *J Neuropsychiatry Clin Neurosci.* 2018;30(1):51–57. doi:10.1176/appi.neuropsych.17030065

18. Kalvas LB, Monroe TB. Structural brain changes in delirium: An integrative review. *Biol Res Nurs.* 2019;21(4):355–365. doi:10.1177/1099800419849489

19. FitzGerald JM. Delirium clinical motor subtypes: A narrative review of the literature and insights from neurobiology. *Aging Ment Health.* 2018;22(4):431–443. doi:10.1080/13607863.2017.1310802

20. Smith T, Cooper A, Peryer G, Griffiths R, Fox C, Cross J. Factors predicting incidence of post-operative delirium in older people following hip fracture surgery: A systematic review and meta-analysis. *Int J Geriatr Psychiatry.* 2017;32(4):386–396. doi:10.1002/gps.4655

21. Watt CL, Momoli F, Ansari MT, et al. The incidence and prevalence of delirium across palliative care settings: A systematic review. *Palliat Med.* 2019;33(8):865–877. doi:10.1177/0269216319854944

22. Inouye SK, Charpentier PA. Precipitating factors for delirium in hospitalized elderly persons. *JAMA.* 1996;275(11):852–857.

23. Davis DH, Muniz Terrera G, Keage H, et al. Delirium is a strong risk factor for dementia in the oldest-old: A population-based cohort study. *Brain.* 2012;135(Pt 9):2809–2816. doi:10.1093/brain/aws190

24. Shenvi C, Kennedy M, Austin CA, Wilson MP, Gerardi M, Schneider S. Managing delirium and agitation in the older emergency department patient: The adept tool. *Ann Emerg Med.* 2020;75(2):136–145. doi:10.1016/j.annemergmed.2019.07.023

25. Oh ES, Fong TG, Hshieh TT, Inouye SK. Delirium in older persons: Advances in diagnosis and treatment. *JAMA.* 2017;318(12):1161–1174. doi:10.1001/jama.2017.12067

26. Harrison A, Smith R, Champagne M, Martin B, Pursley J, Hendrix C. Implementation of a delirium assessment protocol in an inpatient hospice setting. *J Hospice Palliat Nurs.* 2016;18(3):227–232.

27. White J, Hammond L. Delirium assessment tool for end of life: CHIMBOP. *J Palliat Med.* 2008;11(8):1069. doi:10.1089/jpm.2008.9851

28. Schreier A. Nursing care, delirium, and pain management for the hospitalized older adult. *Pain Manag Nurs.* 2010;11(3):177–185. doi:10.1016/j.pmn.2009.07.002

29. McCusker J, Cole M, Abrahamowicz M, Han L, Podoba J, Ramman-Haddad L. Environmental risk factors for delirium in hospitalized older people. *J Am Geriatr Soc.* 2001;49(10):1327–1334. doi:10.1046/j.1532-5415.2001.49260.x

30. Van Rompaey B, Elseviers M, Schuurmans M, Shortridge-Baggett L, Truijen S, Bossaert L. Risk factors for delirium in intensive care patients: A prospective cohort study. *Crit Care.* 2009;13(3):R77. doi:10.1186/cc7892

31. Pandharipande PP, Ely EW, Arora RC, et al. The intensive care delirium research agenda: A multinational, interprofessional perspective. *Intensive Care Med.* 2017;43(9):1329–1339. doi:10.1007/s00134-017-4860-7

32. Duceppe MA, Williamson DR, Elliott A, et al. Modifiable risk factors for delirium in critically ill trauma patients: A multicenter prospective study. *J Intensive Care Med.* 2019;34(4):330–336. doi:10.1177/0885066617698646

33. Zhu Y, Wang G, Liu S, et al. Risk factors for postoperative delirium in patients undergoing major head and neck cancer surgery: A meta-analysis. *Jpn J Clin Oncol.* 2017;47(6):505–511. doi:doi:10.1093/jjco/hyx029

34. Magny E, Le Petitcorps H, Pociumban M, et al. Predisposing and precipitating factors for delirium in community-dwelling older adults admitted to hospital with this condition: A prospective case series. *PLoS One.* 2018;13(2):e0193034. doi:10.1371/journal.pone.0193034

35. Hshieh TT, Inouye SK, Oh ES. Delirium in the elderly. *Psychiatr Clin North Am.* 2018;41(1):1–17. doi:10.1016/j.psc.2017.10.001

36. Hshieh TT, Saczynski J, Gou RY, et al. Trajectory of functional recovery after postoperative delirium in elective surgery. *Ann Surg.* 2017;265(4):647–653. doi:10.1097/SLA.0000000000001952

37. Pandharipande PP, Girard TD, Jackson JC, et al. Long-term cognitive impairment after critical illness. *N Engl J Med.* 2013;369(14):1306–1316. doi:10.1056/NEJMoa1301372

38. Fong TG, Davis D, Growdon ME, Albuquerque A, Inouye SK. The interface between delirium and dementia in elderly adults. *Lancet Neurol.* 2015;14(8):823–832. doi:10.1016/s1474-4422(15)00101-5

39. Witlox J, Eurelings L, de Jonghe J, Kalisvaart K, Eikelenboom P, van Gool W. Delirium in elderly patients and the risk of postdischarge mortality, institutionalization, and dementia: A meta-analysis. *JAMA.* 2010;304(4):443–451. doi:10.1001/jama.2010.1013

40. Mosk CA, Mus M, Vroemen JP, et al. Dementia and delirium, the outcomes in elderly hip fracture patients. *Clin Interv Aging.* 2017;12:421–430. doi:10.2147/CIA.S115945

41. Brummel NE, Boehm LM, Girard TD, et al. Subsyndromal delirium and institutionalization among patients with critical illness. *Am J Crit Care.* 2017;26(6):447–455. doi:10.4037/ajcc2017263

42. Salluh JI, Wang H, Schneider EB, et al. Outcome of delirium in critically ill patients: Systematic review and meta-analysis. *BMJ.* 2015;350:h2538. doi:10.1136/bmj.h2538

43. Dani M, Owen LH, Jackson TA, Rockwood K, Sampson EL, Davis D. Delirium, frailty, and mortality: Interactions in a prospective study of hospitalized older people. *J Gerontol A Biol Sci Med Sci.* 2018;73(3):415–418. doi:10.1093/gerona/glx214

44. Israni J, Lesser A, Kent T, Ko K. Delirium as a predictor of mortality in us medicare beneficiaries discharged from the emergency department: A national claims-level analysis up to 12 months. *BMJ Open.* 2018;8(5):e021258. doi:10.1136/bmjopen-2017-021258

45. Krewulak KD, Stelfox HT, Ely EW, Fiest KM. Risk factors and outcomes among delirium subtypes in adult icus: A systematic review. *J Crit Care.* 2020;56:257–264. doi:10.1016/j.jcrc.2020.01.017

46. Gual N, Inzitari M, Carrizo G, et al. Delirium subtypes and associated characteristics in older patients with exacerbation of chronic conditions. *Am J Geriatr Psychiatry.* 2018;26(12):1204–1212. doi:10.1016/j.jagp.2018.07.003

47. Hosie A, Davidson PM, Agar M, Sanderson CR, Phillips J. Delirium prevalence, incidence, and implications for screening in specialist palliative care inpatient settings: A systematic review. *Palliat Med.* 2013;27(6):486–498. doi:10.1177/0269216312457214

48. Inouye S, van Dyck C, Alessi C, Balkin S, Siegal A, Horwitz R. Clarifying confusion: The confusion assessment method. A new method for detection of delirium. *Ann Intern Med.* 1990;113(12):941–948. doi:10.7326/0003-4819-113-12-941

49. Trzepacz PT, Baker R, Greenhouse J. A symptom rating scale for delirium. *Psychiatry Res.* 1988;23(1):89–97. doi:10.1016/0165-1781(88)90037-6

50. Quispel-Aggenbach DWP, Holtman GA, Zwartjes HAHT, Zuidema SU, Luijendijk HJ. Attention, arousal and other rapid bedside screening instruments for delirium in older patients: A systematic review of test accuracy studies. *Age Ageing.* 2018;47(5):644–653. doi:10.1093/ageing/afy058

51. Breitbart W, Rosenfeld B, Roth A, Smith M, Cohen K, Passik S. The Memorial Delirium Assessment Scale. *J Pain Symptom Manage.* 1997;13(3):128–137. doi:10.1016/s0885-3924(96)00316-8

52. Leonard MM, Nekolaichuk C, Meagher DJ, et al. Practical assessment of delirium in palliative care. *J Pain Symptom Manage.* 2014;48(2):176–190. doi:10.1016/j.jpainsymman.2013.10.024

53. De J, Wand AP. Delirium screening: A systematic review of delirium screening tools in hospitalized patients. *Gerontologist.* 2015;55(6):1079–1099. doi:10.1093/geront/gnv100

54. Klankluang W, Pukrittayakamee P, Atsariyasing W, et al. Validity and reliability of the Memorial Delirium Assessment Scale-Thai Version (MDAS-T) for assessment of delirium in palliative care patients. *Oncologist.* 2020;25(2):e335–e340. doi:10.1634/theoncologist.2019-0399

55. Jones RN, Cizginer S, Pavlech L, et al. Assessment of instruments for measurement of delirium severity: A systematic review. *JAMA Intern Med.* 2019;179(2):231–239. doi:10.1001/jamainternmed.2018.6975

56. Inouye SK, Kosar CM, Tommet D, et al. The CAM-S: Development and validation of a new scoring system for delirium severity in 2 cohorts. *Ann Intern Med.* 2014;160(8):526–533. doi:10.7326/M13-1927

57. Robertsson B, Karlsson I, Styrud E, Gottfries CG. Confusional State Evaluation (CSE): An instrument for measuring severity of delirium in the elderly. 1997;170(6):565–570. doi:10.1192/bjp.170.6.565

58. de Jonghe JF, Kalisvaart KJ, Timmers JF, Kat MG, Jackson JC. Delirium-o-Meter: A nurses' rating scale for monitoring delirium severity in geriatric patients. *Int J Geriatr Psychiatry.* 2005;20(12):1158–1166. doi:10.1002/gps.1410

59. Schuurmans MJ, Shortridge-Baggett L, Duursma SA. The delirium observation screening scale: A screening instrument for delirium. *Res Theor Nurs Pract.* 2003;17(1):31–50. doi:10.1891/rtnp.17.1.31.53169

60. Neelon V, Champagne M, Carlson J, Funk S. The Neecham confusion scale: Construction, validation, and clinical testing. *Nurs Res.* 1996;45(6):324–330. doi:10.1097/00006199-199611000-00002I

61. Grover S, Kate N. Assessment scales for delirium: A review. *World J Psychiatry.* 2012;2(4):58–70. doi:10.5498/wjp.v2.i4.58

62. Gaudreau JD, Gagnon P, Harel F, Roy MA. Impact on delirium detection of using a sensitive instrument integrated into clinical practice. *Gen Hosp Psychiatry.* 2005;27(3):194–199. doi:10.1016/j.genhosppsych.2005.01.002

63. Scholtens RM, van Munster BC, Adamis D, de Jonghe A, Meagher DJ, de Rooij SE. Variability of delirium motor subtype scale-defined delirium motor subtypes in elderly adults with hip fracture: A longitudinal study. *J Am Geriatr Soc.* 2017;65(2):e45–e50. doi:10.1111/jgs.14582

64. Perez-Ros P, Martinez-Arnau FM. Delirium assessment in older people in emergency departments. A literature review. *Diseases.* 2019;7(1). doi:10.3390/diseases7010014

65. Ryan K, Leonard M, Guerin S, Donnelly S, Conroy M, Meagher D. Validation of the confusion assessment method in the palliative care setting. *Palliat Med.* 2009;23(1):40–45. doi:10.1177/0269216308099210

66. Ely EW, Inouye SK, Bernard GR, et al. Delirium in mechanically ventilated patients: Validity and reliability of the Confusion Assessment Method for the Intensive Care Unit (CAM-ICU). *JAMA.* 2001;286(21):2703–2710. doi:10.1001/jama.286.21.2703

67. Meagher D, Adamis D, Leonard M, et al. Development of an abbreviated version of the Delirium Motor Subtyping Scale (DMSS-4). *Int Psychogeriatr.* 2014;26(4):693–702. doi:10.1017/S1041610213002585

68. Boettger S, Nunez DG, Meyer R, et al. Brief assessment of delirium subtypes: Psychometric evaluation of the Delirium Motor Subtype Scale (DMSS)-4 in the intensive care setting. *Palliat Support Care.* 2017;15(5):535–543. doi:10.1017/S147895151600105X

69. NIDUS: Network for Investigation of Delirium: Unifying Scientists. Measurement and harmonization core. No date. https://deliriumnetwork.org/measurement/

70. Borson S, Scanlan J, Brush M, Vitaliano P, Dokmak A. The Mini-Cog: A cognitive "vital signs" measure for dementia screening in multi-lingual elderly. *Int J Geriatr Psychiatry.* 2000;15(11):1021–1027. doi:10.1002/1099-1166(200011)15:11<1021::aid-gps234>3.0.co;2-6

71. Pfeiffer E. A short portable mental status questionnaire for the assessment of organic brain deficit in elderly patients. *J Am Geriatr Soc.* 1975;23(10):433–441. doi:10.1111/j.1532-5415.1975.tb00927.x

72. Guthrie P, Rayborn S, Butcher H. Evidence-based practice guideline: Delirium. *J Gerontol Nurs.* 2018;44(2):14–24.t. doi:10.3928/00989134-20180110-04

73. Portela Millinger F, Fellinger M. Clinical characteristics and treatment of delirium in palliative care settings. memo. 2020;14:48-52. https://doi.org/10.1007/s12254-020-00641-w

74. Yesavage J, Brink T, Rose T, et al. Development and validation of a geriatric depression screening scale: A preliminary report. *J Psychiatr Res.* 1982;17(1):37–49. doi:10.1016/0022-3956(82)90033-4

75. Volland J, Fisher A, Drexler D. Preventing and identifying hospital-acquired delirium. *Nursing.* 2020;50(1):32–37. doi:10.1097/01.NURSE.0000615072.68682.f0

76. Weng C, Lin K, Lu F, et al. Effects of depression, dementia, and delirium on activities of daily living in elderly patients after discharge. *BMC Geriatr.* 2019 Oct 11;19(1):261. doi:10.1186/s12877-019-1294-9

77. Loving, N, Dahlin C. Anxiety, depression, and delirium. In: Matzo M, Sherman D, eds. *Palliative Care Nursing.* 5th ed. New York: Springer; 2019: 545-580.

78. Milisen K, Braes T, Fick DM, Foreman M. Cognitive assessment and differentiating the 3 Ds (dementia, depression, delirium). *Nurs Clin North Am.* 2006 Mar;41(1):1–22. doi:10.1016/j.cnur.2005.09.001

79. Lawlor PG, Gagnon B, Mancini I, et al. Occurrence, causes, and outcome of delirium in patients with advanced cancer: A prospective study. *Arch Intern Med.* 2000;160(6):786–794. doi:10.1001/archinte.160.6.786

80. Finucane AM, Lugton J, Kennedy C, Spiller JA. The experiences of caregivers of patients with delirium, and their role in its management in palliative care settings: An integrative literature review. *Psychooncology.* 2017;26(3):291–300. doi:10.1002/pon.4140

81. Bush SH, Marchington KL, Agar M, Davis DHJ, Sikora L, Tsang TWY. Quality of clinical practice guidelines in delirium: A systematic appraisal. *BMJ Open.* 2017;7(3):e013809. doi:10.1136/bmjopen-2016-013809

82. Schmitt EM, Gallagher J, Albuquerque A, et al. Perspectives on the delirium experience and its burden: Common themes among older patients, their family caregivers, and nurses. *Gerontologist.* 2019;59(2):327–337. doi:10.1093/geront/gnx153

83. Bush SH, Lawlor PG, Ryan K, et al. Delirium in adult cancer patients: ESMO clinical practice guidelines. *Ann Oncol.* 2018;29:iv143–iv165. doi:10.1093/annonc/mdy147

84. Inouye SK, Bogardus ST, Baker D, Leo-Summers L, Cooney LM. The hospital elder life program: A model of care to prevent cognitive and functional decline in older hospitalized patients. *J Am Geriatr Soc.* 2000;48(12):1697–1706. doi:10.1111/j.1532-5415.2000.tb03885.x

85. Inouye SK, Bogardus ST, Charpentier PA, et al. A multicomponent intervention to prevent delirium in hospitalized older patients. *New Engl J Med.* 1999;340(9):669–676. doi:10.1056/nejm199903043400901

86. Hshieh TT, Yue J, Oh E, et al. Effectiveness of multicomponent nonpharmacological delirium interventions. *JAMA Intern Med.* 2015;175(4):512. doi:10.1001/jamainternmed.2014.7779

87. Siddiqi N, Harrison JK, Clegg A, et al. Interventions for preventing delirium in hospitalised non-ICU patients. *Cochrane Database Syst Rev.* 2016;3:CD005563. Published 2016 Mar 11. doi:10.1002/14651858.CD005563.pub3

88. National Institute for Health and Care Excellence (NICE). Delirium: Prevention, diagnosis and management [CG 103]. Published 28 July 2010. Updated March 14, 2019. https://www.nice.org.uk/guidance/cg103

89. Hosker CMG, Bennett MI. Delirium and agitation at the end of life. *BMJ.* 2016;353(i3085):1–6. doi:10.1136/bmj.i3085

90. American Geriatrics Society (AGS). AGS CoCare®: Help. 2021. https://www.americangeriatrics.org/programs/ags-cocare-helptmy

91. American Society of Addiction Medicine. The ASAM clinical practice guideline on alcohol withdrawal management. Adopted

January 23, 2020. Rockville, MD: American Society of Addiction Medicine https://www.asam.org/Quality-Science/quality/guideline-on-alcohol-withdrawal-management

92. Santos C, Olmedo RE. Sedative-hypnotic drug withdrawal syndrome: Recognition and treatment. *Emerg Med Pract.* 2017;19(3):1–20.

93. Finucane AM, Jones L, Leurent B, et al. Drug therapy for delirium in terminally ill adults. *Cochrane Database Syst Rev.* 2020;1:CD004770. Published 2020 Jan 21. doi:10.1002/14651858.CD004770.pub3

94. Beller EM, van Driel ML, McGregor L, Truong S, Mitchell G. Palliative pharmacological sedation for terminally ill adults. *Cochrane Database Syst Rev.* 2015;1:CD010206. Published 2015 Jan 2. doi:10.1002/14651858.CD010206.pub2

95. Partridge JS, Martin FC, Harari D, Dhesi JK. The delirium experience: What is the effect on patients, relatives and staff and what can be done to modify this? *Int J Geriatr Psychiatry.* 2013;28(8):804–812. doi:10.1002/gps.3900

96. Grassi L, Caraceni A, Mitchell AJ, et al. Management of delirium in palliative care: A review. *Curr Psychiatry Rep.* 2015;17(3):550. doi:10.1007/s11920-015-0550-8

97. Kishi T, Hirota T, Matsunaga S, Iwata N. Antipsychotic medications for the treatment of delirium: A systematic review and meta-analysis of randomised controlled trials. *J Neurol Neurosurg Psychiatry.* 2016;87(7):767–774. doi:10.1136/jnnp-2015-311049

98. Neufeld KJ, Yue J, Robinson TN, Inouye SK, Needham DM. Antipsychotic medication for prevention and treatment of delirium in hospitalized adults: A systematic review and meta-analysis. *J Am Geriatr Soc.* 2016;64(4):705–714. doi:10.1111/jgs.14076

99. Cerveira CCT, Pupo CC, Santos SDSD, Santos JEM. Delirium in the elderly: A systematic review of pharmacological and non-pharmacological treatments. *Dement Neuropsychol.* 2017;11(3):270–275. doi:10.1590/1980-57642016dn11-030009

100. Lawley H, Hewison A. An integrative literature review exploring the clinical management of delirium in patients with advanced cancer. *J Clin Nurs.* 2017;26(23–24):4172–4183. doi:10.1111/jocn.13960

101. Burry L, Mehta S, Perreault MM, et al. Antipsychotics for treatment of delirium in hospitalised non-icu patients. *Cochrane Database Syst Rev.* 2018;6:CD005594. Published 2018 Jun 18. doi:10.1002/14651858.CD005594.pub3

102. Wu Y-C, Tseng P-T, Tu Y-K, et al. Association of delirium response and safety of pharmacological interventions for the management and prevention of delirium. *JAMA Psychiatry.* 2019;76(5):526. doi:10.1001/jamapsychiatry.2018.4365

103. Hui D, De La Rosa A, Wilson A, et al. Neuroleptic strategies for terminal agitation in patients with cancer and delirium at an acute palliative care unit: A single-centre, double-blind, parallel-group, randomised trial. *Lancet Oncol.* 2020;21(7):989–998. doi:10.1016/s1470-2045(20)30307-7

104. Li Y, Ma J, Jin Y, et al. Benzodiazepines for treatment of patients with delirium excluding those who are cared for in an intensive care unit. *Cochrane Database Syst Rev.* 2020(2):CD012670. Published 2020 Feb 28. doi:10.1002/14651858.CD012670.pub2

105. van der Vorst M, Neefjes ECW, Boddaert MSA, et al. Olanzapine versus haloperidol for treatment of delirium in patients with advanced cancer: A phase III randomized clinical trial. *Oncologist.* 2020;25(3):e570–e577. doi:10.1634/theoncologist.2019-0470I

106. Camber Pharmaceuticals, Inc. Aripiprazole [package insert]. U.S. National Library of Medicine, Dailymed website. https://daily med.nlm.nih.gov/dailymed/drugInfo.cfm?setid=2d8d574b-fbf4-4d2c-a37c-25556ecbf1aa. Updated June 18, 2021.

107. Lannett Company, Inc. Chlorpromazine hydrochloride [package insert]. U.S. National Library of Medicine, Dailymed website. https://dailymed.nlm.nih.gov/dailymed/drugInfo.cfm?setid=10495 38a-c012-41bf-932e-3c85f57f9577. Updated February 19, 2020.

108. Aurobindo Pharma Limited. Olanzapine [package insert]. U.S. National Library of Medicine, Dailymed website. https://daily med.nlm.nih.gov/dailymed/drugInfo.cfm?setid=636665be-9d7e-443a-8134-e8cc47e6ba24. Updated May 4, 2020.

109. AvKare. Risperidone [package insert]. U.S. National Library of Medicine, Dailymed website. https://dailymed.nlm.nih.gov/daily med/drugInfo.cfm?setid=cba7628c-30b2-5d26-e053-2a95a90a3 e57. Updated September 10, 2021.

110. Burel Pharmaceuticals, LLC. Haloperidol [package insert]. U.S. National Library of Medicine, Dailymed website. https://daily med.nlm.nih.gov/dailymed/drugInfo.cfm?setid=43bb14ed-d0c3-43be-92c4-ccb913737390. Updated April 1, 2021.

111. Ascend Laboratories, LLC. Quetiapine fumarate [package insert]. U.S. National Library of Medicine, Dailymed website. https:// dailymed.nlm.nih.gov/dailymed/drugInfo.cfm?setid=3112a006-1c61-47f2-84f5-9a7670d09c9b. Updated July 28, 2021.

112. Maust DT, Kim HM, Seyfried LS, et al. Antipsychotics, other psychotropics, and the risk of death in patients with dementia: Number needed to harm. *JAMA Psychiatry.* 2015;72(5):438–445. doi:10.1001/jamapsychiatry.2014.3018

113. Kheirbek RE, Fokar A, Little JT, et al. Association between antipsychotics and all-cause mortality among community-dwelling older adults. *J Gerontol A Biol Sci Med Sci.* 2019;74(12):1916–1921. doi:10.1093/gerona/glz045

114. Ebersbach G, Ip CW, Klebe S, et al. Management of delirium in Parkinson's disease. *J Neural Transm (Vienna).* 2019;126(7):905–912. doi:10.1007/s00702-019-01980-7

115. McKeith I, Fairbairn A, Perry R, Thompson P, Perry E. Neruoleptic sensitivity in patients with senile dementia of Lewy body type. *BMJ.* 1992;305:673–678. doi:10.1136/bmj.305.6855.673I

116. GoodRx Inc. Haloperidol page. 2021. Available at https://www.goodrx.com/haloperidol

117. GoodRx Inc. Chlorpromazine page. 2021. Available at https://www.goodrx.com/chlorpromazine

118. GoodRx Inc. Risperidone page. 2021. Available at https://www.goodrx.com/risperidone

119. Stinton C, McKeith I, Taylor JP, et al. Pharmacological management of Lewy body dementia: A systematic review and meta-analysis. *Am J Psychiatry.* 2015;172(8):731–742. doi:10.1176/appi.ajp.2015.14121582

120. Good Rx. Olanzapine page. 2021. Available at https://www.goodrx.com/olanzapine

121. Good Rx. Quetiapine page. 2021. Available at https://www.goodrx.com/quetiapine

122. Good Rx. Aripiprazole page. 2021. Available at https://www.goodrx.com/aripiprazole

123. Civica, Inc. Lorazepam [package insert]. U.S. National Library of Medicine, Dailymed website. https://dailymed.nlm.nih.gov/daily med/drugInfo.cfm?setid=5140798d-8571-41fb-84a4-e182aac3f 64c. Updated April 27, 2021.

124. Gland Pharma Limited. Midazolam hydrochloride [package insert]. U.S. National Library of Medicine, Dailymed website. https://daily med.nlm.nih.gov/dailymed/drugInfo.cfm?setid=81b2f48d-a05c-4301-8fee-761af220d44f. Updated October 14, 2017.

125. Good Rx. Lorazepam page. 2021. Available at https://www.goodrx.com/lorazepam

126. Good Rx. Midazolam page. 2021. Available at https://www.goodrx.com/midazolam

127. Morita T, Akechi T, Ikenaga M, et al. Terminal delirium: Recommendations from bereaved families' experiences. *J Pain Symptom Manage.* 2007;34(6):579–589. doi:10.1016/j.jpainsymman.2007.01.012

128. Paulson CM, Monroe T, McDougall GJ, Jr., Fick DM. A family-focused delirium educational initiative with practice and research implications. *Gerontol Geriatr Educ.* 2016;37(1):4–11. doi:10.1080/02701960.2015.1031896

129. Bull MJ, Boaz L, Jermé MG. Educating family caregivers for older adults about delirium: A systematic review. *Worldviews Evid Based Nurs.* 2016;13(3):232–240. doi:10.1111/wvn.12154

130. LaHue SC, James TC, Newman JC, Esmaili AM, Ormseth CH, Ely EW. Collaborative delirium prevention in the age of COVID-19. *J Am Geriatr Soc.* 2020;68(5):947–949. doi:10.1111/jgs.16480

50.

DEPRESSION AND SUICIDE

John Chovan

KEY POINTS

- National guidelines require the interdisciplinary team to address the psychological and psychiatric aspects of care for patients and families in palliative care.

- Adjusting to the news of a life-limiting disease requires drawing on past experiences and developed coping mechanisms that may be maladaptive. Every individual is different in their adjustment.

- Not all instances of a depressed mood constitute a diagnosable depressive disorder.

- The palliative advanced practice registered nurse (APRN) uses evidence-based practices and patient-centered care to support their patients and families across the trajectory of their disease, including complementary and alternative therapies as well as referrals to psychiatric and mental health specialists as needed.

- Assessing for patient safety includes evaluating for self-harm in depressed palliative care patients and their families at every encounter.

CASE STUDY: THE PATIENT WITH DEPRESSION

Theresa is a 41-year-old African American transgender female who lives with her wife of 10 years Regina, in a mid-sized Midwestern city. Regina is a stay-at-home mother and cares for their 9-year-old twin boys, Asa and Jeremy. Theresa has been living with sickle-cell disease since her diagnosis when she was 4 years old. She describes her infrequent pain crises as "worse than knives being stuck into me." During Theresa's last admission, Regina asked her if she had noticed that her pain episodes were starting to get closer together. Theresa told Regina to stop worrying about it and that she was imagining things. But Theresa suspected that was indeed the case and that she might be getting worse.

INTRODUCTION

Per the National Consensus Project for Quality Palliative Care *Clinical Practice Guidelines for Quality Palliative Care*, the interdisciplinary palliative care team must address the psychological and psychiatric aspects of care that can occur across the spectrum of a diagnosis of a life-limiting illness. This includes screenings, the psychological and psychiatric aspects of setting goals of care as part of the treatment plan, supporting the patient and family, and delivering and assessing interventions (Domain 3: Psychological and Psychiatric Aspects of Care).[1]

The initial response by patients and families to learning such a diagnosis varies. Disbelief, needing time to let the news sink in, shock, sadness, anger, and denial are all potential psychological responses. Yet not all the psychological responses are pathological. This chapter focuses on feelings associated with depression that accompany patients and their family members (as defined by the patient) throughout the trajectory of a chronic, life-threatening illness. Because symptoms associated with depression can emerge at any time throughout the course of the illness, the framework used to examine the symptoms associated with depression involves the four stages of the illness trajectory: (1) at the time of diagnosis; (2) during treatment, including initial treatments and subsequent planned or unplanned treatments; (3) after treatment, including when the planned course of treatment is completed or when the goals shift away from treatment; and (4) during active dying.[2,3]

DEFINITION OF DEPRESSION

The term "depression" has a technical definition but is often used colloquially in healthcare. When a person says, "I'm depressed," in all likelihood the person has not assessed and diagnosed themselves according to evidence-based standards. It often means that they are feeling blue, have low spirits, or are unhappy. It may also mean that they are lonely, having physical or psychic pain, or are angry and need to talk.[4] Motivating a person to the point of being able to report "I'm depressed" may be a very complex challenge. For clarity, the terms used in this chapter are

- *Mood*: One's perceived emotional state.

- *Sadness*: The feeling of being unhappy or in low spirits, also called a depressed mood.[5]

- *Depressive symptoms*: The behavioral indicators associated with a depressed mood include sleep changes, anhedonia, guilt, helplessness, hopelessness, changes in energy level, reduced ability to concentrate, appetite changes, psychomotor slowing, and suicidal ideation or attempts.

Depressive symptoms can worsen over time in frequency, severity, duration, and impact on functioning to the point of causing disability, thus meeting criteria for a depressive disorder.

- *Dysthymia*: A condition of persistent depressive symptoms of insufficient severity and frequency to meet criteria for a depressive episode.[6]

- *Depressive episode*: A pathological state that meets predefined criteria based on the existence of a depressed mood or anhedonia as well as five of nine defined depressive symptoms for at least 2 weeks.[6] Most encounters in palliative care and hospice in which the patient says "I'm depressed" will present a constellation of symptoms that very likely do not meet the criteria for a depressive episode.[7]

- *Depressive disorder*: One of the constellations of pathological mood syndromes in which the hallmark feature is severe and persistent depressed mood and associated pathology that limits one's ability to function in social, occupational, or other important settings. These include major depressive disorder, pervasive depressive disorder, premenstrual dysphoric disorder, substance-induced depression, and depression due to another medical condition.[6] Some palliative care and hospice patients will have a depressive disorder in addition to a chronic, life-threatening somatic illness.[8–10]

To provide optimal care, the palliative advanced practice registered nurse (APRN) must understand the symptomatology of both somatic and psychiatric illness and the interplay between them.[11–13]

DEPRESSED MOOD AND LIFE-THREATENING ILLNESS

CASE STUDY: THE PATIENT WITH DEPRESSION (CONTINUED)

Three months after her last admission, Theresa was sleeping in later during the day and calling off work because she did not feel like going in. One Saturday, while Regina was out shopping with Jeremy, Theresa was walking up the stairs to go back to bed and found it more difficult to breathe, so she stopped midflight. Asa came down the stairs and stopped to ask her if she was all right. Trying not to frighten her son, she calmly asked him to call 911 and request an ambulance. She was so proud of Asa's poise while talking on the phone with the operator but was so tired of being in pain and so tired of dealing with these crises. At the hospital, Theresa was evaluated and found to have a pulmonary embolism, likely from a deep vein thrombosis.

Throughout the course of a chronic, life-threatening illness, a patient's response to the illness is often a waxing and waning mood. Patients and their families are often faced with impactful news and difficult decisions that can trigger depressive symptoms and thoughts of suicide. As a member of the multidisciplinary team, the APRN assesses for symptoms, plans interventions, and implements them to alleviate these symptoms.

Prior to diagnosis, patients and their families may be anxious in anticipation of the unknown to come but may not show evidence of depressive symptoms. Patients may find that changes they have observed prior to seeking medical attention or the process of going through diagnostic procedures is stressful, triggering depressive symptoms. Persons with preexisting depressive disorder may find that these stressors will make their depression worse or cause a relapse of depression that had been in remission.[14]

At diagnosis, no matter how prepared the person may be, hearing the news for the first time can be a stressor that triggers feelings of sadness, hopelessness, guilt, pain, regret, and helplessness in patients and families. At any point along the illness trajectory, depressive symptoms can become pathological or preexisting depression can be made worse.[15–18]

As treatment begins and continues, difficulties with side effects from the treatments or intermittent and recurring exacerbations can trigger disappointments and depressive symptoms in patients and their families. Patient's feelings of guilt about the impact the diagnosis and treatment have had on the family can cause a depressed mood. Discussions about code status, naming a healthcare proxy, and decisions about a living will can cause the patient's or family members' moods to sag. Physical symptoms can trigger depressive symptoms as the patient and their family try to cope with a new sense of normal, particularly pain. Spiritual angst can also cause depressive symptoms to emerge.[19–21]

Remissions or return to baseline from exacerbations can offer hope that dangles by a thread. The specter of relapsing or another worse exacerbation is a stressor that can cause depressed mood or make a depressive disorder worse. It can also increase anxiety levels to pathological magnitudes.[22,23]

During end-stage disease and the dying phase, resolution of depressive symptoms prior to the onset of active dying process is ideal. However, patients with depressive symptoms may still have trigger stressors, leaving them at risk for a difficult death. The focus of the palliative APRN is on comfort, which allows for the mood of the family to concomitantly be managed. For the family, the dying process of a loved one can be complex and layered, particularly if there is unfinished business when the patient dies.[24–27]

At the end of a patient's life, family members may be asked about the patient's previously expressed wishes. This is a major stressor to those who have not had difficult conversations about the patient's desires, and it can trigger depressive symptomatology and anxiety in the healthcare proxy and family. Grief is a normal response but can become pathological if it persists and has a negative impact on ability to function.[28]

Emerging research on the neuroendocrine response to grief has shed light on the involvement of the hypothalamic-pituitary-adrenal (HPA) axis in depressive symptoms of loss. Psychological reactions temper the dysfunction of the HPA axis, but increases in mean cortisol levels and flattened diurnal cortisol slopes are seen immediately and long after a loss. Both of these changes are associated with negative health outcomes.[29] The palliative APRN anticipates these potential responses to a life-limiting illness and living with a life-limiting illness and takes into account facets of culture, gender identity, sexual orientation, and other unmodifiable social determinants of mental health and illness.[30]

After comprehensive assessment, the palliative APRN collaborates with the multidisciplinary team to develop a care plan, marshal community resources, and organize supportive information in anticipation of patient and family questions and concerns. Although the scope of practice for a palliative APRN clearly includes psychiatric symptom management, the extent to which APRNs may manage psychiatric and mental health issues varies according to state laws and institutional policies.[12] Psychiatric and mental health specialist colleagues may be necessary to assist in severe and persistent mental illnesses, such as recurrent, refractory major depressive disorder; schizophrenia; and bipolar disorder. As part of primary care, all APRNs screen for depressive symptoms. Many APRNs can provide therapy and prescribe antidepressants as delineated by scope of practice. As appropriate, referral of a patient or family member to a psychiatric or mental health professional may be necessary. Such multidisciplinary team members include a psychiatric and mental health nurse practitioner or a clinical nurse specialist, a social worker, a psychologist, a psychiatrist, an inpatient consultation team, or an outpatient mental healthcare provider.[31,32]

EPIDEMIOLOGY OF DEPRESSION IN CHRONIC ILLNESS

Depression is associated with severe, chronic illness. Table 50.1 lists some types of chronic illnesses and their associated rates of depression.[33] The rate of depression is quite high for cardiac and neurological chronic illnesses. The palliative APRN should be familiar with this epidemiology to anticipate and monitor for depressive symptoms in persons with these chronic illnesses.[33–37]

Table 50.1 DEPRESSION IN CHRONIC ILLNESS

CHRONIC ILLNESS	% EXPERIENCING DEPRESSION
Heart Disease	45–65
Parkinson's disease	40
Multiple sclerosis	40
Cancer	25
Diabetes	25

From WebMD.[33]

HISTORY AND PATHOLOGY

When a person reports depressive symptoms, the APRN should consider reversible physical causes of the symptoms (Box 50.1).[38–42] For example, hypothyroidism causes symptoms that mimic depression and can be corrected medically, often with levothyroxine (Synthroid). It can be detected with a blood test that measures circulating levels of thyroid-stimulating hormone (TSH) and thyroxine (T4).[39] Metastatic disease to the brain can cause mood swings, including depression, as the lesions alter function in mood-related foci of the cerebrum.[40] Normal-pressure hydrocephalus can cause gait and mood changes that mimic depressive symptoms; a consult to neurology or neuropsychiatry is appropriate.[41] Unmanaged pain is a common cause of stress, and subsequent somatic symptoms and depressive symptoms, yet it is correctible. Pain can include distress from insomnia, anorexia, dysphagia, and existential rumination, which can lead the patient to ask, "Why me?"[42] Appropriate total pain management can alleviate these stressors and their comorbid depressive symptoms. If potential physiological causes are ruled out, or detected and treated, but the symptoms remain, the APRN can conclude that the symptoms are psychiatric and not due to a correctible physical cause. A referral to a specialist should be considered.

Acute stress does not always result in maladaptive responses. The diathesis–stress model of mental illness posits that persons may be genetically predisposed to development of a mental illness.[43] Incipient mental illness is expressed only after stressors trigger the symptoms. A family history of depression can point to a genetic predisposition to depression. Genetic markers have been identified for predisposition to depression and subtypes of depression.[44] The palliative APRN's comprehensive history can uncover threads of a genetic predisposition.

The process of taking a history allows the palliative APRN to build rapport with the patient and family when evaluating a new patient for depressive symptoms. Evidence of prior depressive symptoms is the best predictor of future depressive symptoms. Onset, duration, measures that exacerbate it or alleviate it, and amount of debility that the symptoms induce

Box 50.1 PHYSICAL CAUSES OF DEPRESSION

Cardiac surgeries
Dementia
Hypothyroidism
Hypoxia
Neurological malignancies, brain tumors
Normopressure hydrocephalus
Obstructive sleep apnea
Parturition
Seizures
Strokes
Traumatic brain injury

From APA Working Group[38]; Puchalapalli, Mahmood[39]; Pidani et al.[40]; and Israelsson et al.[41]

are all features that give insight into how to approach treatment. The therapeutic use of self allows the APRN to defuse any anxiety or reticence about discussing depression, particularly if the distress is in any way related to fear of rejection and the stigma of mental illness.[45]

Understanding the pathology attributed to depression continues to evolve. For the past 50 years, the *monoamine theory* of depression has been the paradigm to explain symptoms. The theory states that the lack of monoamine neurotransmitters in sufficient quantities to trigger postsynaptic neurons to fire appropriately in the prefrontal cortex and in the limbic system causes depression. The monoamines, primarily norepinephrine, serotonin, and dopamine, are the major neurotransmitters implicated in this theory. The theory holds up in that monoamine therapy, such as the monoamine oxidase inhibitors (MAOIs; e.g., phenelzine [Nardil]), tricyclic antidepressants (TCAs; e.g., amitriptyline [Elavil]), selective serotonin reuptake inhibitors (SSRIs; e.g., citalopram [Celexa]), and serotonin-norepinephrine reuptake inhibitors (SNRIs; e.g., venlafaxine [Effexor]) do offer symptomatic relief. With these therapies there is often a protracted delay between therapy initiation and onset of symptom relief, and their effect on depressive symptoms is inconsistent. When symptoms are detected before permanent neurological changes take effect, the symptoms can be reversed, and treatment eventually can be discontinued. More severe symptoms, however, will require life-long treatment.[46,47]

The *neurotrophic theory* of depression complements the monoamine theory.[48] Stress-induced atrophy and loss of neurons and glia in the structure and function of the cortex, particularly the prefrontal cortex and the limbic system's hippocampal pyramidal neurons, are mechanisms that contribute to depression.[49] Stress causes dendrites to retract in these areas and decreases spine density through inflammatory mechanisms, such as pro-inflammatory cytokines, interleukins, tumor necrosis factor, and peripheral growth factors.[48,50,51] Furthermore, the inflammatory response results in an increase of neurotoxic amyloid-β peptides that can cause cell death, particularly in refractory depression.[52] Changes in glutaminergic signaling have been seen in animal models of depression.[53] These findings serve as emerging evidence linking a history of major depressive disorder with Alzheimer's disease.[54]

An amalgam of these theories results in the *neurodevelopmental theory* of depression.[55,56] This theory underscores the importance of where along the developmental trajectory an insult to normal development might occur to impact on mood regulation.[57] For example, if a mother has an infection during pregnancy, the fetus could experience an insult from the mother's immune system; altering its brain at that point in development that could result in mood dysregulation. Early childhood trauma could impact on the development of the hippocampus and prefrontal cortex, which have been shown to be reduced in size for people with depression. A high fever during late childhood could result in inflammation that has a negative impact on cortical structures that play a role in mood regulation. These theories together continue to expand our knowledge of the mechanisms of depression and its etiology to inform the development of new treatments and explain how current treatments have an effect.

ASSESSMENT

All persons with chronic illness are at risk for depression.[58,59] The palliative APRN uses evidence-based guidelines to inform their nursing practice.[60–64] Risk factors for depression are listed in Table 50.2.[65] A targeted assessment for depression, performed as part of the complete patient and family assessment, provides evidence on which to plan symptom management. In doing the targeted assessment, the APRN looks for evidence that will support or rule out depressive symptoms and depression.[38,60–64] A focused history and physical examination will determine the need for appropriate diagnostic tests and their interpretation.

The palliative APRN should first review the patient's record for prior history of depression. If the patient has a history of depression, the APRN should discover what treatments were initiated and their effectiveness. The APRN should also inquire about other mental health issues, including bipolar disorder, personality disorders, disorders that emerge in childhood, and schizophrenia. The APRN must inquire about physiological conditions that can contribute to or mimic depression. The family history should examine the patient's and family's history of suicide. Exposure to a suicide or suicide attempt is a major risk factor for suicide.

A medication history should help determine interventions for depression. It should include specific medications that were helpful in the past and those that were not and any allergies to medications or products in pharmaceuticals. The medication review should include all current prescription medication, over-the-counter preparations, supplements, and allergies to avoid known sensitivities and reduce the risk of drug–drug interactions. Finally, there should be discussion about the patient's and the family's knowledge and beliefs about psychiatric illness, pharmacotherapy, and complementary and alternative therapies. The reader is referred to *Oxford Textbook of Palliative Nursing 5th ed*, Chapter 4, "Principles of Patient and Family Assessment" for detailed information.[2]

The physical impact of the illness and the treatment can cause depressive symptoms, as can the patient and family response to it. For depression, the examination should be focused on mood and psychomotor changes. A mnemonic for the features of depression is SIG E CAPS, a play on the prescription to "Take (Sig) energy (E) capsules (Caps)," which stands for **S**leep changes, **I**nterest changes, **G**uilt or hopelessness, **E**nergy decreases, **C**oncentration difficulties, **A**ppetite changes, **P**sychomotor changes, **S**uicidal ideation.[66] The assessment and history should include the following:

- *Depressed mood*: A depressed mood is characterized by negative emotions as reported by the patient. Simply asking "How is your mood?" can elicit a response from the

Table 50.2 RISK FACTORS FOR DEPRESSION AND SUICIDE IN ADULTS

DOMAIN	RISK FACTOR	AT RISK FOR DEPRESSION	AT RISK FOR SUICIDE
Mood	Depressed mood	Depression as a child or teen	Feel hopeless, socially isolated, or lonely
Stressors	Stressful life event or experienced trauma	Yes	Yes
Substance abuse	More than socially acceptable use of legal substances. Use of illegal substances	Yes	Yes; May worsen thoughts of suicide and can instill recklessness or impulsivity enough to act on thoughts
Family	Genetic link or environmental exposure to mental illness, substance abuse, or suicide	Family history; also trauma, including verbal physical or sexual abuse	Family history; also trauma, including verbal physical or sexual abuse
Psychiatric	Any psychiatric disorder but especially anxiety, posttraumatic stress disorder, personality disorders	Yes. Plus: • Borderline personality disorder • Certain personality traits, such as having low self-esteem and being overly dependent, self-critical, or pessimistic	Yes. Plus: • Psychosis • Paranoia
Somatic illness	Chronic, life-threatening illness; chronic pain	Yes	Yes
Medications	Taking a substance that can participate in inducing depressive symptoms.	Certain medications, such as some high blood pressure medications or sleeping pills	Beginning initiating an antidepressant for symptoms of depression; child, adolescent, elderly taking SSRI,
Development	Difficulties of developmental stage or insult to brain during developmental periods that impact on future development	Insult to brain from prenatal to mid-twenties.	Identify as LGBTQ+ with an unsupportive family or in a hostile environment. In adolescents and children, being unsure of sexual orientation.
Means	Access to and lethality of means to harm self.	No	Lethality of means increases the risk for harm to self (e.g., firearms, explosives)
History of suicide	Exposure to suicide or experienced a previous attempt	Yes, especially if close to the person who has died.	Previous suicide attempt or exposure to a successful suicide increases the likelihood of a suicide attempt.

From Schaakxs et al.[65]

patient that indicates an unaltered mood (euthymia) or a mood that is not normal for him or her (dysthymia). "Is this a change from your usual mood?" will help distinguish the patient's current state from his or her baseline and will give insight into the duration of a possible depressive episode.

• *Sleep changes*: Decreased need for sleep, early morning wakening, or an increased need for sleep can all indicate depression. Questions can include: "How are you sleeping? Any difficulty falling asleep? Once you fall asleep, do you stay asleep? Once you wake up in the middle of the night, do you have trouble falling asleep? Do you sleep until your planned waking time? Has this changed from your usual sleep schedule?" Changes in sleep patterns are associated with depression, particularly sleep difficulties in the early to the middle part of the sleep cycle.[67]

• *Lack of interests or anhedonia*: The depressed patient may report lack of interest in activities he or she used to enjoy or a general lack of interest in anything. The APRN might ask, "What sorts of activities are you interested in doing? Has this interest changed recently?"

• *Feelings of guilt, hopelessness, or helplessness (Beck's cognitive triad)*[68]: Excessive guilt and feelings of worthlessness indicate thoughts about the self and can be elicited by asking the patient, "Tell me about your feelings of self-worth. Are there things you feel guilty about?" Thinking about the world is captured by asking the patient to describe how others view him or her from their perspective. "Are you feeling helpless and that others do not want to help you?" And finally, the patient may see the future as dim when depressed and may believe that there is no way out of his or her current situation: "Do you feel hopeless?"

• *Energy*: Changes in level of energy, typically decreases, are associated with depression: "How is your energy level? Has this changed recently? For how long have you felt your energy was this way?"

- *Concentration*: Changes in ability to concentrate, typically more difficulty concentrating, are associated with depression: "How is your ability to concentrate? Has this changed recently?"

- *Appetite*: Changes in appetite, either up or down, and significant weight loss without intentional dieting are features associated with depression. The APRN can ask, "How is your appetite? Is that a change from your usual appetite? Have you lost weight? How much? Over what period of time?"

- *Psychomotor slowing*: Moving more slowly than usual, difficulty initiating activity, such as getting out of bed or off the couch, slower gait, and slower speech are symptoms of depression. Self-report is not as reliable as observation by a friend or family member. The nurse can ask the patient whether the friend or family member has mentioned anything unusual about the patient's ability to move or walk.

- *Suicidal thoughts or attempts* are associated with depression.[69,70]

SUICIDE

Risk factors for suicide include exposure to a completed suicide or suicide attempt, thoughts about committing suicide, planning to commit suicide, possessing the means to commit suicide, having access to the means to commit suicide, the potential lethality of the means (e.g., the amount of physical damage that the means could cause), and an unsuccessful attempt at suicide in the past. Other risk factors for suicide are also listed in Table 50.3.[71]

The palliative APRN screens for suicide by asking these questions[72]:

1. Has anyone close to you attempted or completed suicide?
2. Have you ever tried to hurt yourself?
3. Are you currently thinking about hurting yourself?
4. Do you have a plan?
5. How are you planning on doing it?
6. Do you have means to implement such a plan?

Access to means that are of higher lethality (e.g., firearms) contribute to a greater risk of suicide. If the patient or family member reports that the patient has thoughts about committing suicide, along with a plan and access to the means, the palliative APRN should arrange for the patient not to be left alone and then seek advanced psychiatric help.[72]

Suicide can trigger physical or psychiatric illness in the surviving members of the family and friends.[73,74] When someone takes his or her own life, the first question typically asked is, "Why?" Even when a suicide note is left behind, questions remain unanswered. The palliative APRN will be better able to support the survivors if they have previously thought about their own beliefs and attitudes about suicide, and how it fits into their own philosophy of life. Exploring

Table 50.3 DIFFERENTIAL DIAGNOSIS FOR DEPRESSION

DIFFERENTIAL*	DESCRIPTION	COMMENTS
Grief	Normal emotional reaction to a loss	The prominent symptom is emptiness, not anhedonia and depressed mood. Self-esteem is preserved, although feelings of sadness come and go. Persons experiencing grief may express a desire to be with the lost loved one, but they do not think of suicide as a way to make the bad feelings go away. Over time, can evolve into a depressive disorder.
Depressed mood	Sadness or feeling blue; also called intermittent dysthymia	A depressed mood by itself is not a depressive disorder but a stand-alone symptom. It can be debilitating and can progress to a depressive disorder.
Adjustment disorder	Clinical disorder as defined in DSM-5; difficulty adapting to a new sense of normal	The parameters for depressive symptoms (number, severity, duration, and impact) are of a lesser degree and do not meet the criteria for major depressive disorder.
Major depressive disorder	A depressive disorder characterized in DSM-5 by multiple symptoms over a defined period.	In adults, five or more symptoms (*SIG E CAPS*), including depressed mood, for at least 2 weeks with an impact on at least one functional domain (e.g., home, work, school, interacting with others). May be recurrent. For children, symptoms are fewer and can include irritability.
Bipolar disorder	A mood disorder characterized by alternating depression and manic mood states.	Must meet criteria for major depression during depressive episodes and either mania or hypomania as defined in DSM-5 (*DIG FAST*: distractibility, irresponsibility, grandiosity, flight of ideas, activity increases, sleep is decreased, talkative)

DSM-5 depressive disorders include disruptive mood dysregulation disorder, major depressive disorder, persistent depressive disorder, premenstrual dysphoric disorder, substance/medication-induced depressive disorder, and depressive disorder due to another medical condition.

From Franklin et al.[71]

other people's views, including other members of the multidisciplinary team, is beneficial. It allows the APRN to anticipate their own personal reactions and perspectives so they can best help members of the patient's family and other team members.

Medically assisted death may be perceived differently. In this case patients legally obtain and use prescription medications to commit suicide. This typically is not done due to depression; rather, they are exercising their own autonomy in determining when and how their life will end. In many states, medically assisted death is legal.[75] The palliative APRN should support persons who request information about medically assisted death according to the laws of the state in which he or she practices.[76] See Chapter 53, "Navigating Ethical Dilemmas" and Chapter 57, "Palliative Sedation."

ONGOING ASSESSMENT

At the initial encounter, the palliative APRN collects baseline data. At subsequent encounters, the APRN assesses the patient and family for any changes from this baseline, using them to measure progress, emerging issues, and the effectiveness of treatments: "Compared to [before or last time] we met, is it the same, better, or worse?"[77] During each encounter, the palliative APRN builds a trusting relationship with the patient and family to facilitate the sharing of information. This is particularly important when discussing mental health issues because of the sensitive nature of mental illness and the stigma associated with it.

The palliative APRN continues to build the database from which an appropriate plan of care will be derived, including evidence of risk for and symptoms of depression, as well as related substance abuse and risk for suicide. The acuity of each symptom is also determined, as is frequency (e.g., nearly every day, most days, 2 or 3 days per week, weekly, once per month or less), duration (e.g., nonstop, months, days, just that day, a few hours), and impact on daily function (e.g., can or cannot work, can or cannot take care of one's own needs, can or cannot cook for oneself, bedbound).

Several standardized tools are available to screen for depression. There are two items on the Palliative Care Observation Scale (PCOS) that can be used to screen for depression.[78] Other tools may be categorized by the age of the persons they were designed to measure. For example, the Children's Depression Rating Scale (CDRS) is useful for children under the age of 18. With persons over the age of 14, useful tools include the Patient Health Questionnaire-9 (PHQ-9), Beck Depression Inventory (BDI), the Center for Epidemiological Studies Depression Scale (CES-D), and the Hamilton Depression Scale (Ham-D).[79-84] Elderly patients can be evaluated using the Zung Self-Rating Depression Scale, the General Well-Being Schedule Depression (GWB-D) Subscale, the Geriatric Depression Scale (GDS), and others.[85-88]

Newly diagnosed patients without a history of depressive disorder will likely not meet the criteria for a diagnosis of major depressive disorder. They may have fewer symptoms, or their symptoms may not have persisted long enough to meet the criteria. In these cases, adjustment disorder with depressed mood may be an appropriate diagnosis.[89] The palliative APRN must remember that depressive symptoms that persist can evolve into a pathologically significant major depressive disorder diagnosis. Although the labels of the diagnoses themselves may not completely inform treatment, the evaluation of the existence of symptoms and their severity, duration, and impact will provide a baseline to direct evaluation of agreed-upon therapeutic interventions. The *Diagnostic and Statistical Manual of Psychiatric Disorders* (DSM-5) lists the specific criteria for these disorders.[64]

DIFFERENTIAL DIAGNOSIS

The differential diagnosis for depressive symptoms is shown in Table 50.4.[6] When these symptoms are observed, the palliative APRN collects appropriate data to differentiate sub-pathological conditions, such as normal grief, from higher-acuity conditions based on the constellation of signs and symptoms, their characteristics, and the impact on the individual and family. Only then can appropriate interventions be planned and implemented to address the specific needs of the individual or family.

Table 50.4 COMMON PHARMACOTHERAPIES FOR DEPRESSION

CLASS	GENERIC NAME	BRAND NAME
Selective serotonin reuptake inhibitors (SSRIs)	citalopram escitalopram fluoxetine paroxetine sertraline vilazodone	Celexa Lexapro Prozac Paxil Zoloft Viibryd
Serotonin-norepinephrine reuptake inhibitors (SNRIs)	desvenlafaxine duloxetine venlafaxine	Pristiq Cymbalta Effexor
Serotonin and dopamine reuptake inhibitor	bupropion	Wellbutrin
Serotonin and catecholamine reuptake inhibitor	mirtazapine	Remeron
Serotonin modulator	vortioxetine	Trintillex
N-methyl-D-aspartate (NMDA) receptor agonist	esketamine	Spravato

Note: APRNs will also discover that some patients are prescribed older classes of antidepressants, such as tricyclic antidepressants (TCAs) and monoamine oxidase inhibitors (MAOIs). For specific approved drug information including safe prescribing for persons taking these medications, the reader is advised to review information available at FDA.gov.

From US Food and Drug Administration.[100]

MANAGEMENT/INTERVENTIONAL TECHNIQUES

CASE STUDY: THE PATIENT WITH DEPRESSION (CONTINUED)

As a child, Theresa lived as a boy. Her father and uncles had taught her how to hunt and fish along with her male cousins. She enjoyed those time bonding with her family, but she always knew that she was transgender and decided to transition to living as a girl in high school. She was always treated differently before her transition because of her sickle-cell disease. But when she came out as a girl, the bullying worsened. As an adult, she worried about her sons and what was in store for them in their lives, particularly if she were to die young. Her pain crises were getting closer together, and she felt guilty for being hospitalized and debilitated all the time. The thought of committing suicide was happening more frequently, and she found a sort of solace that her father's shotgun and a box of shells were in the bedroom closet.

Evidence-based interventions and approaches for helping patients with depressive symptoms are based on the principles that (a) the patient–clinician relationship is important to the development of a successful plan of care, (b) the patient and the family are at the center of the therapeutic relationship, and (c) an interdisciplinary approach will result in optimal care. Ongoing monitoring of effectiveness is key to managing depression.[12,13]

Within the context of palliative care, the goal is to maximize quality of life by minimizing symptoms and minimizing the impact of symptoms and therapy on the patient.[90] Techniques for treating depression and depressive symptoms include talk therapies, pharmaceutical interventions, and complementary therapies to achieve this goal. The link between the anatomy and physiology of the brain and these processes explains in part the success of various treatment modalities.[91]

PSYCHOTHERAPY

Current evidence for depression shows that management is best when it includes psychotherapy.[92–94] Psychotherapy has been shown to cause changes in the brain and thus result in mood changes. For patients and families with depressive symptoms, processing their feelings aloud can help them find peace, make meaning out of their situation, and develop hope. The challenge for patients with serious illness is finding a supportive and affordable group therapy or therapists at a convenient location. The emergence of telehealth and its rapid expansion during the COVID-19 pandemic has increased familiarization with videoconferencing tools in all areas of our lives. Access to high-quality, professional psychotherapy is now ubiquitous, albeit limited by costs. Early evidence shows that, although a reduction of symptoms and increased coping occurs with teletherapy, patients are more likely to cancel meetings or not be present for their appointments than in a

traditional format.[95,96] The palliative APRN with training in therapy provides opportunities for the person to process his or her feelings. Otherwise, a referral to a professional trained in brief therapy, cognitive-behavioral therapy, or other therapeutic techniques can be made to manage depressive symptoms in palliative settings.[97]

PHARMACOLOGIC MANAGEMENT

Pharmaceutical therapy is the most common technique used for managing depressive symptoms. This choice, however, may depend on the patient's prognosis.[98] For patients who have a prognosis of longer than 2–3 months, there are more options. SSRIs and SNRIs are first-line medications for treating depressive symptoms in adults, children, and adolescents.[99] Table 50.4 lists the generic and brand names of commonly prescribed antidepressants.[100] Table 50.5 lists the side effects of SSRIs and SNRIs.[47]

A common patient concern regarding antidepressants is the sexual side effects of the SSRIs, specifically orgasmic delay in men and women and erectile dysfunction in men. These side effects can be treated with psychotherapy or with the addition of bupropion (Wellbutrin). A referral to an expert in women's or men's health may be in order.[101]

Like any other medication in palliative care, antidepressants are initiated at the lowest therapeutic dose and the dosage is adjusted as needed. Subtherapeutic effects are often observed in the first few weeks, but full therapeutic effect is achieved in 6–8 weeks after pharmacotherapy has started. Citalopram (Celexa) and its levo-isomer escitalopram (Lexapro) have been used to control depressive symptoms while minimizing side effects. Duloxetine (Cymbalta) is used to alleviate depressive symptoms and some somatic symptoms of depression. Mirtazapine (Remeron) has demonstrated a

Table 50.5 COMMON SIDE EFFECTS OF SELECTIVE SEROTONIN REUPTAKE INHIBITORS (SSRIS) AND SEROTONIN-NOREPINEPHRINE REUPTAKE INHIBITORS (SNRIS)

SSRIS	SNRIS
Agitation	Agitation
Anorexia	Discontinuation syndrome
Anxiety	Headache
Constipation	Hypertension (dose-related)
Diarrhea	Nausea
Discontinuation syndrome	Sleep disturbances
Dizziness	Sweating
Dry mouth	Tremor
Headache	
Insomnia	
Nausea	
Sexual dysfunction	
Somnolence	
Sweating	
Tremor	

From Taylor et al.[47]

more rapid onset than SSRIs when used to treat major depression, but the side-effect profile is often debilitating. Off-label uses of mirtazapine include treating anxiety symptoms, nausea, pruritus, insomnia, and anorexia. When either discontinuing an antidepressant or switching to a new antidepressant, a taper or cross-taper over 2 weeks is required to avoid discontinuation effects.[47]

The rise of the neurotrophic theory of depression creates an opportunity for the emergence of new treatments. Esketamine, like its racemic mixture ketamine, shows a rapid antidepressant action by increasing prefrontal cortex spine synapses.[102–104] An N-methyl-D-aspartate (NMDA) receptor antagonist, as is memantine [Namenda], it increases glutamate transmission and relieves some symptoms of depression when combined with an SSRI.[105] Similarly, scopolamine, an anticholinergic agent has an impact on neuroplasticity by modulating NMDA receptor gene expression.[106] Psychostimulants (e.g., methylphenidate [Ritalin]) have rapid onset and treatment effectiveness in the treatment of depression, including short-term effectiveness in palliative care.[107–109] Effectiveness of psychedelic drugs in the treatment of depression is emerging in combination with psychotherapy and as standalone therapy.[110,111]

Long-standing thought has been that the combination of pharmacologic treatment and psychotherapy produced effects that were greater than the use of either modality alone. Recent evidence supports the effectiveness of psychotherapy alone for short-term depressive symptoms and the combination of both modalities if the trajectory of illness is longer term.[112] The European Palliative Care Research Collaborative (EPCRC) derived recommendations for the prevention, detection, and treatment of depression in palliative care patients that include pharmacotherapy and talk therapy. They also recommend open communication, patient involvement in care planning, and regular assessment of symptoms as situations change along the course of illness. For patients with severe depression, the EPCRC recommends a referral to a mental health specialist.[113]

Complex Medication Use

Palliative care patients with long-standing depressive disorders may be taking medications unfamiliar to the palliative APRN. The SSRIs and SNRIs that are used today are third- and fourth-generation medications that manipulate the monoamine neurotransmitters. Earlier medications with similar effects are the MAOIs and TCAs.

If a patient is taking a drug from one of these earlier classes, the palliative APRN needs to be aware of the patient's risk for a life-threatening condition-serotonin syndrome (SS; Box 50.2).[101,114] Of note, one substance commonly taken by patients is St. John's wort, an over-the-counter herbal medication that is used to augment mood and to treat other ailments by increasing serotonin levels. Although not approved by the U.S. Food and Drug Administration as a pharmaceutical, St. John's wort, in combination with other serotonergic drugs, can cause SS.[115]

Box 50.2 SEROTONIN SYNDROME: A LIFE-THREATENING CONDITION

Sustained levels of serotonin in the synaptic cleft alleviate depressive symptoms. Combinations of medications that increase the level of serotonin in the synaptic cleft, however, can be additive and cause concentrations of serotonin to rise to dangerously high levels. When this happens, evidence of serotonin syndrome (SS) emerges.

SS presents as three or more of the following symptoms: agitation; diarrhea; heavy sweating not due to activity; fever; mental status changes, such as confusion or hypomania; muscle spasms (myoclonus); overactive reflexes (hyperreflexia); shivering; tremor; and uncoordinated movements (ataxia).

This is a crisis that is typically treated by stopping the medication and administering benzodiazepines, intravenous fluids, and cyproheptadine, a serotonin antagonist antihistamine.

From Jing, Straw-Wilson[101]; and Tormoehlen, Rusyniak.[114]

MAOIs and TCAs must not be taken with SSRIs and SNRIs. If the patient's depressive symptoms become refractory to his or her older medications, then a washout period of 2 weeks is required before starting the more current medications.[47]

If the patient is taking an MAOI, diet must be restricted to avoid foods high in tyramine, a precursor to serotonin. These foods include some cheeses; beer; dried meats, such as salami and pepperoni; chicken livers; meat bouillons and gravies; and fermented foods, such as kimchi, sauerkraut, tofu, soy sauce, and fish sauce.[116] When liberalizing a diet to affect a goal of improving quality of life, the benefits and burdens of continuing or discontinuing the MAOI in light of the wishes of the patient to eat foods high in tyramine must be weighed. The palliative APRN educates the patient and the family on this tradeoff to inform their decision-making.

Management of Concomitant Diagnoses

The palliative APRN must note the presence of other mental health diagnoses and the effect of medications on other conditions. Some bipolar disorders are characterized by the existence of a depressed mood and are treated with mood stabilizers. The use of an SSRI or SNRI in a patient with bipolar disorder may trigger a manic episode, a pathological state that may have been revealed in the history.[117] If mania is discovered, SSRI and SNRI antidepressants should be avoided. In these cases, mood elevators (e.g., lithium) are the first-line therapy.[47]

Depression can also be accompanied by psychosis, or not being in touch with reality. If psychotic features are also present, the patient requires antipsychotics in addition to, and sometimes instead of antidepressants.[47] These medications can cause metabolic changes (such as hyperlipidemia, hyperglycemia, and prolonged QTc interval) that can precipitate other comorbid conditions. For example, some antipsychotics (e.g., quetiapine [Seroquel]) cause hyperlipidemia, which can lead to coronary artery disease and distributed atherosclerosis. Olanzapine (Zyprexa) causes hyperglycemia that can lead to diabetes mellitus. Cardiac conduction may be affected, such as a prolonged QTc interval (nominally, longer than 400 ms) caused by haloperidol (Haldol), leaving the patient at risk for lethal dysrhythmias. Any side effects should be treated according to evidence-based guidelines.[118]

Of note, the palliative APRN should use caution when attempting to manage agitation or delirium in a patient who is already taking antipsychotics as the patient's illness progresses toward end of life. High levels of antipsychotics can lead to neuroleptic malignant syndrome (NMS), a life-threatening emergency characterized by muscle cramps and tremors, fever, symptoms of autonomic nervous system instability like unstable blood pressure, and alterations in mental status (agitation, delirium, or coma). NMS is treated symptomatically, with ice packs for fever, supportive respiratory and circulatory care, and dantrolene for muscle rigidity.[114]

SS and NMS are life-threatening emergencies. NMS is distinguished from SS by the presence of bradykinesia, muscle rigidity, elevated white blood cell count and plasma creatine kinase level. Prevention of these conditions should include a referral to a mental health professional for alternative approaches to optimal patient care.[114]

Safe Prescribing

Safe prescribing begins with a thorough history that includes diet, allergies, and medications, both historical and current, and herbal supplements.[119] Avoiding concomitant substances (such as St. John's wort) and foods that induce serotonin will decrease the likelihood of SS. Understanding the patient's use of antipsychotics and safe prescribing will help avoid NMS.

Safe prescribing also includes minimizing the availability of lethal doses of any medication that could be used as a means of suicide.[119] For example, consider a patient who has depressive symptoms and is being treated for anxiety with benzodiazepines. The patient has a 30-day supply of lorazepam (Ativan) in 1 mg tablets and the APRN understands that the maximum safe dosage of lorazepam in 24 hours is 10 mg.[120] In a moment of despair due to new-onset depression, this patient could attempt to kill themself by taking all 30 pills at once and, if not found soon enough, would succeed.

A patient who is planning suicide could hoard pills over time to build a lethal stash. Even acetaminophen in large enough quantities can damage an otherwise healthy liver and cause death.[121] The palliative APRN should consider dosages, amounts, and refills of medication to prevent their lethal use. Interventions and therapy for depression can relieve some symptoms, so the patient may start to feel less fatigued and more energetic as the therapeutic effects emerge. But these effects can occur for a time before effecting the patient's suicidal intentions, thus increasing the risk for suicide.[122] The palliative APRN must remain vigilant for depression and assess for and document suicidal ideation, plan, means, and access at every interaction. The challenge is tailoring such practices to

promote a supportive encounter that meets the needs of the patient without enabling a dysfunctional response.[123]

NONPHARMACOLOGIC INTERVENTIONS

Depressive symptoms can be improved with physical activity, such as walking, swimming, and yoga, and with proper nutrition and sleep hygiene.[124] Talk therapies can assist patients and families to find a new sense of normal and create meaning in the patient's situation, which can mitigate depressive symptoms.[10,124]

Evidence for the effectiveness of complementary therapies continues to grow, although accessibility to these therapies is mixed.[125] Various approaches have shown efficacy in reducing psychological symptoms including depression. Table 50.6 summarizes identified evidence.[126-136] Reiki therapy has been shown useful for relieving pain, decreasing anxiety and depression, and improving quality of life.[126] Patients and families reported decreased depressive symptoms when patients participated in an art therapy session. They reported their depression decreased later than did their anxiety.[127] Clinical hypnosis in palliative care has been shown to decrease pain and to lessen stress for the patients and families. It also shows some evidence of controlling somatic, psychiatric, and spiritual symptoms.[128] For patients with metastatic lung cancer, higher levels of mindfulness in patients and in spousal caregivers were associated with less depressive symptoms in both groups, and higher levels of mindfulness of patients was associated with decreased depressive symptoms in the spousal caregivers.[129] Reflexology and relaxation techniques both improved anxiety and depression in patients with cancer. Reflexology also improved pain and physical symptoms.[130] Live music interventions decreased pain, anxiety, and depression and increased feelings of well-being.[131] Animal-involved therapy decreased psychological symptoms in patients who previously owned pets but increased symptoms in patients who had not previously owned pets.[132] Mindfulness approaches were shown to reduce patients' psychological symptoms and to improve quality of life.[133] Treating co-occurring anxiety and depression with chamomile has been effective.[134] Acupuncture has decreased depression and other psychological symptoms as well as shown benefits with cancer-related pain, stress, and nausea.[135,136]

PATIENT AND FAMILY EDUCATION

Palliative APRNs provide quality care by offering patient and family education that includes information about the following:

1. *Stressors trigger depressive symptoms.* Reducing exposure to stressors that can be manipulated will reduce the likelihood of the development of longstanding depressive symptoms. Stress management is healthy.

2. *Sadness is a normal response to loss.* When sadness worsens and impairs functioning over a period of time, seeking help through individual or group therapy or a healthcare provider can assist patients to cope with the sadness.

Table 50.6 COMPLEMENTARY AND ALTERNATIVE MODALITIES FOR DEPRESSION IN PALLIATIVE CARE

STUDY	YEAR	MODALITY	DEPRESSIVE SYMPTOMS	OTHER
Billot et al.[126]	2019	Reiki	Decreased	Decreased anxiety Improved quality of life Pain relief
Collette et al.[127]	2020	Art therapy	Decreased in patients and families	Decreased anxiety
Brugnoli[128]	2016	Hypnosis	Decreased	Decreased pain Controlled physical symptoms Controlled other psychological symptoms Controlled spiritual stress Lessening stress for patients and family
Cho et al.[129]	2020	Mindfulness	Decreased in patients and spousal caregivers	
Mantoudi et al.[130]	2020	Reflexology	Decreased	Decreased anxiety
		Relaxation therapy	Decreased	Decreased anxiety Improved pain Improved physical symptoms
Peng et al.[131]	2019	Music therapy	Decreased	Decreased pain Decreased anxiety Increased feelings of well-being
Sagnetto et al.[132]	2020	Animal-assisted intervention	Decreased depression if patient previously owned pets. Increased depression if patient did not previously own pets.	Decreased anxiety if patient previously owned pets Increased anxiety if patient did not previously own pets
Breitbart et al.[133]	2015	Mindfulness	Decreased	Decreased anxiety Improved overall quality of life.
Amsterdam et al.[134]	2020	Chamomile	Decreased if coexist with anxiety	Decreased anxiety if coexist with depression
Birch et al.[135]	2020	Acupuncture	Decreased	Initial anxiety
Fink et al.[136]	2020	Acupuncture And massage	Decreased	Improved cancer related pain Improved cancer related nausea Improved cancer related stress

3. *Depression and depressive symptoms are evidence of psychiatric illness*, not lack of moral character, and they can be treated with pharmaceutical and nonpharmaceutical interventions.

4. *Taking all medications as prescribed is important.* Symptoms take time to go away. Partial effects of a medication may be felt in 2–4 weeks after initiation, but the full effects might not be felt for 6–8 weeks.

5. *Medications should not be stopped abruptly and only under the direction of the prescriber.* Patients and family members should know the signs and symptoms of dangerous conditions like NMS and SS.

6. *Patients need to be monitored for thoughts of self-harm or harm to others.* This may include identifying a trusted person to whom to disclose such thoughts. Families need to know to trust their instincts and call for help as needed.[137]

7. *The overall strategy for safe treatment is a combination* of medications as prescribed; appropriate diet, exercise, and sleep, and management of alcohol intake to reduce the possibility of side effects and dangerous interactions.

CASE STUDY: THE PATIENT WITH DEPRESSION (CONCLUSION)

Theresa resigned from her job because of her health getting worse, causing her to feel unproductive and useless. She never wanted to rely on welfare, and being on Social Security Disability made her feel worse. Regina took a part-time job at the local bakery to help make ends meet. One day, Regina came home from work to find Theresa unable to talk or move her limbs. At the hospital, Regina learned that Theresa had experienced a severe stroke. Theresa continued to decline and was put on a ventilator. She never breathed on her own again.

SUMMARY

Pain and symptom management for persons with chronic, life-threatening illness is profoundly important. It is the most sacred honor to work with patients and families while they are facing enormous physical, emotional, social, and spiritual challenges. Symptoms of depression are very common in patients and their families in these circumstances. The palliative APRN cares for people with symptoms of depression by being fully present, having done their own psychic and spiritual work; by understanding what to look for during an assessment; by offering treatment options based on sound scientific and nursing evidence; and educating patients and families. Disentangling the causes for the constellation of depression symptoms requires keen insights and a strong base of scientific knowledge. The palliative APRN uses the nursing process to assess patients, diagnose needs, plan interventions, implement care, and evaluate the effectiveness of that care according to professional, legal, and institutional scopes and standards of practice. Helping patients to cope emotionally maximizes their quality of life, the goal of palliative care. As we alleviate the suffering from depressive symptoms and disorders, we improve the quality of life for them, their families, their caregivers, and ourselves as APRNs and fellow human beings.

REFERENCES

1. Ferrell BR, Twaddle ML, Melnick A, Meier DE. National Consensus Project clinical practice guidelines for quality palliative care guidelines, 4th edition. *J Palliat Med.* 2018 Dec;21(12):1684–1689. doi:10.1089/jpm.2018.0431. doi:10.1089/jpm.2018.0431

2. Chovan JD. Principles of patient and family assessment. In: Ferrell B, Paice J, eds. Oxford *Textbook of Palliative Nursing.* 5th ed. New York: Oxford University Press; 2019:32–54.

3. Taylor A, Ritchie Al White C. Psychiatric conditions in palliative medicine. *Medicine.* 2020;48(1):29–32. doi:10.1016/j.mpmed.2019.10.015

4. American Psychiatric Association. *Diagnostic and Statistical Manual of Mental Disorders.* 5th ed. Arlington, VA: American Psychiatric Association; 2013.

5. Tebeka S, Geoffroy PA, Dubertret C, Le Strat Y. Sadness and the continuum from well-being to depressive disorder: Findings from a representative US population sample. *J Psychiatr Res.* 2021 Jan;132:50–54. doi:10.1016/j.jpsychires.2020.10.004. Epub 2020 Oct 3.

6. American Psychiatric Association. Depressive disorders. *Diagnostic and Statistical Manual of Mental Disorders.* 5th ed. Arlington, VA: American Psychiatric Association; 2013; 155–188.

7. Bolstad CJ, Moak R, Brown CJ, Kennedy RE, Buys DR. Neighborhood disadvantage is associated with depressive symptoms but not depression diagnosis in older adults. *Int J Environ Res Public Health.* 2020;17(16):5745. doi:10.3390/ijerph17165745

8. Grotmol KS, Lie HC, Hjermstad MJ, et al. Depression: A major contributor to poor quality of life in patients with advanced cancer. *J Pain Symptom Manage.* 2017;54(6):889–897. doi:10.1016/j.jpainsymman.2017.04.010

9. Lua W, Pikhart H, Peasey A, Lubinova R. Pitman A, Bobak M. Risk of depressive symptoms before and after the first hospitalization for cancer: Evidence from a 16-year cohort study in the Czech republic. *J Affect Disord.* 2020;278:76–83. doi:10.1016/j.jad.2020.06.070

10. Okuyama T, Akechi T, Mackenzie L, Furukawa TA. Psychotherapy for depression among advanced, incurable cancer patients: A systematic review and meta-analysis. *Cancer Treat Rev.* 2017;56:16–27. doi:10.1016/j.ctrv.2017.03.012

11. Trachsel M, Irwin SA, Biller-Andorno N, Hoff P, Riese F. Palliative psychiatry for severe persistent mental illness as a new approach to psychiatry? Definition, scope, benefits, and risks. *BMC Psychiatry.* 2016;16:260. doi:10.1186/s12888-016-0970-y

12. Dahlin C, *Palliative Nursing: Scope and Standards of Practice. 6th ed.* Pittsburgh, PA: Hospice and Palliative Nurses Association; 2021.

13. American Psychiatric Nurses Association, International Society of Psychiatric Mental Health Nurses, American Nurses Association. *Psychiatric Mental Health Nursing: Scope and Standards of Practice.* 2nd ed. Silver Spring, MD: Nursesbooks.org; 2014.

14. Temel JS, Greer JA, El-Jawahri A, et al. Effects of early integrated palliative care in patients with lung and GI cancer: A randomized clinical trial. *J Clin Oncol.* 2017;35(8):834–841. doi:10.1200/JCO.2016.70.5046

15. Davis LE, Gupta V, Allen-Ayodabo C, et al. Patient-reported symptoms following diagnosis in esophagus cancer patients treated with palliative intent. *Dis Esophagus.* 2020;33(8):doz108. doi:10.1093/dote/doz108

16. Julião M, Sobral MA, Calçada P, et al. "Truly holistic?" Differences in documenting physical and psychosocial needs and hope in Portuguese palliative patients. *Palliat Support Care.* 2020:1–6. doi:10.1017/S1478951520000413

17. McMahan RD, Barnes DE, Ritchie CS, et al. Anxious, depressed, and planning for the future: Advance care planning in diverse older adults. *J Am Geriatr Soc.* doi:10.1111/jgs.16754

18. Verduzco-Aguirre HC, Babu D, Mohile SG, et al. Associations of uncertainty with psychological health and quality of life in older adults with advanced cancer. *J Pain Symptom Manage.* 2021;61(2):369–376.e1. doi:10.1016/j.jpainsymman.2020.08.012

19. Lee W, Pulbrook M, Sheehan C, et al. Clinically significant depressive symptoms are prevalent in people with extremely short prognoses: A systematic review. *J Pain Symptom Manage.* 2021;61(1):143–166.e2. doi:10.1016/j.jpainsymman.2020.07.011

20. Oechsle K, Ullrich A, Marx G, et al. Psychological burden in family caregivers of patients with advanced cancer at initiation of specialist inpatient palliative care. *BMC Palliat Care.* 2019;18(1):102. Published 2019 Nov 18. doi:10.1186/s12904-019-0469-7

21. Utne I, Cooper BA, Ritchie C, et al. Co-occurrence of decrements in physical and cognitive function is common in older oncology patients receiving chemotherapy. *Eur J Oncol Nurs.* 2020;48:101823. doi:10.1016/j.ejon.2020.101823

22. Lage DE, El-Jawahri A, Fuh CX, et al. Functional impairment, symptom burden, and clinical outcomes among hospitalized patients with advanced cancer. *J Natl Compr Canc Netw.* 2020;18(6):747–754. doi:10.6004/jnccn.2019.7385

23. Yi JC, Syrjala KL. Anxiety and depression in cancer survivors. *Med Clin North Am.* 2017;101(6):1099–1113. doi:10.1016/j.mcna.2017.06.005

24. Kozlov E, Phongtankuel V, Prigerson H, et al. Prevalence, severity, and correlates of symptoms of anxiety and depression at the very end of life. *J Pain Symptom Manage.* 2019;58(1):80–85. doi:10.1016/j.jpainsymman.2019.04.012

25. Petursdottir AB, Sigurdardottir V, Rayens MK, Svavarsdottir EK. The impact of receiving a family-oriented therapeutic conversation intervention before and during bereavement among family cancer caregivers: A nonrandomized trial. *J Hosp Palliat Nurs.* 2020;22(5):383–391. doi:10.1097/NJH.0000000000000679

26. Knies AK, Zhang Q, Juthani P, et al. Psychological attachment orientations of surrogate decision-makers and goals-of-care decisions for brain injury patients in ICUs. *Crit Care Explor.* 2020;2(7):e0151. Published 2020 Jul 6. doi:10.1097/CCE.0000000000000151

27. von Heymann-Horan A, Bidstrup P, Guldin MB, et al. Effect of home-based specialised palliative care and dyadic psychological intervention on caregiver anxiety and depression: A randomised controlled trial. *Br J Cancer.* 2018;119(11):1307–1315. doi:10.1038/s41416-018-0193-8

28. El-Jawahri A, Greer JA, Park ER, et al. Psychological distress in bereaved caregivers of patients with advanced cancer. *J Pain*

Symptom Manage. 2020;S0885-3924(20)30714-4. doi:10.1016/j.jpainsymman.2020.08.028

29. Hopf D, Eckstein M, Aguilar-Raab C, Warth M, Ditzen B. Neuroendocrine mechanisms of grief and bereavement: A systematic review and implications for future interventions. *J Neuroendocrinol.* 2020;32(8):e12887. doi:10.1111/jne.12887

30. Sutter M, Perrin PB. Discrimination, mental health, and suicidal ideation among LGBTQ people of color. *J Couns Psychol.* 2016;63(1):98–105. doi:10.1037/cou0000126

31. Slipka AF, Monsen KA. Toward improving quality of end-of-life care: Encoding clinical guidelines and standing orders using the Omaha system. *Worldviews Evid Based Nurs.* 2018;15(1):26–37. doi:10.1111/wvn.12248

32. Meier DE, Esch AE, Gualtieri-Reed T, Bowman B. Building effective palliative care teams toolkit. Last reviewed June 20, 2020. https://www.capc.org/toolkits/building-and-supporting-effective-palliative-care-teams/

33. WebMD. Chronic illness and depression. February 12, 2018. Available at https://www.webmd.com/depression/video/chronic-illness-and-depression.

34. Tori K, Kalligeros M, Nanda A, et al. Association between dementia and psychiatric disorders in long-term care residents: An observational clinical study. *Medicine (Baltimore).* 2020;99(31):e21412. doi:10.1097/MD.0000000000021412

35. Hartung T, Brähler E, Faller H, et al. The risk of being depressed is significantly higher in cancer patients than in the general population: Prevalence and severity of depressive symptoms across major cancer types. *Eur J Cancer.* 2017;72:46–53. doi:10.1016/j.ejca.2016.11.017

36. Singer AE, Goebel JR, Kim YS, et al. Populations and interventions for palliative and end-of-life care: A systematic review. *J Palliat Med.* 2016;19(9):995–1008. doi:10.1089/jpm.2015.036

37. van Oorschot B, Ishii K, Kusomoto Y, et al. Anxiety, depression and psychosocial needs are the most frequent concerns reported by patients: Preliminary results of a comparative explorative analysis of two hospital-based palliative care teams in Germany and Japan [published online ahead of print, 2020 may 17]. *J Neural Transm (Vienna).* 2020. doi:10.1007/s00702-020-02186-y

38. APA Work Group on Psychiatric Evaluation. *The American Psychiatric Association Practice Guidelines for the Psychiatric Evaluation of Adults.* 3rd ed. Washington, DC: American Psychiatric Association Publishing; 2016.

39. Puchalapalli A, Mahmood A. Neuropsychiatric comorbidities in hypothyroidism: A systematic review. *Neurol Psychiatry Brain Res.* 2020;37:79–86. doi:10.1016/j.npbr.2020.06.005

40. Pidani AS, Siddiqui AR, Azam I, Shamim MS, Jabbar AA, Khan S. Depression among adult patients with primary brain tumour: A cross-sectional study of risk factors in a low-middle-income country. *BMJ Open.* 2020;10(9):e032748. doi:10.1136/bmjopen-2019-032748

41. Israelsson H, Allard P, Eklund A, Malm J. Symptoms of depression are common in patients with idiopathic normal pressure hydrocephalus: The INPH-CRASH study. *Neurosurgery.* 2016;78(2):161–168. doi:10.1227/NEU.0000000000001093

42. Cluxton C. The challenge of cancer pain assessment. *Ulster Med J.* 2019;88(1):43–46.

43. Colodro-Conde L, Couvy-Duchesne B, Zhu G, et al. A direct test of the diathesis-stress model for depression. *Mol Psychiatry.* 2018;23(7):1590–1596. doi:10.1038/mp.2017.130

44. Kennis M, Gerritsen L, van Dalen M, Williams A, Cuijpers P, Bockting C. Prospective biomarkers of major depressive disorder: A systematic review and meta-analysis. *Mol Psychiatry.* 2020;25(2):321–338. doi:10.1038/s41380-019-0585-z

45. Edwards G, Nuckols T, Herrera N, Danovitch I, Ishak WW. Improving depression management in patients with medical illness using collaborative care: Linking treatment from the inpatient to the outpatient setting. *Innov Clin Neurosci.* 2019;16(11–12):19–24.

46. Maffioletti E, Minelli A, Tardito D, Gennarelli M. Blues in the brain and beyond: Molecular bases of major depressive disorder and relative pharmacological and non-pharmacological treatments. *Genes.* 2020;11(9):E1089. doi:10.3390/genes11091089

47. Taylor DM, Barnes TRE, Young AH. Depression. In: Taylor DM, Barnes TRE, Young AH, eds. *The Maudsley Prescribing Guidelines in Psychiatry.* 13th ed. Hoboken, NJ: Wiley; 2018: 255–382.

48. Khan AR, Geiger L, Wiborg O, Czéh B. Stress-induced morphological, cellular, and molecular changes in the brain-lessons learned from the chronic mild stress model of depression. *Cells.* 2020;9(4):1026. doi:10.3390/cells9041026

49. Rashidi-Ranjbar N, Miranda D, Butters MA, Mulsant BH, Voineskos AN. Evidence for structural and functional alterations of frontal-executive and corticolimbic circuits in late-life depression and relationship to mild cognitive impairment and dementia: A systematic review. *Front Neurosci.* 2020;14:253. doi:10.3389/fnins.2020.00253

50. Nagy EE, Frigy A, Szász JA, Horváth E. Neuroinflammation and microglia/macrophage phenotype modulate the molecular background of post-stroke depression: A literature review. *Exp Ther Med.* 2020;20(3):2510–2523. doi:10.3892/etm.2020.8933

51. Jiao JT, Cheng C, Ma YJ, et al. Association between inflammatory cytokines and the risk of post-stroke depression, and the effect of depression on outcomes of patients with ischemic stroke in a 2-year prospective study. *Exp Ther Med.* 2016;12(3):1591–1598. doi:10.3892/etm.2016.3494

52. Mahgoub N, Alexopoulos GS. Amyloid hypothesis: Is there a role for antiamyloid treatment in late-life depression? *Am J Geriatr Psychiatry.* 2016;24(3):239–247. doi:10.1016/j.jagp.2015.12.003

53. Kadriu B, Musazzi L, Henter ID, Graves M, Popoli M, Zarate CA Jr. Glutamatergic neurotransmission: Pathway to developing novel rapid-acting antidepressant treatments. *Int J Neuropsychopharmacol.* 2019;22(2):119–135. doi:10.1093/ijnp/pyy094

54. Wiels W, Baeken C, Engelborghs S. Depressive symptoms in the elderly-an early symptom of dementia? A systematic review. *Front Pharmacol.* 2020;11:34. Published 2020 Feb 7. doi:10.3389/fphar.2020.00034

55. Gałecki P, Talarowska M. Neurodevelopmental theory of depression. *Prog Neuropsychopharmacol Biol Psychiatry.* 2018;80(Pt C):267–272. doi:10.1016/j.pnpbp.2017.05.023

56. Hughes K, Bellis MA, Hardcastle KA, et al. The effect of multiple adverse childhood experiences on health: A systematic review and meta-analysis. *Lancet Public Health.* 2017, 2, e356–e366. doi:10.1016/S2468-2667(17)30118-4

57. Zhang HH, Meng SQ, Guo XY, et al. Traumatic stress produces delayed alterations of synaptic plasticity in basolateral amygdala. *Front Psychol.* 2019;10:2394. Published 2019 Oct 25. doi:10.3389/fpsyg.2019.02394

58. Mullins AJ, Gamwell KL, Sharkey CM, et al. Illness uncertainty and illness intrusiveness as predictors of depressive and anxious symptomology in college students with chronic illnesses. *J Am Coll Health.* 2017;65(5):352–360. doi:10.1080/07448481.2017.1312415

59. National Institute of Mental Health. Depression. February 28, 2018. https://www.nimh.nih.gov/health/topics/depression/index.shtml

60. Siu AL, US Preventive Services Task Force (USPSTF). Screening for depression in adults: Us preventive services task force recommendation statement. *JAMA.* 2016;315(4):380–387. doi:10.1001/jama.2015.18392

61. APA Work Group on Major Depressive Disorder. *The American Psychiatric Association Practice Guideline for the Treatment of Patients with Major Depressive Disorder.* 3rd ed. Washington, DC: American Psychiatric Association Publishing; 2010.

62. Zuckerbrot RA, Cheung A, Jensen PS, Stein REK, Laraque D; GLAD-PC steering group. Guidelines for adolescent depression in primary care (GLAD-PC): Part I. Practice preparation, identification, assessment, and initial management. *Pediatrics.* 2018;141(3):e20174081. doi:10.1542/peds.2017-4081

63. Lazris A. Geriatric palliative care. *Prim Care.* 2019;46(3):447–459. doi:10.1016/j.pop.2019.05.007

64. Avasthi A, Grover S. Clinical practice guidelines for management of depression in elderly. *Indian J Psychiatry.* 2018;60(Suppl 3):S341–S362. doi:10.4103/0019-5545.224474

65. Schaakxs R, Comijs HC, van der Mast RC, et al. Risk factors for depression: Differential across age? *Am J Geriatr Psychiatry.* 2017;25(9):966–977. doi:10.1016/j.jagp.2017.04.004

66. Carlat DJ. The psychiatric review of symptoms: A screening tool for family physicians. *Am Fam Physician.* 1998;58(7):1617–1624

67. D'Agostino A, Ferrara P, Terzoni S, et al. Efficacy of triple chronotherapy in unipolar and bipolar depression: A systematic review of the available evidence. *J Affect Disord.* 2020;276:297–304. doi:10.1016/j.jad.2020.07.026

68. Mehta MH, Grover RL, DiDonato TE, Kirkhart MW. Examining the positive cognitive triad: A link between resilience and well-being. *Psychol Rep.* 2019;122(3):776–788. doi:10.1177/0033294118773722

69. Akechi T, Okuyama T, Uchida M, et al. Factors associated with suicidal ideation in patients with multiple myeloma. *Jpn J Clin Oncol.* 2020;50(12):1475–1478. doi:10.1093/jjco/hyaa143

70. Belar A, Arantzamendi M, Santesteban Y, et al. Cross-sectional survey of the wish to die among palliative patients in Spain: One phenomenon, different experience]. *BMJ Support Palliat Care.* 2021;11(2):156–162. doi:10.1136/bmjspcare-2020-002234

71. Franklin JC, Ribiero JD, Fox KR, et al. Risk factors for suicidal thoughts and behaviors: A meta-analysis of 50 years of research. *Psych Bull.* 2017;143(2):187–232. doi:10.1037/bul0000084

72. Weber AN, Michail M, Thompson A, Fiedorowicz JG. Psychiatric emergencies: Assessing and managing suicidal ideation. *Med Clin North Am.* 2017;101(3):553–571. doi:10.1016/j.mcna.2016.12.006

73. Spillane A, Larkin C, Corcoran P, Matvienko-Sikar K, Riordan F, Arensman E. Physical and psychosomatic health outcomes in people bereaved by suicide compared to people bereaved by other modes of death: A systematic review. *BMC Public Health.* 2017;17(1):939. doi:10.1186/s12889-017-4930-3

74. Wise J. GPs should provide tailored support to people bereaved by suicide, says NICE. *BMJ.* 2019;366:l5498. doi:10.1136/bmj.l5498

75. ProCon.Org. States with legal physician-assisted suicide. Updated July 25, 2019. https://euthanasia.procon.org/states-with-legal-physician-assisted-suicide/

76. Otte IC, Jung C, Elger B, Bally K. "We need to talk!" Barriers to GPs' communication about the option of physician-assisted suicide and their ethical implications: Results from a qualitative study. *Med Health Care Philos.* 2017;20(2):249–256. doi:10.1007/s11019-016-9744-z

77. Perese EF. Chapter 13: Depressive Disorders. In: Perese EF, ed. *Psychiatric Advanced Practice Nursing: A Biopsychosocial Foundation for Practice.* Philadelphia, PA: FA Davis; 2012: 383–426.

78. Antunes B, Rodrigues PP, Higginson IJ, Ferreira PL. Determining the prevalence of palliative needs and exploring screening accuracy of depression and anxiety items of the Integrated Palliative Care Outcome Scale: A multi-centre study. *BMC Palliat Care.* 2020;19(1):69. Published 2020 May 14. doi:10.1186/s12904-020-00571-8

79. Rodríguez-Mayoral O, Peña-Nieves A, Allende-Pérez S, Lloyd-Williams M. Comparing the hospital anxiety and depression scale to the Brief Edinburgh Depression Scale for identifying cases of major depressive disorder in advanced cancer palliative patients. *Palliat Support Care.* 2020;1–5. doi:10.1017/S1478951520000760

80. Piqueras JA, Martín-Vivar M, Sandin B, San Luis C, Pineda D. The revised child anxiety and depression scale: A systematic review and reliability generalization meta-analysis. *J Affect Disord.* 2017;218:153–169. doi:10.1016/j.jad.2017.04.022

81. Patrick S, Connick P. Psychometric properties of the phq-9 depression scale in people with multiple sclerosis: A systematic review. *PLoS ONE.* 2019;14(2):e0197943. Published 2019 Feb 19. doi:10.1371/journal.pone.0197943

82. von Glischinski M, von Brachel R, Hirschfeld G. How depressed is "depressed"? A systematic review and diagnostic meta-analysis of optimal cut points for the Beck Depression Inventory Revised (BDI-II). *Qual Life Res.* 2019;28(5):1111–1118. doi:10.1007/s11136-018-2050-x

83. Williams MW, Li C-Y, Hay CC. Validation of the 10-item center for epidemiologic studies depression scale post stroke. *J Stroke Cerebrovasc Dis.* 2020;29(12):105334. doi:10.1016/j.jstrokecerebrovasdis.2020.105334

84. Carrozzino D, Patierno C, Fava GA, Guidi J. The Hamilton rating scales for depression: A critical review of clinimetric properties of different versions. *Psychother Psychosom.* 2020;89(3):133–150. doi:10.1159/00050687

85. Jokelainen J, Timonen M, Keinänen-Kiukaanniemi S, Härkönen P, Jurvelin H, Suija K. Validation of the Zung Self-Rating Depression Scale (SDS) in older adults. *Scand J Prim Health Care.* 2019;37(3):353–357. doi:10.1080/02813432.2019.1639923

86. Fish J. General well-being schedule. In: Kreutzer JS, Deluca J, Caplan B, eds. *Encyclopedia of Clinical Neuropsychology.* Springer; 2018: 193. doi:10.1007/978-3-319-57111-9_193

87. Balsamo M, Cataldi F, Carlucci L, Padulo C, Fairfield B. Assessment of late-life depression via self-report measures: A review. *Clin Interv Aging.* 2018;13:2021–2044. doi:10.2147/CIA.S178943

88. American Psychological Association. Geriatric Depression Scale (GDS). Last updated June 2020. Available at https://www.apa.org/pi/about/publications/caregivers/practice-settings/assessment/tools/geriatric-depression

89. O'Donnell ML, Agathos JA, Metcalf O, Gibson K, Lau W. Adjustment disorder: Current developments and future directions. *Int J Environ Res Public Health.* 2019;16(14):2537. doi:10.3390/ijerph16142537

90. Ng F, Crawford GB, Chur-Hansen A. Treatment approaches of palliative medicine specialists for depression in the palliative care setting: Findings from a qualitative, in-depth interview study. *BMJ Support Palliat Care.* 2016;6(2):186–193. doi:10.1136/bmjspcare-2014-000719

91. Greene RD, Cook A, Nowaskie D, Wang S. Neurological changes and depression: 2020 update. *Clin Geriatr Med.* 2020;36(2):297–313. doi:10.1016/j.cger.2019.11.009

92. von Blanckenburg P, Leppin N. Psychological interventions in palliative care. *Curr Opin Psychiatry.* 2018;31(5):389–395. doi:10.1097/YCO.0000000000000441

93. Fulton JJ, Newins AR, Porter LS, Ramos K. Psychotherapy targeting depression and anxiety for use in palliative care: A meta-analysis. *J Palliat Med.* 2018;21(7):1024–1037. doi:10.1089/jpm.2017.0576

94. Teo I, Tan YP, Finkelstein EA, et al. The feasibility and acceptability of a cognitive behavioral therapy-based intervention for patients with advanced colorectal cancer. *J Pain Symptom Manage.* 2020;60(6):1200–1207. doi:10.1016/j.jpainsymman.2020.06.016.

95. Osenbach JE, O'Brien KM, Mishkind M, Smolenski DJ. Synchronous telehealth technologies in psychotherapy for depression: A meta-analysis. *Depress Anxiety.* 2013;30(11):1058–1067. doi:10.1002/da.2216

96. Poletti B, Tagini S, Brugnera A, et al. Telepsychotherapy: A leaflet for psychotherapists in the age of covid-19. A review of the evidence. *Couns Psychol Q.* 2020(May 27). doi:10.1080/09515070.2020.1769557

97. Wheeler K. The nurse psychotherapist and a framework for practice. In: Wheeler K, ed., *Psychotherapy for the Advanced Practice Psychiatric Nurse.* 3rd ed. Springer; 2020: 4–56.

98. Ostuzzi G, Matcham F, Dauchy S, Barbui C, Hotopf M. Antidepressants for the treatment of depression in people with cancer. *Cochrane Database Syst Rev.* 2015;2015(6):CD011006. Published 2015 Jun 1. doi:10.1002/14651858.CD011006.pub2

99. Birmaher B, Brent D; AACAP Work Group on Quality Issues, et al. Practice parameter for the assessment and treatment of children and adolescents with depressive disorders. *J Am Acad Child Adolesc Psychiatry.* 2007;46(11):1503–1526. doi:10.1097/chi.0b013e318145ae1c

100. US Food & Drug Administration. FDA Consumer Updates. Depression: FDA approved medications may help. Updated April

28, 2017. Available at https://www.fda.gov/consumers/consumer-updates/depression-fda-approved-medications-may-help

101. Jing E, Straw-Wilson K. Sexual dysfunction in selective serotonin reuptake inhibitors (SSRIs) and potential solutions: A narrative literature review. *Ment Health Clin.* 2016;6(4):191–196. doi:10.9740/mhc.2016.07.191

102. Peng FZ, Fan J, Ge TT, Liu QQ, Li BJ. Rapid anti-depressant-like effects of ketamine and other candidates: Molecular and cellular mechanisms. *Cell Prolif.* 2020;53(5):e12804. doi:10.1111/cpr.12804

103. Popova V, Daly EJ, Trivedi M, et al. Efficacy and safety of flexibly dosed esketamine nasal spray combined with a newly initiated oral antidepressant in treatment-resistant depression: A randomized double-blind active-controlled study. [published correction appears in Am J Psychiatry. 2019 Aug 1;176(8):669]. *Am J Psychiatry.* 2019;176(6):428–438. doi:10.1176/appi.ajp.2019.19020172

104. Canuso CM, Singh JB, Fedgchin M, et al. Efficacy and safety of intranasal esketamine for the rapid reduction of symptoms of depression and suicidality in patients at imminent risk for suicide: Results of a double-blind, randomized, placebo-controlled study. *Am J Psychiatry.* 2018;175(7):620–630. doi:10.1176/appi.ajp.2018.17060720

105. Krause-Sorio B, Siddarth P, Kilpatrick L, et al. Combined treatment with escitalopram and memantine increases gray matter volume and cortical thickness compared to escitalopram and placebo in a pilot study of geriatric depression. *J Affect Disord.* 2020;274:464–470. doi:10.1016/j.jad.2020.05.092

106. Navarria A, Wohleb ES, Voleti B, et al. Rapid antidepressant actions of scopolamine: Role of medial prefrontal cortex and m1-subtype muscarinic acetylcholine receptors. *Neurobiol Dis.* 2015;82:254–261. doi:10.1016/j.nbd.2015.06.012

107. Candy M, Jones L, Williams R, Tookman A, King M. Psychostimulants for depression. *Cochrane Database Syst Rev.* 2008;(2):CD006722. Published 2008 Apr 16. doi:10.1002/14651858.CD006722.pub2

108. Andrew BN, Guan NC, Jaafar NRN. The use of methylphenidate for physical and psychological symptoms in cancer patients: A review. *Curr Drug Targets.* 2018;19(8):877–887. doi:10.2174/1389450118666170317162603

109. Tsapakis EM, Preti A, Mintzas MD, Fountoulakis KN. Adjunctive treatment with psychostimulants and stimulant-like drugs for resistant bipolar depression: A systematic review and meta-analysis. [published online ahead of print, 2020 Jul 9]. *CNS Spectr.* 2020;1–12. doi:10.1017/S109285292000156X

110. Byock I. Taking psychedelics seriously. *J Palliat Med.* 2018;21(4):417–421. doi:10.1089/jpm.2017.0684

111. Reiff CM, Richman EE, Nemeroff CB, et al. Psychedelics and psychedelic-assisted psychotherapy. *Am J Psychiatry.* 2020;177(5):391–410. doi:10.1176/appi.ajp.2019.19010035

112. Leichsenring F, Steinert C, Hoyer J. Psychotherapy versus pharmacotherapy of depression: What's the evidence? *Z Psychosom Med Psychother.* 2016;62(2):190–195 doi:10.13109/zptm.2016.62.2.190.

113. Rayner L, Price A, Hotopf M, Higginson IJ. The development of evidence-based European guidelines on the management of depression in palliative cancer care. *Eur J Cancer.* 2011; 47(5): 702–712. doi:10.1016/j.ejca.2010.11.027

114. Tormoehlen LM, Rusyniak DE. Neuroleptic malignant syndrome and serotonin syndrome. In: Romanovsky AA, ed. *Handbook of Clinical Neurology.* 2018;(157), 663–675. doi:10.1016/B978-0-444-64074-1.00039-2

115. Maher AR, Hempel S, Apaydin E, et al. St. John's wort for major depressive disorder: A systematic review. *Rand Health Q.* 2016;5(4):12. Published 2016 May 9.

116. Durak-Dados A, Michalski M, Osek J. Histamine and other biogenic amines in food. *J Vet Res.* 2020;64(2):281–288. doi:10.2478/jvetres-2020-0029

117. O'Donovan C, Alda M. Depression preceding diagnosis of bipolar disorder. *Front Psychiatry.* 2020;11:500. doi:10.3389/fpsyt.2020.00500

118. Stroup TS, Gray N. Management of common adverse effects of antipsychotic medications. *World Psychiatry.* 2018;17(3):341–356. doi:10.1002/wps.20567

119. Brown MA, Kaplan L. *The Advanced Practice Registered Nurse as Prescriber.* 2nd ed. Hoboken, NJ: Wiley; 2021

120. US Food & Drug Administration. Ativan© C-IV, (lorazepam). Medication guide. Updated December 16, 2016. Available at https://www.accessdata.fda.gov/drugsatfda_docs/label/2016/017794s044lbl.pdf#page=9

121. US Food and Drug Administration. Drug Safety and Availability. FDA drug safety communication: Prescription acetaminophen products to be limited to 325 mg per dosage unit; boxed warning will highlight potential for severe liver failure. Updated February 7, 2018. Available at http://www.fda.gov/drugs/drugsafety/ucm239821.htm#aihp

122. US Food and Drug Administration. Postmarket Drug Safety Information for Patients And Providers. FDA drug safety communication: Suicidality in children and adolescents being treated with antidepressant medications. Drug safety and availability. Updated February 5, 2018. Available at https://www.fda.gov/drugs/postmarket-drug-safety-information-patients-and-providers/suicidality-children-and-adolescents-being-treated-antidepressant-medications/

123. Boaden K, Tomlinson A, Cortese S, Cipriani A. Antidepressants in children and adolescents: Meta-review of efficacy, tolerability and suicidality in acute treatment. *Front Psychiatry.* 2020;11:717. Published 2020 Sep 2. doi:10.3389/fpsyt.2020.00717

124. Rolin D, Fox I, Jain R, Cole SP, Tran C, Jain S. Interventions in psychiatrically ill patients: Impact of wild 5 wellness, a five-domain mental health wellness intervention on depression, anxiety, and wellness. *J Am Psychiatr Nurses Assoc.* 2020;26(5):493–502. doi:10.1177/1078390319886883

125. Chiaramonte DR, Adler SR. Integrative palliative care: A new transformative field to alleviate suffering. *J Altern Complement Med.* 2020;26(9):761–765. doi:10.1089/acm.2019.0366

126. Billot M, Daycard M, Wood C, Tchalla A. Reiki therapy for pain, anxiety and quality of life. *BMJ Support Palliat Care.* 2019;9(4):434–438. doi:10.1136/bmjspcare-2019-001775

127. Collette N, Güell E, Fariñas O, Pascual A. Art therapy in a palliative care unit: Symptom relief and perceived helpfulness in patients and their relatives. *J Pain Symptom Manage.* 2020;S0885-3924(20)30639-4. doi:10.1016/j.jpainsymman.2020.07.027

128. Brugnoli MP. Clinical hypnosis for palliative care in severe chronic disease: A review and procedures for relieving physical, psychological, and spiritual symptoms. *Ann Palliat Med.* 2016;5:280–97. doi:10.21037/apm.2016.09.04

129. Cho D, Kim S, Durrani S, Liao Z, Milbury K. Associations between spirituality, mindfulness, and psychological symptoms among advanced lung cancer patients and their spousal caregivers. *J Pain Symptom Manage.* 2020. Epub 16 October 2020. doi:10.1016/j.jpainsymman.2020.10.001

130. Mantoudi A, Parpa E, Tsilika E, et al. Complementary therapies for patients with cancer: Reflexology and relaxation in integrative palliative care: A randomized controlled comparative study. *J Altern Complement Med.* 2020;26(9):792–798. doi:10.1089/acm.2019.0402

131. Peng CS, Baxter K, Lally KM. Music intervention as a tool in improving patient experience in palliative care. *Am J Hosp Palliat Care.* 2019;3 6(1):45–49. doi:10.1177/1049909118788643

132. Sagnetto F, Poles G, Guadagno C, Notari V, Giacopini N. Animal-assisted intervention to improve end-of-life care: The moderating effect of gender and pet ownership on anxiety and depression. *J Altern Complement Med.* 2020;26(9):841–842. doi:10.1089/acm.2019.0034

133. Breitbart W, Rosenfeld B, Pessin H, Applebaum A, Kulikowski J, Lichtenthal WG. Meaning-centered group psychotherapy: An

effective intervention for improving psychological well-being in patients with advanced cancer. *J Clin Oncol.* 2015;33(7):749–754. doi:10.1200/JCO.2014.57.2198

134. Amsterdam JD, Li QS, Xie SX, Mao JJ. Putative antidepressant effect of chamomile (Matricaria chamomilla l.) Oral extract in subjects with comorbid generalized anxiety disorder and depression. *J Altern Complement Med.* 2020;26(9):815–821. doi:10.1089/acm.2019.0252

135. Birch S, Bovey M, Alraek T, Robinson N, Kim T-H, Lee MS. Acupuncture as a treatment within integrative health for palliative care: A brief narrative review of evidence and recommendations. *J Altern Complement Med.* 2020;26(9):786–793. doi:10.1089/acm.2019. 0032

136. Fink J, Burns J, Moreno ACP, et al. A quality brief of an oncological multisite massage and acupuncture therapy program to improve cancer-related outcomes. *J Altern Complement Med.* 2020;26(9):822–826. doi:10.1089/acm.2019.0371

137. Fulginiti A, Frey LM. Are the "right" people selected for first disclosures about suicidal thoughts? Exploring what we know about advance care planning in the context of safety planning. *Community Ment Health J.* 2020;56(1):174–185. doi:10.1007/s10597-019-00457-x

51.

PALLIATIVE EMERGENCIES

Ann Quinn Syrett, Marcia J. Buckley, and Beth Carlson

KEY POINTS

- Hemorrhage is a frightening experience for both patient and family. The palliative advanced practice registered nurse (APRN) should screen for and discuss potential for hemorrhage in high-risk patients, reassuring them and their families that if a significant bleed occurs, a plan of action exists and needs to be promptly initiated.

- Spinal cord compression remains a presenting symptom for 20% of cancer patients. The palliative APRN should maintain vigilance for its probability and symptoms of potential onset. With the exception of steroids, the palliative APRN must consider the patient's overall prognosis before initiating therapy.

- Seizures are a medical emergency. Brain metastases are the most common etiology of seizures in palliative care and increases risk of sudden death. Education and planning is needed to urgently treat seizures when they occur and use antiepileptic medications to prevent recurrence.

- Superior vena cava syndrome is a true medical emergency if the airway becomes obstructed. Lung cancer accounts for more than 70% of all cases annually. Early diagnosis and management can lead to a longer time between recurrences.

CASE STUDY: HEMORRHAGE

Karl was a 63-year-old man with anaplastic thyroid cancer status post total thyroidectomy, total neck dissection, and extensive radiotherapy and chemotherapy. He continued to show progression of disease. Karl had a laryngeal ulceration and was followed by the palliative care team for symptom management. He had episodes of bleeding thought to be secondary to weakening of the arterial wall due to radiation. The palliative advanced practice registered nurse (APRN) met with Karl and his wife to discuss his significant risk for life-threatening bleeding. Karl expressed his wishes regarding no resuscitation and adamantly stated he wanted to die at home, not in the hospital. Karl was admitted to home hospice. Karl's opioid medications were liberalized for as-needed usage to be given both sublingually as well as subcutaneously in the case of a major bleed. The family was instructed on measures to take in the event of a terminal hemorrhage incorporating nonpharmacologic measures (such as using dark towels, bedding, a basin at the bedside, moist towelettes). Karl enjoyed 2 months at home surrounded by his family before having a catastrophic gastrointestinal hemorrhage. He was given opioid and anxiolytic medications to ensure he was comfortable when he died.

INTRODUCTION

This chapter discusses four palliative emergencies: hemorrhage, spinal cord compression, seizures, and superior vena cava syndrome. Each emergency has different ramifications for the patient because all of these conditions can result in terminal event. It should be noted that each symptom may be terrifying for family to witness, both as a symptom and as a dying event. Therefore, though rare, the palliative advanced practice registered nurse (APRN) must assess for their potential occurrence and then plan accordingly. With proactive planning, patients may still be managed in both the acute and community setting. However, there must always be a plan for planned sedation for a crisis situation or palliative sedation if the conditions become a terminal event. Palliative sedation is a special therapy that requires a particular expertise; discussion is beyond the scope of this chapter but it is covered in Chapter 57.

HEMORRHAGE

Hemorrhage as a cause of death is relatively rare. Akinola et al.[1] defined major hemorrhage as "that [which] is likely to rapidly result in a patients' death due to a massive loss of circulating volume." There is a consensus in the literature on the importance of identifying at-risk patients. The pathophysiology of a bleed is related to the underlying cause or type of cancer a patient has, thereby creating insight into who may be susceptible. Often patients may have a slight bleed before a major bleed, allowing time for planning. Table 51.1 depicts etiology and risk according to tumor type.[1-4]

Treatment will depend on the underlying cause of the bleed, extent of the bleed, patient risk factors, and prognosis, as well as goals of care and where the patient is located. The focus here will be on patients who experience catastrophic bleeding as a result of malignancy. Consider two patients. The first is an older patient with dementia and a neck mass with occasional bleeding. This patient lives at a skilled facility with a do-not-transfer order in place. The plan for the potential bleed from the neck mass is for management with a small

Table 51.1 RISK AND ETIOLOGY OF HEMORRHAGE IN ADVANCED MALIGNANCIES

TUMOR TYPE	AT RISK FOR	ETIOLOGY
Head and neck cancer	Carotid artery rupture	Direct invasion of arterial wall, damage to the wall due to radiation
Lung tumors	Catastrophic hemoptysis	Tumor erosion into a vessel wall. Irritation, tumor necrosis
Gastrointestinal (GI)	Hematemesis, melena	Erosion or ulceration through the bowel wall; esophageal varices; Coagulopathies due to liver involvement
Genitourinary (GU)	Hematuria, clots	Sloughing of the tumor mass
Gynecologic (GYN)	Vaginal bleeding	Direct invasion, tumor erosion
Hematologic	Petechiae, ecchymosis, sentinel bleed	Disruption in platelet function; disseminated intravascular coagulopathy (DIC); Idiopathic thrombocytopenia purpura (ITP)

From Akinola et al.[1]; Gershman et al.[2]; Smith, Jackson[3]; and Abt et al.[4]

sandbag, liquid morphine, dark towels, and psychosocial support to the nursing assistant staff to key her at the facility. The second patient is an older adult in the hospital with a bleeding esophageal mass. The plan for the potential bleed from the neck mass is for management with packing and IV opioids. In both situations, preparation and support is given to staff, and medications are used to ensure comfort with imminent death related to hemorrhage.

INCIDENCE

In people with cancer, approximately 10% will experience at least one episode of bleeding, and 6–14% will experience a significant bleed during their cancer course. If hemorrhaging occurs suddenly, there is a short window of time in which to support the patient and try to control the bleed.[1–4]

MANAGEMENT

Early discussion with patients at risk for hemorrhage can help guide overall treatment decisions as do an individual's prognosis, comorbidities, and quality of life.[5] The palliative APRN has a role in clarifying goals of care and developing a realistic management plan, which are essential.[5,6] Prevention of hemorrhage is the first goal. The APRN should review the patients' medications and herbal supplements to identify any that may potentiate bleeding (Table 51.2).[7] A pharmacist can

Table 51.2 MEDICATIONS AND HERBAL SUPPLEMENTS THAT MAY POTENTIATE BLEEDING

Medications	Anticoagulants (warfarin, heparin), anti-inflammatory medication (steroids); Cox-2 inhibitors (celecoxib), non-steroidals (ibuprofen, naproxen, aspirin)
Herbal supplements	Arnica, turmeric celery, chamomile, clove, garlic, ginger, ginkgo biloba, ginseng, horse chestnut, licorice root, onion, and willow bark

From Pori.[7]

be invaluable in identifying culpable medications, drug interactions, and the effects of complementary substances (such as herbs) in patients on multiple medications and noncontrolled substances. An assessment and discussion of the benefit-to-burden ratio of anticoagulants is critical.

If bleeding occurs via the nose, rectum, or vagina, careful packing of the orifice may help. Acetone, a hemostatic agent, may be used for vaginal packing; gauze soaked in tranexamic gauze can be used with nasal packing. Nonadherent saline-soaked dressings provide a compression dressing and may slow or stop even arterial bleeding. Bleeding surface wounds can be treated with hemostatic dressings such as alginates and hemostatic agents such as epinephrine or tranexamic acid syrup.[8] The palliative APRN should consult a wound ostomy certified nurse (WOCN) whenever possible. The WOCN can assess the patient in their setting of care to determine the best dressing regimen and necessary supplies. There may be a need for multiple dressing and supplies that are often expensive.[9]

Hematuria is initially often treated with a three-way Foley catheter to decompress the bladder and allow for saline irrigation. Intravesically administered agents have been tried but lack supportive studies for use.[10] However, administering anti-fibrinolytic agents can be effective for refractory bleeding. Endovascular techniques are quite effective but not without risks. Cystoscopy with laser coagulation is a favored strategy, as is radiation therapy.[9–11]

Severity of hemoptysis in the patient with lung cancer will determine initial management. The integrity of the airway, the patient's ability to manage secretions, and a review of realistic outcomes and goals of care will guide these steps. More aggressive therapies would include bronchial airway embolization, ablation, and tumor debulking. Surgical intervention is rarely an option for palliation.[2]

Acute onset of an upper gastrointestinal (GI) bleed carries a high mortality rate in people with advanced disease. Endoscopic interventions, saline gastric irrigation using a nasogastric tube (NGT), or initiation of argon plasma and laser therapies can be employed, but the success rate is variable. Transcutaneous arterial embolization may be effective in select situations, as is external beam radiotherapy with or without chemotherapy.[10,12] The overall performance status of the patient, as well as prognosis, play key roles in determining if they are surgical candidate and what treatment will be employed.

There are systemic therapies available to treat hemorrhage. Phytonadione (vitamin K) is important in aiding the liver to produce multiple clotting factors (II, VII, XI, X). It can be given orally, subcutaneously, or intravenously (IV). In one study, oral phytonadione was shown to be as effective as IV administration in returning a patient's International Normalized Ratio (INR) to an acceptable level.[13] Vasopressin has been shown to slow upper GI bleeds. Octreotide, a somatostatin analog, is also effective in the management of upper GI bleeding, usually given either subcutaneously twice to three times or as a continuous IV infusion.

The continued use of platelet and blood transfusions becomes an ethical discussion. On one hand, transfusions may help for a while, but their effect becomes shorter and shorter. One the other hand, without these transfusions, death will come sooner. Moreover, even with a change of focus to comfort, the majority of hospice programs will not admit patients still pursuing transfusions because they see them as curative therapies. Quality of life appraisal is highly personal and should be part of the ongoing goals of care discussions.[14,15]

A terminal hemorrhage may cause death within minutes, often before any sedating medicine administered takes full effect. Depending on where a patient receives care (i.e., the hospital, residential settings, or long-term care settings) frontline caregivers and families need education and support. The palliative APRN should provide a description of what the potential bleeding will look like and how it will occur, with an emphasis on the low probability of survival from bleeding out. Nonetheless, the APRN should make a plan for patient comfort. In addition, the plan should include measures to support family and caregivers. Box 51.1 describes tips to prepare for hemorrhage.

MALIGNANT SPINAL CORD COMPRESSION

CASE STUDY: MALIGNANT SPINAL CORD COMPRESSION

Jean was a 68-year-old female with history of tobacco smoking, osteoarthritis, and gastric reflux. She was admitted to the hospital from her chiropractor's office presenting with progressive back pain and new onset of left leg weakness and bladder/bowel incontinence. Imaging revealed a large left lung mass and bony metastatic lesions to her ribs, thoracic and lumbar spine, and pelvis. Jane was started on high-dose steroids with improved neurological symptoms. Pathology results from an ileum bone biopsy revealed metastatic high-grade neuroendocrine tumor. Jean underwent palliative radiation to her lumbar-sacral spine and pelvis to improve motor function and reduce pain. Due to her poor functional status, she was not a candidate for chemo- or immunotherapy. She was admitted to inpatient hospice, receiving long-acting oxycodone and scheduled lorazepam to control her pain and anxiety. Jean enjoyed some quality time with family and friends before dying peacefully a few weeks later.

Box 51.1 PREPARATIONS FOR A TERMINAL HEMORRHAGE

1. Identify patients at risk for significant bleed.

2. Mitigate risk factors.
   a. Eliminate nonsteroidal and anticoagulant medications.
   b. Consider therapies if in accordance with patient wishes.

3. Develop a plan of action depending on whether the patient is home, in a skilled nursing facility, in a hospital.

4. Prepare family and caregivers for the possibility.
   a. Take into consideration that herald (or initial) bleeding episodes often indicate a major bleed within 24–48 hours.

5. Have appropriate medications available. If patient is at home, consider prefilled syringes near the bedside. Instruct and coach family regarding use of
   a. Opioids
   b. Anxiolytics

6. Prepare the bedside.
   a. Encourage use of darker bed linens.
   b. Place dark towels particularly under potential site of bleed and have extras nearby.
   c. Have a small sandbag to apply pressure, as appropriate.
   d. Have supplies such as a basin, gloves, wash clothes.
   e. Have suction available if appropriate for patient situation.

INCIDENCE

Malignant spinal cord compression (MSCC) is a fairly common sequelae of malignancy and is considered a medical emergency. Approximately 20% of all patients diagnosed with a malignancy present with a MSCC as their presenting symptom.[16–19] As many as 85–90% are due to metastatic disease to vertebral bones. Often, as the tumor grows, it surrounds the thecal sac, obstructing the venous plexus. Vasogenic edema ensues, and, if left unchecked, the patient will sustain a spinal infarction.[17] Prompt diagnosis of MSCC can have profound effects on outcomes for the patient. Outcomes for people who develop a spinal cord compression for reasons other than cancer (infections, rheumatoid arthritis, neurological diseases/insults including primary astrocytomas/ependymomas) will often have better outcomes.[17,20]

The majority of MSCCs are due to metastases to the vertebral bone, with the spine being the third most common site. The neurological deficits that occur can be permanent due to direct compression of the cord or cauda equina, interruption of the vascular supply to the cord, or actual fracture of the vertebra. Less common etiologies of MSCC would be direct extension of the tumor through the intervertebral foramina or via leptomeningeal spread.[17,21,22]

SIGNS AND SYMPTOMS

Recognition of the signs and symptoms of MSCC is crucial to avoid complete and irreversible paralysis. A patient's overall

Table 51.3 SIGNS AND SYMPTOMS OF MALIGNANT SPINAL CORD COMPRESSION

Back pain (localized, mechanical, radicular)	80–95% of patients present with back pain Often worse at night Often felt when coughing or sneezing Described as aching and constant
Motor deficits	35–75% of patients present with motor deficits Weakness of lower extremities Cauda equina syndrome: Lower extremity weakness in a patchy distribution
Sensory deficits	Multiple dermatomes can be involved Urinary retention Overflow incontinence Bowel incontinence Gait abnormalities

From Laufer et al.[17]; and Wänman et al.[18]

functional status, which correlates to survival, can be diminished greatly by MSCC. Twenty-three percent of people with a MSCC do not have any history of cancer. Back pain is common and can precede other symptoms by several weeks, causing an important delay in the diagnosis and treatment of MSCC.[17,20]

These symptoms may be missed in older adults, particularly those individuals who live in skilled facilities and already have musculoskeletal pain and bowel and bladder conditions.

If worsening back pain is present and varies with position changes, MSCC should be presumed until ruled out. MSCC should be considered in the differential diagnosis in patients presenting with thoracic pain, since this portion of the spine rarely produces pain from other conditions. Pain that only occurs with movement can be an important indicator of spinal instability, which may need rapid surgical intervention. Weakness with ambulation, the inability to walk, and increased deep tendon reflexes are the most significant predictors of MSCC.[16] Bladder and bowel dysfunction are later signs of cord compression, and history should include questions of sexual function. Table 51.3 lists presenting signs and symptoms.[17,18]

DIAGNOSTICS

Magnetic resonance imaging (MRI) of the entire spine, with and without contrast, remains the gold standard of diagnosis. The palliative APRN should first order this imaging immediately when MSCC is suspected. MRI of entire spine has replaced all radiologic modalities as the diagnostic of choice and needs to be done as soon as a MSCC is suspected.[16,17,19,23] It produces the most accurate anatomical image of intraforaminal and leptomeningeal disease and shows clear definition of the adjacent bone and soft tissue structures. Plain spinal films are not useful in patients with suspected MSCC.

MANAGEMENT

When a MSCC is identified, prompt treatment is essential for preservation or restoration of a person's function. It also promotes quality of life, most notably relief of pain. The APRN must consider a patient's predicted prognosis along with their values and goals prior to any treatment decision. Standard treatments for managing MSCC include corticosteroids, radiotherapy, and/or decompressive surgery. Even prior to MSCC being diagnosed, many providers initiate therapy with the use of a glucocorticosteroid. Dexamethasone decreases vasogenic edema by inhibiting prostaglandin E_2, along with inhibiting vascular endothelial growth factor.[24,25] This decrease in edema and inflammation reduces pain. There must be consideration of the benefits of steroids versus the burden of possible distressing GI and mental side effects from moderate to high-dose steroids including propensity to infection.[26]

Radiation therapy (XRT), used as a single-modality treatment, has been shown to improve ambulation, improve neurologic status, and decrease or even eliminate pain, thereby improving quality of life and sometimes lengthening survival. In a study of 688 patients were randomly assigned to receive either a single dose of 8 Gy or a 5-day course totaling 20 Gy with evaluation of post radiation ambulatory status. There were no statistically significant differences between the two groups either in function or survival.[27] A study looking at pain management as well as neurological improvement found short-course (1, 5, or 10 days) XRT had significant improvement in pain scores and supported the fact that the patient benefits from the shortest course possible based on extent of tumor.[28]

While XRT remains the mainstay of treatment, Le et al.[22] recognized that, for some individuals, surgical approaches can actually be more effective. It is the treatment of choice for patients with either high-grade MSCC or those with an unstable spine. It is often combined with either XRT or stereotactic radiation therapy (SRS) based on whether the tumor is radiosensitive, the degree of cord compression, and overall stability of the spine. Pain control is not achieved with an unstable spine or with bracing. The 2017 update of Bone Metastases Guidelines concluded that surgery, radionuclides, bisphosphonates, and kyphoplasty/vertebroplasty do not replace the need for external beam radiation therapy and these therapies can be done in tandem.[29]

SUPPORTIVE THERAPIES

In a select group of patients who have MSCC, there appears to be a role for physical medicine and rehabilitation.[30,31] Physical therapy consultation may be warranted to optimize function and safety for both the patient and their care providers. If a patient with a short prognosis develops an MSCC, the palliative APRN can order a trial of steroids with a course XRT to alleviate pain, optimize quality of life, and try to preserve some modest function and dignity.

SEIZURES

CASE STUDY: SEIZURES

Ms. K was a 74-year-old woman brought to the emergency department (ED) by ambulance after family witnessed a sustained tonic-clonic seizure at home, relieved by 10 mg intramuscular midazolam. Past medical history was significant for metastatic breast cancer; her status was post mastectomy, chemo, and radiation. Labs revealed liver dysfunction and a repeat positron emission tomography (PET) scan revealed disease widely metastatic to liver, spine, and brain. A head MRI revealed a parieto-occipital lesion. Ms. K experienced another seizure while transferring to the ICU and received 4 mg of IV lorazepam for seizure cessation. Oral levetiracetam 750 mg twice a day and oral dexamethasone 6 mg twice a day were initiated to decrease cerebral edema and risk of seizure. Ms. K improved mentally and physically. An electroencephalogram (EEG) revealed no seizure activity. The palliative APRN met with Ms. K and her family to review her understanding of options, determine her goals for care, and provide support. Ms. K chose to prioritize her comfort with the goal of home hospice. The patient and family were educated about the risk of seizure recurrence. Ms. K was prescribed an antiepileptic medication, a steroid, and an as-needed benzodiazepines in the event of another seizure. She was surrounded by her loved ones when she peacefully died at home.

Epilepsy is a disorder characterized by recurrent unprovoked seizures and categorized by its related etiology of onset as focal, generalized, or unknown.[32] Experiencing a seizure is considered a medical emergency.[33] Basic knowledge of seizure presentation, predisposing factors, and anticipatory management is crucial to expediting resolution or relief of the symptoms and preventing recurrences.

INCIDENCE

Approximately 1.2% of the US population or 3.4 million have been affected by epileptic episodes.[34] Seizure prevalence is highest in those younger than 1 year and older than 65 years. Nearly 50% of seizures occur in persons without a prior history of epilepsy.[35] After two initial unprovoked seizures, approximately 30–50% of patients will experience a seizure recurrence and become epileptic.[36]

The most common cause of seizures in the older adult (>65 years) is stroke. The risk of epilepsy due to unprovoked seizure is at its highest more than 7 days after the initial stroke.[37] It is estimated that 60% of patients with brain metastases will experience seizure depending on the primary tumor.[38] The actual incidence of seizures in dying patients is unknown.[39] Many studies establish that patients with brain tumors are at risk for seizure, and this is associated with a higher risk of sudden death, thus highlighting the goal of proactively working to minimize seizures and their negative impact on quality of life.[40–44]

PATHOPHYSIOLOGY

The International League Against Epilepsy updated the operational classification of seizure types in 2017. Seizures are divided into focal, generalized, or unknown onset, with subcategories of motor, nonmotor, with retained or impaired awareness for focal seizures (Table 51.4).[32] The expanded terminology for focal or generalized onset allows greater

Table 51.4 INTERNATIONAL LEAGUE AGAINST EPILEPSY (ILAE) CLASSIFICATION OF SEIZURE TYPES, EXPANDED VERSION

Focal onset *Aware vs. impaired awareness*	Motor onset: Nonmotor onset:	Automatisms, atonic, clonic, epileptic spasms, hyperkinetic, myoclonic, tonic Autonomic, behavior arrest, cognitive, emotional, sensory
Generalized onset	Motor: Nonmotor (absence)	Tonic-clonic, clonic, tonic, myoclonic, myoclonic-tonic-clonic, myoclonic-atonic, atonic, epileptic spasms Typical, atypical, myoclonic, eyelid myoclonia
Unknown onset	Motor Nonmotor Unclassified	Tonic-clonic, epileptic spasms Behavior arrest

From Fisher et al.[32]

transparency in naming seizure types.[32] Status epilepticus focal seizures occur with or without loss of consciousness. Generalized status epilepticus (tonic-clonic, absence, myoclonic) are always associated with loss of consciousness, and these have a greater incidence of associated mortality. When a seizure involves loss of consciousness, there will be a postictal state that may include somnolence, confusion, and/or headache; it may last several hours.[33]

CLINICAL FEATURES

Factors influencing the risk of seizure recurrence include a history of long seizure duration and failure to respond to other medications.[45] Table 51.5 outlines predisposing factors for seizures. Mortality from these underlying predisposing factors resulting in acute symptomatic status epilepticus is six times greater compared to chronic epilepsy. Death may occur from metabolic stress related to muscular convulsions, rhabdomyolysis, lactic acidosis, aspiration pneumonitis, neurogenic pulmonary edema, and respiratory failure.[46]

DIAGNOSIS

Status epilepticus of any type is determined by a neurological examination and involves repeated seizures lasting at least 5 minutes without a recovery period of greater than 30 minutes.[35] Therefore, witnesses' accounts of activity prior to a seizure and description of seizure activity, including any incontinence or loss of consciousness, are crucial in determining the seizure type. Suspect a structural cause if aura or heightened sensory experience occurs before the seizure. Versive eye movements (deviation to one side) are associated with focal seizures. An electroencephalogram (EEG) is helpful in determining status epilepticus in an unresponsive patient. Adults present with an abnormal EEG finding with first unprovoked seizure about 51% of the time.[36] A

Table 51.5 PREDISPOSING FACTORS FOR SEIZURES

FACTOR	EXAMPLES
Structural	Brain tumor, metastasis, stroke, head trauma, subarachnoid hemorrhage
Degenerative	Cerebral palsy in young patients, Alzheimer's disease in older patients
Systemic	Cerebral anoxia/hypoxia or infections (such as encephalitis, meningitis, abscess), fever, sleep deprivation
Metabolic	Hepatic encephalopathy, uremia, electrolyte abnormalities, such as sodium, calcium, magnesium, phosphorus, or glucose metabolism
Drug treatments	Use of seizure threshold–lowering drugs, such as antibiotics, antiarrhythmics, chemotherapy, opioids, or psychotropics
Withdrawal	Rapid withdrawal from alcohol intoxication or antiseizure medication

From Lee et al.[34]; Khan et al.[47]; and Buckley MJ, Syrett A, Palliative emergencies. In: Dahlin C, Coyne P, Ferrell B, eds. *Advance Practice Palliative Nursing.* Oxford: Oxford Unity Press, 2016: 362.

Table 51.6 SUGGESTED POST-SEIZURE LAB TESTING

TEST	EVALUATION
CBC	Leukocytosis, thrombocytopenia, plethora
Blood chemistries	Ammonia, urea, sodium, calcium, magnesium, phosphorus, or glucose abnormalities
TSH	Low TSH indicates hyperthyroidism-associated seizures
Urinalysis	Increased glucose, infection
C-reactive protein	Inflammatory marker, increased after tonic-clonic seizures
Coagulation studies	Increased risk of intracranial bleeding
Vitamin B_{12}, folate	Vitamin B_{12} deficiency, folate deficiency
Prolactin	Elevated levels seen after seizure
Blood cultures	Infectious cause
Blood gas	Hypoxia and metabolic imbalances
Toxicology	Overdose of tricyclic antidepressants, cocaine
Pregnancy test	Possible eclampsia

From Buckley MJ, Syrett A, Palliative emergencies. In: Dahlin C, Coyne P, Ferrell B, eds. *Advance Practice Palliative Nursing.* Oxford: Oxford Unity Press, 2016: 363.

computed tomography (CT) head scan without IV contrast is appropriate in emergent situations to evaluate new-onset seizures in the setting of trauma. MRI is the study of choice for determining structural lesions that are triggering seizures and is indicated for patients considering palliative surgery and/or radiation.[34]

MANAGEMENT

Primary management when a seizure occurs includes the ABCs: patent airway, effective breathing, and adequate circulation. The workup involves a thorough history from the patient and witnesses to the seizure, a full neurological exam and individualized neuroimaging, and lab studies appropriate to the patient's goals of care.[35] Table 51.6 summarizes suggested post-seizure laboratory testing and the rationale.

The American Academy of Neurology guidelines suggest prudent consideration of testing on an individual basis because there has not been strong evidence to support or refute the recommendations.[36] When seizure etiology is unknown, glucose and thiamine should be given together immediately to rule out treatable causes.[33] Knowledge of seizure type is helpful in determining if neuroimaging is warranted.[34]

Treatment of seizures should be initiated after 5 minutes of sustained seizure activity because it is unlikely to stop spontaneously.[35] In a hospice situation, 5 minutes can seem like 5 hours to a loved one, and every effort should be made to treat the seizure, with the goal of comfort. If the patient has an IV in place, this route is preferable, although this is not always possible in palliative/hospice settings. Antiseizure medications may be administered subcutaneously, sublingually, or rectally. Table 51.7 reviews commonly used antiseizure medications used to stop status epilepticus.[33,35,48]

In the palliative setting, it may be desirable to use lower doses of benzodiazepines with frequent repeat doses available as needed when the goal is to avoid long periods of unconsciousness.[39] If in the acute setting, regardless of the response to these first-line benzodiazepines, initiate a conventional antiepileptic drug (AED). The preferred nonsedating, fast-acting antiepileptic with minimal drug interactions is levetiracetam.[39,49] Third-line treatment for status epilepticus includes valproate and general anesthesia (phenobarbital, propofol, ketamine) inducing chemical coma, with the goal to alleviate suffering while accepting the risk of respiratory failure.[33,45,46] Clinical pharmacists may be helpful to evaluate medication regimens to optimize seizure control and improve quality of life.[50]

The decision to initiate long-term empiric treatment with antiseizure medication is individualized based on the risk of seizure recurrence, the consequences of seizure recurrence, and potential interactions.[36,37] The European Stroke Organisation has issued guidelines based on an assessment and evaluation approach due to lack of reliable evidence. There is weak support to recommend routine prophylaxis with antiseizure medications after one post-stroke unprovoked seizure.[37] A study of 225 people found evidence that oral cannabidiol can decrease seizure incidence in Lennox-Gastaut syndrome.[51]

After two or more unprovoked seizures on separate days, empiric monotherapy with a long-term antiseizure agent should be initiated to prevent recurrences. In cases of seizures

Table 51.7 COMMONLY USED ANTIEPILEPTIC MEDICATIONS (AEDS) FOR STATUS EPILEPTICUS (SE) CESSATION

First line, early SE:	Common dosing	
Lorazepam	0.1 mg/kg bolus IV (at least 4 mg)	Benzodiazepines are first-line treatment for seizure cessation
Midazolam	10 mg IM or buccal	Repeat bolus every 5 minutes
Diazepam	10 mg bolus, rectal	Sedation; SE is considered refractory if starting midazolam continuous infusion
Second line, established SE:		
Levetiracetam	250–4,000 mg/d; 30 mg/kg IV bolus over 10 min	Nonsedating, low side-effect profile
Phenytoin/fosphenytoin	18–20 mg/kg bolus/4–6 mg/kg/d	Administer fosphenytoin at rate of 50 mg/min
Valproic acid	500–2,500 mg/d; 15–45 mg/kg bolus 6–10 mg/kg/min	Nonsedating, mild hypotension
Phenobarbital	30–180 mg/d; bolus 10 mg/kg, infuse max 100 mg/min	Alcohol withdrawal; sedating, respiratory depression, hypotension
Third line, refractory SE:		
Propofol	Goal <48 hours and not >5 mg/kg/h	Associated with higher mortality and morbidity.
Ketamine	1–3 mg/kg IV bolus; 6–10 mg/kg/h	Ketamine has less respiratory depression;
Pentobarbital/thiopental	5–15 mg/kg IV bolus then continuous infusion to maintain burst suppression on electroencephalogram (EEG)	pentobarbital has the most and is reserved for severe cases of refractory SE

From Douglas, Aminoff[33]; Grönheit et al.[39]; Alkhachroum et al.[46]; Daly, Lugassy[48]; and Trinka et al.[52]

caused by a brain lesion, consider increasing or initiating steroids in addition to starting an anticonvulsant. Patients undergoing cerebral radiation should receive steroids (dexamethasone 4 mg to maximum 16 mg daily) to prevent seizures associated with cerebral edema.[53] If undergoing surgical resection of the brain tumor, consider weaning off antiseizure medications after surgery. If palliative chemotherapy is an option, preference should be given to antiseizure medications that do not induce cytochrome P450 activity; these include levetiracetam, gabapentin, lamotrigine, and pregabalin.[36,51] The benefits of prophylaxis in primary brain tumor patients should be considered on an individual basis, taking into consideration the known risk of psychomotor slowing and general cognitive decline.[43,54] Compared to older generation AEDs (phenytoin, carbamazepine, and valproic acid), the newer generation AEDs (levetiracetam) have fewer adverse cognitive side effects.[36,53,55]

The palliative APRN has a large role in planning for seizure management in the hospice setting. First, the APRN needs to assess the cause of seizures and the use of medications. If the cause of the seizure is reversible, then long-term anticonvulsant treatment is not warranted. Although anticonvulsants are often initiated on diagnosis of a brain tumor, they have not been shown to prevent seizures in patients with no seizure history.[53] In addition, current guidelines do not recommend the use of anticonvulsants prophylactically in stroke patients. Therefore, it is recommended to consider stopping prophylactic dosing of antiseizure medications in patients with no seizure history.[53] If medications are continued, the APRN should consider the appropriate medication, with the preference being to avoid enzyme-inducing medications or those that require frequent blood draws to monitor medication levels.[39]

Experiencing and witnessing a seizure can be terrifying for both patient and family, necessitating proactive planning to avoid recurrence. In the hospice and home setting, benzodiazepines. should be available for suppression of seizures if they occur. These should be administered sublingually, subcutaneously, or via a gastronomy tube. The rectal route may cause more distress for patients and families in the event of terminal seizures. Family instruction should include avoiding putting anything in the mouth and protecting the seizing person from falls or injury. Families need reassurance that if seizures become refractory, palliative sedation is warranted for patients to allow for a peaceful death.

SUPERIOR VENA CAVA SYNDROME

CASE STUDY: SUPERIOR VENA CAVA SYNDROME

Mr. P was a 62-year-old male tobacco smoker with history of diabetes and hypertension. He presented with progressive difficulty swallowing for weeks and acute shortness of breath with stridor. On exam, Mr. P had a short neck and edematous upper extremities. He was tachycardic and hypoxic. Chest CT revealed a right-sided mediastinal mass encroaching on his laryngopharynx. Thoracic surgery emergently placed a stent to open his airway and obtained a tissue biopsy of the mass. Mr. P's respiratory status stabilized immediately, and his swallowing improved. Pathology results revealed non-small cell cancer. He underwent surgical resection followed by radiation to the mass. Mr. P required hospitalization a few months later with aspiration pneumonia requiring ICU-level care. Imaging revealed progression of his cancer and recurrent superior vena cava syndrome (SVCS). The palliative APRN met with Mr. P and his family to discuss his wishes regarding restenting, intubation, and resuscitation. Mr. P opted to forgo further procedures and transitioned to a comfort-measures-only plan of care. As his breathing became more labored, Mr. P received opioid and anxiolytic medications to ensure his comfort until his peaceful death.

INCIDENCE

Superior vena cava syndrome (SVCS) is a group of symptoms resulting from an obstruction of blood flow from the upper body to the right atrium. It is considered an emergency in the presence of neurological symptoms or respiratory distress.[56] This relatively rare syndrome was first described in 1757, by Scottish surgeon William Hunter, in a patient suffering from syphilis aortitis. In most cases, it is caused by a carcinoma of the bronchus or metastases to paratracheal or paracarinal lymph nodes compressing on the SVC.[56] The common use of implantable intravenous devices such as central line catheters and pacemakers has increased the prevalence of thrombosis-related SVCS. In rare cases, SVCS develops from infections, such as tuberculosis or histoplasmosis, which increase pleural thickening and cause significant systemic-to-pleural venous shunting.[57]

In the United States, approximately 15,000 cases of SVCS occur annually. Lung cancer is responsible for approximately 72% of SVCS cases, with an estimated 50% related to non-small cell lung cancer (NSCLC) and 22% caused by small cell lung cancer (SCLC). Median survival after cancer-related SVCS symptom presentation is about 6 months, although many patients undergoing treatment survive past 2 years. An estimated 35% of SVCS cases are caused by thrombosis or nonmalignant causes.[58]

PATHOPHYSIOLOGY

The SVC is a thin-walled blood vessel. The brachiocephalic veins feed into the SVC, which terminates in the right atrium. An extrinsic chest mass generally to the right of midline (i.e., enlarged lymph nodes, lymphoma, thymoma, inflammatory process, or aortic aneurysm) or internal thrombus compressing on the SVC can easily cause obstruction of blood flow because the chest wall and surrounding organs leave little movement for compensation. Increased venous pressure caused by the obstruction leads to increased flow through collateral blood vessels.

CLINICAL FEATURES

SVCS classically presents as progressive swelling of the head and neck. Symptoms associated with increased venous pressure of the upper body usually develop over a period of 2 weeks and include edema of the face, neck, and arms. Symptoms are severe when the obstruction occurs rapidly or below the level of the azygos vein.[57] A blanching rash represents the excess development and dilation of compensatory subcutaneous vessels of neck and anterior chest. SVCS can also manifest with cerebral edema, causing headaches, dizziness, and syncope, or laryngopharynx-related compression, causing dysphagia, dyspnea, hoarseness, and cough.[58–59]

DIAGNOSIS

Chest CT imaging with contrast is the most useful study to detect an impeding SVC compression, such as aortic aneurysm or thrombosis, before symptoms present. MRI can be used when contrast medium is contraindicated. A tissue biopsy is recommended to definitely diagnose malignancy.[54] In approximately 65% of cases, SVCS is the clinical presentation with malignancy of the lung or mediastinum.[58]

MANAGEMENT STRATEGIES

The American College of Chest Physicians and the National Comprehensive Cancer Network have made general recommendations supporting radiation and stent placement for symptomatic SVC obstruction due to NSCLC.[60] If thrombus is related to an indwelling catheter, anticoagulation is the primary treatment. Removal of the catheter and balloon dilation or stenting should be considered if fibrosis remains and the procedure is deemed clinically appropriate.[58] Management of SVCS related to malignancy is guided by the severity of symptoms and anticipated response to the cancer. The prognosis for SVCS correlates with the underlying diagnosis, with better outcomes for hematological malignancies versus solid tumors.[59] In all cases, the goal of treatment should be to alleviate the bothersome symptoms of the obstruction.

In cases of SCLC and lymphoma, treatment with radiation or chemotherapy alone have been found to be equally effective in relieving symptoms of SVCS. Radiation is best for well-defined tumors that are less chemo-sensitive, such as NSCLC. SVCS symptoms usually show improvement within 72 hours of radiation and resolve within 1–2 weeks after chemotherapy or radiation therapy.[56]

Placement of a stent relieves symptoms within hours and is optimal for recurrent SVCS related to malignancy when the goal is to avoid the toxic effects of repeating chemotherapy or radiation.[61] While rare, complications with stenting the SVC are related to stent misplacement.[58] Once a stent is placed, consideration should be given to anticoagulation and implications for management of SVCS recurrence, which occurs in an estimated 20–50% of patients. Researchers have used oral aspirin as antiplatelet preventative maintenance therapy after 3–4 days of complete heparinization after stent placement.[59]

The palliative APRN should be vigilant for SVCS in patients with implanted devices, those with malignant conditions, or those with predisposing risks for cancer (smoking, asbestos exposure). Management is focused on determining and treating the root cause of SVCS. Palliative therapy is focused on addressing symptoms and may include elevating the head, diuretics, steroids, stenting, or surgical removal of the offending mass or intravascular device.

SUMMARY

The National Consensus Project for Quality Palliative Care *Clinical Practice Guidelines* Domain 2: Physical Aspects of Care focuses on expert assessment and management of physical aspects of care and screening for and relieving distressing physical symptoms, which includes palliative emergencies.[62]

The palliative APRN must have knowledge about disease trajectories with the potential for hemorrhage, MSCC, seizures, and SVCS. Caring for patients with these diagnoses, the APRN must understand the assessment, physical examination, and diagnostic procedures that lead to their diagnosis and create a care plan that includes anticipatory management which may depend on the care setting.

When these palliative emergencies do occur, the palliative APRN must collaborate with the palliative interdisciplinary team and other specialties to support the patient and family. Of course, educating the patient, family, and other healthcare staff is critical to understanding the necessity for a proactive rapid response. In cases where emergently distressing symptoms are intractable, the care plan should include medications to relieve suffering and ensure a peaceful, dignified death, including palliative sedation.

REFERENCES

1. Akinola O, Baru J, Marks S. Terminal hemorrhage preparation and management #297. *J Palliat Med.* 2015;18(12):1074–1075. doi:10.1089/jpm.2015.0244

2. Gershman E, Guthrie R, Swiatek K, Shojaee S. Management of hemoptysis in patients with lung cancer. *Ann Transl Med.* 2019;7(15):358. doi:10.21037/atm.2019.04.91

3. Smith LN, Jackson VA. How do symptoms change for patients in the last days and hours of life. In: Goldstein N, Morrison R, eds. *Evidence-Based Practice of Palliative Medicine.* Philadelphia, PA: Elsevier Saunders; 2013: 218–224.

4. Abt D, Bywater M, Engeler DS, Schmid HP. Therapeutic options for intractable hematuria in advanced bladder cancer. *Int J Urol.* 2013;20(7):651–660. doi:10.1111/iju.12113

5. McGrath P, Leahy M. Catastrophic bleeds during end-of-life care in haematology: Controversies from Australian research. *Support Care Cancer.* 2009;17(5):527–537. doi:10.1007/s00520-008-0506-1

6. Johnstone C, Rich SE. Bleeding in cancer patients and its treatment: A review. *Ann Palliat Med.* 2018;7(2):265–273. doi:10.21037/apm.2017.11.01

7. Pori D. Herbs and clotting. Eat Right to Fight Cancer. Oncology Nutrition. Academy of Nutrition and Dietetics 2021. https://www.oncologynutrition.org/erfc/healthy-nutrition-now/dietary-supplements/herbs-blood-clotting

8. Sood R, Mancinetti M, Betticher D, Cantin B, Ebneter A. Management of bleeding in palliative care patients in the general internal medicine ward: A systematic review. *Ann Med Surg (Lond).* 2019 Dec 18;50:14–23. doi:10.1016/j.amsu.2019.12.002

9. Leigh A, Tucker R. What techniques can be used in the hospital or home setting to best manage uncontrollable bleeding. In: Goldstein N, Morrison R, eds. *Evidence-Based Practice of Palliative Medicine.* Philadelphia, PA: Elsevier Saunders; 2013: 398–401.

10. Ghahestani SM, Shakhssalim N. Palliative treatment of intractable hematuria in context of advanced bladder cancer: A systematic review. *Urol J.* 2009;6(3):149–156.

11. Groninger H, Phillips JM. Gross hematuria: Assessment and management at the end of life. *J Hosp Palliat Nurs.* 2012 12;14(3):184–188. doi:10.1097/NJH.0b013e31824fc169

12. Alberti LR, Santos RS, Castro AFD, et al. Upper gastrointestinal bleeding in oncological patients. *Gastroenterol Hepatol Open Access.* 2016;4(6):00123. doi:10.15406/ghoa.2016.04.00123

13. Green B, Cairns S, Harvey R, Pettit M. Phytomenadione or menadiol in the management of an elevated international normalized ratio (prothrombin time). *Aliment Pharmacol Ther.* 2000;14(12):1685–1689. doi:10.1046/j.1365-2036.2000.00880.x

14. Gergi M, Soriano-Pisaturo MA. Palliative care issues for transfusion-dependent patients #359. *J Palliat Med.* 2018;21(9):1359–1360. doi:10.1089/jpm.2018.0347

15. LeBlanc TW, Litzow MR. Are transfusions a barrier to high-quality-end-of-life care in hematology. *Hematologist.* 2018;15;13. https://ashpublications.org/thehematologist/article/doi/10.1182/hem.V17.3.10356/461798/Hematology-Advocates-Raise-Palliative-Care-Issues

16. Singleton JM, Hefner M. Spinal cord compression. *StatPearls [Internet].* Treasure Island, FL: StatPearls Publishing. 2021 Jan-. Available from: https://www.ncbi.nlm.nih.gov/books/NBK557604/

17. Laufer I, Schiff D, Kelly H, Bilsky M. In: Drews R, Wen P. ed. Clinical features and diagnosis of neoplastic epidural spinal cord compression. *UpToDate.* Waltham, MA: UptoDate. Updated Feb 9, 2021. https://www.uptodate.com/contents/clinical-features-and-diagnosis-of-neoplastic-cpidural-spinal-cord-compression

18. Wänman J, Grabowski P, Nyström H, et al. Metastatic spinal cord compression as the first sign of malignancy. *Acta Orthop.* 2017;88(4):457–462. doi:10.1080/17453674.2017.1319179

19. Savage P, Sharkey R, Kua T, et al. Malignant spinal cord compression: NICE guidance, improvements and challenges. *QJM.* 2014;107(4):277–282. doi:10.1093/qjmed/hct244

20. da Silva GT, Bergmann A, Santos Thuler LC. Prognostic factors in patients with metastatic spinal cord compression secondary to lung cancer: A systematic review of the literature. *Eur Spine J.* 2015;24(10):2107–2113. doi:10.1007/s00586-015-4157-x

21. Robertson Q, Gershon K. Urgent syndromes at end of life. In: Ferrell B, Paice J eds. *Oxford Textbook of Palliative Nursing.* 5th ed. New York: Oxford University Press; 2019: 344–355.

22. Le R, Tran JD, Lizaso M, Beheshti R, Moats A. Surgical intervention vs. radiation therapy: The shifting paradigm in treating metastatic spinal disease. *Cureus.* 2018;10(10):e3406. Published 2018 Oct 3. doi:10.7759/cureus.3406

23. Loblaw DA, Perry J, Chambers A, Laperriere NJ. Systematic review of the diagnosis and management of malignant extradural spinal cord compression: The Cancer Care Ontario Practice Guidelines Initiative's Neuro-Oncology Disease Site Group. *J Clin Oncol.* 2005;23(9):2028–2037. doi:10.1200/JCO.2005.00.067

24. Abrahm JL, Banffy MB, Harris MB. Spinal cord compression in patients with advanced metastatic cancer: "All I care about is walking and living my life". *JAMA.* 2008;299(8):937–46. doi:10.1001/jama.299.8.937

25. Mehta RS, Arnold R. Fast facts and concepts #238: Management of spinal cord compression. Appleton, WI: Palliative Care Network of Wisconsin. Updated Nov 2015. https://www.mypcnow.org/fast-fact/management-of-spinal-cord-compression/

26. National Collaborating Centre for Cancer (UK). *Metastatic Spinal Cord Compression: Diagnosis and Management of Patients at Risk of or with Metastatic Spinal Cord Compression.* Cardiff, UK: National Collaborating Centre for Cancer; Nov 2008.

27. Hofland P. Single dose radiation therapy may help relieve debilitating spinal cord compression. *ASCO.* Onco'Zine. Jun 6, 2017. https://www.oncozine.com/single-dose-radiation-therapy-may-help-relieve-debilitating-spinal-cord-compression/

28. Abdelmunim L, Elanabi M, gafer N. Study of radiation therapy treatment effect in pain management for metastatic breast cancer in RICK. *Open Acc J Oncol Med.* 2019; 2(5). doi:10.32474/OAJOM.2019.02.000147

29. Lutz S, Balboni T, Jones J, et al. Palliative radiation therapy for bone metastases: Update of an ASTRO Evidence-Based Guideline. *Pract Radiat Oncol.* 2017;7(1):4–12. doi:10.1016/j.prro.2016.08.001

30. Fortin CD, Voth J, Jaglal SB, Craven BC. Inpatient rehabilitation outcomes in patients with malignant spinal cord compression compared to other non-traumatic spinal cord injury: A population based study. *J Spinal Cord Med.* 2015;38(6):754–764. doi:10.1179/2045772314Y.0000000278

31. Ruff RL, Adamson VW, Ruff SS, Wang X. Directed rehabilitation reduces pain and depression while increasing independence and satisfaction with life for patients with paraplegia due to

epidural metastatic spinal cord compression. *J Rehabil Res Dev.* 2007;44(1):1–10. doi:10.1682/jrrd.2005.10.0168

32. Fisher RS, Cross JH, Fisher RS, et al. Operational classification of seizure types by the International League Against Epilepsy: Position Paper of the ILAE Commission for Classification and Terminology. *Epilepsia,* 2017;58(4):522–530. doi:10.1111/epi.13670

33. Douglas VC, Aminoff MJ. Nervous system disorders: Epilepsy. In: Papadakis MA, McPhee SJ, Rabow MW. eds. *Current Medical Diagnosis & Treatment.* New York: McGraw-Hill; 2020;24(03): 1–9. https://accessmedicine.mhmedical.com/content.aspx?bookid=2449&sectionid=194575853

34. Lee RK, et al. ACR appropriateness criteria seizures and epilepsy. *J Am Coll Radiol,* 17(5S): S293–S304. doi:10.1016/j.jacr.2020.01.037

35. Benedict M, St Louis EK. Status epilepticus. In: Ebell MH, Lin K, Shaughnessy AF, eds. Essential Evidence Plus. Wiley. 2021:1–6. Last updated July 10, 2021. https://www.essentialevidenceplus-com/content/eee/459

36. Louis EK, Benedict M. Seizure disorder (adult). In: Ebell MH, Lin K, Ferenchick G, eds. Essential Evidence Plus. Wiley. 2021:1–12. Last updated July 10, 2021. https://www.essentialevidenceplus-com/

37. Holtkamp M, Beghi E, Benninger F, et al. European Stroke Organization guidelines for the management of post-stroke seizures and epilepsy. *Eur Stroke J.* 2017;2(2):103–115. doi:10.1177/2396987317705536

38. Bénit CP, Vecht CJ. Seizures and cancer: Drug interactions of anticonvulsants with chemotherapeutic agents, tyrosine kinase inhibitors and glucocorticoids. *Neurooncol Pract.* 2016;3(4):245–260. doi:10.1093/nop/npv038

39. Grönheit W, Popkirov S, Wehner T, Schlegel U, Wellmer J. Practical management of epileptic seizures and status epilepticus in adult palliative care patients. *Front Neurol.* 2018;9:595. Published 2018 Aug 2. doi:10.3389/fneur.2018.00595

40. Harden C, Tomson T, Gloss D, et al. Practice guideline summary: Sudden unexpected death in epilepsy incidence rates and risk factors: Report of the Guideline Development, Dissemination, and Implementation Subcommittee of the American Academy of Neurology and the American Epilepsy Society. *Epilepsy Curr.* 2017;17(3):180–187. doi:10.5698/1535-7511.17.3.180

41. Their K, Calabek B, Tinchon A, Grisold W, Oberndorfer S. The last 10 days of patients with glioblastoma. *Am J Hosp Palliat Med.* 2016;33(10):985–988. doi:10.1177/1049909115609295

42. Shin JY, Kizilbash SH, Robinson SI, et al. Seizures in patients with primary brain tumors: What is their psychosocial impact?. *J Neurooncol.* 2016;128(2):285–291. doi:10.1007/s11060-016-2108-y

43. Wasilewski A, Serventi J, Kamalyan L, Wychowski T, Mohile N. Acute care in glioblastoma: The burden and the consequences. *Neuro-Oncology Practice.* 2017;4(4):248–254. doi:10.1093/nop/npw032

44. Shin JY, et al. Incidence, characteristics, and implications of seizures in patients with glioblastoma. *Am J Hosp Palliat Med.* 2017;34(7):650–651. doi:10.1177/1049909116647405

45. Wiss AL, Samarin M, Marler J, Jones GM. Continuous infusion antiepileptic medications for refractory status epilepticus. *Crit Care Nurs Q.* 2017;40(1):67–85. doi:10.1097/CNQ.0000000000000143

46. Alkhachroum A, Der-Nigoghossian CA, Rubinos C, Claassen J. Markers in status epilepticus prognosis. *J Clin Neurophysiol.* 2020;37(5):422–428. doi:10.1097/WNP.0000000000000761

47. Khan TV, Alkire S, Chirunomula S. Neurology. In: David JA, eds. *Current Practice Guidelines in Inpatient Medicine.* 2019;4:1–14. New York: McGraw-Hill. https://accessmedicine-mhmedical-com.ezp.lib.rochester.edu/content.aspx?bookid=2378&sectionid=186647316

48. Daly FN, Lugassy MM. Hospice and end of life care in neurologic disease. In: Creutzfeldt CJ, Kluger BM, Holloway RG, eds. *Neuropalliative Care: A Guide to Improving the Lives of Patients and Families Affected by Neurologic Disease.* Cham: Springer; 2019: 221–236.

49. Lyttle MD, Rainford NEA, Gamble C, et al. Levetiracetam versus phenytoin for second-line treatment of paediatric convulsive status epilepticus (EcLiPSE): A multicentre, open-label, randomised trial. *Lancet.* 2019;393(10186):2125–2134. doi:10.1016/S0140-6736(19)30724-X

50. Maguire MJ, Jackson CF, Marson AG, Nevitt SJ. Treatments for the prevention of Sudden Unexpected Death in Epilepsy (SUDEP). *Cochrane Database Syst Rev* 2020;4(4):CD011792. Published 2020 Apr 2. doi:10.1002/14651858.CD011792.pub3

51. Devinsky O, Patel AD, Cross JH, et al. Effect of cannabidiol on drop seizures in the Lennox-Gastaut syndrome. *N Engl J Med.* 2018;378(20):1888–1897. doi:10.1056/NEJMoa1714631

52. Trinka E, Höfler J, Leitinger M, Brigo F. Pharmacotherapy for status epilepticus. *Drugs.* 2015;75(13):1499–1521. doi:10.1007/s40265-015-0454-2 53. Sharma A, Taylor LP. Malignant brain tumors. In: Creutzfeldt CJ, Kluger BM, Holloway RG, eds. *Neuropalliative Care: A Guide to Improving the Lives of Patients and Families Affected by Neurologic Disease.* Cham: Springer; 2019, 117–134.

54. Stocksdale B, Nagpal S, Hixson JD, et al. Clinical debate: Long-term antiepileptic drug prophylaxis in patients with glioma. *Neurooncol Pract.* 2020;7(6):583–588. doi:10.1093/nop/npaa026

55. Bergo E, Lombardi G, Guglieri I, Capovilla E, Pambuku A, Zagone V. Neurocognitive functions and health-related quality of life in glioblastoma patients: A concise review of the literature. *Eur J Cancer Care (Engl).* 2019;28(1):e12410. doi:10.1111/ecc.12410

56. Yeung S, Manzullo EF. Oncologic emergencies. In: Kantarjian HM, Wolff RA, eds. *The MD Anderson Manual of Medical Oncology.* 3rd ed. New York: McGraw-Hill; 2016:53(3). https://accessmedicine.mhmedical.com/content.aspx?bookid=1772&sectionid=121903052

57. Straka C, Ying J, Kong FM, Willey CD, Kaminski J, Kim DW. Review of evolving etiologies, implications and treatment strategies for the superior vena cava syndrome. *Springerplus.* 2016;5:229. Published 2016 Feb 29. doi:10.1186/s40064-016-1900-7

58. Murrow J, Talluri SK, Besur SV. *Superior vena cava syndrome. Essential Evidence Plus.* Wiley. 2021:1–4. Last updated March 22, 2021. https://www-essentialevidenceplus-com/content/eee/54

59. Morin S, Grateau A, Reuter D, et al. Management of superior vena cava syndrome in critically ill cancer patients. *Support Care Cancer.* 2018;26(2):521–528. doi:10.1007/s00520-017-3860-z

60. Simoff MJ, Lally B, Slade MG, et al. Symptom management in patients with lung cancer: Diagnosis and management of lung cancer, 3rd ed.: American College of Chest Physicians evidence-based clinical practice guidelines. *Chest.* 2013;143(5 Suppl):e455S–e497S. doi:10.1378/chest.12-2366

61. Ameli-Renani S, Belli AM, Chun JY, Morgan RA. Peripheral vascular disease intervention. In: Adam A, Dixon A, Gilliard J, Schaefer-Prokop C. eds. *Grainger & Allison's Diagnostic Radiology.* 7th ed. Philadelphia: Elsevier; 2021:80, 2094–2112.

62. Dy SM, Kiley KB, Ast K, et al. Measuring what matters: Top-ranked quality indicators for hospice and palliative care from the American Academy of Hospice and Palliative Medicine and Hospice and Palliative Nurses Association. *J Pain Symptom Manage.* 2015;49(4):773–781. doi:10.1016/j.jpainsymman.2015.01.012

52.

CHALLENGING SYMPTOMS

PRURITUS, HICCUPS, DRY MOUTH, FEVERS, AND SLEEP DISORDERS

Barton T. Bobb and Devon S. Wojcikewych

KEY POINTS

- The palliative advanced practice registered nurse (APRN) must have a working knowledge of the symptoms of pruritus, hiccups, dry mouth, fever, and sleep disorders so they can be effectively managed.

- Pruritus can be challenging to treat; determining the cause when possible can help tailor treatment.

- Hiccups are a common symptom; though seemingly benign, they can affect quality of life.

- Dry mouth is a common symptom among palliative care patients, especially cancer patients.

- Fever may require scheduled antipyretic treatment at end of life if it is believed to be distressing.

- Sleep disorders can also cause distress. The most common one, primary insomnia, has a variety of potential treatment options that may require titration/rotation.

CASE STUDY: CHALLENGING SYMPTOMS

Ms. B was a 60-year-old woman with advanced cirrhosis and hepatocellular carcinoma with associated pain. She had been followed by a palliative advanced practice registered nurse (APRN) in a palliative care clinic. The short-acting opioid that best managed her pain after multiple attempts at opioid rotation, immediate-release morphine, unfortunately caused some pruritus. The palliative APRN prescribed oral hydroxyzine 25 mg every 6 hours, as needed.

Ms. B also complained of ongoing dry mouth as well as difficulty sleeping at night. She used sugar-free chewing gum and was prescribed 5 mg oral pilocarpine three times a day to stimulate saliva production. Saliva substitutes were prescribed as well. A variety of sleep hygiene measures were suggested to help her sleep. Oral mirtazapine 7.5 mg nightly was prescribed. With sleep medications, pain medications, changes in sleep hygiene, and improved pain control, Ms. B reported more consecutive hours of uninterrupted sleep. Cholestyramine was added for worsening pruritus that was likely caused by cholestasis.

After several months, Ms. B's disease progressed, and she was actively dying at home with hospice. Because she was running high fevers that appeared to be distressing to her and her family,

the attending hospice APRN ordered scheduled acetaminophen rectal suppositories every 6 hours. Her oral pain medications were switched to home IV fentanyl patient-controlled analgesia (PCA). The palliative APRN made a home visit to check on her and her family. She appeared to be very comfortable. Her family expressed appreciation for all the care the APRN had provided for her and them over the past several months. Ms. B died peacefully 3 days later.

PRURITUS

The word *pruritus* comes from the Latin *prurire*, meaning "to itch." Pruritus causes a desire to scratch. This scratch reflex is meant to be a protective mechanism, but when this sensation becomes chronic, there can be significant emotional and physical consequences.[1-5] The impact of itch on quality of life, sleep, anxiety, and depression can be very distressing, and this symptom must not be overlooked.

The physiology of the itch sensation has been increasingly studied over recent years but is proving to be a diverse and complex symptom that is still not completely understood. The mechanism of itch was initially thought to be a subset of the pain transmission pathway but is now thought to be significantly more complicated than this and may differ depending on the underlying cause.[6-12] Chronic pruritus can also lead to neural sensitization, like that found in chronic pain.[13] There are increasingly identified neuropeptide targets associated with itch, and, as the understanding of these mechanisms improve, so do the potential targets for its treatment.[11-14]

ETIOLOGY

Determining the trigger for the itch reflex can be challenging and cannot always be identified. Often patients may have overlapping or multiple causes of pruritus as well. When possible, however, determining the cause can help direct the choice of treatment, especially as different molecular pathways of itch for specific disease states are further identified. As with any assessment, a detailed history and physical exam should be performed because teasing out any primary dermatologic conditions, systemic disease, or neurologic or psychiatric/psychosomatic diseases may help determine referral and treatment options.[15-18]

Primary Dermatologic Causes

Pruritus is the most commonly reported symptom in dermatologic disorders as a whole.[19] Often itch-producing stimuli are short-lived or self-limiting and usually can be treated effectively by a primary care provider or other first-line providers. Causes of primary dermatologic conditions can range from dry skin and insect bites to dermatologic malignancies. Atopic dermatitis and prurigo nodularis are known to be especially associated with pruritus.[4] Depending on the severity of the symptoms, the advanced practice registered nurse (APRN) may need to refer to a dermatology specialist.

Systemic Diseases

Pruritus can manifest in many systemic diseases (Table 52.1). A large percentage of patients with cholestatic liver disease report pruritus. Bile salt accumulation was previously thought to be the underlying cause, but more recent studies have increased knowledge of the mechanism of itch in cholestatic liver disease. There are now thought to be multiple potential targets to interrupt the itch pathways in cholestatic liver disease, including endogenous opioid receptors.[8,17,20–22]

Chronic renal insufficiency is another systemic disease with a high symptom burden from pruritus, especially in patients on chronic hemodialysis.[19,23–25] As in cholestatic liver disease, activation of endogenous opioid receptors are thought to be important mediators of itch in this patient population.[23–25] Metabolic derangements in renal disease, such as hypercalcemia, hyperphosphatemia, and hypermagnesemia, seem to contribute independently to pruritus as well.[17] Endocrinopathies such as hyperparathyroidism, both hypothyroidism and hyperthyroidism, and diabetes are all associated with itching as well.[17,19,26,27]

Multiple hematopoietic disorders, ranging from the more benign iron deficiency anemia and polycythemia vera to malignancies such as lymphoma and multiple myeloma, can cause itching or chronic pruritus. T-cell lymphomas, such as Sézary syndrome, are characterized by a high incidence of pruritus and commonly require the assistance of a palliative provider for more advanced interventions.[17,28,29]

Multiple infectious diseases can also cause local and systemic pruritus, including hepatitis and herpetic infections. Chronic pruritus is recognized in HIV-positive patients; it appears to be independent of primary dermatologic sources of itch.[5,30]

Medications

Any medication can cause itching from an allergic reaction or sensitivity. Certain medications or illicit drugs commonly known to cause itching include opiates, amphetamines, cocaine, heparin, niacin, aspirin, certain antibiotics, calcium channel blockers, and angiotensin-converting enzyme (ACE) inhibitors.[19,31]

Neurologic

Patients with stroke or brain tumor (either primary or due to metastatic disease) can have a centrally mediated itch. There are also peripheral neuropathic itch syndromes, such as postherpetic itch and notalgia paresthetica.[15,32]

Psychiatric

Pruritus is reported to be common in psychiatric conditions, such as psychosis, delirium, and delusional parasitosis, but epidemiologic data on the actual prevalence are lacking.[19,33,34] In addition, anxiety and depression are thought to worsen the patient's ability to cope with pruritus of other etiologies.[34] The palliative APRN may need to collaborate with psychiatric colleagues to manage these causes for effective treatment.

TREATMENT

Treatment of systemic pruritus is often difficult, likely in part due to its complex and overlapping signaling pathways. Balancing the side effects against the benefit of a treatment is always at the core of the palliative APRN's decision to administer or prescribe therapeutic agents. If the pruritus is from a disease process or a medication that cannot be removed, then treatment modalities range from topical therapies and

Table 52.1 SYSTEMIC CAUSES OF PRURITUS

Autoimmune	Endocrinopathy	Hematologic/oncologic
Dermatitis herpetiformis	Hyper/hypothyroid	Lymphoma/Leukemia
Dermatomyositis	Hyperparathyroid	Systemic mastocytosis
Linear immunoglobulin A	Diabetes mellitus	Multiple myeloma
	Carcinoid syndrome	Polycythemia vera
		Iron-deficiency anemia
Infectious diseases	Medications	Biliary and hepatic disease
HIV/AIDS	Opioids	
Infectious hepatitis	Amphetamines	Chronic renal insufficiency/uremia
Parasitic disease	Cocaine	
Prion disease	Niacin	
Herpetic	Aspirin	
	Heparin	
	Calcium channel blockers	
	ACE inhibitors	

systemic medications to invasive interventions in which the symptom burden should outweigh the risk of treatment. The evidence basis for treatment of pruritus is varied based on cause of pruritus and may be difficult to generalize. The palliative APRN should be prepared for a stepwise trial approach to determine what interventions are effective at relieving pruritus.

Initial nonpharmacologic interventions include patient and family education on methods to decrease itching, such as wearing lightweight clothing and lowering the room temperature and keeping the skin moisturized. The palliative APRN should also continue to monitor the patient's skin for excoriation and secondary infections from scratching as well.[1,15]

Topical Treatments

Topical barrier creams are often recommended for most causes of itch (Box 52.1). Topical treatments are less likely to be helpful when pruritus is due to a systemic cause, however.[15,19] Prescription topical therapies include steroids, calcineurin inhibitors such as pimecrolimus and tacrolimus, and crisaborole, a phosphodiesterase-4 inhibitor.[12]

Systemic Treatments

Systemic therapies are varied (Table 52.2), and, when possible, systemic therapy should be directed toward the source of pruritus. Understanding the multiple itch-inducing mechanisms, often different for varying diseases, has led to further targets for symptom management of pruritus in these systemic diseases. Some of the newer targets for pruritus treatment include opioid receptors, tropomyosin receptor kinase A antagonists, voltage-gated sodium channel (Nav 1.7) antagonists, phosphodiesterase-4 inhibitors, interleukin antagonists, janus kinase inhibitors, histamine-4 receptor antagonists, ileal bile acid transporter (IBAT) inhibitors, aryl hydrocarbon receptor (AhR) agonists, and monoclonal Anti-IgE antibodies. There has been an extensive increase in research into this troubling symptom in the past decade, but further understanding is still needed.[11–13,15,35]

Antihistamines are generally trialed for all types of pruritus at some point due to a relatively benign side-effect profile but are particularly helpful for pruritus that is known to be histamine-mediated, such as that seen in allergy-mediated

---

Box 52.1 TOPICAL TREATMENTS OF PRURITUS

Calamine
Menthol
Oatmeal bath
Antihistamines
Steroids
Capsaicin
Lidocaine
Calcineurin inhibitors
Crisaborole

Table 52.2 SYSTEMIC TREATMENTS OF PRURITUS

Antihistamines Diphenhydramine Doxylamine Hydroxyzine	Bile sequestrants Cholestyramine Colestipol	μ-Opioid antagonists Naloxone Naltrexone
Mixed μ-opioid antagonists/κ-opioid agonists Butorphanol Nalbuphine	Neuroleptics Gabapentin Pregabalin	Antidepressants SSRIs Mirtazapine Doxepin
Neurokinin receptor-1 (NK-1) antagonist Aprepitant	Immunosuppressants Steroids Cyclosporin A Methotrexate Azathioprine Mycophenolate mofetil	Cannabinoids Rifampicin

---

skin diseases. A non-histaminergic mechanism is more commonly seen in chronic pruritus, however.[36] Side effects of antihistamines commonly include drowsiness and dry mouth; the former can be helpful if the patient is experiencing pruritus at night affecting sleep but can limit use if causing sedation during the day.[35] The second-generation antihistamines may be less sedating.

Opiate rotation should be considered for patients experiencing pruritus associated with opiate use. If this is not possible, the use of an opioid receptor antagonist such as naloxone or naltrexone may be helpful. Intravenous naloxone is not a realistic treatment option for outpatient, home management or long-term use because its half-life is too short, but it can be given by intravenous infusion for acute symptoms.[13,37] Opiate antagonism can produce side effects similar to opiate withdrawal, and patients should be warned of this prior to use; opiates may not be appropriate for palliative patients on chronic opiate therapy for pain control.[36] The increasing understanding of μ- and κ-opioid receptors in the pathologic itch of cholestatic liver disease and chronic kidney disease and the improved symptoms seen with naltrexone warrants consideration of this treatment in certain situations, however.[23,24,38,39] Newer mixed μ-opioid antagonists/κ-opioid agonists are also helpful for treatment of opiate-induced pruritus and uremic pruritus specifically.[24,37,40] κ-opioid receptor antagonists are not available in the United States currently, but some initial studies in other countries and clinical trials are promising, especially for uremia associated pruritus, but potentially for other etiologies as well.[12,13,35]

Bile sequestrant medications, such as cholestyramine and colestipol, are often used as first-line agents to control pruritus in cholestatic liver disease. Cholestyramine is the only medication approved by the US Food and Drug Administration (FDA) for cholestatic pruritus.[41] It is of note that levels of bile acids do not always correlate with intensity of itch, however, and often these medications are not helpful.[36,41] Compliance difficulties can arise for these medications because they can be unpleasant to swallow, and there should be a 4-hour interval before taking other oral medications. Ileal bile acid transporter inhibitors are another class under investigation for treatment of pruritus in cholestatic liver disease.[36]

Rifampicin has been found to be helpful for pruritus in hepatic cholestasis as a second-line agent. Its utility is limited due to potential hepatotoxicity, but continued studies suggest it may be considered in certain cases.[42,43]

Neuroleptics like gabapentin, an α-2-δ calcium channel ligand, seem to be effective for neurologic causes of itching. Both gabapentin and pregabalin have increasing data supporting their use in the treatment of pruritus associated with uremia. Both medications can be associated with drowsiness, among other side effects.[44–46]

Serotonin reuptake inhibitors, such as sertraline, paroxetine, and fluvoxamine, as well as mirtazapine, a tetracyclic antidepressant, and doxepin, a tricyclic antidepressant, have all shown some benefit in pruritus caused by various etiologies.[35,47–49]

Antiemetics, such as ondansetron, a type 3 (5-HT3) serotonin receptor antagonist, were previously used to relieve itch because serotonin was thought to play a role in the mechanism of pruritus, but this is controversial and further randomized controlled trials suggest ondansetron may not be as helpful for pruritus related to hepatic cholestatic disease and chronic renal disease.[44,50]

Aprepitant, a neurokinin receptor-1 (NK-1) antagonist used as an antiemetic, blocks the binding of substance P and has been shown to be helpful in patients with treatment-refractory pruritus from T-cell lymphoma and nodular prurigo, and it does seem to have relatively minimal side effects.[51] Several newer NK-1 receptor antagonists are being researched and show promise for the treatment of pruritus as well.[52] Due to NK-1 receptor antagonist's cost, the utility in comparison to established treatments for pruritus needs further studies, however, and it may not be superior to these older treatments.[53]

Due to continued legalization of marijuana in the United States and the potential use for cannabinoids in treating multiple symptoms encountered by the palliative APRN, it is important to be aware of ongoing evaluations of the efficacy and safety of cannabinoids for pruritus, including for topical use.[36,54,55]

Immunosuppressants such as topical steroids are frequently used for allergic or immune-induced dermatologic disorders, and oral steroids are thought to help reduce itch only if an inflammatory component is present. Because of the side effects of long-term steroid use, providers should exhaust other treatments before using steroids for systemic pruritus. Other immunosuppressants and monoclonal antibodies are not typically used by the palliative APRN, but it is important to be aware of evolving research of the uses for these treatments against pruritus. The APRN may need specialty consultation from subspecialists who regularly use these treatment modalities.[12,13,15]

Interventional Treatments

Several interventions for pruritus, mostly pruritus caused by liver disease, have been developed for patients with symptoms refractory to less invasive treatments (Box 52.2). A

Box 52.2 INTERVENTIONAL TREATMENTS FOR PRURITUS

Acupuncture
Biliary drainage
Hemodialysis
Liver transplantation
Parathyroidectomy
Phototherapy
Plasmapheresis
Transcutaneous nerve stimulation

---

patient's ability to withstand these interventions depends on overall prognosis and clinical status. Patients with primary biliary cirrhosis with cholestatic disease may be liver transplant candidates based on severe pruritus symptoms alone.[56] Phototherapy seems to have an increasing evidence basis for treating a variety of primary dermatologic and systemic causes of pruritus.[17,57–59] Extracorporeal albumin dialysis, nasobiliary drainage, plasmapheresis, and charcoal hemoperfusion may be beneficial in relieving chronic pruritus, but their benefit seems to be short lived and likely the risk and burden of these treatments would outweigh the benefit.[36] Therapies such as acupuncture[60] and transcutaneous nerve stimulation[61] have shown some promise and may be worth exploring; however, currently there is relatively little evidence to support their use.

HICCUPS

Hiccup, or *singultus* in medical terms, is derived from the Latin word *singult*, which means "the act of catching one's breath while sobbing."[62] Most people experience hiccups periodically, but when hiccups are persistent (>48 hours) or intractable (>1 month), they can become a burdensome symptom, severely affecting quality of life.[62,63]

Epidemiologic studies of prevalence are limited, although it is believed that persistent or intractable hiccups are relatively uncommon; as a result, minimal research has been done to test the effectiveness of treatments.[64] The actual number of patients suffering from hiccups affecting quality of life may be higher in the palliative care population, but it is thought that nearly one-third of patients with esophageal cancer may report this symptom[65] and by some estimates, hiccups may affect up to 9% of patients treated in palliative care settings.[66,67] Despite this statistic there are very few palliative-specific studies to help guide management, and most evidence for treatment is derived from non-palliative patient studies.[66,68,69]

ETIOLOGY

Hiccups represent an involuntary spasm of the diaphragm and accessory respiratory muscles. The hiccup reflex involves the afferent vagal, phrenic, and sympathetic nerves; the brainstem; and the efferent phrenic nerve to the glottis, diaphragm, and inspiratory respiratory muscle. The causes of hiccups can be varied, but they generally result from an irritation of the diaphragm directly or of the nervous system controlling these muscles.[62]

Causes of hiccups can be divided into several broad categories (Box 52.3), and identifying the cause can often help treat the symptom. Hiccups can result from direct irritation of the vagus or phrenic nerve reflexes by various causes such intubation, endoscopy, surgery, radiation, cancer infiltration, or esophageal stenting, as a few examples.[70,71] Gastric distention and gastroesophageal reflux are among the more common causes of persistent hiccups and should be treated if suspected.[62,64,71,72] Ruling out serious pathology in cases of persistent hiccups is important. Hiccups have been shown to be the initial presenting symptom for a gastrointestinal malignancy, such as esophageal cancer.[62] Hiccups have also been reported as a symptom in myocardial infarction and pulmonary embolism.[65,73,74] Toxic and metabolic causes such as alcohol, infections, and uremia are also reported causes. Central nervous system disorders such as head trauma, stroke,

and intracranial malignancies are thought to be causes of intractable hiccups, with an especially high frequency (20%) in patients with Parkinson's disease.[75-77] Medications such as corticosteroids, opiates, benzodiazepines, and chemotherapeutic agents have all been linked with hiccups.[66,69,78] This knowledge may be beneficial for palliative APRNs working with patients who are often exposed to some or all of these medications for treatment of cancer or end-of-life–related symptoms. Once organic pathology has been ruled out, psychogenic hiccups becomes a potential cause in the differential diagnosis.

TREATMENT

Nonpharmacologic Treatments

Although there are limited prospective studies on the topic, attempting vagal maneuvers and other nonpharmacologic maneuvers have minimal side effects and can potentially be effective so should be tried prior to medication management.[71,79] Valsalva maneuvers, nasopharyngeal stimulation, and inducing hypercapnia with hyperventilation and potentially even positive pressure ventilation are among the initial physical interventions that may be successful.[80,81] These maneuvers are potentially less helpful for prolonged or intractable episodes of hiccups, however.[82]

Pharmacologic Treatments

If symptoms persist or recur at a frequency where the benefit of interventions outweighs the potential side effects, several medications have been tried with some success, although no one medication has been demonstrated to consistently manage hiccups. The exact mechanism of neurotransmitters involved in intractable hiccups is not well understood, and there are many conflicting case reports and studies; therefore, directing pharmacologic treatments has been difficult.[82,83] Chlorpromazine is the only medication approved by the FDA for the treatment of persistent hiccups. Baclofen, gabapentin, and metoclopramide are the only agents that have been studied in a prospective manner, and only baclofen and metoclopramide have been studied in randomized controlled trials. Due to this, definitive recommendations are difficult to make. Thus, the APRN must consider the patient, the current medication profile, comorbidities, other medications being taken, and goals of care.[83-86]

As GI-related pathology is frequently related to recurrent or chronic hiccups, including simple gastrointestinal reflux, use of a proton pump inhibitor as an initial medication is relatively low risk and should be tried if a GI source is in the differential diagnosis as a cause of the hiccups.[81]

Metoclopramide, a prokinetic agent with central dopamine receptor antagonist properties, has the strongest evidence basis, although still limited, for treatment of intractable hiccups caused by gastric distention. Side effects include sedation, extrapyramidal symptoms and tardive dyskinesia, elevation in blood pressure, and arrhythmias due to QT prolongation.[84]

Box 52.3 CAUSES OF INTRACTABLE HICCUPS

Gastrointestinal
Esophageal distention, stenting
Gastroesophageal reflux disease (GERD)
Gastric ulcer
Gastric distention
Pancreatitis
Cholelithiasis/cystitis

Cardiovascular
Myocardial infarction
Pericarditis

Local nerve compression
Goiter
Tumor
Mediastinal lymph nodes
Abscess/infection (intubation, catheters, stents)

Pulmonary
Pneumonia
Asthma
Lung tumors
Pulmonary embolism

Central nervous system
Vascular
Tumor
Inflammation
Trauma
Infection

Systemic
Medications
Electrolyte disturbances
Infection

From Kaneishi, Kawabata.[90]

Chlorpromazine, a phenothiazine first-generation antipsychotic, is the only medication approved by the FDA for the treatment of persistent hiccups, based on older studies.[85] It is thought to potentially be effective for hiccup management due to its dopamine antagonism, but this is not well understood. Side effects include drowsiness, agitation, tardive dyskinesia, dizziness, and confusion, which may limit its use in certain patient populations. QTc prolongation may occur, and monitoring may be indicated, especially if the patient is using other medications that may also prolong QTc and increase the risk of arrhythmias.[64,83]

Baclofen, a γ-aminobutyric acid (GABA) analog used as a muscle relaxant, is emerging as the first-line treatment for central nervous system (CNS)–related intractable hiccups.[64,66,86] Baclofen's potential side effects include respiratory depression, sedation, and asthenia but are most common in patients with impaired renal function, and the APRN must take care to avoid withdrawal symptoms.

Gabapentin, an α-2-δ calcium channel ligand, has also been identified as a relatively low-burden therapy for intractable hiccups, including in advanced cancer patients.[66,72] When choosing an agent for treatment of hiccups, gabapentin is thought to be more helpful for hiccups with a CNS cause.[65] Gabapentin does not have as strong evidence as baclofen to support its use, but it may be worth considering in palliative patients for whom gabapentin may additionally be helpful for an alternative symptom, such as peripheral neuropathy. Sedation and dizziness have been identified as the major potential side effect, and titrating slowly can help avoid these. Pregabalin, another α-2-δ calcium channel ligand, may potentially be helpful for hiccups as well. Emerging concerns regarding the abuse potential and respiratory suppression of both these agents warrants close monitoring, especially if they are used in conjunction with opiates.[87]

Multiple other medications have case reports or case series to support their use, although it is of note that some are contradictory. Despite this, it is helpful to know these alternatives in case first-line medications are not helpful, as even these have relatively limited data for their use. These medications include but are not limited to olanzapine, haloperidol, risperidone, nifedipine, nimodipine, cisapride, carvedilol, midazolam, valproic acid, phenytoin, carbamazepine, amantadine, methylphenidate, and lidocaine.[64,66,69,72,75,82,88–91]

Interventional Treatments

If hiccups are persisting and affecting quality of life significantly despite the just discussed pharmacologic and nonpharmacologic interventions, several invasive therapeutic interventions have been proposed as alternatives when needed. These include surgical interventions, nerve blocks, ablations,[66,92–95] and, potentially, diaphragmatic pacing.[96] Studies evaluating acupuncture as a treatment for hiccups suggest its possible effectiveness as well, but due to the quality of evidence, conclusive recommendations for its use cannot be given; however, it may be worth considering if the burden from intractable hiccups is high.[64,97]

Dry mouth, or *xerostomia*, is common in cancer patients and patients at the end of life.[98–100] The differential diagnosis can be broadly divided into decreased saliva secretion and erosion of the buccal mucosa.[100]

Saliva secretion is regulated by both sympathetic and parasympathetic processes and involves a number of different pathways, so the pathophysiology of hyposalivation can be traced to several potential causes, including a slight disruption of the muscarinic receptors to outright obliteration of parenchymal tissue.[101] The parotid, submandibular, and sublingual glands work together to produce saliva and maintain proper consistency, so damage to any of them will affect not only the amount but also the viscosity of the saliva.[100]

Decreased saliva secretion can be caused by radiation to the head and neck, chemotherapy, a variety of medications (e.g., anticholinergics, antihistamines, tricyclic antidepressants, opioids, and sedatives), and some medical conditions (e.g., autoimmune disorders, infections, and sarcoidosis).[99,100]

Erosion of the buccal mucosa can also be caused by a variety of medical conditions (e.g., HIV/AIDS, Sjögren syndrome, systemic lupus erythematosus, and diabetes mellitus) plus chemotherapy and radiation, where higher doses and more radiation treatments also directly affect the extent and length of impairment in saliva production.[99,100] Xerostomia from dehydration can occur as a result of vomiting, diarrhea, dysphagia, oxygen use, and fever, while mental health issues, such as depression or anxiety, are potential miscellaneous causes of xerostomia.[98,100]

For the assessment of xerostomia, the palliative APRN can use several precise ways to make the diagnosis, such as measuring salivary flow or salivary gland scintigraphy, but these are usually not appropriate to the palliative care population.[98,102] A basic clinical history and focused exam should be sufficient to make the diagnosis and determine the likely etiology.[98] The inside of the mouth can be examined for signs of xerostomia, such as dry mucosa and tongue and ulceration. Two simple bedside tests to evaluate for xerostomia are the cracker biscuit test, where the patient is diagnosed to have xerostomia if unable to eat a cracker or biscuit without drinking something, and the tongue depressor test, which diagnoses xerostomia if the tongue depressor sticks to the tongue after placement.[100] There are also certain assessment tools, such as the University of Michigan Xerostomia tool, that allow patients to rate their symptoms.[100]

The management of xerostomia relies on potentially complex medication use as well as nonpharmacologic interventions (Table 52.3, Box 52.4). A general approach to management involves treating any underlying conditions (e.g., candidiasis), reviewing medications and changing those that may be contributing to xerostomia, finding ways to stimulate salivation, using saliva substitutes to replace lost saliva, and managing the xerostomia holistically in general.[100]

Mucin-based saliva substitutes appear to be better tolerated than carboxymethyl-cellulose-based ones, and sprays overall better than gels.[98,100] Contraindications to taking

Table 52.3 PHARMACOLOGIC XEROSTOMIA TREATMENTS

SALIVA STIMULANTS	SALIVA SUBSTITUTES
Pilocarpine 5–10 mg tid (primarily muscarinic agonist)	Mucin-based (e.g., Saliva Orthana)
Cevimeline 15–30 mg tid (muscarinic)	Carboxymethyl-cellulose-based (e.g., BioXtra)

From Davies[98]; Klinedinst et al.[100]; and Millsop et al.[102]

pilocarpine include asthma, bronchitis/chronic obstructive pulmonary disease, glaucoma, and heart, kidney, or liver disease.[98,100] Cevimeline should not be used in patients with acute iritis, uncontrolled asthma, or narrow-angle glaucoma.[102]

Preventative oral care interventions for patients with xerostomia should be encouraged. This includes brushing teeth regularly with fluoridated toothpaste, rinsing with a cup of warm water containing ½ teaspoon of baking soda, and using an antimicrobial rinse daily.[101] Potential interventional techniques to treat xerostomia are acupuncture and intraductal gene therapy, which is inserted via the parotid gland, but acupuncture does not have sufficient evidence to recommend it and gene therapy is in its early stages of research.[102]

The palliative APRN should focus patient and family education on good preventive and nonpharmacologic measures. Oral care is especially important throughout the disease course, including at end of life for continued comfort.[100] Ensure that the patient and family know how to use any prescription medications or over-the-counter medications. They should also understand any potential side effects, precautions, contraindications, or drug interactions.

FEVERS

Fever is generally defined as a rise in oral body temperature above 38°C (100.4°F).[1] The pathophysiology of fever is based on the presence of *pyrogens*, substances that produce fever, inducing the hypothalamus to reset the body temperature set point.[103] Pathogens release exogenous pyrogens, and the destruction of pathogens causes the body to produce endogenous pyrogens, namely interleukin-1 and -6, interferons, and tumor necrosis factor, but both types of pyrogens can ultimately induce fever.[103]

Box 52.4 NONPHARMACOLOGIC XEROSTOMIA TREATMENTS

Sugar-free chewing gum
Organic acids (ascorbic acid, citric acid, malic acid)
Water/peppermint water
Electrostimulation (embedded in a custom-made mouthguard)
Diet modifications (e.g., soft foods, increased fluid intake with meals, avoiding sugary and spicy foods)

From Davies[98]; Klinedinst et al.[100]; and Millsop et al.[102]

Clinically, fever often presents in three stages: chill, fever, and flush.[1] During the chill phase, the body is reacting to the body's new temperature set point and generates heat through shivering and tries to prevent heat loss through vasoconstriction.[1] During the fever phase, the body raises its temperature to meet the new set point, resulting in a warm feeling, lethargy, and possible dehydration or even seizures. In the flush stage, the body tries to acclimate to the new set point through diaphoresis and vasodilation.[1] Certain populations, such as immunocompromised patients, older adults, newborns, and those taking steroids, may not mount a fever response to an infection.[104]

The assessment of patients with fever usually begins with a detailed history and exam, but the extent of evaluation and further workup may vary greatly depending on the patient's prognosis and established goals.[104] When appropriate, the APRN conducts a thorough examination, looking for signs of infection and possible disease progression in cancer patients, and reviews the patient's medications; this may be followed by laboratory (e.g., blood and urine cultures, complete blood count) and radiographic (e.g., chest radiograph, computed tomography [CT] scan) testing.[104]

Some of the most common differential diagnoses of fever in palliative care patients include infection (by far the most common etiology), medications, paraneoplastic-related fevers, neurologic damage, and inflammation.[103] Neutropenic patients are particularly susceptible to infections; some common sources include wounds, the bloodstream and urinary tract, implanted vascular access devices, pneumonia, and the gastrointestinal tract.[103]

The palliative APRN must decide whether to treat the source of the fever in the first place. How much workup to pursue will depend on the patient's prognosis, potential burden versus benefit, and overall goals of care. If a workup is pursued and the source of the fever is identified, treatment of the underlying condition may involve both interventional techniques (e.g., drainage of an abscess) and complex medication options (e.g., intravenous antibiotics). In some instances, the APRN could initiate empiric antibiotics without further workup. This may be appropriate when patients have a colonized infection and antibiotics curb the infection just enough to ward off fevers.

However, when patients are actively dying, even empiric antibiotics are usually no longer indicated.[1] In fact, even symptomatic treatment of fever is not always necessary or appropriate. Fevers may not cause discomfort, but breaking the fever, and the likely resulting sweats, could cause discomfort.[103] There is also some indication that low-level fevers can have a protective function. It is ultimately the patient's decision whether the fever is bothering him or her; if the patient can no longer communicate, then the patient's family can help the palliative APRN with decision-making.[103]

For symptomatic treatment of fever, the major medication options include acetaminophen 325 to 650 mg every 4–6 hours (orally, intravenously, or rectally), nonsteroidal anti-inflammatories (NSAIDs; e.g., naproxen 225–500 mg orally every 12 hours, intravenous ketorolac 15–30 mg every 6 hours, ibuprofen 200–400 mg orally every 4–6 hours, or indomethacin 50 mg orally or rectally every 8 hours), or aspirin 325–650 mg orally or rectally every 6 hours plus corticosteroids.[103] Generally speaking, antipyretics' action centers on preventing the production of prostaglandin E2.[104] When antipyretics are administered for symptomatic relief, it is best to schedule them around the clock to avoid fluctuations in body temperature and diaphoresis with fever.[1]

Nonpharmacologic interventions to treat fevers need to be chosen carefully. Many of the treatments historically used to bring down fevers, such as ice packs, cooling blankets, cold sponge baths, or a fan blowing directly on the patient, can cause more discomfort by making the patient too cold and inducing shivering.[1] Instead, some measures that can be safely implemented to help maintain patient comfort include keeping the room temperature at a comfortable level, ensuring that the patient's bed linen and clothing are clean and dry, offering cool liquids to drink for those who can drink, and ensuring that the patient's lips are kept moist.[1,103]

The palliative APRN should be aware of the very severe side effects that can occur with excessive use of acetaminophen (liver failure) or NSAIDs (kidney failure, gastrointestinal bleed—a much higher risk with ketorolac). The patient's prognosis and goals of care could once again affect the risk-benefit ratio of administering either of these medications for symptomatic management of fever. In the actively dying patient who is believed to have discomfort from persistent fevers, the potential benefit of giving either medication on a scheduled basis should outweigh the potential risks. The treatment of any underlying infection with antibiotics may also involve careful evaluation of any potential side effects or drug interactions when prescribing them.

When the palliative APRN is treating a fever in a patient with advanced illness, especially one who is actively dying, careful patient and family education is vital. The APRN must ensure that the approach to treatment is properly established and that the patient does not accidentally receive some of the aforementioned nonpharmacologic interventions that may cause more harm than benefit (e.g., cold packs). Cool, not cold, cloths may help, as well as light bedding. Mouth care should be continued since fever causes dry mouth.[1] Patients and family members may need frequent reinforcement when the decision is made not to treat the underlying cause of a fever or its symptoms if it does not appear to be causing discomfort to the dying patient. However, if family members insist that their loved one receive symptomatic fever treatment, it may be an appropriate and palliative measure to do so.[103] When patients require symptomatic treatment for fevers earlier in the course of their disease, patients and families may require extensive education and reminders about the potential dangers of excessive NSAID or acetaminophen use.

SLEEP DISORDERS

Sleep disorders, and the associated insomnia or lack of quality sleep, are a potentially very disturbing issue for palliative patients and a challenge for the APRNs treating them. Broadly speaking, the American Academy of Sleep Medicine classifies sleep disorders into four categories: disorders of extreme somnolence; disorders of the sleep–wake cycle; difficulty initiating or maintaining sleep; and dysfunction of sleep, sleep stages, or incomplete arousal.[105] More specifically, the differential diagnoses among the major sleep disorders include primary insomnia (e.g., acute, life-long or chronic, psychological, or poor sleep hygiene), sleep apnea, restless leg syndrome, parasomnia, and narcolepsy.[106] A workup to differentiate primary insomnia from another specific sleep disorder may include the Epworth Sleepiness Scale questionnaire; an overnight polysomnogram, followed by daytime multiple sleep latency testing if evaluating for narcolepsy; use of an actigraph to study sleep–wake patterns; and other miscellaneous tests.[107] A polysomnogram positive for sleep apnea would likely be followed by a trial of continuous positive airway pressure (CPAP), possibly even done halfway through the night of a polysomnogram if the results are blatantly positive. A survey of 76 palliative care clinic patients indicated that about 40% met criteria for restless leg syndrome that reduced their quality of life negatively[108] (Box 52.5).

The most common sleep disorder is some form of simple/primary insomnia (occurs in 23–61% of cancer patients); it will be the focus of the rest of this section.[105] The normal architecture of sleep involves two major phases, rapid eye movement (REM) and non-rapid eye movement sleep (NREM).[105] During REM sleep, sometimes also called "dream sleep," the brain is very active, while NREM sleep consists of four increasingly deep, quiet, and restorative periods of sleep that together make up one sleep cycle of approximately 90 minutes.[105] The pathophysiology of insomnia is potentially quite complex involving as it does an increased level of arousal of the brain, including higher activity during NREM sleep. Genetic factors may predispose individuals to be more sensitive to external factors, such as caffeine or stress, that can subsequently disrupt the sleep–wake cycle.[105] Some other biological differences found in patients with chronic insomnia include higher levels of adrenocorticotropic hormone (ACTH), cortisol, and adrenaline release and increased body temperature compared to patients who sleep normally.[105]

The assessment of insomnia begins by obtaining a thorough sleep history from the patient and any sleeping partner and involves an evaluation of sleep chronology, environment, and hygiene in addition to any physical symptoms, medical conditions, and spiritual concerns.[106] The sleep assessment questionnaires that have been used most frequently in research include the Epworth Sleepiness Scale, the Insomnia

---

Box 52.5 **DIFFERENTIAL DIAGNOSIS OF MAJOR SLEEP DISORDERS**

Primary insomnia

Sleep apnea

Restless leg syndrome

Narcolepsy

Parasomnia

From Arnold et al.[106]

Severity Index, and the Pittsburgh Sleep Quality Index; the Insomnia Severity Index appears to have the most consistency and reliability regarding cancer patients in particular.[109]

The palliative APRN should determine whether the patient follows generally accepted sleep hygiene behaviors: (a) a regular sleep time and wake time, (b) using the bed only for sleep and sexual activity, (c) not lying in bed awake for more than about 30 minutes if unable to fall asleep at night, and (d) subsequently not returning to bed again until sleepy. The APRN should ask whether the patient takes naps during the day. Naps should be avoided, except possibly a short one between 2 and 4 PM. The APRN should assess the patient's caffeine intake in food and beverages or the use of alcoholic beverages. Finally, the APRN should assess the patient's activity level. Usually, strenuous exercise from late afternoon on should be avoided unless the patient has a very different sleep cycle. The sleep environment, such as the lighting, an unfamiliar bed, and noises, can also affect the patient's ability to sleep in a strange environment (e.g., a hospital, child's/relative's home).[106]

By assessing the sleep chronology, the course of the patient's insomnia can be determined in more detail and the palliative APRN can pinpoint whether the main issue involves sleep onset, maintenance, or both.[106] If the insomnia is an ongoing problem, there is often a medical, psychological, or neurological disorder that is at least partially responsible.[106] Medications may cause frequent awakening throughout the night, and early morning awakening is often related to depression.[106]

Medical conditions can also contribute to insomnia, including worsening of a chronic problem, such as chronic obstructive pulmonary disease or congestive heart failure; a recent or deepening depression that may also be accompanied by anxiety; a variety of medications to treat such conditions (e.g., corticosteroids, stimulants); or previously mentioned sleep disorders like restless leg syndrome.[106] Physical symptoms such as pain, shortness of breath, or cough may interfere with sleep initiation or maintenance. Spiritual distress associated with the fear of dying while asleep, together with other anxiety and the fear of uncertainty, may precipitate reluctance to fall asleep and nightmares.[106] The only sleep disorder that routinely uses an interventional technique for management is obstructive sleep apnea, which may be treated with use of a CPAP machine at night or, in some cases, can improve with uvulopalatopharyngoplasty surgery.

The management of insomnia generally consists of complex medication management and nonpharmacologic interventions. The major classes of medications approved by the FDA to treat insomnia are benzodiazepines, benzodiazepine receptor agonists, non-benzodiazepine receptor agonists, and melatonin-receptor agonists.[105] Some of the other major classes of drugs frequently used to treat insomnia include antidepressants, atypical antipsychotics, and antihistamines.[110]

Benzodiazepine and non-benzodiazepine agonists both act on the GABA receptor complex. The APRN should use caution if a patient already taking opioids is started on benzodiazepines. For some patients, a synergistic effect may occur and more sedation may ensue. Non-benzodiazepine agonists do not affect the sleep architecture and tend to have fewer side effects, especially longer lasting ones (e.g., less risk for abuse, dependence, and lingering oversedation).[105] Melatonin-receptor

Table 52.4 PHARMACOLOGIC OPTIONS TO MANAGE INSOMNIA

MEDICATION AND DOSAGE	MAJOR SIDE EFFECTS
Benzodiazepine receptor agonists	
Temazepam 7.5–15 mg	Drowsiness, confusion
Triazolam 0.125 mg	Amnesia, drowsiness
Lorazepam 0.5–4 mg	Respiratory depression, sedation
Non-benzodiazepine receptor agonists	
Zolpidem 5–10 mg (IR), 6.25–12.5 mg (ER)	Sedation, dizziness
Eszopiclone 1–3 mg	Headache, drowsiness, dizziness
Antidepressants	
Trazodone 25–100 mg	Sedation, confusion, headache
Mirtazapine 7.5–30 mg	Constipation, sedation, xerostomia
Melatonin-receptor agonist	
Ramelteon 8 mg	Central nervous system (CNS) depression, headache
Atypical antipsychotics	
Olanzapine 5–10 mg	Extrapyramidal side effects, drowsiness
Antihistamines	
Diphenhydramine 25–50 mg	Dizziness, headache, sedation
Doxylamine 25 mg	Paradoxical CNS arousal, dizziness, sedation

ER, extended release; IR, immediate release.

From Schroeder[105]; Wijemanne, Ondo[107]; and Arnold et al.[110]

agonists act on MT_1 and MT_2 receptors, are believed to be involved in normal sleep–wake cycle regulation, and have fewer side effects and no risk for abuse or dependence; only ramelteon has FDA approval.[105] The other classes of drugs are used due to their sedating properties[105,110] (Table 52.4).

SUMMARY

Pruritus, hiccups, dry mouth, fevers, and sleep disorders are all distressing and difficult to treat symptoms that negatively impact quality of life. Consistent assessment is essential. While there is often a lack of consensus on evidence-based management, the palliative APRN should be familiar with treatments for these less common and often treatment resistant symptoms. Continued investigation into the mechanisms of action of these symptoms will help guide improved management, and evaluation of novel approaches to treatment is needed and under way.

REFERENCES

1. Smothers A. Pruritus, fever, and sweats. In: Ferrell BR, Paice J, eds. *Oxford Textbook of Palliative Nursing.* 5th ed. Oxford: Oxford University Press; 2019: 285–290. doi:10.1093/med/9780190862374.001.0001

2. Jin XY, Khan TM. Quality of life among patients suffering from cholestatic liver disease-induced pruritus: A systematic review. *J Formos Med Assoc.* 2016;115(9):689–702. doi:10.1016/j.jfma.2016.05.006

3. Marron SE, Tomas-Aragones L, Boira S, Campos-Rodenas R. Quality of life, emotional wellbeing and family repercussions in dermatological patients experiencing chronic itching: A pilot study. *Acta Derm Venereol.* 2016;96(3):331–335. doi:10.2340/00015555-2263

4. Blome C, Radtke MA, Eissing L, Augustin M. Quality of life in patients with atopic dermatitis: Disease burden, measurement, and treatment benefit. *Am J Clin Dermatol.* 2016;17(2):163–169. doi:10.1007/s40257-015-0171-3

5. Kaushik SB, Cerci FB, Miracle J, et al. Chronic pruritus in HIV-positive patients in the southeastern United States: Its prevalence and effect on quality of life. *J Am Acad Dermatol.* 2014;70(4):659–664. doi:10.1016/j.jaad.2013.12.015

6. Mu D, Deng J, Liu KF, et al. A central neural circuit for itch sensation. *Science.* 2017;357:695–699. doi:10.1126/science.aaf4918

7. Meng J, Steinhoff M. Molecular mechanisms of pruritus. *Curr Res Transl Med.* 2016;64:203–206. doi:10.1016/j.retram.2016.08.006

8. Tajiri K, Shimizu Y. Recent advances in the management of pruritus in chronic liver diseases. *World J Gastroenterol.* 2017;23(19):3418–3426. doi:10.3748/wjg.v23.i19.3418

9. Green D, Dong X. The cell biology of acute itch. *J Cell Biol.* 2016;213:155–161. doi:10.1083/jcb.201603042

10. Kuraishi Y. Recent advances in the study of itching: Potential new therapeutic targets for pathological pruritus. *Biol Pharm Bull.* 2013;36(8):1228–1234. doi:10.1248/bpb.b13-00343

11. Helge Meyer N, Kotnik N, Meyer V, et al. The complexity of pruritus requires a variety of treatment strategies. *Curr Treat Options Allergy.* 2019;6:189–199. doi:10.1007/s40521-019-00217-y

12. Fowler E, Yosipovitch G. A new generation of treatments for itch. *Acta Derm Venereal.* 2020;100(2):Adc00027. doi:10.2340/00015555-3347

13. Pereira MP, Stander S. Novel drugs for the treatment of chronic pruritus. *Expert Opin Investig Drugs.* 2018;27(12):981–988. doi:10.1080/13543784.2018.1548606

14. Oetjen LK, Mack MR, Feng J, et al. Sensory neurons co-opt classical immune signaling pathways to mediate chronic itch. *Cell.* 2017;171:217–228. doi:10.1016/j.cell.2017.08.006

15. Golpanian RS, Gonzalez JM, Yosipovitch G. Practical approach for the diagnosis and treatment of chronic pruritus. *J Nurse Pract.* 2020;16:590–596. doi:10.1016/j.nurpra.2020.05.002

16. Dalgard FJ, Svensson Å, Halvorsen JA, et al. Itch and mental health in dermatological patients across Europe: A cross-sectional study in 13 countries. *J Investig Dermatol.* 2020;140(3):568–573. doi:10.1016/j.jid.2019.05.034

17. Tarikci N, Kocatürk E, Güngör S, Ilteris OT, Pelin Ülkümen C, Singer R. Pruritus in systemic diseases: A review of etiological factors and new treatment modalities. *Sci World J.* 2015:803752. doi:10.1155/2015/803752

18. Weisshaar E. Epidemiology of itch. *Curr Probl Dermatol.* 2016;50:5–10. doi:10.1159/000446010

19. Nowak D, Yeung J. Diagnosis and treatment of pruritus. *Can Fam Physician.* 2017;63(12):918–924. PMID: 29237630

20. Düll MM, Kremer AE. Newer approaches to the management of pruritus in cholestatic liver disease. *Curr Hepatology Rep.* 2020;19:86–95. doi:10.1007/s11901-020-00517-x

21. Bergasa NV. The pruritus of cholestasis: From bile acids to opiate agonists: Relevant after all these years. *Med Hypotheses.* 2018;110:86–89. doi:10.1016/j.mehy.2017.11.002

22. Pederson M, Mayo MJ. Therapeutics for pruritus in cholestatic liver disease: Many treatments but few cures. *Curr Hepatology Rep.* 2018;17:143–151. doi:10.1007/s11901-018-0397-7

23. Verduzco HA, Shirazian S. CKD-associated pruritus: New insights into diagnosis, pathogenesis, and management. *Kidney Int Rep.* 2020;5(9):1387–1402. doi:10.1016/j.ekir.2020.04.027

24. Swarna SS, Aziz K, Zubair T, Qadir N, Khan M. Pruritus associated with chronic kidney disease: A comprehensive literature review. *Cureus.* 2019;11(7):e5256. doi:10.7759/cureus.5256

25. Altınok Ersoy N, Akyar İ. Multidimensional pruritus assessment in hemodialysis patients. *BMC Nephrol.* 2019;20(1):42. doi:10.1186/s12882-019-1234-0

26. Serrano L, Martinez-Escala ME, Zhou XA, Guitart J. Pruritus in cutaneous T-cell lymphoma and its management. *Dermatol Clin.* 2018;36:245–258. doi:10.1016/j.det.2018.02.011

27. Jiménez Gallo D, Albarrán Planelles C, Linares Barrios M, Fernández Anguita MJ, Márquez Enríquez J, Rodríguez Mateos ME. Treatment of pruritus in early-stage hypopigmented mycosis fungoides with aprepitant. *Dermatol Ther.* 2014;27(3):178–182. doi:10.1111/dth.12113

28. Cheng SP, Lee JJ, Liu TP, et al. Parathyroidectomy improves symptomatology and quality of life in patients with secondary hyperparathyroidism. *Surgery.* 2014;155(2):320–328. doi:10.1016/j.surg.2013.08.013

29. Tăranu T, Toader S, Eşanu I, Toader MP. Pruritus in the elderly: Pathophysiological, clinical, laboratory and therapeutic approach. *Rev Med Chir Soc Med Nat.* 2014;118(1):33–38. PMID: 24741772

30. Serling SLC, Leslie K, Maurer T. Approach to pruritus in the adult HIV-positive patient. *Semin Cutan Med Surg.* 2011;30:101–106. doi:10.1016/j.sder.2011.04.004

31. Huang AH, Kaffenberger BH, Reich A, Szepietowski JC, Ständer S, Kwatra SG. Pruritus associated with commonly prescribed medications in a tertiary care center. *Medicines (Basel).* 2019;6(3):84. Published 2019 Aug 4. doi:10.3390/medicines6030084

32. Dhand A, Aminoff MJ. The neurology of itch. *Brain.* 2014;137(2):313–322. doi:10.1093/brain/awt158

33. Misery L, Dutray S, Chastaing M, Schollhammer M, Consoli SG, Consoli SM. Psychogenic itch. *Transl Psychiatry.* 2018;8(1):52. Published 2018 Mar 1. doi:10.1038/s41398-018-0097-7

34. Lee HE, Stull C, Carolyn BS, Yosipovitch G. Psychiatric disorders and pruritus. *Clin Dermatol.* 2017;35(2):273–280. doi:10.1016/j.clindermatol.2017.01.008

35. Reszke R, Krajewski P, Szepietowski JC. Emerging therapeutic options for chronic pruritus. *American J ClinDermat.* 2020;21(5):601–618. doi:10.1007/s40257-020-00534-y

36. Patel SP, Vasavda C, Ho B, Meixiong J, Dong X, Kwatra SG. Cholestatic pruritus: Emerging mechanisms and therapeutics. *J Am Acad Dermatol.* 2019;81(6):1371–1378. doi:10.1016/j.jaad.2019.04.035

37. Jannuzzi RG. Nalbuphine for treatment of opioid-induced pruritus: A systematic review of literature. *Clin J Pain.* 2016 Jan;32(1):87–93. doi:10.1097/AJP.0000000000000211

38. Siemens W, Xander C, Meerpohl JJ, Buroh S, Antes G, Schwarzer G, Becker G. Pharmacological interventions for pruritus in adult palliative care patients. *Cochrane Database Syst Rev.* 2016;16(11):CD008320. Published 2016 Nov 16. doi:10.1002/14651858.CD008320.pub3

39. Yosipovitch G, Rosen JD, Hashimoto T. Itch: From mechanism to (novel) therapeutic approaches. *J Allergy Clin Immunol.* 2018;142(5):1375–1390. doi:10.1016/j.jaci.2018.09.005

40. Mathur VS, Kumar J, Crawford PW, Hait H, Sciascia T. A multicenter, randomized, double-blind, placebo-controlled trial of nalbuphine ER tablets for uremic pruritus. *Am J Nephrol.* 2017;46(6):450–458. doi:10.1159/000484573

41. Patel AD, Katz K, Gordon KB. Cutaneous manifestations of chronic liver disease. *Clinics in Liver Disease.* 2020;24(3):351–360. doi:10.1016/j.cld.2020.04.003

42. Bachs L, Pares A, Elena M, et al. Effects of long-term rifampicin administration in primary biliary cirrhosis. *Gastroenterology.* 1992;102(6):2077–2080. doi:10.1016/0016-5085(92)90335-v

43. Webb GJ, Rahman SR, Levy C, Hirschfield GM. Low risk of hepatotoxicity from rifampicin when used for cholestatic pruritus: A cross-disease cohort study. *Aliment Pharmaco Ther.* 2018;47(8):1213–1219. doi:10.1111/apt.14579

44. Yue J, Jiao S, Xiao Y, Ren W, Zhao T, Meng J. Comparison of pregabalin with ondansetron in treatment of uraemic pruritus in dialysis patients: A prospective, randomized, double-blind study. *Int Urol Nephrol.* 2015;47(1):161–167. doi:10.1007/s11255-014-0795-x

45. Kremer M, Salvat E, Muller A, et al. Antidepressants and gabapentinoids in neuropathic pain: Mechanistic insights. *Neuroscience.* 2016;338:183–206. doi:10.1016/j.neuroscience.2016.06.057

46. Mohammadi Kebar S, Sharghi A, Ghorghani M, Hoseininia S. Comparison of gabapentin and hydroxyzine in the treatment of pruritus in patients on dialysis. *ClinExp Dermatol.* 2020;45(7):866–871. doi:10.1111/ced.14270

47. Kouwenhoven TA, van de Kerkhof PC, Kamsteeg M. Use of oral antidepressants in patients with chronic pruritus: A systematic review. *J Am Acad Dermatol.* 2017;77(6):1068–1073.e7. doi:10.1016/j.jaad.2017.08.025

48. Pereira MP, Kremer AE, Mettang T, Stander S. Chronic pruritus in the absence of skin disease: Pathophysiology, diagnosis and treatment. *Am J Clin Dermatol.* 2016;17(4):337–348. doi:10.1007/s40257-016-0198-0

49. Brasileiro LE, Barreto DP, Nunes EA. Psychotropics in different causes of itch: Systematic review with controlled studies. *An Bras Dermatol.* 2016;91(6):791–798. doi:10.1590/abd1806-4841.20164878

50. Clark K, Lam L, Shelby-James T, Currow DC. The role of ondansetron in the management of cholestatic or uremic pruritus: Systematic review. *J Pain Symptom Manage.* 2012;44(5):725–730. doi:10.1016/j.jpainsymman.2011.11.007

51. Tsianakas A, Zeidler C, Riepe C et al. Aprepitant in antihistamine-refractory chronic nodular prurigo: A multicentre, randomized, double-blind, placebo-controlled, cross-over, phase-II trial (APREPRU). *Acta Derm Venereol.* 2019;99(4):379–385. doi:10.2340/00015555-3120

52. Ständer S, Spellman MC, Kwon P, Yosipovitch G. The NK1 receptor antagonist serlopitant for treatment of chronic pruritus. *Expert Opin Investig Drugs.* 2019;28(8):659–666. doi:10.1080/13543784.2019.1638910

53. Lonndahl L, Holst M, Bradley M, et al. Substance P antagonist aprepitant shows no additive effect compared with standardized topical treatment alone in patients with atopic dermatitis. *Br J Dermatol.* 2019;181(5):932–938. doi:10.2340/00015555-2852

54. Avila C, Massick S, Kaffenberger BH, Kwatra SG, Bechtel M. Cannabinoids for the treatment of chronic pruritus: A review. *J Am Acad Dermatol.* 2020;82(5):1205–1212. doi:10.1016/j.jaad.2020.01.036

55. Mounessa JS, Siegel JA, Dunnick CA, Dellavalle RP. The role of cannabinoids in dermatology. *J Am Acad Dermatol.* 2017;77(1):188–190. doi:10.1016/j.jaad.2017.02.056

56. Janmohamed A, Trivedi PJ. Patterns of disease progression and incidence of complications in primary biliary cholangitis (PBC). *Best Pract Res Clin Gastroenterol.* 2018;34–35:71–83. doi:10.1016/j.bpg.2018.06.002

57. Hussain AB, Samuel R, Hegade VS, et al. Pruritus secondary to primary biliary cholangitis: A review of the pathophysiology and management with phototherapy. *Br J Dermatol.* 2019;181(6):1138–1145. doi:10.1111/bjd.17933

58. Maul JT, Kretschmer L, Anzengruber F, et al. Impact of UVA on pruritus during UVA/B phototherapy of inflammatory skin diseases: A randomized double-blind study. *J Eur Acad Dermatol Venereol.* 2017;31(7):1208–1213. doi:10.1111/jdv.13994

59. Nakamura M, Koo JY. Phototherapy for the treatment of prurigo nodularis: A review. *Dermatol Online J.* 2016;22(4):13030/qt4b07778z. Published 2016 Apr 18. PMID: 27617458

60. Aval SB, Ravanshad Y, Azarfar A, Mehrad-Majd H, Torabi S, Ravanshad S. A systematic review and meta-analysis of using acupuncture and acupressure for uremic pruritus. *Iran J Kidney Dis.* 2018;12(2):78–83. PMID: 29507269

61. Mohammad Ali BM, Hegab DS, El Saadany MH. Use of transcutaneous electrical nerve stimulation for chronic pruritus: Transcutaneous electrical nerve stimulation for pruritus. *Dermatol Ther.* 2015;28(4):210–215. doi:10.1111/dth.12242

62. Reichenbach ZW, Piech GM, Malik Z. Chronic hiccups. *Curr Treat Options Gastroenterol.* 2020;18:43–59. doi:10.1007/s11938-020-00273-3

63. Kohse EK, Hollmann MW, Bardenheuer HJ, Kessler J. Chronic hiccups: An underestimated problem. *Anesth Analg.* 2017;125(4):1169–1183. doi:10.1213/ANE.0000000000002289

64. Moretto EN, Wee B, Wiffen PJ, Murchison AG. Interventions for treating persistent and intractable hiccups in adults. *Cochrane Database Syst Rev.* 2013;31:1. Published 2013 Jan 31. doi:10.1002/14651858.CD008768.pub2

65. Steger M, Schneemann M, Fox M. Systemic review: The pathogenesis and pharmacological treatment of hiccups. *Aliment Pharmacol Ther.* 2015;42(9):1037–1050. doi:10.1111/apt.13374

66. Jeon YS, Kearney AM, Baker PG. Management of hiccups in palliative care patients. *BMJ Support Palliat Care.* 2018;8(1):1–6. doi:10.1136/bmjspcare-2016-001264

67. Calsina-Berna A, García-Gómez G, González-Barboteo J, Porta-Sales J. Treatment of chronic hiccups in cancer patients: A systematic review. *J Palliat Med.* 2012;15(10):1142–1150. doi:10.1089/jpm.2012.0087

68. Adam E. A systematic review of the effectiveness of oral baclofen in the management of hiccups in adult palliative care patients. *J Pain Palliat Care Pharmacother.* 2020;34(1):43–54. doi:10.1080/15360288.2019.1705457

69. Smith HS, Busracamwongs A. Management of hiccups in the palliative care population. *Am J Hosp Palliat Care.* 2003;20(2):149–154. doi:10.1177/104990910302000214

70. Arsanious D, Khoury S, Martinez E. Ultrasound-guided phrenic nerve block for intractable hiccups following placement of esophageal stent for esophageal squamous cell carcinoma. *Pain Physician.* 2016;19(4):E653–6. PMID: 27228533

71. Bredenoord AJ. Management of belching, hiccups, and aerophagia. *Clin Gastroenterol Hepatol.* 2013;11(1):6–12. doi:10.1016/j.cgh.2012.09.006

72. Marinella MA. Diagnosis and management of hiccups in the patient with advanced cancer. *J Support Oncol.* 2009;7(4):122–130. PMID: 19731575

73. Bryer E, Bryer J. Persistent postoperative hiccups. *Case Rep Anesthesiol.* 2020;2020:8867431. Published 2020 Jul 4. doi:10.1155/2020/8867431

74. Kao CC, Yen DH, Lee YT. Hiccups as the only symptom of acute myocardial infarction. *Am J Emerg Med.* 2019;37(7):1396.e1–1396.e3. doi:10.1016/j.ajem.2019.04.023

75. Rouse S, Wodziak M. Intractable hiccups. *Curr Neurol Neurosci Rep.* 2018;18(8):51. Published 2018 Jun 22. doi:10.1007/s11910-018-0856-0

76. Lertxundi U, Marquinez AC, Domingo-Echaburu S, et al. Hiccups in Parkinson's disease: An analysis of cases reported in the European pharmacovigilance database and a review of the literature. *Eur J Clin Pharmacol.* 2017;73(9):1159–1164. doi:10.1007/s00228-017-2275-6

77. Nausheen F, Mohsin H, Lakhan SE. Neurotransmitters in hiccups. *Springerplus.* 2016;5(1):1357. Published 2016 Aug 17. doi:10.1186/s40064-016-3034-3

78. Kang JH, Hui D, Kim MJ, et al. Corticosteroid rotation to alleviate dexamethasone-induced hiccup: A case series at a single institution. *J Pain Symptom Manage.* 2014;43(3):625–630. doi:10.1016/j.jpainsymman.2011.04.011

79. Orlovich DS, Brodsky JB, Brock-Utne JG. Nonpharmacologic management of acute singultus (hiccups). *Anesth Analg.* 2018 Mar 1;126(3):1091. doi:10.1213/ANE.0000000000002789

80. Byun SH, Jeon YH. Treatment of idiopathic persistent hiccups with positive pressure ventilation: A case report-. *Korean J Pain.* 2012;25(2):105–107. doi:10.3344/kjp.2012.25.2.105

81. Gonella S, Gonella F, Gonella S, et al. Use of vinegar to relieve persistent hiccups in an advanced cancer patient. *J Palliat Med.* 2015 May;18(5):467–470. doi:10.1089/jpm.2014.0391

82. Petroianu GA. Treatment of hiccup by vagal maneuvers. *J Hist Neurosci.* 2015;24(2):123–136. doi:10.1080/0964704X.2014.897133

83. Nausheen F, Mohsin H, Lakhan SE. Neurotransmitters in hiccups. *Springerplus.* 2016;5(1):1357. Published 2016 Aug 17. doi:10.1186/s40064-016-3034-3

84. Wang T, Wang D. Metoclopramide for patients with intractable hiccups: A multi-center, randomized, controlled pilot study. *Intern Med J*. 2014;44(12a):1205–1209. doi:10.1111/imj.12542

85. Friedgood CE, Ripstein CB. Chlorpromazine (Thorazine) in the treatment of intractable hiccups. *JAMA*. 1955;157(4):309–310. doi:10.1001/jama.1955.02950210005002

86. Ramírez FC, Graham DY. Treatment of intractable hiccup with baclofen: Results of a double-blind randomized, controlled, cross-over study. *Am J Gastroenterol* 1992;87(12):1789–1791. PMID: 1449142

87. Grononger H, Cheng M A Case of persistent hiccups successfully managed with pregabalin. *Progress Palliative Care*. 2015;23(4):224–226. doi:10.1179/1743291X14Y.0000000117

88. Nishikawa T, Araki Y, Hayashi T. Intractable hiccups (singultus) abolished by risperidone, but not by haloperidol. *Ann Gen Psychiatry*. 2015;14:13. Published 2015 Mar 5. doi:10.1186/s12991-015-0051-5

89. Thompson AN, Ehret Leal J, Brzezinski WA. Olanzapine and baclofen for the treatment of intractable hiccups. *Pharmacotherapy*. 2014;34(1):e4–8. doi:10.1002/phar.1378

90. Kaneishi K, Kawabata M. Continuous subcutaneous infusion of lidocaine for persistent hiccup in advanced cancer. *Palliat Med*. 2013;27(3):284–285. doi:10.1177/0269216312448508

91. Hernandez SL, Fasnacht KS, Sheyner I, King JM, Stewart JT. Treatment of refractory hiccups with amantadine. *J Pain Palliat Care Pharmacothery*. 2015;29(40):374–377. doi:10.3109/15360288.2015.1101640

92. Arsanious D, Khoury S, Martinez E, et al. Ultrasound-guided phrenic nerve block for intractable hiccups following placement of esophageal stent for esophageal squamous cell carcinoma. *Pain Physician*. 2016;19(4):E653–6. PMID: 27228533

93. Lee AR, Cho YW, Lee JM, Shin YJ, Han IS, Lee HK. Treatment of persistent postoperative hiccups with stellate ganglion block: Three case reports. *Medicine (Baltimore)*. 2018;97(48):e13370. doi:10.1097/MD.0000000000013370

94. Kim JE, Lee MK, Lee DH, Choi SS, Park JS. Continuous cervical epidural block: Treatment for intractable hiccups. *Medicine*. 2018;97(6):e9444. doi:10.1097/MD.0000000000009444

95. Pittman T, DiStephano A, Chow R, Samet R Ultrasound-guided phrenic nerve block for intractable hiccups in patients with metastatic colon cancer: A case report. *J Palliat Care Med*. 2017;7:302. Published April 7, 2017. doi:10.4172/2165-7386.1000302

96. Andres D. Transesophageal diaphragmatic pacing for treatment of persistent hiccups. *Anesthesiology*. 2005;102(2):483. doi:10.1097/00000542-200502000-00040

97. Yue J, Liu M, Li J, et al. Acupuncture for the treatment of hiccups following stroke: A systematic review and meta-analysis. *Acupunct Med*. 2017;35(1):2–8. doi:10.1136/acupmed-2015-011024

98. Davies A. Oral care. In: Cherny N, Fallon M, Kaasa S, et al., eds. *Oxford Textbook of Palliative Medicine*. 6th ed. Oxford: Oxford University Press; 2021.

99. Reisfield G, Rosielle D, Wilson. Palliative care fast facts and concepts #182: Xerostomia. Appleton, WI: Palliative Care Network of Wisconsin. 2015. https://www.mypcnow.org/fast-fact/xerostomia/.

100. Klinedinst R, Cohen A, Dahlin C. Dysphagia, xerostomia, and hiccups. In: Ferrell BR, Paice J, eds. *Oxford Textbook of Palliative Nursing*. 5th ed. Oxford: Oxford University Press; 2019: 163–185. doi:10.1093/med/9780199332342.001.0001

101. Talha B, Swarnkar SA. Xerostomia. StatPearls [Internet]. Treasure Island, FL: StatPearls Publishing; 2021 Jan-. Available from: https://www.ncbi.nlm.nih.gov/books/NBK545287/

102. Millsop JW, Wang EA, Fazel N. Etiology, evaluation, and management of xerostomia. *Clin Dermatol*. 2017;35(5):468–476. doi:10.1016/j.clindermatol.2017.06.010

103. Bobb B, Lyckholm L, Coyne P. Fever and sweats. In: Walsh D, Caraceni AT, Fainsinger R, et al., eds. *Palliative Medicine*. Philadelphia, PA: Saunders Elsevier; 2009: 890–893.

104. Strickland M, Stovsky E. Palliative care fast facts and concepts #256: Fever near the end of life. Appleton, WI: Palliative Care Network of Wisconsin. 2015. https://www.mypcnow.org/fast-fact/fever-near-the-end-of-life/

105. Schroeder K. Insomnia. In: Ferrell BR, Paice J, eds. *Oxford Textbook of Palliative Nursing*. 5th ed. Oxford: Oxford University Press; 2019: 330–336. doi:10.1093/med/9780199332342.001.0001

106. Arnold R, Miller M, Mehta R. Palliative care fast facts and concepts # 101: Insomnia: Patient assessment. Appleton, WI: Palliative Care Network of Wisconsin. 2015.https://www.mypcnow.org/fast-fact/insomnia-patient-assessment/

107. Wijemanne S, Ondo W. Restless legs syndrome: Clinical features, diagnosis and a practical approach to management. *Pract Neurol*. 2017;17(6):444–452. doi:10.1136/practneurol-2017-001762

108. Walia HK, Shalhoub G, Ramsammy V, Thornton JD, Auckley D. Symptoms of restless leg syndrome in a palliative care population: Frequency and impact. *J Palliat Care*. 2013;29(4):201–216. PMID: 24601071

109. Yennurajalingam S, Barla S, Arthur J, Chisholm G, Bruera E. Frequency and characteristics of drowsiness, somnolence, or daytime sleepiness in patients with advanced cancer. *Palliat Support Care*. 2019 Aug;17(4):459–463. doi:10.1017/S1478951518000779

110. Arnold R, Miller M, Mehta R. Palliative care fast facts and concepts # 105: Insomnia: Drug therapies. Appleton, WI: Palliative Care Network of Wisconsin. 2011. https://www.mypcnow.org/fast-fact/insomnia-drug-therapies/

SECTION IX

ETHICAL CONSIDERATIONS

53.

NAVIGATING ETHICAL DILEMMAS

Nessa Coyle and Timothy W. Kirk

KEY POINTS

- The palliative advanced practice registered nurse (APRN) is uniquely trained and situated within palliative care teams to navigate ethical discussions.

- Professional codes of ethics, bioethical principles, and the defining aims of palliative care are the foundation for such discussions.

- An ethical framework of advocacy, truthfulness, and accommodation guides discussions, highlighting that *process* rather than *outcome* is the appropriate focus.

- Three skill sets—communication, empathy, and moral reflection/deliberation—aid the palliative APRN in facilitating discussions.

- Curiosity, an open mind, and humility are necessary components.

CASE STUDY: THE CASE OF MR. S (PART I)

This case will be used to illustrate key principles and skills for navigating ethical discussions.

Mr. S was a 69-year-old Jewish man with refractory leukemia. He was critically ill with bacteremia, multiple organ failure, and hemodynamic instability. Although earlier in his illness he had been considered a candidate for a research protocol, he was no longer eligible. There were no further disease-focused treatment options available.

Mr. S was married with three adult children—two daughters and a son. Shortly after admission to hospital, his medical condition deteriorated. In a discussion with a covering physician, he agreed to a do-not-attempt-resuscitation (DNAR) code status. No family member was present during this conversation. Shortly thereafter, Mr. S lost decision-making capacity.

The following day, in a discussion with the attending physician, the patient's family learned that Mr. S had agreed to a DNAR code status on admission. Despite the wife reporting the patient's decision was consistent with prior conversations between them, there was dissension within the family. Because of this dissension, the patient's wife recused herself from being spokesperson for her husband. The son, with family agreement, assumed this responsibility. After consultation with an outside rabbi, the son revoked his father's DNAR code status. The patient's attending physician honored the son's decision and removed the DNAR order.

The nursing staff were concerned that Mr. S's wishes regarding end-of-life care were being overridden by his son. A palliative APRN consult was requested to bring clarity to the situation and help with communication. After talking with the nursing staff and other members of the interdisciplinary team, a family meeting was arranged. Mr. S's wife opted not to attend the meeting, stating that her son was the spokesperson for the family. The son, as well as one of the two daughters (a social worker), participated in the meeting alongside involved members of the team. The second daughter opted not to participate in the meeting but to remain with her mother. The palliative APRN led the discussion.

INTRODUCTION

What is an ethical discussion? When the question "What is the 'right' thing to do in this situation?" is asked, it is an ethical question.[1] When a discussion touches on one or more core values of the participants involved, or the core values of their respective traditions or professions, it is likely ethically significant. The context of palliative care, in which patients and their families are faced with many choices and decisions throughout the disease trajectory, but especially during transitions from curative or life-prolonging therapy to end-of-life care, makes such discussions commonplace.[2] Effective communication skills, empathy, and moral reflection and deliberation are essential ingredients in such conversations. Progressive illness with a long trajectory provides both the opportunity and the obligation for the palliative advanced practice registered nurse (APRN) to have ongoing conversations with patients and their families about their preferences for present and future healthcare interventions.[3] The importance of having these conversations and clearly documenting them becomes even more urgent when patients present with advanced disease.[4]

The Institute of Medicine's 2011 report, *The Future of Nursing: Leading Change, Advancing Health*, states that, although physicians have traditionally been responsible for end-of-life conversations, with the advancement of nursing practice, nurses are now taking the lead.[5] The Hospice and Palliative Nurses Association emphasizes that, due to their advanced training, visibility, and presence at the bedside, APRNs are ideally placed to create an ethical environment in which staff, patients, and families can navigate the difficult decisions to be made.[6] The palliative APRN's influence in creating an ethical environment is seen not only in the inpatient setting but also in outpatient clinics, as a clinical palliative care consultant, in home hospice care, and in long-term care facilities. By serving on ethics committees and clinical ethics consultation teams, palliative APRNs can help create ethical environments across their care organizations. By participating in the creation and review of institutional policies and procedures guiding palliative care interventions, APRNs ensure that the perspective of nurses helps to shape such documents. An ethical environment is one in which interactions are characterized by trust and respect, where there is encouragement to "speak up" and psychological safety in doing so, and where differences of opinion are welcomed and discussed.[7,8]

As you read this chapter, we would like you to reflect on ethical discussions you have navigated with patients, families, or staff. What was it about these discussions that left you with a feeling of satisfaction or failure? Was it in the process, or was it in the outcome? If in the process, what elements of the process contributed to success? If in the outcome, how was success or failure measured? This chapter addresses these questions by providing the palliative APRN with the structure and language that complement the classic patient-centered care model of autonomy, beneficence, nonmaleficence, and justice. The chapter builds on the ethical foundation already inherent in the practice of the palliative APRN, explaining ethical principles and skills to facilitate and guide navigation of ethical discussions. Throughout, the palliative APRN is recognized as being uniquely well-trained and situated within palliative care teams to be an advocate to ensure that the values, goals, perspectives, and concerns of patients, families, and fellow clinicians are appropriately heard in patient care conversations.

The tools and principles we present in this chapter function as guides. However, just as clinicians use their clinical judgment to apply best practice standards in each case, we invite readers to use their ethical judgment when applying the tools and principles in our model. The uncertainty in which clinical practice occurs, and which makes diagnostic and treatment decisions subject to constant revision as new information unfolds, extends to the ethics of clinical situations. How best to apply principles and tools—which principles are most applicable and how to weigh their relative importance—is necessarily (a) specific to the context of each case and (b) subject to interpretation, error, and revision. With this in mind we have included an appendix to provide the APRN with common definitions and distinctions in palliative care ethics. Each of these definitions and distinctions is followed by four questions for the APRN to consider, to be challenged by, and to challenge her team with. Included are decision-making capacity, foregoing medical interventions, discontinuing life-sustaining therapy, palliative sedation, the doctrine of double effect, medically hastened death, moral distress, and conscientious objection.

THE FOUNDATION OF ETHICAL DISCUSSIONS

This section briefly reviews nursing codes of ethics, core principles in healthcare ethics, and the defining aims of palliative care. All three provide important background knowledge and set the foundation for the ethical framework explained in the fourth part of the chapter.

NURSING CODES OF ETHICS

Nursing codes of ethics articulate defining values that unite individual nurses into a caregiving community with ideals of professional conduct. While ideals cannot always be realized, they nonetheless give nurses a direction toward which practice aspires. The International Council of Nurses (ICN) *Code of Ethics for Nurses*[9] states in its preamble, "Nurses have four fundamental responsibilities: to promote health, to prevent illness, to restore health and to alleviate suffering."[(9, p. 1)] In addition, the American Nurses Association (ANA) *Code of Ethics* has its tenets consisting of nine statements that describe the commitment of nurses to patients, duty to self and others, and duties beyond individual patient encounters.[3] These codes are a reminder to nurses of their special responsibilities in caring for the sick, and they highlight the use of knowledge and skills to help individuals and families when they are at their most vulnerable. We encourage palliative APRNs to familiarize themselves with the both the ICN and the ANA code and the applicable national nursing association codes in their practice locations. The palliative APRN works toward realizing the ideals outlined in these codes at the individual, unit, and institutional levels.

BASIC ETHICAL PRINCIPLES

These four ethical principles inform the broad landscape of nursing ethics[10,11]:

1. *Autonomy.* This principle is rooted in the notion of self-governance—the belief that individuals should have the strongest voice in making their own healthcare decisions because such decisions have a significant impact on their lives. Respecting autonomy allows persons with decision-making capacity to make healthcare decisions for themselves by giving them the support and information necessary to integrate their values, beliefs, and preferences into the decision-making process.[10,12] Autonomy has a relational component. Most people live in a cultural and familial context involving obligations, reciprocal relationships, and interdependence. Patients commonly incorporate the impact of their decisions on others into their deliberative process and seek the assistance of loved ones in formulating care preference.[13]

2. *Beneficence.* This principle asserts that a primary ethical obligation of all clinicians is to do good—to provide care and support that enhances patients' well-being and offers benefit consistent with their goals and values.[10] While clinicians are strongly positioned to determine what biomedical benefits may accrue from certain treatments, patients and family members know

best which outcomes are beneficial in light of patients' goals and values. As such, honoring beneficence requires knowledge about what each patient values in his or her life and discussion with each patient of which treatment options align best with those values. In this setting *non-abandonment*—whether or not clinicians agree with a patient's decision—is a key element of beneficence.

3. *Nonmaleficence.* Minimizing the risk of harm, mitigating or removing preventable harm, and ensuring care interventions have a favorable benefit-harm ratio grounded in the values of the patient are the hallmarks of nonmaleficence.[12] Many treatments cause a degree of harm, but the benefit to patients, on their terms, should outweigh the harm. When a patient's values and preferences are not able to be known, nonmaleficence requires teams to craft plans of care which prioritize minimization of pain and suffering.

4. *Justice.* This principle refers to providing care that is equitable and fair to all and includes the fair distribution of scarce resources. Two types of justice are referred to here, *procedural justice* and *distributive justice*. Procedural justice requires that clinicians engage care processes that elicit the goals and preferences of patients and respect the values and rights of all involved in giving and receiving care. Such processes are considered "fair" when all appropriate voices are heard and considered. Family meetings, for example, benefit from being guided by procedural justice so that patients' and family members' voices are at the forefront when decisions about the type and site of care are made. Distributive justice requires that resources be allocated fairly and equitably, using transparent and appropriate criteria. The availability of palliative care is a good example: all patients and families should have access to palliative care services, interventions, and support, and access to care should be based on transparent, appropriate criteria applied equally to all regardless of socioeconomic state or social status.[11,12,14] The significance of distributive justice was underscored in the COVID-19 pandemic, when allocation of scarce life-saving resources became a reality.

While discrete conceptually, in practice, these four principles often overlap. Nonmaleficence works in concert with beneficence and autonomy. The patient, family, and clinicians partner together to discern (a) which values and goals of care are most important to the patient and (b) how best to support these values and achieve these goals while at the same time maximizing benefit and minimizing harm. Procedural justice requires that clinicians engage the moral agency of all stakeholders, thereby implicating autonomy. Equitably distributing care resources requires assessing procedural and outcomes-based harms and benefits. When one principle is insufficiently engaged, other principles are often similarly at risk of violation. All four principles resonate strongly with the defining aims of palliative care.

DEFINING AIMS OF PALLIATIVE CARE

Palliative care is an approach that improves the quality of life of patients (adults and children) and their families who are facing problems associated with life-threatening illness. It prevents and relieves suffering through the early identification, correct assessment and treatment of pain and other problems, whether physical, psychosocial or spiritual.[15]

As we have written elsewhere,[16] palliative care is an inherently moral enterprise because it seeks to empower the agency of patients and families through the relief of suffering, thereby strengthening their ability to make decisions consistent with their moral values. Agency is a concept that describes one's ability to develop and exercise a sense of self—engaging with the world in a manner that sets and achieves goals by doing what one can for oneself. It is linked to concepts like self-efficacy and autonomy and is predictive of improved health outcomes via variables like treatment adherence, self-care, hope, and ability to cope.[17] A person's *moral* agency is the ability to identify and embrace guiding values in life and to execute decisions, participate in actions, and develop character traits that reflect and express those values.[18] For persons who need assistance, moral agency can be respected by ensuring that the actions of caregivers are consistent with the values and preferences of patients, even if patients are not able to exercise their agency independently.

Suffering that arises in the context of life-limiting illness can constitute a threat to the agency of patients and families.[19,20] One important way that palliative APRNs can address the suffering of their patients while concurrently honoring the four ethical principles of autonomy, beneficence, nonmaleficence and justice is to offer support and interventions that restore and engage patients' moral agency. Doing so resonates strongly with the philosophy underpinning palliative care as a model of care.[21,22] Therefore, relieving suffering and empowering moral agency should be primary aims in advanced practice palliative nursing, informing how palliative APRNs navigate ethical discussions.

AN ETHICAL FRAMEWORK FOR NAVIGATING ETHICAL DISCUSSIONS

Advocacy, truthfulness, and accommodation provide an ethical framework to guide the palliative APRN in navigating ethical discussions informed by the ultimate goal of palliative care: reducing suffering by supporting and engaging moral agency.[22] The unique balance among these principles will vary in each discussion, paralleling the unique blend of persons, goals, and values involved.

ADVOCACY

Advocacy is frequently cited as the primary—perhaps even the defining—role of the nurse in the context of healthcare ethics.[23] Two models of advocacy are presented in this section: existential advocacy and advocacy as rights protection.

EXISTENTIAL ADVOCACY

Gadow's model of *existential advocacy* is an apt model for the palliative APRN when a patient has decision-making capacity and is able to participate in the decision-making process.[24] This chapter adapts the model to include patients and families, insofar as palliative care is patient- and family-centered care. The nurse as advocate offers care focused on restoring and empowering patients' moral agency as well as fostering and respecting the agency of family members. This is done through providing therapeutic presence to create conditions in which a patient and family can partner with clinicians to (a) discern the meaning of clinical changes in the patient's condition, (b) explore how such changes interact with their values and goals, and (c) appreciate together which care options might best honor those values and goals.

Explaining the role of existential advocacy in nursing care, Gadow writes:

> The ideal which existential advocacy expresses is this: that individuals be assisted by nursing to authentically exercise their freedom of self-determination. By authentic is meant a way of reaching decisions which are truly one's own decisions that express all that one believes important about oneself and the world, the entire complexity of one's values.
>
> Individuals can express their wholeness and uniqueness as valuing beings only if their full complexity of values—including contradictions and conflicts—is clearly in mind, having been reexamined and clarified in the new context. Yet, that clarification is the most difficult precisely when it is most needed, when a situation arises which threatens to overturn previously stable values. In such situations, of which health impairment is a paradigm, individuals face the necessity of either recreating their values or recreating their situation according to their existing hierarchy of values.[24 (p. 85)]

As Gadow makes clear, the goal in existential advocacy is not for the nurse to put herself in the place of *speaking for* patients. Rather, it is to provide the supportive presence and facilitate the empowering conditions necessary for patients to restore their sense of self by (a) understanding the facts and experiences of their illness, (b) appreciating what they mean in the larger context of their lives, (c) reconnecting to the values that are most important to them and most directly relevant to the situation at hand, and (d) engaging in a decision-making process that integrates such understanding, appreciation, and reconnection. The palliative APRN as a moral advocate directs attention not toward specific decisions or outcomes, but to the ongoing discussion *process* itself—a process that promotes and engages the moral agency of all involved. Humility,

openness, and an ability to listen and to let go of preconceived ideas are key components.

ADVOCACY AS RIGHTS PROTECTION

A *rights protection* model of advocacy is a common approach to nursing advocacy in which the nurse represents the wishes of the patient when he or she is in danger of being subsumed to the wishes of someone else—most commonly clinicians or family members.[3] In this model, the nurse functions in the healthcare system in a manner similar to that of a legal advocate in the legal system—protecting the rights of his or her client. This notion of advocacy has two main elements: (a) speaking up for others who cannot speak for themselves (a process element) and (b) seeking to achieve a particular outcome, presumed to be in the best interest of the party being spoken for (an outcome element).[23] These elements also imply a context in which advocacy occurs: there is some threat in the environment that increases the risk of (a) the voice of the patient or family not being heard and (b) an outcome consistent with the patient's best interest not being prioritized. In other words, the assumed condition in which this model of advocacy is needed is when there is an imbalance of power that creates vulnerability. The role of the nurse advocate is to protect the rights of the vulnerable. Again humility, openness, letting go of preconceived ideas, and an ability to listen are key components.

The rights protection model assumes that the patient needs someone else to speak *for* him or her and that the primary ethical risk in such discussions is that the patient's preferences will be overridden by the preferences of others. Such risks may well be present for certain palliative care patients for whom this model of advocacy is appropriate. An example is when a patient loses decision-making capacity and his or her advance directive is not being honored, as is seen in our case study. Another example is advocating for an unrepresented patient whose values and preferences may be unknown despite extensive attempts to do so.

Discerning the best way to advocate for patients and families requires curiosity, empathy, and good communication skills. We know so little about the full and many-faceted lives of our patients and families and we may make assumptions that cloud our ability to listen—especially when faced with a stressed family whose actions seem counterproductive to the wishes and best interests of the patient.

TRUTHFULNESS

The dominant model of truth-telling in healthcare ethics is the *disclosure model*.[25] The disclosure model begins with the assumption that healthcare providers have access to important information—a diagnosis or prognosis, for example—that patients need to make decisions about their care. Telling the truth, then, focuses on effectively communicating this information to patients so that it can be used in the decision-making process. Hallmarks of truth-telling in this model are (a) accuracy (Is what is communicated to the patient consistent with what is known by the provider?), (b) sufficiency (Is the provider telling the patient all of the relevant information?), (c) coherence (Is what is being communicated by the provider integrated with other relevant facts and circumstances such that the patient understands the context of the disclosure?), (d) timeliness (Is the disclosure shared with the patient at a point in time when it can be effectively integrated into the decision-making process?), and (e) uncertainty (How is the relative certainty/uncertainty of the situation being communicated to the patient)?

It is a common but misinformed belief among healthcare providers that telling a patient the truth is harmful. In fact, in research primarily done with cancer patients, the opposite has been found to be true.[26,27] Telling the truth fosters trust and demonstrates respect when it is told in a compassionate and sensitive manner and titrated to the patient's ability to absorb the information.[28] The purpose of sharing information with patients and families is to enable the kind of understanding, reflection, and deliberation necessary to make informed care decisions that resonate with their goals, values, and beliefs.

While the spirit of the disclosure model of truth telling is important, we have intentionally opted for the term "truthfulness." As noted earlier, palliative care is family-centered care that seeks to support the moral agency of patients by acknowledging and caring for the web of intimate relationships through which patients already find and create meaning. That relational structure is all the more important in times of distress and serious illness. Patients, loved ones, and clinicians work together in palliative care to interpret the meaning of clinical developments and integrate that meaning into the larger life horizon of the patient.[29] Truth, in other words, is not something possessed by clinicians and disclosed to patients. Rather, the truth of patients' situations is discerned through a shared process of enquiry, discovery, and meaning making.[30,31]

Truthfulness promotes patterns of engagement that create a supportive environment in which all parties can explore, share, and integrate their points of view. The goal is to achieve the fullest understanding of a patient's situation and develop a plan of care driven by the values of the patient. Such integration is likely to require some accommodation—the final element of the ethical framework.

ACCOMMODATION

Originally developed in the context of home care, the principle of accommodation is a very helpful guide in palliative care.[32] Palliative care clinicians are frequently invited into the circle of care for patients whose clinical care is managed by other primary teams. Patients are often in the late stages of progressive illness and may have become dependent on loved ones for rides to appointments, upkeep of their homes, and activities of daily living. As their ability to live independently has slowly eroded, patients have had to accommodate the schedules, preferences, and abilities of others, even when conflicting with their own. Families, in turn, have had to accommodate in similar ways. This is an example of a mutual and reciprocal process that the principle of accommodation acknowledges and promotes.

Sometimes, however, accommodation can be one-sided or gradually erode into one-sidedness. Collopy and colleagues, in addressing this phenomenon, strive to correct ways in which one-sided accommodation by patients can gradually erode their autonomy:

> In practice, such erosion of autonomy is often incremental. Caregivers intervene when clients function slowly and imperfectly. In the basic, repeated routine of care clients' preferences are not elicited; their efforts to be autonomous are waved aside by paternalistic soothing or efficient impatience on the part of caregivers. The dominant interactive pattern is frequently one in which progressive physical and mental incapacity is expected in clients and is equated with progressive inability to be autonomous.[32 (p. 8)]

These words may seem lacking in sensitivity to the needs of family members, discounting the significant accommodations they have had to make in their lives to care for the sick person. Indeed, family members may have many responsibilities to self and others that have been set aside to meet the needs of a seriously ill loved one. It may seem intuitive that healthy family members must do all of the accommodating because they are well. However, this one-sided approach can be destructive for both patients and families. It can be harmful for patients because failing to ask them to accommodate the needs and abilities of loved ones can constitute a significant departure from their usual role in relationships. This can result in a loss of self as a responsible member of a family, with the give and take that such a role entails. Similarly, a one-sided model of accommodation can harm family members and their relationships with a sick loved one—they may become overwhelmed and resentful.

Accommodation in the palliative care arena is complex. Many different players are involved, including the patient, family members, friends, and members of the healthcare team. Sensitivity and awareness of the ethical issues and complexities implicit in the principle of accommodation will allow the palliative APRN to navigate discussions and make visible the accommodation each person or group is making or being asked to make. This acknowledgment allows people to feel heard and to believe that what they say matters. Because people with advanced disease can be so frail, their voice and agency may be lost inadvertently to the strength of others. It is important that their agency is recognized and re-engaged.

In sum, advocacy, truthfulness, and accommodation constitute an ethical framework guiding palliative APRNs in navigating ethical discussions. While there are surely other principles that would be helpful guides, we have chosen these three because they (a) explicitly and effectively support the moral agency of patients, families, and clinicians and (b) are particularly well matched to the training and role of the palliative APRN.

SKILLS TO NAVIGATE ETHICAL DISCUSSIONS

COMMUNICATION SKILLS

Principles of communication (discussed in depth in Chapter 32, "Advance Care Planning"; Chapter 33, "Family Meetings"; and Chapter 34, "Communication Near End of Life"), are essential for the palliative APRN's approach when navigating ethical discussions. They include where possible (1) making sure that the patient's symptoms are under control and that some privacy has been provided; (2) eliciting, understanding, and validating the patient's perspective of the situation (concerns, feelings, expectations, goals, and values); (3) understanding the patient within his or her own psychological, cultural, social, and spiritual context; (4) reaching a shared understanding of the patient's situation; and (5) supporting the patient or surrogate in the decision made.[33-35] These principles of communication are enhanced by certain APRN behaviors, both nonverbal and verbal. Nonverbal behaviors include maintaining eye contact if culturally appropriate, leaning forward to indicate attentiveness, avoiding interrupting the patient, tolerating silence, and refraining from distracting behavior such as glancing at a cellphone. Verbal behaviors include soliciting the beliefs, values, and preferences of the patient; exploring the family's social and spiritual context and their explanatory model of health and disease; checking the patient's understanding of what has been said; validating the patient's emotions; and offering reassurance, non-abandonment, and support.[34-36]

Understanding the patient's explanatory model of disease—for example, the patient's beliefs about what has caused the illness and, therefore, what kinds of treatments may or may not work—is important as it may shape the patient's response to illness.[37,38] Such an explanatory model may be learned from multiple sources, including culture, mass media, friends, and family. However, the patient is the best source of such information.

EMPATHY SKILLS

Empathy is a skill that can be taught.[39] Empathy has three components: affective, cognitive, and behavioral.[40,41] Affectively, empathy enables us to have a sense of fellow-feeling with others; to appreciate their lived experience by using imagination to connect it to our own. This fellow-feeling can be a valuable motivator to respond to the suffering of patients and families. The affective component of empathy also carries with it the risk of projective identification. A palliative APRN's emotional response to a patient's situation can become overwhelming, directing attention to the APRN's emotional activation rather than the patient and family. Risk of distortion can be reduced by emphasizing the cognitive and behavioral elements of empathy.

Cognitively, empathy enables the palliative APRN to understand conceptually (a) the elements of others' experiences and circumstances—the "facts of the matter" and

(b) the *meaning* of those experiences and circumstances *for them*. Such meaning can be elicited through exploration with patients and families of the psychosocial implications of their situations.[42] Attentive listening, engaging all relevant parties, and facilitation of shared discussion among all those involved contribute to obtaining a fuller understanding of the situation at hand.

Behaviorally, palliative APRNs can communicate with empathy by demonstrating to patients and families that "We have heard and appreciate the significance of what you are going through." Verbal and nonverbal behaviors which acknowledge patients' and families' experience validate and normalize the feelings and significance of that experience and praise their efforts to engage and cope with serious illness. These are key components of behavioral empathy.[41] Active listening and engaging the communication skills explained in the previous section help shape behaviors which create a supportive presence with patients and families.

CASE STUDY: THE CASE OF MR. S (PART II: APPLYING THE FRAMEWORK)

The circumstances of Mr. S were as follows: soon after admission to the hospital, when he was gravely ill and medically unstable, Mr. S's code status was discussed with him by the admitting physician—no family member was present. He agreed to a DNAR code status. The following day, Mr. S was found to be delirious and without decision-making capacity. His son, who was the family spokesperson and surrogate decision-maker, learned of his father's code status and asked that the DNAR order be rescinded. The request was honored, and the patient reverted to a full code.

Mr. S's care team asked the palliative APRN to address this primary question: *How do you proceed when a healthcare agent or surrogate decision-maker challenges a patient's advance directive after decision-making capacity has been lost?*

Although the team was clear that autonomy, beneficence, and nonmaleficence all support continuing to honor a patient's documented preferences after decision-making capacity is lost, the reality was that Mr. S's decision about his code status had been reversed after he lost capacity and the validity of his decision was challenged by his son.

With this as a background, the palliative APRN used communication and empathy skills to engage a process guided by advocacy, accommodation, and truthfulness. In modeling this process the APRN also created a template for a pattern of engagement between the team and the patient's son that could be used going forward.

Listening to the Narratives

The palliative APRN wanted to have a context within which to frame and understand the son's position regarding his father's code status. She therefore needed to hear the narratives of the son and other members of the family. In addition, although the teams' question to her was quite specific, she wanted to learn more about their concerns.

In this first step, the APRN attentively listened to separate narratives—that of the primary team and that of the family. The patient was unable to participate. It was understood that there might be different narratives among the family members and among the team members. If that were the case, the different narratives would need to be heard.

The Team's Narrative

The patient has far-advanced disease, no further disease-focused treatment options were available to him, and he had agreed to a DNAR code status on admission. No family member had been present at the time of the discussion. The following day after Mr. S had lost decision-making capacity, the physician was challenged by Mr. S's son saying that his father was a religious Jew, had not understood what he was agreeing to, had not consulted with his rabbi, and that his mind had been clouded by pain medications. The DNAR code status was rescinded at the son's request.

The team was concerned that the patient's autonomy and right to self-determination was being violated. At the same time, they fully acknowledged that their knowledge of Jewish law around end-of-life care was limited. The team expressed ambivalence as to whether or not to be guided by the son's knowledge in this area, specifically how it applied to his father's end-of-life care as death drew near. The team wanted to respect the patient's autonomy; they were unsure how best to integrate the patient's stated preferences with the son's knowledge of his father. This concern reflected patient- and family-centered care.

The Wife's Narrative

There was dissension among the family about the patient's code status. The dissension was unsettling to all of them and would have been distressing to her husband. Having the family united had always been important to Mr. S. The family was in agreement that the son should be their spokesperson and surrogate decision-maker.

The Son's Narrative

His father was a Jew and lived his life according to a Jewish code of ethics. His father's consent to a DNAR code status on time of admission was not authentic. He had been under the influence of opioid medications when the discussion had taken place and had not understood the implications of the decision in the context of Jewish law. In addition, no family member had been present at the time the code status discussion took place. He stated that his father would want his care at the end of life to be consistent with Jewish law—guided by his rabbi.

Integrating the Narratives

Eliciting and integrating narratives from key participants in a patient's care provides a background through which the APRN can guide discussions within the framework and ethical principles previously outlined.

What was Mr. S's authentic preference regarding resuscitation? Perceptions and claims by different parties may conflict. Respect for autonomy strongly favors privileging the values and preferences of the patient unless there is a compelling reason to do otherwise. The son's claims that the father's expressed preferences were not authentic challenged the team's commitment to honor Mr. S's DNAR code status. They were conflicted as to what was the "right" thing to do. They took seriously several of the son's points: (a) that Mr. S had been medically unstable and receiving opioids for pain when the code discussion took place; (b) that he had not had a formal capacity assessment at the time (as his capacity had not been called into question); and (c) that, in an ideal situation, a family member would have been present for the discussion. The team was uncertain if they should honor Mr. S's advance directive in the face of his son's challenge, conceding the preceding points, and aware that their knowledge of the patient and his values was limited compared to the decades-long relationship between Mr. S and his family.

Because the patient's DNAR code status had already been rescinded, the team made the decision to accept in good faith the son's report that his father would want his end-of-life care to conform with Jewish law as directed by the rabbi, swiftly moving forward with the son and rabbi to clarifying the care parameters.

The Family Meeting

Having integrated the narratives, the palliative APRN led a family meeting. The attending physician provided a clear and candid review of Mr. S's medical situation, rapid deterioration, and likely end-of-life scenario with and without attempted resuscitation. The son indicated that he understood the clinical situation, did not want his father to suffer, but wanted his father's death to conform with Jewish law. He again stated it was "what his father would want." The son asked for very specific medical information that he could share with the rabbi: evidence of his father's progressive deterioration, evidence of progressive organ failure, and evidence that death was imminent. Although both Mr. S's attending physician and the palliative APRN offered to speak directly with the consulting rabbi, the son said that he preferred to do so. The requested information was provided to the son both verbally and in written form. Based on this information, the rabbi stated that, according to Jewish law, it was appropriate for Mr. S's code status to be DNAR—but that all other life-sustaining treatments should be continued[43,44] (see also Chapter 33, "Family Meetings").

By taking such an intentional approach to the *process* of eliciting and integrating everyone's narrative—using the skills and principles outlined in this chapter—the APRN facilitated a discussion notable for its mutual respect, careful listening, and ability to find common ground. Mr. S's care plan was modified to reinstate the DNAR order and maintain other life-sustaining interventions. He died peacefully 48 hours later.

Moral Reflection and Deliberation

Following Mr. S's death, the team and the APRN set aside time for moral reflection and deliberation. Reflection and deliberation can be an important way for team members to maintain connection with each other, restoring focus on the moral foundation and framework of their work.[7] This approach is grounded on the assumption that good care is defined and redefined in concrete situations wherein a dialogue occurs involving ethical principles, professional standards, constraints, and the unique circumstances of each narrative.

Although the team expressed relief at the eventual outcome of the case, they described the tension, conflict, and moral distress they had experienced. By accommodating Mr. S's son as an advocate for his father, were they violating the patient's autonomy by negating his advance directive? As they struggled with this tension a question arose: Was it possible that Mr. S's long-standing value of living and dying according to Jewish law had changed when faced with the immediacy of death and associated suffering? Had this change in values led to his agreeing to a DNAR code status without consulting his rabbi? In addition, they wondered if there was some validity to the son's claim that his father's judgment had been impaired by pain and/or opioid administration and that he had not realized the implications of what he was agreeing to. Should they have performed or requested a formal decision-making capacity assessment? Had they been lacking in not doing so?

Creating space for moral reflection and deliberation provided the palliative APRN with a format for educating, debriefing, and supporting the staff following their challenging interactions with the patient's son.

SUMMARY

This chapter has provided the APRN with a structure and language that complement the classic patient-centered care model of autonomy, beneficence, nonmaleficence, and justice. It articulated the ethical foundation of palliative care, explaining further ethical principles and skills to navigate ethical discussions. Throughout, the palliative APRN was recognized as being uniquely well-trained and situated to be an advocate to ensure that the values, goals, perspectives, and concerns of patients, families, and fellow clinicians are appropriately heard in patient care conversations.

APPENDIX A-COMMON DEFINITIONS AND DISTINCTIONS IN PALLIATIVE CARE ETHICS

DECISION-MAKING CAPACITY

Decision-making capacity is a situation-specific clinical determination that a patient is able to make their own healthcare decisions. Capacity has four elements. A patient must be able to

(a) understand the relevant information,

(b) appreciate the current situation and its consequences,

(c) reason about treatment choices; and

(d) communicate a consistent choice.

The assumption is that a patient has capacity unless indications suggest otherwise.[45,46] If a patient is found not to have capacity and an immediate decision is not required, clinicians must make a good faith attempt to restore the patient's capacity. If restoring capacity is not possible, a surrogate decision-maker—appointed by the patient or identified per applicable law—makes decisions on behalf of the patient. Any treatment decisions made on behalf of the patient must be shared with the patient. If the patient objects to the determination of incapacity or the surrogate's decision, the care team must seek additional assistance before proceeding.

Questions to consider:

1. What ethical principles are embedded in the concept of decision-making capacity?

2. What are the triggers for a capacity assessment?

3. Does our responsibility end with the initial capacity assessment?

4. How do we mitigate the risk that the initial capacity assessment is inappropriately expanded to all decisions?

FOREGOING MEDICAL INTERVENTIONS

The correlate of a capable patient's right to consent to a medical intervention is the right to refuse such an intervention. It is an established principle of law and ethics that capable patients have the right to refuse any proposed medical treatment.[10] Respecting the patient's treatment refusal, like seeking the patient's consent, is an aspect of honoring the patient's autonomy. For patients to make informed decisions to accept or refuse healthcare interventions, special attention should be given to (a) the adequacy of the information presented and the quality of the explanation; (b) possible language or cultural barriers to understanding; and (c) the patient's appreciation of the consequences, both positive and negative, of all options available to them. When a patient lacks decision-making capacity, surrogates may exercise a patient's right to refuse treatment consistent with the patient's known wishes.

WITHHOLDING AND DISCONTINUING LIFE-SUSTAINING THERAPIES

Palliative APRNs are often part of discussions about starting and stopping life-sustaining treatment. In the ethics literature, decisions to limit life-sustaining treatment are often categorized as either (a) withholding treatment or (b) discontinuing (or withdrawing) treatment. *Withholding* such treatment is a decision "not to start or increase a life-sustaining treatment."[47] (p. 859) Whereas *discontinuing* such treatment is a decision "to actively stop a life-sustaining treatment presently being given."[47] (p. 860) The prevailing position in the ethics literature is that decisions to withhold and discontinue life-sustaining treatment are considered ethically equivalent, meaning that the same ethical reasoning that would justify withholding a treatment also justifies withdrawing that treatment after it has begun.[48] However, actions that are conceptually equivalent in the ethics literature don't always feel equivalent in clinical practice. Some clinicians—especially those new to the field—report that discontinuing a life-sustaining treatment after it has been initiated "feels" different from never beginning such a treatment. Rules may differ among religions in regard to withholding and discontinuing life-prolonging therapy.[43,44]

Questions to consider:

1. Which ethical principles and values are most helpful when making decisions about withholding or discontinuing life-sustaining treatment with patients and families?

2. How is withdrawing or discontinuing life-sustaining treatment ethically distinct from medical aid in dying?

3. Does a decision to discontinue a life-sustaining treatment require a stronger/different ethical justification than a decision to withhold a life-sustaining treatment? Why or why not?

4. If a palliative APRN has a personal moral objection to discontinuing life-sustaining treatments, is she obliged to explain the option of discontinuing treatment to the patient even if she is not willing, personally, to participate in such discontinuation? (See also the later discussion on conscientious objection.)

PALLIATIVE SEDATION

Palliative sedation is the administration of sedative medications to reduce awareness of suffering which has been refractory to other interventions.[49,50] While there is some variation across regions and institutions regarding the conditions in which sedation is administered,[51] the defining element of palliative sedation is that it targets a patient's conscious awareness of distress because more precise targeting of the cause of distress via other interventions has not worked. Sedation can be appropriate for patients who are imminently dying and patients who are not close to death. Considerations for both groups of patients are offered here.

Informed consent for sedation includes discussion of whether concurrently administered treatments—including nutrition and hydration—will continue. There remains a lack of consensus in the literature regarding whether sedation is an appropriate intervention for symptoms which are primarily non-physical, such as existential distress.[52,53] Some guidelines indicate that sedation is only appropriate when patients are imminently dying—in a matter of days. Others posit that the aim of reducing refractory suffering is sufficient justification for initiating sedation regardless of a patient's projected time until death. The most prevalent concern regarding timing is that sedation of patients who are not imminently dying may hasten their death if sedation precludes oral intake and nutrition and/or hydration are not concurrently administered via an alternate route.[54] Sedation is a distinct intervention from resuscitation; code status for patients considering sedation must be clarified. Palliative APRNs are encouraged to consult their institutional policies and procedures regarding sedation.

PALLIATIVE SEDATION AT END OF LIFE

Palliative sedation is a medical therapy for the imminently dying. The intent is to relieve intractable pain and other symptoms where pain and suffering are intolerable. All parties agree that, because palliative interventions which compromise consciousness have been ineffective, reducing consciousness to reduce awareness of symptoms is acceptable. This is with the consent of the patient or surrogate decision-maker. Sedation is increased until the patient is without evidence of distress and then no further. Clear parameters for increasing the level of sedation are set and documentation is specific. The intent is not to hasten death but to control symptoms. Indeed, when carefully titrated there is no evidence that imminently dying patients who are sedated die more quickly that those who are not sedated.[55]

SEDATION FOR INTRACTABLE SYMPTOMS

In contrast to palliative sedation in the imminently dying, some patients may have intractable symptoms but are not within the last few days of life. At the same time an intensive effort is made to find other means for controlling the symptoms with the patient remaining awake and alert. As previously described, sedation is increased until the patient is without evidence of distress and then no further. Clear parameters for increasing the level of sedation are set and documentation is specific. The intent is to control symptoms while other means to control the symptoms with the patient remaining more awake and alert are sought. All life-preserving measures continue. In contrast to palliative sedation in the imminently dying, there is the luxury of time to explore different approaches to manage the patient's symptoms.

Questions to consider:

1. How does one determine the harm-benefit ratio of sedation?

2. What are important elements of consent for sedation?

3. Does sedation hasten death? How does one engage this question?

4. How does one ensure that sedation is for the treatment of the patient's suffering and not the suffering of family/clinicians?

DOCTRINE OF DOUBLE EFFECT

Though there is considerable debate as to its usefulness,[56,57] the doctrine of double effect remains commonly used and taught in healthcare ethics, especially in end-of-life decision-making.[58] Rooted in Catholic moral theology, the doctrine presents conditions in which interventions that carry the likelihood of both good and bad effects (outcomes) may be morally justified. Mangan's[59] formulation of the conditions is most frequently cited, modified here for clarity and simplicity.

A. The good effects are intended. The bad effects are foreseen but not intended.

B. The act itself is morally good or neutral.

C. The bad effect is not the means of producing the good effect.

D. The good of the good effect must proportionately outweigh the bad of the bad effect.

The doctrine has been used in discussion of opioid titration, palliative sedation, and discontinuation of some burdensome life-sustaining treatments to argue that relief of suffering (intended effect) can justify a perceived risk of hastened death (foreseen effect). Careful use of the doctrine requires (a) engaging all four conditions in the doctrine, (b) agreement regarding which actions and effects are "good" and "bad," (c) ability to discern which effects of an action are intended and which are merely foreseen, and (d) careful clinical assessment of the likely effects of an intervention, ensuring that any possible steps to mitigate the bad effects have been taken.

Questions to consider:

1. Is it necessary to evoke the doctrine of double effect when titrating treatments in response symptom distress?

2. Does proportionality (balancing benefits and harms) and the relationship between beneficence and non-maleficence render the doctrine of double effect unnecessary?

3. How does one identify interventions which are and are not intrinsically good or neutral?

4. How does one distinguish between intended and foreseen effects?

MEDICALLY HASTENED DEATH

Physician-assisted dying (PAD), physician-assisted suicide (PAS), or medical aid-in-dying (MAID) is a practice whereby a physician provides a capacitated, terminally ill patient with a prescription for a lethal dose of medication, upon the patient's request, to end their own life.[60] Patients self-administer the lethal dose of medication at a time of their choosing. (In some countries, the term also includes lethal doses of a medication directly administered by a clinician, a practice currently not legal in the United States.) The intended goal is to prevent or relieve intractable suffering through the person's death. As of 2021, the legality of this practice varies across jurisdictions. There is considerable debate over whether PAD/PAS/MAID should be considered a "palliative" intervention. Given societal trends and the leadership role of APRNs in healthcare, it is likely that in the future palliative APRNs (as is the case in Canada) will be authorized to be the prescribing clinician, making knowledge about and careful consideration of the practice essential.

Questions to consider:

1. How does one determine the harm-benefit ratio of medically hastened dying?

2. What are important elements of informed consent for medically hastened dying?

3. How does one ensure that medically hastened dying intended to relieve patients' suffering is not primarily directed by the suffering of family/clinicians?

4. In jurisdictions where the practice is legal, can palliative APRNs morally opposed to medically hastened dying refuse to provide information about the practice to eligible patients?

MORAL DISTRESS

Moral distress can be experienced by clinicians when their ability to practice in accordance with accepted professional values and standards is compromised by factors perceived as outside of their control.[61] It is a relational experience shaped by multiple contexts, including the sociopolitical and cultural context of the workplace environment.[62] For example, a nurse follows a medical order to increase administration of vasopressors, all the while believing that (a) doing so is violating nonmaleficence and (b) she has no choice but to administer the prescribed treatment. Common causes of moral distress are lack of clarity about goals of care among family members and healthcare providers, disagreement within the team about goals of care, voice not heard, fragmentation of care, and inadequate communication. By identifying the existence of moral distress and talking about it—giving a name to the phenomenon, recognizing it as a multidisciplinary problem—reduces the threat to the individual clinician's moral integrity and can be an instigator for change.[63]

Questions to consider:

1. Is the experience and acknowledgment of moral distress ethically significant in healthcare, and, if so, why?

2. What are the personal ramifications to the nurse of repeated exposure to situations causing moral distress?

3. Does the experience of moral distress always indicate the patient is receiving inappropriate care? If yes, why? If not, why not?

4. If, as stated earlier, palliative APRNs have a responsibility as clinical leaders to create an ethical climate, how can palliative APRNs help teams identify and address conditions which lead to repeated episodes of moral distress?

CONSCIENTIOUS OBJECTION

Conscientious objection in healthcare refers to a situation where a clinician opts out of participating in a plan of care or providing a particular medical service on personal moral or religious grounds.[64] The intent of recognizing the right of clinicians to engage conscientious objection is to protect clinicians' ability to practice professionally without damaging their personal moral integrity.[3,65] Individual moral and religious convictions represent what a clinician stands for on a deep level, constituting their identity as responsible individuals accountable for their actions. To violate such convictions can damage clinicians' moral and religious identities; to bar an individual from engaging in conscientious objection is to put him or her in the position either of resigning or violating his or her conscience.[3] As conscientious objection is grounded in personal moral beliefs, it is distinct from a palliative APRN refusing to participate in a clinical intervention because such an intervention is contrary to best practice. When clinicians object to participating in a clinical intervention on personal moral grounds, several conditions must be met to ensure that exercising such objection does not violate the rights of the patient and the accepted norms of nursing practice.[66]

Questions to consider:

1. What are the key differences in refusing to participate in a clinical intervention when based on a personal moral belief or on professional judgment?

2. Are both valid grounds for conscientious objection?

3. If a nurse objects to participating in a clinical intervention based on personal moral grounds, what conditions must be met to ensure that the rights of the patient and accepted norms of nursing practice are not violated?

4. Is it important that an organization has a transparent process/formal policy for engaging conscientious objection? If so, why?

COMMON QUESTIONS FROM PATIENTS AND FAMILIES

Sometimes opportunities for ethical engagement arise not in the form of full discussion but in short—perhaps unforeseen—questions from patients and families. Box 53.1 lists some difficult questions and statements from the patient and/or family that the APRN may be confronted with and on which it can be useful to reflect. Common fears associated with these, and pitfalls to avoid, are also included.

Box 53.1 QUESTIONS TO EXPECT AND PITFALLS TO AVOID

Questions/statements that may arise while navigating ethical discussions:

1. How long do I have to live?

2. Tell me that everything is going to be all right.

3. Are you saying that I am going to die?

4. Is there no hope for me?

5. Don't tell XX (the patient) that he is dying.

6. If you don't feed her, she will starve to death.

7. If this were your mother, what would you do?

8. There must be something you can do.

9. She is going to die anyway, so why not give more chemo?

10. Withdrawing the machine is the same as killing her—euthanasia. Call it what it is.

11. Why can't you just dial up the morphine? Why does she have to linger this way? Why does she have to suffer?

12. How can I tell my children that I am dying?

13. How will I die?

14. What is it like to die?

15. I don't like Dr. Q; is he always so rude?

Common fears when navigating ethical discussions:

1. Being blamed—"shooting the messenger"

2. Saying the wrong thing

3. Eliciting strong emotional responses

4. Not knowing the answer—not being comfortable saying "I don't know"

5. Expressing one's own emotions (crying)

6. Anxiety about one's own mortality

Pitfalls to avoid:

1. Making promises you can't keep

2. Giving information when you don't have the facts

3. Giving premature reassurance

There is an abundance of literature suggesting phrases to use in responding to such questions and statements, and the reader is referred to this literature.[25,31,67–69]

REFERENCES

1. Tarzian AJ. Ethical aspects of palliative care. In: Matzo M, Witt Sherman D, eds. *Palliative Care Nursing: Quality Care to the End of Life*. 5th ed. New York: Springer; 2018: 49–78. doi:10.1891/9780826127198.0004

2. Cheon J, Coyle N, Wiegand DL, Welsh S. Ethical issues experienced by hospice and palliative nurses. *J Hosp Palliat Nurs*. 2015;17(1):7–13. doi:10.1097/NJH.0000000000000129

3. American Nurses Association (ANA). *Code of Ethics for Nurses with Interpretive Statements*. 2nd ed. Silver Spring, MD: ANA; 2015. https://www.nursingworld.org/coe-view-only

4. Etkind SN, Bone AE, Lovell N, Higginson IJ, Murtagh FEM. Influences on care preferences of older people with advanced illness: A systematic review and thematic synthesis. *J Am Geriatr Soc*. 2018;66(5):1031–1039. doi:10.1111/jgs.15272

5. Institute of Medicine (IOM). *The Future of Nursing: Leading Change, Advancing Health*. Washington, DC: National Academies Press; 2011. https://www.nap.edu/catalog/12956/the-future-of-nursing-leading-change-advancing-health

6. Russo M, Wiegand D. Ethical considerations. In: Dahlin C, Moreines Tycon L, Root M, eds. *Core Curriculum for the Hospice and Palliative Advanced Practice Registered Nurse*. 3rd ed. Pittsburgh, PA: HPNA; 2020: 739–763.

7. Altilio T, Coyle N. The interdisciplinary team: Integrating moral reflection and deliberation. In: Kirk TW, Jennings B, eds. *Hospice Ethics: Policy and Practice in Palliative Care*. New York: Oxford University Press; 2014: 103–117. doi:10.1093/acprof:oso/9780199944941.003.0006

8. Rushton CH. Creating a culture of ethical practice in health care delivery systems. *Hastings Cent Rep*. 2016;46(Suppl 1):S28–S31. doi:10.1002/hast.628

9. International Council of Nurses (ICN). *Code of Ethics for Nurses*. Geneva: ICN; 2012. https://www.icn.ch/sites/default/files/inline-files/2012_ICN_Codeofethicsfornurses_%20eng.pdf

10. Yeo M, Moorhouse A, Khan P, Rodney P, eds. *Concepts and Cases in Nursing Ethics*. 4th ed. Peterborough, ONT: Broadview Press; 2020.

11. Coyle N. Palliative care, hospice care, and bioethics: A natural fit. *J Hosp Palliat Nurs*. 2014;6(1):6–14. doi:10.1097/NJH.0000000000000032

12. Beauchamp TL, Childress JF. *Principles of Biomedical Ethics*. 8th ed. New York: Oxford University Press; 2019.

13. Walter JK, Ross LF. Relational autonomy: Moving beyond the limits of isolated individualism. *Pediatrics*. 2014;133(Suppl 1):S16–S23. doi:10.1542/peds.2013-3608D

14. National Health and Medical Research Council. An Ethical Framework for Integrating Palliative Care Principles into the Management of Advanced Chronic or Terminal Conditions. Canberra, ACT: National Health and Medical Research Council; 2011. https://pallcarevic.asn.au/wp-content/uploads/2015/11/Ethical-Framework-for-Integrating-Palliative-Care-Principles-.pdf

15. World Health Organization. Palliative Care. Key Facts. Aug 5, 2020. Geneva, Available at https://www.who.int/news-room/fact-sheets/detail/palliative-care

16. Kirk TW. Hospice care as a moral practice: Exploring the philosophy and ethics of hospice care. In: Kirk TW, Jennings B, eds. *Hospice Ethics: Policy and Practice in Palliative Care*. New York: Oxford University Press; 2014: 35–56. doi:10.1093/acprof:oso/9780199944941.003.0003

17. O'Hair D, Villigran MM, Wittenberg E, et al. Cancer survivorship and agency model: Implications for patient choice, decision making, and influence. *Health Commun*. 2003;15(2):193–202. doi:10.1207/S15327027HC1502_7

18. Manning RC. Toward a thick theory of moral agency. *Soc Theory Pract*. 1994;20(2):203–220.

19. Cassell EJ. *The Nature of Suffering and the Goals of Medicine*. 2nd ed. New York: Oxford University Press; 2004.

20. Ferrell BR, Coyle N. *The Nature of Suffering and the Goals of Nursing*. New York: Oxford University Press; 2008.

21. National Consensus Project for Quality Palliative Care. *The Clinical Practice Guidelines for Quality Palliative Care*. 4th ed. Richmond, VA: National Consensus Project for Quality Palliative Care; 2018. https://www.nationalcoalitionhpc.org/ncp/

22. Coyle N, Kirk TW, Coyle N, Doolittle M. Communication ethics. In: Wittenberg E, Ferrell B, Goldsmith J, Smith T, Glajchen M, Handzo GF, eds. *Textbook of Palliative Care Communication*. New York: Oxford University Press; 2016: 27–34. doi:10.1093/med/9780190201708.003.0005

23. Coyle N, Kirk TW. Advocacy in palliative nursing: A conceptual model. In: Ferrell BF, Paice JE, eds. *Oxford Textbook of Palliative Nursing*. 5th ed. Oxford: Oxford University Press; 2019: 861–867. doi:10.1093/med/9780190862374.003.0074

24. Gadow S. Existential advocacy: Philosophical foundation of nursing. In: Gadow S, Spicker SF, eds. *Nursing: Images and Ideals*. New York: Springer; 1980: 79–101.

25. Surbone A. Telling the truth to patients with cancer: what is the truth? *Lancet Oncol*. 2006;7(11):944-50. doi:10.1016/S1470-2045(06)70941-X

26. Trice ED, Prigerson HG. Communication in end-stage cancer: Review of the literature and future research. *J Health Commun*. 2009;14(Supp 1):95–108. doi:10.1080/10810730902806786

27. Zhang B, Nilsson ME, Prigerson HG. Factors important to patients' quality of life at end of life. *Arch Intern Med*. 2012;172(15):1133–1142. doi:10.1001/archinternmed.2012.2364

28. Siminoff LA, Thomson MD. The ethics of communication in cancer and palliative care. In: Kissane DW, Bultz BD, Butow PM, Bylund CL, Noble S, Wilkinson S, eds. *Oxford Textbook of Communication in Oncology and Palliative Care*. 2nd ed. Oxford: Oxford University Press; 2017: 28–32. doi:10.1093/med/9780198736134.003.0005

29. Becker G, Jors K, Block S. Discovering the truth beyond the truth. *J Pain Symptom Manage*. 2015;49(3):646–649. doi:10.1016/j.jpainsymman.2014.10.016

30. Hallenbeck J, Arnold R. A request for nondisclosure: Don't tell mother. *J Clin Oncol*. 2007;25(31):5030–5034. doi:10.1200/JCO.2007.11.8802

31. Lamas D, Rosenbaum L. Freedom from the tyranny of choice: Teaching end-of-life conversation. *N Engl J Med*. 2012;366(18):1655–1657. doi:10.1056/NEJMp1201202

32. Collopy B, Dubler N, Zuckerman C. The ethics of home care: Autonomy and accommodation. *Hastings Cent Rep*. 1990;20(2):S1–S16.

33. Epstein RM, Street RL Jr. *Patient-Centered Communication in Cancer Care*: Promoting Healing and Reducing Suffering. NIH Publication No. 07-6225. Bethesda, MD: National Cancer Institute; 2007. https://cancercontrol.cancer.gov/sites/default/files/2020-06/pcc_monograph.pdf

34. Wittenberg-Lyles E, Goldsmith J, Ferrell B, Ragan SL. *Communication in Palliative Nursing*. Oxford: Oxford University Press; 2013.

35. Dahlin C, Wittenberg E. Communication in palliative care: An essential competency for nurses. In: Ferrell BR, Paice J, eds. *Oxford Textbook of Palliative Nursing*. 5th ed. Oxford: Oxford University Press; 2019: 55–78. doi:10.1093/med/9780190862374.003.0005

36. Baile W, Buckman R, Lenzi R, Glover G, Beale EA, Kudelka AP. SPIKES: A six-step protocol for delivering bad news: Application to the patient with cancer. *Oncologist*. 2000;5(4):302–311. doi:10.1634/theoncologist.5-4-302

37. Helman CG. Communication in primary care: The role of patient and practitioner explanatory models. *Soc Sci Med*. 1985;20(9):923–931. doi:10.1016/0277-9536(85)90348-x

38. Kleinman A. *Patients and Healers in the Context of Culture*. Berkeley CA: University of California Press; 1980.

39. Kelm Z, Womer J, Walter JK, Feudtner C. Interventions to cultivate physician empathy: A systematic review. *BMC Med Educ*. 2014;14:219. doi:10.1186/1472-6920-14-219

40. Derksen F, Bensing J, Lagro-Janssen A. Effectiveness of empathy in general practice: A systematic review. *Brit J Gen Pract*. 2013;63(606):76–84. doi:10.3399/bjgp13X660814

41. Pehrson C, Banerjee SC, Manna R et al. Responding empathetically to patients: Development, implementation, and evaluation of a communication skills training module for oncology nurses. *Patient Educ Couns*. 2016;99(4):610–616. doi:10.1016/j.pec.2015.11.021

42. Irving P, Dickson D. Empathy: Towards a conceptual framework for health professionals. *Int J Health Care Qual Assur*. 2004;17(4):212–220. doi:10.1108/09526860410541531

43. Pan CX, Almeida Costa B, Yushuvayev EK, Gross L, Kawai F. Can Orthodox Jewish patients undergo palliative extubation? A challenging ethics case study. *J Pain Symptom Manage.* 2020;60(6):260–265. doi:10.1016/j.jpainsymman.2020.08.027

44. Loike J, Gillick M, Mayer S, et al. The critical role of religion: Caring for the dying patient from an Orthodox Jewish perspective. *J Palliat Med.* 2010;13(10):1267–1271. doi:10.1089/jpm.2010.0088

45. Applebaum PS. Assessment of patients' competence to consent to treatment. *N Engl J Med.* 2007;357(18):1834–1840. doi:10.1056/NEJMcp074045

46. McFarland DC, Blackler L, Hlubocky FJ, et al. Decisional capacity determination in patients with cancer. *Oncology (Willston Park).* 2020;34(6):203–210. https://www.cancernetwork.com/view/decisional-capacity-determination-in-patients-with-cancer

47. Sprung CL, Truog RD, Curtis JR, et al. Seeking worldwide professional consensus on the principles of end-of-life care for the critically ill. *Am J Respir Crit Care Med.* 2014;190(8):855–966. doi:10.1164/rccm.201403-0593CC

48. Sprung CL, Paruk F, Kissoon N, et al. The Durban World Congress ethics roundtable report: I. Differences between withholding and withdrawing life-sustaining treatments. *J Crit Care.* 2014;29(6):890–895. doi:10.1016/j.jcrc.2014.06.022

49. Cherny NI, Radbruch, EAPC. European Association for Palliative Care (EAPC) recommended framework for the use of sedation in palliative care. *Palliat Med.* 2009;23(7):581–593. doi:10.1177/0269216309107024

50. Imai K, Morita T, Akechi T, et al. The principles of revised clinical guidelines about palliative sedation of the Japanese Society for Palliative Medicine. *J Palliat Med.* 2020;23(9):1184–1190. doi:10.1089/jpm.2019.0626

51. Abarshi E, Rietjens J, Robijn L, et al. International variations in clinical practice guidelines for palliative sedation: A systematic review. *BMJ Support Palliat Care.* 2017;7(3):223–229. doi:10.1136/bmjspcare-2016-001159

52. Rodrigues P, Crokaert J, Gastmans G. Palliative sedation for existential suffering: A systematic review of argument-based ethics literature. *J Pain Symptom Manage.* 2018;55(6):1577–1590. doi:10.1016/j.jpainsymman.2018.01.013

53. Ciancio AL, Mirza RM, Ciancio AA, Klinger CA. The use of palliative sedation to treat existential suffering: A scoping review on practices, ethical considerations, and guidelines. *J Palliat Care.* 2020;35(1):13–20. doi:10.1177/0825859719827585

54. Gurschick L, Mayer DK, Hanson LC. Palliative sedation: An analysis of international guidelines and position statements. *Am J Hosp Palliat Care.* 2015;32(6):660–671. doi:10.1177/1049909114533002

55. Maltoni M, Scarpi E, Rosati M, et al. Palliative sedation in end-of-life care and survival: A systematic review. *J Clin Oncol.* 2012;30(12):1378–1383. doi:10.1200/JCO.2011.37.3795

56. Spielthenner G. The principle of double effect as a guide for medical decision making. *Med Health Care and Phil.* 2008;11(4):465–473. doi:10.1007/s11019-008-9128-0

57. Quill TE, Dresser R, Brock DW. The rule of double effect: A critique of its role in end-of-life decision making. *N Engl J Med.* 1997;337(24):1768–1771. doi:10.1056/NEJM199712113372413

58. Macauley R. The role of the principle of double effect in ethics education in US medical schools and its potential impact on pain management at the end of life. *J Med Ethics.* 2012;38(3):174–178. doi:10.1136/medethics-2011-100105

59. Mangan JT. An historical analysis of the principle of double effect. *Theol Stud.* 1949;10(1):41–61. doi:10.1177/004056394901000102

60. Suva G, Penney T, McPherson CJ. Medical assistance in dying: A scoping review to inform nurses' practice. *J Hosp Palliat Nurs.* 2019;21(1):46–53. doi:10.1097/NJH.0000000000000486

61. Epstein EG, Hamric AB. Moral distress, moral residue, and the crescendo effect. *J Clin Ethics.* 2009;20(4):330–342.

62. Varcoe C, Pauly B, Webster G, Storch J. Moral distress: Tensions as springboards for action. *HEC Forum.* 2012;24(1):51–62. doi:10.1007/s10730-012-9180-2

63. Ruston CH, Kazniak AW, Halifax JS. Addressing moral distress: Application of a framework to palliative care practice. *J Palliat Med.* 2013;16(9):1080–1088. doi:10.1089/jpm.2013.0105

64. Lamb C, Evans M, Babenko-Mould Y, Wong CA, Kirkwood KW. Conscience, conscientious objection, and nursing: A concept analysis. *Nurs Ethics.* 2019;26(1):37–49. doi:10.1177/0969733017700236

65. Wicclair M. Conscientious objection in healthcare and moral integrity. *Camb Q Healthc Ethics.* 2017;26(1):7–17. doi:10.1017/S096318011600061X

66. Wicclair M. Preventing conscientious objection in medicine from running amok: A defense of reasonable accommodation. *Theor Med Bioeth.* 2019;40(6):539–564. doi:10.1007/s11017-019-09514-8

67. Back AL, Arnold RM. Dealing with conflict in caring for the seriously ill: "It was just out of the question." *JAMA.* 2005;293(11):1374–1381. doi:10.1001/jama.293.11.1374

68. Borowske D. Straddling the fence: ICU nurses advocating for hospice care. *Crit Car Nurs Clin North Am.* 2012;24(1):105–116. doi:10.1016/j.ccell.2012.01.006

69. Quill TE, Arnold R, Back A. Discussing treatment preferences with patients who want "everything." *Ann Intern Med.* 2009;151(5):345–349. doi:10.7326/0003-4819-151-5-200909010-00010

54.

DISCONTINUATION OF CARDIAC THERAPIES

Patricia Maani Fogelman and Janine A. Gerringer

KEY POINTS

- Heart failure and cardiac advanced practice registered nurses (APRNs) are vital members of the management team for patients with heart failure. APRNs are primarily the providers following patients through trajectories of long-term chronic disease management and progression.

- The heart failure and cardiac APRN is often the primary provider who maintains responsibility for managing the treatment of complex and advancing heart failure.

- Ongoing assessment, medication management, symptom management, care planning, goals-of-care discussions, and end-of-life planning are all under the purview of the APRN.

- Heart failure, cardiac, and palliative APRNs provide medical care and disease management, education, patient and family counseling, and overall health promotion for patients with advancing and/or terminal heart failure.

CASE STUDY: A PATIENT WITH HEART FAILURE

Mrs. X was a 73-year-old woman with an extensive history of heart disease with resulting severe heart failure, chronic kidney disease Stage III, diabetes, hypothyroidism, and osteoporosis. She underwent triple-vessel coronary artery bypass graft (CABG) surgery 15 years prior with two myocardial infarctions in the past 3 years. Her quality of life was deteriorating due to her increasing need for assistance with her daily activities. Mrs. X was not a candidate for heart transplantation. She resided with her husband in their home, and two adult children lived nearby. Approximately 5 months prior, her doctors implanted a left ventricular assist device (LVAD) as destination therapy for her very debilitating Stage IV heart failure, with the hopes that this device would maximize the volume of blood pumped by her heart into her body.

Following device implantation, Mrs. X was in the intensive care unit (ICU) for approximately 2 months due to complications of chronic wound infections, kidney failure, and sepsis. She was discharged from the hospital to a nursing home for short-term rehabilitation and returned home 8 weeks later. Her quality of life did not appreciably improve. After 3 weeks, Mrs. X was readmitted due to significant weakness, fatigue, air hunger, pain, nausea, anorexia, and declining performance status bordering on a performance status of 4. Palliative care was consulted as she began to ask questions about device deactivation. In a family

meeting including the palliative advanced practice registered nurse (APRN), cardiology, Mrs. X and family were informed that once the LVAD was disabled, death would occur within hours. Mrs. X verbalized understanding of these implications and emphasized her poor quality of life. She was particularly distressed by her continued weakness, air hunger, and loss of dignity. Mrs. X declared her desire for deactivation of her device with the transition to comfort care. Her family was tearful but supportive, acknowledging she had struggled for a long time and wanted to avoid prolonging her suffering. The heart failure and palliative APRNs reviewed the procedure for device discontinuation. They planned the deactivation and medications were administered to relieve any respiratory distress or anxiety. Later that afternoon, her LVAD was disabled. The palliative APRN and ICU nurses provided supportive care for Mrs. X, ensuring that her dyspnea, anxiety, and agitation were well controlled. She died peacefully 2 hours later, surrounded by her family.

INTRODUCTION

There are many challenges to the integration of palliative care in the care of heart failure patients, likely due in part to the difficulty of prognostication in a population with exacerbations and a high risk for sudden death, as well as deficits in provider knowledge. Patients with advanced heart failure have demonstrated preferences to discontinue therapies or procedures they deem to be ineffective or burdensome, and they may ask about deactivating devices that had been placed earlier in their disease course, when there was more benefit to be gained. As their disease trajectory evolves, patients demonstrate a desire and willingness to discuss end-of-life planning, redefine the goals of care, and establish a plan for pain and symptom management when their disease can no longer be controlled or managed by their present medical regimen. Healthcare providers, often perceiving death as a "failure," tend to avoid these discussions. The key to breaking down these barriers is continued promotion of palliative care education and awareness. Palliative advanced practice registered nurses (APRNs) can facilitate the delivery of palliative care to heart failure patients by promoting educational activities on their units and using resources from the American Association of the Colleges of Nursing's End of Life Nursing Education Consortium (AACN-ELNEC). This national education initiative strives to enhance the delivery of palliative care by providing education and development tools for nursing staff. The ELNEC project provides APRNs with education in palliative care and advanced disease management and allows these nurse educators to "teach it forward" to their staff, peers, and healthcare colleagues.

DISCONTINUATION OF VASOPRESSORS

Vasopressors are medications delivered intravenously to support blood pressure during periods of hemodynamic instability in the acute care setting, most notably in the treatment of shock. Examples of vasopressors are epinephrine, norepinephrine, phenylephrine, and vasopressin.[1] Vasopressors induce vasoconstriction and elevate arterial pressure.

The general practice is to stop these medications when their desired effects are no longer elicited. Vasopressors are generally discontinued when other forms of life support, such as ventilator support or renal dialysis, are discontinued after the patient, patient's family, and medical teams have deemed their use to have no further benefit. The role of the palliative APRN is to offer treatment to relieve and anticipate distressing symptoms before discontinuing vasopressors and other forms of life support. In the acute care setting, medications are often stopped either at the same time or before or after ventilator support. It is critical to anticipate the provision of palliative management of terminal heart failure symptoms (pain, dyspnea, nausea, anxiety). To ensure a peaceful death, palliative APRNs should educate the patient and family about the dying process, including signs and symptoms and how they will be managed. This includes sudden cardiac death, hypotension with loss of perfusion (skin changes, mottling, and cyanosis), somnolence, disorientation when awake, restlessness, diminished senses and inability to respond to stimulus (although awareness remains intact longer), coma, changes in body temperature, respiratory pattern changes, and changes in oral secretions.

Palliative APRNs should refer to organizational policies regarding discontinuation of vasopressors. Heart failure and palliative APRNs are often critical players in developing these protocols. If there are complicated circumstances, an ethics consultation should be initiated. The heart failure APRN should rapidly assess the patient to ensure that appropriate care is provided. The palliative care team is especially important in situations where the patient's acute decline was not expected, thereby exacerbating the period of crisis. Palliative care consultation will help family members decide what the patient would want under the circumstances and will help the family understand the discontinuation process, including how they can keep the patient comfortable during the dying process (see Box 54.1 for discontinuation steps).

DISCONTINUATION OF INOTROPES

Intravenous inotropic agents are used in acutely ill, hospitalized heart failure patients with a severely reduced ejection fraction. In the acute setting, inotropes are used to establish

---

Box 54.1 DISCONTINUATION OF VASOPRESSORS AND INOTROPES

1. Patient and family discussion regarding goals of care
   a. Include who would like to be present with the patient during discontinuation

2. Team meeting
   a. Sequence of medication discontinuation if more than one
   b. Any other life-saving measures that need to be addressed

3. Room preparation
   a. Clearing of unnecessary or distracting items
   b. Prepare the patient; reposition for comfort

4. Interdisciplinary team presence (e.g., spiritual care, respiratory therapy for ventilator)

5. Premedication

6. Discontinuation of medication

7. Monitor until death
   a. Treat any perceived patient discomfort

8. Death pronouncement per facility guidelines

9. Support for the family and staff

10. Care of the body per facility guidelines

---

hemodynamic stability by increasing systemic perfusion and preserving end-organ function. The use of inotropes focuses on clinical improvement or as a bridge to a more permanent treatment, such as surgery, cardiac transplant, or left ventricular assist device (LVAD) placement. In rare circumstances, patients at home may receive short-term initiation of inotropes under palliative home care or hospice.

In an acute situation, a discussion should be held with the patient and family regarding the limited options available should inotrope therapy be unsuccessful. Treatment goals should be discussed so that appropriate steps can be taken regarding the patient's plan of care.[2] Inotropes may also be used as a long-term palliative treatment in patients whose advanced heart failure is refractory to other guideline-directed oral medications and who are not candidates for a ventricular assist device (VAD) or a cardiac transplant. The goal of chronic inotropic therapy is symptom relief. Inotrope treatment is initiated based on hemodynamic evidence of clinical benefit and on the patient's wishes. Goals of care and possible end-of-life scenarios should be discussed before starting continuous inotrope therapy.[2]

The most common inotropes used in the home setting are milrinone, dobutamine, and dopamine. These inotropes can be administered intravenously through a small pump, which allows the patient to remain at home during treatment.[3] Palliative APRNs should monitor patients for the risks of continuous inotropic therapy, such as central line infection, hypotension, and arrhythmias.[4] To minimize the risk of adverse effects such as arrhythmias, the lowest dose needed for symptom relief should be used.[2] Inotropes can help reduce hospitalizations and reduce symptoms in advanced heart failure patients. It is important to note that chronic inotrope therapy in patients who are not candidates for cardiac transplant or LVAD results in poor survival outcomes.[5]

APRNs should monitor the patient for changes in clinical status and goals of care. If the patient is no longer benefiting from inotrope therapy, the palliative APRN should revisit the goals of care. APRNs can manage heart failure patients with the right medications and can perform the tasks associated with discontinuation (if allowed in their practice setting), including writing orders to discontinue medications. Again, the palliative APRN should discuss the signs and symptoms of the dying process and should establish mutual goals with the family regarding a peaceful death for the patient. Many patients express their desire to be at home during the final stages of dying. Taitel and colleagues[6] found that patients who participated in a home inotrope infusion program were more likely to die at home than in the hospital. Patients may be discharged to hospice as well.

DISCONTINUATION OF VENTRICULAR ASSIST DEVICES

Mechanical circulatory support is becoming a widely accepted treatment for patients with advanced (stage D) heart failure with a reduced ejection fraction refractory to guideline-directed oral medications and cardiac device intervention. VADs are designed to assist the patient's failing native ventricle by improving cardiac output.

VADs can serve patients in both the short term, when patients are acutely decompensated and hemodynamically unstable, and in the long term, when patients have chronic advanced heart failure. VADs can stabilize the patient so decisions can be made regarding the plan of care, such as the need for surgical intervention (e.g., revascularization, correction of valve abnormalities, permanent pump placement, or, when appropriate, pump explant).[2]

Patients who are waiting for a cardiac transplant and need additional support until a donor heart becomes available can receive an LVAD as a bridge to transplant. If the patient's heart failure is severe and irreversible and the patient is not a cardiac transplant candidate, he or she can receive an LVAD as destination therapy. Destination therapy with an LVAD has proved to prolong survival and improve both quality of life and functional status in select patients with end-stage heart failure.[7]

Long-term LVADs are surgically implanted pumps that connect from the left ventricle to the ascending aorta to assist with systemic circulation. Blood exits the left ventricle through the inflow cannula, enters the pump, and is then directed through an outflow cannula to the aorta. An external driveline and power source are connected to the body to power the pump.[8]

Hospitals that offer LVAD therapy have an interdisciplinary team that participates in the patient's pre-implant and long-term care. In October 2014, the Joint Commission mandated that certified destination therapy VAD programs have a palliative care representative who has experience with the VAD population on the institution's interdisciplinary team.[9] Palliative care services should be initiated early on, when the patient is undergoing evaluation prior to implantation. The role of the palliative care team is to promote goals-of-care discussions, ensuring the inclusion of both the patient and the surrogate decision-makers. Palliative care should be available to support patients who have decided to undergo LVAD implantation, as well as patients who have been deemed ineligible for an LVAD or who decline implantation in favor of optimal medical management alone. The palliative APRN provides ongoing assessment of quality of life, goals of care, and health status. Major changes in health status due to device-related complications or other comorbidities not related to the device may lead to revisiting end-of-life discussions. Potential complications that may result in death include stroke, infection, and multiple-organ failure.[8] Again, partnership with the palliative care team is vital in managing patients with an LVAD and approaching the end of life.[10]

When deactivating an LVAD, many issues need to be considered. Of primary importance is the patient's wishes, expressed either directly or through advance care planning documents such as a living will or surrogate decision-maker. The medical team must agree on the lack of benefit and a minimal chance of meaningful recovery to continuing device therapy. APRNs are integral members of this team as they develop an intimate relationship with heart failure patients and families due to the chronicity of the disease. Caring for these patients at the end of life is just as important as caring for them through their life. If the interdisciplinary medical team cannot reach a consensus regarding device discontinuation, consultation with a hospital ethicist or ethics committee may be necessary.[11]

Swetz and colleagues[12] found that consultation with palliative care before patients received an LVAD for destination therapy was conducive to developing *personal preparedness plans*, which are expanded advance directives for patients with LVADs. Personal preparedness planning focuses on points unique to treatment with an LVAD, including situations where the heart can be supported by the device but other medical conditions or functional limitations may have a significant negative effect on the patient's health status and quality of life. Preparedness planning can be particularly advantageous if a major adverse event or change in quality of life occurs because palliative care already established a rapport with the patient and family and can focus on the situation at hand.

Various models have evolved for addressing ethical concerns in the treatment of VAD patients.[13] Key elements note that advance directives are particularly important in VAD patients because most patients and families are not aware of the issues that may arise while the patient is supported with a VAD. For example, the VAD can continue to mechanically support the blood pressure in an otherwise fatal situation.

1. The APRN should be familiar with the system's alarms and how to turn them off, so as not to cause any additional distress to the patient and the patient's family members.

2. The APRN should order, assist in administration of, and monitor the efficacy of medications directed toward patient comfort prior to LVAD device deactivation because the cardiovascular circulation may significantly decrease when the LVAD ceases to function.

3. Removal of the power sources and the driveline from the controller will cause the LVAD to stop functioning. As with ventilator discontinuation, the APRN should be prepared to act quickly to prevent and treat signs and symptoms of discomfort.

1. Patient and family discussion regarding goals of care[14]
   a. Include who would like to be present with the patient during deactivation

2. Team meeting
   a. Who will deactivate the device?
   b. Any other life-saving measures that need to be addressed

3. Room preparation
   a. Clearing of unnecessary or distracting items
   b. Prepare the patient; reposition for comfort

4. Interdisciplinary team presence (e.g., spiritual care, respiratory therapy for ventilator)

5. Premedication[15]

6. Deactivation of LVAD[14]
   a. Attempt to limit device noise to decrease anxiety for patient and family

7. Monitor until death[15]

8. Death pronouncement per facility guidelines

9. Support for the family and staff

10. Care of the body per facility guidelines

Discussion should be based on the type of support the VAD will offer, either as destination therapy or a bridge to transplant, keeping in mind that the patient can transition between the two types of support under certain circumstances. The model further states that discussion should occur before an advance directive is formulated regarding complications related to the implant procedure and to VAD therapy, such as bleeding, neurological events, and infection. This is the time to address any major conflicts between the patient and designated decision-makers.

Prior to deactivation of the LVAD, the following points should be discussed with the patient and a surrogate decision-maker: current condition and prognosis, change in benefit of current therapy, how the device will be halted, how symptoms will be treated, patient and surrogate decision-maker's readiness to proceed, and the anticipated outcome.[14] There are models of LVADs which have different steps for deactivation. Healthcare professionals should first refer to any institutional protocols regarding VAD deactivation. In the absence of a formal institutional protocol, Gafford and colleagues[15] have outlined key points for LVAD withdrawal so that the patient can die peacefully (Box 54.2).

Deactivation can occur in the hospital or at home, depending on the patient's medical condition, preference and wishes for site of death, and whether the event is acute or chronic. In the hospital, the APRN can oversee the process and be available to support the patient, the patient's family, and the staff. This includes writing orders for discontinuation of the device and administering medications for comfort. If deactivation is to occur at home, the process will depend on whether hospice is involved and state advanced practice nurse statutes. The palliative APRN may be responsible for overseeing the deactivation from start to finish. Or they may teach the patient's family or hospice staff how to deactivate the device and how to administer medication for the patient's comfort to ensure a peaceful death. Both in the hospital and at home, the palliative APRN acts as a liaison between the patient and the heart failure team to determine how to dispose of the external LVAD equipment according to local regulations for biological medical equipment (see Box 54.3).

DISCONTINUATION OF EXTRACORPOREAL MEMBRANE OXYGENATION

Extracorporeal membrane oxygenation (ECMO) is a form of temporary mechanical circulatory support used in critically ill patients with respiratory and/or cardiac failure. It is connected to the patient via cannulas in the large arteries and veins, removing blood from the body and transporting it to an oxygenator that adds oxygen and removes carbon dioxide (lung function). It then returns blood to the heart through a pump with the same force as the heart (cardiac function).[16]

Venoarterial (VA)- ECMO is used in patients with acute cardiogenic shock and/or cardiac arrest as either a bridge to recovery or other treatment. It does not cure the patient of the underlying condition. It provides time for the patient to heal or acts as a bridge to another long-term solution such as LVAD or heart transplant, staying in place for days to weeks until a decision can be made.[17] Ethically, it may be more beneficial to discontinue ECMO support after a prognosis becomes clear instead of withholding treatment under acute clinical conditions in which the outcome is uncertain.[18]

Critically ill patients requiring ECMO are usually cared for by a multidisciplinary team including critical care, cardiology cardiothoracic surgery, perfusion, and anesthesia. Core ECMO teams usually consist of specially trained physicians, an ECMO coordinator, nurse practitioners, staff nurses, perfusionists, and respiratory therapists.[19] Potential complications can include pulmonary edema, limb ischemia, ischemic stroke, intracranial bleed, severe bleeding, and infection.[20]

The acute need associated with ECMO can leave little time for detailed discussions regarding goals of care. The patient being placed on ECMO may not be able to participate in decision-making. In this case, the medical team and surrogate decision-maker often need to make complex decisions based on clinical outcomes that are not entirely clear.[21] If recovery becomes unlikely, the palliative APRN can support both the clinical team and family as the goals of care are discussed and plans for termination of therapy are made. If discontinuation of ECMO is likely to result in immediate death, surrogate decision-makers and even staff members may perceive this decision-making as a profound burden.[22]

The palliative APRN can support the ECMO patient and families as they would any other acutely ill patient at a high risk of dying by continually assessing and clarifying the patient's and family's understanding, providing emotional and spiritual care, supporting conversations regarding patient-centered goals of care, and helping to provide comfort to the dying patient.[23] They also collaborate with their interdisciplinary team members, such as social work and chaplaincy, to provide support to patients, families, and health colleagues.

Often, the patient does not have the capacity to request or participate in the decision to discontinue ECMO support.[24] The palliative APRN may facilitate communication between the surrogate decision-makers and clinical team by organizing and leading family meetings to discuss clinical progress and goals of care. When patients are transitioning from a process of living to a process of dying, they or their family may decide to stop life-prolonging measures, and direct communication with the decision-makers is important to decrease the burden associated with making decisions for a patient unable to participate. Again, the palliative APRN can oversee the process and support the patient, surrogate decision-makers, and staff by writing orders for discontinuation of the device and administering medications for comfort.

DISCONTINUATION OF PACEMAKERS/ AUTOMATIC IMPLANTABLE CARDIOVERTER-DEFIBRILLATORS

Implantable pacemakers are commonly used to treat patients with symptomatic bradycardia and sinus node dysfunction. Current pacing systems have one or two leads that are positioned in the right atrium and right ventricle and a small computerized pulse generator that is placed under subcutaneous tissue in the shoulder area. The pacemaker can deliver an electrical pulse to the heart, leading to cardiac muscle contraction.[25]

Implantable cardioverter-defibrillators (ICDs) are devices that increase survival by terminating life-threatening arrhythmias. ICDs do not treat heart failure by improving cardiac function or decreasing symptom burden, but they decrease the risk of sudden cardiac death.[26] The 2017 American College of Cardiology Foundation/American Heart Association/Heart Rhythm Society *Guidelines for the Management of Patients with Ventricular Arrhythmias and Prevention of Sudden Cardiac Death* address the specific criteria, determined through clinical trials, to identify those patients most at risk and make recommendations for the proper use of ICD devices.

Cardiac resynchronization therapy (CRT), on the other hand, synchronizes segmental and global contraction of the left as well as the right ventricle in patients with systolic heart failure who have a left bundle-type wide QRS complex and clinical symptoms of heart failure despite optimal medical therapy.[27] CRT can be combined with a pacemaker or ICD.[28]

CRT and ICD therapy may be available in the same device, but they offer very different options. CRT reduces the altered electrical activation of the left and right ventricles. This sometimes leads to favorable reverse remodeling and decreased severity of mitral regurgitation and left ventricular hypertrophy. CRT has been shown to improve survival and can significantly reduce symptoms and improve quality of life in end-stage heart failure patients. ICDs treat life-threatening tachyarrhythmias but do not improve symptoms. CRT-D (CRT with an ICD) implantation should prompt discussion regarding deactivation of either or both functions.[29]

The patient's goals of care should be assessed prior to implantation of a cardiovascular implantable electronic device (CIED), such as a pacemaker or ICD. The healthcare provider is responsible for discussing both the risks and benefits of CIED therapy. The palliative APRN can initiate discussion regarding deactivation and scenarios for the end of life prior to CIED implantation. The APRN may recommend that the patient complete an advance directive to outline his or her wishes at the end of life and designate a surrogate decision-maker. Deactivation should be readdressed should any major changes occur in the patient's health status,[30] as when prompted for a generator change, notification of device recall, diagnosis of another life-limiting illness, and when a decision is made for hospice care.[31] Sometimes, it is necessary to remove a CIED system, the generator, or the leads due to complications such as a CIED infection or structure failure of the CIED (e.g., lead fracture). When a pacemaker is removed, the indication for pacing versus risks of reimplantation should be discussed. When an ICD is removed, the patient is no longer protected from sudden cardiac death and a discussion regarding if and when to place a new ICD should occur.[32]

Prior to device deactivation, the patient should understand his or her prognosis, any treatment options, and what will happen when the device is discontinued. For example, the palliative APRN should discuss with the patient how deactivation of an automatic ICD may lead to death if a life-threatening arrhythmia occurs.[33]

Any provider or institution that implants CIEDs should have a protocol in place that clearly outlines the process for deactivating CIEDs when withdrawal of such care is appropriate. Palliative care professionals can facilitate discussions regarding deactivation of CIEDs, including the patient's and family's wishes as well as expected symptom management.[34] The final decision as to whether an ICD is burdensome should be made by the patient or a surrogate decision-maker.[33] A study by Buchhalter and colleagues[35] of patients who underwent cardiac device deactivation revealed that more than half of the requests for device deactivation came from surrogate decision-makers.

Whenever possible, deactivation should be performed by healthcare professionals with electrophysiology experience. This may include physicians and device-trained APRNs or technologists. In the absence of a device-trained specialist, deactivation can be performed by a healthcare professional such as a physician or an APRN under the guidance of an industry representative.[36] When a patient is at home with hospice or home health, a pacemaker magnet can be used to deactivate an ICD generator if a programmer is unavailable.[34] These general steps can be followed in any setting in which deactivation occurs, including acute care hospitals, patient care facilities, or the patient's home. Pacemakers may be discontinued by changing the programming mode, or the rate may be lowered and the output adjusted so that the device is no longer functional. ICD deactivation can be performed by changing the programming or, for certain pulse generators, constant application of a magnet over the device. Placement of a magnet over a pulse generator of most ICDs will temporarily cease the anti-tachycardia therapies while not affecting the pacemaker function. To spare the patient from multiple painful shocks, a doughnut magnet and instructions for use should be provided to patients with a terminal diagnosis.[2] The patient should be reassured that deactivation of the ICD through reprogramming is not painful.[37] The defibrillator function of an ICD is separate from the pacing function. Pacing does not need to be disabled when the ICD is reprogrammed. Pacing may treat bradyarrhythmias and cardiac resynchronization at the end of life for symptomatic relief in patients without causing discomfort (Box 54.4).[38]

Box 54.4 AUTOMATIC IMPLANTABLE CARDIOVERTER-DEFIBRILLATOR (AICD) DEACTIVATION STEPS

1. Patient and family discussion regarding goals of care
   a. Discussion regarding potential consequences of device deactivation
   b. Include who would like to be present with the patient during deactivation

2. Team meeting
   a. Who will deactivate the device?
   b. How will the device be deactivated (magnet vs. program change)?[38]

3. Deactivation of the AICD

4. Support for the patient, family, and staff

PALLIATIVE CARE AND THE ADVANCED HEART FAILURE PATIENT

Patients with advanced heart failure are living longer and with far more advanced modalities than once thought possible. Medical innovation highlights its intention to prolong life, but without attention to the truth that, for all of us, the natural endpoint of all life—death—will eventually arrive. APRNs are often the primary providers for these patients over their disease continuum, and it is the time-tested strength of this patient–APRN partnership that builds trust and therapeutic rapport and facilitates discussions about difficult but necessary end-of-life topics. The APRN can initiate the discussion about advance illness planning and revisit this discussion during clinic appointments throughout the disease management trajectory.

APRNs can initiate the referral to palliative care for early, upstream involvement to ensure comprehensive, patient-focused care that is not solely "disease-focused" but involves critically assessing the overall needs of the patient, family, and caregivers while allowing for periodic reassessment of needs and preferences. Considerable discussion and attention tends to be given to life-sustaining treatment while end-of-life issues are often considered the bane of patient–provider dialogue.[26] Advanced illness discussions are often deferred or avoided for a multitude of reasons including provider discomfort, patient fears, and inconsistent prognostication, as well as a shortage of trained palliative care clinicians. For this latter reason, earlier integration of palliative care principles into medical school, residency, and fellowship education will increase awareness of and understanding about palliative care in advanced diseases, with the hopeful goal of leading to earlier utilization of palliative care in the trajectory of chronically, progressive heart failure.[39,40] Advanced illness management requires ongoing goals-of-care discussions and shared decision-making as crucial to navigating the divergence between patient and provider ideals on perceived quality of care. For patients with advanced heart failure, especially those with assistive devices, early palliative care discussions and interventions are critical.[40,41]

Thanks to progress in bioengineering, devices can be used as destination therapy, aiming for stable provision of cardiac function; to this end, devices are now able to be successfully implanted in the human body. With this advanced technology, however, comes the responsibility to ensure that patients are aware of the risks, complications, and adverse outcomes. Medical technology fosters the conviction that one does not have to die "yet," which further solidifies an existing resistance or reluctance to discuss advanced illness planning, symptom management needs, goals of care, end-of-life care preferences, and code status.[42,43] National nursing and medical professional organizations have taken up the call to advocate for earlier and more appropriate involvement of palliative care in the care of patients with advanced disease.[44–47]

In palliative care, these challenging discussions provide the foundation for optimizing comprehensive "whole-person" care of the cardiac failure patient, especially those with implanted devices. Withdrawal of device support is an issue rampant with ethical and moral conflict, further emphasizing the need for early involvement of palliative care in partnership with cardiology so that effective, comprehensive care can be delivered to patients with advanced heart failure.[48] Palliative care assists patients across their continuum of illness, regardless of whether therapy is curative in intent, offering clinician and patient/family centered perspectives on a barrier-breaking approach to care with education, resources for support, frank but compassionate conversations about symptoms, advance illness planning and a framework for re-evaluation of goals as the disease progresses over time which integrates teaching from national models of care such as ELNEC.[49-54]

SYMPTOM MANAGEMENT

The predominant symptoms of distress for most dying patients, and especially those with cardiopulmonary organ failure, are pain, anxiety, and dyspnea. The goal of therapy for these symptoms is to ensure relief from suffering while allowing the desired level of interaction for as long as possible. Opioids such as morphine have been foundational medications to providing relief from the more severe symptoms of end-stage heart failure, such as dyspnea and pain.[55] It is important to bear in mind that there is no maximum dose of opioids for patients with end-of-life symptoms: patients must receive the dose that controls and relieves their distress and suffering and provides maximal comfort—sometimes in the necessary form of palliative sedation. Stronger medications may be necessary (see Chapter 43, "Pain" and Chapter 44, "Respiratory Symptoms" for more information).

The American Pain Society provides excellent guidelines and dosing recommendations for opioid medication management for end-stage or advanced illness.[55,56] *Principles of Analgesic Use in the Treatment of Acute Pain and Cancer Pain*[43] is a clinical resource that provides well-established guidelines for opioid initiation and management. This publication provides a solid framework and guidance for safe medication administration that can be useful for all practitioners.

The palliative APRN's goals for palliative care of the end-stage heart failure patient are to ensure clear patient and family communication, provide psychosocial support, and, when indicated, relieve pain, dyspnea, nausea, and any other distress. The APRN facilitates discussions to determine the goals of care by direct communication with the patient and family, by arranging a family meeting with palliative care and medical teams, or perhaps, if early in the disease trajectory, by simply initiating the referral to palliative care, with a preliminary patient discussion about the importance of planning for advanced illness and the services offered by additional consultants. Common symptoms to anticipate include chest pain, shortness of breath/dyspnea, air hunger, anxiety, nausea, and, later in the process, hallucinations. For patients with an LVAD, one of the most serious risk factors is a traumatic brain bleed leading to death. For these patients, control of neurotrauma-related symptoms is of utmost importance as

they can often be most distressing to the family. Symptoms can include increased secretions, agitation, and myoclonic or seizure-like activity.

PAIN AND DYSPNEA

Pain and dyspnea are best relieved using a multimodal approach: relief of pain and dyspnea with opioid therapy,[55-56] mindful breathing practice,[57] and the additional control of air hunger via enhanced air movement modalities such as a ceiling or oscillating fan because air movement across one's face often reduces the sensation of breathlessness, leading to a decreased sense of air hunger/dyspnea and anxiety.[54] A cooler temperature may also add to comfort and provide relief, as the reduction of humidity can remove it as a trigger for shortness of breath. The primary goal is to always assure the temperature of the room is comfortable for the patient. For patients who are awake and alert, the use of oral opioids for pain and dyspnea is preferred; for those with refractory or uncontrolled symptoms, escalation to intravenous or continuous therapy is preferred.[55-57]

MEDICATIONS USED AT END OF LIFE FOR PATIENTS WITH END-STAGE CARDIAC DISEASE

Patients with end stage cardiac diagnoses struggle with symptoms that may be physical, psychological, and spiritual. The APRN should bear in mind that not all suffering is physical, but the physical symptoms may often cause the most initial distress to the patient and will be what the family members remember after death. In heart failure, the symptom prevalence is as follows: pain (78%), dyspnea (61%), depression (59%), insomnia (45%), anorexia (43%), anxiety (30%), constipation (37%), nausea/vomiting (32%), fatigue, difficulty ambulating, and edema.[53,54] The APRN should continue to evaluate the patient's comfort and symptom burden and determine when/if additional interventions are warranted.

Diuretics: Furosemide (Lasix) and Torsemide (Demadex)

Heart failure patients at the end of life often have fluid overload, and diuretics are the core treatment of hypervolemia in these patients. Fluid status should be assessed prior to device removal. If a volume overload state is assessed, additional diuretic should be provided prior to withdrawal. Doses will vary because heart failure patients through the course of their illness tend to tolerate relatively high doses of diuretics; it is recommended that dosing be –initiated at the patient's last known dose and increased in 10–20 mg increments from their baseline dose. Advanced heart failure patients develop diuretic resistance over time, which requires rotation to a new diuretic (e.g., from furosemide to torsemide, which has been shown to have a better reduction in brain natriuretic peptide [BNP] level, collagen volume fraction [CVF], and edema). However, no meaningful difference between the agents concerning glomerular filtration rate (GFR), water extraction, and sodium excretion was demonstrated.[58] Regarding side effects, no significant difference among diuretics was observed in terms of hospital readmission and mortality rates. Therefore, there is no "correct" dose, but instead there is a "right dose for the patient." A urinary catheter should be in place for comfort, as frequent urination could create more distress than relief. To further reduce fluid overload, the palliative APRN should stop therapies that do not provide or contribute to comfort (e.g., intravenous fluids, continuous infusions). Opioids, when given as an infusion, can be concentrated to limit unnecessary fluids: the pharmacy can assist with this higher concentration.[55]

Lorazepam (Ativan)

Patients with end-stage cardiac diagnoses become more dyspneic with disease progression, leading to increasing levels of anxiety. Lorazepam is used to treat anxiety due to disease progression, uncontrolled dyspnea, or fear of dying. In addition, heart failure patients experience nausea from the effects of hypoperfusion and hypotension, for which lorazepam may also provide relief.[46] It can be given as an elixir, subcutaneously, intravenously, or as a continuous infusion for management of nausea, agitation, anxiety, myoclonus, or seizures. Dosing varies based on the patient's history and needs. Begin at 0.5 mg intravenously or orally every 4 hours as needed and rapidly titrate up to an effective dose; doses may be needed every hour for some patients.

Olanzapine (Zyprexa)

Olanzapine is a second-generation atypical antipsychotic that has shown off-label efficacy for the treatment of nausea, delirium, anxiety, insomnia, and cachexia in adults. This capacity for multisymptom relief allows it to be preferable to other alternatives such as haloperidol because it has a less significant impact on QTc intervals. Dosing begins at 2.5 mg daily and can be increased in 2.5 mg increments up to 20 mg daily.[59, 60]

Hyoscyamine (Levsin)

As their level of consciousness decreases, dying patients lose their ability to swallow and clear oral secretions. As air moves over the secretions, which have pooled in the oropharynx and bronchi, the resulting turbulence produces noisy ventilation with each breath, described as "gurgling" or "rattling" noises. While there is no evidence that patients find this "death rattle" disturbing, the noises may be disturbing to family, visitors, or caregivers, who worry the patient is choking to death. The death rattle is a good predictor of approaching death; one study indicated that the median time from onset of the death rattle to death was 16 hours.

Hyoscyamine should be given as an intravenous or subcutaneous injection for the management of oral secretions and is preferred over suctioning, which can cause further damage, swelling, edema, and secretions in the posterior airway and

increase patient distress. Dosing generally begins at 0.125 mg given intravenously every 4 hours.[61]

Scopolamine (Transderm Scop)

An option for oral secretion management is scopolamine. Scopolamine patches decrease secretions over a longer period of time. Scopolamine should not be used for acute symptoms because it takes an hour or so to take effect, but it does have the benefit of a steady state of symptom management. The usual dose for scopolamine is a 1.5 mg patch placed on the hairless area of skin just behind one ear. The patch needs to be replaced every 72 hours.[62]

Glycopyrrolate (Robinul)

Glycopyrrolate is an anticholinergic agent with approximately five times the anti-secretory potency of medications such as atropine, but it can have issues with erratic absorption. When administered intravenously, its onset of action is usually noted within a few minutes; dosing begins at 0.2 mg and can be increased to 0.4 mg every 1–4 hours as needed. It is especially helpful when administered 15 minutes prior to extubation in cases of compassionate extubation with transition to comfort care. For this reason, it can be a highly effective option for rapid improvement of distressing death rattle secretions for the patient's family and caregivers.[63]

Haloperidol (Haldol)

Haloperidol can be given as a liquid or as a subcutaneous or intravenous injection for management of agitation, restlessness, nausea, or terminal delirium. Delirium can be seen in a disproportionate amount of patients in end-of-life care;. Terminal delirium is an acute change in the level of arousal; features include an altered sleep–wake cycle, mumbling speech, disturbance of memory and attention, and perceptual disturbances accompanied by delusions and hallucinations. Haloperidol is commonly used for sedation. Haloperidol is administered in a dose-escalation process similar to that used to treat pain: the starting dose is 0.5–2 mg given orally or intravenously every hour as needed.[64]

Medical Cannabis

There is an increasing interest in the use of medical cannabis largely due to its potential to help reduce opioid dose requirements. There are variations in state and federal regulations as well as global views. It may not be available in the acute care setting but rather in the home setting. The data remain mixed, with no irrefutable evidence that medical cannabis diminished pain severity or yielded an opioid-sparing effect. Systematic reviews show doubt and bias, and conclusions had Grading of Recommendations, Assessment, Development and Evaluations (GRADE) rating of low- to very-low-quality evidence. As medical cannabis use increases, it is vital that well-constructed clinical trials, inclusive of patients with complex comorbidities, be performed (Table 54.1).[65–67]

Table 54.1 SYMPTOM MANAGEMENT MEDICATIONS

MEDICATION	PURPOSE	ROUTES	DOSE RANGES
Furosemide, Torsemide[58]	Fluid volume management, relief of swelling, dyspnea/	IV, oral	Begin at patient's baseline dose and increase by 10–20 mg increments.
Lorazepam[46]	Anxiety	IV, oral	0.5 mg IV or PO q4h as needed; rapidly titrate up to an effective dose. Doses may be needed every hour for some patients.
Olanzapine[59, 60]	Nausea	Oral	Begin 2.5 mg PO daily, increase in 2.5 mg increments to max dose of 20 mg/day.
Hyoscyamine[61]	Anti-secretory	IV	Dosing generally begins at 0.125 mg given IV q4h
Scopolamine[62]	Long-acting drug for secretion management	Transdermal	1.5 mg patch placed on the hairless area of skin just behind one ear and changed ever q72h. May be increased to 2 patches (one behind each ear) if no improvement in 72 hours.
Glycopyrrolate[63]	Anti-secretory	IV: Onset of action is usually noted within a few minutes.	0.2 to >0.4 mg every 1–4 hours as needed *or* start 15 min prior to compassionate extubation.
Haloperidol[64]	Agitation, restlessness, nausea, or terminal delirium	IV, SQ, or oral	0.5–2 mg PO, IV, or SQ every hour as needed
Medical Cannabis	Pain, nausea	Edibles, inhalational, tinctures	Availability varies with state policies governing use. Check your state's rules.

CARE TO PROMOTE HUMAN DIGNITY

Many nonpharmacological yet therapeutic options promote human dignity in caring for patients who are dying with end-stage cardiac diagnoses.

- *If a patient is feeling warm or uncomfortable*: Cool mouth swabs, cool compress to forehead. Families can be encouraged to participate in this care.

- *For mild dyspnea*: An oscillating fan, promoting air movement across the face can be helpful. Facilities may not allow fans if there is the potential to spread viruses and bacteria, particulary with new procedures with the onset of COVID-19. However, in the home setting, this is a preferred strategy to ameliorate shortness of breath

- *For increased oral secretions (or those not yet controlled by medications like hyoscyamine)*: Position or instruct the family to position the patient on his or her side or in a semi-prone position to facilitate postural drainage.

- *Encourage a peaceful atmosphere and family participation*: Use gentle massage, soft music, comforting stimuli (e.g., reading favorite poems or stories, religious music, aromatherapy).

- *Promote a calm environment and healing environment*: Food, support of a vigil volunteer, continued presence, and ask the family members or caregivers "What helps you relax? What would help you feel more comfortable?" (Try to meet their requests whenever possible within the means and resources of your organization.)[40]

SUMMARY

Mark Lazenby, APRN, once wrote: "Nursing imagination establishes the hope of health promoted, health restored, or life safely passing. When we are able to help our patients achieve that, through our imagination, we have resisted the threat of becoming an automaton. This is the ethical significance of imagination in our everyday lives as nurses. Through the habit of imagination, we preserve our patients' humanity in the world of automation and technology. We preserve our own as well."[68]

The management of heart failure begins with advance care planning: for patients with advanced heart failure, early palliative care intervention embodies an alliance between cardiology and palliative care with the shared goal of optimizing heart failure patients' care and well-being. Ongoing supportive care, with multimodality approaches including telephonic support, counseling, or medication management for effective symptom relief will all contribute to reducing both patient and caregiver burden and improving their quality of life.[69] Truly patient-centered planning entails timely referral to and partnership with palliative care so that the plan of care can be customized. Early and ongoing discussions with patients and families are vital elements to assuring ongoing, goal-concordant care. As heart failure worsens, the patient's needs will change as existing symptoms will intensify and new symptoms develop, and the goals of care need to be modified.

The palliative APRN can advocate for patients with heart failure and their families to ensure they receive excellent care throughout the illness and at the end of life. Palliative APRNs can manage cardiac medications and partner with palliative care for advanced modalities when the symptom burden intensifies or becomes refractory. Palliative APRNs caring for these patients must remember that end-of-life care is an art as well as a science, balancing the needs of the patient and effective symptom management.

REFERENCES

1. Gamper G, Havel C, Arrich J, et al. Vasopressors for hypotensive shock. *Cochrane Database Syst Rev.* 2016;2(2):CD003709. Published 2016 Feb 15. doi:10.1002/14651858.CD003709.pub4

2. Yancy CW, Jessup M, Bozkurt B, et al. 2013 ACCF/AHA guideline for the management of heart failure: A report of the American College of Cardiology Foundation/American Heart Association Task Force on Practice Guidelines. *J Am Coll Cardiol.* 2013;62(16):e147–e239. doi:10.1016/j.jacc.2013.05.019

3. Murthy S, Lipman HI. Management of end-stage heart failure. *Prim Care.* 2011;38(2):265–268. doi:10.1016/j.pop.2011.03.007

4. Kazory A, Ross EA. Emerging therapies for heart failure: Renal mechanisms and effects. *Heart Fail Rev.* 2012;17(1):1–16. doi:10.1007/s10741-010-9191-5

5. Hashim T, Sanam K, Revilla-Martinez M, et al. Clinical characteristics and outcomes of intravenous inotropic therapy in advanced heart failure. *Circ Heart Fail.* 2015;8(5):880–886. doi:10.1161/CIRCHEARTFAILURE.114.001778.

6. Taitel M, Meaux N, Pegus C, Valerian C, Kirkham H. Place of death among patients with terminal heart failure in a continuous inotropic infusion program. *Am J Hosp Palliat Care.* 2012;29(4):249–253. doi:10.1177/1049909111418638

7. Slaughter MS, Rogers JG, Milano CA, et al. Advanced heart failure treated with continuous-flow left ventricular assist device [published correction appears in *N Engl J Med.* 2018 Aug 16;379(7):697]. *N Engl J Med.* 2009;361(23):2241–2251. doi:10.1056/NEJMoa0909938

8. Slaughter MS, Pagani FD, Rogers JG, et al. Clinical management of continuous-flow left ventricular assist devices in advanced heart failure. *J Heart Lung Transplant.* 2010;29(4 Suppl):S1–S39. doi:10.1016/j.healun.2010.01.011

9. Lockard KL, Weimer A, O'Shea G, et al. The Joint Commission's disease-specific care certification for destination therapy ventricular assist devices. *Prog Transplant.* 2010;20(2):155–162. doi:10.7182/prtr.20.2.k52764070580v516

10. Goldstein NE, May CW, Meier DE. Comprehensive care for mechanical circulatory support: A new frontier for synergy with palliative care. *Circ Heart Fail.* 2011;4(4):519–527. doi:10.1161/CIRCHEARTFAILURE.110.957241

11. Feldman D, Pamboukian SV, Teuteberg JJ, et al. The 2013 International Society for Heart and Lung Transplantation Guidelines for mechanical circulatory support: Executive summary. *J Heart Lung Transplant.* 2013;32(2):157–187. doi:10.1016/j.healun.2012.09.013

12. Swetz KM, Freeman MR, AbouEzzeddine OF, et al. Palliative medicine consultation for preparedness planning in patients receiving left ventricular assist devices as destination therapy. *Mayo Clin Proc.* 2011;86(6):493–500. doi:10.4065/mcp.2010.0747

13. Cai A, Eisen HJ. Ethical considerations in the long-term ventricular assist device patient. *Curr Heart Fail Rep.* 2017;14(1):7–12. doi:10.1007/s11897-017-0313-4

14. Allen LA, Stevenson LW, Grady KL, et al. Decision making in advanced heart failure: A scientific statement from the American Heart Association. *Circulation.* 2012;125(15):1928–1952. doi:10.1161/CIR.0b013e31824f2173

15. Gafford EF, Luckhardt AJ, Swetz KM. Palliative care fast facts and concepts #269: Deactivation of a left ventricular assist device at the end-of-life. Sept 2015. Appleton, WI: Palliative Care Network of Wisconsin. https://www.mypcnow.org/fast-fact/deactivation-of-a-left-ventricular-assist-device-at-the-end-of-life/

16. White A, Fan E. American Thoracic Society "What is ECMO?" Patient Education Information series. *Am J Respir Crit Care Med.* 2016;193:9–10. Online version updated Mar 2020. https://www.thoracicorg/patients/patient-resources/resources/what-is-ecmo.pdf

17. Guglin M, Zucker MJ, Bazan VM, et al. Venoarterial ECMO for adults: JACC scientific expert panel. *J Am Coll Cardiol.* 2019;73(6):698–716. doi:10.1016/j.jacc.2018.11.038

18. DeMartino ES, Braus NA, Sulmasy DP, et al. Decisions to withdraw extracorporeal support: Patient characteristics and ethical considerations. *Mayo Clin Proc.* 2019;(94)4:620–627. doi:10.1016/j.mayocp.2018.09.020.

19. Salna M, Chicotka S, Biscotti M 3rd, et al. Management of surge in extracorporeal membrane oxygenation transport. *Ann Thorac Surg.* 2018;105(2):528–534. doi:10.1016/j.athoracsur.2017.07.019

20. Pineton de Chambrun M, Bréchot N, Combes A. Venoarterial extracorporeal membrane oxygenation in cardiogenic shock: indications, mode of operation, and current evidence. *Curr Opin Crit Care.* 2019 Aug;25(4):397–402. doi:10.1097/MCC.0000000000000627. PMID: 31116109.

21. Makdisi T, Makdisi G. Extra corporeal membrane oxygenation support: Ethical dilemmas. *Ann Transl Med.* 2017;5(5):112. doi:10.21037/atm.2017.01.38

22. Bein T, Brodie D. Understanding ethical decisions for patients on extracorporeal life support. *Intensive Care Med.* 2017;43(10):1510–1511. doi:10.1007/s00134-017-4781-5

23. Feinstein E, Rubins J, Rosielle DA. Palliative care fast facts and concepts #339: Extracorporeal membrane oxygenation in adults. Appleton, WI: Palliative Care Network of Wisconsin. 2017. https://www.mypcnow.org/fast-fact/extracorporeal-membrane-oxygenation-in-adults/

24. Godfrey S, Sahoo, A Sanchez J, et al. The role of palliative care in consultation in withdrawal of veno-arterial extracorporeal membrane oxygenation support for cardiogenic shock. *J Heart Lung Transplant.* 2020;39 (4):Supplement S417. doi:10.1016/j.healun.2020.01.190).

25. Kusumoto FM, Goldschlager N. Device therapy for cardiac arrhythmias. *JAMA.* 2002;287(14):1848–1852. doi:10.1001/jama.287.14.1848

26. Bardy GH, Lee KL, Mark DB, et al. Amiodarone or an implantable cardioverter-defibrillator for congestive heart failure [published correction appears in *N Engl J Med.* 2005 May 19;352(20):2146]. *N Engl J Med.* 2005;352(3):225–237. doi:10.1056/NEJMoa043399

27. Jarcho JA. Biventricular pacing [published correction appears in *N Engl J Med.* 2006 Sep 14;355(11):1184]. *N Engl J Med.* 2006;355(3):288–294. doi:10.1056/NEJMct055185

28. Kramer DB, Reynolds MR, Mitchell SL. Resynchronization: Considering device-based cardiac therapy in older adults. *J Am Geriatr Soc.* 2013;61(4):615–621. doi:10.1111/jgs.12174

29. Allen LA, Stevenson LW, Grady KL, et al. Decision making in advanced heart failure: A scientific statement from the American Heart Association. *Circulation.* 2012;125(15):1928–1952. doi:10.1161/CIR.0b013e31824f2173

30. Lampert R, Hayes DL, Annas GJ, et al. HRS expert consensus statement on the management of cardiovascular implantable electronic devices (CIEDs) in patients nearing end of life or requesting withdrawal of therapy. *Heart Rhythm.* 2010;7(7):1008–1026. doi:10.1016/j.hrthm.2010.04.033

31. Morgenweck CJ. Ethical considerations for discontinuing pacemakers and automatic implantable cardiac defibrillators at the end-of-life. *Curr Opin Anaesthesiol.* 2013;26(2):171–175. doi:10.1097/ACO.0b013e32835e8349

32. Garlitski AC. In: Morrison S. Ed. Management of cardiac implantation electronic devices in patients receiving palliative care. UpToDate. Waltham, MA: UptoDate. Updated Jan 24, 2020. https://www.uptodate.com/contents/management-of-cardiac-implantable-electronic-devices-in-patients-receiving-palliative-care

33. Wiegand DL, Kalowes PG. Withdrawal of cardiac medications and devices. *AACN Adv Crit Care.* 2007 Oct-Dec;18(4):415–425. doi:10.1097/01.AACN.0000298634.45653.81.

34. Wan D, Chakrabarti S. Deactivation of implantable cardioverter-defibrillators. *CMAJ.* 2021;193(23):E852. doi:10.1503/cmaj.210327

35. Buchhalter LC, Ottenberg AL, Webster TL, Swetz KM, Hayes DL, Mueller PS. Features and outcomes of patients who underwent

cardiac device deactivation. *JAMA Intern Med*. 2014;174(1):80–85. doi:10.1001/jamainternmed.2013.11564

36. Lindsay BD, Estes NA 3rd, Maloney JD, Reynolds DW; Heart Rhythm Society. Heart Rhythm Society policy statement update: Recommendations on the role of industry employed allied professionals (IEAPs). *Heart Rhythm*. 2008;5(11):e8–e10. doi:10.1016/j.hrthm.2008.09.023

37. Goldstein N, Carlson M, Livote E, Kutner JS. Brief communication: Management of implantable cardioverter-defibrillators in hospice: A nationwide survey. *Ann Intern Med*. 2010;152(5):296–299. doi:10.7326/0003-4819-152-5-201003020-00007

38. Murthy S, Lipman HI. Management of end-stage heart failure. *Prim Care*. 2011 Jun;38(2):265–276, viii. doi:10.1016/j.pop.2011.03.007

39. Chang YK, Kaplan H, Geng Y, et al. Referral criteria to palliative care for patients with heart failure: A systematic review. *Circ Heart Fail*. 2020;13(9):e006881. doi:10.1161/CIRCHEARTFAILURE.120.006881

40. Verdoorn BP, Luckhardt AJ, Wordingham SE, Dunlay SM, Swetz KM. Palliative medicine and preparedness planning for patients receiving left ventricular assist device as destination therapy: Challenges to measuring impact and change in institutional culture. *J Pain Symptom Manage*. 2017;54(2):231–236. doi:10.1016/j.jpainsymman.2016.10.372

41. Wordingham SE, McIlvennan CK. Palliative care for patients on mechanical circulatory support. *AMA J Ethics*. 2019 May 1;21(5):E435–442. doi:10.1001/amajethics.2019.435

42. SUPPORT Principal Investigators. A controlled trial to improve care for seriously ill hospitalized patients. The study to understand prognoses and preferences for outcomes and risks of treatments (SUPPORT). [published correction appears in *JAMA*.1996 Apr 24;275(16):1232]. *JAMA*. 1995;274(20):1591–1598.

43. Ben Gal T, Jaarsma T. Self-care and communication issues at the end of life of recipients of a left-ventricular assist device as destination therapy. *Curr Opin Support Palliat Care*. 2013;7(1):29–35. doi:10.1097/SPC.0b013e32835d2d50.

44. Ferrell BR, Twaddle ML, Melnick A, Meier DE. National Consensus Project clinical practice guidelines for quality palliative care guidelines, 4th edition. *J Palliat Med*. 2018;21(12):1684–1689. doi:10.1089/jpm.2018.0431

45. Mularski RA, Reinke LF, Carrieri-Kohlman V, et al. An official American Thoracic Society workshop report: Assessment and palliative management of dyspnea crisis. *Ann Am Thorac Soc*. 2013;10(5):S98–S106. doi:10.1513/AnnalsATS.201306-169ST

46. Lanken PN, Terry PB, Delisser HM, et al. An official American Thoracic Society clinical policy statement: Palliative medicine for patients with respiratory diseases and critical illnesses. *Am J Respir Crit Care Med*. 2008;177(8):912–927. doi:10.1164/rccm.200605-587ST

47. Whellan DJ, Goodlin SJ, Dickinson MG, et al.; Quality of Care Committee, Heart Failure Society of America. End-of-life care in patients with heart failure. *J Card* Fail. 2014;20(2):121–134. doi:10.1016/j.cardfail.2013.12.003

48. McKenna M, Wrightson N, Regnard C, Clark S. Life-sustaining medical devices at the end of life. *BMJ Support Palliat Care*. 2013;3(1):5–7. doi:10.1136/bmjspcare-2012-000364

49. Crimmins RM, Elliott L, Absher DT. Palliative Care in a Death-Denying Culture: Exploring Barriers to Timely Palliative Efforts for Heart Failure Patients in the Primary Care Setting. *Am J Hosp Palliat Care*. 2021;38(1):77–83. doi:10.1177/1049909120920545

50. Gelfman LP, Bakitas M, Warner Stevenson L, Kirkpatrick JN, Goldstein NE. The state of the science on integrating palliative care in heart failure. *J Palliat Med*. 2017 Jun;20(6):592–603. doi:10.1089/jpm.2017.0178. Epub 2017 May 12.

51. Pham R, McQuade C, Somerfeld A, Blakowski S, Hickey GW. Palliative care consultation affects how and where heart failure patients die [published online ahead of print, 2020 Oct 5]. *Am J Hosp Palliat Care*. 2020;1049909120963565. doi:10.1177/1049909120963565

52. Sullivan MF, Kirkpatrick JN. Palliative cardiovascular care: The right patient at the right time. *Clin Cardiol*. 2020;43(2):205–212. doi:10.1002/clc.23307

53. American Association of Colleges of Nursing. End-of-Life Nursing Education Consortium (ELNEC), ELNEC Curricula. APRN. 2021. https://www.aacnnursing.org/ELNEC/About/ELNEC-Curricula

54. Nguyen Q, Wang K, Nikhanj A, et al. Screening and initiating supportive care in patients with heart failure. *Front Cardiovasc Med*. 2019;6:151. doi:10.3389/fcvm.2019.00151

55. Manchikanti L, Kaye AM, Knezevic NN, et al. Responsible, safe, and effective prescription of opioids for chronic non-cancer pain: American Society of Interventional Pain Physicians (ASIPP) guidelines. *Pain Physician*. 2017;20(2S):S3–S92.

56. Paice JA. Cancer pain management and the opioid crisis in America: How to preserve hard-earned gains in improving the quality of cancer pain management. *Cancer*. 2018;124(12):2491–2497. doi:10.1002/cncr.31303

57. Ng DL, Chai CS, Tan KL, et al. The efficacy of a single session of 20-minute mindful breathing in reducing dyspnea among patients with acute decompensated heart failure: A randomized controlled trial [published online ahead of print, 2020 Jun 26]. *Am J Hosp Palliat Care*. 2021;38(3):246–252. doi:10.1177/1049909120934743

58. Eid PS, Ibrahim DA, Zayan AH, et al. Comparative effects of furosemide and other diuretics in the treatment of heart failure: A systematic review and combined meta-analysis of randomized controlled trials [published online ahead of print, 2020 Aug 11]. *Heart Fail Rev*. 2020. doi:10.1007/s10741-020-10003-7

59. Simon ST, Higginson IJ, Booth S, Harding R, Weingärtner V, Bausewein C. Benzodiazepines for the relief of breathlessness in advanced malignant and non-malignant diseases in adults. *Cochrane Database Syst Rev*. 2016;10(10):CD007354. doi:10.1002/14651858.CD007354.pub3

60. Washington NB, Brahm NC, Kissack J. Which psychotropics carry the greatest risk of QTc prolongation? *Curr Psychiatry*. 2012 Oct;11(10):36–39.

61. Hirsch CA, Marriott JF, Faull CM. Influences on the decision to prescribe or administer anticholinergic drugs to treat death rattle: A focus group study. *Palliat Med*. 2013;27(8):732–738. doi:10.1177/0269216312464407

62. Bailey FA, Williams BR, Woodby LL, et al. Intervention to improve care at life's end in inpatient settings: The BEACON trial. *J Gen Intern Med*. 2014;29(6):836–843. doi:10.1007/s11606-013-2724-6

63. Murtagh FE, Thorns A, Oliver DJ. Hyoscine and glycopyrrolate for death rattle. *Palliat Med*. 2002;16(5):449–450. doi:10.1191/0269216302pm601xx

64. Vella-Brincat J, Macleod AD. Haloperidol in palliative care. *Palliat Med*. 2004;18(3):195–201. doi:10.1191/0269216304pm881oa

65. Okusanya BO, Asaolu IO, Ehiri JE, Kimaru LJ, Okechukwu A, Rosales C. Medical cannabis for the reduction of opioid dosage in the treatment of non-cancer chronic pain: A systematic review. *Syst Rev*. 2020;9(1):167. doi:10.1186/s13643-020-01425-3

66. Fisher E, Moore RA, Fogarty AE, et al. Cannabinoids, cannabis, and cannabis-based medicine for pain management: A systematic review of randomised controlled trials [published online ahead of print, 2020 May 18]. *Pain*. 2020. doi:10.1097/j.pain.0000000000001929

67. Alonso-Coello P, Schünemann HJ, Moberg J, et al. GRADE Evidence to Decision (EtD) frameworks: A systematic and transparent approach to making well informed healthcare choices. 1: Introduction. *BMJ*. 2016;353:i2016. doi:10.1136/bmj.i2016

68. Lazenby M. *Caring Matters Most: The Ethical Significance of Nursing*. Oxford: Oxford University Press; 2017. https://oxford-medicine.com/view/10.1093/med/9780199364541.001.0001/med-9780199364541

69. Bakitas MA, Dionne-Odom JN, Ejem DB, et al. Effect of an early palliative care telehealth intervention vs usual care on patients with heart failure: The ENABLE CHF-PC Randomized Clinical Trial [published online ahead of print, 2020 Jul 27]. *JAMA Intern Med*. 2020;180(9):1203–1213. doi:10.1001/jamainternmed.2020.2861

55.

DISCONTINUATION OF RESPIRATORY THERAPIES

Brenna Winn

KEY POINTS

- The palliative advanced practice registered nurse (APRN) must have clinical knowledge of respiratory conditions that warrant advanced respiratory support.

- The palliative APRN must understand the importance of mastering effective communication with the family and/or patient regarding decisions to discontinue respiratory support/technology.

- The palliative APRN should anticipate and proactively manage symptoms associated with discontinuing respiratory support/technology at end of life.

- The palliative APRN must have an understanding of and take necessary precautions for withdrawing respiratory support in the setting of COVID-19.

- The palliative APRN must understand the clinical, ethical, and legal aspects of discontinuing respiratory support/technology.

CASE STUDY: DISCONTINUING RESPIRATORY SUPPORT

LM was an 81-year-old man with a past medical history significant for chronic obstructive pulmonary disease (COPD); diabetes type 2; coronary artery disease, status post double coronary artery bypass surgery in 1994; and a cerebrovascular accident (CVA) in 2013, leaving him with right-sided weakness and mild dysphagia. His dysphagia and right-sided weakness improved after his stay in inpatient rehabilitation. LM was recently admitted to the hospital with acute respiratory distress and fever. He was found to have pneumonia on chest radiograph and was started on oxygen as well as intravenous antibiotics.

LM had a rapid response called early the next morning: he was tachycardic, hypoxic, and minimally responsive. He was transferred to the intensive care unit (ICU) and emergently intubated for airway protection. LM's morning labs revealed a significant drop in his hemoglobin. A gastroenterology consult was placed. Further lab tests were ordered which raised concern for possible leukemia. An esophagogastroduodenoscopy revealed a gastrointestinal bleed. Hematology-oncology were consulted for further workup. Further testing confirmed an acute leukemia diagnosis. The palliative care team was consulted on hospital Day 11, intubation Day 10. LM lived with his wife of 63 years, and they had two grown children; all family members were involved in his care. The palliative advanced practice registered nurse (APRN)

was in daily communication with the intensivist in the ICU as well as the hematology/oncology team. Both ICU and hematology/oncology had discussed the patient's new diagnosis with the family as well as LM's overall prognosis.

Unfortunately, LM had difficulty weaning from the ventilator due to severe delirium and agitation thought to have been encephalopathy secondary to his acute pneumonia infection. The weaning process went on for several days during which the palliative APRN met daily with the family and continued ongoing discussions regarding their goals of care. LM's wife expressed that LM "would never want to live like this nor would he ever want to go through any sort of chemo treatment. I know he would rather just be comfortable. His only request has only ever been that he does not die in the hospital. Do you think he can make it home?" LM's wife was elderly herself and taking care of him at home would have been incredibly difficult for her.

The discussion regarding transitioning to comfort care was held with the goal being to transfer to the hospice house nearby. As part of the conversation of transitioning to comfort care, the procedure of palliatively extubating LM was described in detail to the family. There was emphasis placed on ensuring that LM would be calm and comfortable prior to beginning the procedure and throughout the end of his life.

The family made the decision to stay in the room for the procedure, the palliative APRN was present for emotional support and to assist in expert symptom management during extubation and afterward. LM received a bolus of morphine 2 mg IV and lorazepam 1 mg IV prior to extubating. He remained comfortable during the procedure. He received an additional three doses of morphine 2 mg IV and one additional dose of lorazepam 1 mg IV prior to transferring to the hospice house later that afternoon. His symptoms were well-managed at the hospice house by the hospice nurses. LM died 2 days later with his entire family at his bedside.

INTRODUCTION

Discontinuation of respiratory technology is a frequent occurrence in intensive care units (ICUs) all over the world. This procedure may be referred to as *compassionate extubation* or *palliative extubation*. In fact, 40% of ICU deaths typically involve palliative extubation, removal, or discontinuation of respiratory support.[1] *Respiratory technology* is a broad term that includes mechanical ventilation, noninvasive positive-pressure ventilation (NPPV), extracorporeal membrane oxygenation (ECMO), and high-flow nasal

> ### Box 55.1 ACRONYMS FOR TYPES OF
> ### SUPPLEMENTAL OXYGEN
>
> AIRVO: High-flow nasal oxygen
> NPPV: Noninvasive positive-pressure ventilation
> ECMO: Extracorporeal membrane oxygenation
> BIPAP: Bilevel positive airway pressure
> CPAP: Continuous positive airway pressure

oxygen (AIRVO). NPPV includes modalities such as continuous positive airway pressure (CPAP), bilevel positive airway pressure (BiPAP), and delivered oxygen (see Box 55.1). There are very few standards or protocols for discontinuing respiratory technology.[2] However, there are a multitude of research and case studies to guide APRNs when faced with patients in respiratory failure.

Discontinuing advanced respiratory technology is a carefully planned process that can occur when all efforts of weaning ventilation have failed, treatments may be nonbeneficial, and death is expected. When discussions regarding discontinuation of respiratory support arise, palliative advanced practice registered nurses (APRNs) and care team members have acknowledged that death is probable and that continuation of life-sustaining treatment may be prolonging the patient's dying process.[3] Typically, multiorgan failure is also a common factor that further validates poor prognosis and further warrants these discussions with families.[4] This chapter promotes a better understanding of the clinical, ethical, and legal aspects of discontinuing respiratory technology as well as improving symptom management skills associated with end of life in these patients.

RESPIRATORY FAILURE AND TYPES OF RESPIRATORY SUPPORT/TECHNOLOGY

Acute respiratory distress syndrome (ARDS), also known as hypoxic respiratory failure (AHRF), is one of the most common causes of critical illness requiring intensive care unit (ICU)-level care and advanced respiratory support.[4] ARDS is defined clinically as acute arterial hypoxemia, with a minimum requirement of 5 cm H_2O positive end-expiratory pressure (PEEP). Patients who meet this criteria typically exhibit signs on chest radiograph (CXR) such as bilateral opacities not exclusive to fluid overload[5] or cardiogenic pulmonary edema.[4]

OXYGEN

Oxygen is often used in patients with chronic obstructive pulmonary disease (COPD) or ARDS to alleviate dyspnea. However, there is little evidence proving that the addition of medical oxygen alleviates feelings of breathlessness. Supplemental oxygen is often part of palliative care or comfort care order sets, but it may not always be helpful. Some patients can report subjective improvement in symptoms

with addition of oxygen, and it can also lend psychological benefit to some patients and their families. However, oxygen can be uncomfortable for some patients, causing discomfort to the patient's nose; it can interfere with eating and talking and can cause dryness as well as bleeding. Opioids are proved to be more effective in relieving severe dyspnea than is higher flow oxygen. In fact, oxygen may prolong the patient's dying process. At end of life, the body's oxygen requirements change as the body begins to slow down.[6] High-flow oxygen may be discontinued as a way to improve a patient's comfort at end of life.

MECHANICAL VENTILATION

Mechanical ventilation includes respiratory support from an external machine to help patients in respiratory failure effectively breathe. This can be done using aggressive measures such as an endotracheal (ET) tube and ventilator or through less invasive methods involving NPPV. Any decision involving the need to initiate any form of mechanical ventilation warrants a conversation with the patient and/or family to review the medical condition, establish goals of care, discuss risks and benefits, and discuss alternative options to proceeding with aggressive measures.

NONINVASIVE POSITIVE-PRESSURE VENTILATION

NPPV includes AIRVO, CPAP, and BiPAP. Patients who require mechanical ventilation are typically in acute hypercapnic respiratory failure,[2] having difficulty adequately oxygenating and eliminating carbon dioxide. Common conditions that support use of NPPV include acute exacerbations of COPD, hypoxic respiratory failure in immunocompromised patient, acute respiratory failure with cardiogenic pulmonary edema, and neuromuscular diseases.[7] Patients who are on NPPV are generally able to have a conversation with the palliative APRN. Ideally, goals of care should be established prior to initiating NPPV.[2] It is important to address goals of care and ask questions regarding quality of life and if this type of intervention is causing discomfort or undesirable life prolongation. NPPV can be bothersome to patients, causing claustrophobia and anxiety, and, over time, it can lead to skin breakdown. It also negatively impacts goals of comfort at end of life. NPPV is used in both home and critical care settings, and the option of discontinuing this therapy presents itself in both settings. When death is expected, the palliative APRN should continuously assess the advantages and disadvantages of NPPV and the patient's physical symptoms and determine if these interventions are prolonging the patient's dying process.[2]

There are differing perspectives regarding NPPV at end of life; some suggest that offering NPPV can give the patient time with family or to finalize personal affairs.[7] Another perspective is that if a patient has decided to forgo intubation and mechanical ventilation, NPPV can prolong the dying process because NPPV is considered a form of life support.[7] The Society of Critical Care Medicine Task Force developed an approach for providers considering initiating NPPV in critical care settings using three categories.[7]

Category 1: NPPV as life support with no limitations on life-sustaining treatment, including escalation of care to ET intubation and ventilation.[7]

Category 2: NPPV as life support with the limitation of "do not intubate." The patient's goals of care are consistent with alleviating dyspnea, improving comfort, and restoring health. Improved oxygenation and little discomfort are signs of success. The patient will be able to wean from the machine and breathe on their own, or the patient will have difficulty tolerating NPPV. If there is difficulty tolerating, discussion should be initiated and transitioning to comfort care should be recommended.[7]

Category 3: NPPV as a comfort measure only in patients who are dying. The goal in this category is palliation of the patient's work of breathing.[5] This can minimize usage of opioids and increase wakefulness at end of life, which some patients prefer.[5,7] If the patient is unable to tolerate NPPV, symptoms should continue to be managed and NPPV should be discontinued.

There are no evidence-based guidelines for weaning NPPV at end of life. However, for quality and consistency, it is helpful for an organization to develop a policy and procedure. It should include medicine, nursing, respiratory therapy, social work, and chaplaincy to ensure that all the domains of care are met. If the decision is made to discontinue NPPV, symptoms should be closely monitored because severe dyspnea and anxiety can occur after removing NPPV. Initiating opioids and/or anxiolytics prior to discontinuing NPPV may help ensure the patient's comfort. Table 55.1 provides dosing details on opioids and anxiolytics.

INVASIVE MECHANICAL VENTILATION

Invasive mechanical ventilation refers to an artificial airway via an endotracheal or a tracheal tube that is then attached to a ventilator which in turn provides proper gas exchange and ventilation for the patient. ET tubes are meant to be temporary: the goal is to continue working with the patient to wean from the ventilator as their condition improves.[8] When attempts at weaning begin to fail and continued ventilator support becomes medically nonbeneficial, the option of palliative extubation should be presented to the patient, if able to speak for themselves, or to the family as surrogate decision-makers.[8] The palliative APRN should reinforce that mechanical ventilatory support is a treatment that can be forgone or discontinued. Moreover, palliative extubation is not hastening death. Rather, the process allows a dignified death consistent with a patient's values, preferences, and beliefs as stated in advance care planning documents. As well, palliative extubation may be viewed as promoting a more natural death without technology rather than a prolonged dying process (see Chapter 53, "Navigating Ethical Dilemmas"). The outcome

Table 55.1 SYMPTOM MANAGEMENT GUIDE OPIOIDS: MODERATE TO SEVERE DYSPNEA IN OPIOID-NAÏVE PATIENTS

MEDICATION	GUIDELINES
Morphine	2–5 mg IV q10–15 min PRN If two doses in an hour are providing little relief but are tolerated well, double the dose. Consider initiating continuous infusion if 2 bolus doses are required in 1 hour after increasing bolus dose. Typical starting continuous infusion rate is 4 mg/h. If the patient receives 2 bolus doses in an hour after initiating infusion, consider doubling the infusion rate. (Same titration rules apply to hydromorphone and fentanyl.)
Hydromorphone	0.5–1 mg IV q10–15 min PRN Typical starting continuous infusion rate is 0.5 mg/h
Fentanyl	50–100 μg IV q30min–1 h Typical starting continuous infusion rate is 25 μg/h

BENZODIAZEPINES: MODERATE TO SEVERE ANXIETY

MEDICATIONS	GUIDELINES
Lorazepam	1–2 mg IV q4h PRN If infusion is needed, typical starting infusion rate is 0.5–1 μg/h
Midazolam	2 mg q4h PRN 0.02–0.1 mg/kg/h infusion Patients can receive 1–2× the hourly infusion rate as bolus dose

From Yeow, Chen[1]; Coradazzi et al.[8]; Blinderman[9]; and Dudgeon.[10]

of palliative extubation is reduced unnecessary suffering on behalf of the patient as well as the family.[8]

EXTRACORPOREAL MEMBRANE OXYGENATION

ECMO is a type of aggressive respiratory support that is typically reserved for the most severe cases of respiratory failure.[5] This is a temporary and aggressive form of life support technology that allows a patient's failing heart or lungs to fully rest and hopefully recover during a life-threatening illness.[11] ECMO has advanced over the past several years from being primarily used in the pediatric population to use among adults as well.[12] ECMO is initiated in addition to mechanical ventilation and should only be considered in the most severe cases.[5] Patients who are on ECMO are already at high risk of death based on their clinical condition. ECMO should fully be discussed in detail with the patient's family prior to initiating the therapy: this communication should involve the purpose and goals of ECMO, the risks and potential benefits, and the possibility of needing to discontinue ECMO. There are two different types of ECMO, *venovenous* (VV), which is used in patients with severe respiratory failure, and *venoarterial* (VA), which is used for patients with combined respiratory and cardiac failure or post-cardiac arrest.[13]

ECMO functions to remove blood from the venous system through a negative pressure machine outside the body which oxygenates the blood and circulates it back to either the venous or arterial system (VV or VA, respectively). The flow rate of the blood determines the oxygenation and CO_2 removal. Vascular access is obtained via two large-bore cannulas, typically placed in the groin or neck depending on the type of ECMO being done.[11] The ECMO circuit functions as a heart-lung bypass machine, allowing the patient's heart and lungs to rest with the intention of recovery. Life-threatening complications may occur with ECMO such as bleeding, thromboembolism, infection, cerebral hemorrhage, and neurological devastation.[11]

Patients can be on ECMO for days to long weeks (>14 days); prolonged ECMO support is associated with a lower hospital survival rate.[14] If organ recovery fails or other serious complications arise, discontinuing ECMO should be considered and discussed open and honestly with the family or surrogate decision-maker if the patient lacks decision-making capacity. Discussions surrounding discontinuing ECMO can be complex and emotional given the technology of ECMO itself. The decision requires the care team to work together in determining what is best for the patient. The Extracorporeal Life Support Organization (ELSO) has a set criteria for determining medical futility; this includes little hope for survival, severe brain damage, no hope for heart or lung transplant, no hope for heart or lung recovery or transplant, and/or fixed pulmonary hypertension.[15] There are slight differences in end-of-life symptom management for patients on ECMO because ECMO can slightly alter the pharmacokinetics of certain medications, causing the need for dose adjustments. The ECMO circuit can also affect the lipophilicity of a drug and extend its absorption time. Morphine may be preferred over fentanyl in these patients because it is a hydrophilic drug.[16]

Discontinuing invasive mechanical ventilation is a complex process that requires careful planning by the palliative APRN and the care team. Table 55.2 outlines this process.

Table 55.2 PROCESS OF DISCONTINUATION OF RESPIRATORY SUPPORT

Prepare When continued aggressive medical interventions are unlikely to reverse the patient's condition and death is expected	Meetings: Ensure interdisciplinary meetings are occurring days prior and the day of with the palliative team as well as with the medical team prior to having discussions with the patient and/or family; this is *key* to ensuring that a consistent message is being relayed. Discuss terminal weaning vs. palliative or compassionate extubation and decide which process is right for the patient based on their clinical condition. Support: Offer social work or spiritual support services to the patient and/or family. Prepare the room: Clear the room of any unnecessary medical devices, ensure the patient is clean, sheets are clean and straight, and that the environment is as comfortable as possible. Ensure all comfort care orders are in place and the bedside RN has comfort medications readily available in the room.
Pre-Medication Anxiety Dyspnea Pain	If dyspnea is anticipated (dosages can vary based on patient's opioid tolerance): Morphine 2–5 mg IV ×1 *or* Hydromorphone 0.5–1 mg IV ×1 *or* Fentanyl 50–100 μg IV ×1 *or* If anxiety is anticipated: Lorazepam 1 mg IV ×1 for pre-medication
Discontinuation of Respiratory Support Removal mechanical ventilation	Ensure patient's surroundings are peaceful and comfortable; turn off all alarms and monitors. Ensure that family is present if they request. *Terminal weaning*: Slowly reduce the ventilator settings over the course of 10–30 minutes. *Palliative/compassionate extubation*: Stop ventilator support and remove ET tube all in one process. The patient may be at higher risk for rapid respiratory distress, but this option may offer a more natural, peaceful death. Offer support to the family by staying close by the room or at bedside if appropriate.
Post-Discontinuation of Respiratory Support	Monitor patient's condition closely. If appropriate, consider transfer to private room or hospice inpatient facility. If death occurs shortly after discontinuation of respiratory support, follow proper institutional/state guidelines for pronouncement process and communicate with the family. Pronouncement of death occurs by assessing that respirations and heartbeat have ceased via auscultation as well as noting the time. Communicating the death of a loved one demands sensitivity, a calm presence, comfort, and kindness. Conduct postmortem care per unit/RN guidelines. If present, offer to assist the RN in bathing the body and making the environment comfortable and peaceful for the family. If necessary, provide education to the family regarding things to anticipate immediately following death (muscles relax, relaxation of the jaw) so that they are assured that things they might observe are normal. Offer spiritual support at time of death.

From Yeow, Chen[1]; Coradazzi et al.[8]; Blinderman[9]; Dudgeon[10]; White et al.[17]; and Kok.[19]

SYMPTOM CONTROL DURING DISCONTINUATION OF RESPIRATORY TECHNOLOGY AND SUPPORT

It is essential that the palliative APRN have expert symptom management skills at end of life, especially in the situation where respiratory technology is being discontinued or withdrawn. Common symptoms include dyspnea, anxiety, increased pulmonary secretions, and dry mouth. Many patients will not be able to express discomfort or distressing symptoms, so it is recommended that the palliative APRN uses validated assessment tools to effectively assess and manage symptoms. Table 55.3 outlines validated tools that are commonly used in the ICU setting to assess pain, dyspnea, agitation, and delirium.

It is imperative that the patient's symptoms are effectively managed for their own comfort but also for the family's comfort. Observing signs of suffering can be distressing for the family. For pain, the use of the Behavioral Pain Scale, Critical Care Pain Observation Tool, or Pain Assessment Behavior Scale is recommended. The palliative APRN assesses the presence of pain behaviors including grimacing, rigidity, squinting of the eyes, clenching of fists, and moaning. The Richmond Agitation Sedation Scale (RASS) or Sedation Agitation Scale (SAS) is recommended in assessing agitation. The CAM-ICU tool is recommended when assessing degree of delirium. The Respiratory Distress Observation Scale is suggested for dyspnea.[1] To accurately assess the patient, discontinuation of neuromuscular blocking agents is recommended. These medications can interfere with the ability to accurately assess patient comfort and could result in unnecessary suffering.[1,23]

Opioids are considered first-line therapy for managing dyspnea. No opioid is superior to another in managing dyspnea.[1,2,23] However, morphine, fentanyl, and hydromorphone are the most commonly used opioids in the critical care setting.[24] There are many guidelines and protocols available for symptom control at end of life and during discontinuation of respiratory support. Many institutions and healthcare systems have their own versions of these orders sets that are initiated when the decision has been made to transition to comfort care. Many guidelines suggest premedicating the patient with an opioid and benzodiazepine prior to extubation.[1,23,25] Opioids and benzodiazepines assist in minimizing the degree of respiratory distress and anxiety as extubation occurs. Table 55.1 outlines opioid and benzodiazepine usage and dosages.

The dose requirement will vary from patient to patient based on their previous opioid usage. In an opioid-naïve patient, a starting bolus dose of IV morphine is 2 mg. Bolus dosing of morphine is typically is 2–4 mg IV every 10–15 minutes as needed. Initiating a continuous infusion may be necessary. Consider starting a continuous infusion if the patient is expected to survive after the discontinuation of ventilatory support or two or more bolus doses are given in 1 hour with little relief.[1,8,9,10] Patients may continue to require bolus dosing of an opioid for dyspnea and/or pain. If dyspnea continues and opioid doses are providing little efficacy, initiating an opioid infusion should be considered. Anxiety is another common symptom at end of life, especially in patients who also are suffering from severe dyspnea. If anxiety is anticipated, lorazepam 1 mg IV often is recommended prior to extubation and can be additionally be given at 1–2 mg IV every 4 hours as needed.[25] Midazolam is another appropriate alternate benzodiazepine that can be started at 2 mg IV, followed by an infusion of 1 mg per hour if necessary, based on the patient's response to the initial dose.[1] Once the patient is extubated, careful symptom management should continue.

COVID-19: IMPLICATIONS AND PRECAUTIONS

CASE STUDY: COVID 19 COMPASSIONATE EXTUBATION

KT was a 41-year-old African American man with a relatively negative past medical history except for obesity (body mass index [BMI] 31). He was admitted to the hospital for respiratory distress and tested positive for COVID-19. On Day 5, KT became increasingly hypoxic; he was transferred to the medical ICU and required emergent intubation. Over the course of the next 21 days he failed weaning trials and eventually required transfer to the cardiovascular ICU (CVICU), where he was placed on VV ECMO. KT was closely monitored and treated for COVID-19 per hospital protocols. The palliative care team was consulted on Day 16 to begin assisting with family communication and goals-of-care conversations.

KT was married and had three children ages 12, 16, and 20. He also had a brother and sister who lived out of state and were involved in the telephone conferences. The palliative APRN organized and led multiple family conferences via telephone as well as video conference with KT's family. She explained that KT

Table 55.3 DISTRESS ASSESSMENT TOOLS

SYMPTOM	TOOL
Pain	Behavioral Pain Scale (BPS) Critical care pain observation tool Pain can be objectively assessed based on signs of tachypnea, tachycardia, diaphoresis, facial grimacing, clenching fists, and moaning.[1]
Dyspnea	Respiratory Distress Observation Scale (RDOS) Objective assessments include tachypnea, increased respiratory rate (sometimes double from baseline), tachycardia, use of accessory muscles, nasal flaring, paradoxical breathing.[1]

Agitation	Sedation-Agitation Score (SAS)
	Ramsay Agitation Sedation Scale (RASS)
	    10-point scale used to assess patient's agitation level ranging from −5 to +4.
	    −1 to −5 ranges from awake to unarousable
	    +1 to +4 ranges from anxious to combative[20,21]

Delirium	CAM-ICU Assesses for acute changes in mental status, inattentiveness, disorganized thoughts, and altered level of consciousness[22]

was not showing any signs of improvement on Day 67 of ECMO. She reviewed the goals of care and his poor outcomes. She asked what KT's wishes would be, knowing he was in a situation with such a poor prognosis.

The family was offered the option of transitioning to comfort care. KT's family verbalized their understanding but wanted a couple of days to process and finalize a decision. During this time, KT was noted to have severe neurological dysfunction and was eventually found to have suffered a stroke while on ECMO. The family decided it was time to transition to comfort care.

On Day 81, KT had his ECMO discontinued. He was placed on comfort care and symptoms were managed appropriately per the hospital's comfort care order set. KT was compassionately extubated with the proper COVID-19 precautions. Although the family was unable to be at KT's bedside when he died, the family greatly appreciated the palliative APRN's compassion and extra time spent arranging family phone conferences to update them and provide them with additional options when things seemed to be getting worse.

The coronavirus disease 2019 (COVID-19) pandemic has without a doubt disrupted every aspect of our country's healthcare system and has affected every healthcare provider, especially palliative care providers and teams. The need for palliative care in the inpatient setting, especially in ICUs, has substantially increased during the COVID pandemic.[26] Patients who are critically ill and hospitalized with COVID-19 typically have an exceptionally long course of illness and, if intubated, a prolonged need for mechanical ventilation.[26]

All previously described advanced respiratory treatment modalities pose an extremely high risk for COVID-19 transmission. AIRVO, CPAP, BiPAP, and tracheal mechanical ventilation are all considered to be high-risk aerosolizing procedures. It is important to note that bronchoscopy and nebulizer treatments expose clinicians to the same risk of exposure, transmission, and infection.[27] It is imperative that the palliative APRN takes proper precautions when present in a room with a patient who is COVID-19–positive.

Goals-of-care conversations are necessary with any hospitalized COVID-19 patient due to the uncertainty of their disease trajectory.[26] The conversations are no longer theoretical but are part of the care plan. Patients and family may not understand the high respiratory support necessary for severe cases of COVID-19. They may also be unaware that it is common that no visitors are allowed in the clinical setting.

Prior to extubation, the palliative APRN should have the same goals-of-care discussions with the patient's family as previously discussed when considering discontinuation of respiratory support. It is important to identify who is the patient's surrogate decision-maker for health as well a backup decision-maker in case the surrogate falls ill.[28] Due to the strict visitor restrictions most institutions have in place, the palliative APRN must often perform this virtually. Ideally, it is important to have goals-of-care discussions upon hospital admission because COVID-19 is unpredictable.

All clinicians should be aware of the necessary special precautions with palliative or compassionate extubation. The procedure of extubating a patient poses significant risk of COVID-19 transmission due to the high risk of cough aerosolization.

Most hospital systems will have their own protocols for extubating a COVID-19–positive patient based on current research. Excess coughing should be kept to a minimum if possible due to the aerosolization risk. If possible, extubation should occur in a negative-pressure room with minimal staff present for the procedure to minimize transmission risk. There have been reports that the COVID-19 virus can remain airborne in aerosols for up to 3 hours.[27] Staff present in the room must be wearing all appropriate personal protective equipment (PPE) including an N-95 mask or powered air-purifying respiratory (PAPR), a gown, gloves, and eye protection.[29] To date, no consensus guidelines for extubation of COVID-19 patients have been developed.[29] However, oxygen via nasal cannula or mask should be placed on the patient following extubation. There are some centers that are using barrier hoods made from PVC or clear rigid plastic. The one principle is that NPPV should be avoided post extubation due to risk of aerosolization.

In some cases, traditional ventilatory support fails, eventually requiring patients to receive ECMO support. There is little research at this point regarding COVID-19 and ECMO efficacy.[30] The studies that have been done so far demonstrate an extremely poor survival rate.[30] This scenario further supports the need for earlier palliative care consults in COVID patients to assist in goals-of-care discussions with the patient before their condition deteriorates so rapidly that they are intubated and placed on ECMO.

ETHICAL CONSIDERATIONS

Discontinuation of life-sustaining therapies, including respiratory technology, often raises ethical concerns. Palliative APRNs, along with their team, have a duty to ensure patients are comfortable and that their dying process is not prolonged. There is also the legal obligation to avoid hastening a patient's death.[23] The following ethical issues surround palliative or compassionate extubation or discontinuing or withdrawing respiratory ventilation (see also Chapter 53, "Navigating Ethical Dilemmas," for further discussion).

1. *Abandonment*: The ability to breathe is seen as a core requirement of life. There may be the perspective that discontinuation of ventilatory support is a form of patient abandonment. The perception arises from the concern that the palliative APRN will stop caring for the patient and that the established patient–provider relationship has ceased without notice. Discontinuation of mechanical ventilation at end of life is not considered abandonment because the APRN continues a therapeutic relationship and will provide proper symptom management.[17,18]

2. *Beneficence*: The best interest and well-being of a patient is the core of healthcare. There are limitations to what

medicine can accomplish, and allowing the patient to die in a controlled manner consistent with their values, wishes, and goals of care is promoting beneficence.[17] Beneficence requires the palliative APRN to facilitate the patient's best interest in considering the benefits and burdens of treatments. In patients who are critically ill, it is important to acknowledge that continued mechanical ventilation and other aggressive therapies may not be in the patient's best interest.

3. *Hastening death*: Patient have a choice to decline or stop treatments that are life-sustaining. Patients, families, and even some clinicians believe that providing sedatives or opioids at the end of life unnecessarily hastens death. The palliative APRN has ethical obligation to alleviate uncontrolled symptoms at end of life. Severe dyspnea can cause tremendous suffering at end of life that is distressing for families to witness at the bedside. In this situation, managing potential suffering of end-of-life symptoms is paramount even if death occurs as a consequence.[17,30] This leads to the principle of the *double effect*, which differentiates intended "good" versus unintended "bad" effects. The discussion of intentions and goals with the use of medications is imperative with patients, families, and staff and should be documented.[30]

4. *Nonbeneficial care/futility*: Medical technology has advanced to the point where there is always something that can be done. The question is whether it should be. *Nonbeneficial care* or *futility* refers to the failure of a specific intervention to lead to the intended outcome. This may be gauged by unintended consequences or suffering. There may be situations in which the palliative APRN is faced with discussing therapies or interventions with patients and/or family members that are providing little to no benefits to the patient and some that may potentially cause a great deal of harm.[30]

Ethics and legal consults should be considered in particularly challenging cases. It is critical to know the institution's guidelines, policies, and resources as well as one's state regulations. There are many resources for the palliative APRN (Box 55.2).

SUMMARY

All palliative care teams will be involved in the discontinuation of respiratory technology. The palliative APRN is an integral member of the palliative care team in this process. It is essential that care teams understand the ethical principles behind discontinuation. Moreover, the team must develop a collaborative process delineating each member's roles, responsibilities, and process consistent with the resources of the setting. The palliative APRN can lead the development in policies and procedures appropriate to the acute care, rehabilitation, and home settings. Procedures should include clarity of the role of each team member, medications to use, who orders medications, and who discontinues oxygen therapy. To ensure a dignified end of life for a patient, the APRN is responsible for

---

Box 55.2 ETHICAL CONSIDERATIONS: ADDITIONAL RESOURCES

1. American Nurses Association. *Position Statement: Nurses' Roles and Responsibilities in Providing Care and Support at the End of Life.*[31]

2. Hospice and Palliative Nurses Association. *Position Statement on Withdrawal of Life-Sustaining Therapies.*[32]

3. National Consensus Project for Quality Palliative Care. *Clinical Practice Guidelines Domain 8: Ethical and Legal Aspects of Care.*[33]

4. American Academy of Hospice and Palliative Medicine. *Statement on Withholding and Withdrawing Nonbeneficial Medical Interventions.*[34]

5. American Thoracic Society/American College of Chest Physicians. *Official Executive Summary. Clinical Practice Guideline: Liberation from Mechanical Ventilation in Critically Ill Adults.*[34]

6. American Medical Association. *Ethics: Withholding or Withdrawing Life-Sustaining Treatment.*[35]

7. Center for Practical Bioethics. *Considerations Regarding Withholding/Withdrawing Life-Sustaining Treatment.* Reviewed and Revised 2015.[36]

8. Palliative Care Network of Wisconsin Fast Facts and Concepts.

Number 33: Ventilator Withdrawal Protocol
Number 34: Symptom Control for Ventilator Withdrawal in the Dying Patient.[25]

---

collaboratively developing a proactive care plan that supports the needs of the patient and family. The care plan requires effective communication to plan the event with the team members; pre-meet prior to the event to consider how dyspnea, anxiety, and secretions will be managed; prepare the family and the patient (as able) for the process; support the staff involved with the process; facilitate the process as necessary; and debrief the event afterward. The palliative APRN can offer resources to support the family in their bereavement as well.

REFERENCES

1. Yeow M-E, Chen E. Ventilator withdrawal in anticipation of death: The simulation lab as an educational tool in Palliative Medicine. *J Pain Symptom Management.* 2020;59(1):165–171. doi:10.1016/j.jpainsymman.2019.09.025

2. Kapo. *Unipac Four: Management of Selected Nonpain Symptoms of Life-Limiting Illness.* 5th ed. Chicago: American Academy of Hospice and Palliative Medicine; 2017.

3. Daly BJ, Newlon B, Montenegro HD, Langdon T. Withdrawal of mechanical ventilation: Ethical principles and guidelines for terminal weaning. *Am J Crit Care.* 1993;2(3):217–223.

4. Ketcham SW, Sedhai YR, Miller HC, et al. Causes and characteristics of death in patients with acute hypoxemic respiratory failure and acute respiratory distress syndrome: A retrospective cohort study. *Crit Care.* 2020;24(1):391. doi:10.1186/s13054-020-03108-w

5. Chiumello D, Brochard L, Marini JJ, et al. Respiratory support in patients with acute respiratory distress syndrome: An expert opinion. *Crit Care*. 2017;21(1):240. Published 2017 Sep 12. doi:10.1186/s13054-017-1820-0

6. Yeow M-E, Mehta RS, White DB, Szmuilowicz E. Using noninvasive ventilation at the end of life #230. *J Palliat Med*. 2010;13(9):1149–1150. doi:10.1089/jpm.2010.9788

7. Curtis JR, Cook DJ, Sinuff T, et al. Noninvasive positive pressure ventilation in critical and palliative care settings: Understanding the goals of therapy. *Crit Care*. 2007;35(3):932–939. doi:10.1097/01.CCM.0000256725.73993.74

8. Coradazzi AL, Inhaia CLS, Santana MT, et al. Palliative withdrawal ventilation: Why, when and how to do it? *Hosp Palliat Med Int J*. 2019;3(1). doi:10.15406/hpmij.2019.03.00141

9. Blinderman CD. Comfort care for patients dying in the hospital. *N Engl J Med*. 2016;374(17):1693. doi:10.1056/NEJMra1411746

10. Dudgeon D, IN; Bruera E, ed. Assessment and management of dyspnea in palliative care. UpToDate. Waltham, MA: UptoDate. Reviewed June 21, 2021. https://www.uptodate.com/contents/assessment-and-management-of-dyspnea-in-palliative-care

11. Williams SB, Dahnke MD. Clarification and mitigation of ethical problems surrounding withdrawal of extracorporeal membrane oxygenation. *Crit Care Nurse*. 2016;36(5):56–65. doi:10.4037/ccn2016504.

12. Klinedinst R, O'Connor N, Farabelli J. Walking across the bridge to nowhere: The role of palliative care in the support of patients on ECMO (FR400). *J Pain Symptom Manage* 2017;53(2):350. doi.org/10.1016/j.painsymman.2016.12.096.

13. Vieira J, Frakes M, Cohen J, Wilcox S. Extracorporeal membrane oxygenation in transport part 1: Extracorporeal membrane oxygenation configurations and physiology. *Air Med J*. 2020;39(1):56–63. doi:10.1016/j.amj.2019.09.008.

14. Posluszny J, Rycus PT, Bartlett RH, et al. Outcome of adult respiratory failure patients receiving prolonged (≥14 days) ECMO. *Ann Surg*. 2016;263(3):573–581. doi:10.1097/SLA.0000000000001176.

15. Extracorporeal Life Support Organization. Extracorporeal Life Support Organization guidelines. Version 1.4. 2017. Ann Arbor, MI: ELSO. https://www.elso.org/Portals/0/ELSO%20Guidelines%20For%20Adult%20Respiratory%20Failure%201_4.pdf

16. Shekar K, Fraser JF, Smith MT, Roberts JA. Pharmacokinetic changes in patients receiving extracorporeal membrane oxygenation. *J Crit Care*. 2012;27(6):741.e9–18. doi:10.1016/j.jcrc.2012.02.013

17. White D. In: Arnold R, Parsons P, (ed). Withholding and withdrawing ventilatory support in adults in the intensive care unit. UpTodate. Waltham, MA: Uptodate. July 30, 2021. http://www.uptodate.com/contents/withholding-and-withdrawing-ventilatory-support-in-adults-in-the-intensive-care-unit

18. Efstathiou N, Vanderspank-Wright B, Vandyk A, et al. Terminal withdrawal of mechanical ventilation in adult intensive care units: A systematic review and narrative synthesis of perceptions, experiences and practices. *Palliat Med*. 2020;34(9):1140–1164. doi:10.1177/0269216320935002

19. Kok VC. Compassionate extubation for a peaceful death in the setting of a community hospital: A case-series study. *Clin Interv Aging*. 2015;10:679–685. doi:10.2147/CIA.S82760

20. Trivedi V, Iyer VN. Utility of the Richmond Agitation-Sedation Scale in evaluation of acute neurologic dysfunction in the intensive care unit. *J Thorac Dis*. 2016;8(5):E292–294. doi:10.21037/jtd.2016.03.71

21. Ely EW, Truman B, Shintani A, et al. Monitoring sedation status over time in ICU patients: Reliability and validity of the Richmond Agitation-Sedation Scale (RASS). *JAMA*. 2003;289(22):2983–2991. doi:10.1001/jama.289.22.2983

22. Khan BA, Perkins AJ, Gao S, et al. The confusion assessment method for the ICU-7 delirium severity scale: A novel delirium severity instrument for use in the ICU. *Crit Care Med*. 2017;45(5):851–857. doi:10.1097/CCM.0000000000002368.

23. Delaney JW, Downar J. How is life support withdrawn in intensive care units: A narrative review. *J Crit Care*. 2016;35:12–18. doi:10.1016/j.jcrc.2012.02.013.

24. Fuchs B, Bellmay, C. In: Parsons, P, O'Connor, M. Sedative-analgesic medications in critically ill adults: Selection, initiation, maintenance, and withdrawal. UpToDate. Waltham, MA: UptoDate. September 23, 2020. https://www.uptodate.com/contents/sedative-analgesic-medications-in-critically-ill-adults-selection-initiation-maintenance-and-withdrawal

25. von Gunten MD David E Weissman CF. Palliative care fast facts and concepts: Symptom control for ventilator withdrawal in the dying patient. Appleton, WI: Palliative Care Network of Wisconsin. 2015. https://www.mypcnow.org/fast-fact/symptom-control-for-ventilator-withdrawal-in-the-dying-patient/

26. Schoenherr LA, Cook A, Peck S, et al. Proactive identification of palliative care needs among patients with COVID-19 in the ICU. *J Pain Symptom Manage*. 2020;60(3):e17–e21. doi:10.1016/j.jpainsymman.2020.06.008

27. Sullivan EH, Gibson LE, Berra L, Chang MG, Bittner EA. In-hospital airway management of COVID-19 patients. *Crit Care*. 2020;24(1):292. doi:https://doi.org/10.1186/s13054-020-03018-x

28. Rao A, Kelemen A. Lessons learned from caring for patients with COVID-19 at the end of life. *J Palliat Med*. 2020;(jpm.2020.0251). doi:10.1089/jpm.2020.0251

29. Kangas-Dick AW, Swearingen B, Wan E, Chawla K, Wiesel O. Safe extubation during the COVID-19 pandemic. *Respir Med*. 2020;170:106038. doi:10.1016/j.rmed.2020.106038

30. Prince-Paul M, Daly B. Ethical considerations in palliative care. In: Ferrell BR, Paice J, eds. *Oxford Textbook of Palliative Nursing*, 5th ed. New York: Oxford University Press; 2019: 824–835.

31. American Nurses Association. Position statement: Nurses' roles and responsibilities in providing care and support at the end of life. Silver Spring, MD: ANA. 2016. https://www.nursingworld.org/~4af078/globalassets/docs/ana/ethics/endoflife-positionstatement.pdf

32. Hospice and Palliative Nurses Association. Position statement: Withdrawal of life-sustaining therapies. Pittsburgh, PA: HPNA. 2016. https://advancingexpertcare.org/position-statements/

33. National Consensus Project for Quality Palliative Care. *Clinical Practice Guidelines for Quality Palliative Care*, 4th edition. Richmond, VA: National Coalition for Hospice and Palliative Care; 2018. https://www.nationalcoalitionhpc.org/ncp

34. Schmidt GA, Girard TD, Kress JP, et al. Official executive summary of an American Thoracic Society/American College of Chest Physicians clinical practice guideline: Liberation from mechanical ventilation in critically ill adults. *Am J Respir Crit Care Med*. 2017;195(1):115–119. doi:10.1164/rccm.201610-2076ST

35. American Medical Association. Ethics: Withholding or withdrawing life-sustaining treatment. Code of Medical Ethics Opinion 5.3. Chicago, IL: AMA. Available at https://www.ama-assn.org/delivering-care/ethics/withholding-or-withdrawing-life-sustaining-treatment

36. Center for Practical Bioethics. Considerations regarding withholding/withdrawing life-sustaining treatment. Kansas City, MO: Center for Practical Ethics. Reviewed and Revised 2015. https://www.practicalbioethics.org/files/ethics-consortium-guidelines/Withholding-Withdrawing-Life-Sustaining-Treatment.pdf

37. American Academy of Hospice and Palliative Medicine. Statement on withholding and withdrawing nonbeneficial medical interventions. Chicago, IL: AAHPM. Nov 2011. http://aahpm.org/positions/withholding-nonbeneficial-interventions

DISCONTINUATION OF OTHER LIFE-SUSTAINING THERAPIES

Kathy Plakovic and Jennifer Donoghue

KEY POINTS

- Withholding, withdrawing, and discontinuing antibiotics, blood products, dialysis, and medically administered nutrition are important topics that require the palliative advanced practice registered nurse (APRN) to provide information and participate in shared decision-making.

- The APRN should explain the benefits and burdens of treatment versus no treatment to the patient and family, along with the ethical framework that supports them.

- If treatment is withheld, withdrawn, or discontinued, discussions should include the expected course of the dying process.

- Although the phrase "withdrawal of care" is often heard, it is important to distinguish between the withdrawal of life-sustaining interventions and the withdrawal of care. While the former is common, the latter should never occur. Language is important, particularly to patients and their families,[1 (p. 956)] which is why more teams are using the term discontinuation.

CASE STUDY: CONSENSUS WITH COVID-19 PROGNOSIS

Mr. R is a 78-year-old man with advanced dementia who presented to the hospital from a local nursing home with shortness of breath. A rapid COVID-19 test was positive. The palliative APRN was consulted immediately upon admission to discuss goals of care with his family because Mr. R did not have any advance directives. He was decompensating quickly and required high-flow oxygen via nasal cannula for respiratory support. He was alert to voice but lethargic and did not appear to be in any distress.

Prior to calling the family, the palliative APRN reviewed the case with the attending physician and intensive care specialist. The APRN, attending, and intensivist agreed that, given Mr. R's underlying terminal diagnosis and frail state, intubation was not recommended. This multidisciplinary medical team was unable to meet in person due to COVID-19 restrictions but held a phone consultation to reach consensus.

The palliative APRN called the Mr. R's daughter and primary surrogate, Betty, to discuss next steps in care. Betty was informed of Mr. R's positive COVID-19 status along with the best and worst case outcomes. In addition, the APRN conveyed

the medical team's recommendation for comfort-focused care. Betty verbalized her inability to make such a difficult decision without the input of her two siblings. The palliative APRN coordinated a virtual call with the Mr. R's three children to achieve consensus. After much discussion, the family agreed that quality of life was more important and gave permission for no resuscitation or intubation. Mr. R's family requested visitation to see their father before he died. Due to COVID-19 visitor restrictions within the intensive care unit (ICU) and Betty and her sibling's own health issues, the decision was made to coordinate video visitation with Mr. R.

The evening of Mr. R's hospital admission, a video call was held at his bedside where his children were able to say goodbye and play his favorite hymns. The patient was started on a morphine drip for respiratory distress and any potential pain and discomfort. The palliative APRN continued to monitor him, and Mr. R died within 24 hours. The palliative care team provided bereavement follow-up to the family.

INTRODUCTION

Technological and medical advancements have led to dilemmas surrounding decisions to withhold, withdraw, or discontinue life-sustaining treatment. For patients with advanced illness, technology has often served to only prolong the dying process. While many patients and loved ones see medical intervention as a human right, it is important to remember that the first obligation of a provider is to do no harm. The ethical principles of *beneficence* and *nonmaleficence* support a provider's right to refuse treatment that may cause harm. *Autonomy* is the ethical principle that allows patients or their assigned decision-maker the right to accept or refuse any treatment that may not align with their personal health wishes.[2]

While withholding, withdrawing, or discontinuing interventions are legally and ethically equivalent, withdrawal or discontinuation of life-sustaining interventions, especially in the intensive care unit (ICU), is harder for both providers and family members. Family members are often burdened with "what ifs" and feel greater responsibility for the outcome when treatment is withdrawn or discontinued versus withheld.[3] Families often associate withdrawal with active participation in death, misunderstanding that the true intention is to allow for a natural dying process. Palliative advanced practice registered nurses (APRNs) ease patient and family distress when decisions on withdrawal or discontinuation of life-sustaining treatments are indicated. Specifically, palliative APRNs can help patients and families better understand the dying process by discussing the nature of the underlying illness, including the expected prognosis and the benefits and burdens of treatment. This allows patients and families to make informed decisions about treatments.

While withdrawal of treatment is most often associated with removal of mechanical ventilation, there are several other life-sustaining interventions that should be addressed in the dying patient. This chapter focuses on the withdrawal or discontinuation of antibiotics, blood products, dialysis, and medically administered nutrition in the terminally ill. It will provide case scenarios for each intervention to aid in understanding and discuss the burdens and benefits of continuing treatment versus stopping. The normal dying process when these therapies are discontinued will be reviewed.

Decisions regarding life-sustaining treatments regularly happen in the ICU. The aim of ICU-level care is to treat acute illness with the goal of returning patients to a level of function that offers an acceptable quality of life. Unfortunately, ICU admissions tend to be prolonged, complex, and often delay death instead of supporting life in patients with terminal illness. With a mortality rate of up to 20%, it is important for palliative care providers not only to be present, but also skilled at navigating end-of-life discussions in this setting.[4]

Conversations surrounding life-sustaining treatments are often difficult and emotionally charged even for the most skilled providers. Prognostic uncertainty in the ICU has made it challenging for palliative APRNs to navigate end-of-life discussions with patients and family members. The current recommendations support a multidisciplinary approach to family meetings.[5] While multiple prognostic scoring systems are available, they are not often applied in the ICU setting. Prognosis tends to be overestimated, and there are commonly conflicting opinions on prognosis from different specialty groups.[4] When the multidisciplinary team is not on the same page, the palliative APRN plays an important role in bringing the team together prior to meeting with the family to present a united front. Consensus among the medical team regarding prognosis is key to effective end-of-life discussions. The team must also have an understanding of how the patient's and family's culture, religion, and ethnicity may affect decisions (see Chapter 35, "Culturally Respectful Palliative Care," and Chapter 53, "Navigating Ethical Dilemmas").

The coronavirus pandemic has forced medical providers to face end-of-life conversations in a rapidly changing environment. It has highlighted the important role that palliative APRNs play in critical care situations and helped medical providers understand why the "big picture" of patient care is just as important as managing the acute illness, especially when it comes to clinical outcomes and accurate prognostication. COVID-19 has forced providers to question the almost 20 years of research that has gone into improving patient and provider communication at the end of life. It has physically separated the patient, provider, and family and led many to question their ethical beliefs.[6] Navigating goals-of-care discussions with providers and family members via telehealth has proved challenging for palliative APRNs, especially in environments where access to smart devices and training for patients, loved ones, and providers is limited. Consensus and a team-based approach have been more important now than ever.

The ability to navigate complex, interdisciplinary patient- and family-centered goals-of-care conversations is a key skill that palliative APRNs must possess. Family members often rely on palliative APRNs as the primary source of information and support when loved ones are terminally ill. Building rapport with patients and families allows palliative providers to lead effective team meetings once consensus among the team has been established. Palliative APRNs play a key role in educating patients and loved ones on prognosis and expectations with and without treatment. They ensure that decisions made by loved ones for patients who are incapacitated have the patient's preferences for care as the primary focus. When the decision is made to withdraw or discontinue life-sustaining treatment, the palliative APRN should also discuss expectations for the dying process.

ANTIBIOTICS

Antibiotic use is common for infections and is considered the standard of care. As patients near the end of life, antibiotic use may become a life-sustaining or a death-prolonging treatment. Using antimicrobial medications at the end of life is a common practice.[7,8] Albrecht and colleagues evaluated 3,884 hospice patients and found that 27% received antibiotics in the last week of life, but only 15% of those patients had a documented infectious diagnosis.[9] Merel et al. reported that 15–20% of patients remained on antibiotics after comfort care was started.[7] As with other life-sustaining treatments, the decision to either withhold or withdraw or discontinue antibiotics requires informed decision-making based on the goals of care for the individual patient.

Many families and healthcare professionals fail to see dementia as a terminal illness, however, patients with all types of dementia have a median survival of 5 years from diagnosis to death.[10] Dementia is the sixth leading cause of death in the United States for all ages and the fifth leading cause of death for those 65 and older.[11,12] As dementia progresses, patients lose their ability to swallow food and manage their own secretions, which can lead to aspiration pneumonia. In a study of nursing home patients with dementia (FAST 6e and above), 42% had swallowing issues at the start of the study. Of the patients that died, 20% had aspiration and 47% had breathing difficulties at the end of life.[13] Several studies have shown pneumonia to be one of the leading causes of death in patients with dementia.[14,15] Manabe and colleagues reported that patients with dementia are two times more likely to die of pneumonia.[16] Patients with Lewy body dementia are twice as likely as those with Alzheimer's disease to have a respiratory death.[17]

Patients with other disease processes, such as advanced cancer, are at risk for infection due to immune suppression from the disease or neutropenia as a result of cancer treatment. Among hospitalized advanced cancer patients, nearly 90% received antibiotics in their last week of life.[18] Even when patients are transitioned to comfort-focused care, many patients continue to receive antimicrobial therapy.[19,20] One study showed that almost 80% of dying patients received antimicrobial therapy in the 24 hours before and after being transitioned to comfort care. That number decreased to 20% when patients had been on comfort measures for more than 24 hours.[7]

A growing body of evidence suggests that antibiotic prescribing frequently occurs at end of life and often is nonbeneficial.[21,22] However, many healthcare providers believe that because infection is a reversible problem, it should always be treated. Decisions to withhold, withdraw, or discontinue antibiotics at the end of life can also be stressful for families. A study looking at antimicrobial use when patients are transitioned to hospice showed that 19% of patients were sent with a prescription because of a family request.[23]

A common belief is that the treatment of an infection provides comfort by decreasing fever and other distressing symptoms, such as shortness of breath. Symptoms like confusion, dyspnea, fever, and hypotension can also occur. However, a study conducted by Givens and colleagues[24] showed that comfort scores for patients receiving antibiotics were worse than those for patients not receiving treatment in pneumonia patients with severe dementia. Data from another study showed that antimicrobial use in hospice patients had little effect in relieving symptoms for patients with infections, including bacteremia and pneumonia, although it did decrease symptoms in patients with urinary tract infections.[25] Interestingly, that study also showed no difference in median survival in those patients with an infection versus those without infection: 29.1 and 30.5 days, respectively. Survival was the same for patients treated with antibiotics and those with no antibiotics: 29.3 and 30.7 days, respectively. For patients near the end of life, there is little evidence that survival is prolonged with antibiotic therapy.[14] Palliation of infection-related symptoms at the end of life, such as dyspnea, can be managed by opioids and other, nonpharmacologic treatments (see Section VIII, "Symptoms").[26]

The burdens of using antimicrobial therapy should also be considered when choosing whether to treat an infection. Antibiotic stewardship programs seek to improve appropriate use in an effort to decrease adverse effects and antimicrobial resistance. Pasay and colleagues implemented a stewardship program that significantly reduced urine culture testing and antimicrobial prescriptions with no increase in hospital admission or mortality.[21] Other potential harms include the potential for *Clostridium difficile* infection, side effects or adverse reactions to the medication, and the need for intravenous access, which can be difficult to obtain in patients near the end of life. The volume of fluid required to deliver intravenous antibiotics can also place a burden on patients with impaired kidney function or with edema due to hypoalbuminemia. Tamma et al. reported that 20% of hospitalized patients experienced an adverse event related to antimicrobial therapy.[27] The healthcare cost, especially for patients on newer antimicrobial medications or those prescribed multiple agents, can place a financial burden on patients, healthcare institutions, and society.[28]

Ethical considerations can assist in guiding decision-making. Eliciting the patient and family perspective of quality versus quantity of life, including their belief system and other values, supports patient autonomy.[29] When the expressed goal is comfort at the end of life, antibiotic use should be reduced. Figure 56.1[8] proposes an algorithm for antibiotic use at the end of life. Sinert and colleagues recommend using a decision support tool to help guide use of antibiotics for patients in hospice care (see Table 56.1).[30]

Palliative APRNs can explain that most symptoms can be successfully managed at the end of life. They can also educate families that hypotension in the dying patient is normal and that giving medications like vasopressors or fluid boluses will only prolong the dying process and potentially prolong suffering,

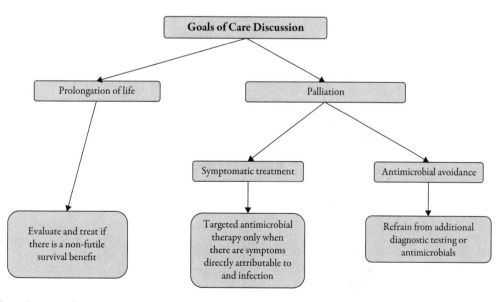

Figure 56.1 Goals of care discussion.[8]

Table 56.1 STAMPS: A HOSPICE DECISION SUPPORT TOOL FOR ANTIBIOTIC USE

	DESCRIPTION	ACTION
S	Symptom assessment	When infection is suspected, determine symptoms impacting comfort or quality of life. If asymptomatic or if symptoms do not significantly impair comfort/quality of life, no antibiotic is indicated.
T	Targets/goals of therapy	Review specific goals for infection and symptom management with the patient and caregiver.
A	Alternative treatment options	Based on patient-specific goals, determine what other nonantibiotic treatment options exist and compare expected outcomes.
M	Medication factors	Review drug allergies, drug interactions, and anticipated adverse effect/risks. Assess swallowing function and other factors that affecting antibiotic selection and administration.
P	Prognosis	Evaluated estimated prognosis versus necessary treatment duration and anticipated time to symptom resolution.
S	Stewardship	Avoid bug-drug, infection-drug, or patient-drug mismatch. If antibiotic therapy is chosen, ensure the use of correct drug, dose, route of administration, and therapy duration.

From Sinert et al.[30] (table 2)

which is not recommended. The decision to proceed with, withhold, withdraw, or discontinue treatment should be individualized for each patient based on the goals of care. Determining the goals of care for patients with advanced disease can help guide antibiotic use. If the goal is to prolong life at any cost, then family members may elect to proceed with antimicrobial therapy. However, if comfort is the primary focus, families should be educated on the burdens of antibiotic treatment, including a prolonged dying process and potentially worse symptoms.

CASE STUDY: USE OF ANTIBIOTICS

Mrs. F was an 87-year-old woman with Parkinson's disease, chronic obstructive pulmonary disease (COPD), and Alzheimer's disease. The patient and family had decided to proceed with enteral feeding after multiple admissions for aspiration pneumonia and a percutaneous endoscopic gastrostomy (PEG) tube was placed. Mrs. F was admitted to a long-term care facility when her care needs became too much for her family.

The palliative APRN at the nursing home met with the patient and family to address goals of care. They completed a provider/physician's orders for life-sustaining treatment (POLST) form indicating (a) do not attempt resuscitation, (b) selective medical treatments with no intubation, and (c) long-term medically administered nutrition. The palliative APRN discussed that the risk for aspiration was still a concern as the patient could aspirate her tube feeding or her own secretions. She discussed that Mrs. F may continue to have frequent cases of pneumonia. The family insisted on continued hospitalizations and antibiotics because "you can treat an infection." They remained hopeful that Mrs. F would make it to her 90th birthday.

Mrs. F was hospitalized three more times over the next 5 weeks for aspiration pneumonia. With each admission her functional and cognitive status declined. The palliative APRN met with the family again after the third discharge and recommended comfort-focused care. While there was disagreement among family members initially, they were able to come to a consensus with guidance from the APRN to discontinue antibiotics. The patient's orders for life sustaining treatments or POLST form was updated to reflect the goal of comfort care. Mrs. F was admitted to hospice care and died 1 week later.

BLOOD PRODUCTS

Transfusions of blood products, including red blood cells and platelets, are life-sustaining treatments for patients with anemia and thrombocytopenia caused by the disease process or treatment-related cytopenias. Many patients with advanced disease become transfusion-dependent due to bone marrow infiltration or chronic bleeding from tumor invasion. For these patients, continued transfusions are used not as a bridge to wellness but as a temporizing measure.

Many providers, especially ones with a long-term relationship with a patient, have difficulty discussing goals of care when there are no further treatment options. Aggressive care is often continued when patients are actively dying. This can lead to patients and families not having the time to attend to unfinished business prior to death. While some patients and families will continue to request ongoing care despite a poor prognosis,[31,32] they must receive honest, direct information about treatment options—including no treatment—so they can make informed decisions about the goals of care.

Advances in medicine have improved survival rates for patients with hematological malignancies, but some patients will succumb to their disease despite aggressive management.[33,34] Many of these patients are transfusion-dependent due to bone marrow failure or infiltration. These patients often die on the hematology ward or in the ICU.[35,36,37,38] Forty-eight percent of hospitalized patients who died with hematological malignancies received a blood transfusion during their terminal admission.[38]

Patients with hematological cancers are commonly referred to palliative care too late when they are actively dying even though treatment of their disease entails a high symptom burden and psychosocial and spiritual distress.[39] Reasons for the late referral to palliative care include the aggressive nature of treatment, including chemotherapy, transfusions, and antibiotics until the end of life. Blood and platelet transfusions become a "normal" part of the patient's life; stopping them is a difficult decision, not only for the patient but also for the hematologist.

Transfusions are often not allowed in hospice programs, which makes providers reluctant to refer patients who are transfusion-dependent.[37,40] Patients with multiple myeloma who were transfusion-dependent were three times more likely to be referred late to hospice.[41] Patients with hematologic malignancies are often symptomatic and could benefit from the services provided by hospice. Of those patients who are referred, they are significantly sicker and usually have a hospice length of stay measured in days.[34,36]

Patients with acute myelocytic leukemia (AML) in particular appear to use hospice services less, and those that do often transfer in and out of hospice care in order to receive disease-directed care such as transfusions.[42] A small study of patients with AML showed that most patients continue cancer-related care until the end of life.[43] Older adults diagnosed with AML spent more than a quarter of their life in the hospital.[39] These patients have a much greater likelihood of dying hospitalized.[44]

Recognizing when patients are near the end of life becomes particularly important in this patient population. Kripp and colleagues[45] looked at five factors—low performance status, low platelet count, opioid therapy, high lactate dehydrogenase (LDH), and low albumin—that would identify patients with a high risk of death (Box 56.1). Patients with four or five risk factors had a median survival of 10 days. Median survival for those with two or three risk factors was 63 days. This information can assist healthcare providers in identifying patients at risk of death so they can have in-depth discussions with patients and families regarding goals of care. Other factors associated with mortality in hematologic malignancies include declining performance, treatment limitations of the hematological malignancy, relapse, refractory or persistent disease, presence of two or more comorbidities, invasive fungal infections, and persistent infections.[46] Most studies looking at prognostication in hematologic malignancies have focused on patients who are receiving aggressive ICU-level care. There is little information to help guide clinicians on predicting survival for patients receiving palliative-focused care.[47]

It is important to look at patient and family goals of care in regard to continued transfusions. The patient's perceived and desired quality of life should be considered.[46] Transfusions can palliate symptoms, but the benefit is usually not durable.[48,49] The risks and benefits should be carefully weighed. Continuing transfusions in terminally ill patients can place a tremendous burden on the patient and family and usually requires frequent clinic visits for laboratory tests and transfusions, which can also result in unplanned hospitalizations. Patients requiring frequent transfusions are at risk for fluid overload, transfusion reactions, and alloimmunization, making matched transfusions more difficult. Routine transfusions based on complete blood count results showing anemia or thrombocytopenia should be discouraged. Given the national shortage of blood products, thoughtful consideration should be given before transfusing patients in the terminal phase of their disease.[50] Suggested guidelines for transfusions at the end of life can be found in Box 56.2. Symptomatic treatment for fatigue or active bleeding should guide clinical practice.

Box 56.1 PROGNOSTIC FACTORS IN PATIENTS WITH HEMATOLOGIC MALIGNANCIES

Eastern Cooperative Oncology Group (ECOG) status >2
Platelet count <90 × 10^{-9}/L
Lactate dehydrogenase (LDH) >248 U/L
Opioid use per World Health Organization (WHO) level 3
Albumin <30 g/L
Median survival with no or one risk factor is 440 days; two or three risk factors, 63 days; four or five risk factors, 10 days.

Adapted from Kripp et al.[45]

Box 56.2 GUIDELINES FOR BLOOD PRODUCT USE AT END OF LIFE

1. Exceedingly scarce resources, such as cross-matched and HLA-matched platelets, granulocytes, and rare units of blood should not be used in patients who have transitioned to palliative or comfort care. Routine blood products should be used sparingly, and requests should be reviewed by the transfusion medicine service.

2. Transfusions in medically nonbeneficial situations should be avoided if possible and limited to the minimum number of red blood cell transfusions necessary to ameliorate symptoms of anemia. Platelets should also be limited to the minimum necessary to control bleeding (if it is causing significant patient distress, such as upper airway bleeding). If the frequency of transfusions has an impact on the resources available for other patients (i.e., more than twice a week), the request should be reviewed by the transfusion medicine service.

3. If shortages of blood products arise, attempts should be made to defer transfusion in patients at the end of life so the products can be used for other patients. Unusual requests, such as massive transfusion in a nonbeneficial situation, should not be filled. If agreement cannot be reached on this, an ethics consult should be requested.

4. Transfusion in stable, terminally ill patients requires a careful analysis of the goals of care. Transfusions should not be discouraged in patients for whom an occasional transfusion is likely to alleviate primary symptoms, such as extreme fatigue. Large numbers of transfusions, however, should be reviewed by the transfusion medicine service.

Adapted from Smith, Cooling.[50]

Mr. J was a 59-year-old man with relapsed AML with complex cytogentics. He had failed to obtain remission with multiple chemotherapy regimens and opted for best supportive care, including ongoing blood transfusions. He had many short- and long-term goals including making it to his birthday (2 months away), wedding anniversary (3 months away), and birth of his first grandchild (6 months away). Mr. J met with the outpatient palliative APRN to discuss goals of care.

The palliative APRN outlined options for care with Mr. J and his family, including continued aggressive care or comfort-focused care with home hospice. She explained to Mr. J and his family the risks and benefits of continued transfusions versus stopping transfusions, and they decided to continue transfusions as long as the benefits outweighed the burdens.

Mr. J was able to celebrate his milestone birthday and anniversary. His transfusion requirement increased to needing platelets once a week and blood twice a week. He became increasingly more fatigued and was not getting the "bump" in energy that he previously did after receiving blood. The palliative APRN readdressed goals of care, and Mr. J elected to continue as he was still able to spend quality time with his family.

After the birth of his grandson, he decided to forgo further transfusions. The palliative APRN facilitated a referral to hospice. Over the next 2 weeks, Mr. J became increasingly fatigued and somnolent. His family reported he died peacefully at home with hospice care.

DIALYSIS

The primary goal of renal replacement therapy (RRT) is to prolong life. Initially, dialysis was used to either bridge patients to transplant or allow time for renal recovery in patients with acute kidney injury (AKI).[51] Due to the aging population and advancements in technology, dialysis has now become a destination therapy. According to the US Renal Data System, in 2017, there were 746,557 patients with end-stage renal disease (ESRD). Roughly 70% of these patients received either peritoneal or hemodialysis, and the majority of these patients were older than 65.[52] With the number of patients over 65 expected to triple in the next 30 years, there is rising concern about the burden such treatment places on an already fragile patient population.[53]

The mortality rate of patients with Stage 5 chronic kidney disease (CKD) in the first year of maintenance of dialysis exceeds 20%.[54] For patients older than 75, the risk of death in the first year is 40%.[55] Elderly patients on dialysis experience higher rates of hospitalizations, intensive care admissions, invasive procedures, and death in a hospital setting in the last month of their life as compared to cancer or heart failure patients.[55] A study by Brown and colleagues showed that elderly patients with CKD who choose not to initiate dialysis survived a median of 16 months past the time dialysis was recommended and had marked improvements in symptom management with the initiation of palliative care.[56] While

dialysis may be an option for elderly CKD patients, it is not the only option. When RRT is initiated in this population, it has a significant negative impact on quality of life.[53]

A reported 60% of dialysis patients feel regret after initiating treatment.[55] Patients often feel ill-prepared for the physical and psychological toll dialysis takes on the body.[54] The lack of conversations on realistic expectations both with and without dialysis contribute to this problem. Only 10% of ESRD patients report having goals-of-care conversations with their nephrologist while up to 90% wanted them.[55] Prognostic uncertainty and unfamiliarity in leading complex discussions contribute to miscommunications between ESRD patients and their providers. While dialysis is meant to lower the symptom burden associated with advanced kidney disease, research has shown that patients undergoing maintenance dialysis suffer from a symptom burden comparable to patients who have not yet started treatment.[54]

Dialysis survival rates have increased in the past 2 years, leading to more uncertainty on prognosis in patients who have initiated treatment.[51] Discussing short-term prognosis with patients and family members can aid in decision-making. Several risk factors have been linked to increased mortality in ESRD patients. These risk factors have been used to develop prognostication tools that help providers determine which patients should initiate dialysis versus conservative management. One system, shown in Table 56.2 and developed by Santos and colleagues,[57] uses readily available clinical and laboratory data to predict which elderly patients have the highest 6-month mortality. Points are assigned based on five common risk factors. The higher the score, the greater the mortality risk. Patients with a score of 2 had a 10% risk of death in the first 6 months, while patients with a score of 6 had a 70% risk. Prognostication tools such as this can be useful to palliative APRNs as they identify which patients are at risk of death so they can help patients and families navigate difficult decisions surrounding initiation of dialysis.[57]

Withdrawal or discontinuation of RRT also occurs in patients with acute kidney injury (AKI). AKI affects up to 57% of patients in the ICU with 10–15% of these patients

Table 56.2 PREDICTORS OF 6-MONTH MORTALITY IN PATIENTS WITH END-STAGE RENAL DISEASE (ESRD)

RISK FACTOR		POINTS
Age >75		2
Coronary artery disease		2
Cerebrovascular disease with hemiplegia		2
Time of nephrology care before dialysis	< 3.0 months	2
	> 3.0 to < 12 months	1
Serum albumin	3.0–3.49 g/dL	1
	< 3.0 g/dL	2

The higher the score, the greater the mortality risk. Patients with a score of 2 had a 10% risk of death in the first 6 months, while patients with a score of 6 had a 70% risk.

From Santos et al.[57 (fig. 2)]

requiring RRT. The mortality rate in this population is high. Only 50% of AKI patients who start dialysis survive to discharge and of those who do, up to 14% require it long term.[58] Current guidelines recommend withholding dialysis in acutely ill patients who have an underlying terminal condition, advanced dementia, and in patients older than 75 years. Unfortunately, these guidelines are often ignored as the acute illness takes precedence, which leads to prolonged suffering in terminally ill patients in the ICU.[59] Palliative APRNs play an important role in educating patients, families, and collaborating providers on prognosis with and without dialysis. This type of informed discussion allows patients and families to better understand the burdens of dialysis in the final days to weeks of life and can lead to reduced initiation in this population or increased discontinuation of dialysis.

At this time, there are no standardized criteria for withdrawal or discontinuation of RRT. Research suggests dialysis should be stopped when the burdens of treatment outweigh the benefits, when the goals of treatment are not being met, and when a competent patient or surrogate decision-maker decide to forgo treatment.[59] Conversations regarding withdrawal and discontinuation should start prior to initiation of RRT and continue throughout treatment, as recommended by the American Society of Nephrology.[60] When the recommendations are followed, patients and their loved ones feel more prepared for the end of life and have realistic expectations after withdrawal or discontinuation. Unfortunately, lack of training on serious illness conversations for nephrologists often leaves these conversations to the last minute, when they are most difficult.[55] Palliative APRNs can help fill this gap in knowledge to ensure that all ESRD patients are making the most informed decisions.

Palliative APRNs play an important role in educating patients and families on the normal dying process. While many fear cessation of dialysis will lead to increased symptoms, death from uremia is often peaceful. Withdrawal or discontinuation from dialysis is the third leading cause of death in ESRD patients. The mean survival after withdrawal or discontinuation is approximately 7 days in this population.[61] Survival is even shorter for AKI patients in the ICU setting. Approximately 50% of deaths after withdrawal or discontinuation occur in a hospital setting without hospice care, which has been shown to increase patient and family suffering at the end of life.[55,62] Schmidt and colleagues linked early palliative referrals and advance care planning to a higher use of hospice in ESRD patients and improved quality of death.[62]

Discussions on withdrawal or discontinuation of life-sustaining treatment are difficult. Advance directives, when completed early, can help guide patient, family, and provider conversations on end of life. While advance directives appoint a decision-maker and give guidance on patient's preferences for resuscitation, intubation, and medically administered nutrition, they do not address dialysis at the end of life.[55] This is one reason that palliative APRNs are so important to this population. Patients who utilize palliative services in coordination with RRT report a lower symptom burden, improved quality of life, and better coping with the stressors associated with treatment.[51] Because palliative APRNs are skilled in complex discussions and prognostication, they can initiate discussions on withdrawal or discontinuation of RRT early and help patients and families understand kidney failure as a normal part of the dying process.

CASE STUDY 4: DIALYSIS

Mrs. M was a 66-year-old woman with a history of hypertension and triple negative Stage IV breast cancer. Her course is complicated by bilateral hydronephrosis with bilateral ureteral stents. She was currently on palliative chemotherapy and presented to the hospital after falling at home. Mrs. M was found to have lower extremity cellulitis on admission and was initiated on IV antibiotics. Her hospitalization was complicated by persistent hypotension not responsive to fluid resuscitation, worsening leukocytosis, and increasing blood urea nitrogen (BUN) and creatinine levels with decreased urine output. She was transferred to the ICU for further care and initiation of vasopressors. Her renal function continued to fluctuate throughout a prolonged ICU course, but it was ultimately unable to recover despite maximal treatment. Mrs. M required initiation of dialysis 2 weeks after hospital admission.

Prior to initiation of dialysis, palliative care was consulted. Mrs. M and her brother, John, met with the palliative APRN, Amy, to discuss next steps in care. The discussion included risks and benefits of dialysis, expectations given her advanced cancer diagnosis, and advance directives including power of attorney for healthcare (POAHC) and provider order for life-sustaining treatment (POLST) forms. She identified her brother as her chosen agent, and the POAHC form was completed with assistance from the social worker. At that time, Mrs. M was not interested in limiting any life-sustaining interventions. Her goals were to recover her renal status and work on regaining her functional status with intense physical therapy, hoping she could continue palliative chemo in the near future. However, Mrs. M did state that she would not want her life prolonged if she was going to be dependent on machines long term.

Mrs. M took a turn for the worse during her third week in the hospital. She became progressively thrombocytopenic, intermittently confused, and unable to meaningfully participate in therapy. Her body was unable to maintain fluid balance without IV supplementation. Mrs. M also became less tolerant of dialysis and required premedication with midodrine. Amy suggested a family meeting to readdress goals of care.

Mrs. M and her brother met with Amy, and the oncologist, hospitalist, and nephrologist. Mrs. M was alert and oriented enough to participate in the meeting. Both she and her brother were updated on her current status, prognosis, and goals of care were readdressed. Amy, with consensus from the multidisciplinary team, expressed concern that further dialysis would only prolong suffering and not enhance quality of life. Mrs. M and her family were informed that renal recovery was not possible and discontinuation of dialysis was recommended. Mrs. M and her brother were reminded of her previously verbalized wish to not be dependent on machines if there was no meaningful chance of recovery. It was eventually decided to move Mrs. M into inpatient hospice, where dialysis would be discontinued. Mrs. M died comfortably 3 days later with her brother at her bedside.

NUTRITION

Medically administered nutrition is a medical intervention used in patients who have difficulty swallowing or maintaining adequate nutrition as a result of a number of medical conditions. For patients with functioning gastrointestinal (GI) tracts, nutrition can be administered through a percutaneous endoscopy gastrostomy (PEG) tube or a nasogastric tube (NG). For patients without a functioning GI tract, total parenteral nutrition (TPN) is usually indicated. While all methods of medically administered nutrition carry risks and benefits, as a whole it has not been shown to prolong patients' lives as they near the end of life regardless of the route of administration or cause.[63]

Nearly 50 million people worldwide are suffering from dementia with an expected 10 million new cases each year.[64] Dementia is characterized by a progressive decline in mental, functional, and nutritional status ultimately leading to the end of life. Because anorexia is a normal part of the disease process, the risks and benefits of medically administered nutrition in this population have been widely researched. At this time, there are no prospective randomized control trials that demonstrate that artificial nutrition benefits patients with advanced dementia.[65] Consensus statements from both the American Geriatric Society and American Academy of Hospice and Palliative Medicine recommend against medically administered nutrition in advanced dementia. The Hospice and Palliative Nurses Association (HPNA) does not recommend medically administered nutrition in patients with a prognosis of 6 months or less but acknowledges the right for competent patients and family members to choose it with guidance from palliative APRNs.[66]

Placement of feeding tubes in advanced dementia patients remains controversial despite the overwhelming evidence against the benefits and clear recommendations.[2] This can be attributed to cultural and familial beliefs, lack of advance directives in this population, and misinterpretation of preferences by loved ones. Medically administered nutrition is often seen as a necessity and not a life-prolonging intervention. Family members tend to separate interventions for nutrition and hydration from "more invasive" end-of-life interventions such as mechanical ventilation and intubation.[67,68] A study by Tsai and colleagues showed that only 35–45% of patients with dementia had disclosed their preferences on end-of-life decisions. Of the patients who had, almost 50% of caregivers disagreed with or misunderstood the patient's preference. This, in turn, led to a high percentage of caregiver distress. Their research showed that comprehensive education on advanced dementia starting at diagnosis significantly reduced caregiver depression and use of medically administered nutrition in this patient population.[67]

Malnutrition impacts between 40% and 80% of cancer patients. It most commonly occurs in patients with late-stage disease and/or disease affecting the GI tract, lung, head, neck, and liver. While medically administered nutrition is recommended in cancer patients who are unable to meet 60% of nutritional needs despite nutritional counseling, there is no evidence that supports its use in advanced cancer patients, especially in the last weeks of life.[69] Though malnutrition in cancer patients is linked to higher mortality, oral feeding is recommended over medically administered nutrition and has been shown to provide just as much benefit without the risks.[70] Much like dementia, research has shown that early palliative care referrals significantly decreased the use of medically administered nutrition in this population.[71]

TPN is most commonly used in cancer patients suffering from radiation enteritis, chronic bowel obstruction, peritoneal carcinomatosis, and short bowel syndrome. While evidence on the benefit of such intervention is lacking, the current recommendation is to only initiate TPN in patients who are expected to be cured or live longer than 2–3 months.[69] When anorexia is caused by cancer cachexia syndrome rather than decreased oral intake, medically administered nutrition will not change the course and is associated with higher treatment-related complications, including sepsis. TPN has also been linked to poor quality of life and disruption in sleep, work, travel, fluid balance, and electrolyte abnormalities. Because TPN requires close monitoring both in the hospital and out, it is often seen as a burden for patients with advanced malignancies.[72]

Communication plays an important role in the patient's and family's understanding of nutrition at the end of life, regardless of the diagnosis. There is overwhelming evidence that early screening for malnutrition, consistent discussion on expectations throughout the disease course, and early advance directives reduce the use of artificial nutrition in patients with end-stage disease.[2,65,66,70] When families understand anorexia as a normal, natural part of the disease process, there is less report of suffering and improved promotion of patient-centered care.[2,65] One barrier to education and effective communication is lack of provider and nursing experience caring for terminally ill patients and overestimation of prognosis.[71,73,74] Palliative services have been demonstrated to break down these barriers, reduce the use of medically administered nutrition, improve overall quality of life, and reduce suffering associated with cessation of feeding for terminally ill patients.[67,70]

The role of the palliative APRN is to ensure providers, patients, and loved ones understand that medically administered nutrition is a medical intervention and not a basic provision of comfort. Withdrawal or discontinuation of medically administered nutrition is ethically justified when continuing treatment cannot achieve the intended benefit, the burdens of treatment outweigh the benefits, and/or when a competent patient or designated decision-maker chooses to discontinue treatment.[75] The dying process is characterized by diminished oral intake, diminished awareness, and decreased perception of hunger.[2] When the dying process has begun, medically administered nutrition has not been shown to provide benefit regardless of the cause. Despite the evidence, conversations regarding withdrawal, discontinuation, or withholding medically administered nutrition remain highly charged. Palliative care programs not only improve patient, caregiver, and provider understanding and acceptance of withdrawing, withholding, or discontinuing medically administered nutrition at end of life, but also protect patients from harm and ensure that patients' advance health wishes are respected.[2] Once a patient or family member has decided to withdraw or discontinue it, it is important that advance directives are updated accordingly.

CASE STUDY 5: MEDICALLY ADMINISTERED NUTRITION

Mrs. D was an 82-year-old Cantonese-speaking woman with history of cerebrovascular accident, coronary artery disease, COPD on 2 L nasal cannula, type 2 diabetes, CKD Stage IV, and hypertension who presented from a nursing home with hyperkalemia and hypoxia, her fifth admission for abnormal blood values. She was bedbound and could not provide any care for herself at baseline. On admission, Mrs. D was awake and alert to voice, oriented only to herself. She received nutrition through a PEG tube. While her hyperkalemia was quickly resolved, her hospitalization was complicated by worsening respiratory failure unresponsive to IV diuresis and requiring noninvasive ventilatory support.

Palliative APRN Sarah was consulted to discuss goals of care with Mrs. D's family. Sarah began working with Mrs. D and her five children after she was admitted a year ago for a stroke. Mrs. D did not have any advance directives in place. During one of the previous palliative meetings, her son Huang was established as the primary surrogate decision-maker and a POLST form was completed. With consensus among her children, the decision was for no resuscitation or intubation; however, long-term medically administered nutrition could be initiated. Because Mrs. D could no longer safely take oral nutrition, discussion turned to a feeding tube. Despite discussions on risks and benefits of a feeding tube, her family decided to proceed with placement in hopes it would aid in her recovery. Unfortunately, the last year of Mrs. D's care had been marked by progressive functional, cognitive, and nutritional decline; opportunistic infections; and repeated hospitalizations. Up to this point, Mrs. D's family have declined

discussions on end of life and hospice care and have verbalized preferences to continue hospitalizations.

Given Mrs. D's clinical condition, another family meeting was held to discuss next steps in her care. Palliative APRN Sarah knew this was Mrs. D's last hospitalization because she was unresponsive, hypotensive, and her breathing was irregular. Given COVID-19 restrictions, only two of her five children were allowed in the meeting room. The rest of the family joined via videoconference. Mrs. D's prognosis of hours to days was discussed, as well as discontinuation of medically administered nutrition and hydration and expectations for a normal dying process. Initially, Mrs. D's family was hesitant to withhold food and fluids. They were concerned that she would starve, die faster, and be more uncomfortable without nutrition. Sarah educated the family on the harms of nutrition at the end of life and addressed concerns about the cessation of food and fluids. Ultimately, her family agreed to withdrawal of further life-sustaining interventions, including tube feedings, and Mrs. D was moved to the inpatient hospice unit. Her POLST form was updated to reflect the new goals of comfort care. Mrs. D died 2 days later, comfortably, with family at her side.

SUMMARY

Life-sustaining treatments, such as antibiotics, blood products, dialysis, and medically administered nutrition, can prolong the dying process in critically and terminally ill patients. These treatments may provide little benefit, and the burdens of these interventions can increase suffering. Families are often faced with decisions regarding withholding, withdrawing, or discontinuing life-sustaining treatment as patients near the end of life. Recommendations regarding withholding, withdrawing, or discontinuing treatments should be made based on medical knowledge and evidence-based practice.

The palliative APRN must be adept at using communication skills to navigate these often emotionally charged conversations. Careful attention should be paid to avoid using

Table 56.3 SUGGESTED PALLIATIVE APRN COMMUNICATION REGARDING LIFE-SUSTAINING THERAPIES AT END OF LIFE

CLINICAL SITUATION	SUGGESTED WORDING AND/OR MESSAGES
Infection in advanced disease	Your father is dying from advanced cancer and has no further treatment options. Antibiotics may prolong the dying process and cause unnecessary suffering. I recommend withholding or discontinuing antibiotic therapy.
Blood products in advanced hematological malignancies	Your loved one is anemic because the disease has worsened and is no longer responding to treatment. Transfusions may sustain or prolong life for some time but will not help the underlying disease.
Kidney failure in sepsis with underlying terminal illness	Your mother's kidneys are shutting down as a part of the dying process, and dialysis will not be beneficial. As the toxins she normally urinates out build up in her system, she will become more sleepy, then comatose. It is usually a peaceful death.
Total parenteral nutrition (TPN) for malignant gastrointestinal failure	TPN is not likely to prolong life or improve quality of life. Medically administered nutrition is not recommended. Most patients with advanced disease do not feel hunger. We can offer pleasure feeds if the patient wants to eat.

judgmental terms such as "inappropriate" and "futile." The current terminology is the wording "nonbeneficial care," which implies less judgment. Sensitivity to cultural and religious beliefs is also key (see Section VI, "Communication"). Suggested messaging and wording for these conversations can be found in Table 56.3.

Palliative APRNs can play a key role in explaining the underlying disease process and prognosis to patients and families. They must also educate colleagues about prognostic tools that enable clinicians to identify patients who are nearing the end of life. Their role includes facilitating team and family meetings to encourage informed decision-making. Palliative APRNs can also educate colleagues, patients, and families regarding what to expect during the normal process of dying when treatments are discontinued.

REFERENCES

1. Truog RD, Campbell ML, Curtis JR, et al. Recommendations for end-of-life care in the intensive care unit: A consensus statement by the American College of Critical Care Medicine. *Crit Care Med.* 2008;36(3);953–963. doi:10.1097/CCM.0B013E3181659096

2. Danis M. UpToDate. Arnold R, ed. Stopping artificial nutrition and hydration at the end of life. Waltham, MA: UpToDate. March 21, 2021. https://www.uptodate.com/contents/stopping-nutrition-and-hydration-at-the-end-of-life

3. Breslin J. The status quo bias and decisions to withdraw life-sustaining treatment. *CMAJ.* 2018;190(9): E265–E267. doi:10.1503/cmaj.171005

4. Cosgrove J, Baruah R, Bassford C, et al. Care at the end of life: A guide to best practice, discussion, and decision-making in and around critical care. Critical Futures. London, UK: The Faculty of Intensive Care Medicine.September 2019. https://www.ficm.ac.uk/critical-futures-initiative/care-end-life

5. Coelho CBT, Yankaskas JR. New concepts in palliative care in the intensive care unit. *Rev Bras Ter Intensiva.* 2017;29(2):222–230. doi:10.5935/0103-507X.20170031

6. Robert R, Kentish-Barnes N, Boyer A, Laurent A, Azoulay E, Reignier J. Ethical dilemmas due to the Covid-19 pandemic. *Ann Intensive Care.* 2020;10(1):84. doi:10.1186/s13613-020-00702-7

7. Merel, SE, Meier CA, McKinney CM, Pottinger PS. Antimicrobial use in patients on a comfort care protocol: A retrospective cohort study. *J Palliat Med.* 2016;19(11):121–124. doi:10.1089/jpm.2016.0094

8. Baghban A, Juthani-Mehta M. Antimicrobial use at the end of life. *Infect Dis Clin North Am.* 2017;31(4):639–647. doi:10.1016/j.idc.2017.07.009

9. Albrecht JS, McGregor JC, Fromme EK, Bearden DT, Furuno JP. A nationwide analysis of antibiotic use in hospice care in the final week of life. *J Pain Symptom Manage.* 2013;46(4):483–490.

10. Joling KJ, Janssen O, Francke AL, et al. Time from diagnosis to institutionalization and death in people with dementia. *Alzheimers Dement.* 2020;16(4):662–671. doi:10.1002/alz.12063

11. Kochanek KD, Murphy SL, Xu JQ, Arias E. Deaths: Final data for 2017. National Vital Statistics Reports;68(9). Hyattsville, MD: National Center for Health Statistics. 2019. https://www.cdc.gov/nchs/data/nvsr/nvsr68/nvsr68_09-508.pdf

12. Kramarow EA, Tejada-Vera B. Dementia mortality in the United States, 2000–2017. National Vital Statistics Reports;68(2). Hyattsville, MD: National Center for Health Statistics. 2019. https://www.cdc.gov/nchs/data/nvsr/nvsr68/nvsr68_02-508.pdf.

13. Sampson EL, Candy B, Davis S, et al. Living and dying with advanced dementia: A prospective cohort study of symptoms, service use and care at the end of life. *Palliat Med.* 2018;32(3):668–681. doi:10.1177/0269216317726443

14. Brunnström HR, Englund EM. Cause of death in patients with dementia disorders. *Eur J Neurol.* 2009;16(4):488–492. doi:10.1111/j.1468-1331.2008.02503.x

15. Armstrong MJ, Alliance S, Corsentino P, DeKosky ST, Taylor A. Cause of death and end-of-life experiences in individuals with dementia with Lewy Bodies. *J Am Geriatr Soc.* 2019;67(1):67–73. doi:10.1111/jgs.15608

16. Manabe T, Fujikura Y, Mizukami K, Akatsu H, Kudo K. Pneumonia-associated death in patients with dementia: A systematic review and meta-analysis. *PLoS One.* 2019;14(3):e0213825. doi:10.1371/journal.pone.0213825

17. Garcia-Ptacek S, Kåreholt I, Cermakova P, Rizzuto D, Religa D, Eriksdotter M. Causes of death according to death certificates in individuals with dementia: A cohort from the Swedish Dementia Registry. *J Am Geriat Soc.* 2016;64(11):e137–e142. doi:10.1111/jgs.14421

18. Juthani-Mehta M, Malani PN, Mitchell SL. Antimicrobials at the end of life: An opportunity to improve palliative care and infection management. *JAMA.* 2015;314(19):2017–2018. doi:10.1001/jama.2015.13080

19. Thompson AJ, Silveria MJ, Vitale CA, Malani PN. Antimicrobial use at the end of life among hospitalized patients with advanced cancer. *Am J Hospice Palliat Care.* 2012;29(8):599–603.

20. Vallard A, Morisson S, Tinquaut F, et al. Drug management in end-of-life hospitalized palliative care cancer patients: The RHESO Cohort Study. *Oncology.* 2019;97(4):217–227. doi:10.1159/00050078

21. Pasay DK, Guirguis MS, Shkrobot RC, et al. Antimicrobial stewardship in rural nursing homes: Impact of interprofessional education and clinical decision tool implementation on urinary tract infection treatment in a cluster randomized trial. *Infect Control Hosp Epidemiol.* 2019;40(4):432–437. doi:10.1017/ice.2019.9

22. Wilder-Smith A, Gillespie T, Taylor DR. Antimicrobial use and misuse at the end of life: A retrospective analysis of a treatment escalation/limitation plan. *J R Coll Physicians Edinb.* 2019;49(3):188–192. doi:10.4997/JRCPE.2019.304

23. Servid SA, Noble BN, Fromme EK, Furuno JP. Clinical intentions of antibiotics prescribed upon discharge to hospice care. *J Am Geriatr Soc.* 2018;66(3):565–569. doi:10.1111/jgs.15246

24. Givens JL, Jones RN, Shaffer ML, Kiely DK, Mitchell SL. Survival and comfort after treatment of pneumonia in advanced dementia. *Arch Intern Med.* 2010;170(13):1102–1107. doi:10.1001/archinternmed.2010.181

25. Reinbolt RE, Shenk AM, White PH, Navari RM. Symptomatic treatment of infections in patients with advanced cancer receiving hospice care. *J Pain Symptom Manage.* 2005;30(2):175–182. doi:10.1016/j.jpainsymman.2005.03.006

26. Blinderman CD, Billings JA. Comfort care for patients dying in the hospital. *N Engl J Med.* 2015;373(26):2549–2561. doi:10.1056/NEJMra1411746

27. Tamma PD, Avdic E, Li DX, Dzintars K, Cosgrove SE. Association of adverse events with antibiotic use in hospitalized patients. *JAMA Int Med.* 2017;177(9):1308–1315. doi:10.1001/jamainternmed.2017.1938

28. Duncan I, Ahmed T, Dove H, Maxwell TL. Medicare cost at end of life. *Am J Hosp Palliat Care.* 2019;36(8):705–710. doi:10.1177/1049909119836204

29. Vaughan L, Duckett AA, Adler M, Cain J. Ethical and clinical considerations in treating infections at the end of life. *J Hosp Palliat Nurs.* 2019;21(2):110–115. doi:10.1097/NJH.0000000000000541

30. Sinert M, Stammet Schmidt MM, Lovell AG, Protus BM. Guidance for safe and appropriate use of antibiotics in hospice using a collaborative decision support tool. *J Hospice Palliat Nurs.* 2020;22(4):276–282. doi:10.1097/NJH.0000000000000655

31. Wright AA, Keating NL, Ayanian JZ, et al. Family perspectives on aggressive cancer care near the end of life. *JAMA.* 2016;315(3):284–292. doi:10.1001/jama.2015.18604

32. Mack JW, Weeks JC, Wright AA, Block SD, Prigerson HG. End-of-life discussions, goal attainment and distress: Predictors and

outcomes for receipt of care consistent with preferences *J Clin Oncol.* 2010;28(7):1203–1208. doi:10.1200/JCO.2009.25.4672

33. Manitta VJ, Philip JAJAM, Cole-Sinclair MF. Palliative care and the hemato-oncological patient: Can we live together?: A review of the literature. *J Palliat Med.* 2010;13(8):1021–1025. doi:10.1089/jpm.2009.0267

34. LeBlanc TW, Abernethy AP, Casarett DJ. What is different about patients with hematologic malignancies? A retrospective cohort study of cancer patients referred to a hospice research network. *J Pain Symptom Manage.* 2015;49(3):505–512. doi:10.1016/j.jpainsymman.2014.07.003

35. Hill QA. Intensify, resuscitate or palliate: Decision-making in the critically ill patient with haematological malignancy. *Blood Rev.* 2010;24(1):17–25. doi:10.1016/j.blre.2009.10.002

36. Egan PC, LeBlanc TW, Olszewski AJ. End-of-life care quality outcomes among Medicare beneficiaries with hematologic malignancies. *Blood Adv.* 2020;4(15):3606–3614. doi:10.1182/bloodadvances.2020001767

37. Fletcher SA, Cronin AM, Zeidan AM, et al. Intensity of end-of-life care for patients with myelodysplastic syndromes: Findings from a large national database. *Cancer.* 2016;122(8):1209–1215. doi:10.1002/cncr.29913

38. Beaussant Y, Daguindau E, Chauchet A, et al. Hospital end-of-life care in haematological malignancies. *BMJ Support Palliat Care.* 2018;8(3):314–324. doi:10.1136/bmjspcare-2017-001446

39. El-Jawahri AR, Abel GA, Steensma DP, et al. Health care utilization and end-of-life care for older patients with acute myeloid leukemia. *Cancer.* 2015;121(16):2840–2848. doi:10.1002/cncr.29430

40. Odejide OO, Cronin AM, Earle CC, Tulsky JA, Abel GA. Why are patients with blood cancers more likely to die without hospice? *Cancer.* 2017;123(17):3377–3384. doi:10.1002/cncr.30735

41. Odejide OO, Li L, Cronin AM, et al. Meaningful changes in end-of-life care among patients with myeloma. *Haematologica.* 2018;103(8):1380–1389. doi:10.3324/haematol.2018.187609

42. Wang R, Zeidan AM, Halene S, et al. Health care use by older adults with acute myeloid leukemia at the end of life. *J Clin Oncol.* 2017;35(30):3417–3424. doi:10.1200/JCO.2017.72.7149

43. Lowe JR, Yu Y, Wolf S, Samsa G, LeBlanc TW. A cohort study of patient-reported outcomes and healthcare utilization in acute myeloid leukemia patients receiving active cancer therapy in the last six months of life. *J Palliat Med.* 2018;21(5):592–597. doi:10.1089/jpm.2017.0463

44. LeBlanc TW, Egan PC, Olszewski AJ. Transfusion dependence, use of hospice services, and quality of end-of-life care in leukemia. *Blood.* 2018;132(7):717–726. doi:10.1182/blood-2018-03-842575

45. Kripp M, Willer A, Schmidt C, et al. Patients with malignant hematological disorders treated on a palliative care unit: Prognostic impact of clinical factors. *Ann Hematol.* 2014;93(2):317–325. doi:10.1007/s00277-013-1861-7.

46. Button E, Gavin NC, Chan RJ, Chambers S, Butler J, Yates P. Clinical indicators that identify risk of deteriorating and dying in people with a hematological malignancy: A case–control study with multivariable analysis. *J Palliat Med.* 2018;21(12):1729–1740. doi:10.1089/jpm.2018.0033

47. Button E, Chan RJ, Chambers S, Butler J, Yates P. A systematic review of prognostic factors at the end of life for people with a hematological malignancy. *BMC cancer.* 2017;17(1):213. doi:10.1186/s12885-017-3207-7

48. Chin-Yee N, Taylor J, Rourke K, et al. Red blood cell transfusion in adult palliative care: A systematic review. *Transfusion.* 2018;58(1):233–241. doi:10.1111/trf.14413

49. Wang WS, Ma JD, Nelson SH, et al. Transfusion practices at end of life for hematopoietic stem cell transplant patients. *Support Care Cancer.* 2018;26(6):1927–1931. doi:10.1007/s00520-017-4023-y

50. Smith LB, Cooling L, Davenport R. How do I allocate blood products at the end of life? An ethical analysis with suggested guidelines. *Transfusion.* 2013;53(4):696–700. doi:10.1111/j.1537-2995.2012.03656.x

51. Castro MCM. Reflections on end-of-life dialysis. *J Bras Nefrol.* 2018;40(3):233–241. doi:10.1590/2175-8239-jbn-3833

52. United States Renal Data System. USRDS 2019 Annual Data Report: Epidemiology of kidney disease in the United States. Executive Summary. National Institutes of Health, National Institute of Diabetes and Digestive and Kidney Diseases, Bethesda, MD. 2019. https://www.usrds.org/media/2371/2019-executive-summary.pdf

53. Rak A, Raina R, Suh TT, et al. Palliative care for patients with end-stage renal disease: Approach to treatment that aims to improve quality of life and relieve suffering for patients (and families) with chronic illnesses. *Clin Kidney J.* 2017;10(1):68–73. doi:10.1093/ckj/sfw105

54. Rivara MB, Mehrotra R. Timing of dialysis initiation: What has changed since IDEAL? *Semin Nephrol.* 2017;37(2):181–193. doi:10.1016/j.semnephrol.2016.12.008

55. Mandel EI, Bernacki RE, Block SD. Serious illness conversations in ESRD. *Clin J Am Soc Nephrol.* 2017;12(5):854–863. doi:10.2215/CJN.05760516

56. Brown MA, Collett GK, Josland EA, Foote C, Li Q, Brennan FP. CKD in elderly patients managed without dialysis: Survival, symptoms, and quality of life. *Clin J Am Soc Nephrol.* 2015;10(2):260–268. doi:10.2215/CJN.03330414

57. Santos J, Oliveira P, Malheiro J, et al. Predicting 6-month mortality in incident elderly dialysis patients: A simple prognostic score. *Kidney Blood Press Res.* 2020;45(1):38–50. doi:10.1159/000504136

58. Hoste EA, Bagshaw SM, Bellomo R, et al. Epidemiology of acute kidney injury in critically ill patients: The multinational AKI-EPI study. *Intensive Care Med.* 2015;41(8):1411–1423. doi:10.1007/s00134-015-3934

59. Shin SJ, Lee JH. Hemodialysis as a life-sustaining treatment at the end of life. *Kidney Res Clin Pract.* 2018;37(2):112–118. doi:10.23876/j.krcp.2018.37.2.112

60. Renal Physicians Association. *Shared Decision-Making in the Appropriate Initiation of and Withdrawal from Dialysis,* 2nd ed. Rockville, MD: Renal Physicians Association; 2010. https://cdn.ymaws.com/www.renalmd.org/resource/resmgr/ESRD_Guidelines/Recommendations_Summary.pdf.

61. Findlay MD, Donaldson K, Doyle A, et al. Factors influencing withdrawal from dialysis: A national registry study. *Nephrol Dial Transplant.* 2016;31(12):2041–2048. doi:10.1093/ndt/gfw074

62. Schmidt RJ, Weaner BB, Long D. The power of advance care planning in promoting hospice and out-of-hospital death in a dialysis unit. *J Palliat Med.* 2015;18(1):62–66. doi:10.1089/jpm.2014.0031

63. Masaki S, Kawamoto T. Comparison of long-term outcomes between enteral nutrition via gastrostomy and total parenteral nutrition in older persons with dysphagia: A propensity-matched cohort study. *PLoS One.* 2019;14(10):e0217120. doi:10.1371/journal.pone.0217120

64. World Health Organization. Key Facts. Sep 2, 2021. https://www.who.int/en/news-room/fact-sheets/detail/dementia.

65. Volkert D, Chourdakis M, Faxen-Irving G, et al. ESPEN guidelines on nutrition in dementia. *Clin Nutr.* 2015;34(6):1052–1073. doi:10.1016/j.clnu.2015.09.004

66. Hospice and Palliative Nurses Association. Position statement: Medically administered nutrition and hydration. Pittsburgh, PA: HPNA. Jan 2020. https://advancingexpertcare.org/position-statements/

67. Marcolini EG, Putnam AT, Aydin A. History and perspectives on nutrition and hydration at the end of life. *Yale J Biol Med.* 2018;91(2):173–176.

68. Tsai CF, Lee YT, Lee WJ, Hwang JP, Wang SJ, Fuh JL. Depression of family caregivers is associated with disagreements on life-sustaining preferences for treating patients with dementia. *PLoS One.* 2015;10(7):e0133711. doi:10.1371/journal.pone.0133711

69. De Las Peñas R, Majem M, Perez-Altozano J, et al. SEOM clinical guidelines on nutrition in cancer patients (2018). *Clin Transl Oncol.* 2019;21(1):87–93. doi:10.1007/s12094-018-02009-3

70. Arends J, Bachmann P, Baracos V, et al. ESPEN guidelines on nutrition in cancer patients. *Clin Nutr.* 2017;36(1):11–48. doi:10.1016/j.clnu.2016.07.015

71. Baumstarck K, Boyer L, Pauly V, et al. Use of artificial nutrition near the end of life: Results from a French national population-based study of hospitalized cancer patients. *Cancer Med.* 2020;9(2):530–540. doi:10.1002/cam4.2731

72. Jatoi A, Loprinzi C. In. Hesketh P, Seres D, eds. The role of parenteral and enteral/oral nutritional support in patients with cancer. UpToDate. Waltham, MA: UptoDate. Aug 19, 2020. https://www.uptodate.com/contents/the-role-of-parenteral-and-enteral-oral-nutritional-support-in-patients-with-cancer

73. Heuberger R, Wong H. Knowledge, attitudes, and beliefs of physicians and other health care providers regarding artificial nutrition and hydration at the end of life. *J Aging Health.* 2019;31(7):1121–1133. doi:10.1177/0898264318762850

74. White KR, Roczen ML, Coyne PJ, Wiencek C. Acute and critical care nurses' perceptions of palliative care competencies: A pilot study. *J Cont Ed Nurs.* 2014;45(6):265–277. doi:10.3928/00220124-20140528-01

75. Kirsch RE, Balit CR, Carnevale FA, Latour JM, Larcher V. Ethical, cultural, social, and individual considerations prior to transition to limitation or withdrawal of life-sustaining therapies. *Pediatr Crit Care Med.* 2018;19(8S Suppl 2):S10–S18. doi:10.1097/PCC.0000000000001488

57.

PALLIATIVE SEDATION

David Collett and Kelly Baxter

KEY POINTS

- Palliative sedation is an important therapy of last resort to relieve suffering in patients who have intractable pain and/or other symptoms.

- The palliative advanced practice registered nurse (APRN) must understand the ethical framework of palliative sedation as well their institutional and jurisdiction's context.

- The palliative APRN should be familiar with the various medications and monitoring guidelines that are used to provide safe and effective sedation.

- Palliative sedation necessitates interdisciplinary team involvement, utilization of evidence-based practice, and knowledge of ethical principles, as well as practice guidelines.

CASE STUDY

Miguel is a 30-year-old man who was diagnosed 2 years prior with metastatic osteosarcoma. He had recently finished business school and was advancing in his company when he was diagnosed. Miguel had initially presented to his family nurse practitioner with a history of persistent and worsening knee pain, weight loss, and fatigue that was interfering with his workouts as well as his daily activities. After being ruled out for other causes, he underwent imaging that showed a femur mass concerning for malignancy, and a subsequent biopsy confirmed metastatic sarcoma involving bone, soft tissue, and liver.

Miguel underwent several lines of chemotherapy and radiation with ongoing progression of disease. Because of his continued high functional status and tolerance of treatment, he was able to continue to receive disease-directed treatment. However, he continued to have neuropathic and somatic right lower extremity pain. His medical oncologist referred him to the palliative nurse practitioner who was embedded as part of the oncology practice. She initiated a pain regimen of morphine and gabapentin, although, over the next several months, he required increases in doses and initiation of long-acting morphine.

Miguel continued to be followed by palliative care, who also engaged him in advance care planning and referred him for chaplaincy for spiritual support. The palliative social worker also held sessions with both Miguel as well as his parents to help them process his advanced illness. As his disease progressed, he required rotation to methadone due to tolerance at significantly higher doses of opioids, and he received some benefit from a short course of palliative radiation. Several months later, his oncologist asked palliative care to participate in a goals-of-care meeting to share that Miguel's disease had continued to progress and that there were no further treatments. A recommendation for home hospice services was provided, and a prognosis of 6 months was given. Miguel initially declined home hospice services, stating that he was hopeful to continue to receive disease-directed treatment.

Miguel enrolled in a Phase I clinical trial at a nearby academic medical center. However, he had an adverse reaction to one of the trial drugs and was forced to disenroll in the trial. A week later, he presented to the oncology center's emergency department with severe pain, nausea, and failure to thrive. He was admitted by the oncology hospitalist team, and palliative care was consulted. His clinical status continued to decline, with continued severe pain. Miguel's nausea interfered with his ability to take oral medications, and his oral methadone was converted to intravenous (IV) form. Eventually, he required the addition of patient-controlled analgesia with hydromorphone, and he also received ketamine as an adjuvant analgesic.

Miguel continued to have moderate-severe pain, though the pain was tolerable. He preferred to remain as alert as possible to spend time with his friends and family who were frequently at bedside. He continued to decline, and there were multiple discussions regarding goals of care. Miguel elected to have a do-not-resuscitate (DNR) order placed. Though Miguel shared he would prefer to be at home, he expressed understanding that his opioid regimen and IV requirement would require inpatient services. Social work was involved, and a referral was made for a local inpatient hospice that had an adequate supply of the opioids Miguel required.

Unfortunately, the inpatient hospice had a waitlist. Miguel declined further, with increasing pain and frequent pain crises that required extensive titration under the guidance of the palliative care team's pharmacist. It was shared with him and his family that his prognosis was likely short – death was probable within days. Miguel's intractable pain was distressing to him as well as his family, as he would often wake up screaming and boluses were providing less and less relief. The palliative care team discussed the potential of using palliative sedation as a way to control his refractory pain. Miguel expressed interest in this, although he shared that he was hopeful to see his brother who was traveling to the hospital to see him. After discussion, it was decided by Miguel to pursue palliative sedation until his brother was able to be present bedside. A clinical meeting was held with Miguel's primary hospital team, nursing staff, and the palliative care interdisciplinary team. One nurse shared that he felt ethically uncomfortable with palliative sedation because of religious beliefs, and a change in nursing staff was made. An overview was provided to Miguel and his family, and his DNR code status was reconfirmed. Later that evening, a midazolam infusion was started that relieved Miguel's symptoms, with his family staying close. His opioid regimen was continued concurrently, and he was monitored closely for signs of pain.

His family stayed at his bedside. The next night, Miguel's brother arrived, and sedation was paused. Miguel awoke in severe pain and again received boluses for breakthrough pain with minimal relief. He was able to spend an hour with his brother and family and say goodbye to them. The palliative chaplain provided prayers and spiritual support before Miguel requested that sedation be restarted. The infusion was restarted and Miguel continued to be monitored by nursing and his medical teams, with his family present at bedside until he died the following afternoon.

INTRODUCTION

Every individual hopes for a peaceful death. When a serious illness becomes a terminal illness, the goals of care may shift from curative or life-prolonging to an exclusive focus on comfort. When someone transitions to the end of life, physical comfort can be achieved for many people. With physical symptoms controlled, the dying experience may become a time for personal growth, reconciliation, strengthening of relationships, and spiritual enrichment. However, there are rare circumstances when, despite best efforts, distressing symptoms may not be fully managed. This results in not only physical suffering but can also cause psychological and existential suffering that may interfere with a peaceful death. When patients have intractable symptoms, palliative sedation is offered as a treatment of last resort when all other expert palliative care treatments have failed.[6] The process of deciding to offer palliative sedation is multifaceted, but its intention—to relieve suffering and not to hasten death—is clear.[1]

Critical and systematic review of the palliative sedation literature reveals differences in the concepts and practice of palliative sedation.[6] The lack of consensus among experts demonstrates that even experienced palliative care clinicians may be uncomfortable with palliative sedation—whether based on personal beliefs, unfamiliarity, or a lack of guidelines. The focus of this chapter is the role of the palliative advanced practice registered nurse (APRN) in palliative sedation based on expert opinion and evidence-based practice.

TERMS AND PREVALENCE OF USE

Palliative sedation has also been described as "controlled sedation" "terminal sedation," "sedation for intractable symptoms," "continuous sedation," "sedation at end of life," "total sedation," and "prolonged sedation."[1,6,7] The Hospice and Palliative Nurses Association uses the term "palliative sedation" rather than "terminal sedation" in its position statement regarding the practice because "the name was modified to more accurately reflect the intent and application of its use—to palliate the patient's experience of symptoms rather than to cause or hasten death."[1]

Even though there is no universal terminology of palliative sedation, and even some disagreement on its conceptual foundation, there is some agreement that it involves the monitored use of medications to induce controlled sedation to the point of unconsciousness in a dying patient to relieve distress caused by otherwise uncontrolled pain and symptoms and that it is used as a last resort.[8,9] It is typically continued until the patient dies. Palliative sedation is different from *procedural sedation* or *conscious sedation*, in which time-limited use of sedation decreases awareness and pain during an anticipated painful procedure in a patient who is going to survive. Palliative sedation also includes *respite sedation* and *emergency sedation*. Respite sedation is a time-limited use of sedative medications in dying patients with the goal of providing reprieve from distress and suffering for a period of time and then returning the patient to consciousness. Emergency sedation is utilized in patients who experience an emergent, symptomatic crisis at the end of life that causes severe distress—such as a hemorrhage or profound hemoptysis.

Palliative sedation is not a veiled type of euthanasia or aid in dying. Clearly, the intent and practice of palliative sedation are to reduce suffering by inducing an altered consciousness, not by precipitating death. *Voluntary active euthanasia* is when a clinician *administers* a lethal dose of medication in response to a request from a competent patient for help in ending life.[2] *Assisted death* (i.e., medical aid in dying or physician-assisted dying) is when a patient is prescribed a lethal dose of medication that is self-administered by a patient who has requested the means to end their own life (Table 57.1). The American Nurses Association (ANA) position statement, *The Nurse's Role When a Patient Requests Medical Aid in Dying*, states that nurses are "ethically prohibited from administering medical aid in dying medication." However, the statement also states that nurses need to "remain objective when discussing end-of-life options with patients who are exploring medical aid in dying" and to also advocate for palliative care[3] (see Chapter 53, "Navigating Ethical Dilemmas").

The literature reports wide variation in the use of palliative sedation, although, when it is utilized, it is often in cancer patients.[10] Frequency of palliative sedation is broad, with studies showing use ranging from 1% to 80% of study population patients.[7] The lack of consensus on the definition of palliative sedation, the retrospective nature of palliative sedation studies, and the settings that palliative sedation takes place in may contribute to this variation.[11] Other hypotheses for the wide deviation in its reported use include varied cultural, religious, and ethnic values and beliefs about the ethics and appropriateness of its use. Research has found an increase in the use of palliative sedation in recent years in some countries, which may be a result of increased recognition of palliative sedation by clinicians and/or by patients and families.[7]

Table 57.1 COMMON TERMS RELATED TO PALLIATIVE SEDATION

INTERVENTION	DEFINITION	TYPICAL SCENARIO	LEGALITY
Palliative sedation	Sedation provided to a terminally ill patient near end of life with goal of reducing suffering. The controlled induction of sedation to the point of unconsciousness in a patient at end of life to relieve otherwise refractory pain, symptoms, and emotional suffering (though this is more controversial).	End of life with intractable symptoms continued through death Could be planned or emergent	Legal in the United States
Respite sedation	Temporary or time-limited sedation provided to a terminally ill patient with goal of giving respite from symptoms for a period of time and then returning the patient to consciousness.	End of life with intractable symptoms	Legal in the United States
Urgent or emergency palliative sedation	An emergent use of palliative sedation medications provided in a crisis for patients at end of life with the goal of giving respite from urgently arising symptoms.	End of life with a symptomatic crisis (e.g., hemorrhage, acute respiratory distress from lung shift)	Legal in the United States
Procedural sedation	The time-limited or temporary use of sedation to decrease awareness and prevent pain during a medical procedure or surgery in a patient who is going to survive.	Surgical settings, other procedures (e.g., intubation, wound packing for ENT issues)	Legal in the United States
Voluntary active euthanasia	Administration of an agent by a third party to a patient by request with goal of ending life.	Varies depending on locale, typically in terminally ill patients	Not legal in the United States and not recognized by most discipline-specific organizations in the United States (i.e., American Medical Association, American Nurses Association)
Assisted death	Self-administration of an agent prescribed by a medical provider with goal of ending own life	Varies depending on locale, typically in terminally ill patients	Legal in some states throughout the United States. In most states, APRNs are not authorized to prescribe medications for this procedure

From Hospice and Palliative Nurses Association[1], Billings[2], American Nurses Association[3], Cherny[4].

LEGAL JUSTIFICATION FOR THE USE OF PALLIATIVE SEDATION

Several important legal cases set the support and precedent for the use of palliative sedation. In the 1997 US Supreme Court decisions in *Vacco v. Quill* and *Washington v. Glucksberg*, Justice O'Connor stated that "a patient who is suffering from a terminal illness and who is experiencing great pain has no legal barriers to obtaining medication, from qualified physicians, to alleviate that suffering, even to the point of causing unconsciousness and hastening death."[12,13] O'Connor went further to describe the end of life: "Death will be different for each of us. For many, the last days will be spent in physical pain and perhaps the despair that accompanies physical deterioration and a loss of control of basic bodily and mental functions. Some will seek medication to alleviate that pain and other symptoms." Justice O'Connor affirmed the distinction between intentionally hastening death and the justifiable use of medication to alleviate suffering, even to the point of unconsciousness and hastening death.

Multiple ethical concepts support the use of palliative sedation. Principles of dignity, autonomy, fidelity, beneficence, nonmaleficence, and the rule of double effect are often used. A palliative APRN must be familiar with how these concepts relate to decision-making about palliative sedation and be able to counsel, educate, and support their team. The ANA's *Code of Ethics for Nurses* states that "A fundamental principle that underlies all nursing practice is respect for the inherent dignity, worth, unique attributes and human rights of all individuals."[14] Palliative sedation frees a patient from suffering and thereby preserves his or her dignity and self-worth. The ANA's *Nurses' Roles and Responsibilities in Providing Care and Support at the End of Life* exhorts all nurses to have a basic understanding of palliative care, how to advocate for palliative care for patients, and basic symptom recognition and management. Nurses are also to be able to engage with patients and their families on advance care planning and discussing with them their goals and values in the context of their medical care, including do-not-resuscitate orders.[15,16] By respecting the values, beliefs, goals, privacy, actions, priorities, and body of an autonomous adult, the palliative APRN respects the dignity of that person.[14]

Autonomy or self-determination is derived from the principle of respect for persons. It is the right of a capable person to decide their own course of action based on their own personal values and goals of life.[17] Informed consent derives from self-determination. It requires that the patient has the capacity and sufficient information to understand the risks and potential benefits of palliative sedation before it is started. The patient without the capacity to make decisions has the same right to informed consent before treatment, but decisions should be made through a surrogate decision-maker who is substituting for the patient.[18]

The principle of fidelity is also an ethical imperative that ensures that healthcare providers keep promises and faithfully act in the correct manner toward the patient. The commitment to not abandon our patients or their families at the end of life, even in the face of great suffering, is based on fidelity. Beneficence is the ethical duty to act to the benefit or good for the person under our care.[17] Treating physical and psychological distress, promoting comfort, and honoring the wishes of our patients are perceived as beneficial. Nonmaleficence is historically linked to the Hippocratic Oath and its stated imperative of doing no harm.[17] This principle is often used as a moral argument against the practice of palliative sedation, as some believe that harm is incurred in the potential for hastening death. The validity of this argument is contradicted by Maltoni and colleagues who reviewed 30 years of data in patient cohorts matched for prognostic variables. They demonstrated that patients receiving palliative sedation did not die sooner than those not receiving sedation.[19] Moreover, careful use of the therapy in terms of patient selection and close monitoring limit potential harm.

The ANA's *Code of Ethics for Nurses* states that "the nurse should provide interventions to relieve pain and other symptoms in the dying patient even if those interventions entail the risk of hastening death. However, nurses may not act with the sole intent to end a patient's life even if motivated by compassion, respect for patient autonomy, and quality of life considerations."[14] This reflects the principle of double effect. Billings points out that solely relying on this precept ignores the issue that although the intended effect of palliative sedation is to reduce suffering, it often involves withholding fluids and other life-supporting measures and that death from the underlying disease or condition is actually inevitable[2,20] (Table 57.2).

The Hospice and Palliative Nurses Association, the American Academy of Hospice and Palliative Medicine, the National Hospice and Palliative Care Organization, and other professional organizations endorse palliative sedation for intractable symptoms to relieve suffering.[1,21–24] Despite this general acceptance in the healthcare community for the use of palliative sedation, it is important to understand and acknowledge the concerns of those who do not agree that the practice is morally acceptable. Objections include the fear that the practice is part of a slippery slope that will lead to hastening death or euthanasia, violating the sanctity of life, or a belief that a higher power or deity alone should choose when a patient dies. Also, the withdrawal of life support or withholding of nutrition, although legally permissible and ethically supported in nursing and medicine, may be unacceptable for someone's moral framework.[2] Team members, patients, and families may differ in their opinions based on their cultural norms and religious beliefs. The palliative APRN must explore these values while offering nonjudgmental support and negotiating a care plan that is respectful of these other opinions but consistent with the patient's wishes and codes of professional conduct. This may result in the APRN assuming the responsibility of care for others who are uncomfortable with palliative sedation. Such actions include offering to take the lead in care, writing orders, directly initiating the medication administration, and providing ongoing support of the family and staff.

In the final analysis, each team member must create his or her own personal ethical and moral framework to work

Table 57.2 PALLIATIVE SEDATION AND DOUBLE EFFECT

DOUBLE EFFECT	PALLIATIVE SEDATION
The act itself is morally good or indifferent.	Giving medication to relieve suffering is good.
The intent of the act is only to cause a good effect.	The intent is to alleviate suffering and distress from intractable pain and suffering.
A bad effect may be foreseen but is not intended and would have been avoided if a satisfactory alternative method to achieve the good effect could be found.	Death is foreseen but is not intended with palliative sedation.
The desirable effect follows from the intended effect and not from the bad effect (death).	Relief of pain and symptoms and the subsequent suffering is achieved through sedation, not death.
A proportionately grave reason exists for seeking the good effect and thus compensates for risking or permitting the bad effect.	The use of palliative sedation to relieve intolerable suffering from intractable pain and symptoms outweighs the risk of hastening death.

Adapted from Billings[2]; and Billings, Churchill.[20]

with the patient, family, and other team members to come to a mutually supportive plan that is respectful of each person's values. The use of palliative sedation, although supported by the law and leading organizations in the science, will not be morally or ethically permissible to some patients and families and some members of the healthcare team. Thus, the palliative APRN needs to understand the legal and ethical doctrines that support and challenge the use of palliative sedation as well as the institution's guidelines while simultaneously initiating and participating in discussions about its use, with sensitivity to the concerns and perspectives of all: patients, families, and members of the healthcare team.

CREATING A MODEL OF CARE FOR PALLIATIVE SEDATION THERAPY

There are three types of sedation: palliative sedation for symptoms, palliative sedation for existential issues, and respite sedation. To create a model of safe, effective, high-quality care, best practice in the following six areas listed in must be delineated:

- Patient eligibility

- Clinician/team member competence, involvement, and care

- Informed consent and decision-making about continued treatments (including the use of life support and nutrition and hydration)

- Team preplanning: who will lead the process, who will write orders, who will support the family and the care team

- Family involvement and care

- Medications and procedure of palliative sedation

- Post-sedation debrief

PATIENT ELIGIBILITY

For the use of palliative sedation to be considered, the patient must have a terminal condition with imminent death anticipated and must be experiencing severe symptoms and suffering, often described as intolerable, intractable, or refractory to aggressive standard palliative interventions. Imminent death is defined as a life expectancy of hours to days based on the person's physical exam, the progression of disease, and the symptom constellation.[25,26]

Cherny and Portenoy define a refractory symptom as having these attributes: (1) aggressive palliative care interventions short of sedation fail to provide relief, (2) additional invasive or noninvasive treatments are unlikely to provide relief, and (3) additional therapies are likely to be associated with excessive or unacceptable morbidity or are unlikely to provide relief within a reasonable timeframe[4] (e.g., a patient in the last few days of life with severe neoplasm-related pain unrelieved by escalating multidrug analgesic regimens despite the involvement and evaluation of palliative specialists).

The type of refractory patient suffering (physical vs. existential) for which palliative sedation therapy may be considered is another factor. The term "existential suffering" can also include spiritual suffering and typically relates to nonphysical symptoms, including the inability to find meaning, purpose, and fulfillment in one's life, a loss of dignity, fear of death, hopelessness, and loneliness.[27,28] Prevalence of existential distress for patients with terminal illness is 13–18%, and potential risk factors for existential distress include lack of social support, uncontrolled physical symptoms, reduced physical activity, and coping through blaming oneself.[29,30] Additionally, it is important to consider posttraumatic stress disorder (PTSD) as a precipitating factor in existential distress as well as physical symptoms and to identify patients who are at increased risk.[31]

For some patients, such existential distress can be intolerable. The use of palliative sedation for existential distress is controversial and views vary widely, even among palliative care providers.[32] One argument against its use is the difficulty of defining the intractability of existential distress. While there are objective criteria for quantifying and treating physical distress, evaluating existential distress is more difficult and exposed to clinician subjectivity.[33] Additionally, there is a lack of research to provide evidence and evolving guidelines for patients with existential distress.[34] Some experts argue that it is not about the cause of the suffering. It is the degree of the distress and the proximity of death that should be considered when determining whether to use palliative sedation. Nonetheless, many clinicians find the idea of sedation for existential suffering to be morally and ethically challenging.[33] Refractory psychological distress must be distinguished from other treatable problems, such as depression, anxiety, delirium, other psychiatric illness, and family conflict. The American Medical Association's Opinion *2.201: Sedation to Unconsciousness in End-of-Life Care* recommends against the use of palliative sedation for existential distress.[23] The Veterans' Administration (VA) Ethics Committee report explores this issue and concludes, "When the patient's suffering is interpersonal, existential, or spiritual, the tasks of the clinician are to remain present, to 'suffer with' the patient in compassion, and to enlist the support of clergy, social workers, family, and friends in healing the aspects of suffering that are beyond the legitimate scope of medical care."[24]

Specific clinical guidelines for the use of palliative sedation in the patient with existential suffering include[5,35]:

- Ensuring it is utilized in a patient with advanced terminal disease, with informed consent from the patient or surrogate decision-maker.

- Exhausting all palliative treatments, including treatment for depression, delirium, anxiety, and any other contributing psychiatric illnesses.

- Completing a psychological assessment by a skilled clinician. If applicable, spiritual assessment should also be done by a skilled clinician or clergy member.

- Initially starting with a trial of respite sedation, ranging from 6 to 24 hours, with ongoing re-evaluation prior to continuous sedation.

Respite palliative sedation has been found to be helpful for the patient, family, and healthcare team in re-evaluating the decision for and benefit of palliative sedation. Some patients who were provided with short periods of sedation have been found to be able to break the cycle of anxiety and distress that created the request for palliative sedation in the first place—as a result, further palliative sedation was unnecessary.[36] These criteria seem prudent and appropriate for evaluating the use of palliative sedation not only in patients with existential distress but also in all patients with severe uncontrolled symptoms who are considering palliative sedation.

In practice, some clinicians and protocols limit the use of palliative sedation to only physical distress (or symptoms that are somatic in nature), whereas others include existential and psychological distress, though typically only under special circumstances or for short periods (respite sedation). Although only the patient can determine if a symptom is intolerable, and although the patient has a right to request sedation, the clinician does not have to act to provide sedation. Severe distress in itself should always create urgency for palliative care clinicians to attempt to reduce the suffering. If the treatment of severe symptoms is not successful, the team may consider palliative sedation as an option only if the patient's condition, in terms of both the immediacy of expected death and the intractability of the symptoms and distress, meets established criteria for palliative sedation (Box 57.1).

There is general acceptance that when palliative sedation is considered, whether continuously or intermittently, there should be specific policies, procedures, and protocols for its use.[28] All treatment and diagnostic options for the previously discussed problems must be addressed adequately before palliative sedation is considered and provided. The decision to begin sedation is often difficult for clinicians, requiring thorough patient assessment and discussions with the patient, family, and other team members.

The literature cites many different reasons palliative sedation has been used. While Muller-Busch, in their analysis of 7 years of data, found anxiety and existential distress (40% anxiety/psychological distress, 35% dyspnea, and 14% delirium/agitation) to be the most commonly cited reason for the use of palliative sedation, another study that looked at 30 years of palliative sedation practice reported delirium as the most common reason for its use (54%), followed by dyspnea (30%), psychological distress (19%), pain (17%), and vomiting (5%).[37] They also reported that some programs never provided palliative sedation for patients with existential psychological distress while others included it, and it was one of the most often-cited reasons for its use. A recent systematic review found dyspnea, agitation/delirium, and pain to be the most common reasons for use.[7]

INTERDISCIPLINARY TEAM MEMBER COMPETENCE, INVOLVEMENT, AND CARE

Interdisciplinary assessment determines the refractory nature of the symptoms. Key roles of the palliative APRN, along with the physician, pharmacist, and nurse, include (1) a thorough review that all potential treatments have been pursued and all other potential specialties have offered an opinion, thus ensuring that all standard treatments have been aggressively used, and (2) determining that the symptom is truly refractory despite adjustments in regimens. The involvement of a pharmacist, optimally a palliative care–trained pharmacist, can help with symptom assessment and recommendations for regimen changes or alternative therapeutics.[38] Involving the social worker and the chaplain assists with the assessment and management of the patient's psychological, existential, and spiritual distress (which also affects their physical distress) and family and patient well-being and coping.[39,40] The importance of addressing and treating the nonphysical distress that contributes to the patient's total pain expression cannot be overemphasized. A multidimensional approach is important to prevent, detect, and manage risk factors for intractable pain, including psychosocial distress, addictive behavior, and delirium in patients with terminal disease.

Even with specialist-level palliative care, pain and other distress can be difficult to treat, especially when complicated by profound suffering. Interdisciplinary collaboration among the primary care providers, the palliative care interdisciplinary experts, and other team members confirms the patient's condition and assists in the essential aspects of care planning, including assessment (making sure patients meet the conditions of imminently dying, refractory symptoms, assessment of distress), goals-of-care establishment, and care delivery during the sedation period.

An additional aspect has to do with the competence of the palliative APRN and their team in performing the palliative sedation, including their knowledge, critical thinking, and experience. A team should be part of developing a protocol and discussing their personal comfort with the process, ethically and morally. It can be difficult if this is not done and a team member surprises the team by opting out at the last minute. Most protocols involve the interdisciplinary team in decision-making about palliative sedation. This includes the attending or primary care physician who consults and/or receives advice from a palliative care clinical expert (typically an experienced palliative physician and/or a palliative APRN), a pain specialist who has interventional expertise, a palliative pharmacist, or another expert specialty clinician as appropriate to the symptoms being managed (e.g., pulmonary or cardiology for dyspnea, psychiatry for delirium and to assess for depression and anxiety). The palliative APRN and bedside nurses are critical in the support and coaching of other direct-care providers and each other to ensure that the patient and family members are given the psychosocial care they need.

Collaboration with the interdisciplinary team not only validates the appropriateness of palliative sedation and facilitates the informed consent process but also reduces the emotional burden for the healthcare providers. Palliative care team members work in a specialty that has significant factors for burnout.[41] Team members have said that one of the worst aspects of their jobs is when they cannot treat a patient's symptoms, especially pain and existential suffering.[5] For care team members, managing the multiple, complex, and overlapping aspects of palliative sedation—from recognizing symptoms to managing family distress and interdisciplinary team dynamics—can be emotionally challenging.[42]

One study found that palliative sedation caused team members to have doubts about their professional competence and that bedside nurses were especially susceptible, due to their role in palliative sedation.[43] Ongoing care of all members of the team is crucial and should be part of the formal protocols for providing palliative sedation. During the process of palliative sedation, as well as before and after, there should be opportunities for team members to debrief, share concerns, and discuss personal distress. Debriefing models may vary based on type of setting but are typically voluntary, led

by a trained facilitator (often a palliative care social worker), and allow team members to talk through their emotional experiences as they relate to the clinical situation; debriefing discussions have the added benefit of helping build clinician resilience.[44,45]

In addition to ongoing team support, policies must also state how to handle conscientious objection by any member of the team to participating in palliative sedation and give procedures to transfer care to another available team member of equal competence while ensuring ongoing patient care. There should be mechanisms to discuss and resolve conflicts or concerns raised by anyone involved, along with consistent consultation with ethics committees and legal counsel. This promotes open communication within the organization.

Care of patients with life-limiting illness has always been at the core of the practice of professional nursing. Florence Nightingale observed that nursing relieves a patient's suffering from an illness, even when the disease itself cannot be treated, and that suffering includes more than the physical body's response to disease.[46] Ferrell and Coyle further describe a patient's suffering as a personal and multidimensional experience that is expressed in many ways, including grief, loss, pain, discomfort, loss of control or helplessness, hopelessness, inability to cope, loneliness, isolation, and loss of meaning.[47]

Thus, the palliative APRN may first recognize the need to consider palliative sedation in the face of intractable suffering. Collaboration with other clinicians ensures that all reasonable treatment options to manage the distress have been exhausted and that the patient truly is near death. Depending on institution and state regulations, the palliative APRN may initiate the sedation, which means that they must have knowledge of the medications commonly used to ensure safe and effective therapy and understand monitoring requirements. For safe and consistent practice, the palliative APRN should follow a palliative sedation policy, collaborating with other clinicians. They must inform and educate colleagues and team members about the process of decision-making and implementing palliative sedation. The palliative APRN must collaborate with the interdisciplinary team to support the patient, family, and other team members. When palliative sedation is part of a treatment plan, the palliative APRN often leads and/or participates in multiple meetings with staff before, during, and after the procedure to ensure the success of the intervention and to provide ongoing support to team members.

INFORMED CONSENT AND DECISION-MAKING

Informed consent requires the clinician to provide key information to the patient so that the patient can weigh the risks and benefits of a procedure or treatment before reaching a voluntary decision about its use in the individual's care.[48] The palliative APRN has an essential role in explaining palliative sedation to patients, family, and staff. It is important to review prior symptom management regimes trialed and to be certain that all other options have been explored. Once this has been determined, an agreement between provider, patient, and family is required to proceed with palliative sedation. Some palliative sedation protocols require written consent and some accept verbal consent, but all require that the discussion must occur before palliative sedation starts and must be documented in detail. This discussion should include acknowledgment of the terminal disease, review of the patient's goals of care, identification of the intractable symptom/symptoms and regimes trialed, education surrounding the option of palliative sedation, medication selection, and a review of the side-effect profile and plan for titration (respite sedation or continuous).

When discussing the option of palliative sedation, it is very important to determine the patient's capacity to make informed decisions—that the patient is able to receive information, understand and apply the information to their context, and communicate this decision.[49] If a patient is deemed to lack decision-making capacity, the surrogate decision-maker or healthcare proxy becomes the voice for the patient. Even if the patient is capable of making a decision, most protocols mention the importance of family members' being involved with the informed consent discussion along with the patient. Some protocols even require consent from the family.[50] Specific benefits of palliative sedation are relief of suffering and distress and a controlled environment. Burdens include loss of consciousness and awareness and an inability to relate to family and others. As discussed earlier in the chapter, the distinction between palliative sedation and euthanasia is subtle but real. It relies on the intention of the provider who is administering treatment. The goal of palliative sedation is to relieve suffering. The goal of euthanasia is to cause death. Causation is not the key issue, intent is. Clinicians have the moral obligation to do no harm and relieve suffering.[21]

Before palliative sedation is to be initiated, decisions regarding the use of life support, resuscitation, and medically administered nutrition and hydration need to be determined separately from the decision for palliative sedation. Since palliative sedation is only used for the imminently dying, there should be a clear understanding that no attempt at cardiopulmonary resuscitation will occur and that the appropriate order (do-not-resuscitate [DNR], do-not-intubate [DNI], do-not-attempt-resuscitation [DNAR]) will be in place before palliative sedation is provided. Other life-prolonging treatments, such as medically administered nutrition and hydration, are typically also withdrawn before beginning palliative sedation, except for cases when respite sedation is being considered. Refer to Box 57.2 for guidelines for a comprehensive approach regarding the use of palliative sedation.

FAMILY INVOLVEMENT AND CARE

The palliative APRN should seek to elicit an understanding of the suffering of family members and provide careful, compassionate, and ongoing communication with them. Interdisciplinary care is critical during this time. Clear, comprehensive communication detailing the purpose of palliative sedation, the risks and benefits of therapy, and the plan

---

Box 57.2 GUIDELINES FOR A COMPREHENSIVE APPROACH REGARDING THE USE OF PALLIATIVE SEDATION

1. Multidimensional evaluation and determination of refractory suffering and consultation procedures and consult to palliative care for palliative sedation.

2. Palliative care team discusses on role of sedation in end-of-life care and contingency planning, and clarification of indications in which sedation may or should be considered.

3. Palliative care team engages with the patient and family, and education about the option of palliative sedation and purpose of its use. Promote shared decision-making.

4. Palliative care team ensures a do-not-resuscitate order is in place with documented decisions regarding hydration, nutrition, and concomitant medications.

5. Palliative care team elicits and documents patient/family consent.

6. Palliative care team convenes clinical meeting about selection of the sedation method, staff education regarding guidelines and protocol.

7. Palliative care team initiates therapy, dose titration, patient monitoring, and care.

8. Palliative care team provides information, care, and support to the patient, the patient's family, and the staff.

9. Post procedure, provide support and debrief with staff and interdisciplinary team.

Adapted from Cherny et al.[35]

---

for assessing comfort and titrating sedation should be clearly outlined to both family and staff. When patients are considering or undergoing palliative sedation, family distress may stem from many factors, including inability to interact with patient, anticipatory grief, disagreement or confusion regarding the use of sedation, perceptions that the use of sedation was precipitous or inappropriately delayed, and impressions that sedation hastened or actually caused the death or that death did not follow sedation as quickly as hoped.[51-53] Communication and trust building are essential. Experts in palliative nursing stress the importance of deliberate, careful, and compassionate communication. Successful communication involves the principles listed in Chapter 33, "Family Meetings" and Chapter 53, "Navigating Ethical Dilemmas."

MEDICATIONS AND PROCEDURE OF SEDATION

Palliative sedation is an option of last resort when treating refractory symptoms. Refractory symptoms differ from difficult or "difficult-to-treat" symptoms in that, despite the multiple efforts of clinical experts, they cannot be adequately treated without compromising the consciousness of the patient.[54] Indications for palliative sedation may include delirium, dyspnea, pain, agitation, nausea, vomiting, and existential suffering. Administering palliative sedation to alleviate psycho-existential suffering remains a controversial issue partly because it is difficult to determine when this type of suffering is refractory.[34]

Drug selection is based on the type of suffering present, current medications, response to past medications, the patient's medical problems, and the drug's efficacy, side-effect profile, and potential for success.[50] Consultation with a palliative care pharmacist, if available, is recommended. Although the intravenous (IV) route is preferred because it allows for quick titration and safety, subcutaneous (SC) and rectal administration (PR) are acceptable alternatives for some of the common medications. The clinical, ethical, and legal decision-making for the use of palliative sedation includes determining the best type of sedative to use.

In 1958, Dame Cecily Saunders advocated for the use of non-opioid sedative therapy to reduce anxiety and induce a sense of relaxation.[55] She was clear that the use of opioids as analgesia was beneficial but advised against their use to induce drowsiness.[56] Even today, opioids are not recommended as a sedative drug. However, they are often used alongside sedatives as part of the management of pain or dyspnea, and it is recommended that they not be stopped prior to palliative sedation and they should be continued.[57] The most common medications used for palliative sedation are benzodiazepines, barbiturates, and anesthetics. Patient assessment and clinical protocols developed by the interdisciplinary team, including pharmacists, guide drug selection, initial dosing, dose titration, and route of administration.[38,50] Additionally, complications of the sedation process may include respiratory depression, aspiration, or hemodynamic compromise. Although patients who are candidates for palliative sedation are imminently dying and in severe distress, the palliative APRN must discuss death as a potential effect.

Benzodiazepines are the most common medications used for palliative sedation. Midazolam is the drug of choice due to its rapid onset and shorter duration, allowing for greater flexibility in dosing than other benzodiazepines. Also, it can be combined with other drugs used in palliative care. The typical starting dose of midazolam in an acute care setting is 1–5 mg IV bolus every 5 minutes until the patient is comfortable or a maximum of 20 mg. Continuous infusion is started generally at 0.5–1 mg/h. Usual effective dose range is 1–20 mg/h SC or IV.[58] In the community setting, midazolam can be given SC as a 1–5 mg bolus every 5 minutes until the patient is comfortable, followed by a continuous infusion of 0.5–1 mg/h, or diazepam suppositories given PR may be used. Clinical trials show that midazolam is safe to give with opiates for the treatment of dyspnea in advanced illness.[58] Other drugs used either alone or in combination with midazolam are haloperidol, phenobarbital, and opioids.

Barbiturates have been used for many years for palliative sedation. Thiopental, pentobarbital, and phenobarbital also have quick onsets of action and short durations so they can be easily titrated. The starting dose for thiopental is an IV bolus of 5–7 mg/kg and then 20 mg/h as a continuous infusion. The usual maintenance dose is 70–180 mg/h. Pentobarbital can be given rectally at 60–200 mg every 2-4 hours in the community setting or IV in the inpatient setting at 1–3 mg/kg bolus followed by a continuous infusion of 1 mg/kg/h. Titrate for appropriate level of sedation. Pentobarbital may offer antiemetic and anticonvulsant effects, making it more advantageous in patients at risk for vomiting and seizures. Phenobarbital is given as an IV/SC bolus of 200 mg and then with a continuous infusion of 600 mg/day. Usual maintenance dose is 600–1,600 mg/day. Side effects include the irritant nature of the injection.[59] For home use, phenobarbital or pentobarbitol may be compounded into a suppository.

Anesthetics such as propofol (Diprivan) are considered excellent agents for palliative sedation.[60] This classification of medications can only be used in the acute care setting because they require frequent monitoring. Propofol can be used safely in patients who have renal or liver disease; it has an extremely short onset of action, duration of action, and half-life (shorter than the benzodiazepines and barbiturates), and is very easy to titrate. It provides anxiolytic, antiemetic, antipruritic, anticonvulsant, antimyoclonic, and muscle relaxant effects.[60] Dosing for propofol is initially based on weight; a continuous infusion of 2.5–5 μg/kg/min can be increased by 2.5–5 μg/kg/min every hour to the desired level of sedation. During the infusion, the palliative APRN may also give bolus doses of propofol (2.5–5 μg/kg) by IV push every 10 minutes as needed for rapid control of severe symptoms.[60] This is a suggested option for respite or temporary palliative sedation because the sedation effects can be reversed quickly with decreased titrations or discontinuation of the medication.

Dexmedetomidine (Precedex) is a newer sedative agent that could be beneficial in palliative sedation, although it has not been studied extensively for this indication. It is an α-2 agonist that may induce unconsciousness without causing respiratory depression.[61] It is a potent sedative that also possesses analgesic and opioid-sparing properties. Its sedative effects induce a state of non-rapid eye movement (NREM)-like sleep that fosters easy awakening if desired.[62] It may reduce the likelihood of delirium in comparison to benzodiazepines. Moreover, it is reported to possess anxiolytic and anti-sialagogue properties.[61] The dosing range is typically 0.2–1.4 μg/kg/h. Loading or IV push doses are not needed. Avoiding a loading dose minimizes the risk of developing hypotension or bradycardia. The onset of effect for dexmedetomidine after beginning infusion is 5–10 minutes, with action lasting for approximately 60 minutes once the infusion is discontinued.[58,63]

Ketamine (Ketalar) is classified as an anesthetic and centrally acting non-opiate. It is an N-methyl-D-aspartase (NMDA) receptor antagonist known for its analgesic and anesthetic properties. It is used in the inpatient setting for the management of pain and refractory symptoms related to terminal illness. Starting dose is 1–4.5 mg/kg/dose IV; 3–5mg/kg/dose IM; infusion 0.5–2 mg/kg/h. An adjuvant anti-sialagogue and benzodiazepine are recommended. Oral, sublingual, and intranasal doses of ketamine are available but not indicated by this route for palliative sedation purposes.[64,65]

Antipsychotics are not traditionally used for initiation of palliative sedation, but they play an important role as adjuvants in the treatment of terminal delirium. Haloperidol is not a sedative and therefore should not be used to induce sedation. However, studies show that it is used in combination with benzodiazepines in the treatment of refractory agitated delirium.[54] Suggested starting dose for haloperidol is 0.5–5 mg PO/SC every 2–4 hours or 1–5 mg bolus IV/SC followed by continuous infusion totaling 5–15 mg/day.[59] In the community setting, PO, SL, SC routes are used with similar dosing patterns as in the inpatient setting.

Although many patients are on opioids prior to the initiation of palliative sedation, opioids are not effective at producing sustained sedation. However, opioids should be continued, along with the sedating drug, to avoid opioid withdrawal and to treat unobserved pain (Table 57.3).

CONTINUOUS VERSUS INTERMITTENT SEDATION

A modified Delphi study concluded that experts agreed to the use of sedatives, continuous or temporary, for patients with refractory dyspnea and delirium at end of life. Conversely, there was wide variation in opinions on the appropriateness of sedation in dementia patients and existential suffering.[66] Continuous versus intermittent sedation are suggested depending on the refractory symptom and goals of care. *Proportional sedation* is suggested as the best description for sedation types.[67] Sedation should be performed proportionately, appropriate to the patient's situation. The intensity and nature of the suffering determines which form of sedation and, more specifically, whether it will be intermittent versus continuous sedation and what dosage of sedatives will be administered to the patient. Thus, palliative sedation does not

Table 57.3 RECOMMENDED MEDICATIONS FOR PALLIATIVE SEDATION

MEDICATION	ACUTE CARE	COMMUNITY
Benzodiazepines	*Midazolam* (SC/IV) 1–5 mg bolus q 5min until comfortable or maximum of 20 mg Continuous infusion is started generally 0.5–1 mg/h Usual effective dose range is 1–20 mg/h	*Midazolam* (SC) 1–5 mg bolus q5min until comfortable or maximum of 20 mg Continuous SC infusion is started generally at 0.5–1 mg/h Midazolam is available in IM and intranasal formulations (limited data support these formulations for palliative sedation purposes)
	Lorazepam (SC/IV) 2–5 mg bolus Continuous infusion is 0.5–1.0 mg/h	*Lorazepam* (SC) 2–5 mg bolus; continuous infusion 0.5–1.0 mg/h
Barbiturates	*Thiopental* (IV) 5–7 mg/kg bolus and then 20 mg/h as a continuous infusion Usual maintenance dose is 70–180 mg/h.	
	Pentobarbital (IV) 1–3 mg/kg bolus and then continuous infusion of 1 mg/kg/h.	*Pentobarbital* (PR) 60–200 mg q4–8h
	Phenobarbital (IV/SC) 200 mg bolus (can repeat q10–15min) then continuous infusion of 25 mg/h (or 600 mg/day) Usual maintenance dose is 600–1,600 mg/day.	*Phenobarbital* (SC) 200 mg bolus (can repeat q10–15min) then continuous infusion of 25 mg/h (or 600 mg/day)
Anesthetics	*Diprivan* (IV) 20–50 mg bolus (may repeat) then a continuous infusion of 2.5–5 μg/kg/min can be increased by 2.5–5 μg/kg/min every hour to the desired level of sedation. During the infusion, the palliative APRN may also give bolus doses of propofol (2.5–5 μg/kg) by IV push every 10 minutes as needed for rapid control of severe symptoms	This class of medications is not recommended for use in the home or community setting
	Dexmedetomidine (IV) 0.2–1.4 μg/kg/h. Loading or IV push doses are not needed.	
	Ketamine (IV) 1–4.5 mg/kg/dose IV; 3–5 mg/kg/dose IM; infusion 0.5–2 mg/kg/h. Adjuvant anti-sialagogue and benzodiazepine are recommended. Oral, sublingual, and intranasal doses of ketamine are available but not indicated by this route for palliative sedation purposes.	
Antipsychotics	*Haldol* (should not be used to induce sedation, but as an adjuvant in the treatment of terminal delirium) Haldol (IV/SC) 0.5–5 mg bolus followed by continuous infusion totaling 5–15 mg/day	*Haldol** (PO, SL, SC) 0.5–5 mg loading dose, followed by 1–5 mg q4h scheduled *or* 1–5 mg/h by continuous SC infusion * doses are the same despite route

Adapted from Prommer[58]; Rousseau[59]; O'Hara et al.[61]; and Jackson et al.[63]

presuppose that a patient is sedated until unconscious; palliative sedation means that sedative drugs are administered in dosages and combinations required to reduce consciousness as much as necessary to adequately relieve one or more refractory symptom.[67] This illustrates how important the principle of proportionality is in the decision-making process.

Once the palliative medication has been chosen, generally the infusion is initiated and then titrated to a point where the patient appears to be comfortable. Care should be taken to make further adjustments when necessary to facilitate palliative nursing care. Other reported strategies include varying the depth of sedation during the day, providing deeper sedation at night to ensure peaceful rest.[68] Sedation should not be increased unless the patient shows signs of distress, such as restlessness, grimacing, or findings that could reasonably be interpreted as evidence of suffering (including tachypnea and tachycardia). Invasive assessment tools to monitor conscious sedation in hospitals are not appropriate for the dying patient, though frequent assessment of pain and consciousness is recommended. Two tools, the Critical Care Pain Observation Tool (CPOT) and the Richmond Agitation Sedation Scale, are frequently used, though other tools exist in the literature.[69] The level of sedation needed varies with each patient and is based on the achievement of comfort and predetermined goals.

Once palliative sedation is initiated, survival can be quite variable but generally is brief because it is utilized for patients who are already at the end of life. Muller-Busch and colleagues reported survival of 58–63 hours after initiation of sedation; Sykes reported that 56% of patients survived less than 48 hours.[37,70] Another study showed that the mean survival of patients after the onset of palliative sedation ranged from 1 to 6 days.[54] A prospective multicenter study of 518 patients found that the overall survival between a cohort receiving palliative sedation and a cohort not receiving palliative sedation was not statistically significant, providing evidence that the intervention does not hasten death.[19] Additionally, a secondary analysis of a prospective cohort study found that palliative sedation did not hasten death for oncology patients receiving palliative care services.[71] Given the lack of uniformity surrounding the process around palliative sedation, outcomes remain quite variable.

EFFICACY

More than 80% of families stated that palliative sedation resulted in adequate relief of their loved one's suffering.[72] Eighty-eight percent of families felt that palliative sedation helped to considerably decrease symptom distress.[72] Morita et al. reported that palliative sedation adequately relieved symptoms in 83% of the cases studied.[53]

CARE OF THE DYING PATIENT RECEIVING PALLIATIVE SEDATION

As the patient nears death, all members of the clinical team apply their own special skills and abilities to guiding the family and supporting the patient on this final journey.[73] End-of-life care for the dying is an interdisciplinary effort that includes anticipatory counseling, symptom management, and comprehensive psychosocial, spiritual, and bereavement care.[74] Although basic to nursing care, the care of the imminently dying is a fundamental element of the total care of a patient undergoing palliative sedation. Since most palliative sedation is done in the impersonal often sterile environment of a facility, the use of favorite music, special clothes, colorful blankets, supportive aromas, and personal mementos in the room can create an environment that supports the patient's comfort, is unique to the individual, and is soothing to the family and patient (see Chapter 38, "Grief and Bereavement").

In addition to addressing and acknowledging the family's grief, it is equally important to debrief the patient case with staff. This provides an opportunity to emphasize moral reflectiveness and the impact of nursing practice in end-of-life care.[75] Allowing time to process, reflect on, and review the experience is essential to supporting the clinical aspects of care we provide, as well as the emotional and moral components.

The case study at the beginning of the chapter illustrates the mixed physical and existential components of suffering that patients often experience and the palliative APRN's role in advocating for the patient while providing physical, psychological, spiritual, and emotional support.

SUMMARY

Although palliative sedation is used only when patients experience the most extreme distress, it is a therapy that is a core competency of the palliative APRN. A palliative APRN must be able to demonstrate how he or she uses the fundamental elements of the safe and effective provision of palliative sedation in practice. This begins with a basic competency in understanding the complex issues surrounding palliative sedation decision-making. Ideally, palliative sedation is done with the support of a palliative care team and follows a policy or protocol. Development of policies and procedures around the use of palliative sedation is recommended in your practice setting. Refer to Boxes 57.1 and 57.2 for a framework for procedural guidelines. If one does not exist, the palliative APRN must garner support from a team to develop a policy for palliative sedation. The salient points of each step of palliative sedation can be used to develop these protocols and policies and will assist in the provision of palliative sedation.

In addition, the palliative APRN will need to gain trust from the staff. This often begins with education and requires an individual commitment to be present with nursing and other team members during the often-complex process of considering and delivering palliative sedation. Finally, although palliative care exists to ensure the comfort of patients at the end of their lives and their families, even an experienced APRN may never be wholly comfortable with palliative sedation. Open dialogue and collaboration with all team members will reduce the emotional burden and create an environment of mutual support and personal growth. Palliative sedation is an option of last resort for patients experiencing the most suffering, and it requires the skills and commitment of the palliative APRN.

REFERENCES

1. Hospice and Palliative Nurses Association. Position statement: Palliative sedation. Pittsburgh, PA: Hospice and Palliative Nurses Association. 2016. https://advancingexpertcare.org/position-statements
2. Billings J. Palliative sedation. In: Quill T, Miller F, eds. *Palliative Care and Ethics*. New York: Oxford University Press; 2014: 209–230.
3. American Nurses Association. Position statement: The nurse's role when a patient requests medical aid in dying. Silver Spring, MD: American Nurses Association; 2019. https://www.nursingworld.org/~49e869/globalassets/practiceandpolicy/nursing-excellence/ana-position-statements/social-causes-and-health-care/the-nurses-role-when-a-patient-requests-medical-aid-in-dying-web-format.pdf
4. Cherny NI, Portenoy RK. Sedation in the management of refractory symptoms: Guidelines for evaluation and treatment. *J Palliat Care*. 1994;10(2):31–38. doi:10.1177/082585979401000207
5. Rousseau P. *Existential Suffering and Palliative Sedation: A Brief Commentary with a Proposal for Clinical Guidelines*. Thousand Oaks, CA: Sage; 2001.
6. Abarshi E, Rietjens J, Robijn L, Caraceni A, Payne S, Deliens L, International variations in clinical practice guidelines for palliative sedation: A systematic review. *BMJ Support Palliat Care*. 2017;7(3):223–229. doi:10.1136/bmjspcare-2016-001159
7. Heijltjes MT, van Thiel GJMW, Rietjens JAC, van der Heide A, de Graeff A, van Delden JJM. Changing practices in the use of continuous sedation at the end of life: A systematic review of the literature. *J Pain Symptom Manage*. 2020;60(4):828–846.e3. doi:10.1016/j.jpainsymman.2020.06.019
8. Twycross R. Reflections on palliative sedation. *Palliat Care*. 2019;12:1178224218823511. Published 2019 Jan 27. doi:10.1177/1178224218823511
9. Kremling A, Schildmann J. What do you mean by "palliative sedation"?: Pre-explicative analyses as preliminary steps towards better definitions: Pre-explicative analyses as preliminary steps towards better definitions. *BMC Palliat Care*. 2020;19(1):147. doi:10.1186/s12904-020-00635-9
10. Beller EM, van Driel ML, McGregor L, Truong S, Mitchell G. Palliative pharmacological sedation for terminally ill adults. *Cochrane Database Syst Rev*. 2015;1(1):CD010206. Published 2015 Jan 2. doi:10.1002/14651858.CD010206.pub2
11. Garetto F, Cancelli F, Rossi R, Maltoni M. Palliative sedation for the terminally ill patient. *CNS Drugs*. 2018;32(10):951–961. doi:10.1007/s40263-018-0576-7
12. *Vacco v. Quill 521 US 793*. October Term 1996. ertiorari to the united states court of appeals for the second circuit No. 95–1858. Argued January 8, 1997—Decided June 26, 1997. https://supreme.justia.com/cases/federal/us/521/793/case.pdf
13. *Washington v. Glucksberg 521 US 702*, 736. October Term 1996. certiorari to the united states court of appeals for the ninth circuit No. 96–110. Argued January 8, 1997—Decided June 26, 1997. https://supreme.justia.com/cases/federal/us/521/702/case.pdf
14. American Nurses Association. Code of ethics for nurses with interpretive statements. 2nd ed. Silver Spring, MD: American Nurses Association; 2015. https://www.nursingworld.org/practice-policy/nursing-excellence/ethics/code-of-ethics-for-nurses/coe-view-only/
15. American Nurses Association. Position Statement. Nurses roles and responsibilities in providing care and support at the end of life. Silver Spring, MD: American Nurses Association. 2016. https://www.nursingworld.org/~4af078/globalassets/docs/ana/ethics/endoflife-positionstatement.pdf
16. American Nurses Association. Position Statement. Nursing care and do-not-resuscitate (DNR) decisions. Silver Spring, MD:
American Nurses Association. 2020. https://www.nursingworld.org/~494a87/globalassets/practiceandpolicy/nursing-excellence/ana-position-statements/social-causes-and-health-care/nursing-care-and-do-not-resuscitate-dnr-decisions-final-nursingworld.pdf
17. Beauchamp T, Childress J. *Principles of Biomedical Ethics*. 8th ed. New York: Oxford University Press; 2019.
18. President's Commission for the Study of Ethical Problems in Medicine and Biomedical and Behavioral Research. *Making Healthcare Decisions: A Report on the Ethical and Legal Implications of Informed Consent in the Patient–Practitioner Relationship. Volume Three Appendices of the Foundations of Informed Consent*. Washington, DC: US Government Printing Office; 1982. https://www.google.com/books/edition/Making_Health_Care_Decisions/8ldLZyKxXr0C?hl=en&gbpv=0
19. Maltoni M, Pittureri C, Scarpi E, et al. Palliative sedation therapy does not hasten death: Results from a prospective multicenter study. *Ann Oncol*. 2009;20(7):1163–1169. doi:10.1093/annonc/mdp048
20. Billings JA, Churchill LR. Monolithic moral frameworks: How are the ethics of palliative sedation discussed in the clinical literature? *J Palliative Med*. 2012;15(6):709–713. doi:10.1089/jpm.2011.0157
21. Kirk TW, Mahon MM. National Hospice and Palliative Care Organization (NHPCO) position statement and commentary on the use of palliative sedation in imminently dying terminally ill patients. *J Pain Symptom Manage*. 2010;39(5):914–923. doi:10.1016/j.jpainsymman.2010.01.009
22. American Academy of Hospice and Palliative Medicine. Statement on palliative sedation. Chicago: American Academy of Hospice and Palliative Medicine. Dec 5, 2014. http://aahpm.org/positions/palliative-sedation
23. American Medical Association. Code of Medical Ethics' Opinions on Sedation at the End of Life. Opinion 2.201 - Sedation to Unconsciousness in End-of-Life Care. https://journalofethics.ama-assn.org/article/ama-code-medical-ethics-opinions-sedation-end-life/2013-05
24. Veterans Administration. The ethics of palliative sedation as a therapy of last resort. 2006. http://www.ethics.va.gov/docs/net/NET_Topic_20060726_National_Ethics_Committee_Report_Ethics_of_Palliative_Sedation_as_a_Therapy_of_Last_Resort.doc
25. Schneiderman H, Marks S. Physical examination of the dying patient #392. *J Palliat Med*. 2020;23(5):721–722. doi:10.1089/jpm.2020.0180
26. Von Gunten CF. Palliative care fast facts and concepts. #149: Teaching the family what to expect when the patient is dying. Appleton, WI: Palliative Care Network of Wisconsin. 2015. https://www.mypcnow.org/fast-fact/teaching-the-family-what-to-expect-when-the-patient-is-dying/ https://www.mypcnow.org/fast-fact/existential-suffering-part-1-definition-and-diagnosis/
27. Bobb B. A review of palliative sedation. *Nurs Clin North Am*. 2016;51(3):449–457. doi:10.1016/j.cnur.2016.05.008
28. Gurschick L, Mayer DK, Hanson LC. Palliative sedation: An analysis of international guidelines and position statements. *Am J Hosp Palliat Med*. 2015;32(6):660–671. doi:10.1177/1049909114533002
29. Grech T, Marks A. Palliative care fast facts and concepts #319: Existential suffering: Part 1: Definition and diagnosis. Appleton, WI: Palliative Care Network of Wisconsin. 2016. https://www.mypcnow.org/fast-fact/existential-suffering-part-1-definition-and-diagnosis/
30. Robinson S, Kissane DW, Brooker J, Burney S. A systematic review of the demoralization syndrome in individuals with progressive disease and cancer: A decade of research. *J Pain Symptom Manage*. 2015;49(3):595–610. doi:10.1016/j.jpainsymman.2014.07.008
31. Cordova MJ, Riba MB, Spiegel D. Post-traumatic stress disorder and cancer. *Lancet Psychiatry*. 2017;4(4):330–338. doi:10.1016/S2215-0366(17)30014-7
32. Voeuk A, Nekolaichuk C, Fainsinger R, Huot A. Continuous palliative sedation for existential distress? A survey of Canadian palliative care physicians' views. *J Palliat Care*. 2017;32(1):26–33. doi:10.1177/0825859717711301
33. Rodrigues P, Crokaert J, Gastmans C. Palliative sedation for existential suffering: A systematic review of argument-based

ethics literature. *J Pain Symptom Manage*. 2018;55(6):1577–1590. doi:10.1016/j.jpainsymman.2018.01.013

34. Ciancio AL, Mirza RM, Ciancio AA, Klinger CA. The use of palliative sedation to treat existential suffering: A scoping review on practices, ethical considerations, and guidelines. *J Palliat Care*. 2020;35(1):13–20. doi:10.1177/0825859719827585

35. Cherny NI, Radbruch L, Care BotEAfP. European Association for Palliative Care (EAPC) recommended framework for the use of sedation in palliative care. *Palliat Med*. 2009;23(7):581–593. doi:10.1177/0269216309107024

36. Cherny NI. Commentary: Sedation in response to refractory existential distress: Walking the fine line. *J Pain Symptom Manage*. 1998;16(6):404–406. doi:0.1016/S0885-3924(98)00114-6

37. Muller-Busch HC, Andres I, Jehser T. Sedation in palliative care: A critical analysis of 7 years experience. *BMC Palliat Care*. 2003;2(1):2. doi:10.1186/1472-684X-2-2

38. Herndon CM, Nee D, Atayee RS, et al. ASHP guidelines on the pharmacist's role in palliative and hospice care. *Am J Health Syst Pharm*. 2016;73(17):1351–1367. doi:10.2146/ajhp160244

39. Middleton A, Head B, Remke S. Palliative care fast facts and concept #390: Role of the hospice and palliative care social worker. Appleton, WI: Palliative Care Network of Wisconsin. 2019. https://www.mypcnow.org/fast-fact/role-of-the-hospice-and-palliative-care-social-worker/

40. Schmidt R. Palliative care fast facts and concepts #347: The role of chaplaincy in caring for the seriously ill. Appleton, WI: Palliative Care Network of Wisconsin. 2017. https://www.mypcnow.org/fast-fact/the-role-of-chaplaincy-in-caring-for-the-seriously-ill/

41. Blust L. Palliative care fast facts and concepts. #167: Health professional burnout—Part 1. Appleton, WI: Palliative Care Network of Wisconsin. 2015. https://www.mypcnow.org/fast-fact/health-professional-burnout-part-1/

42. Ziegler S, Merker H, Schmid M, Puhan MA. The impact of the inpatient practice of continuous deep sedation until death on healthcare professionals' emotional well-being: A systematic review. *BMC Palliat Care*. 2017;16(1):30. doi:10.1186/s12904-017-0205-0

43. Leboul D, Aubry R, Peter J-M, Royer V, Richard J-F, Guirimand F. Palliative sedation challenging the professional competency of health care providers and staff: A qualitative focus group and personal written narrative study. *BMC Palliat Care*. 2017;16(1):25. doi:10.1186/s12904-017-0198-8

44. McIntosh R. The benefits of debriefing. *Kai Tiaki: Nursing New Zealand*. 2019;25(11):22–24. http://eresources.mssm.edu/login?url=https://www.proquest.com/docview/2327862430?accountid=41157

45. Weiner SB. Creating and implementing a resident emotional wellness initiative in an acute care setting: The role of the palliative care social worker. *J Soc Work End Life Palliat Care* 2020:1–10. doi:10.1080/15524256.2020.1745730

46. Nightingale F. *Notes on Nursing: What It Is and What It Is Not*. London: Gerald Duckworth; 1970.

47. Ferrell B, Coyle N. *The Nature of Suffering and the Goals of Nursing*. New York: Oxford University Press; 2008.

48. Weissman DE, Derse A. Palliative care fast facts and concepts #164: Informed consent in palliative care—Part 1. Appleton, WI: Palliative Care Network of Wisconsin. 2015. https://www.mypcnow.org/fast-fact/informed-consent-in-palliative-care-part-1/

49. Arnold R. Palliative care fast facts and concepts. #55: Decision making capacity. Appleton, WI: Palliative Care Network of Wisconsin. 2015. https://www.mypcnow.org/fast-fact/decision-making-capacity/

50. Schildmann E, Schildmann J. Palliative sedation therapy: A systematic literature review and critical appraisal of available guidance on indication and decision making. *J Palliat Med*. 2014;17(5):601–611. doi:10.1089/jpm.2013.0511

51. Higgins PC, Altilio T. Palliative sedation: An essential place for clinical excellence. *J Soc Work End Life Palliat Care*. 2007;3(4):3–30. doi:10.1080/15524250802003240

52. Brajtman S. The impact on the family of terminal restlessness and its management. *Palliat Med*. 2003;17(5):454–460. doi:10.1191/0960327103pm779oa

53. Morita T, Ikenaga M, Adachi I, et al. Concerns of family members of patients receiving palliative sedation therapy. *Support Care Cancer*. 2004;12(12):885–889. doi:10.1007/s00520-004-0678-2

54. Claessens P, Menten J, Schotsmans P, Broeckaert B. Palliative sedation: A review of the research literature. *J Pain Symptom Manage*. 2008;36(3):310–333. doi:10.1016/j.jpainsymman.2007.10.004

55. Saunders C. Dying of cancer. *St Thomas Hospital Gazette*. 1958;56(2):37–47.

56. Saunders C. Management of patients in the terminal stage. In: Raven R, ed. *Cancer*. Oxford: Butterworth; 1960: 403–417.

57. Cherny NI. In Smith, T, ed. Palliative sedation. UpToDate. Waltham, MA: UptoDate. Last updated March 3, 2021. https://www.uptodate.com/contents/palliative-sedation

58. Prommer E. Midazolam: An essential palliative care drug. *Palliat Care Soc Pract*. 2020;14:1–12. doi:10.1177/2632352419895527.

59. Rousseau P. Palliative sedation in the management of refractory symptoms. *J Support Oncol*. 2004;2(2):181–186. PMID: 15328821

60. Cherny NI, Fallon M, Kaasa S, Portenoy RK, Currow D. *Oxford Textbook of Palliative Medicine*. 5th ed. New York: Oxford University Press; 2015.

61. O'Hara C, Tamburro RF, Ceneviva GD. Dexmedetomidine for sedation during withdrawal of support. *Palliat Care Res Treat*. 2015;9:15–18. Published 2015 Aug 25. doi:10.4137/PCRT.S27954

62. Malotte K, Walker K, Roiselle DA. Palliative care fast facts and concepts. #280: Dexmedetomidine. Appleton, WI: Palliative Care Network of Wisconsin. 2015. https://www.mypcnow.org/fast-fact/dexmedetomidine/

63. Jackson KC, Wohlt P, Fine PG. Dexmedetomidine: A novel analgesic with palliative medicine potential. *J Pain Palliat Care Pharmacother*. 2006;20(2):23–27. doi:10.1080/J354v20n02_05

64. Noreika DM, Coyne P. Discontinuance of life sustaining treatment utilizing ketamine for symptom management. *J Pain Palliat Care Pharmacother*. 2015/01/02 2015;29(1):37–40. doi:10.3109/15360288.2014.1003686

65. Epocrates Website. Ketamine adult dosing. 2021 https://online.epocrates.com/drugs/196901/ketamine/Adult-Dosing

66. Benítez-Rosario M, Morita T. Palliative sedation in clinical scenarios: Results of a modified Delphi study. *Support Care Cancer*. 2019;27(5):1647–1654. doi:10.1007/s00520-018-4409-5

67. Claessens P, Menten J, Schotsmans P, Broeckaert B, Consortium P. Palliative sedation, not slow euthanasia: A prospective, longitudinal study of sedation in Flemish palliative care units. *J Pain Symptom Manage*. 2011;41(1):14–24. doi:10.1016/j.jpainsymman.2010.04.019

68. Salacz ME, Weissman DE. Controlled sedation for refractory suffering: Part I. *J Palliat Med*. 2015;8(1):136–138.

69. Arantzamendi M, Belar A, Payne S, et al. Clinical aspects of palliative sedation in prospective studies. A systematic review. *J Pain Symptom Manage*. 2020. doi:10.1016/j.jpainsymman.2020.09.022

70. Sykes N, Thorns A. Sedative use in the last week of life and the implications for end-of-life decision making. *Arch Int Med*. 2003;163(3):341–344. doi:10.1001/archinte.163.3.341

71. Maeda I, Morita T, Yamaguchi T, et al. Effect of continuous deep sedation on survival in patients with advanced cancer (J-Proval): A propensity score-weighted analysis of a prospective cohort study. *Lancet Oncology*. 2016;17(1):115–122. doi:10.1007/s00520-018-4497-2

72. Tursunov O, Cherny NI, Ganz FD. Experiences of family members of dying patients receiving palliative sedation. *Oncol Nurs Forum*. 2016;43(6):E226–E232. doi:10.1188/16.ONF.E226-E232

73. Hess D. Integrating spirituality in palliative care goals of care conversations. Palliative Care Network of Wisconsin. October 15, 2018. https://www.mypcnow.org/blog/integrating-spirituality-in-palliative-care-goals-of-care-conversations/

74. Johnson L-M, Frader J, Wolfe J, Baker JN, Anghelescu DL, Lantos JD. Palliative sedation with propofol for an adolescent with a DNR order. *Pediatrics*. 2017;140(2):1–6. doi:10.1542/peds.2017-0487

75. Wright DK, Gastmans C, Vandyk A, de Casterlé BD. Moral identity and palliative sedation: A systematic review of normative nursing literature. *Nurs Ethics*. 2020;27(3):868–886. doi:10.1177/0969733019876312

APPENDIX I
Palliative APRN Billing and Coding

Constance Dahlin

Palliative advanced practice registered nurses (APRNs) are eligible for reimbursement based on the requirements of their graduate education coursework, as set forth in Chapter 3, "Credentialing, Certification, and Scope of Practice Issues for the Palliative APRN." Palliative services performed by APRNs are a valuable commodity in financial and business planning and healthcare savings in settings including the home, long-term care facilities, clinics, hospitals, and prisons and via telehealth. Optimizing reimbursement through effective billing and coding supports the financial sustainability of

the palliative care program and the palliative APRN's utilization within a team specifically since a portion of their salary can be recaptured through reimbursement.

It is essential for palliative APRNs to have a working knowledge of billing and coding and the necessary documentation. It is also important to keep abreast of the Centers for Medicare and Medicaid Services (CMS) updates on Medicare and Medicaid billing. Commercial insurers will often follow suit. Finally, it is in the best interest of the palliative APRN to meet with their organizational biller and

Table I.1 PALLIATIVE APRN CHECKLIST FOR ELIGIBILITY FOR REIMBURSEMENT

Education and certification	*Graduate Nursing Education—Master's or clinical doctorate* with coursework in advanced health assessment, advanced pharmacology, and advanced pathophysiology in one of the four roles: clinical nurse specialist (CNS), nurse practitioner (NP), certified midwife (CNM), or certified nurse anesthetist (CRNA). For palliative care, it is a CNS or NP.
	National primary certification from a nationally recognized certification organization related to population focus of graduate education as specified by the National Council of State Boards of Nursing in either the acute care or primary care setting: (1) family/individual across the lifespan, (2) adult/gerontology, (3) neonatal, (4) pediatrics, (5) women's health/gender-related, and (6) psychiatric/mental health.
	Note: Speciality certification in palliative nursing (ACHPN) as a primary certification is rare and only possible in two areas (New York, District of Columbia).
Authority to practice in the APRN role	*State license* to practice as APRN (most commonly NP or CNS)
	State APRN practice act, statutes, or regulations within state APRN practices that grant authority to practice in the advanced role
Role delineation of the APRN	*A job description* that delineates APRN practice
	For APRNs in states where there is no independent practice, it is helpful to have a *collaborative agreement* or *joint protocol*, which is a practice agreement outlining tasks the palliative APRN may perform in a particular setting, under what circumstances the palliative APRN would refer to a physician, and the level of physician involvement or oversight. This can be part of the palliative APRN's job description.
Basis of the APRN's salary	All or a *percentage of salary* (usually percentage of patient care hours) must not be part of a Medicare Part A Cost Report from an organization (i.e., the APRN cannot be under the organization's nursing department where their care would be included as part of Medicare payment for nursing services).
	Note: The palliative APRN can have a percentage of their salary be part of a physician group and a percentage of a health system to account for clinical care and education to the organization.
Healthcare employer organizational credentialing	Occurs at organization or *institution where APRN will provide services*. For hospitals, this must be through a medical staff office, not a human resources department.
	National Provider Identification (NPI) number
	Acceptance on Medicare, Medicaid, and commercial panels
APRN prescriptive authority	*State* prescribing license and/or state-controlled substances registration
	Drug Enforcement Administration (DEA) registration for controlled substances.

From Dahlin.[1-4]

Box I.1 PALLIATIVE APRN SCOPE OF PRACTICE FOR ADULTS AND CHILDREN

I. A professional scope of practice delineates the legal limits of the services the palliative APRN can provide. Specific regulatory elements include graduate nursing education, licensure as an APRN, certification for practice, professional credentialing and privileging within an organization, and the specific description of the level of patient care the palliative APRN can provide.

A. Regulatory elements delineated by both the Centers for Medicare and Medicaid Services (CMS) and the National Council of State Boards of Nursing (NCSBN): The APRN must have education beyond a bachelor's degree; specifically a master's, post-master's, or doctorate in nursing. The APRN Consensus Model implements population-based specialty areas: (i) family/individual across the life span, (ii) adult/gerontology, (iii) neonatal, (iv) pediatrics, (v) women's health/gender-related, and (vi) psychiatric/mental health.[5,6]

B. Legal Authority: In order for the palliative APRN to seek reimbursement from the CMS, the state scope of practice where the palliative APRN delivers patient care must allow the APRN to practice in the advanced role. This means:

   1. The palliative APRN must have the legal authority within the state, where service occurs, to practice beyond the RN level and have the legal authority to practice at the level of a physician. Specifically, this means the work of the palliative APRN would be performed by an MD/DO in his or her absence, not by a hospice or palliative RN.

   2. Advanced tasks and services include the ability to take a patient history, complete a review of systems, perform physical examinations, diagnose, and treat according to Medicare guidelines.

   3. Prescriptive authority is an aspect of advanced practice. In many states, palliative APRNs are permitted to practice at the physician level except related to prescriptive privileges for the various classifications of pharmacotherapeutics and controlled substances.

C. Licensure: The palliative APRN must have a license beyond an RN level of practice (i.e., licensed as NP or CNS).

D. Certification: The palliative APRN must have passed an advanced practice nursing examination through a recognized national body, demonstrating competence within a specific population of advanced nursing practice.

   1. This means the APRN must take a certification examination that matches the area of specialty previously mentioned in regulatory areas.

E. Credentialing (the process of privileging to practice at a setting): The CMS requires that the palliative APRN must have applied for and been granted institutional privileges to practice at a healthcare organization. The Joint Commission requires that APRNs be credentialed through medical credentialing offices for advanced practice, rather than nursing offices (76 Fed. Reg. 210, 2011).

F. Scope of Practice: If the palliative APRN is able to practice to the full scope of their practice, then the federal guidelines delineate:

   1. How the palliative APRN provides services for Medicare patients;

   2. How the palliative APRN provides services for Medicaid patients (if allowable in a particular state);

   3. How the palliative APRN can provide services for hospitalized patients;

   4. Whether the palliative APRN can prescribe controlled substances or different levels of controlled substances;

   5. How Medicare billing and reimbursement should occur; and

   6. The use of electronic prescriptive privileges

From Dahlin.[1–4]

Table I.2 PALLIATIVE CARE ESSENTIAL COMPONENTS OF DOCUMENTATION FOR REIMBURSEMENT

The purpose of documentation is to establish the health record and chronicle important facts, findings, and observations pertinent to the patient's health and illness. Documentation of the medical record promotes communication and continuity between healthcare providers and highlights the work of the palliative care team. Last, it is a legal document that serves to verify care and support billing and coding. The following is the *who, what, where, when, why,* and *how,* of documentation, but in the order of hierarchy.

ELEMENT	DESCRIPTION	IDENTIFYING DATA
Who	Who was the patient that was seen? Who was the clinician who saw the patient?	*Patient identification:* Name, medical record number, date of birth *Palliative APRN identification:* Name, credentials, contact information Identify service line: Palliative care and hospice team Affiliation Attestation of a note through a legible electronic or written signature
Why	Why was the palliative care consult requested (specifically explaining the medical reason for a consult request or a follow-up visit)?	Medical reason, such as pain or symptom Clarification of goals of care Potential for rapid change New diagnosis Referring clinician Palliative trigger
How	How was the time spent for the palliative care visit?	History-taking Physical examination Review of procedures, diagnostic testing, and laboratory testing Family meeting * Counseling* Goals of care* Advance care planning* Out-of-hospital orders for life-sustaining treatments or provider/ physician orders for life-sustaining treatment (POLST) forms * Need to document start and stop time of these elements within a comprehensive visit * Need to specific the topics covered
What	What type of in-person visit occurred (a consultation/initial visit vs. a subsequent or follow-up visit)? What was done during the palliative care visit? What type of non–face-to-face work was done?	Consultation versus ongoing management *Elements of visit:* history, physical examination, medication review, review of systems Discussion with other health providers, review of records, review of diagnostics, care plan development
Where	Where or in what setting did the palliative care visit occur?	Inpatient: Acute care or rehabilitation hospital Clinic, ambulatory, or outpatient setting Residential home Skilled nursing facility, subacute or long-term care Assisted-living facility Hospice setting Telehealth
When	When did the palliative care visit occur, and how long was it?	Date, time, and year Start and end time of visit: Assists in determining the level Start and end time of in-person visit: Assists in determining whether goals-of-care discussion is added to diagnosis codes Total time of counseling and topics discussed in that time: Determines time-based billing Total Time (see Table for more explanation of coding)

From Dahlin.[2,3]

Box I.2 DOCUMENTATION

A. Effective documentation is essential to support optimal coding and billing by the APRN. With electronic health records, there are often templates and prompts for notes to assure that all the work done is captured.

B. It is helpful to understand necessary documentation elements prior to a visit to assure a comprehensive review, history, physical examination, and treatment plan.

C. General documentation includes[2,3]:

1. Identifying data: Patient name, medical record number

2. Requesting provider for consultation

3. Specialty code of APRN (e.g., hospice, palliative care)

4. Service or procedural codes (evaluation and management codes)

5. Diagnoses: Diagnosis by International Classification of Diseases (ICD); ICD-10 codes (10th version of the codes)

D. Documentation demonstrates evaluation and management[7]:

1. Chief concern/nature of presenting problem

2. History of present illness, with a focus on a symptom(s) and the description capturing as many as possible of the following details:
   a. Location
   b. Quality
   c. Severity
   d. Duration
   e. Timing
   f. Context
   g. Modifying factors
   h. Associated signs and symptoms.

3. Review of Systems (ROS), delineated in one of the following categories:
   a. Problem: Based on 1–5 problems within an organ specific system;
   b. Extended: Based on specific problem and 2–9 other organ systems;
   c. Comprehensive: Based on the specific issue and a minimum of 10 other organ systems, or critical care billing as per Centers for Medicare and Medicaid Services (CMS) guidelines

4. Past medical, family, and social history: This includes social determinants of health and a cultural history (one line from each):
   a. Past history, including experiences with illnesses and treatments
   b. Past surgeries, injuries, and treatments
   c. Family history including a review of medical events, diseases, and hereditary conditions that may place the patient at risk
   d. Social history including an age-appropriate review of past and current activities

5. Examination: 2–8 systems (constitutional; eyes; ear, nose, mouth, and throat [EENMT]; cardiovascular; respiratory; gastrointestinal; genitourinary; musculoskeletal; skin; neurologic; hematologic/lymph/immunologic; psychiatric) depending on level of visit

Palliative care observation alone: Includes constitutional (1 system), HEENT (5 systems), respiratory, neuro, psychiatric

6. Medical decision-making
   a. Diagnoses managed
   b. Data reviewed: Laboratory, radiology, chart review, medications
   c. Risk: Methadone, opioid infusions, benzodiazepines, code status discussion and DNR, de-escalation of care

7. Counseling

8. Coordination of care

9. Time spent on the visit

From Dahlin[1–3] National Council of State Boards of Nursing.[7]

Box I.3 PALLIATIVE CARE CONSULTATIONS

Although initial palliative care visits are reimbursed as "consultations" per the Centers for Medicare and Medicaid Services (CMS), there are four elements of documentation to attend to within an initial palliative care visit that are part of best practice.

I. *Request*: This is the request for a palliative care consultation. It can be a verbal or written request via a specific order or note in the chart. More often, these are now placed as orders within a healthcare record as non-medication orders. Remember, the CMS allows a variety of providers to request a palliative consult including osteopaths, APRNs, physician assistants, rehabilitation therapists, psychologists, and social workers, as well as physicians. The requesting provider must be identified and documented in the APRN consultation or initial evaluation note.

II. *Reason*: The reason for the palliative consult should accompany the request. The most common reasons are pain and symptom management, advance care planning, goals of care, considerations of treatments, psychosocial or spiritual support, or discharge planning. The reason for the request should be documented in the palliative APRN's initial consultation note.

III. *Render service*: The palliative care consultation must be rendered. Thus, the APRN preforms the patient consultation, documents the examination and findings, and offers suggestions to managing the problem. This includes the development of diagnoses and a recommended individualized treatment plan.

IV. *Report*: The palliative APRN must complete a written record or report of the consultation for the requesting provider. There are several ways this can occur. If within the same health organization, the consult note can be completed in the shared electronic health record. If out of a health system, this can be a consultative note or letter, available to the referring provider who made the original request.

From Dahlin.[1,2]

Table I.3 PALLIATIVE BILLING AND CODING 101: PRINCIPLES

TYPE OF CODE	DESCRIPTION
ICD-10 codes: Diagnosis International Classification of Disease and Health-Related Conditions, 10th revision	Codes for diseases, signs and symptoms, abnormal findings, complaints, social circumstances, educational needs, and external causes of injury or diseases
ICD-10 code: Palliative Care Identifier: Z51.5	The Z51.5 is the code for all palliative care encounters, regardless of setting. Other ICD-10 codes speak to the symptoms the palliative care provider is addressing within the diagnosis on which the palliative care provider is focused.
Current Procedural Technology (CPT) codes: Level of service provided The CPT code set is a medical code set maintained by the American Medical Association and designed to communicate uniform information about medical services and procedures. CPT codes apply to any type of care and delineate location, intensity, and duration of services. Billing can be complexity-based or time-based	1. Location of service a. Acute care setting b. Office or clinic c. Home d. Nursing home e. Assisted living f. Skilled nursing facility g. Telehealth, telephonic 2. Type of patient: New vs. established 3. Type of visit: Initial vs. subsequent 4. Duration of visit: Time period of visit 5. Complexity of service: Medical decision-making aspect of visit Most palliative care visits meet the criteria for the visit levels at 3, 4, 5.
Evaluation and Management (E/M) codes: Level of complexity	Documentation of key components: 1. History 2. Exam 3. Level of complexity of medical decision-making • Number and complexity of problems addressed • Amount of data to be reviewed and analyzed • Risk of complications, morbidity, and/or mortality 4. Time (time of beginning and end of encounter)

(continued)

Table I.3 CONTINUED

TYPE OF CODE	DESCRIPTION

Time codes: These now include total time for date of encounter (preparation, review, history, counseling, examination, orders, coordination, etc.).

Palliative care subsequent visits:
If less than 20 minutes, bill on medical decision-making
If greater than 20 minutes, give exact time and start and end times

Prolonged Physician Service with Direct Patient Contact series	*Prolonged service* involving direct (face-to-face) patient contact beyond the usual service (typical time) in setting.
	Criteria include:
	   1. Specific time intervals that qualify for these codes
	   2. Documentation that includes the exact start and stop time for the visit
	   3. Specific codes for the prolonged time intervals
	Outpatient time applies to day of service (same or different) with face-to-face and non–face-to-face contact.
	Includes the following activities, when performed:
	• Preparing to see the patient (e.g., review of tests)
	• Obtaining and/or reviewing separately obtained history
	• Performing a medically appropriate examination and/or evaluation
	• Counseling and educating the patient/family/caregiver
	• Ordering medications, tests, or procedures
	• Referring and communicating with other healthcare professionals (when not separately reported)
	• Documenting clinical information in the electronic or other health record
	• Independently interpreting results (not separately reported) and communicating results to the patient/family/caregiver
	• Care coordination (not separately reported)

Point of Service (POS) codes: Setting
POS codes are used only by coders and billers, however, the APRN must indicate in the documentation where the patient was located during the encounter.

Telehealth codes[8]	Available for: Video visits (vVisit): Connecting via video Telephone call (tVisit): Call via the telephone Secure messaging (eVisit): Connecting via secure patient portal or telehealth platform Remote patient monitoring (RPM)

Care coordination codes

Care Plan Oversight (CPO) codes apply to the supervision of patients under either the home health or hospice benefit where the patient requires complex or multidisciplinary care requiring ongoing physician involvement.	Billed by physicians and advanced practice providers who are part of the same team. Occurs for patients under home health or hospice: Home health (GO181) Hospice (GO182) Includes: • 30 minutes of time • Frequent update and review of patient status • Frequent review of laboratory and other studies • Frequent adjustment of medical therapies • Frequent revision of care plans or development of new plans with integration of updated information and ongoing laboratory studies • Communication with other health providers involved in the patient's care who are outside the practice (e.g., physical therapy, pharmacy regarding pharmaceutical options)

Transitional Care Management (TCM) codes represent the clinical interactive process in which there is consistent coverage in the "home" setting to help prevent hospital readmission. For patients being discharged or returned to home/ assisted living facility/domiciliary or other community-based setting. Patient cannot be in an inpatient setting such as hospital or skilled nursing facility.	THREE COMPONENTS		
	A required interactive contact with patient or other providers: • Phone • Telehealth • Direct exchange of information	Certain non–face-to-face services: • Obtain and review discharge information • Review diagnostic tests and treatments • Referrals • Interaction with other health providers	A face-to-face visit: • A first visit is required but not reported or billed separately • This first visit is made within required 7- or 14-day period • Cannot be billed during same period of care plan oversight or chronic care management

Table I.3 CONTINUED

TYPE OF CODE	DESCRIPTION
Chronic Care Management (CCM) codes and Chronic and Complex Management (CCCM) codes	CCM and CCCM: Multiple chronic conditions expected to last 12 months or until death. Chronic conditions place the patient at significant risk of death, acute exacerbation, decompensation, or functional decline. CCCM: Moderate or high decision-making Requires: • Patient consent • Comprehensive plan of care • 24/7 access • Use of Centers for Medicare and Medicaid Services (CMS) certified electronic health record (EHR)
ACP Codes[9]	Advance care planning includes the explanation and discussion of advance directives, which is in conjunction with another visit—whether inpatient, outpatient, home, or telehealth. • 99498: Codes added to E/M when performing initial consultations, follow-up visits, or care coordination codes for more than 16 minutes or when there is specific discussion on surrogate decision-makers, living wills, advance directives, out-of-hospital orders for life-sustaining treatment, provider/physician orders for life sustaining treatments (POLST) Time is longer than 16 minutes with a threshold of 16–45 min • 99497: Second 30 minutes Time over 45 minutes with a threshold of 46–74 min (See Chapter 32, "Advance Care Planning")
Non–Face-to-Face Codes[10]	Non–face-to-face codes • Greater than 31 minutes spent on patient care • In preparation of seeing the patients • Does not require face-to-face contact; could include a telephone call • Review of records, phone calls to other providers, coordinating care • Doesn't need to be continuous

There are general principles to the skill of billing and coding. However, billing and coding varies based on organization and region of the country. It is important to understand billing and coding concepts, as well as the regional environment of billing and coding. Most important is to work with the billers and coders of your organization.

From Dahlin[2]; American Medical Association[11]; and Acevado.[12]

Box I.4 SUMMARY OF PALLIATIVE APRN REIMBURSEMENT BY TYPE AND SETTING

I. Palliative APRNs have the potential to bill for visits across settings.

  A. Community settings

    1. Home visits: Consult for palliative care services or initial palliative care visit
      a. A palliative APRN may bill independently for these services.
      b. A palliative APRN may not bill a consult as a shared visit for a consult (i.e., patient is seen by both an MD and APRN).

    2. Subsequent home visits for palliative care follow-up
      a. A palliative APRN may bill independently for these services.
      b. A palliative APRN may bill incident to the visit if a physician was present at the visit.
      c. Shared visits are not allowed in the home setting.

    3. Ambulatory setting: Outpatient clinics
      a. Outpatient clinic consult for palliative care services or initial palliative care visit
        i. A palliative APRN may bill independently for these services.
        ii. A palliative APRN may not bill a new patient consult as a shared visit (i.e., patient is seen by both an MD and APRN).
      b. Subsequent clinic outpatient visit for a palliative care follow-up
        i. A palliative APRN may bill independently for these services.
        ii. A palliative APRN may bill subsequent care with a shared visit (i.e., patient is seen by both an MD and an APRN) if the plan of treatment has been established by the physician.

B. Hospital care

   1. Acute inpatient setting

      a. Consult for palliative care services or initial palliative care visit

         i. A palliative APRN may bill independently for these services.

         ii. A palliative APRN may not bill a consult as a shared visit for a consult (i.e., patient is seen by both an MD and APRN).

      b. Initial hospital care for patient admitted as a palliative care patient

         i. A palliative APRN may not bill a hospital admission visit independently unless serving as the Attending of Record.

         ii. A palliative APRN may bill an admission with a shared visit (i.e., patient is seen by both an MD and APRN).

      c. Subsequent hospital visit for a palliative care follow-up

         i. A palliative APRN may bill independently for these services.

         ii. A palliative APRN may bill subsequent care as a shared visit (i.e., patient is seen by both an MD and APRN).

      d. Critical care for a palliative care symptom

         i. A palliative APRN may bill independently for these services as a palliative care consultant.

         ii. A palliative APRN may not bill critical care as a shared visit (i.e., patient is seen by both an MD and APRN).

      e. Discharge services for a palliative care patient

         i. A palliative APRN may bill independently for these services if the APRN is the Attending of Record and admitted the patient to the facility.

         ii. A palliative APRN may bill discharge services as a shared visit (i.e., patient is seen by both an MD and APRN).

         iii. Both of these scenarios are submitted under the discharge management code.

      f. Death pronouncement and certification of a palliative care patient

         i. A palliative APRN may bill independently for these services under the discharge management code if state statute allows the APRN to perform a death pronouncement and complete a death certificate.

         ii. If allowed by state statutes to perform these services and the APRN performs the "final examination" to pronounce the death and complete a death certificate, services would be billed under the discharge management code.

   2. Acute rehabilitation settings

      a. Consult for palliative care services or initial palliative care visit

         i. A palliative APRN may bill independently for these services.

         ii. A palliative APRN may not bill a consult as a shared visit (i.e., patient is seen by both an MD and APRN).

      b. Initial hospital care for a palliative care patients

         i. A palliative APRN may not bill an admission independently unless serving as Attending of Record.

         ii. A palliative APRN may bill an admission as a shared visit (i.e., patient is seen by both an MD and APRN).

      c. Subsequent hospital visit for palliative care follow-up

         i. A palliative APRN may bill independently for these services.

         ii. A palliative APRN may bill subsequent care as a shared visit (i.e., patient is seen by both an MD and APRN).

      d. Discharge services of a palliative patient

         i. A palliative APRN may bill independently for these services if the APRN is the Attending of Record and admitted the patient to the facility.

         ii. A palliative APRN may bill discharge services as a shared visit (i.e., patient is seen by both an MD and APRN).

      e. Death pronouncement and certification of a palliative patient

         i. A palliative APRN may bill independently for these services under the discharge management code if state statute allows the APRN to perform a death pronouncement and complete a death certificate.

         ii. If allowed by state statutes to perform these services and the APRN performs the "final examination" to pronounce the death and complete a death certificate, services would be billed under the discharge management code.

C. In-patient hospice units with the APRN serving as the Attending of Record

   1. The hospice APRN may bill for the initial admission as the admitting Attending of Record.

   2. The hospice APRN may bill for subsequent visits independently as the Attending of Record

   3. The hospice APRN may bill for discharge services under the discharge management code, if the APRN admitted the patient to the unit.

   4. The hospice APRN may bill for death pronouncement and certification, under the discharge management code, if allowed by state statutes to do so and if she or he performs the "final examination" to pronounce the death.

D. Telehealth codes

    1. The palliative APRN in the acute care setting, clinic setting, or home setting may bill for initial palliative consultations.

    2. The Palliative APRN in the acute care setting, clinic setting, or home setting may bill for subsequent visits.

From Dahlin.[1-3]

Table I.4 THE FOUR PARTS OF MEDICARE

MEDICARE BENEFIT	PART A HOSPITAL INSURANCE	PART B MEDICAL INSURANCE	PART C MEDICARE ADVANTAGE PLANS	PART D PRESCRIPTION DRUG COVERAGE
Type of services	Hospital/Inpatient coverage	Professional outpatient services	Health programs that replace Medicare (Medicare Advantage plans)	Prescription drug programs
Universal or voluntary	Universal coverage	Voluntary; premium payment	Voluntary; premium payment	Voluntary; premium
Coverage	Fully covered: However, there may be a deductible amount per admission.	Covered 80%: However, there may be an annual deductible	Varies by plan	Varies by plan: May have a premium and limits of dollar amounts of medications

From Centers for Medicare and Medicaid Services[13,14,16]; and Bunis.[15]

Table I.5 MEDICARE PART A AND PART B

PART A	PART B
Institutional services	Professional services of clinicians
Eligibility: Universal coverage for people ≥65 years and people with certain disabilities. No copayments.	*Eligibility*: Voluntary. Coinsurance. People ≥65 years and people with certain disabilities. Copayments required.
Sites of care where services are covered:	Types of services covered:
Hospital care	Physicians, APRNs, PAs, psychologists, clinical social workers
Skilled nursing facility	Durable Medical Equipment
Nursing home care (above custodial care)	Outpatient dialysis
Hospice	Mental health services
Home healthcare	Outpatient hospital
Inpatient rehabilitation	Ambulance services
Inpatient dialysis	Rural health clinic and federally qualified health center services

From Centers for Medicare and Medicaid Services.[13,14,16]

coder to understand the culture of billing at their organization. Quality metrics would also support quarterly meetings that include all eligible healthcare providers who can bill and the organization billers and coders to ensure common understanding and consistency of billing and coding within the palliative care service. The following tables and boxes summarize the billing and coding requirements for palliative APRNs.

REFERENCES

1. Dahlin C. Reimbursement and Billing. In: Dahlin C, Lynch M, eds. *Core Curriculum for the Advanced Practice Hospice and Palliative Registered Nurse.* 2nd ed. Pittsburgh, PA: Hospice and Palliative Nurses Association; 2013: 25–38.

2. Dahlin C. *A Primer of Reimbursement. Billing, and Coding: Essential Information for the Hospice and Palliative Advanced Practice Nurse (APRN).* Pittsburgh, PA: Hospice and Palliative Nurses Association; 2015.

3. Dahlin C. Reimbursement for the palliative advanced practice registered nurse. In: Dahlin C, Coyne P, Ferrell B, eds. *Advanced Practice Palliative Nursing.* New York: Oxford University Press; 2016: 31–40.

4. Dahlin C. *The Hospice and Palliative APRN Professional Practice Guide.* Pittsburgh, PA: Hospice and Palliative Nurses Association; 2017.

5. APRN Consensus Work Group, National Council of State Boards of Nursing APRN Advisory Committee. Consensus model for APRN regulation: Licensure, accreditation, certification, and education. Chicago, IL: NCSBN. 2008. www.nursingworld.org/ConsensusModelforAPRN

6. National Council of State Boards of Nursing, APRN Advisory Committee. APRN regulation: Licensure, accreditation, certification, and education. Chicago, IL; NCSBN. 2008. https://www.ncsbn.org/Consensus_Model_for_APRN_Regulation_July_2008.pdf

7. Centers for Medicare and Medicaid Services, Medicare Learning Network. *Evaluation and Management Services Guide.* Baltimore, MD: Centers for Medicare and Medicaid Services; February 2021. https://www.cms.gov/outreach-and-education/medicare-learning-network-mln/mlnproducts/downloads/eval-mgmt-serv-guide-icn006764.pdf

8. American Academy of Family Physicians, Manett Health. *A Toolkit for Building and Growing a Sustainable Telehealth Program in Your Practice.* Leawood, KS: American Academy of Family Physicians; September 2020. https://www.aafp.org/dam/AAFP/documents/practice_management/telehealth/2020-AAFP-Telehealth-Toolkit.pdf

9. American College of Physicians, High Value Care Task Force. Advanced care planning: Implementation for practices. 2015. https://www.acponline.org/system/files/documents/running_practice/payment_coding/medicare/advance_care_planning_toolkit.pdf

10. Department of Health and Human Services, Centers for Medicare & Medicaid Services. MLN Matters. Transmittal R3678CP: Prolonged services without direct face-to-face patient contact separately payable under the physician fee schedule (manual update). December 16, 2016. https://www.cms.gov/Outreach-and-Education/Medicare-Learning-Network-MLN/MLNMattersArticles/Downloads/MM9905.pdf

11. American Medical Association. CPT® Evaluation and Management (E/M) Office or Other Outpatient (99202-99215) and Prolonged Services (99354, 99355, 99356, 99XXX) code and guideline change. Medical decision-making (MDM). 2021. https://www.ama-assn.org/system/files/2019-06/cpt-office-prolonged-svs-code-changes.pdf

12. Acevado J. *Documentation and Coding Handbook: Palliative Care.* Sacramento, CA: California Health Care Foundation; 2019. https://www.chcf.org/wp-content/uploads/2019/05/DocumentationCodingHandbookPalliativeCare.pdf

13. Centers for Medicare and Medicaid Services. Medicare.gov. What part A covers? 2021. www.medicare.gov/what-medicare-covers/part-a/what-part-a-covers.html.

14. Centers for Medicare and Medicaid Services. Medicare.gov. What part B covers? 2021. www.medicare.gov/what-medicare-covers/part-b/what-medicare-part-b-covers.html

15. Bunis D. What is Medicare? Understanding Medicare's options: Parts A, B, C, and D. AARP. 2021. https://www.aarp.org/health/medicare-insurance/info-01-2011/understanding_medicare_the_plans.html

16. Centers for Medicare and Medicaid Services, Medicare Learning Network. *Medicare and Medicaid Basics.* Baltimore, MD: Centers for Medicare and Medicaid Services; 2018. https://www.cms.gov/Outreach-and-Education/Medicare-Learning-Network-MLN/MLNProducts/Downloads/ProgramBasics.pdf

17. AANP Forum. CARES Act bolsters access to home health care services. *J Nurse Pract.* 2020;*16*(6):A11–A14.

18. Department of Health and Human Services, Centers for Medicare and Medicaid Services. Transmittal 246: Manual updates related to payment policy changes affecting the hospice aggregate cap calculation and the designation of hospice attending physicians. *CMS manual system: Pub 100-02 Medicare benefit policy.* 2018. https://www.cms.gov/Regulations-and-Guidance/Guidance/Transmittals/2018Downloads/R246BP.pdf

APPENDIX II
Perinatal and Pediatric Pain and Symptom Tables

Maggie C. Root, Mallory Fossa, Gina Santucci, Nicole Sartor, Faith Kinnear, Alice Bass,

Jaime Hensel, Amy Corey Haskamp, Joanne M. Greene, Cheryl Ann Thaxton,

Joan "Jody" Chrastek, Vanessa Battista, and Constance Dahlin

Infants, children, and adolescents with serious illnesses experience a myriad of pain syndromes and symptoms. It is essential that the pediatric palliative APRN evaluate each symptom through exquisite assessment, physical examination, and review of diagnostic information. To understand the pathophysiology of pain and symptoms, the reader is referred to the Section VIII "Symptoms" in this book. Chapters 39 through 44 provide information on the etiology, pathophysiology, assessment, and management of pain, anorexia and cachexia, bowel symptoms, fatigue, nausea and vomiting, and respiratory symptoms. Chapters 45 through 50 provide information on the etiology, pathophysiology, assessment, and management of anxiety, delirium, and other challenging symptoms. This appendix offers suggestions for the medical management of common infant and pediatric palliative care symptoms. However, it is not meant as medical advice. The pediatric palliative APRN should always review the literature and consult pharmacology databases and palliative care colleagues to ensure that the most current information on medication use and dosages is being used. Additionally, the pediatric palliative APRN should consider consulting other specialists, which may include anesthesia/pain management, psychiatry, neurology, and gastroenterology to name a few.

There are few guidelines for pediatric medications in palliative care. Most of the literature focuses on the adaptation of medications used in the adult population to the pediatric population.[1] Per the World Health Organization (WHO) and the US Centers for Disease Control and Prevention (CDC), when treating pediatric patients, it is wise to avoid the unnecessary use of medications and be aware of the potential for medication overdoses.[2,3] Therefore, a step-wise approach to management is appropriate.

Step 1 is the use of nonpharmacological strategies listed in Table II.1.[4,5,6] This includes a range of interventions. For the infant, the focus is often on adjusting the environment of care to maximize comfort and reduce overstimulation. For the child and adolescent, it moves beyond managing the environment to initiating cognitive, rehabilitative, expressive, and integrative therapies, as available and affordable to families.

Step 2 is pharmacological management of pain and symptoms (Table II.2). Although there are guidelines for the use of medications in the pediatric population (see Table 10), there are limited randomized trials specifically in this population. In children, medication use is frequently based on the opinions and guidelines of experts. Medication management must be individualized to the infant, child, and adolescent based on age, weight, metabolism, and development. Dosing of medications is based on either weight or age. The pediatric palliative APRN should always consult the most recent literature for dosing guidelines. In addition, the APRN must consider regional access to medications, health organization formularies, and the insurance coverage of any therapeutics. The

Table II.1 NONPHARMACOLOGICAL INTERVENTIONS

ENVIRONMENTAL STRATEGIES	COGNITIVE THERAPIES	REHABILITATIVE THERAPIES	EXPRESSIVE THERAPIES	INTEGRATIVE
Swaddling/cuddling	Cognitive-behavioral therapy	Physical therapy	Art therapy	Acupuncture
Heating pads	Hypnosis	Massage	Music therapy	Yoga
Cold packs	Guided imagery	Occupational therapy	Dance and movement therapy	Reiki
Distraction	Counseling		Bibliotherapy or poetry therapy	Biofeedback

From Davis[5]; and Wren et al.[6]; Friedrichsof & Goubert[7]

Table II.2 NOCICEPTIVE AND NEUROPATHIC PAIN: CAUSES AND DESCRIPTORS

CAUSES	DESCRIPTORS
Nociceptive: Somatic tissues	
Increased pressure, bony invasion or metastases, mucositis, skin breakdown, radiation skin burns, vaso-occlusive crisis in sickle cell disease	Well-localized, sharp/stabbing (if superficial) or dull/throbbing (if deep tissue), constant but worse with movement, point tenderness common
Nociceptive: Visceral organs	
Tumor invasion resulting in organ distention, infiltration, necrosis, or obstruction such as intestine, kidneys, liver, or peritoneum	Poorly localized, dull, deep pressure, spasm or cramping
Neuropathic: Peripheral or central nervous system	
Nerve compression or injury due to tumor or metastatic invasion to the brain, spinal cord, or nerve roots; peripheral neuropathy caused from chemotherapy such as vincristine, phantom limb pain	Difficult to describe or localize, associated with paresthesia or dysesthesia. Tingling, burning, shooting, electric/shooting, prickly

From Postovsky et al.[8]; and Hauer.[9]

Table II.3 PAIN MANAGEMENT: SUGGESTED DOSING FOR INITIATION OF OPIOIDS IN OPIOID-NAÏVE INFANTS AND CHILDREN

OPIOID	COMMON DOSING BASED ON WEIGHT AND AGE

Oxycodone	*Weight-based dosing*
	Infants <6 months:
	    Not recommended due to wide variability in drug conversion and clearance[10]
	Children >6 months[8,10,11,12]:
	    <50 kg: 0.1–0.2 mg/kg q4–6h PO prn, maximum 5–10 mg/dose
	    >50 kg: 5–10 mg q4–6h PO prn

Morphine	*Weight-based dosing*
	Neonates <1 month[9]: Use preservative-free formulation.
	    0.025–0.05 mg/kg/dose IV q4–8h prn
	    or
	    0.08 mg/kg/dose PO q4–6h prn
	Infants >1 month and ≤6 months[3]:
	    Nonventilated:
	        0.025–0.03 mg/kg IV q4h prn
	        or
	        0.08–0.1 mg/kg PO q4h prn
	    Ventilated:
	        0.05 mg/kg/dose q2–4h prn
	        Continuous IV infusion (initial dosing):
	        0.008–0.02 mg/kg/hr, titrate carefully to effect
	
	Infants >6 months, children and adolescents[3,8]:
	    <50 kg:
	        0.05–0.1 mg/kg/dose IV q4h prn maximum 1–2 mg/dose
	        or
	        0.15–0.3 mg/kg PO q4h prn usual maximum 7.5–15 mg every 4 hours
	    >50 kg:
	        2–5 mg IV q4h prn
	        or
	        15–20 mg PO q4h prn

Table II.3 CONTINUED

OPIOID	COMMON DOSING BASED ON WEIGHT AND AGE

Fentanyl	*Weight-based dosing*
	Infants ≤12 months[11]:
	Infants 0–5 months
	    0.5–1 mcg/kg/hr with the bolus dose being the same
	    1–2 mcg/kg IV/SC q2–4h prn
	Children and adolescents:[2,3,8]
	    <50 kg: 0.5–1 mcg/kg IV q1–2h prn (maximum 25–50 mcg)
	      administer slowly over 3–5 minutes)
	    >50 kg: 25–50 mcg /dose IV q1– 2 h prn
	    Continuous infusion 0.5–1 mcg/kg/hr (maximum 25–50 mcg/h)
	    Transdermal Patch 12 mcg/hr patch
	    *Must be using minimum of 30 mg oral morphine/24 hours
	      before initiating patch.

Hydromorphone	*Age- and weight-based dosing*[12]:
	Infants 6 months and >10 kg:
	    0.01 mg/kg/dose IV q3–6h prn
	    or
	    0.03 mg/kg/dose PO q4h prn
	Children and adolescents <50 kg[8]:
	    0.015 mg/kg IV q4h prn *or* 0.04–0.06 mg/kg PO q4h prn
	Children and adolescents 50 kg[7]:
	    0.2–0.6 mg IV q4h prn *or* 1–2 mg PO q4h prn

Methadone	*Opioid-naïve children and adolescents*[8,11]:
	    Wide dosing ranges:
	    0.05–0.1 mg/kg/dose (maximum 2.5–5 mg PO q8–12h)

Note: Best practice is to cross check dosing with a palliative care colleague or a pharmacist.

Infants are at high risk of respiratory depression from opioids. Metabolism and excretion can vary widely in infants. Use caution when prescribing in this population.

From Wren et al.[6]; Hauer[8]; Friedrichsdorf[11]; and Taketomo, Hodding.[13]

Table II.4 MANAGEMENT OF NEUROPATHIC PAIN

MEDICATION	COMMON DOSING BASED ON WEIGHT AND AGE
	ANTICONVULSANTS

Gabapentin	*Age- and weight-based dosing*:
	    Infants[14–17]:
	      2.5–5 mg/kg/day PO, titrate every 3–5 days
	    Children and adolescents (neuropathic pain)[11]:
	    2 mg/kg PO qhs
	      Slow titration to initial target dose of 6 mg/kg/dose tid (maximum 300 mg/dose tid)
	      Titrate to effect (maximum dose 24 mg/kg/dose tid or 1,200 mg/dose tid)
	    *Children and adolescents with severe neurologic impairment (dosing for peripheral and central
	      neuropathic pain, spasticity and visceral hyperalgesia)*[9,16,18]:
	    Days 1–2: 2 mg/kg (100 mg maximum) PO tid
	    Days 4–6: 4 mg/kg PO tid
	      Titrate to effect every 2–4 days by 5–6 mg/kg/day until any of the following:
	      Analgesia is effective (often noted at 30–45 mg/kg/day)
	      Side effects experienced (nystagmus, sedation, tremor, ataxia, swelling)
	      Maximum dose per day is reached (50–72 mg/kg/day *or* 2,400–3,600 mg/day)
	Note: Younger children (<5 years) may require a 30% higher mg/kg/day dosing, such as a total dose of
	45–60 mg/kg/day
	Sedation is more common with rapid titration. Adjust dose in renal impairment.

Pregabalin	*Weight-based dosing*:
	    Children[18]:
	      Days 1–3: 1 mg/kg (maximum 50 mg), enterally, every night
	      Days 4–6: 1 mg/kg, enterally, bid
	      Increase every 2–4 days up to 3 mg/kg/dose, enterally, given 2 or 3 times daily
	        (maximum 6 mg/kg/dose)

(continued)

Table II.4 CONTINUED

MEDICATION	COMMON DOSING BASED ON WEIGHT AND AGE

TRICYCLIC ANTIDEPRESSANTS

Amitriptyline	*Age-based dosing*
	Children and Adolescents <50 kg[18]:
	    Days 1–4: 0.2 mg/kg (maximum 10 mg), enterally, qhs
	    Days 5–8: 0.4 mg/kg, enterally, every night
	    Increase every 4–5 days by 0.2 mg/kg/day until desired effect (maximum 50 mg/day)
	    OR
	    Initial: 0.1 mg/kg at bedtime, may advance as tolerated over 2–3 weeks to 0.5–2 mg/kg at bedtime.
	      Max: 50 mg/day
	Adolescents and adults >50 kg[9,18]:
	    Oral: Initial: 10–25 mg qhs; gradually increase dose based on response and tolerability in 10–25 mg
	      increments at intervals ≥1 week up to 150 mg/day given once daily at bedtime or in 2 divided doses

CENTRALLY ACTING A-AGONIST

Clonidine	*Weight-based dosing*
	For children and adolescents[3,7–18]:
	    Day 1–3: 0.002 mg/kg (maximum 0.1 mg), enterally at night
	    Days 4–6: 0.002 mg/kg (maximum 0.1 mg), enterally, bid
	    Days 7–9: 0.002 mg/kg (maximum 0.1 mg), enterally tid
	    Increase every 2–4 days by 0.002 mg/kg to effect
	    Can consider clonidine patch when at stable enteral dosing
	    For episodic dosing - 0.002–0.004 mg/kg every 4 hours as needed for autonomic storm events
	      (suggested by facial flushing, muscle stiffening and tremors, hyperthermia)

From Hauer[9]; Friedrichsdorf[11]; and Taketomo, Hodding.[13]

Table II.5 MANAGEMENT OF CONSTIPATION

MEDICATION	COMMON DOSING BASED ON WEIGHT AND AGE[3]
Docusate	*Age-based dosing*: *Children*: Docusate alone is not an effective bowel regimen[19]

Docusate and senna	*Age-based dosing*:
	Infants:
	    No recommendations
	Children:
	    2–6 years: ½ tablet (25 mg docusate/4.3 mg sennosides) PO qhs maximum 1 tab bid
	    6–12 years: 1 tablet (50 mg docusate/8.6 mg sennosides) PO qhs maximum 2 tabs bid
	    > 12 years: 2 tablets (100 mg docusate/17.2 mg sennosides) PO qhs maximum 4 tabs bid

Senna	*Age-based dosing*:
	Infants:
	    No recommendations
	Children:
	    2–6 years: 2.5–3.75 mL PO qhs, maximum 3.75 mL bid
	    6–12 years: 5–7.5 mL PO qhs, maximum 7.5 mL bid
	    >12 years: 10–15 mL PO qhs, maximum 15 mL bid

Lactulose	*Infants*:
	    Use caution with infants as they are at risk for dehydration and hyponatremia[20]
	Children:
	    Weight-based dosing: 1–2 g/kg/day (1.5–3 mL/kg/day) PO divided 1–2 times per day, maximum 60 mL/day

Methylnaltrexone	*Infants*:
	    Little evidence exists on the use of methylnaltrexone in infants and neonates.[21]
	Children:
	    Consultation with a neonatal pharmacist is recommended for use in children under 2 years old.[22]
	    Weight-based dosing[22,23]:
	    < 38 kg: 0.15 mg/kg SC every other day, maximum 8–12 mg, once daily
	    38–62 kg: 8 mg SC every other day, maximum once daily
	    62–114 kg: 12 mg SC every other day maximum once daily
	    >114 kg: 0.15 mg/kg SC every other day maximum once daily

Polyethylene glycol	*Children*:
	    Weight-based dosing:
	    ≥6 months: 0.2–0.8 g/kg PO Q day, starting dose 17 g/day to maximum dose of 32 g/day

From Komatz, Carter.[24]

Table II.6 MANAGEMENT OF DELIRIUM

MEDICATION	COMMON DOSING BASED ON WEIGHT AND AGE
Risperidone	*Age-based dosing* *Infants >6 months*[25]: Oral: 0.05 mg PO qhs *Children <5 yrs. of age*[26]: Oral: Initial: 0.1–0.2 mg qhs; doses may be increased based upon response *Children >5 yr. and adolescents*[26]: Oral: Initial: 0.2–0.5 mg once daily at bedtime May titrate every 1–2 days; usual range: 0.2–2.5 mg/day in divided doses 2–4 times daily Some have suggested maximum daily dose depending on patient weight: <20 kg: 1 mg/day; 20–45 kg: 2.5 mg/day; >45 kg: 3 mg/day
Olanzapine	*Age-based dosing* (very limited data) *Infants*[27]: Olanzapine 0.625 mg PO qhs *Infants ≥7 months to children <3 years*[26]: Oral disintegrating tablet (ODT): Reported range: 0.625–1.25 mg once daily qhs or bid *Children ≥3 years and adolescents*: <30 kg: 1.25 mg po q hs 30–60 kg: 2.5 mg po q hs >60 kg: 5 mg po q hs ODT: Usual initial range: 1.25–5 mg once daily qhs or bid; should be initiated at low dose and then titrated as needed (maximum 10 mg).
Quetiapine	*Age- and weight-based dosing* (very limited data) *Infants*[28]: Ventilated infants: Quetiapine 0.5 mg/kg PO q8h *Children and adolescents <50 kg*[26–28]: Initial dose range 0.43–0.7 mg/kg/dose *Adolescents >50 kg*[26]: Initial: 50 mg bid; suggested increase by 100 mg at intervals ≥1 day up to a maximum dose of 400 mg/day

From Taketomo, Hodding.[13]

Table II.7 TREATMENT OF NAUSEA AND VOMITING

MEDICATION	COMMON DOSING BASED ON WEIGHT AND AGE
Benzodiazepines	
Lorazepam	*Weight-based dosing:* *Infants and children:* 0.025–0.05 mg/kg/dose PO or IV q6h, maximum 2 mg/dose
Dopamine antagonists: Atypical antipsychotic	
Olanzapine	*Weight-based dosing:* *Infants and children*[29]: 0.1–0.14 mg/kg/dose PO every day, maximum 10 mg/dose
Serotonin (5-HT3) antagonists	
Ondansetron	*Weight-based dosing:* *Infants and children:* 0.15 mg/kg/dose IV or PO q8h, maximum 8 mg/dose
Granisetron	*Age- and weight-based dosing* *Infants:* No guidelines for infants with nausea for non–chemotherapy-related vomiting For infants and children receiving highly emetogenic chemotherapy *Infants ≤ 6 months:* 40 mcg/kg IV once daily prior to chemotherapy *Children:* >6 months: 40 mcg/kg IV or PO q12h, maximum 1 mg/dose

(continued)

Table II.7 CONTINUED

MEDICATION	COMMON DOSING BASED ON WEIGHT AND AGE
Antimuscarinics	
Scopolamine patch	Age-based dosing based on prevention of postop nausea[3]: *Children <2 years*: Apply 1/4 patch *Children ≥2 to 6 years*: Apply 1/2 patch *Children ≥6 to 12 years*: Apply 1/2 to 1 patch *Children ≥12 years and adolescents*: Apply 1 patch *Weight-based dosing*: >40 kg: 1.5 mg transdermal patch q72h *Note*: Patches should not be cut. A reduced dose may be achieved by the placement of an impermeable material under the scopolamine patch.
Neurokinin-1 antagonists	

Aprepitant	*Age-based dosing:*
	6 months—12 years (6–30 kg):
	    Day 1: 3 mg/kg PO, maximum 125 mg
	    Days 2 and 3: 2 mg/kg PO, maximum 80 mg
	12 years or >30 kg:
	    Day 1: 125 mg PO
	    Days 2 and 3: 80 mg PO once daily

Corticosteroids	
Dexamethasone for chemotherapy-induced nausea and vomiting (CINV)	*Age-based dosing:* *Infants*: No dosing guidelines exist for <6 months *Child <1 year*: 250 mg to 1 mg, enterally tid[14] *6 months*: 6–10 mg/m² IV or PO every day; maximum 20 mg/dose *Note*: Reduce dose by 50% if administered concomitantly with aprepitant.
Cannabinoids	
Dronabinol	*Age-based dosing:* Recommend use in age *≥6 years*: 2.5 mg/m²/dose PO q4–6h *Adolescents*: 2.5 mg PO q6–8h 0.05–0.1 mg/kg PO q 12hr (2.5-5 mg) May increase if tolerated to maximum of 10 mg bid

From Taketomo, Hodding.[13]

Table II.8 TREATMENT OF FATIGUE AND INSOMNIA IN PEDIATRICS

MEDICATION	COMMON DOSING BASED ON WEIGHT AND AGE
Sleep agents	

Melatonin	*Age-based dosing:*
	Infants ≥ 6 months[20]:
	    1 mg
	Children:
	    Initially 2–3 mg PO qhs, increase every 1–2 weeks by 1 mg to a maximum of 10 mg/day[14]

Trazodone	*Age-based dosing:* *> 5 years*: 0.75–1 mg/kg/dose (25–50 mg) PO qhs (maximum 200 mg/day)
Zolpidem	*Age-based dosing:* *2–18 years limited data*: 0.25 mg/kg PO qhs (maximum 10 mg/dose) *>18 years*: 5 mg (females) or 5–10 mg (males) PO qhs (maximum 10 mg/dose)
Psychostimulants	
Methylphenidate	*Age-based dosing:* *Infants*: No indication for use *Children*: 2.5–5 mg PO 1–4 times/day prn up to 20 mg twice daily

From Taketomo, Hodding.[13]

Table II.9 TREATMENT FOR ANOREXIA/CACHEXIA IN PEDIATRICS

MEDICATION	COMMON DOSING BASED ON WEIGHT AND AGE
Megestrol acetate	*Weight-based dosing:* *>8 months—Adolescents*: 7.5–10 mg/kg/day PO in 1–2 divided doses (maximum 800 mg/day)
Dexamethasone	*Weight-based dosing:* 0.05–0.5 mg/kg/day PO (maximum 4 mg/day)
Dronabinol	*Adolescents*: 2.5 mg PO 1–2 times/day, may increase to 5 mg/dose

From Anekar, Cascalla[3]; Davis[5]; Taketomo, Hodding[13]; Flank et al.[29]; Loprinzi & Jatoi[30] and Schack, Wholihan.[31]

Table II.10 SECRETION MANAGEMENT

MEDICATIONS	COMMON DOSING BASED ON WEIGHT AND AGE
Atropine ophthalmic drops	*Weight-based dosing*: ≤*10 kg*: 1 drop SL of 0.25% solution q6h prn >*10 kg*: 1 drop SL of 0.5% solution q6h prn >*25 kg or adolescents*: 1 drop of SL 1% solution q6h prn
Glycopyrrolate	*Weight-based dosing*: 4–10 mg/kg/dose IV q3–4h 20–100 mg/kg/dose PO q6–8h 0.05–0.1 mg/kg PO q 12 hr (2.5–5 mg). May increase if tolerated to maximum of 10 mg bid
Scopolamine transdermal patch	*Weight-based dosing*: >40 kg or >12 years: 1.5 mg transdermal patch q72h; may consider partial patch for younger populations to titrate as needed *Note*: Scopolamine patch takes approximately 12 hours to peak effect

From Hunt et al.[20]

Table II.11 AGITATION MANAGEMENT

MEDICATION	COMMON DOSING BASED ON WEIGHT AND AGE
Lorazepam	*Weight-based dosing*: 0.05 mg/kg IV/PO for agitation (consult with neurology in an infant with known neurological condition/seizure disorder; maximum 2 mg)
Diazepam	*Weight-based dosing*: >*6 months*: 0.12–0.8 mg/kg/day divided PO (long-acting) >*13 years*: 2–10 mg PO bid-qid
Midazolam	*Weight-based dosing*: >*6 months*: Intranasal 0.2 mg/kg (divided between nares) PO/PR: 0.2–0.5 mg/kg IV: 0.05 mg/kg Rarely used for agitation; infants <6 months at higher risk for airway obstruction and hypoventilation
Haloperidol	*Weight-based dosing* (limited data available): *Children ≥3 years and adolescents*: 0.01 mg/kg/dose PO/IV tid prn; To manage new-onset acute episode: 0.025–0.05 mg/kg once; may repeat 0.025 mg/kg/dose in 1 hour prn
Gabapentin	For use in chronic agitation in children with severe neurologic impairment See dosing recommendations under "Pain"

From Taketomo, Hodding[13]; and Hunt et al.[20]

---

following tables offer evidence-based medications to use for common symptoms based on both age and weight.

REFERENCES

1. Matson KL, Johnson PN, Tran V, Horton ER, Sterner-Allison J. Advocacy committee on behalf of pediatric pharmacy advocacy group. *J Pediatr Pharmacol Ther.* 2019;24(1):72–75.
2. U. S. Department of Health and Human Services. Center for Disease Control and Prevention. Opioids. Improve opioid prescribing. Guideline for Prescribing Opioids for Chronic Pain: 2019. https://www.cdc.gov/opioids/overdoseprevention/prescribing.html
3. Anekar AA, Cascella M. WHO Analgesic Ladder. [Updated 2021 May 18]. In: StatPearls [Internet]. Treasure Island (FL): StatPearls Publishing; 2021 Jan-. Available from: https://www.ncbi.nlm.nih.gov/books/NBK554435/
4. Pillai Riddell RR, Racine NM, Gennis HG, et al. Non-pharmacological management of infant and young child procedural pain. *Cochrane Database Syst Rev.* 2015;12:CD006275.
5. Davis K. Nonpharmacological Pain Management for Children. Palliative Care Resource Series. Alexandria, VA: National Hospice and Palliative Care Organization; 2017. https://www.nhpco.org/wp-content/uploads/2019/04/PALLIATIVECARE_Nonpharmacological.pdf Accessed September 17, 2021
6. Friedrichsdorf SJ, Goubert L. Pediatric pain treatment and prevention for hospitalized children. *Pain Rep.* 2019;5(1):e804. Published 2019 Dec 19. doi:10.1097/PR9.0000000000000804
7. Wren AA, Ross AC, D'Souza G, et al. Multidisciplinary pain management for pediatric patients with acute and chronic pain: A foundational treatment approach when prescribing opioids. *Children (Basel).* 2019;6(2):33. Published 2019 Feb 21. doi:10.3390/children6020033
8. Postovsky S, Lehavi A, Attias O, Hershman E. Easing of physical distress in pediatric cancer. In: Wolfe J, Jones BL, Kreicbergs U, Jankovic M, eds. *Palliative Care in Pediatric Oncology.* New York: Springer; 2018: 119–157.
9. Hauer J. Jones B. In: Poplack D, eds. Evaluation and management of pain in children UptoDate. Waltham, MA; UptoDate. Updated February 6, 2020. https://www.uptodate.com/contents/evaluation-and-management-of-pain-in-children
10. Thigpen JC OB, Harirforoosh S. Opioids: A review of pharmacokinetics and pharmacodynamics in neonates, infants, and children. *Eur J Drug Metab Pharmacokinet.* 2019;44(5):591–609. doi:10.1007/s13318-019-00552-0
11. Friedrichsdorf SJ. From tramadol to methadone: Opioids in the treatment of pain and dyspnea in pediatric palliative care. *Clin J Pain.* 2019;36(6):501–508. doi:10.1097/AJP.0000000000000704
12. Zernikow B, Michel E, Craig F, Anderson BJ. Pediatric palliative care: Use of opioids for the management of pain. *Paediatr Drugs.* 2009;11(2):129–151. doi:10.2165/00148581-200911020-00004
13. Taketomo C, Hodding J. *Lexicomp Pediatric and Neonatal Dosage Handbook.* 27th ed. Philadelphia, PA: American Pharmacists Association and Wolters Kluwer; 2020–2021.
14. Burnsed JC, Heinan K, Letzkus L, Zanelli S. Gabapentin for pain, movement disorders, and irritability in neonates and infants. *Dev Med Child Neurol.* 2020;63(3):386–389. doi:10.1111/dmcn.14324
15. Edwards LE, Hutchison LB, Hornik CD, Smith PB, Cotten CM, Bidegain M. A case of infant delirium in the neonatal intensive care unit. *J Neonatal Perinatal Med.* 2017;10(1):119–123. doi:10.3233/NPM-1637
16. Hauer JM, Solodiuk JC. Gabapentin for management of recurrent pain in 22 nonverbal children with severe neurological impairment:

A retrospective analysis. *J Palliat Med.* 2015;18(5):453–456. doi:10.1089/jpm.2014.0359

17. Sacha GL, Foreman MG, Kyllonen K, Rodriguez RJ. The use of gabapentin for pain and agitation in neonates and infants in a neonatal ICU. *J Pediatr Pharmacol Ther.* 2017;22(3):207–211. doi:10.5863/1551-6776-22.3.207

18. Hauer J, Houtrow AJ. Section on Hospice and Palliative Medicine, Council on Children with Disabilities. Pain assessment and treatment in children with significant impairment of the central nervous system. *Pediatrics.* 2017;139(6):e20171002. doi:10.1542/peds.2017-1002

19. Canadian Agency for Drugs and Technologies in Health. Dioctyl sulfosuccinate or docusate (calcium or sodium) for the prevention or management of constipation: A review of the clinical effectiveness. Summary of evidence. June 26, 2014. Available from: https://www.ncbi.nlm.nih.gov/books/NBK259247/

20. Dana Farber Cancer Institute/Boston Children's Hospital Pediatric Advanced Care Team. Pediatric Palliative Care Approach to Pain & Symptom Management, 3rd ed. Boston, MA: DFCI. 2020. https://pinkbook.dfci.org/assets/docs/blueBook.pdf

21. Garten L, Degenhardt P, Bührer C. Resolution of opioid-induced postoperative ileus in a newborn infant after methylnaltrexone. *J Pediatr Surg.* 2011;46(3):e13–e15. doi:10.1016/j.jpedsurg.2010.10.015

22. López J, Fernández SN, Santiago MJ, et al. Methylnaltrexone for the treatment of constipation in critically ill children. *J Clin Gastroenterol.* 2016;50(4):351–352. doi:10.1097/MCG.0000000000000483

23. Flerlage JE, Baker JN. Methylnaltrexone for opioid-induced constipation in children and adolescents and young adults with progressive incurable cancer at the end of life. *J Palliat Med.* 2015;18(7): 631–633. doi:10.1089/jpm.2014.0364

24. Komatz K, Carter B. Pain and symptom management in pediatric palliative care. *Pediatr Rev.* 2015;36(12):527–534. doi:10.1542/pir.36-12-527

25. Turkel SB, Jacobson JR, Tavaré CJ. The diagnosis and management of delirium in infancy. *J Child Adolesc Psychopharmacol.* 2013;23(5):352–356. doi:10.1089/cap.2013.0001

26. Capino AC, Thomas AN, Baylor S, Hughes KM, Miller JL, Johnson PN. Antipsychotic use in the prevention and treatment of intensive care unit delirium in pediatric patients. *J Pediatr Pharmacol Ther.* 2020;25(2):81–95. doi:10.5863/1551-6776-25.2.81

27. Sassano-Higgins S, Freudenberg N, Jacobson J, Turkel SB. Olanzapine reduces delirium symptoms in the critically ill pediatric patient. *J Pediatr Intensive Care.* 2013;2(2):49–54. doi:10.3233/PIC-13049

28. Groves A, Traube C, Silver G. Detection and management of delirium in the neonatal unit: A case series. *Pediatrics.* 2016;137(3):e20153369. doi:10.1542/peds.2015-3369

29. Flank J, Thackray J, Nielson D, et al. Olanzapine for treatment and prevention of acute chemotherapy-induced vomiting in children: A retrospective, multi-center review. *Pediatr Blood Cancer.* 2015;62(3):496–501. doi:10.1002/pbc.25286

30. Loprinzi C, Jatoi A. IN Hesleth, P (ed). Management of cancer anorexia/cachexia. UptoDate. Waltham, MA: UptoDate. August 17, 2021. https://www.uptodate.com/contents/management-of-cancer-anorexia-cachexia

31. Schack E, Wholihan D. Anorexia and cachexia. In: Ferrell BPJ, ed. *Oxford Textbook of Palliative Nursing.* 5th ed. New York: Oxford University Press; 2019: 140–148.

INDEX

Tables, figures, and boxes are indicated by an italic t, f, and b following the page number.

modafinil, 507*t*
Modified Caregiver Strain Index, 587
Moller, David Wendell, 249, 253, 254
MOLST. *See* medical orders for life-sustaining treatment
monoamine oxidase inhibitor (MAOI), 658
monoamine theory of depression, 653
Montreal Cognitive Assessment (MOCA), 576
mood stabilizers, 598, 658
moral agency, 69, 69*b*, 693
moral distress, 700–701
moral injury, 275, 339
morphine
    for cardiac symptoms, 164
    for cough, 565–566
    in discontinuation of respiratory technology, 719
    for dyspnea, 555–556, 717*t*
    in end-of-life care, 710
    for neonatal pain, 337, 761*t*
    for pain, 541*t*
Morrow Assessment of Nausea and Vomiting (MANE), 522–523
motor neuron disease, 581
mourning, defined, 469
Movantik, 493*t*
MPI (Multidimensional Prognostic Index), 150*b*
MPOA (Medical Power of Attorney), 319*t*
MSAS (Memorial Symptom Assessment Scale), 554
MSAs (metropolitan statistical areas), 217–218
MSCC (malignant spinal cord compression), 668–669, 669*t*
MST (Malnutrition Screening Tool), 483
MST (military sexual trauma), 273
Multidimensional Fatigue Symptom Inventory-Short Form (MFSI-SF), 504
Multidimensional Prognostic Index (MPI), 150*b*
multisite palliative care, 174
muscle loss, 483
music therapy, 659, 660*t*
myalgic encephalomyelitis (ME), 502
Mydirectives.com, 152*b*
My Wishes, 387

N

nabilone, 484, 529*t*
NACNS (National Association of Clinical Nurse Specialist), 50
naloxegol, 493*t*
naloxone, 547, 613, 613*b*
Namenda, 582
National Academy of Medicine (NAM), 89–90
National Academy of Sciences, Engineering, and Medicine, 11*t*, 13, 54
National Association of Clinical Nurse Specialist (NACNS), 50
National Center on Caregiving, 624
National Coalition for Cancer Survivorship (NCCS), 286
National Comprehensive Cancer Network (NCCN), 11*t*, 148, 361, 502
National Consensus Project for Quality Palliative Care (NCP), 11*t*, 147, 189, 447, 448*b*. *See also Clinical Practice Guidelines for Quality Palliative Care*
National Council of State Boards of Nursing (NCSBN), 10*t*, 35, 67*t*
National Framework and Preferred Practices for Palliative and Hospice Care Quality, A (NQF Preferred Practices), 20
National Hospice and Palliative Care Organization (NHPCO), 175, 232, 304*t*

definition of palliative care, 62
    educational opportunities, 28*t*
    leadership training, 50
    resources, 194
    Standards of Practice for Hospice Programs, 192, 192*t*
National Institute for Health and Care Excellence (NICE), 643*t*
National Institute of Nursing Research (NINR), 7, 11*t*, 25, 26*t*, 88*t*, 95*b*
National Institutes of Health (NIH), 7, 88*t*
National LGBT Cancer Network, 267*t*
National LGBTQIA+ Health Education Center, 267*t*
National Nursing Home Quality Initiative (NHQI), 230
National Organization of Nurse Practitioner Faculty (NONPF), 21, 30, 30*t*, 50
National POLST, 399*t*
National Prescription Drug Take-Back Program, 545
National Priorities Partnership (NPP), 7
National Quality Forum, 7, 11*t*, 20
Nausea and Emesis Module, 522–523
nausea and vomiting, 519–532
    assessment of, 522–523, 523*t*
    in bowel obstruction, 531
    in cannabinoid hyperemesis syndrome, 531
    case study, 519, 524, 531–532
    chemotherapy-induced, 358–359, 520, 531, 765*t*
    defined, 519–520
    etiology of, 521–522, 522*t*
    gastroparesis-induced, management of, 530
    management approaches to, 524, 525*t*
    nonpharmacologic interventions for, 524–526
    opioid-induced, management of, 530–531
    overview, 519
    in pediatric cancer, 358–359
    in pediatric palliative care, 764*t*
    pharmacologic interventions for, 526–530, 527*t*
    physiology of, 520–521
    prevalence of, 520, 520*t*
    risk factors in, 520
NCCN (National Comprehensive Cancer Network), 11*t*, 148, 361, 502
NCCS (National Coalition for Cancer Survivorship), 286
NCP. *See* National Consensus Project for Quality Palliative Care
NCSBN (National Council of State Boards of Nursing), 10*t*, 35, 67*t*
nebulized medications, 114
nebulized opioids, 556
needs assessments, 56–57
Neelon-Champagne Confusion Scale (NEECHAM), 634, 635*t*
Nefazodone, 274*t*
negative adjustment, 620
negotiation skills, 307
neonatal ICU (NICU)
    care of team in, 338–339
    consult etiquette in, 336
    education and support to team in, 340
neonatal palliative care
    bereavement care in, 340
    care of family in, 338
    care of infants in, 336–338
    care of NICU team in, 338–339
    consult etiquette in NICU, 336
    current state of, 336
    end-of-life care in, 339–340

history of, 335–336
    overview, 328–329
    versus perinatal palliative care, 329*f*
netupitant, 528*t*
neurodevelopmental theory of depression, 653
neuroirritability, 322
neurokinin-1 receptor antagonists, 528*t*, 530, 531, 765*t*
neuroleptic malignant syndrome (NMS), 659
neurological disease
    in ambulatory pediatric palliative care, 346*t*
    pruritus from, 677
    rehabilitation care for, 204
neurological impairment
    advance care planning for children with, 323, 324*b*
    end-of-life communication in, 422*b*
neuromodulatory agents, 566
neuromuscular electrical stimulation (NMES), 559
neuropathic pain, 537, 761*t*, 762*t*
Neuropsychiatric Inventory–Questionnaire (NPI-Q), 584, 587
neurotrophic theory of depression, 653, 658
NHPCO. *See* National Hospice and Palliative Care Organization
NHQI (National Nursing Home Quality Initiative), 230
NICE (National Institute for Health and Care Excellence), 643*t*
NICU. *See* neonatal ICU
NIH (National Institutes of Health), 7, 88*t*
NINR (National Institute of Nursing Research), 7, 11*t*, 25, 26*t*, 88*t*, 95*b*
nitrates, 160*t*
NIV (noninvasive ventilation), 556*t*, 558
NK$_1$-receptor antagonist, 359, 679
NMES (neuromuscular electrical stimulation), 559
N-methyl-d-aspartate (NMDA) receptor agonists, 582, 656*t*
N-methyl-d-aspartate (NMDA) receptor antagonists, 543*t*, 658, 743
NMS (neuroleptic malignant syndrome), 659
nociceptive pain, 761*t*
non-abandonment, 693
non-APRN practice models, 231
nonasthmatic eosinophilic bronchitis, 562
nonbeneficial care/futility, 721
non-benzodiazepine agonists, 684, 684*t*
noncardiac pain, in heart disease, 164–165
non–face-to-face codes, 755*t*
non-Hodgkin's lymphoma, 288*t*
noninvasive positive-pressure ventilation (NPPV), 715–717
noninvasive ventilation (NIV), 556*t*, 558
nonmaleficence, 693, 723, 738
nonmalignant fatigue, 502
nonmedical use, defined, 605*t*
non-opioids for pain management, 539
NONPF (National Organization of Nurse Practitioner Faculty), 21, 30, 30*t*, 50
nonpharmacological interventions for, 626, 626*t*, 627*t*
non-small cell lung cancers (NSCLC), 104–106, 673
nonsteroidal anti-inflammatory drugs (NSAIDs), 164–165, 484, 539, 682–683
nonverbal patients
    end-of-life communication in, 422
    pain management for, 111–112
    pediatric pain management for, 321,

321*b*, 322*b*
normal adjustment, 619, 620*t*
norming state of teams, 57
nortriptyline, 625*t*
notification of death, 127–130
    via virtual platform or telephone, 129*t*, 423*b*, 424, 424*b*
NPI-Q (Neuropsychiatric Inventory–Questionnaire), 584, 587
NPP (National Priorities Partnership), 7
NPPV (noninvasive positive-pressure ventilation), 715–717
NRS (Nutritional Risk Screening), 483
numeracy, health, 440
numeric rating scale (NRS), 554
NURSE mnemonic, 409*b*, 414
nurse–patient relationship, 419
nurse practitioner (NP), 10*t*, 12–13, 35, 229
Nurse Practitioner Core Competencies Content (NONPF), 21
Nurses on Boards Coalition, 51
Nurses' Roles and Responsibilities in Providing Care and Support at the End of Life, 737
Nurse's Role When a Patient Requests Medical Aid in Dying, 736
NURSE statements, 384
Nursing Delirium Screening Scale (Nu-Desc), 634, 635*t*
nursing home palliative care, 227–234
    ABCDE mnemonic for care in, 230, 230*t*
    case study, 227–228
    clinical practice considerations, 232–233
    current implications and future opportunities, 233–234
    defined, 228–229, 228*t*
    models of care delivery in, 231–232
    overview, 228
    role of APRN in, 229
    state and federal regulations for, 229–231, 231*t*
Nursing Home Reform Act, 229
Nursing Leadership Consortium on End-of-Life Care, 8
Nursing Scope and Standards of Practice (ANA), 47, 48*b*, 67*t*, 433
nutrition. *See also* medically administered nutrition and hydration
    for cancer-related anorexia/cachexia, 359
    discontinuation of, 730–731
    discussing withdrawal in family meetings, 412–413
    end-of-life care of infants, 334, 339
Nutritional Risk Screening (NRS), 483
nutritionists, 203

O

occupational therapists, 202, 510
octreotide, 496*t*, 498*t*, 529*t*, 668
OEND (Opioid Overdose Education and Naloxone Distribution) Program, 276
OIC (opioid induced constipation), 490
olanzapine
    for anxiety, 625*t*
    for delirium, 644*t*
    for end-stage cardiac disease, 711, 712*t*
    for nausea and vomiting, 526, 527*t*
    for pediatric delirium, 764*t*
    for pediatric nausea and vomiting, 359, 764*t*
Omnibus Budget Reconciliation Act, 229
oncology. *See also* cancer; pediatric palliative care, in oncology
    in ambulatory pediatric palliative care, 346*t*, 347
    palliative care in acute setting, 104–105
    palliative care within, 13–14